a LANGE medical book

Smith's
General Urology

fifteenth edition

Edited by

Emil A. Tanagho, MD
Professor of Urology
University of California School of Medicine
San Francisco

and

Jack W. McAninch, MD
Professor of Urology
University of California School of Medicine
San Francisco

Chief of Urology
San Francisco General Hospital
San Francisco

Lange Medical Books/McGraw-Hill
Health Professions Division

New York   St. Louis   San Francisco   Auckland   Bogotá   Caracas   Lisbon
London   Madrid   Mexico City   Milan   Montreal   New Delhi   San Juan
Singapore   Sydney   Tokyo   Toronto

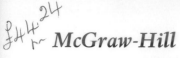

McGraw-Hill

A Division of The McGraw·Hill Companies

Smith's General Urology, 15/e

Copyright © 2000 by **The McGraw-Hill Companies,** Inc. All Rights Reserved. Printed in the United States of America. Except as permitted under the United States Copyright Act of 1976, no part of this publication may be reproduced or distributed in any form or by any means, or stored in a data base or retrieval system, without the prior written permission of the publisher.

Previous edition copyright © 1995 by Appleton & Lange

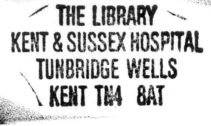

234567890 HPCHPC 99

ISBN 0-8385-8607-4
ISSN 0892-1245

Notice

Medicine is an ever changing science. As new research and clinical experience broaden our knowledge, changes in treatment and drug therapy are required. The authors and the publisher of this work have checked with sources believed to be reliable in their efforts to provide information that is complete and generally in accord with the standards accepted at the time of publication. However, in view of the possibility of human error or changes in medical sciences, neither the authors nor the publisher nor any other party who has been involved in the preparation or publication of this work warrants that the information contained herein is in every respect accurate or complete, and they are not responsible for any errors or omissions or for the results obtained from use of such information. Readers are encouraged to confirm the information contained herein with other sources. For example and in particular, readers are advised to check the product information sheet included in the package of each drug they plan to administer to be certain that the information contained in this book is accurate and that changes have not been made in the recommended dose or in the contraindications for administration. This recommendation is of particular importance in connection with new or infrequently used drugs.

This book was set in Times Roman by Pine Tree Composition.
The editors were Janet Foltin, Harriet Lebowitz, and Jeanmarie Roche.
The production supervisor was Phil Galea.
The cover designer was Elizabeth Schmitz.
The manager of art services was Eve Siegel.
The illustrators were Teshin Associates.
The index was prepared by Katherine Pitcoff.

Hamilton Printing Company was printer and binder.

This book is printed on acid-free paper.

Contents

Authors

William J.C. Amend, Jr., MD
Professor of Clinical Medicine and Surgery, University of California, San Francisco.

Susan Barbour, RN, MS, CETN
Clinical Nurse Specialist, Department of Nursing, The Medical Center at the University of California, San Francisco.

Timothy G. Berger, MD
Chief, Department of Dermatology, San Francisco General Hospital; Clinical Professor, Residency Program, Department of Dermatology, University of California, San Francisco.

Allan I. Bloom, MD
Clinical Fellow, Vascular and Interventional Radiology, San Francisco General Hospital, San Francisco.

Damien M. Bolton, MD, FRACS
Senior Associate, Department of Surgery, University of Melbourne, Australia.

Peter N. Bretan, Jr., MD
Clinical Professor, University of California Medical Center, San Francisco.

Peter R. Carroll, MD
Professor and Chair, Department of Urology, University of California School of Medicine, San Francisco.

Felix A. Conte, MD
Professor of Pediatrics, University of California, San Francisco.

Jeffrey A. Cooper, MD
Professor, Department of Radiology, Director, Nuclear Medicine, Albany Medical College, Albany, New York.

Robert Dreicer, MD, MS, FACP
Assistant Professor, Departments of Internal Medicine and Urology, University of Iowa, Iowa City.

Christian P. Gilfrich, MD
Department of Urology, Johannes Gutenberg University Medical School, Mainz, Germany.

Roy L. Gordon, MD
Professor and Chief of Interventional Radiology, University of California, San Francisco.

Melvin M. Grumbach, MD, DM (hon)
Edward B. Shaw Professor of Pediatrics and Chairman Emeritus, Department of Pediatrics, University of California School of Medicine, San Francisco.

Robert S. Hattner, MD
Associate Professor and Senior Attending Nuclear Physician, Department of Radiology, University of California School of Medicine, San Francisco.

Hedvig Hricak, MD, PhD
Professor of Radiology, Urology, and Radiation Oncology, and Obstetrics, Gynecology and Reproductive Sciences, University of California, San Francisco.

Barry A. Kogan, MD
Professor, Departments of Surgery and Pediatrics; Chief, Division of Urology, Albany Medical College, Albany, New York.

Karl J. Kreder, Jr., MD
Professor, Department of Urology, University of Iowa Hospitals and Clinics, Iowa City.

John N. Krieger, MD
Professor of Urology, University of Washington School of Medicine; Chief of Urology, VA Puget Sound Health Care System, Seattle.

Marcus A. Krupp, AB, MD
Clinical Professor of Medicine, Emeritus, Stanford University School of Medicine, Stanford, California.

Tom F. Lue, MD
Professor of Urology, University of California, San Francisco; Chief of Urology, Mount Zion Medical Center, University of California, San Francisco.

Michael Malone, MD
Senior Staff Consultant, Department of Urology, Lahey Clinic, Burlington, Massachusetts.

Shelley R. Marder, MD
Assistant Clinical Professor, Department of Radiology, San Francisco General Hospital, San Francisco.

Jack W. McAninch, MD
Professor, Department of Urology, University of California School of Medicine, San Francisco; Chief of Urology, San Francisco General Hospital, San Francisco.

Simon N. McRae, MD
Resident, Department of Urology, Stanford University School of Medicine, Stanford, California.

Willaim Okuno, MD
Clinical Instructor, Department of Radiology, University of California, San Francisco.

Joseph C. Presti, Jr., MD
Assistant Professor, Department of Urology, University of California, San Francisco; Chief, Urology Section, San Francisco VA Medical Center, San Francisco.

Mack Roach, III, MD
Assistant Professor, Departments of Radiation Oncology, Medical Oncology, and Urology, University of California, San Francisco.

Linda M. Dairiki Shortliffe, MD
Professor and Chair of Urology, Stanford University School of Medicine; Chief of Pediatric Urology, Lucile Packard Children's Hospital, Stanford, California.

Eric J. Small, MD
Associate Clinical Professor of Medicine and Urology, University of California, San Francisco.

R. Ernest Sosa, MD
Associate Professor of Urology, The New York Presbyterian Hospital, New York.

Joycelyn L. Speight, MD, PhD
Clinical Fellow, Department of Radiation Oncology, University of California, San Francisco.

Marshall L. Stoller, MD
Assistant Professor, Department of Urology, University of California, San Francisco.

Emil A. Tanagho, MD
Professor, Department of Urology, University of California School of Medicine, San Francisco.

Joachim W. Thüroff, MD
Professor and Chairman, Department of Urology, Johannes Gutenberg University Medical School, Mainz, Germany.

Paul J. Turek, MD
Assistant Professor of Urology; Director, Male Reproductive Laboratory, University of California, San Francisco.

J. Blake Tyrrell, MD
Clinical Professor of Medicine, Chief, Clinical Endocrinology and Metabolism, University of California, San Francisco.

E. Darracott Vaughan, Jr., MD, FACS
Chairman, Department of Urology; James J. Colt Professor of Urology, Department of Urology, The New York Presbyterian Hospital, Weill Medical College of Cornell University, New York.

Flavio G. Vincenti, MD
Professor of Clinical Medicine, Transplant Service, University of California, San Francisco.

Richard D. Williams, MD
Professor and Head, Rubin H. Flocks Chair, Department of Urology, University of Iowa, Iowa City.

Howard N. Winfield, MD, FRCS, FACS
Associate Professor of Urology, Stanford University School of Medicine, Stanford; Chief of Urology, Palo Alto VA Health Care, Palo Alto, California.

Stuart Wolf, Jr., MD
Assistant Professor of Surgery, University of Michigan; Director, Michigan Center for Minimally Invasive Urology, University of Michigan.

Preface

Smith's General Urology, 15th Edition, provides in a concise format the information necessary for the understanding, diagnosis, and treatment of diseases managed by urologic surgeons. Our goal has been to keep the book current, to the point, and readable.

Medical students will find this book useful because of its concise, easy-to-follow format and organization and its breadth of information. Interns and residents, as well as practicing physicians in urology or general medicine, will find it an efficient and current reference, particularly because of its emphasis on diagnosis and treatment.

The 15th edition is a thorough revision and updating of the book, incorporating the following new chapters: Laparoscopic Surgery (Howard Winfield) and Bacterial Infections of the Genitourinary Tract (Simon McRae and Linda Dairiki Shortliffe). In addition, the following contributors have assumed authorship of existing, newly revised chapters: John Krieger, Sexually Transmitted Diseases; Eric Small, Immunology and Immunotherapy of Urologic Cancers; Joseph Presti, Jr., Neoplasms of the Prostate Gland as well as Genital Tumors; Stuart Wolf, Jr., Urologic Laser Surgery; Joycelyn Speight and Mack Roach, III, Radiotherapy of Urologic Tumors; and Paul Turek, Male Infertility. To these, and to all our ongoing contributors, we are deeply indebted.

The book has been reviewed and updated throughout, with emphasis on current references. The several hundred illustrations have been further modernized and improved, including many fine anatomic drawings and the latest imaging techniques.

Smith's General Urology is currently available in Japanese, Polish, Portuguese, Italian, and Spanish editions. The book has also been recorded in English on tape for use by the blind. The tape recording is available from Recording for the Blind, Inc., 20 Roszel Road, Princeton, NJ 08540.

We greatly appreciate the assistance of our sponsoring editor, Shelley Reinhardt, whose expertise and patience have been instrumental in bringing this edition to completion.

Emil A. Tanagho, MD
Jack W. McAninch, MD

San Francisco, California
November 1999

Anatomy of the Genitourinary Tract

1

Emil A. Tanagho, MD

Urology deals with diseases and disorders of the male genitourinary tract and the female urinary tract. Surgical diseases of the adrenal gland are also included. These systems are illustrated in Figures 1–1 and 1–2.

ADRENALS

Gross Appearance

A. Anatomy: Each kidney is capped by an adrenal gland, and both organs are enclosed within Gerota's (perirenal) fascia. Each adrenal weighs about 5 g. The right adrenal is triangular in shape; the left is more rounded and crescentic. Each gland is composed of a cortex, chiefly influenced by the pituitary gland, and a medulla derived from chromaffin tissue.

B. Relations: Figure 1–2 shows the relation of the adrenals to other organs. The right adrenal lies between the liver and the vena cava. The left adrenal lies close to the aorta and is covered on its lower surface by the pancreas; superiorly and laterally, it is related to the spleen.

Histology

The adrenal cortex is composed of 3 distinct layers: the outer zona glomerulosa, the middle zona fasciculata, and the inner zona reticularis. The medulla lies centrally and is made up of polyhedral cells containing eosinophilic granular cytoplasm. These chromaffin cells are accompanied by ganglion and small round cells.

Blood Supply

A. Arterial: Each adrenal receives 3 arteries: one from the inferior phrenic artery, one from the aorta, and one from the renal artery.

B. Venous: Blood from the right adrenal is drained by a very short vein that empties into the vena cava; the left adrenal vein terminates in the left renal vein.

Lymphatics

The lymphatic vessels accompany the suprarenal vein and drain into the lumbar lymph nodes.

KIDNEYS

Gross Appearance

A. Anatomy: The kidneys lie along the borders of the psoas muscles and are therefore obliquely placed. The position of the liver causes the right kidney to be lower than the left (Figures 1–2 and 1–3). The adult kidney weighs about 150 g.

The kidneys are supported by the perirenal fat (which is enclosed in the perirenal fascia), the renal vascular pedicle, abdominal muscle tone, and the general bulk of the abdominal viscera. Variations in these factors permit variations in the degree of renal mobility. The average descent on inspiration or on assuming the upright position is 4–5 cm. Lack of mobility suggests abnormal fixation (eg, perinephritis), but extreme mobility is not necessarily pathologic.

On longitudinal section (Figure 1–4), the kidney is seen to be made up of an outer cortex, a central medulla, and the internal calices and pelvis. The cortex is homogeneous in appearance. Portions of it project toward the pelvis between the papillae and fornices and are called the columns of Bertin. The medulla consists of numerous pyramids formed by the converging collecting renal tubules, which drain into the minor calices at the tip of the papillae.

B. Relations: Figures 1–2 and 1–3 show the relations of the kidneys to adjacent organs and structures. Their intimacy with intraperitoneal organs and the autonomic innervation they share with these organs explain, in part, some of the gastrointestinal symptoms that accompany genitourinary disease.

Histology

A. Nephron: The functioning unit of the kidney is the nephron, which is composed of a tubule that has both secretory and excretory functions (Figure 1–4). The secretory portion is contained largely within the

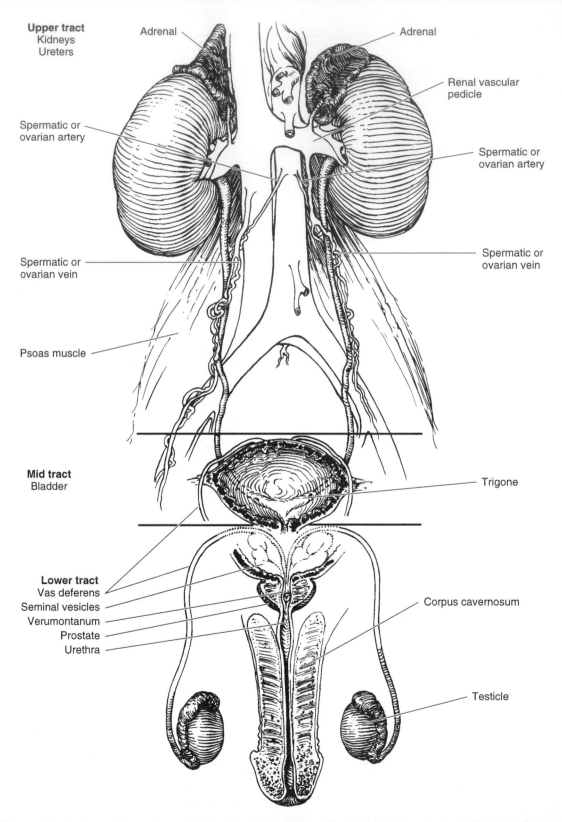

Upper tract
Kidneys
Ureters

Adrenal

Adrenal

Renal vascular
pedicle

Spermatic or
ovarian artery

Spermatic or
ovarian artery

Spermatic or
ovarian vein

Spermatic or
ovarian vein

Psoas muscle

Mid tract
Bladder

Trigone

Lower tract
Vas deferens
Seminal vesicles
Verumontanum
Prostate
Urethra

Corpus cavernosum

Testicle

Figure 1–1. Anatomy of the male genitourinary tract. The upper and mid tracts have urologic function only. The lower tract has both genital and urinary functions.

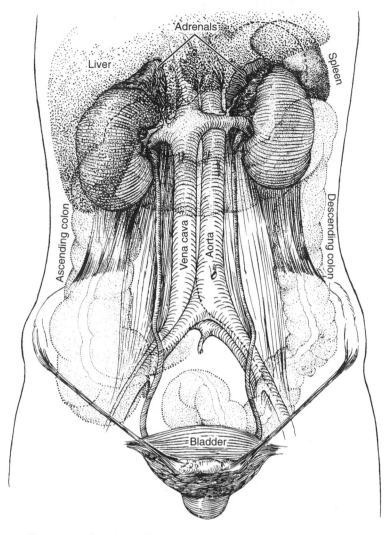

Figure 1–2. Relations of kidney, ureters, and bladder (anterior aspect).

cortex and consists of a renal corpuscle and the secretory part of the renal tubule. The excretory portion of this duct lies in the medulla. The renal corpuscle is composed of the vascular glomerulus, which projects into Bowman's capsule, which, in turn, is continuous with the epithelium of the proximal convoluted tubule. The secretory portion of the renal tubule is made up of the proximal convoluted tubule, the loop of Henle, and the distal convoluted tubule.

The excretory portion of the nephron is the collecting tubule, which is continuous with the distal end of the ascending limb of the convoluted tubule. It empties its contents through the tip (papilla) of a pyramid into a minor calyx.

B. Supporting Tissue: The renal stroma is composed of loose connective tissue and contains blood vessels, capillaries, nerves, and lymphatics.

Blood Supply
(Figures 1–2, 1–4, and 1–5)

A. Arterial: Usually there is one renal artery, a branch of the aorta, that enters the hilum of the kidney between the pelvis, which normally lies posteriorly, and the renal vein. It may branch before it reaches the kidney, and 2 or more separate arteries may be noted. In duplication of the pelvis and ureter, it is usual for each renal segment to have its own arterial supply.

The renal artery divides into anterior and posterior branches. The posterior branch supplies the mid segment of the posterior surface. The anterior branch supplies both upper and lower poles as well as the entire anterior surface. The renal arteries are all end arteries.

The renal artery further divides into interlobar ar-

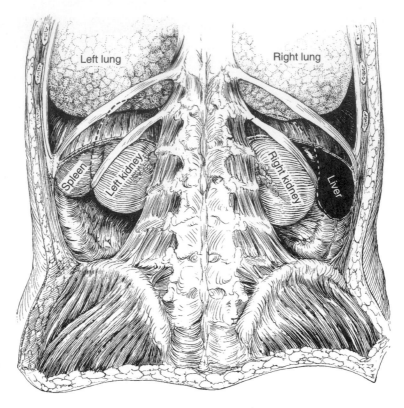

Figure 1–3. Relations of kidneys (posterior aspect). The dashed lines represent the outline of the kidneys where they are obscured by overlying structures.

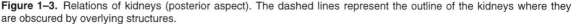

teries, which ascend in the columns of Bertin (between the pyramids) and then arch along the base of the pyramids (arcuate arteries). The renal artery then ascends as interlobular arteries. From these vessels, smaller (afferent) branches pass to the glomeruli. From the glomerular tuft, efferent arterioles pass to the tubules in the stroma.

B. Venous: The renal veins are paired with the arteries, but any of them will drain the entire kidney if the others are tied off.

Although the renal artery and vein are usually the sole blood vessels of the kidney, accessory renal vessels are common and may be of clinical importance if they are so placed to compress the ureter, in which case hydronephrosis may result.

Nerve Supply

The renal nerves derived from the renal plexus accompany the renal vessels throughout the renal parenchyma.

Lymphatics

The lymphatics of the kidney drain into the lumbar lymph nodes.

CALICES, RENAL PELVIS, & URETER

Gross Appearance

A. Anatomy:

1. Calices–The tips of the minor calices (8–12 in number) are indented by the projecting pyramids (Figure 1–4). These calices unite to form 2 or 3 major calices, which join to form the renal pelvis.

2. Renal pelvis–The pelvis may be entirely intrarenal or partly intrarenal and partly extrarenal. Inferomedially, it tapers to form the ureter.

3. Ureter–The adult ureter is about 30 cm long, varying in direct relation to the height of the individual. It follows a rather smooth S curve. Areas of relative narrowing are found (1) at the ureteropelvic junction, (2) where the ureter crosses over the iliac vessels, and (3) where it courses through the bladder wall.

B. Relations:

1. Calices–The calices are intrarenal and are intimately related to the renal parenchyma.

2. Renal pelvis–If the pelvis is partly extrarenal, it lies along the lateral border of the psoas muscle and on the quadratus lumborum muscle; the renal vascular pedicle is placed just anterior to it. The

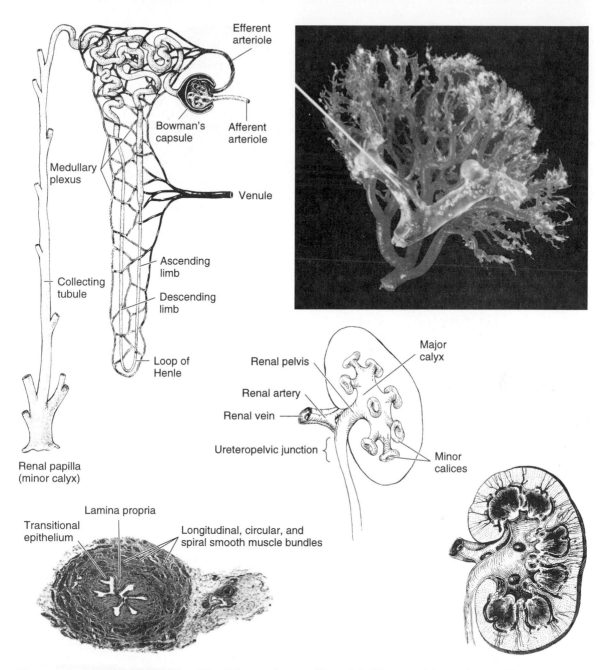

Figure 1–4. Anatomy and histology of the kidney and ureter. **Upper left:** Diagram of the nephron and its blood supply (Courtesy of Merck, Sharp, & Dohme: Seminar: 1947;9[3].) **Upper right:** Cast of the pelvic caliceal system and the arterial supply of the kidney. **Middle:** Renal calices, pelvis, and ureter (posterior aspect). **Lower left:** Histology of the ureter. The smooth-muscle bundles are arranged in both a spiral and a longitudinal manner. **Lower right:** Longitudinal section of kidney showing calices, pelvis, ureter, and renal blood supply (posterior aspect).

left renal pelvis lies at the level of the first or second lumbar vertebra; the right pelvis is a little lower.

3. Ureter–As followed from above downward, the ureters lie on the psoas muscles, pass medially to the sacroiliac joints, and then swing laterally near the ischial spines before passing medially to penetrate the base of the bladder (Figure 1–2). In females, the uterine arteries are closely related to the juxtavesical portion of the ureters. The ureters are covered by the posterior peritoneum; their lowermost portions are

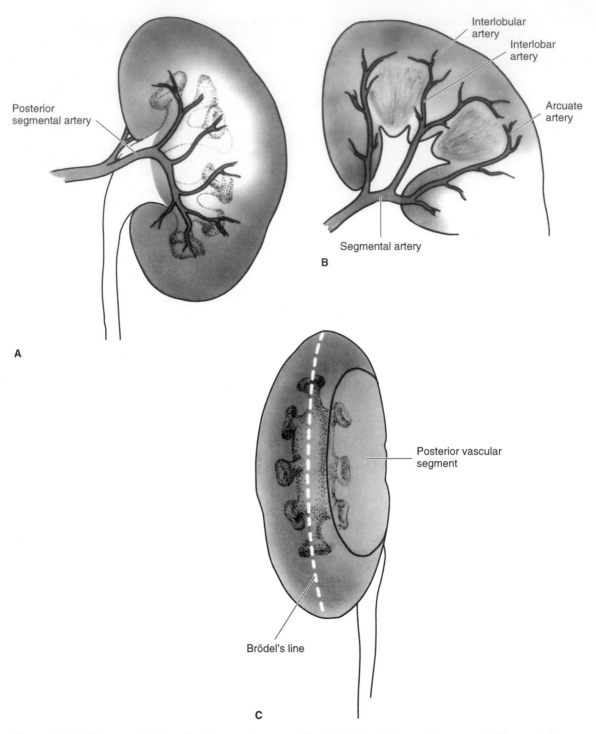

Figure 1–5. A: The posterior branch of the renal artery and its distribution to the central segment of the posterior surface of the kidney. **B:** Branches of the anterior division of the renal artery supplying the entire anterior surface of the kidney as well as the upper and lower poles at both surfaces. The segmental branches lead to interlobar, arcuate, and interlobular arteries. **C:** The lateral convex margin of the kidney. Brödel's line, which is 1 cm from the convex margin, is the bloodless plane demarcated by the distribution of the posterior branch of the renal artery.

closely attached to it, while the juxtavesical portions are embedded in vascular retroperitoneal fat.

The vasa deferentia, as they leave the internal inguinal rings, sweep over the lateral pelvic walls anterior to the ureters (Figure 1–6). They lie medial to the latter before joining the seminal vesicle and penetrating the base of the prostate to become the ejaculatory ducts.

Histology
(Figure 1–4)

The walls of the calices, pelvis, and ureters are composed of transitional cell epithelium under which lies loose connective and elastic tissue (lamina propria). External to these are a mixture of helical and longitudinal smooth muscle fibers. They are not arranged in definite layers. The outermost adventitial coat is composed of fibrous connective tissue.

Blood Supply

A. Arterial: The renal calices, pelvis, and upper ureters derive their blood supply from the renal arteries; the mid ureter is fed by the internal spermatic (or ovarian) arteries. The lowermost portion of the ureter is served by branches from the common iliac, internal iliac (hypogastric), and vesical arteries.

B. Venous: The veins of the renal calices, pelvis, and ureters are paired with the arteries.

Lymphatics

The lymphatics of the upper portions of the ureters as well as those from the pelvis and calices enter the lumbar lymph nodes. The lymphatics of the mid ureter pass to the internal iliac (hypogastric) and common iliac lymph nodes; the lower ureteral lymphatics empty into the vesical and hypogastric lymph nodes.

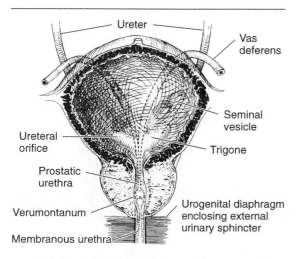

Figure 1–6. Anatomy and relations of the ureters, bladder, prostate, seminal vesicles, and vasa deferentia (anterior view).

BLADDER

Gross Appearance

The bladder is a hollow muscular organ that serves as a reservoir for urine. In women, its posterior wall and dome are invaginated by the uterus. The adult bladder normally has a capacity of 400–500 mL.

A. Anatomy: When empty, the adult bladder lies behind the pubic symphysis and is largely a pelvic organ. In infants and children, it is situated higher. When it is full, it rises well above the symphysis and can readily be palpated or percussed. When overdistended, as in acute or chronic urinary retention, it may cause the lower abdomen to bulge visibly.

Extending from the dome of the bladder to the umbilicus is a fibrous cord, the median umbilical ligament, which represents the obliterated urachus. The ureters enter the bladder posteroinferiorly in an oblique manner and at these points are about 5 cm apart (Figure 1–6). The orifices, situated at the extremities of the crescent-shaped interureteric ridge that forms the proximal border of the trigone, are about 2.5 cm apart. The trigone occupies the area between the ridge and the bladder neck.

The internal sphincter, or bladder neck, is not a true circular sphincter but a thickening formed by interlaced and converging muscle fibers of the detrusor as they pass distally to become the smooth musculature of the urethra.

B. Relations: In males, the bladder is related posteriorly to the seminal vesicles, vasa deferentia, ureters, and rectum (Figures 1–8 and 1–9). In females, the uterus and vagina are interposed between the bladder and rectum (Figure 1–10). The dome and posterior surfaces are covered by peritoneum; hence, in this area the bladder is closely related to the small intestine and sigmoid colon. In both males and females, the bladder is related to the posterior surface of the pubic symphysis, and, when distended, it is in contact with the lower abdominal wall.

Histology
(Figure 1–7)

The mucosa of the bladder is composed of transitional epithelium. Beneath it is a well-developed submucosal layer formed largely of connective and elastic tissues. External to the submucosa is the detrusor muscle, which is made up of a mixture of smooth muscle fibers arranged at random in a longitudinal, circular, and spiral manner without any layer formation or specific orientation except close to the internal meatus, where the detrusor muscle assumes 3 definite layers: inner longitudinal, middle circular, and outer longitudinal.

Blood Supply

A. Arterial: The bladder is supplied with blood by the superior, middle, and inferior vesical arteries,

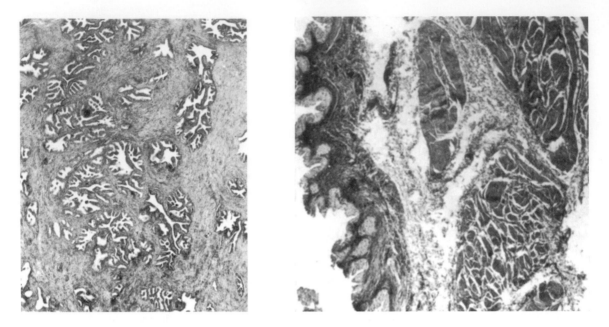

Figure 1–7. Left: Histology of the prostate. Epithelial glands embedded in a mixture of connective and elastic tissue and smooth muscle. **Right:** Histology of the bladder. The mucosa is transitional cell in type and lies on a well-developed submucosal layer of connective tissue. The detrusor muscle is composed of interlacing longitudinal, circular, and spiral smooth-muscle bundles.

which arise from the anterior trunk of the internal iliac (hypogastric) artery, and by smaller branches from the obturator and inferior gluteal arteries. In females, the uterine and vaginal arteries also send branches to the bladder.

B. Venous: Surrounding the bladder is a rich plexus of veins that ultimately empties into the internal iliac (hypogastric) veins.

Lymphatics

The lymphatics of the bladder drain into the vesical, external iliac, internal iliac (hypogastric), and common iliac lymph nodes.

PROSTATE GLAND

Gross Appearance

A. Anatomy: The prostate is a fibromuscular and glandular organ lying just inferior to the bladder (Figures 1–6 and 1–8). The normal prostate weighs about 20 g and contains the posterior urethra, which is about 2.5 cm in length. It is supported anteriorly by the puboprostatic ligaments and inferiorly by the urogenital diaphragm (Figure 1–6). The prostate is perforated posteriorly by the ejaculatory ducts, which pass obliquely to empty through the verumontanum on the floor of the prostatic urethra just proximal to the striated external urinary sphincter (Figure 1–11).

According to the classification of Lowsley, the prostate consists of 5 lobes: anterior, posterior, median, right lateral, and left lateral. According to Mc-Neal (1972), the prostate has a peripheral zone, a central zone, and a transitional zone; an anterior segment; and a preprostatic sphincteric zone (Figure 1–12). The segment of urethra that traverses the prostate gland is the prostatic urethra. It is lined by an inner longitudinal layer of muscle (continuous with a similar layer of the vesical wall). Incorporated within the prostate gland is an abundant amount of smooth musculature derived primarily from the external longitudinal bladder musculature. This musculature represents the true smooth involuntary sphincter of the posterior urethra in males.

Prostatic adenoma develops from the periurethral glands at the site of the median or lateral lobes. The posterior lobe, however, is prone to cancerous degeneration.

B. Relations: The prostate gland lies behind the pubic symphysis. Located closely to the posterosuperior surface are the vasa deferentia and seminal vesicles (Figure 1–8). Posteriorly, the prostate is separated from the rectum by the 2 layers of Denonvilliers' fascia, serosal rudiments of the pouch of Douglas, which once extended to the urogenital diaphragm (Figure 1–9).

Histology
(Figure 1–7)

The prostate consists of a thin fibrous capsule

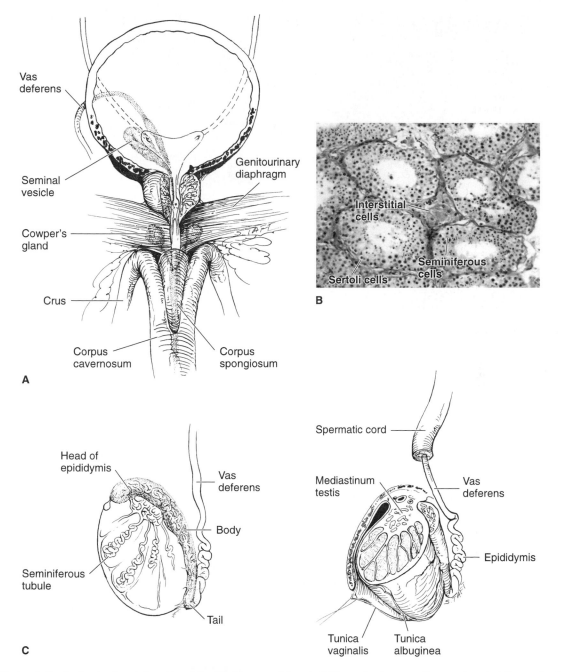

Figure 1–8. A: Anatomic relationship of the bladder, prostate, prostatomembranous urethra, and root of the penis. **B:** Histology of the testis. Seminiferous tubules lined by supporting basement membrane for the Sertoli and spermatogenic cells. The latter are in various stages of development. **C:** Cross sections of the testis and epididymis. (**A** and **C** are reproduced, with permission, from Tanagho EA: Anatomy of the lower urinary tract. In: Walsh PC et al [editors]: *Campbell's Urology,* 6th ed., vol. 1. Saunders, 1992.)

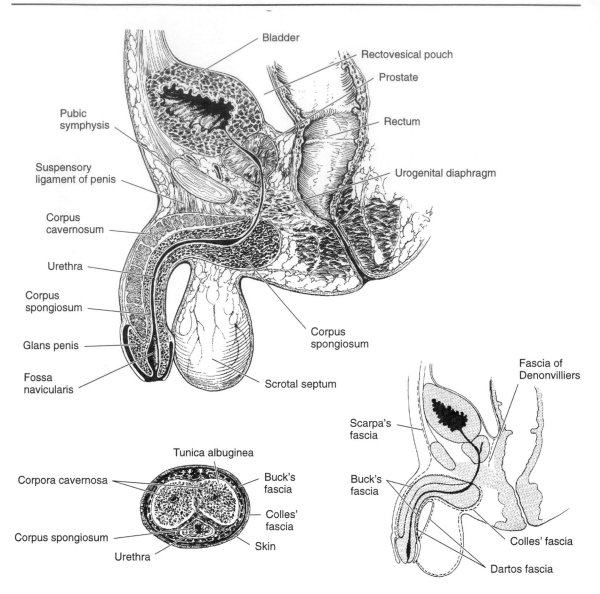

Figure 1–9. Top: Relations of the bladder, prostate, seminal vesicles, penis, urethra, and scrotal contents. **Lower left:** Transverse section through the penis. The paired upper structures are the corpora cavernosa. The single lower body surrounding the urethra is the corpus spongiosum. **Lower right:** Fascial planes of the lower genitourinary tract. (After Wesson.)

under which are circularly oriented smooth muscle fibers and collagenous tissue that surrounds the urethra (involuntary sphincter). Deep to this layer lies the prostatic stroma, composed of connective and elastic tissues and smooth muscle fibers in which are embedded the epithelial glands. These glands drain into the major excretory ducts (about 25 in number), which open chiefly on the floor of the urethra between the verumontanum and the vesical neck. Just beneath the transitional epithelium of the prostatic urethra lie the periurethral glands.

Blood Supply

A. Arterial: The arterial supply to the prostate is derived from the inferior vesical, internal pudendal, and middle rectal (hemorrhoidal) arteries.

B. Venous: The veins from the prostate drain into the periprostatic plexus, which has connections with the deep dorsal vein of the penis and the internal iliac (hypogastric) veins.

Nerve Supply

The prostate gland receives a rich nerve supply from the sympathetic and parasympathetic nerve plexuses.

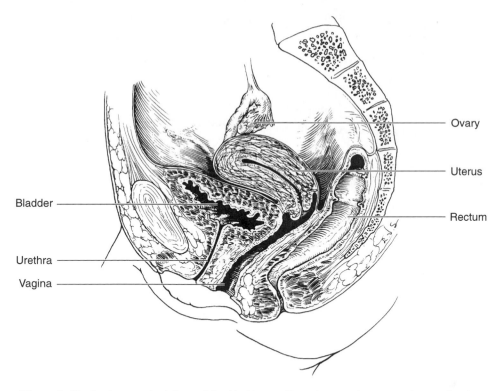

Figure 1–10. Anatomy and relations of the bladder, urethra, uterus and ovary, vagina, and rectum.

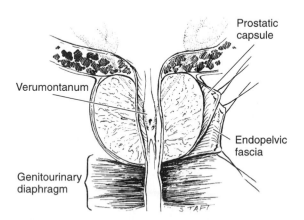

Figure 1–11. Section of the prostate gland shows the prostatic urethra, verumontanum, and crista urethralis, in addition to the opening of the prostatic utricle and the 2 ejaculatory ducts in the midline. Note that the prostate is surrounded by the prostatic capsule, which is covered by another prostatic sheath derived from the endopelvic fascia. The prostate is resting on the genitourinary diaphragm. (Reproduced, with permission, from Tanagho EA: Anatomy of the lower urinary tract. In: Walsh PC et al [editors]: *Campbell's Urology,* 6th ed., vol. 1. Saunders, 1992.)

Lymphatics

The lymphatics from the prostate drain into the internal iliac (hypogastric), sacral, vesical, and external iliac lymph nodes.

SEMINAL VESICLES

Gross Appearance

The seminal vesicles lie just cephalic to the prostate under the base of the bladder (Figures 1–6 and 1–8). They are about 6 cm long and quite soft. Each vesicle joins its corresponding vas deferens to form the ejaculatory duct. The ureters lie medial to each, and the rectum is contiguous with their posterior surfaces.

Histology

The mucous membrane is pseudostratified. The submucosa consists of dense connective tissue covered by a thin layer of muscle that in turn is encapsulated by connective tissue.

Blood Supply

The blood supply is similar to that of the prostate gland.

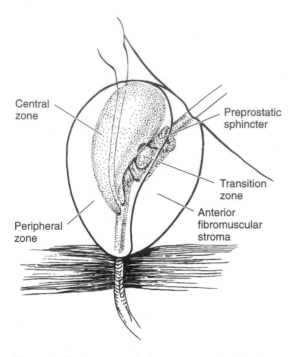

Figure 1–12. Anatomy of the prostate gland (adapted from McNeal). (Reproduced, with permission, from Tanagho EA: Anatomy of the lower urinary tract. In: Walsh PC et al [editors]: *Campbell's Urology,* 6th ed., vol. 1. Saunders, 1992.)

Nerve Supply

The nerve supply is mainly from the sympathetic nerve plexus.

Lymphatics

The lymphatics of the seminal vesicles are those that serve the prostate.

SPERMATIC CORD

Gross Appearance

The 2 spermatic cords extend from the internal inguinal rings through the inguinal canals to the testicles (Figure 1–8). Each cord contains the vas deferens, the internal and external spermatic arteries, the artery of the vas, the venous pampiniform plexus (which forms the spermatic vein superiorly), lymph vessels, and nerves. All of the preceding are enclosed in investing layers of thin fascia. A few fibers of the cremaster muscle insert on the cords in the inguinal canal.

Histology

The fascia covering the cord is formed of loose connective tissue that supports arteries, veins, and lymphatics. The vas deferens is a small, thick-walled tube consisting of an internal mucosa and submucosa surrounded by 3 well-defined layers of smooth muscle encased in a covering of fibrous tissue. Above the testes, this tube is straight. Its proximal 4 cm tends to be convoluted.

Blood Supply

A. Arterial: The external spermatic artery, a branch of the inferior epigastric, supplies the fascial coverings of the cord. The internal spermatic artery passes through the cord on its way to the testis. The deferential artery is close to the vas.

B. Venous: The veins from the testis and the coverings of the spermatic cord form the pampiniform plexus, which, at the internal inguinal ring, unites to form the spermatic vein.

Lymphatics

The lymphatics from the spermatic cord empty into the external iliac lymph nodes.

EPIDIDYMIS

Gross Appearance

A. Anatomy: The upper portion of the epididymis (globus major) is connected to the testis by numerous efferent ducts from the testis (Figure 1–8). The epididymis consists of a markedly coiled duct that, at its lower pole (globus minor), is continuous with the vas deferens. An appendix of the epididymis is often seen on its upper pole; this is a cystic body that in some cases is pedunculated but in others is sessile.

B. Relations: The epididymis lies posterolateral to the testis and is nearest to the testis at its upper pole. Its lower pole is connected to the testis by fibrous tissue. The vas lies posteromedial to the epididymis.

Histology

The epididymis is covered by serosa. The ductus epididymidis is lined by pseudostratified columnar epithelium throughout its length.

Blood Supply

A. Arterial: The arterial supply to the epididymis comes from the internal spermatic artery and the artery of the vas (deferential artery).

B. Venous: The venous blood drains into the pampiniform plexus, which becomes the spermatic vein.

Lymphatics

The lymphatics drain into the external iliac and internal iliac (hypogastric) lymph nodes.

TESTIS

Gross Appearance

A. Anatomy: The average testicle measures about 4 × 3 × 2.5 cm (Figure 1–8). It has a dense fascial covering called the tunica albuginea testis, which, posteriorly, is invaginated somewhat into the body of the testis to form the mediastinum testis. This fibrous mediastinum sends fibrous septa into the testis, thus separating it into about 250 lobules.

The testis is covered anteriorly and laterally by the visceral layer of the serous tunica vaginalis, which is continuous with the parietal layer that separates the testis from the scrotal wall.

At the upper pole of the testis is the appendix testis, a small pedunculated or sessile body similar in appearance to the appendix of the epididymis.

B. Relations: The testis is closely attached posterolaterally to the epididymis, particularly at its upper and lower poles.

Histology
(Figure 1–8)

Each lobule contains 1–4 markedly convoluted seminiferous tubules, each of which is about 60 cm long. These ducts converge at the mediastinum testis, where they connect with the efferent ducts that drain into the epididymis.

The seminiferous tubule has a basement membrane containing connective and elastic tissue. This supports the seminiferous cells, which are of 2 types: (1) Sertoli (supporting) cells and (2) spermatogenic cells. The stroma between the seminiferous tubules contains connective tissue in which the interstitial Leydig cells are located.

Blood Supply

The blood supply to the testes is closely associated with that to the kidneys because of the common embryologic origin of the two organs.

A. Arterial: The arteries to the testes (internal spermatics) arise from the aorta just below the renal arteries and course through the spermatic cords to the testes, where they anastomose with the arteries of the vasa deferentia that branch off from the internal iliac (hypogastric) artery.

B. Venous: The blood from the testis returns in the pampiniform plexus of the spermatic cord. At the internal inguinal ring, the pampiniform plexus forms the spermatic vein.

The right spermatic vein enters the vena cava just below the right renal vein; the left spermatic vein empties into the left renal vein.

Lymphatics

The lymphatic vessels from the testes pass to the lumbar lymph nodes, which in turn are connected to the mediastinal nodes.

SCROTUM

Gross Appearance

Beneath the corrugated skin of the scrotum lies the dartos muscle. Deep to this are the 3 fascial layers derived from the abdominal wall at the time of testicular descent. Beneath these is the parietal layer of the tunica vaginalis.

The scrotum is divided into 2 sacs by a septum of connective tissue. The scrotum not only supports the testes but, by relaxation or contraction of its muscular layer, helps to regulate their environmental temperature.

Histology

The dartos muscle, under the skin of the scrotum, is unstriated. The deeper layer is made up of connective tissue.

Blood Supply

A. Arterial: The arteries to the scrotum arise from the femoral, internal pudendal, and inferior epigastric arteries.

B. Venous: The veins are paired with the arteries.

Lymphatics

The lymphatics drain into the superficial inguinal and subinguinal lymph nodes.

PENIS & MALE URETHRA

Gross Appearance

The penis is composed of 2 corpora cavernosa and the corpus spongiosum, which contains the urethra, whose diameter is 8–9 mm. These corpora are capped distally by the glans. Each corpus is enclosed in a fascial sheath (tunica albuginea), and all are surrounded by a thick fibrous envelope known as Buck's fascia. A covering of skin, devoid of fat, is loosely applied about these bodies. The prepuce forms a hood over the glans.

Beneath the skin of the penis (and scrotum) and extending from the base of the glans to the urogenital diaphragm is Colles' fascia, which is continuous with Scarpa's fascia of the lower abdominal wall (Figure 1–9).

The proximal ends of the corpora cavernosa are attached to the pelvic bones just anterior to the ischial tuberosities. Occupying a depression of their ventral surface in the midline is the corpus spongiosum, which is connected proximally to the undersurface of the urogenital diaphragm, through which emerges the membranous urethra. This portion of the corpus spongiosum is surrounded by the bulbospongiosus muscle. Its distal end expands to form the glans penis.

The suspensory ligament of the penis arises from

the linea alba and pubic symphysis and inserts into the fascial covering of the corpora cavernosa.

Histology

A. Corpora and Glans Penis: The corpora cavernosa, the corpus spongiosum, and the glans penis are composed of septa of smooth muscle and erectile tissue that enclose vascular cavities.

B. Urethra: The urethral mucosa that traverses the glans penis is formed of squamous epithelium. Proximal to this, the mucosa is transitional in type. Underneath the mucosa is the submucosa, which contains connective and elastic tissue and smooth muscle. In the submucosa are the numerous glands of Littre, whose ducts connect with the urethral lumen. The urethra is surrounded by the vascular corpus spongiosum and the glans penis.

Blood Supply

A. Arterial: The penis and urethra are supplied by the internal pudendal arteries. Each artery divides into a deep artery of the penis (which supplies the corpora cavernosa), a dorsal artery of the penis, and the bulbourethral artery. These branches supply the corpus spongiosum, the glans penis, and the urethra.

B. Venous: The superficial dorsal vein lies external to Buck's fascia. The deep dorsal vein is placed beneath Buck's fascia and lies between the dorsal arteries. These veins connect with the pudendal plexus, which drains into the internal pudendal vein.

Lymphatics

Lymphatic drainage from the skin of the penis is to the superficial inguinal and subinguinal lymph nodes. The lymphatics from the glans penis pass to the subinguinal and external iliac nodes. The lymphatics from the deep urethra drain into the internal iliac (hypogastric) and common iliac lymph nodes.

FEMALE URETHRA

The adult female urethra is about 4 cm long and 8 mm in diameter. It is slightly curved and lies beneath the pubic symphysis just anterior to the vagina.

The epithelial lining of the female urethra is squamous in its distal portion and pseudostratified or transitional in the remainder. The submucosa is made up of connective and elastic tissues and spongy venous spaces. Embedded in it are many periurethral glands, which are most numerous distally; the largest of these are the periurethral glands of Skene, which open on the floor of the urethra just inside the meatus.

External to the submucosa is a longitudinal layer of smooth muscle continuous with the inner longitudinal layer of the bladder wall. Surrounding this is a heavy layer of circular smooth muscle fibers extending from the external vesical muscular layer. They constitute the true involuntary urethral sphincter. External to this is the circular striated (voluntary) sphincter surrounding the middle third of the urethra; this constitutes an intensive element in the musculature of the urethra.

The arterial supply to the female urethra is derived from the inferior vesical, vaginal, and internal pudendal arteries. Blood from the urethra drains into the internal pudendal veins.

Lymphatic drainage from the external portion of the urethra is to the inguinal and subinguinal lymph nodes. Drainage from the deep urethra is into the internal iliac (hypogastric) lymph nodes.

Nerve Supply to the Genitourinary Organs

See Figures 3–2 and 3–3.

REFERENCES

ADRENALS

Chang A et al: Adrenal gland: MR imaging. Radiology 1987;163:123.

Peppercorn PD, Reznek RH: State-of-the-art C and MRI of the adrenal gland. Eur Radiol 1997;7:822.

KIDNEYS

Aizenstein RI et al: The perinephric space and renal fascia: Review of normal anatomy, pathology, and pathways of disease spread. J Magn Reson Imaging 1998;8:517.

Amis ES Jr, Cronan JJ: The renal sinus: An imaging review and proposed nomenclature for sinus cysts. J Urol 1988;139:1151.

Chestbrough RM et al: Gerota versus Zuckerkandl: The renal fascia revisited. Radiology 1989;173:845.

Cockett ATK: Lymphatic network of kidney. 1. Anatomic and physiologic considerations. Urology 1977;9:125.

Emamian SA et al: Kidney dimensions at sonography: Correlation with age, sex, and habitus in 655 adult volunteers. AJR 1993;160:83.

Hoeltl W, Hruby W, Aharinejad S: Renal vein anatomy and its implications for retroperitoneal surgery. J Urol 1990;143:1108.

Kikinis R et al: Normal and hydronephrotic kidney:

Evaluation of renal function with contrast-enhanced MR imaging. Radiology 1987;165:837.

Korobkin M et al: CT of the extraperitoneal space: Normal anatomy and fluid collections. AJR 1992;159:933.

Mandell J et al: Structural genitourinary defects detected in utero. Radiology 1991;178:193.

Ohlson L: Normal collecting ducts: Visualization at urography. Radiology 1989;170:33.

Patten RM et al: The fetal genitourinary tract. Radiol Clin North Am 1990;28:115.

Potter EL: Development of the human glomerulus. Arch Pathol 1965;80:241.

Prince MR: Renal MR angiography: A comprehensive approach. J Magn Reson Imaging 1998;8:511.

Resnick MI, Pounds DM, Boyce WH: Surgical anatomy of the human kidney and its applications. Urology 1981;17:367.

Sampaio FJ: Anatomical background for nephron-sparing surgery in renal cell carcinoma. J Urol 1992;147:999.

Sampaio FJ, Aragao AH: Anatomical relationship between the intrarenal arteries and the kidney collecting system. J Urol 1990;143:679.

Sampaio FJ, Aragao AH: Inferior pole collecting system anatomy: Its probable role in extracorporeal shock wave lithotripsy. J Urol 1992;147:322.

Sampaio FJ et al: Intrarenal access: 3-dimensional anatomical study. J Urol 1992;148:1769.

Schlesinger AE et al: Normal standards for kidney length in premature infants: Determination with US. Work in progress. Radiology 1987;164:127.

CALICES, RENAL PELVIS, & URETERS

Dillard JP, Talner LB, Pinckney L: Normal renal papillae simulating caliceal filling defects on sonography. AJR 1987;148:895.

Elbadawi A, Amaku EO, Frank IN: Trilaminar musculature of submucosal ureter: Anatomy and functional implications. Urology 1973;2:409.

Hanna MK et al: Ureteral structure and ultrastructure. 1. Normal human ureter. J Urol 1976;116:718.

Kay R: Ureterocalicostomy. Urol Clin North Am 1988;15:129.

Kneeland JB et al: Perirenal spaces: CT evidence for communication across the midline. Radiology 1987;164:657.

Koff SA et al: Pathophysiology of ureteropelvic junction obstruction: Experimental and clinical observations. J Urol 1986;136:336.

Osathanondh V, Potter EL: Development of human kidney shown by microdissection. 2. Renal pelvis, calyces, and papillae. 3. Formation and interrelationships of collecting tubules and nephrons. 4. Formation of tubular portions of nephrons. 5. Development of vascular pattern of glomerulus. Arch Pathol 1963;76:277, 290 and 1966;82:391, 403.

Rizzo M et al: Ultrastructure of the urinary tract muscle coat in man: Calices, renal pelvis, pelviureteric junction and ureter. Eur Urol 1981;7:171.

Tanagho EA: The ureterovesical junction: Anatomy and physiology. In: Chisholm GD, Williams DI (editors): Scientific Foundations of Urology. Heinemann, 1982.

Weiss RM, Bassett AL, Hoffman BF: Adrenergic innervation of the ureter. Invest Urol 1978;16:123.

BLADDER & URETHRA

Andersson KE: Neurotransmitters and neuroreceptors in the lower urinary tract. Curr Opin Obstet Gynecol 1996;8:361.

Banson ML: Normal MR anatomy and techniques for imaging of the male pelvis. Magn Reson Imaging Clin North Am 1996;4:481.

Chai TC, Steers WD: Neurophysiology of micturition and continence. Urol Clin North Am 1996;23:221.

Crowe R, Burnstock G: A histochemical and immunohistochemical study of the autonomic innervation of the lower urinary tract of the female pig: Is the pig a good model for the human bladder and urethra? J Urol 1989;141:414.

Elbadawi A: Functional anatomy of the organs of micturition. Urol Clin North Am 1996;23:177.

Elbadawi A: Ultrastructure of vesicourethral innervation. 1. Neuroeffector and cell junctions in male internal sphincter. J Urol 1982;128:180.

Gosling JA, Dixon DS: The structure and innervation of smooth muscle in the wall of the bladder neck and proximal urethra. Br J Urol 1975;47:549.

Hakky SI: Ultrastructure of the normal human urethra. Br J Urol 1979;51:304.

Hutch JA: Anatomy and Physiology of the Bladder, Trigone and Urethra. Appleton-Century-Crofts, 1972.

Hutch JA: The internal urinary sphincter: A double loop system. J Urol 1971;105:375.

Juenemann KP et al: Clinical significance of sacral and pudendal nerve anatomy. J Urol 1988;139:74.

Klosterman PW, Laing FC, McAninch JW: Sonourethrography in the evaluation of urethral stricture disease. Urol Clin North Am 1989;16:791.

Lee JK, Rholl KS: MRI of the bladder and prostate. AJR 1986;147:732.

Olesen KP, Grau V: The suspensory apparatus of the female bladder neck. Urol Int 1976;31:33.

Sandler CM, Corriere JN Jr: Urethrography in the diagnosis of acute urethral injuries. Urol Clin North Am 1989;16:283.

Schlegel PN, Walsh PC: Neuroanatomical approach to radical cystoprostatectomy with preservation of sexual function. J Urol 1987;138:1402.

Tanagho EA: Anatomy of the lower urinary tract. In: Walsh PC et al (editors): Campbell's Urology, 6th ed., vol. 1, p. 40. Saunders, 1992.

Tanagho EA, Miller ER: Functional considerations of urethral sphincteric dynamics. J Urol 1973;109:273.

Tanagho EA, Pugh RCB: The anatomy and function of the ureterovesical junction. Br J Urol 1963;35:151.

Tanagho EA, Schmidt RA, de Araujo CG: Urinary striated sphincter: What is its nerve supply? Urology 1982;20:415.

Tanagho EA, Smith DR: The anatomy and function of the bladder neck. Br J Urol 1966;38:54.

Tanagho EA et al: Observations in the dynamics of the bladder neck. Br J Urol 1966;38:72.

PROSTATE

Allen KS et al: Age-related changes of the prostate: Evaluation by MR imaging. AJR 1989;152:77.

Bruschini H, Schmidt RA, Tanagho EA: The male genitourinary sphincter mechanism in the dog. Invest Urol 1978;15:284.

Greene DR, Fitzpatrick JM, Scardino PT: Anatomy of the prostate and distribution of early prostate cancer. Semin Surg Oncol 1995;11:9.

Hricak H et al: MR imaging of the prostate gland: Normal anatomy. AJR 1987;148:51.

Hutch JA, Rambo ON Jr: A study of the anatomy of the prostate, prostatic urethra and the urinary sphincter system. J Urol 1970;104:443.

McNeal JE: The prostate and prostatic urethra: A morphologic study. J Urol 1972;107:1008.

Myers RP: Anatomical variation of the superficial preprostatic veins with respect to radical retropubic prostatectomy. J Urol 1991;145:992.

Myers RP: Male urethral sphincteric anatomy and radical prostatectomy. Urol Clin North Am 1991;18:211.

Myers RP, Goellner JR, Cahill DR: Prostate shape, external striated urethral sphincter and radical prostatectomy: The apical dissection. J Urol 1987;138:543.

Older RA, Watson LR: Ultrasound anatomy of the normal male reproductive tract. J Clin Ultrasound 1996;24:389.

Rifkin MD, Dahnert W, Kurtz AB: State of the art: Endorectal sonography of the prostate gland. AJR 1990;154:691.

Vaalsti A, Hervonen A: Autonomic innervation of the human prostate. Invest Urol 1980;17:293.

Villers A et al: Ultrasound anatomy of the prostate: The normal gland and anatomical variations. J Urol 1990;143:732.

Wein AJ, Benson Gs, Jacobowitz D: Lack of evidence for adrenergic innervation of external urethral sphincter. J Urol 1979;121:324.

Wheeler TM: Anatomic considerations in carcinoma of the prostate. Urol Clin North Am 1989;16:623.

SPERMATIC CORD

Baker LL et al: MR imaging of the scrotum: Normal anatomy. Radiology 1987;163:89.

Bergman LL: The regional anatomy of the inguinal canal. GP (Oct) 1962;26:114.

Gooding GA: Sonography of the spermatic cord. AJR 1988;151:721.

Wishahi MM: Anatomy of spermatic venous plexus (pampiniform plexus) in men with and without varicocele: Intraoperative venographic study. J Urol 1992; 147:1285.

TESTIS

Busch FM, Sayegh ES: Roentgenographic visualization of human testicular lymphatics: A preliminary report. J Urol 1963;89:106.

Mills JL et al: Early growth predicts timing of puberty in boys: Results of a 14-year nutrition and growth study. J Pediatr 1986;109:543.

Takihara H et al: Significance of testicular size measurement in andrology: 2. Correlation of testicular size with testicular function. J Urol 1987;137:416.

Wollin M et al: Aberrant epididymal tissue: A significant clinical entity. J Urol 1987;138:1247.

FEMALE URETHRA

DeLancey JO: Structural aspects of the extrinsic continence mechanism. Obstet Gynecol 1988;72:296.

Klutke C et al: The anatomy of stress incontinence: Magnetic resonance imaging of the female bladder neck and urethra. J Urol 1990;143:563.

Lindner HH, Feldman SE: Surgical anatomy of the perineum. Surg Clin North Am 1962;42:877.

Mostwin JL: Current concepts of female pelvic anatomy and physiology. Urol Clin North Am 1991;18:175.

Ulmsten U: Some reflections and hypotheses on the pathophysiology of female urinary incontinence. Acta Obstet Gynecol Scand Suppl 1997;166:3.

Zacharin RF: The anatomic supports of the female urethra. Obstet Gynecol 1968;32:754.

Embryology of the Genitourinary System

2

Emil A. Tanagho, MD

At birth, the genital and urinary systems are related only in the sense that they share certain common passages. Embryologically, however, they are intimately related. Because of the complex interrelationships of the embryonic phases of the 2 systems, they are discussed here as 5 subdivisions: the nephric system, the vesicourethral unit, the gonads, the genital duct system, and the external genitalia.

NEPHRIC SYSTEM

The nephric system develops progressively as 3 distinct entities: pronephros, mesonephros, and metanephros.

Pronephros

The pronephros is the earliest nephric stage in humans, and it corresponds to the mature structure of the most primitive vertebrate. It extends from the fourth to the 14th somites and consists of 6–10 pairs of tubules. These open into a pair of primary ducts that are formed at the same level, extend caudally, and eventually reach and open into the cloaca. The pronephros is a vestigial structure that disappears completely by the fourth week of embryonic life (Figure 2–1).

Mesonephros

The mature excretory organ of the higher fish and amphibians corresponds to the embryonic mesonephros. It is the principal excretory organ during early embryonic life (4–8 weeks). It, too, gradually degenerates, although parts of its duct system become associated with the male reproductive organs. The mesonephric tubules develop from the intermediate mesoderm caudal to the pronephros shortly before pronephric degeneration. The mesonephric tubules differ from those of the pronephros in that

they develop a cuplike outgrowth into which a knot of capillaries is pushed. This is called Bowman's capsule, and the tuft of capillaries is called a glomerulus. In their growth, the mesonephric tubules extend toward and establish a connection with the nearby primary nephric duct as it grows caudally to join the cloaca (Figure 2–1). This primary nephric duct is now called the mesonephric duct. After establishing their connection with the nephric duct, the primordial tubules elongate and become S-shaped. As the tubules elongate, a series of secondary branchings increase their surface exposure, thereby enhancing their capacity for interchanging material with the blood in adjacent capillaries. Leaving the glomerulus, the blood is carried by one or more efferent vessels that soon break up into a rich capillary plexus closely related to the mesonephric tubules. The mesonephros, which forms early in the fourth week, reaches its maximum size by the end of the second month.

Metanephros

The metanephros, the final phase of development of the nephric system, originates from both the intermediate mesoderm and the mesonephric duct. Development begins in the 5- to 6-mm embryo with a budlike outgrowth from the mesonephric duct as it bends to join the cloaca. This ureteral bud grows cephalad and collects mesoderm from the nephrogenic cord of the intermediate mesoderm around its tip. This mesoderm with the metanephric cap moves, with the growing ureteral bud, more and more cephalad from its point of origin. During this cephalic migration, the metanephric cap becomes progressively larger, and rapid internal differentiation takes place. Meanwhile, the cephalic end of the ureteral bud expands within the growing mass of metanephrogenic tissue to form the renal pelvis (Figure 2–1). Numerous outgrowths from the renal pelvic dilatation push radially into this growing mass and form hollow ducts that branch and rebranch as they push toward the periphery. These form the primary collecting ducts of the kidney. Mesodermal cells become arranged in small

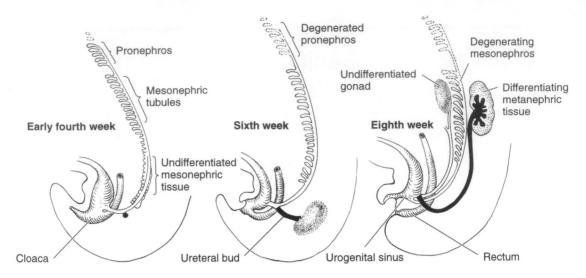

Figure 2–1. Schematic representation of the development of the nephric system. Only a few of the tubules of the pronephros are seen early in the fourth week, while the mesonephric tissue differentiates into mesonephric tubules that progressively join the mesonephric duct. The first sign of the ureteral bud from the mesonephric duct is seen. At 6 weeks, the pronephros has completely degenerated and the mesonephric tubules start to do so. The ureteral bud grows dorsocranially and has met the metanephrogenic cap. At the eighth week, there is cranial migration of the differentiating metanephros. The cranial end of the ureteric bud expands and starts to show multiple successive outgrowths. (Adapted from several sources.)

vesicular masses that lie close to the blind end of the collecting ducts. Each of these vesicular masses will form a uriniferous tubule draining into the duct nearest to its point of origin.

As the kidney grows, increasing numbers of tubules are formed in its peripheral zone. These vesicular masses develop a central cavity and become S-shaped. One end of the S coalesces with the terminal portion of the collecting tubules, resulting in a continuous canal. The proximal portion of the S develops into the distal and proximal convoluted tubules and into Henle's loop; the distal end becomes the glomerulus and Bowman's capsule. At this stage, the undifferentiated mesoderm and the immature glomeruli are readily visible on microscopic examination (Figure 2–2). The glomeruli are fully developed by the 36th week or when the fetus weighs 2500 g (Osathanondh and Potter, 1964). The metanephros arises opposite the 28th somite (fourth lumbar segment). At term, it has ascended to the level of the first lumbar or even the 12th thoracic vertebra. This ascent of the kidney is due not only to actual cephalic migration but also to differential growth in the caudal part of the body. During the early period of ascent (seventh to ninth weeks), the kidney slides above the arterial bifurcation and rotates 90 degrees. Its convex border is now directed laterally, not dorsally. Ascent proceeds more slowly until the kidney reaches its final position.

Certain features of these 3 phases of development must be emphasized: (1) The 3 successive units of the system develop from the intermediate mesoderm. (2) The tubules at all levels appear as independent primordia and only secondarily unite with the duct system. (3) The nephric duct is laid down as the duct of the pronephros and develops from the union of the ends of the anterior pronephric tubules. (4) This pronephric duct serves subsequently as the mesonephric duct and as such gives rise to the ureter. (5) The nephric duct reaches the cloaca by independent caudal growth. (6) The embryonic ureter is an outgrowth of the nephric duct, yet the kidney tubules differentiate from adjacent metanephric blastema.

ANOMALIES OF THE NEPHRIC SYSTEM

Failure of the metanephros to ascend leads to **ectopic kidney.** An ectopic kidney may be on the proper side but low (simple ectopy) or on the opposite side (crossed ectopy) with or without fusion. Failure to rotate during ascent causes a **malrotated kidney.**

Fusion of the paired metanephric masses leads to various anomalies—most commonly **horseshoe kidney.**

The ureteral bud from the mesonephric duct may bifurcate, causing a **bifid ureter** at various levels depending on the time of the bud's subdivision. An accessory ureteral bud may develop from the mesonephric duct, thereby forming a **duplicated ureter,** usually meeting the same metanephric mass.

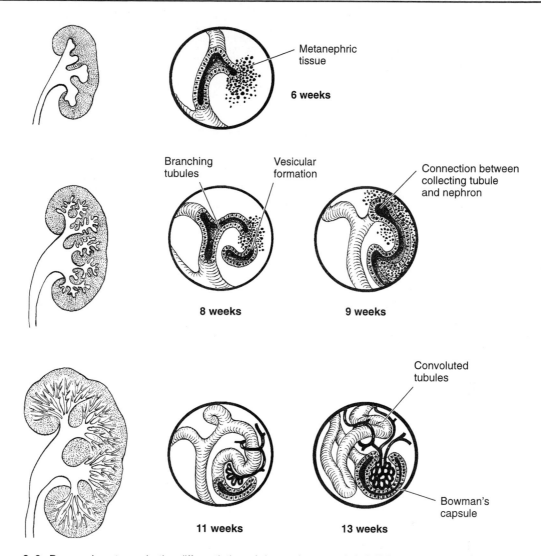

Figure 2–2. Progressive stages in the differentiation of the nephrons and their linkage with the branching collecting tubules. A small lump of metanephric tissue is associated with each terminal collecting tubule. These are then arranged in vesicular masses that later differentiate into a uriniferous tubule draining into the duct near which it arises. At one end, Bowman's capsule and the glomerulus differentiate; the other end establishes communication with the nearby collecting tubules.

Rarely, each bud has a separate metanephric mass, resulting in **supernumerary kidneys.**

If the double ureteral buds are close together on the mesonephric duct, they open near each other in the bladder. In this case, the main ureteral bud, which is the first to appear and the most caudal on the mesonephric ducts, reaches the bladder first. It then starts to move upward and laterally and is followed later by the second accessory bud as it reaches the urogenital sinus. The main ureteral bud (now more cranial on the urogenital sinus) drains the lower portion of the kidney. The 2 ureteral buds reverse their relationship as they move from the mesonephric duct

to the urogenital sinus. This is why double ureters always cross (Weigert-Meyer law). If the 2 ureteral buds are widely separated on the mesonephric duct, the accessory bud appears more proximal and ends in the bladder with an ectopic orifice lower than the normal one. This ectopic orifice could still be in the bladder close to its outlet, in the urethra, or even in the genital duct system (Figure 2–3). A single ureteral bud that arises higher than normal on the mesonephric duct can also end in a similar ectopic location.

Lack of development of a ureteral bud results in a **solitary kidney** and a hemitrigone.

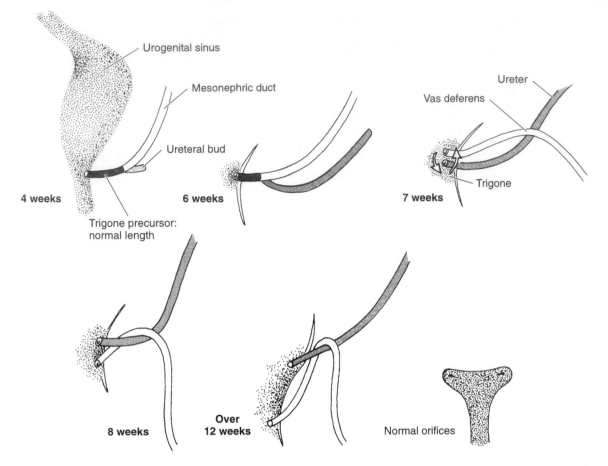

Urogenital sinus

Mesonephric duct

Ureteral bud

4 weeks

Trigone precursor:
normal length

6 weeks

Ureter

Vas deferens

Trigone

7 weeks

8 weeks

**Over
12 weeks**

Normal orifices

Figure 2–3. The development of the ureteral bud from the mesonephric duct and the relationship of both to the urogenital sinus. The ureteral bud appears at the fourth week. The mesonephric duct distal to this ureteral bud is gradually absorbed into the urogenital sinus, resulting in separate endings for the ureter and the mesonephric duct. The mesonephric tissue that is incorporated into the urogenital sinus expands and forms the trigonal tissue.

VESICOURETHRAL UNIT

The blind end of the hindgut caudal to the point of origin of the allantois expands to form the cloaca, which is separated from the outside by a thin plate of tissue (the cloacal membrane) lying in an ectodermal depression (the proctodeum) under the root of the tail. At the 4-mm stage, starting at the cephalic portion of the cloaca where the allantois and gut meet, the cloaca progressively divides into 2 compartments by the caudal growth of a crescentic fold, the urorectal fold. The 2 limbs of the fold bulge into the lumen of the cloaca from either side, eventually meeting and fusing. The division of the cloaca into a ventral portion (urogenital sinus) and a dorsal portion (rectum) is completed during the seventh week. During

the development of the urorectal septum, the cloacal membrane undergoes a reverse rotation, so that the ectodermal surface is no longer directed toward the developing anterior abdominal wall but gradually is turned to face caudally and slightly posteriorly. This change facilitates the subdivision of the cloaca and is brought about mainly by development of the infraumbilical portion of the anterior abdominal wall and regression of the tail. The mesoderm that passes around the cloacal membrane to the caudal attachment of the umbilical cord proliferates and grows, forming a surface elevation, the genital tubercle. Further growth of the infraumbilical part of the abdominal wall progressively separates the umbilical cord from the genital tubercle. The division of the cloaca is completed before the cloacal membrane ruptures, and its 2 parts therefore have separate openings. The ventral part is the primitive urogenital sinus, which has the shape of an elongated cylinder and is continuous cranially with the allantois; its external opening is the urogenital ostium. The dorsal part is the rectum, and its external opening is the anus.

The urogenital sinus receives the mesonephric ducts. The caudal end of the mesonephric duct distal to the ureteral bud is progressively absorbed into the urogenital sinus. By the seventh week, the mesonephric duct and the ureteral bud have independent opening sites. This introduces an island of mesodermal tissue amid the surrounding endoderm of the urogenital sinus. As development progresses, the opening of the mesonephric duct (which will become the ejaculatory duct) migrates downward and medially. The opening of the ureteral bud (which will become the ureteral orifice) migrates upward and laterally. The absorbed mesoderm of the mesonephric duct expands with this migration to occupy the area limited by the final position of these tubes (Figure 2–3). This will later be differentiated as the trigonal structure, which is the only mesodermal inclusion in the endodermal vesicourethral unit.

The urogenital sinus can be divided into 2 main segments; the dividing line, the junction of the combined müllerian ducts with the dorsal wall of the urogenital sinus, is an elevation called Müller's tubercle, which is the most fixed reference point in the whole structure and which is discussed in a subsequent section. The segments are as follows:

(1) The ventral and pelvic portion forms the bladder, part of the urethra in males, and the whole urethra in females. This portion receives the ureter.

(2) The urethral, or phallic, portion receives the mesonephric and the fused müllerian ducts. This will be part of the urethra in males and forms the lower fifth of the vagina and the vaginal vestibule in females.

During the third month, the ventral part of the urogenital sinus starts to expand and forms an epithelial sac whose apex tapers into an elongated, narrowed urachus. The pelvic portion remains narrow and tubular; it forms the whole urethra in females and the supramontanal portion of the prostatic urethra in males. The splanchnic mesoderm surrounding the ventral and pelvic portion of the urogenital sinus begins to differentiate into interlacing bands of smooth muscle fibers and an outer fibrous connective tissue coat. By the 12th week, the layers characteristic of the adult urethra and bladder are recognizable (Figure 2–4).

The part of the urogenital sinus caudal to the opening of the müllerian duct forms the vaginal vestibule and contributes to the lower fifth of the vagina in females (Figure 2–5). In males, it forms the inframontanal part of the prostatic urethra and the membranous urethra. The penile urethra is formed by the fusion of the urethral folds on the ventral surface of the genital tubercle. In females, the urethral folds remain separate and form the labia minora. The glandular urethra in males is formed by canalization of the urethral plate. The bladder originally extends up to the umbilicus, where it is connected to the allantois that extends into the umbilical cord. The allantois usually is obliterated at the level of the umbilicus by the 15th week. The bladder then starts to descend by the 18th week. As it descends, its apex becomes stretched and narrowed, and it pulls on the already obliterated allantois, now called the urachus. By the 20th week, the bladder is well separated from the umbilicus, and the stretched urachus becomes the middle umbilical ligament.

PROSTATE

The prostate develops as multiple solid outgrowths of the urethral epithelium both above and below the entrance of the mesonephric duct. These simple, tubular outgrowths begin to develop in 5 distinct groups at the end of the 11th week and are complete by the 16th week (112-mm stage). They branch and rebranch, ending in a complex duct system that encounters the differentiating mesenchymal cells around this segment of the urogenital sinus. These mesenchymal cells start to develop around the tubules by the 16th week and become denser at the periphery to form the prostatic capsule. By the 22nd week, the muscular stroma is considerably developed, and it continues to increase progressively until birth.

From the 5 groups of epithelial buds, 5 lobes are eventually formed: anterior, posterior, median, and 2 lateral lobes. Initially, these lobes are widely separated, but later they meet, with no definite septa dividing them. Tubules of each lobe do not intermingle with each other but simply lie side by side.

The anterior lobe tubules begin to develop simultaneously with those of the other lobes. Although in the early stages the anterior lobe tubules are large and show multiple branches, gradually they contract and lose most of the branches. They continue to shrink, so that at birth they show no lumen and appear as small, solid embryonic epithelial outgrowths. In contrast, the tubules of the posterior lobe are fewer in number yet larger, with extensive branching. These tubules, as they grow, extend posterior to the developing median and lateral lobes and form the posterior aspect of the gland, which may be felt rectally.

ANOMALIES OF THE VESICOURETHRAL UNIT

Failure of the cloaca to subdivide is rare and results in a **persistent cloaca.** Incomplete subdivision is more frequent, ending with **rectovesical, rectourethral,** or **rectovestibular fistulas** (usually with **imperforate anus** or **anal atresia**).

Failure of descent or incomplete descent of the

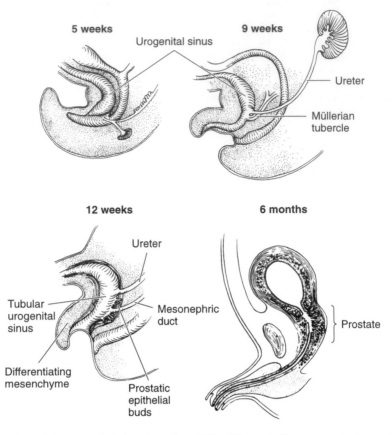

Figure 2–4. Differentiation of the urogenital sinus in males. At the fifth week, the progressively growing urorectal septum is separating the urogenital sinus from the rectum. The former receives the mesonephric duct and the ureteral bud. It retains its tubular structure until the 12th week, when the surrounding mesenchyme starts to differentiate into the muscle fibers around the whole structure. The prostate gland develops as multiple epithelial outgrowths just above and below the mesonephric duct. During the third month, the ventral part of the urogenital sinus expands to form the bladder proper; the pelvic part remains narrow and tubular, forming part of the urethra. (Reproduced, with permission, from Tanagho EA, Smith DR: Mechanisms of urinary continence. 1. Embryologic, anatomic, and pathologic considerations. J Urol 1969;100:640.)

bladder leads to a **urinary umbilical fistula (urachal fistula)**, **urachal cyst**, or **urachal diverticulum** depending on the stage and degree of maldescent.

Development of the genital primordia in an area more caudal than normal can result in formation of the corpora cavernosa just caudal to the urogenital sinus outlet, with the urethral groove on its dorsal surface. This defect results in complete or incomplete **epispadias** depending on its degree. A more extensive defect results in **vesical exstrophy.** Failure of fusion of urethral folds leads to various grades of **hypospadias.** This defect, because of its mechanism, never extends proximal to the bulbous urethra. This is in contrast to epispadias, which usually involves the entire urethra up to the internal meatus.

GONADS

Most of the structures that make up the embryonic genital system have been taken over from other systems, and their readaptation to genital function is a secondary and relatively late phase in their development. The early differentiation of such structures is therefore independent of sexuality. Furthermore, each embryo is at first morphologically bisexual, possessing all the necessary structures for either sex. The development of one set of sex primordia and the gradual involution of the other are determined by the sex of the gonad.

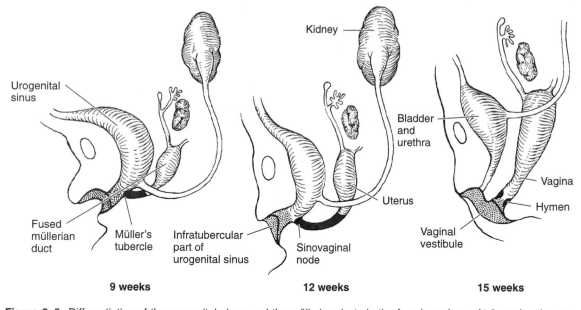

Figure 2–5. Differentiation of the urogenital sinus and the müllerian ducts in the female embryo. At 9 weeks, the urogenital sinus receives the fused müllerian ducts at Müller's tubercle (sinovaginal node; **see p 26**), which is solidly packed with cells. As the urogenital sinus distal to Müller's tubercle becomes wider and shallower (15 weeks), the urethra and fused müllerian duct will have separate openings. The distal part of the urogenital sinus forms the vaginal vestibule and the lower fifth of the vagina (shaded area), and that part above Müller's tubercle forms the urinary bladder and the entire female urethra. The fused müllerian ducts form the uterus and the upper four-fifths of the vagina. The hymen is formed at the junction of the sinovaginal node and the urogenital sinus.

The sexually undifferentiated gonad is a composite structure. Male and female potentials are represented by specific histologic elements (medulla and cortex) that have alternative roles in gonadogenesis. Normal differentiation involves the gradual predominance of one component.

The primitive sex glands make their appearance during the fifth and sixth weeks within a localized region of the thickening known as the urogenital ridge (this contains both the nephric and the genital primordia). At the sixth week, the gonad consists of a superficial germinal epithelium and an internal blastema. The blastemal mass is derived mainly from proliferative ingrowth from the superficial epithelium, which comes loose from its basement membrane.

During the seventh week, the gonad begins to assume the characteristics of a testis or ovary. Differentiation of the ovary usually occurs somewhat later than differentiation of the testis.

If the gonad develops into a testis, the gland increases in size and shortens into a more compact organ while achieving a more caudal location. Its broad attachment to the mesonephros is converted into a gonadal mesentery known as the mesorchium. The cells of the germinal epithelium grow into the underlying mesenchyme and form cordlike masses. These are radially arranged and converge toward the mesorchium, where a dense portion of the blastemal mass

is also emerging as the primordium of the rete testis. A network of strands soon forms that is continuous with the testis cords. The latter also split into 3–4 daughter cords. These eventually become differentiated into the seminiferous tubules by which the spermatozoa are produced. The rete testis unites with the mesonephric components that will form the male genital ducts, as discussed in a subsequent section (Figure 2–6).

If the gonad develops into an ovary, it (like the testis) gains a mesentery (mesovarium) and settles in a more caudal position. The internal blastema differentiates in the ninth week into a primary cortex beneath the germinal epithelium and a loose primary medulla. A compact cellular mass bulges from the medulla into the mesovarium and establishes the primitive rete ovarii. At 3–4 months of age, the internal cell mass becomes young ova. A new definitive cortex is formed from the germinal epithelium as well as from the blastema in the form of distinct cellular cords (Pflüger's tubes), and a permanent medulla is formed. The cortex differentiates into ovarian follicles containing ova.

Descent of the Gonads

A. Testis: In addition to its early caudal migration, the testis later leaves the abdominal cavity and

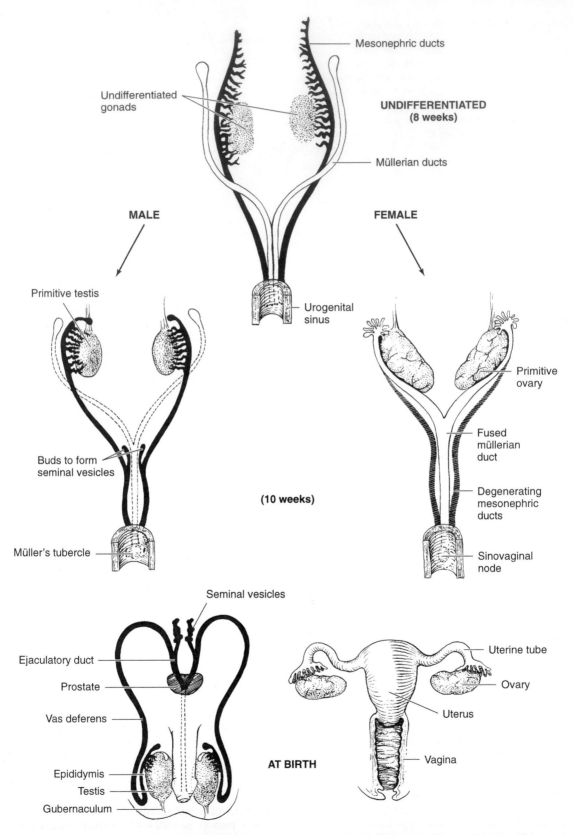

Figure 2–6. Transformation of the undifferentiated genital system into the definitive male and female systems.

descends into the scrotum. By the third month of fetal life, the testis is located retroperitoneally in the false pelvis. A fibromuscular band (the gubernaculum) extends from the lower pole of the testis through the developing muscular layers of the anterior abdominal wall to terminate in the subcutaneous tissue of the scrotal swelling. The gubernaculum also has several other subsidiary strands that extend to adjacent regions. Just below the lower pole of the testis, the peritoneum herniates as a diverticulum along the anterior aspect of the gubernaculum, eventually reaching the scrotal sac through the anterior abdominal muscles (the processus vaginalis). The testis remains at the abdominal end of the inguinal canal until the seventh month. It then passes through the inguinal canal behind (but invaginating) the processus vaginalis. Normally, it reaches the scrotal sac by the end of the eighth month.

B. Ovary: In addition to undergoing an early internal descent, the ovary becomes attached through the gubernaculum to the tissues of the genital fold and then attaches itself to the developing uterovaginal canal at its junction with the uterine (fallopian) tubes. This part of the gubernaculum between the ovary and uterus becomes the ovarian ligament; the part between the uterus and the labia majora becomes the round ligament of the uterus. These ligaments prevent extra-abdominal descent, and the ovary enters the true pelvis. It eventually lies posterior to the uterine tubes on the superior surface of the urogenital mesentery, which has descended with the ovary and now forms the broad ligament. A small processus vaginalis forms and passes toward the labial swelling, but it is usually obliterated at full term.

GONADAL ANOMALIES

Lack of development of the gonads is called **gonadal agenesis.** Incomplete development with arrest at a certain phase is called **hypogenesis. Supernumerary gonads** are rare. The commonest anomaly involves descent of the gonads, especially the testis. Retention of the testis in the abdomen or arrest of its descent at any point along its natural pathway is called **cryptorchidism,** which may be either unilateral or bilateral. If the testis does not follow the main gubernacular structure but follows one of its subsidiary strands, it will end in an abnormal position, resulting in **ectopic testis.**

Failure of union between the rete testis and mesonephros results in a testis separate from the male genital ducts (the epididymis) and azoospermia.

GENITAL DUCT SYSTEM

Alongside the indifferent gonads, there are, early in embryonic life, 2 different yet closely related ducts. One is primarily a nephric duct (wolffian duct), yet it also serves as a genital duct if the embryo develops into a male. The other (müllerian duct) is primarily a genital structure from the start.

Both ducts grow caudally to join the primitive urogenital sinus. The wolffian duct (known as the pronephric duct at the 4-mm stage) joins the ventral part of the cloaca, which will be the urogenital sinus. This duct gives rise to the ureteral bud close to its caudal end. The ureteral bud grows cranially and meets metanephrogenic tissue. The part of each mesonephric duct caudal to the origin of the ureteric bud becomes absorbed into the wall of the primitive urogenital sinus, so that the mesonephric duct and ureter open independently. This is achieved at the 15-mm stage (seventh week). During this period, starting at the 10-mm stage, the müllerian ducts start to develop. They reach the urogenital sinus relatively late—at the 30-mm stage (ninth week)—their partially fused blind ends producing the elevation called Müller's tubercle. Müller's tubercle is the most constant and reliable point of reference in the whole system.

If the gonad starts to develop into a testis (17-mm stage, seventh week), the wolffian duct will start to differentiate into the male duct system, forming the epididymis, vas deferens, seminal vesicles, and ejaculatory ducts. At this time, the müllerian duct proceeds toward its junction with the urogenital sinus and immediately starts to degenerate. Only its upper and lower ends persist, the former as the appendix testis and the latter as part of the prostatic utricle.

If the gonad starts to differentiate into an ovary (22-mm stage, eighth week), the müllerian duct system forms the uterine (fallopian) tubes, uterus, and most of the vagina. The wolffian ducts, aside from their contribution to the urogenital sinus, remain rudimentary.

MALE DUCT SYSTEM

Epididymis

Because of the proximity of the differentiating gonads and the nephric duct, some of the mesonephric tubules are retained as the efferent ductules, and their lumens become continuous with those of the rete testis. These tubules, together with the part of the mesonephric duct into which they empty, will form the epididymis. Each coiled ductule makes a conical mass known as the lobule of the epididymis. The cranial end of the mesonephric duct becomes highly convoluted, completing the formation of the epididymis. This is an example of direct inclusion of a nephric structure into the genital system. Additional mesonephric tubules, both cephalad and caudal to those that were included in the formation of the epididymis, remain as rudimentary structures, ie, the appendix of the epididymis and the paradidymis.

Vas Deferens, Seminal Vesicles, & Ejaculatory Ducts

The mesonephric duct caudal to the portion forming the epididymis forms the vas deferens. Shortly before this duct joins the urethra (urogenital sinus), a localized dilatation (ampulla) develops, and the saccular convoluted structure that will form the seminal vesicle is evaginated from its wall. The mesonephric duct between the origin of the seminal vesicle and the urethra forms the ejaculatory duct. The whole mesonephric duct now achieves its characteristic thick investment of smooth muscle, with a narrow lumen along most of its length.

Both above and below the point of entrance of the mesonephric duct into the urethra, multiple outgrowths of urethral epithelium mark the beginning of the development of the prostate. As these epithelial buds grow, they meet the developing muscular fibers around the urogenital sinus, and some of these fibers become entangled in the branching tubules of the growing prostate and become incorporated into it, forming its muscular stroma (Figure 2–4).

FEMALE DUCT SYSTEM

The müllerian ducts, which are a paired system, are seen alongside the mesonephric duct. It is not known whether they arise directly from the mesonephric ducts or separately as an invagination of the celomic epithelium into the parenchyma lateral to the cranial extremity of the mesonephric duct, but the latter theory is favored. The müllerian duct develops and runs lateral to the mesonephric duct. Its opening into the celomic cavity persists as the peritoneal ostium of the uterine tube (later it develops fimbriae). The other end grows caudally as a solid tip and then crosses in front of the mesonephric duct at the caudal extremity of the mesonephros. It continues its growth in a caudomedial direction until it meets and fuses with the müllerian duct of the opposite side. The fusion is partial at first, so there is a temporary septum between the 2 lumens. This later disappears, leaving one cavity that will form the uterovaginal canal. The potential lumen of the vaginal canal is completely packed with cells. The solid tip of this cord pushes the epithelium of the urogenital sinus outward, where it becomes Müller's tubercle (33-mm stage, ninth week). The müllerian ducts actually fuse at the 63-mm stage (13th week), forming the sinovaginal node, which receives a limited contribution from the uro-

genital sinus. (This contribution forms the lower fifth of the vagina.)

The urogenital sinus distal to Müller's tubercle, originally narrow and deep, shortens, widens, and opens to form the floor of the pudendal or vulval cleft. This results in separate openings for the vagina and urethra and also brings the vaginal orifice to its final position nearer the surface. At the same time, the vaginal segment increases appreciably in length. The vaginal vestibule is derived from the infratubercular segment of the urogenital sinus (in males, the same segment will form the inframontanal part of the prostatic urethra and the membranous urethra). The labia minora are formed from the urethral folds (in males they form the pendulous urethra). The hymen is the remnant of the müllerian tubercle. The lower fifth of the vagina is derived from the portion of the urogenital sinus that combines with the sinovaginal node. The remainder of the vagina and the uterus are formed from the lower (fused) third of the müllerian ducts. The uterine tubes (fallopian tubes, oviducts) are the cephalic two-thirds of the müllerian ducts (Figure 2–6).

ANOMALIES OF THE GONADAL DUCT SYSTEM

Nonunion of the rete testis and the efferent ductules can occur and, if bilateral, causes **azoospermia** and **sterility.** Failure of the müllerian ducts to approximate or to fuse completely can lead to various degrees of **duplication** in the genital ducts. **Congenital absence** of one or both uterine tubes or of the uterus or vagina occurs rarely.

Arrested development of the infratubercular segment of the urogenital sinus leads to its persistence, with the urethra and vagina having a common duct to the outside (**urogenital sinus**).

EXTERNAL GENITALIA

During the eighth week, external sexual differentiation begins to occur. Not until 3 months, however, do the progressively developing external genitalia attain characteristics that can be recognized as distinctively male or female. During the indifferent stage of sexual development, 3 small protuberances appear on the external aspect of the cloacal membrane. In front is the genital tubercle, and on either side of the membrane are the genital swellings.

With the breakdown of the urogenital membrane (17-mm stage, seventh week), the primitive urogenital sinus achieves a separate opening on the undersurface of the genital tubercle.

MALE EXTERNAL GENITALIA

The urogenital sinus opening extends on the ventral aspect of the genital tubercle as the urethral groove. The primitive urogenital orifice and the urethral groove are bounded on either side by the urethral folds. The genital tubercle becomes elongated to form the phallus. The corpora cavernosa are indicated in the seventh week as paired mesenchymal columns within the shaft of the penis. By the 10th week, the urethral folds start to fuse from the urogenital sinus orifice toward the tip of the phallus. At the 14th week, the fusion is complete and results in the formation of the penile urethra. The corpus spongiosum results from the differentiation of the mesenchymal masses around the formed penile urethra.

The glans penis becomes defined by the development of a circular coronary sulcus around the distal part of the phallus. The urethral groove and the fusing folds do not extend beyond the coronary sulcus. The glandular urethra develops as a result of canalization of an ectodermal epithelial cord that has grown through the glans. This canalization reaches and communicates with the distal end of the previously formed penile urethra. During the third month, a fold of skin at the base of the glans begins growing distally and, 2 months later, surrounds the glans. This forms the prepuce. Meanwhile, the genital swellings shift caudally and are recognizable as scrotal swellings. They meet and fuse, resulting in the formation of the scrotum, with 2 compartments partially separated by a median septum and a median raphe, indicating their line of fusion.

FEMALE EXTERNAL GENITALIA

Until the eighth week, the appearance of the female external genitalia closely resembles that of the male genitalia except that the urethral groove is shorter. The genital tubercle, which becomes bent caudally and lags in development, becomes the clitoris. As in males (though on a minor scale), mesenchymal columns differentiate into corpora cavernosa, and a coronary sulcus identifies the glans clitoridis. The most caudal part of the urogenital sinus shortens and widens, forming the vaginal vestibule. The urethral folds do not fuse but remain separate as the labia minora. The genital swellings meet in front of the anus, forming the posterior commissure, while the swellings as a whole enlarge and remain separated on either side of the vestibule and form the labia majora.

ANOMALIES OF THE EXTERNAL GENITALIA

Absence or duplication of the penis or clitoris is very rare. More commonly, the penis remains rudimentary or the clitoris shows hypertrophy. These anomalies may be seen alone or, more frequently, in association with **pseudohermaphroditism.** Concealed penis and transposition of penis and scrotum are relatively rare anomalies.

Failure or incomplete fusion of the urethral folds results in **hypospadias** (see preceding discussion). Penile development is also anomalous in cases of **epispadias** and **exstrophy** (see preceding discussion).

REFERENCES

GENERAL

Allan FD: *Essentials of Human Embryology,* 2nd ed. Oxford Univ Press, 1969.

Arey LB: *Developmental Anatomy: A Textbook and Laboratory Manual of Embryology,* 7th ed. Saunders, 1974.

Blechschmidt E: *The Stages of Human Development Before Birth: An Introduction to Human Embryology.* Saunders, 1961.

Corliss CE: *Patten's Human Embryology,* 4th ed. McGraw-Hill, 1976.

Fine RN: Diagnosis and treatment of fetal urinary tract abnormalities. J Pediatr 1992;121:333.

FitzGerald MJT: *Human Embryology: A Regional Approach.* Harper & Row, 1978.

Gilbert SG: *Pictorial Human Embryology.* University of Washington Press, 1989.

Kjelberg SR, Ericsson NO, Rudhe U: *The Lower Urinary Tract in Childhood: Some Correlated Clinical and Roentgenologic Observations.* Year Book, 1957.

Marshall FF: Embryology of the lower genitourinary tract. Urol Clin North Am 1978;5:3.

Moore KL: *The Developing Human: Clinically Oriented Embryology,* 3rd ed. Saunders, 1982.

Reddy PP, Mandell J: Prenatal diagnosis. Therapeutic implications. Urol Clin North Am 1998;25:171.

Snell RS: *Clinical Embryology for Medical Students,* 3rd ed. Little, Brown, 1983.

Stephens FD: *Congenital Malformations of the Urinary Tract.* Praeger, 1983.

Stephens FD: Embryopathy of malformations. J Urol 1982;127:13.

Tanagho EA: Developmental anatomy and urogenital abnormalities. In: Raz S (editor): *Female Urology.* Saunders, 1983.

Tanagho EA: Embryologic development of the urinary tract. In: Ball TP (editor): *AUA Update Series.* American Urological Association, 1982.

Vaughan ED Jr, Middleton GW: Pertinent genitourinary embryology: Review for practicing urologist. Urology 1975;6:139.

ANOMALIES OF THE NEPHRIC SYSTEM

Avni EF et al: Multicystic dysplastic kidney: Natural history from in utero diagnosis and postnatal followup. J Urol 1987;138:1420.

Bomalaski MD, Hirschl RB, Bloom DA: Vesicoureteral reflux and ureteropelvic junction obstruction: Association, treatment options and outcome. J Urol 1997;157:969.

Chevalier RL: Effects of ureteral obstruction on renal growth. Pediatr Nephrol 1995;9:594.

Churchill BM, Abara EO, McLorie GA: Ureteral duplication, ectopy and ureteroceles. Pediatr Clin North Am 1987;34:1273.

Cole BR, Conley SB, Stapleton FB: Polycystic kidney disease in the first year of life. J Pediatr 1987;111:693.

Corrales JG, Elder JS: Segmental multicystic kidney and ipsilateral duplication anomalies. J Urol 1996;155:1398.

Cox R, Strachan JR, Woodhouse CR: Twenty-year follow-up of primary megaureter. Eur Urol 1990;17:43.

Decter RM: Renal duplication and fusion anomalies. Pediatr Clin North Am 1997;44:1323.

Douglas LL, Pott GA: Congenital ureteral diverticulum and solitary kidney. J Urol 1979;122:401.

Evans WP et al: Association of crossed fused renal ectopia and multicystic kidney. J Urol 1979;122:821.

Gabow PA: Autosomal dominant polycystic kidney disease. N Engl J Med 1993;329:332.

Gibbs T: Genitourinary embryology and congenital malformations. Part 1. The kidneys and ureters. Urol Nurs 1990;10(3):16.

Higashihara E et al: Medullary sponge kidney and hyperparathyroidism. Urology 1988;31:155.

Kaplan BS et al: Polycystic kidney diseases in childhood. J Pediatr 1989;115:867.

Keating MA et al: Changing concepts in management of primary obstructive megaureter. J Urol 1989;142:636.

Lockhard JL, Singer AM, Glenn JF: Congenital megaureter. J Urol 1979;122:310.

Maatman TJ, DeOreo GA Jr, Kay R: Solitary pseudo-crossed renal ectopia. J Urol 1983;129:128.

MacDermot KD et al: Prenatal diagnosis of autosomal dominant polycystic kidney disease (PKD1) presenting in utero and prognosis for very early onset disease. J Med Genet 1998;35:13.

Magee MC: Ureteroceles and duplicated systems: Embryologic hypothesis. J Urol 1980;123:605.

Magee MC: Ureteroceles in single versus duplicated systems: An embryologic hypothesis. Urology 1981;18:365.

Maher ER, Kaelin WG Jr: Von Hippel-Lindau disease. Medicine (Baltimore) 1997;76:381.

Mandell J et al: Ureteral ectopia in infants and children. J Urol 1981;126:219.

Mesrobian HG, Rushton HG, Bulas D: Unilateral renal agenesis may result from in utero regression of multicystic renal dysplasia. J Urol 1993;150:793.

Murphy WK, Palubinskas AJ, Smith DR: Sponge kidney: Report of 7 cases. J Urol 1961;85:866.

Nakada T et al: Unilateral renal agenesis with or without ipsilateral adrenal agenesis. J Urol 1988;140:933.

Nguyen HT, Kogan BA: Upper urinary tract obstruction: Experimental and clinical aspects. Br J Urol 1998;81(Suppl 2):13.

Nunley JR, Sica DA, Smith V: Medullary sponge kidney and staghorn calculi. Urol Int 1990;45:118.

Osathanondh V, Potter EL: Pathogenesis of polycystic kidneys: Survey of results of microdissection. Arch Pathol 1964;77:510.

Osathanondh V, Potter EL: Pathogenesis of polycystic kidneys: Type 4 due to urethral obstruction. Arch Pathol 1964;77:502.

Peters CA et al: Congenital obstructed megaureters in early infancy: Diagnosis and treatment. J Urol 1989;142:641.

Robson WL, Leung AK, Rogers RC: Unilateral renal agenesis. Adv Pediatr 1995;42:575.

Ross JH, Kay R: Ureteropelvic junction obstruction in anomalous kidneys. Urol Clin North Am 1998;25:219.

Scherz HC et al: Ectopic ureteroceles: Surgical management with preservation of continence. Review of 60 cases. J Urol 1989;142:538.

Share JC, Lebowitz RL: Ectopic ureterocele without ureteral and calyceal dilatation (ureterocele disproportion): Findings on urography and sonography. AJR 1989;152:567.

Soderdahl DW, Shiraki IW, Schamber DT: Bilateral ureteral quadruplication. J Urol 1976;116:255.

Tanagho EA: Development of the ureter. In: Bergman H (editor): *The Ureter,* 2nd ed. Springer-Verlag, 1981.

Tanagho EA: Ureteroceles: Embryogenesis, pathogenesis and management. J Cont Educ Urol (Feb) 1979;18:13.

Thomsen HS et al: Renal cystic diseases. Eur Radiol 1997;7:1267.

Tokunaka S et al: Morphological study of ureterocele: Possible clue to its embryogenesis as evidenced by locally arrested myogenesis. J Urol 1981;126:726.

Watson ML, Macnicol AM, Wright AF: Adult polycystic kidney disease. Br Med J 1990;300:62.

Zerres K et al: Autosomal recessive polycystic kidney disease. Contrib Nephrol 1997;122:10.

ANOMALIES OF THE VESICOURETHRAL UNIT

Amar AD, Hutch JA: Anomalies of the ureter. In: *Encyclopedia of Urology,* vol. 7, *Malformations.* Springer, 1968.

Ansell JS: Surgical treatment of exstrophy of bladder with emphasis on neonatal primary closure: Personal experience with 28 consecutive cases treated at University of Washington Hospitals from 1962 to 1977. Techniques and results. J Urol 1979;121:650.

Asopa HS: Newer concepts in the management of hypospadias and its complications. Ann R Coll Surg Engl 1998;80:161.

Austin PF et al: The prenatal diagnosis of cloacal exstrophy. J Urol 1998;160(3 Pt 2):1179.

Bartsch G, Decristoforo A, Schweikert U: Pseudovaginal perineoscrotal hypospadias: Clinical, endocrinological and biochemical characterization of a patient. Eur Urol 1987;13:386.

Begg RC: The urachus, its anatomy, histology and development. J Anat 1930;64:170.

Belman AB: Hypospadias update. Urology 1997;49:166.

Burbige KA et al: Prune belly syndrome: 35 years of experience. J Urol 1987;137:86.

Churchill BM et al: Emergency treatment and long-term follow-up of posterior urethral valves. Urol Clin North Am 1990;17:343.

Chwalle R: The process of formation of cystic dilatations of the vesical end of the ureter and of diverticula at the ureteral ostium. Urol Cutan Rev 1927;31:499.

Connor JP et al: Long-term follow-up of 207 patients with bladder exstrophy: An evolution in treatment. J Urol 1989;142:793.

Dinneen MD, Duffy PG: Posterior urethral valves. Br J Urol 1996;78:275.

Duckett JW: The current hype in hypospadiology. Br J Urol 1995;76 (Suppl 3):1.

Eagle JR Jr, Barrett GS: Congenital deficiency of abdominal musculature with associated genitourinary abnormalities: A syndrome. Report of nine cases. Pediatrics 1950;6:721.

Elmassalme FN et al: Duplication of urethra—case report and review of literature. Eur J Pediatr Surg 1997;7:313.

Escham W, Holt HA: Complete duplication of bladder and urethra. J Urol 1980;123:773.

Goh DW, Davey RB, Dewan PA: Bladder, urethral, and vaginal duplication. J Pediatr Surg 1995;30:125.

Gonzales ET Jr: Alternatives in the management of posterior urethral valves. Urol Clin North Am 1990;17:35.

Greskovich FJ III, Nyberg LM Jr: The prune belly syndrome: A review of its etiology, defects, treatment and prognosis. J Urol 1988;140:707.

Haralson IP: Double bladder and urethra with imperforate anus and ureterorenal reflux: Case presentation with review of literature. J Urol 1980;123:776.

Hinman F Jr: Microphallus: Distinction between anomalous and endocrine types. Trans Am Assoc Genitourin Surg 1979;71:159.

Hinman F Jr: Surgical disorders of the bladder and umbilicus of urachal origin. Surg Gynecol Obstet 1961;113:605.

Jaramillo D, Lebowitz RL, Hendren WH: The cloacal malformation: Radiologic findings and imaging recommendations. Radiology 1990;177:441.

Jeffs RD: Exstrophy, epispadias, and cloacal and urogenital sinus abnormalities. Pediatr Clin North Am 1987;34:1233.

Kroovand RL, Al-Ansari RM, Perlmutter AD: Urethral and genital malformations in prune belly syndrome. J Urol 1982;127:94.

Landes RR, Melnick I, Klein R: Vesical exstrophy with epispadias: Twenty-year follow-up. Urology 1977;9:53.

Lattimer JK: Congenital deficiency of the abdominal musculature and associated genitourinary anomalies: A report of 22 cases. J Urol 1958;79:343.

Loder RT et al: Musculoskeletal aspects of prune-belly syndrome: Description and pathogenesis. Am J Dis Child 1992;146:1224.

Mackie GG: Abnormalities of the ureteral bud. Urol Clin North Am 1978;5:161.

Manzoni GA, Ransley PG, Hurwitz RS: Cloacal exstrophy and cloacal exstrophy variants: A proposed system of classification. J Urol 1987;138:1065.

Massad CA et al: Morphology and histochemistry of infant testes in the prune belly syndrome. J Urol 1991;146:1598.

Mesrobian HG, Kelalis PP, Kramer SA: Long-term followup of 103 patients with bladder exstrophy. J Urol 1988;139:719.

Meyer R: Normal and abnormal development of the ureter in the human embryo: A mechanistic consideration. Anat Rec 1946;96:355.

Morgan RJ, Williams DI, Pryor JP: Müllerian duct remnants in the male. Br J Urol 1979;51:481.

Mouriquand PD, Persad R, Sharma S: Hypospadias repair: Current principles and procedures. Br J Urol 1995;76(Suppl 3):9.

Orvis BR, Bottles K, Kogan BA: Testicular histology in fetuses with the prune belly syndrome and posterior urethral valves. J Urol 1988;139:335.

Parkhouse HF, Woodhouse CR: Long-term status of patients with posterior urethral valves. Urol Clin North Am 1990;7:373.

Peters CA et al: Congenital obstructed megaureters in early infancy: Diagnosis and treatment. J Urol 1989;142:641, 667.

Randall A, Campbell EW: Anomalous relationship of the right ureter to the vena cava. J Urol 1935;34:565.

Reinberg Y et al: Prune belly syndrome in females: A triad of abdominal musculature deficiency and anomalies of the urinary and genital systems. J Pediatr 1991;118:395.

Rosenfeld B et al: Type III posterior urethral valves: Presentation and management. J Pediatr Surg 1994;29:81.

Shapiro E: Embryologic development of the prostate: Insights into the etiology and treatment of benign prostatic hyperplasia. Urol Clin North Am 1990;17:487.

Sharma AK et al: Megalourethra: A report of four cases and review of the literature. Pediatr Surg Int 1997;12:458.

Shima H et al: Developmental anomalies associated with hypospadias. J Urol 1979;122:619.

Sohrabi A et al: Duplication of male urethra. Urology 1978;12:704.

Stephens FD: Congenital Malformations of the Rectum, Anus and Genitourinary Tracts. Livingstone, 1963.

Stephens FD: The female anus, perineum and vestibule: Embryogenesis and deformities. J Obstet Gynaecol Br Commonw 1968;8:55.

Tanagho EA: Embryologic basis for lower ureteral anomalies: A hypothesis. Urology 1976;7:451.

Uehling DT: Posterior urethral valves: Functional classification. Urology 1980;15:27.

Van Savage JG et al: An algorithm for the management of anterior urethral valves. J Urol 1997;158(3 Pt 2):1030.

Wakhlu AK et al: Congenital megalourethra. J Pediatr Surg 1996;31:441.

Wespes E et al: Blind ending, bifid, and double ureters. Urology 1983;21:586.

Woodhouse CR, Reilly JM, Bahadur G: Sexual function and fertility in patients treated for posterior urethral valves. J Urol 1989;142:586.

Workman SJ, Kogan BA: Fetal bladder histology in posterior urethral valves and the prune belly syndrome. J Urol 1990;144:337.

GONADAL ANOMALIES

Bartone FF, Schmidt MA: Cryptorchidism: Incidence of chromosomal anomalies in 50 cases. J Urol 1982;127:1105.

Ben-Chaim J, Gearhart JP: Current management of bladder exstrophy. Scand J Urol Nephrol 1997;31:103.

Borzi PA, Thomas DF: Cantwell-Ransley epispadias repair in male epispadias and bladder exstrophy. J Urol 1994;151:457.

Clinical diagnosis of cryptorchidism. John Radcliffe Hospital Cryptorchidism Study Group. Arch Dis Child 1988;63:587.

Crankson SJ, Ahmed S: Female bladder exstrophy. Int Urogynecol J Pelvic Floor Dysfunct 1997;8:98.

DePalma L, Carter D, Weiss RM: Epididymal and vas deferens immaturity in cryptorchidism. J Urol 1988; 140:1166.

Diez Garcia R et al: Peno-scrotal transposition. Eur J Pediatr Surg 1995;5:222.

Elder JS, Isaacs JT, Walsh PC: Androgenic sensitivity of gubernaculum testis: Evidence for hormonal/mechanical interactions in testicular descent. J Urol 1982; 127:170.

Fallon B, Welton M, Hawtrey C: Congenital anomalies associated with cryptorchidism. J Urol 1982;127:91.

Gad YZ et al: 5 alpha-reductase deficiency in patients with micropenis. J Inherited Metab Dis 1997;20:95.

Hadziselimovic F et al: The significance of postnatal gonadotropin surge for testicular development in normal and cryptorchid testes. J Urol 1986;136:274.

Honoré LH: Unilateral anorchism: Report of 11 cases with discussion of etiology and pathogenesis. Urology 1978;11:251.

Huff DS et al: Postnatal testicular maldevelopment in unilateral cryptorchidism. J Urol 1989;142:546.

Job J-C et al: Hormonal therapy of cryptorchidism with human chorionic gonadotrophin (HCG). Urol Clin North Am 1982;127:508.

Johnson P et al: Inferior vesical fissure. J Urol 1995;154:1478.

Kaplan LM et al: Association between abdominal wall defects and cryptorchidism. J Urol 1986;136:645.

Koff WJ, Scaletscky R: Malformations of the epididymis in undescended testis. J Urol 1990;143:340.

Lustig RH et al: Ontogeny of gonadotropin secretion in congenital anorchism: Sexual dimorphism versus syndrome of gonadal dysgenesis and diagnostic considerations. J Urol 1987;138:587.

Macfarlane FJ: Genitourinary embryology and congenital malformations. Part 2. The lower urinary tract, gonads, and genital duct system. Urol Nurs 1991; 11(1):8.

Marshall FF, Weissman RM, Jeffs RD: Cryptorchidism: Surgical implications of nonunion of epididymis and testis. J Urol 1980;124:560.

McGillivray BC: Genetic aspects of ambiguous genitalia. Pediatr Clin North Am 1992;39:307.

Mollard P, Basset T, Mure PY: Female epispadias. J Urol 1997;158:1543.

Newman K, Randolph J, Anderson K: The surgical management of infants and children with ambiguous genitalia: Lessons learned from 25 years. Ann Surg 1992;215:644.

Pagon RA: Diagnostic approach to the newborn with ambiguous genitalia. Pediatr Clin North Am 1987;34: 1019.

Pujol A et al: The value of bilateral biopsy in unilateral cryptorchidism. Eur Urol 1978;4:85.

Rajfer J, Walsh PC: Testicular descent: Normal and abnormal. Urol Clin North Am 1978;5:223.

Rajfer J et al: Hormonal therapy of cryptorchidism: A randomized, double-blind study comparing human chorionic gonadotropin and gonadotropin-releasing hormone. N Engl J Med 1986;314:466.

Walsh PC: The differential diagnosis of ambiguous genitalia in the newborn. Urol Clin North Am 1978; 5:213.

Zaontz MR, Packer MG. Abnormalities of the external genitalia. Pediatr Clin North Am 1997;44:1267.

Symptoms of Disorders of the Genitourinary Tract

3

Jack W. McAninch, MD

In the workup of any patient, the history is of paramount importance; this is particularly true in urology. It is necessary to discuss here only those urologic symptoms that are apt to be brought to the physician's attention by the patient. It is important to know not only whether the disease is acute or chronic but also whether it is recurrent, since recurring symptoms may represent acute exacerbations of chronic disease.

Obtaining the history is an art that depends on the skill and methods used to elicit information. The history is only as accurate as the patient's ability to describe the symptoms. This subjective information is important in establishing an accurate diagnosis.

SYSTEMIC MANIFESTATIONS

Symptoms of fever and weight loss should be sought. The presence of fever associated with other symptoms of urinary tract infection may be helpful in evaluating the site of the infection. Simple acute cystitis is essentially an afebrile disease. Acute pyelonephritis or prostatitis is apt to cause high temperatures (to 40 °C [104 °F]), often accompanied by violent chills. Infants and children suffering from acute pyelonephritis may have high temperatures without other localizing symptoms or signs. Such a clinical picture, therefore, *invariably* requires bacteriologic study of the urine.

A history of unexplained attacks of fever occurring even years before may represent otherwise asymptomatic pyelonephritis. Renal carcinoma sometimes causes fever that may reach 39 °C (102.2 °F) or more. The absence of fever does not by any means rule out renal infection, for it is the rule that chronic pyelonephritis does not cause fever.

Weight loss is to be expected in the advanced stages of cancer, but it may be noticed also when renal insufficiency due to obstruction or infection supervenes. In children who have "failure to thrive" (low weight and less than average height for age),

chronic obstruction, urinary tract infection, or both should be suspected.

General malaise may be noted with tumors, chronic pyelonephritis, or renal failure.

The presence of many of these symptoms may be compatible with human immunodeficiency virus (HIV; see Chapter 16).

LOCAL & REFERRED PAIN

Two types of pain have their origins in the genitourinary organs: local and referred. The latter is especially common.

Local pain is felt in or near the involved organ. Thus, the pain from a diseased kidney (T10–12, L1) is felt in the costovertebral angle and in the flank in the region of and below the 12th rib. Pain from an inflamed testicle is felt in the gonad itself.

Referred pain originates in a diseased organ but is felt at some distance from that organ. The ureteral colic (Figure 3–1) caused by a stone in the upper ureter may be associated with severe pain in the ipsilateral testicle; this is explained by the common innervation of these two structures (T11–12). A stone in the lower ureter may cause pain referred to the scrotal wall; in this instance, the testis itself is not hyperesthetic. The burning pain with voiding that accompanies acute cystitis is felt in the distal urethra in females and in the glandular urethra in males (S2–3).

Abnormalities of a urologic organ can also cause pain in any other organ (eg, gastrointestinal, gynecologic) that has a sensory nerve supply common to both (Figures 3–2 and 3–3).

Kidney Pain
(Figure 3–1)

Typical renal pain is felt as a dull and constant ache in the costovertebral angle just lateral to the sacrospinalis muscle and just below the 12th rib. This pain often spreads along the subcostal area toward the umbilicus or lower abdominal quadrant. It may be expected in the renal diseases that cause sudden

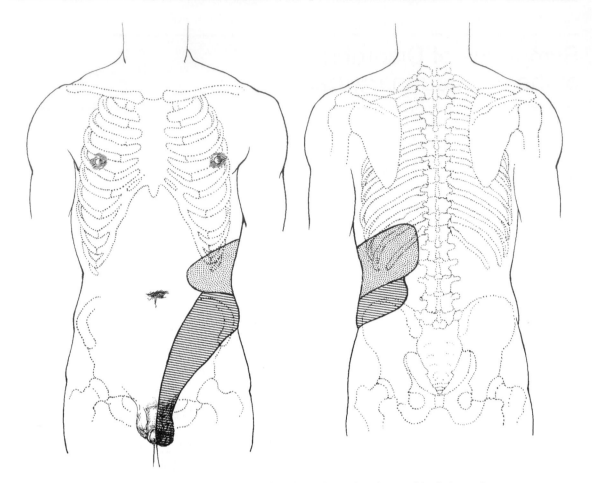

Figure 3–1. Referred pain from kidney (dotted areas) and ureter (shaded areas).

distention of the renal capsule. Acute pyelonephritis (with its sudden edema) and acute ureteral obstruction (with its sudden renal back pressure) both cause this typical pain. It should be pointed out, however, that many urologic renal diseases are painless because their progression is so slow that sudden capsular distention does not occur. Such diseases include cancer, chronic pyelonephritis, staghorn calculus, tuberculosis, polycystic kidney, and hydronephrosis due to chronic ureteral obstruction.

Pseudorenal Pain
(Radiculitis)

Mechanical derangements of the costovertebral or costotransverse joints can cause irritation or pressure on the costal nerves. Disorders of this sort are common in the cervical and thoracic areas, but the most common sites are T10–12. Irritation of these nerves causes costovertebral pain, often with radiation into the ipsilateral lower abdominal quadrant. The pain is positional in nature. Its onset is usually acute, following the lifting of a heavy object, a blow to the cos-

tovertebral area, or a fall on the buttocks from a height. The pain is usually absent on arising from bed; it is apt to increase as the day wears on. It is exacerbated by heavy physical work and is usually increased during an automobile trip over a rough road. It is apt to awaken the patient when a certain position is assumed (eg, lying on the right side) and is relieved by a change of position. Radiculitis may mimic ureteral colic or renal pain. True renal pain is seldom affected by movements of the spine.

Ureteral Pain
(Figure 3–1)

Ureteral pain is typically stimulated by acute obstruction (passage of a stone or a blood clot). In this instance, there is back pain from renal capsular distention combined with severe colicky pain (due to renal pelvic and ureteral muscle spasm) that radiates from the costovertebral angle down toward the lower anterior abdominal quadrant, along the course of the ureter. In men, it may also be felt in the bladder, scrotum, or testicle. In women, it may radiate into the

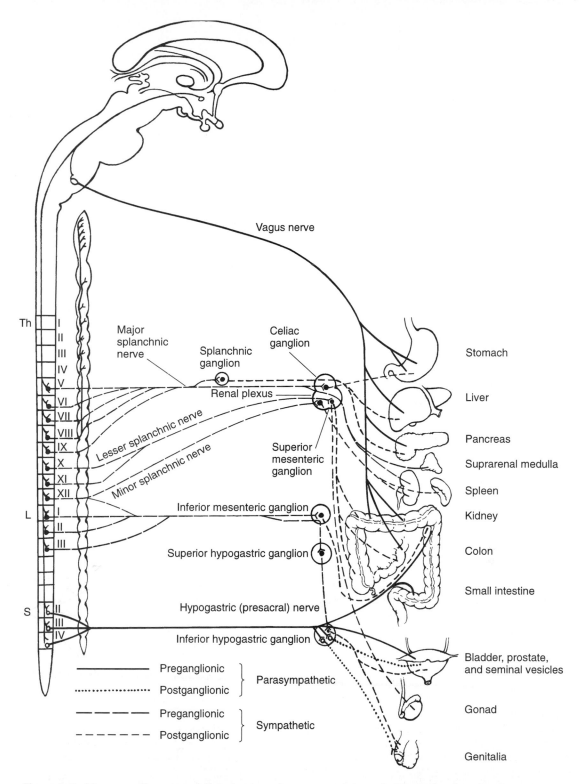

Figure 3–2. Diagrammatic representation of autonomic nerve supply to gastrointestinal and genitourinary tracts.

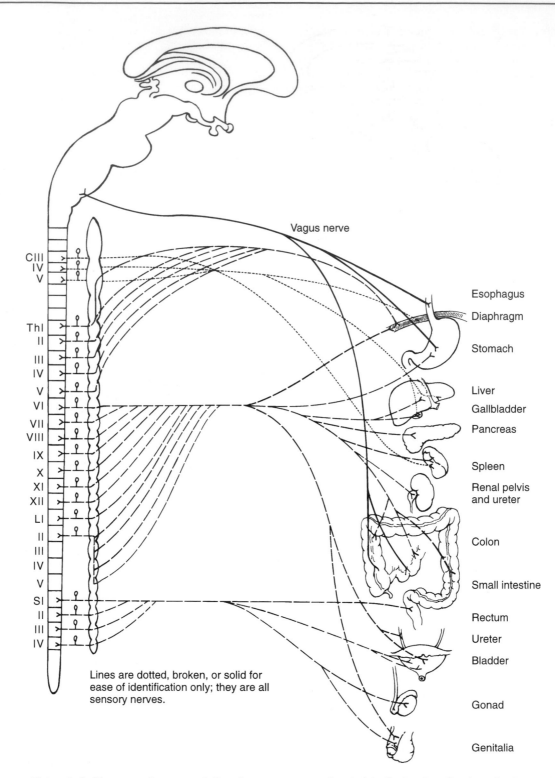

Figure 3–3. Diagrammatic representation of sensory nerves of gastrointestinal and genitourinary tracts.

vulva. The severity and colicky nature of this pain are caused by the hyperperistalsis and spasm of this smooth muscle organ as it attempts to rid itself of a foreign body or to overcome obstruction. It should be remembered that radiculitis may mimic ureteral pain.

The physician may be able to judge the position of a ureteral stone by the history of pain and the site of referral. If the stone is lodged in the upper ureter, the pain radiates to the testicle, since the nerve supply of this organ is similar to that of the kidney and upper ureter (T11–12). With stones in the mid portion of the ureter on the right side, the pain is referred to McBurney's point and may therefore simulate appendicitis; on the left side, it may resemble diverticulitis or other diseases of the descending or sigmoid colon (T12, L1). As the stone approaches the bladder, inflammation and edema of the ureteral orifice ensue, and symptoms of vesical irritability such as urinary frequency and urgency may occur. It is important to realize, however, that in mild ureteral obstruction, as seen in the congenital stenoses, there is usually no pain, either renal or ureteral.

Vesical Pain

The overdistended bladder of the patient in acute urinary retention causes agonizing pain in the suprapubic area. Other than this, however, constant suprapubic pain not related to the act of urination is usually not of urologic origin. The relatively uncommon interstitial cystitis and vesical ulceration caused by tuberculosis or schistosomiasis may cause suprapubic discomfort (usually relieved by urination) when the bladder becomes full.

The patient in chronic urinary retention due to bladder neck obstruction or neurogenic bladder may experience little or no suprapubic discomfort even though the bladder reaches the level of the umbilicus.

The most common cause of bladder pain is infection; the pain is usually not felt over the bladder but is referred to the distal urethra and is related to the act of urination. Terminal dysuria may be a major complaint in severe cystitis.

Prostatic Pain

Direct pain from the prostate gland is not common. Occasionally, when the prostate is acutely inflamed, the patient may feel a vague discomfort or fullness in the perineal or rectal area (S2–4). Lumbosacral backache is occasionally experienced as referred pain from the prostate but is not a common symptom of prostatitis. Inflammation of the gland may cause dysuria, frequency, and urgency.

Testicular Pain

Testicular pain due to trauma, infection, or torsion of the spermatic cord is very severe and is felt locally, although there may be some radiation of the discomfort along the spermatic cord into the lower abdomen. It may involve the costovertebral area as

well. Uninfected hydrocele, spermatocele, and tumor of the testis do not commonly cause pain. A varicocele may cause a dull ache in the testicle that is increased after heavy exercise. At times, the first symptom of an early indirect inguinal hernia may be testicular pain (referred). Pain from a stone in the upper ureter may be referred to the testicle.

Epididymal Pain

Acute infection of the epididymis is the only painful disease of this organ and is quite common. The pain begins in the scrotum, and some degree of neighborhood inflammatory reaction involves the adjacent testis as well, further aggravating the discomfort. In the early stages of epididymitis, pain may first be felt in the groin or lower abdominal quadrant. (If on the right side, it may simulate appendicitis.) This may be a referred type of pain but can be secondary to associated inflammation of the vas deferens. The discomfort associated with epididymitis may reach the costal angle and mimic ureteral stone on rare occasions.

Back & Leg Pain

Pain low in the back and radiating down one or both legs, especially when associated with symptoms of vesical neck obstruction in an older man, suggests metastases to the pelvic bones from cancer of the prostate.

GASTROINTESTINAL SYMPTOMS OF UROLOGIC DISEASES

Whether renal or ureteral disease is painful or not, gastrointestinal symptoms are often present. The patient with acute pyelonephritis suffers not only from localized back pain, symptoms of vesical irritability, chills, and fever but also from generalized abdominal pain and distention. A patient who is passing a stone down the ureter has typical renal and ureteral colic and, usually, hematuria and may experience severe nausea and vomiting as well as abdominal distention. However, the urinary symptoms so far overshadow the gastrointestinal symptoms that the latter are usually ignored. Inadvertent overdistention of the renal pelvis (eg, with opaque material in order to obtain adequate retrograde urograms) may cause the patient to become nauseated, to vomit, and to complain of cramplike pain in the abdomen. This clinical experiment demonstrates the renointestinal reflex, which may lead to confusing symptoms. In the very common "silent" urologic diseases, some degree of gastrointestinal symptomatology may be present, which could mislead the clinician into seeking the diagnosis in the intraperitoneal zone.

Cause of the Mimicry

A. Renointestinal Reflexes: Renointestinal reflexes account for most of the confusion. They arise because of the common autonomic and sensory innervations of the two systems (Figures 3–2 and 3–3). Afferent stimuli from the renal capsule or musculature of the pelvis may, by reflex action, cause pylorospasm (symptoms of peptic ulcer) or other changes in tone of the smooth muscles of the enteric tract and its adnexa.

B. Organ Relationships: The right kidney is closely related to the hepatic flexure of the colon, the duodenum, the head of the pancreas, the common bile duct, the liver, and the gallbladder (Figure 1–3). The left kidney lies just behind the splenic flexure of the colon and is closely related to the stomach, pancreas, and spleen. Inflammations or tumors in the retroperitoneum thus may extend into or displace intraperitoneal organs, causing them to produce symptoms.

C. Peritoneal Irritation: The anterior surfaces of the kidneys are covered by peritoneum. Renal inflammation, therefore, causes peritoneal irritation, which can lead to muscle rigidity and rebound tenderness.

The symptoms arising from chronic renal disease (eg, noninfected hydronephrosis, staghorn calculus, cancer, chronic pyelonephritis) may be entirely gastrointestinal and may simulate in every way the syndromes of peptic ulcer, gallbladder disease, or appendicitis, or other, less specific gastrointestinal complaints. If a thorough survey of the gastrointestinal tract fails to demonstrate suspected disease processes, the physician should give every consideration to study of the urinary tract.

SYMPTOMS RELATED TO THE ACT OF URINATION

Many conditions cause symptoms of "cystitis." These include infections of the bladder, vesical inflammation due to chemical or x-radiation reactions, interstitial cystitis, prostatitis, psychoneurosis, torsion or rupture of an ovarian cyst, and foreign bodies in the bladder. Often, however, the patient with chronic cystitis notices no symptoms of vesical irritability. Irritating chemicals or soap on the urethral meatus may cause cystitislike symptoms of dysuria, frequency, and urgency. This has been specifically noted in young girls taking frequent bubble baths.

Frequency, Nocturia, & Urgency
The normal capacity of the bladder is about 400 mL. Frequency may be caused by residual urine, which decreases the functional capacity of the organ. When the mucosa, submucosa, and even the muscularis become inflamed (eg, infection, foreign body, stones, tumor), the capacity of the bladder decreases sharply. This decrease is due to 2 factors: the pain resulting from even mild stretching of the bladder and the loss of bladder compliance resulting from inflam-

matory edema. When the bladder is normal, urination can be delayed if circumstances require it, but this is not so in acute cystitis. Once the diminished bladder capacity is reached, any further distention may be agonizing, and the patient may urinate involuntarily if voiding does not occur immediately. During very severe acute infections, the desire to urinate may be constant, and each voiding may produce only a few milliliters of urine. Day frequency without nocturia and acute or chronic frequency lasting only a few hours suggest nervous tension.

Diseases that cause fibrosis of the bladder are accompanied by frequency of urination. Examples of such diseases are tuberculosis, radiation cystitis, interstitial cystitis, and schistosomiasis. The presence of stones or foreign bodies causes vesical irritability, but secondary infection is almost always present.

Nocturia may be a symptom of renal disease related to a decrease in the functioning renal parenchyma with loss of concentrating power. Nocturia can occur in the absence of disease in persons who drink excessive amounts of fluid in the late evening. Coffee and alcoholic beverages, because of their specific diuretic effect, often produce nocturia if consumed just before bedtime. In older people who are ambulatory, some fluid retention may develop secondary to mild heart failure or varicose veins. With recumbency at night, this fluid is mobilized, leading to nocturia in these patients.

A very low or very high urine pH can irritate the bladder and cause frequency of urination. In chronic obstructive pulmonary disease, the $Paco_2$ is elevated. Compensation requires increased urinary excretion of chloride, leading to a low pH. With hyperventilation, the urine becomes strongly alkaline.

Dysuria
Painful urination is usually related to acute inflammation of the bladder, urethra, or prostate. At times, the pain is described as "burning" on urination and is usually located in the distal urethra in men. Women usually localize the pain to the urethra. The pain is present only with voiding and disappears soon after micturition is completed. More severe pain sometimes occurs in the bladder just at the end of voiding, suggesting that inflammation of the bladder is the likely cause. Pain also may be more marked at the beginning of or throughout the act of urination. Dysuria often is the first symptom suggesting urinary infection and is often associated with urinary frequency and urgency.

Enuresis
Strictly speaking, enuresis means bedwetting at night. It is physiologic during the first 2 or 3 years of life but becomes troublesome, particularly to parents, after that age. It may be functional or secondary to delayed neuromuscular maturation of the urethrovesical component, but it may present as a symptom

of organic disease (eg, infection, distal urethral stenosis in girls, posterior urethral valves in boys, neurogenic bladder). If wetting occurs also during the daytime, however, or if there are other urinary symptoms—or if the enuresis persists beyond age 5 or 6—urologic investigation is essential. In adult life, enuresis may be replaced by nocturia for which no organic basis can be found.

Symptoms of Bladder Outlet Obstruction

A. Hesitancy: Hesitancy in initiating the urinary stream is one of the early symptoms of bladder outlet obstruction. As the degree of obstruction increases, hesitancy is prolonged and the patient often strains to force urine through the obstruction. Prostate obstruction and urethral stricture are common causes of this symptom.

B. Loss of Force and Decrease of Caliber of the Stream: Progressive loss of force and caliber of the urinary stream is noted as urethral resistance increases despite the generation of increased intravesical pressure. This can be evaluated by measuring urinary flow rates; in normal circumstances with a full bladder a maximal flow of 20 mL/s should be achieved.

C. Terminal Dribbling: Terminal dribbling becomes more and more noticeable as obstruction progresses and is a most distressing symptom.

D. Urgency: A strong, sudden desire to urinate is caused by hyperactivity and irritability of the bladder, resulting from obstruction, inflammation, or neuropathic bladder disease. In most circumstances, the patient is able to control temporarily the sudden need to void, but loss of small amounts of urine may occur (urgency incontinence).

E. Acute Urinary Retention: Sudden inability to urinate may supervene. The patient experiences increasingly agonizing suprapubic pain associated with severe urgency and may dribble only small amounts of urine.

F. Chronic Urinary Retention: Chronic urinary retention may cause little discomfort to the patient even though there is great hesitancy in starting the stream and marked reduction of its force and caliber. Constant dribbling of urine (paradoxic incontinence) may be experienced; it may be likened to water pouring over a dam.

G. Interruption of the Urinary Stream: Interruption may be abrupt and accompanied by severe pain radiating down the urethra. This type of reaction strongly suggests the complication of vesical calculus.

H. Sense of Residual Urine: The patient often feels that urine is still in the bladder even after urination has been completed.

I. Cystitis: Recurring episodes of acute cystitis suggest the presence of residual urine.

Incontinence
(See also Chapter 30.)

There are many reasons for incontinence. The history often gives a clue to its cause.

A. True Incontinence: The patient may lose urine without warning; this may be a constant or periodic symptom. The more obvious causes include exstrophy of the bladder, epispadias, vesicovaginal fistula, and ectopic ureteral orifice. Injury to the urethral smooth muscle sphincters may occur during prostatectomy or childbirth. Congenital or acquired neurogenic diseases may lead to dysfunction of the bladder and incontinence.

B. Stress Incontinence: When slight weakness of the sphincteric mechanisms is present, urine may be lost in association with physical strain (eg, coughing, laughing, rising from a chair). This is common in multiparous women who have weakened muscle support of the bladder neck and urethra. Occasionally, neuropathic bladder dysfunction can cause stress incontinence. The patient stays dry while lying in bed.

C. Urge Incontinence: Urgency may be so precipitate and severe that there is involuntary loss of urine. Urge incontinence not infrequently occurs with acute cystitis, particularly in women, since women seem to have relatively poor anatomic sphincters. Urge incontinence is a common symptom of an upper motor neuron lesion. It is often seen also in tense, anxious women even in the absence of infection.

D. Paradoxic (Overflow or False) Incontinence: Paradoxic incontinence is loss of urine due to chronic urinary retention or secondary to a flaccid bladder. The intravesical pressure finally equals the urethral resistance; urine then constantly dribbles forth.

Oliguria & Anuria

Oliguria and anuria may be caused by acute renal failure (due to shock or dehydration), fluid-ion imbalance, or bilateral ureteral obstruction.

Pneumaturia

The passage of gas in the urine strongly suggests a fistula between the urinary tract and the bowel. This occurs most commonly in the bladder or urethra but may be seen also in the ureter or renal pelvis. Carcinoma of the sigmoid colon, diverticulitis with abscess formation, regional enteritis, and trauma cause most vesical fistulas. Congenital anomalies account for most urethroenteric fistulas. Certain bacteria, by the process of fermentation, may liberate gas on rare occasions.

Cloudy Urine

Patients often complain of cloudy urine, but it is most often cloudy merely because it is alkaline; this causes precipitation of phosphate. Infection can also cause urine to be cloudy and malodorous. A properly performed urinalysis will reveal the cause of cloudiness.

Chyluria

The passage of lymphatic fluid or chyle is noted by the patient as passage of milky white urine. This represents a lymphatic–urinary system fistula. Most often, the cause is obstruction of the renal lymphatics, which results in forniceal rupture and leakage. Filariasis, trauma, tuberculosis, and retroperitoneal tumors have caused the problem.

Bloody Urine

Hematuria is a danger signal that cannot be ignored. Carcinoma of the kidney or bladder, calculi, and infection are a few of the conditions in which hematuria is typically demonstrable at the time of presentation. It is important to know whether urination is painful or not, whether the hematuria is associated with symptoms of vesical irritability, and whether blood is seen in all or only a portion of the urinary stream. Some individuals (particularly if they are anemic) pass red urine after eating beets or taking laxatives containing phenolphthalein, in which case the urine is translucent rather than opaque and contains no red cells. Because of the wide use of rhodamine B as a coloring agent in cookies, cakes, cold drinks, and fruit juices, children commonly pass red urine after ingestion of these foods. This is the so-called Monday morning disorder. The hemoglobinuria that occurs as a feature of the hemolytic syndromes may also cause the urine to be red.

A. Bloody Urine in Relation to Symptoms and Diseases: Hematuria associated with renal colic suggests a ureteral stone, although a clot from a bleeding renal tumor can cause the same type of pain.

Hematuria is not uncommonly associated with nonspecific, tuberculous, or schistosomal infection of the bladder. The bleeding is often terminal (bladder neck or prostate), although it may be present throughout urination (vesical or upper tract). Stone in the bladder often causes hematuria, but infection is usually present, and there are symptoms of bladder neck obstruction, neurogenic bladder, or cystocele. When a tumor of the bladder ulcerates, it is often complicated by infection and bleeding. Thus, symptoms of cystitis and hematuria are also compatible with tumors.

Dilated veins may develop at the bladder neck secondary to enlargement of the prostate. These may rupture when the patient strains to urinate.

Hematuria without other symptoms (silent hematuria) must be regarded as a symptom of tumor of the bladder or kidney until proved otherwise. It is usually intermittent; bleeding may not recur for months. Complacency because the bleeding stops spontaneously must be condemned. Less common causes of silent hematuria are staghorn calculus, polycystic kidneys, solitary renal cyst, sickle cell disease, and hydronephrosis. Painless bleeding is common with acute glomerulonephritis. Recurrent bleeding is occasionally seen in children suffering from focal glomerulitis. Joggers and people who engage in participatory sports frequently develop transient proteinuria and gross or microscopic hematuria (Abarbanel et al, 1990).

B. Time of Hematuria: Learning whether the hematuria is partial (initial, terminal) or total (present throughout urination) is often of help in identifying the site of bleeding. Initial hematuria suggests an anterior urethral lesion (eg, urethritis, stricture, meatal stenosis in young boys). Terminal hematuria usually arises from the posterior urethra, bladder neck, or trigone. Among the common causes are posterior urethritis and polyps and tumors of the vesical neck.

Total hematuria has its source at or above the level of the bladder (eg, stone, tumor, tuberculosis, nephritis).

OTHER OBJECTIVE MANIFESTATIONS

Urethral Discharge

Urethral discharge in men is one of the most common urologic complaints. The causative organism is usually *Neisseria gonorrhoeae* or *Chlamydia trachomatis*. The discharge is often accompanied by local burning on urination or an itching sensation in the urethra (see Chapter 16).

Skin Lesions of the External Genitalia (See Chapters 16 and 43.)

An ulceration of the glans penis or its shaft may represent syphilitic chancre, chancroid, herpes simplex, or squamous cell carcinoma. Venereal warts of the penis are common.

Visible or Palpable Masses

The patient may notice a visible or palpable mass in the upper abdomen that may represent renal tumor, hydronephrosis, or polycystic kidney. Enlarged lymph nodes in the neck may contain metastatic tumor from the prostate or testis. Lumps in the groin may represent spread of tumor of the penis or lymphadenitis from chancroid, syphilis, or lymphogranuloma venereum. Painless masses in the scrotal contents are common and include hydrocele, varicocele, spermatocele, chronic epididymitis, hernia, and testicular tumor.

Edema

Edema of the legs may result from compression of the iliac veins by lymphatic metastases from prostatic cancer. Edema of the genitalia suggests filariasis or chronic ascites.

Bloody Ejaculation

Inflammation of the prostate or seminal vesicles can cause hematospermia.

Gynecomastia

Often idiopathic, gynecomastia is common in elderly men, particularly those taking estrogens for control of prostatic cancer. It is also seen in association with choriocarcinoma and interstitial cell and Sertoli cell tumors of the testis. Certain endocrinologic diseases, eg, Klinefelter syndrome, may also cause gynecomastia.

Size of Penis in Infant or Child

Micropenis is probably due to fetal testosterone deficiency (see Chapter 44). Megalopenis is caused by overactivity of the adrenal cortex (see Chapter 32) and is seen in association with interstitial cell tumor of the testis (see Chapter 24).

Infertility
(See Chapter 46.)

Many men are referred to the urologist for fertility studies. The urologist should explore the patient's sexual habits and investigate diseases and disorders that have affected the scrotal contents (eg, mumps, torsion of the spermatic cord, epididymitis) and exposure to testicular toxins (eg, x-radiation).

COMPLAINTS RELATED TO SEXUAL PROBLEMS

Many people suffer from genitourinary complaints on a purely psychological or emotional basis. In others, organic symptoms may be increased in severity because of tension states. It is important, therefore, to seek clues that might give evidence of emotional stress.

In women, the relationship of the menses to ureteral pain or vesical complaints should be determined, although menstruation may exacerbate both organic and functional vesical and renal difficulties.

Many patients recognize that the state of their "nerves" has a direct effect on their symptoms. They often realize that their "cystitis" develops after a tension-producing or anxiety-producing episode in their personal or occupational environment.

A. Sexual Difficulties in Men: Men may complain directly of sexual difficulty. However, they are often so ashamed of loss of sexual power that they cannot admit it even to a physician. In such cases, they may ask for "prostate treatment" and hope that the physician will understand that they have sexual complaints and that they will be treated accordingly. The main sexual symptoms include impaired quality of erection, premature loss of erection, absence of ejaculate with orgasm, premature ejaculation, and even loss of desire.

B. Sexual Difficulties in Women: Women suffering from the psychosomatic cystitis syndrome almost always admit to an unhappy sex life. They notice that frequency or vaginal-urethral pain often occurs on the day following the incomplete sexual act. Many of them recognize the inadequacy of their sexual experiences as one of the underlying causes of urologic complaints; too frequently, however, the physician either does not ask them pertinent questions or, if patients volunteer this information, ignores it.

C. Sexual Difficulties of Suspected Psychosomatic Origin: In treating sexual difficulties of suspected psychosomatic origin, the physician should explore pertinent facts concerning childhood, adolescence (sex education and experiences), marriage problems, and relationships with relatives, business associates, and others. Even when psychosomatic disease is strongly suspected before history-taking has been completed, a thorough examination and laboratory survey must be done. Both psyche and soma may be involved, and the patient must be assured that there is no serious organic disease. Although sexual interest and activity decline with advancing years, physically healthy men and women may continue to be sexually active into their eighth or ninth decade.

REFERENCES

LOCAL & REFERRED PAIN

Clark AJ, Norman RW: "Mirror pain" as an unusual presentation of renal colic. Urology 1998;51:116.

Hanno P et al: Diagnosis of interstitial cystitis. J Urol 1990;143:278.

Hinman F Jr: Differential diagnosis of flank pain. Probl Urol 1989;3:179.

Paajanen H, Tainio H, Laato M: A chance of misdiagnosis between acute appendicitis and renal colic. Scand J Urol Nephrol 1996;30:363.

Samm BJ, Dmochowski RR: Urologic emergencies. Conditions affecting the kidney, ureter, bladder, prostate, and urethra. Postgrad Med 1996;100(Oct; 4):177, 183.

Walsh A: Renal colic. Probl Urol 1989;3:210.

SYMPTOMS RELATED TO THE ACT OF URINATION

Abarbanel J et al: Sports hematuria. J Urol 1990; 143:887.

Ahn JH, Morey AF, McAninch JW: Workup and management of traumatic hematuria. Emerg Med Clin North Am 1998;16:145.

Andreoli SP: Renal manifestations of systemic diseases. Semin Nephrol 1998;18:270.

Barry MJ: Epidemiology and natural history of benign prostatic hyperplasia. Urol Clin N Am 1990;17:495.

Bartlow BG: Microhematuria: Picking the fewest tests to make an accurate diagnosis. Postgrad Med 1990; 88(4):51, 58, 61.

deVries CR, Freiha FS: Hemorrhagic cystitis: A review. J Urol 1990;143:1.

Edwards BD, Eastwood JB, Shearer RJ: Chyluria as a cause of haematuria in patients from endemic areas. Br J Urol 1988;62:609.

Feld LG et al: Hematuria. An integrated medical and surgical approach. Pediatr Clin North Am 1997;44: 1191.

Friedman RM, King LR: Valve of Guerin as a cause of dysuria and hematuria in young boys: Presentation and difficulties in diagnosis. J Urol 1993;150:159.

Hansson S et al: Lower urinary tract dysfunction in girls with untreated asymptomatic or covert bacteriuria. J Urol 1990;143:333.

Hjalmas K: Nocturnal enuresis: Basic facts and new horizons. Eur Urol 1998;33(Suppl 3):53.

Kirsh GM, et al: Diagnosis and management of vesicoenteric fistulas. Surg Gynecol Obstet 1991;173:91.

Kurowski K: The women with dysuria. Am Fam Physician 1998;57(9):2155.

Lieu TA, Grasmeder HM III, Kaplan BS: An approach to the evaluation and treatment of microscopic hematuria. Pediatr Clin North Am 1991;38:579.

Mann EM: Nocturnal enuresis. West J Med 1991; 155:520.

McCarthy JJ: Outpatient evaluation of hematuria: Locating the source of bleeding. Postgrad Med 1997;101(Feb; 2):125, 131.

Pappas PG: Laboratory in the diagnosis and management of urinary tract infections. Med Clin North Am 1991;75:313.

Payne CK: Epidemiology, pathophysiology, and evaluation of urinary incontinence and overactive bladder. Urology 1998;51(2A Suppl):3.

Punekar SV et al: Surgical disconnection of lymphorenal communication for chyluria: A 15-year experience. Br J Urol 1997;80:858.

Resnick NM, Yalla SV: Management of urinary incontinence in the elderly. N Engl J Med 1985;313:800.

Rockall AG et al: Haematuria. Postgrad Med J 1997;73(Mar; 857):129.

Sayer J, McCarthy MP, Schmidt JD: Identification and significance of dysmorphic versus isomorphic hematuria. J Urol 1990;143:545.

Seeds JW, Mandell J: Congenital obstructive uropathies: Pre- and postnatal treatment. Urol Clin North Am 1986;13:155.

Stalens JP et al: "Milky" urine—a child with chyluria. Eur J Pediatr 1992;151:61.

Tapp AJ, Cardozo L: The postmenopausal bladder. Br J Hosp Med 1986;35:20.

Thrasher JB, Snyder JA: Post-nephrolithotomy chyluria. J Urol 1990;143:578.

Physical Examination of the Genitourinary Tract

4

Emil A. Tanagho, MD

The history will suggest whether a complete or partial examination is indicated. The symptom of urethral discharge usually does not require a thorough physical examination; on the other hand, painless hematuria certainly requires a careful examination of the genitourinary tract. In this chapter the urologic aspects of the physical examination are discussed.

Unusual Findings on General Examination

A. Gynecomastia: Gynecomastia is common and usually of no consequence. Williams (1963) found gynecomastia in 40% of a series of 447 autopsies. Its causes included prostatic carcinoma (treated with estrogen), testicular abnormalities, adrenocortical hyperplasia, adrenocortical tumors, interstitial cell tumors of the testis, certain diseases of the liver and thyroid, cirrhosis, and diabetes. Gynecomastia in a young man suggests to the urologist the presence of a choriocarcinomatous testicular tumor or Klinefelter syndrome.

B. Hemihypertrophy: Hennessy, Cromie, and Duckett (1981) noted abdominal masses associated with this rare phenomenon. The masses were on the side of the hemihypertrophy and, in 7 patients, included 3 Wilms tumors, 2 adrenal tumors, and a neuroblastoma. Saypol and Laudone (1983) have reviewed the literature on this subject.

C. Clues to Renal Anomalies: A child with gross deformity of an external ear and ipsilateral maldevelopment of the facial bones is likely to have a congenital abnormality of the kidney on the same side. Lateral displacement of the nipples has been associated with bilateral renal hypoplasia. Renal abnormalities have also been observed with congenital scoliosis and kyphosis as well as with prelevator imperforate anus.

D. Other Findings: Evidence of endocrinologic changes should be noted, eg, hypertrophy of the external genitalia, hirsutism. The finding of hypertension suggests the possibility of pheochromocytoma or renovascular hypertension.

EXAMINATION OF THE KIDNEYS

Inspection

On occasion, a mass that is visible in the upper abdominal area if soft (eg, as in hydronephrosis), may be difficult to palpate. Fullness in the costovertebral angle may be consistent with cancer (eg, neuroblastoma in children) or perinephric infection. The presence and persistence of indentations in the skin from lying on wrinkled sheets suggest edema of the skin secondary to perinephric abscess. If this disease is suspected, one should have the patient lie on a rough towel and observe for indentations.

Palpation

The kidneys lie rather high under the diaphragm and lower ribs and are therefore well protected from injury. Because of the position of the liver, the right kidney is lower than the left. The kidneys are difficult to palpate in men because of the resistance of abdominal muscle tone and because the kidneys in men are more fixed than those in women and move only slightly with change of posture or respiration. The lower part of the right kidney can sometimes be felt, especially in thin patients, but the left kidney usually cannot be felt unless it is enlarged or displaced.

The most successful method of renal palpation is carried out with the patient lying in the supine position on a hard surface (Figure 4–1). The kidney is lifted by one hand in the costovertebral angle. On deep inspiration, the kidney moves downward; when it is lowest, the other hand is pushed firmly and deeply beneath the costal margin in an effort to trap the kidney below that point. If this is successful, the anterior hand can palpate the size, shape, and consistency of the organ as it slips back into its normal position.

The kidney sometimes can be palpated best with the examiner standing behind the seated patient. At other times, if the patient is lying on one side, the up-

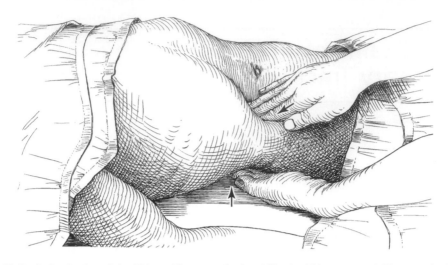

Figure 4–1. Method of palpation of the kidney. The posterior hand lifts the kidney upward. The anterior hand feels for the kidney. The patient then takes a deep breath; this causes the kidney to descend. As the patient inhales, the fingers of the anterior hand are plunged inward at the costal margin. If the kidney is mobile or enlarged, it can be felt between the two hands.

permost kidney drops downward and medially, thereby making it more accessible to palpation.

Perlman and Williams (1976) described a very effective method of identifying renal anomalies in newborns. The fingers are placed in the costovertebral angle, with the thumb anterior. The thumb does the feeling. With this technique, the kidneys can be palpated 95% of the time. Anomalies were found in 0.5% of 11,000 newborns.

An enlarged renal mass suggests compensatory hypertrophy (if the other kidney is absent or atrophic), hydronephrosis, tumor, cyst, or polycystic disease. A mass in this area, however, may be a retroperitoneal tumor, the spleen, a lesion of the bowel (eg, tumor, abscess), a lesion of the gallbladder, or a pancreatic cyst. Tumors may have the consistency of normal tissue; they may also be nodular. Hydronephroses may be firm or soft. Polycystic kidneys are usually nodular and firm.

An acutely infected kidney is tender, but this is difficult to elicit, since marked muscle spasm is usually present. Because normal kidneys are often tender also, this sign is not always helpful.

Although renal pain may be diffusely felt in the back, tenderness is usually well localized just lateral to the sacrospinalis muscle and just below the twelfth rib (costovertebral angle [CVA]). This may be elicited by palpation or, more sharply, by percussion over that area.

Percussion

At times, a greatly enlarged kidney cannot be felt on palpation, particularly if it is soft. This can be true of hydronephrosis. Such masses may be readily out-

lined by percussion, however, both anteriorly and posteriorly; this part of the examination should never be omitted. Percussion is of particular value in outlining an enlarging mass in the flank following renal trauma (progressive hemorrhage), when tenderness and muscle spasm prevent proper palpation.

Transillumination

Transillumination may prove quite helpful in children under age 1 year who present with a suprapubic or flank mass. A 2- or 3-cell flashlight with an opaque flange protruding beyond the lens is an adequate instrument. The flashlight is applied at right angles to the abdomen. The fiberoptic light cord, used to illuminate various optical instruments, is an excellent source of cold light. A dark room is required. A distended bladder or cystic mass will transilluminate; a solid mass will not. Flank masses also may be tested by applying the light posteriorly.

Differentiation of Renal & Radicular Pain

Radicular pain is commonly felt in the costovertebral and subcostal areas. It may spread along the course of the ureter as well and is the most common cause of so-called kidney pain. Every patient who complains of flank pain should be examined for evidence of nerve root irritation. Frequent causes are poor posture (scoliosis, kyphosis), arthritic changes in the costovertebral or costotransverse joints, impingement of a rib spur on a subcostal nerve, hypertrophy of costovertebral ligaments pressing on a nerve, and intervertebral disk disease (Smith and Raney, 1976). Radicular pain may be noted as an aftermath of a flank incision wherein a rib may become dislocated, causing the costal nerve to impinge on the edge of a ligament. Pain experienced during the preeruptive phase of herpes zoster involving any of the segments between T11 and L2 also may simulate pain of renal origin.

Radiculitis usually causes hyperesthesia of the area of skin served by the irritated peripheral nerve. This hypersensitivity can be elicited by means of the pinwheel or by grasping and pinching both skin and fat of the abdomen and flanks. Pressure exerted by the thumb over the costovertebral joints reveals local tenderness at the point of emergence of the involved peripheral nerve.

Auscultation

Auscultation of the costovertebral areas and upper abdominal quadrants may reveal a systolic bruit, which is often associated with stenosis or aneurysm of the renal artery. Bruits over the femoral arteries may be found in association with Leriche syndrome, which may be a cause of impotence.

EXAMINATION OF THE BLADDER

The bladder cannot be felt unless it is moderately distended. In adults, if it is percussible, it contains at least 150 mL of urine. In acute or (more commonly) chronic urinary retention, the bladder may reach or even rise above the umbilicus, in which case its outline may be seen and usually felt. (In chronic retention, in which the bladder wall is flabby, the bladder may be difficult to palpate. In this instance, percussion is of great value.)

In male infants or young boys, palpation of a hard mass deep in the center of the pelvis is compatible with a thickened hypertrophied bladder secondary to obstruction caused by posterior urethral valves.

A sliding inguinal hernia containing some bladder wall can be diagnosed (when the bladder is full) by compression of the scrotal mass. The bladder will be found to distend additionally.

A few instances have been reported wherein marked edema of the legs has developed secondary to compression of the iliac vessels by a distended bladder. Bimanual (abdominorectal or abdominovaginal) palpation may reveal the extent of a vesical tumor. To be successful, it must be done under anesthesia.

EXAMINATION OF THE EXTERNAL MALE GENITALIA

PENIS

Inspection

If the patient has not been circumcised, the foreskin should be retracted. This may reveal tumor or balanitis as the cause of a foul discharge. If retraction is not possible in phimosis, surgical correction (dorsal slit or circumcision) is indicated.

The observation of a poor urinary stream is significant. In newborns, neurogenic (neuropathic) bladder or the presence of posterior urethral valves should be considered. In men, such a finding suggests urethral stricture or prostatic obstruction.

The scars of healed syphilis may be an important clue. An active ulcer requires bacteriologic or pathologic study (eg, syphilitic chancre, epithelioma). Superficial ulcers or vesicles are compatible with herpes simplex; they are often interpreted by the patient as a serious sexually transmitted disease, possibly syphilis. Venereal warts may be observed.

Meatal stenosis is a common cause of bloody spotting in male infants. On rare occasions, it may be of such degree as to cause advanced bilateral hydronephrosis. It is easily corrected by meatotomy.

The position of the meatus should be noted. It may be located proximal to the tip of the glans on either the dorsum (epispadias) or the ventral surface (hypospadias). In either instance, there is apt to be abnormal curvature of the penis—dorsally with epispadias, ventrally with hypospadias. The urethral orifice is often stenotic in the latter.

Micropenis or macropenis may be observed.

Palpation

Palpation of the dorsal surface of the shaft may reveal a fibrous plaque involving the fascial covering of the corpora cavernosa. This is typical of Peyronie disease. Tender areas of induration felt along the urethra may signify periurethritis secondary to urethral stricture.

Urethral Discharge

Urethral discharge is the most common complaint referable to the male sex organ. Gonococcal pus is usually profuse, thick, and yellow or gray-brown. Nongonorrheal discharges may be similar in appearance but are often thin, mucoid, and scanty. Although gonorrhea must be ruled out as the cause of a urethral discharge, a significant percentage of such cases are found to be caused by chlamydiae. Patients with urethral discharge should be examined also for other sexually transmitted diseases; multiple infection is not uncommon.

Bloody discharge should suggest the possibility of a foreign body in the urethra (male or female), urethral stricture, or tumor.

Urethral discharge must always be sought before the patient is asked to void.

SCROTUM

Angioneurotic edema and infections and inflammations of the skin of the scrotum are not common. Small sebaceous cysts are occasionally seen. Malignant tumors are rare. The scrotum is bifid when midscrotal or perineal hypospadias is present.

Elephantiasis of the scrotum is caused by obstruction to lymphatic drainage. It is endemic in the tropics and is due to filariasis. Elephantiasis may result from radical resection of the lymph nodes of the inguinal and femoral areas, in which case the skin of the penis is also involved. Small hemangiomas of the skin are common and may bleed spontaneously.

Scrotal ultrasound is helpful in evaluating scrotal contents.

TESTIS

The testes should be carefully palpated with the fingers of both hands. A hard area in the testis proper must be regarded as a malignant tumor until proved otherwise. Transillumination of all scrotal masses should be done routinely. With the patient in a dark room, a strong flashlight or fiberoptic light is placed against the scrotal sac posteriorly. A hydrocele will cause the intrascrotal mass to glow red. Light is not transmitted through a solid tumor. Tumors are often smooth but may be nodular. Testes seem abnormally heavy. A testis replaced by tumor or damaged by gumma is insensitive to pressure, and the usual sickening sensation is absent. About 10% of tumors are associated with a secondary hydrocele that may have to be aspirated before definitive palpation can be done.

The testis may be absent from the scrotum. This may represent transient (physiologic retractile testis) or true cryptorchidism. Palpation of the groins may reveal the presence of the organ.

The atrophic testis (following postoperative orchiopexy, mumps orchitis, or torsion of the spermatic cord) may be flabby and at times hypersensitive but is usually firm and hyposensitive. Although spermatogenesis may be lost, androgen function is occasionally maintained.

EPIDIDYMIS

The epididymis is sometimes rather closely at-

tached to the posterior surface of the testis, and at other times it is quite free of it. The epididymis should be carefully palpated for size and induration. Induration implies infection (primary tumors are exceedingly rare).

In the acute stage of epididymitis, the testis and epididymis are indistinguishable by palpation; the testicle and epididymis may be adherent to the scrotum, which is usually quite red. Tenderness is exquisite. With few exceptions, the infecting organism is either *Neisseria gonorrhoeae, Chlamydia trachomatis,* or *Escherichia coli.*

Chronic painless induration should suggest tuberculosis or schistosomiasis, although nonspecific chronic epididymitis is also a possibility. Other signs of tuberculosis of the genitourinary tract usually present include "sterile" pyuria, a thickened seminal vesicle, a nodular prostate, and "beading" of the vas deferens.

SPERMATIC CORD & VAS DEFERENS

A swelling in the spermatic cord may be cystic (eg, hydrocele or hernia) or solid (eg, connective tissue tumor). The latter is rare. Lipoma in the investing fascia of the cord may simulate hernia. Diffuse swelling and induration of the cord are seen with filarial funiculitis.

Careful palpation of the vas deferens may reveal thickening (eg, chronic infection), fusiform enlargements (the "beading" caused by tuberculosis), or even absence of the vas. The latter finding is of importance in infertile males; it is rare.

When a male patient stands, a mass of dilated veins (varicocele) may be noted behind and above the testis. The degree of dilatation decreases with recumbency and can be increased by the Valsalva maneuver. The major sequel of varicocele is infertility (see Chapter 46).

TESTICULAR TUNICS & ADNEXA

Hydroceles are usually cystic but on occasion are so tense that they simulate solid tumors. Transillumination makes the differential diagnosis. They may develop secondary to nonspecific acute or tuberculous epididymitis, trauma, or tumor of the testis. The latter is a distinct possibility if hydrocele appears spontaneously between the ages of 18 and 35. It should be aspirated to permit careful palpation of underlying structures.

Hydrocele usually surrounds the testis completely. Cystic masses that are separate from but in the region of the upper pole of the testis are probably spermatoceles. Aspiration reveals the typical thin, milky fluid, which contains sperm.

EXAMINATION OF THE FEMALE GENITALIA

VAGINAL EXAMINATION

Diseases of the female genital tract may involve the urinary organs secondarily, thereby making a thorough gynecologic examination essential. Commonly associated are urethrocystitis secondary to urethral diverticulitis or cervicitis, pyelonephritis during pregnancy, and ureteral obstruction from metastatic nodes or direct extension in cancer of the cervix.

Inspection

In newborns and children especially, the vaginal vestibule should be inspected for a single opening (common urogenital sinus), labial fusion, split clitoris and lack of fusion of the anterior fourchette (epispadias), or hypertrophied clitoris and scrotalization of the labia majora (adrenogenital syndrome).

The urinary meatus may reveal a reddened, tender, friable lesion (urethral caruncle) or a reddened, everted posterior lip, which is often seen with senile urethritis and vaginitis. Biopsy is indicated if a malignant tumor cannot be ruled out. The diagnosis of senile vaginitis (and urethritis) is established by staining a smear of the vaginal epithelium with Lugol's solution. It should be examined immediately after rinsing, because the brown dye in the cells fades quickly. Cells lacking glycogen (hypoestrogenism) do not take up the stain, whereas normal cells do.

Multiple painful small ulcers or blisterlike lesions may be noted; these probably represent herpesvirus type 2 infection, which may have serious sequels.

Smears and cultures of urethral or vaginal discharge should be made. Gonococci are relatively easy to identify; culture of chlamydiae requires techniques seldom available to the physician.

The presence of skenitis and bartholinitis may reveal the source of persistent urethritis or cystitis. The condition of the vaginal wall should be observed. Bacteriologic study of the secretions may be helpful. Urethrocele and cystocele may cause residual urine and lead to persistent infection of the bladder. They are often found in association with stress incontinence. A bulge in the anterior vaginal wall may represent a urethral diverticulum. The cervix should be inspected to detect cancer or infection. Taking biopsy specimens or making Papanicolaou smears may be indicated.

Palpation

At times, the urethra, the base of the bladder, and the lower ureters may be tender on palpation, but little can be deduced from this. Induration of the urethra or trigonal area or a mass involving either may be a clue to an existing tumor. A soft mass found in this area could be a urethral diverticulum. Pressure on such a lesion may cause pus to extrude from the urethra. A stone in the lower ureter may be palpable. Evidence of enlargement of the uterus (eg, pregnancy, myomas) or diseases or inflammations of the colon or adnexa may afford a clue to the cause of urinary symptoms (eg, compression of a ureter by a malignant ovarian tumor, endometriosis, or diverticulitis of the sigmoid colon adherent to the bladder).

Carcinoma of the cervix may invade the base of the bladder, causing vesical irritability or hematuria; its metastases to iliac lymph nodes may compress the ureters.

Rectal examination may afford further information and is the obvious route of examination in children and virgins.

RECTAL EXAMINATION IN MALES

SPHINCTER & LOWER RECTUM

The estimation of sphincter tone is of great importance. Laxity of the muscle strongly suggests similar changes in the urinary sphincters and detrusor and may be a clue to the diagnosis of neurogenic disease. The same is true for a spastic anal sphincter. In addition to the digital prostatic examination, the examiner should palpate the entire lower rectum to rule out stenosis, internal hemorrhoids, cryptitis, rectal fistulas, mucosal polyps, and rectal cancer and should use bidigital palpation for Cowper's glands. Testing perianal sensation is mandatory.

PROSTATE

A specimen of urine for routine analysis should be collected before the rectal examination is made. This is of the utmost importance, since prostatic massage (or even palpation at times) forces prostatic secretion into the posterior urethra. If this secretion contains pus, a specimen of urine voided after the rectal examination will be contaminated by it.

Size

The average prostate is about 4 cm in length and width. It is widest superiorly at the bladder neck. As the gland enlarges, the lateral sulci become relatively deeper and the median furrow becomes obliterated. The prostate may also elongate. The clinical importance of prostatic hyperplasia is measured by the severity of symptoms and the amount of residual urine rather than by the size of the gland. On rectal examination, the prostate may be of normal size and consistency in a patient with acute urinary retention.

Consistency

Normally, the consistency of the gland is similar to that of the contracted thenar eminence of the thumb (with the thumb completely opposed to the little finger). It is rather rubbery. It may be mushy if congested (due to lack of intercourse or to chronic infection with impaired drainage), indurated (due to chronic infection with or without calculi), or stony-hard (due to advanced carcinoma).

The difficulty lies in differentiating firm areas in the prostate: fibrosis from nonspecific infection, granulomatous prostatitis, nodulation from tuberculosis, or firm areas due to prostatic calculi or early cancer. Generally speaking, nodules caused by infection are raised above the surface of the gland. At their edges, the induration gradually fades to the normal softness of surrounding tissue. In cancer, conversely, the suspicious lesion is usually not raised; it is hard and has a sharp edge, ie, there is an abrupt change in

consistency on the same plane. It tends to arise in the lateral sulcus (Figure 4–2).

Even the most experienced clinicians sometimes have trouble making this differentiation. In the absence of other signs of tuberculosis and in the absence of pus in the prostatic secretion, cancer is likely, particularly if an x-ray fails to show prostatic calculi (which are seen just behind or above the symphysis). Serum acid phosphatase determinations and radiograms of bones are of no help in diagnosing early carcinoma of the prostate. The prostate-specific antigen (PSA) level can be helpful if elevated. Transrectal ultrasound-guided biopsy can be diagnostic.

Mobility

The mobility of the gland varies. Occasionally, it has great mobility; at other times, very little. With advanced carcinoma, it is fixed because of local extension through the capsule. The prostate should be routinely massaged in adults and its secretion examined microscopically. It should not be massaged, however, in the presence of an acute urethral discharge, acute prostatitis, or acute prostatocystitis; in men near the stage of complete urinary retention (because it may precipitate complete retention); or in

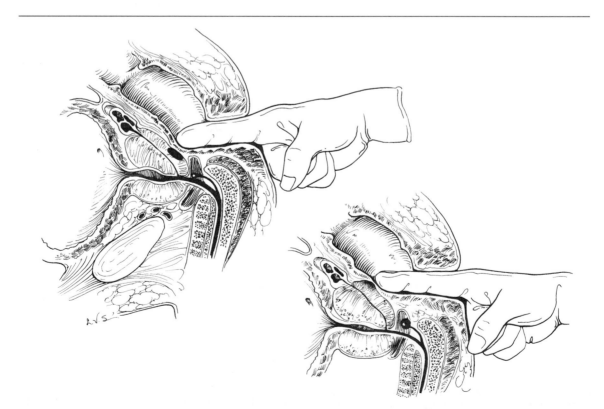

Figure 4–2. Differential diagnosis of prostatic nodules. **A:** Inflammatory area is raised above the surface of the gland; induration decreases gradually at its periphery. **B:** Cancerous nodule is not raised; there is an abrupt change in consistency at its edges.

men suffering from obvious cancer of the gland. Even without symptoms, massage is necessary, for prostatitis is commonly asymptomatic. Diagnosis and treatment of such silent disease is important in preventing cystitis and epididymitis.

Techniques of Massage

The patient should lean over the examining table so that his body is horizontal. His legs should be straight and his feet somewhat apart.

Methods of massage vary, but the basic maneuver is to press the gland substance firmly with the pad of the index finger in order to express secretion into the prostatic urethra. One should start laterally and superiorly, and massage toward the midline. A rolling motion of the finger is less traumatic to the rectal mucosa and prostate gland and is better tolerated by the patient. Finally, the seminal vesicles should be stripped from above downward and medially (Figure 4–3).

Copious amounts of secretion may be obtained from some prostate glands and little or none from others. The amount obtained depends to some extent on the vigor with which the massage is carried out. If no secretion is obtained, the patient should be asked to void even a few drops of urine; these will contain adequate secretion for examination. Microscopic examination of the secretion is done under low-power magnification. Normal secretion contains numerous lecithin bodies, which are refractile, like red cells, but much smaller than red cells. Only an occasional white cell is present. A few epithelial cells and, rarely, corpora amylacea are seen. Sperm may be present, but its absence is of no significance.

The presence of large numbers of pus cells is pathologic and suggests the diagnosis of prostatitis. Stained smears are usually impractical. It is difficult to fix this material on the slide, and even when this is successful, pyogenic bacteria are usually not found. Acid-fast organisms can often be found by appropriate staining methods.

On occasion, it may be necessary to obtain cultures of prostatic secretion in order to demonstrate nonspecific organisms, tubercle bacilli, gonococci, or chlamydiae. After thorough cleansing of the glans and emptying of the bladder (to mechanically cleanse the urethra), massage is done. Drops of secretion are collected in a sterile tube of appropriate culture medium.

SEMINAL VESICLES

Palpation of the seminal vesicles should be attempted. The vesicles are situated under the base of the bladder and diverge from below upward (Figures 1–8 and 4–3). Normal seminal vesicles are usually not palpable, but when the vesicles are overdistended they may feel quite cystic. In the presence of chronic infection (particularly tuberculosis or schistosomiasis) or in association with advanced carcinoma of the prostate, they may be markedly indurated. Stripping of the seminal vesicles should be done in association with prostatic massage, for the vesicles are usually infected when prostatitis is present. Primary tumors of the vesicles are very rare. A cystic mass may rarely be felt over the prostate or just above it. This probably represents a cyst of the müllerian duct or the utricle. The latter is occasionally associated with severe hypospadias.

LYMPH NODES

It should be remembered that generalized lymphadenopathy usually occurs early in human immunodeficiency syndrome (HIV) (see Chapter 16).

Inguinal & Subinguinal Lymph Nodes

With inflammatory lesions of the skin of the penis and scrotum or vulva, the inguinal and subinguinal lymph nodes may be involved. Such diseases include chancroid, syphilitic chancre, lymphogranuloma venereum, and, on occasion, gonorrhea.

Malignant tumors (squamous cell carcinoma) involving the penis, glans, scrotal skin, or distal urethra in women metastasize to the inguinal and subinguinal nodes. Testicular tumors do not spread to these nodes unless they have invaded the scrotal skin or the patient has previously undergone orchiopexy.

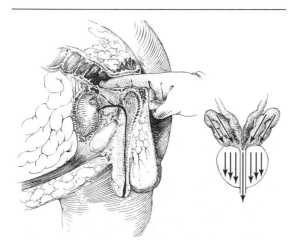

Figure 4–3. Technique of prostatic massage. The glandular substance is compressed from its lateral edges to the urethra, which lies in the center. (Drawing at right shows direction of pressure.) The seminal vesicles are then stripped from above downward.

Other Lymph Nodes

Tumors of the testis and prostate may involve the left supraclavicular nodes. Tumors of the bladder and prostate typically metastasize to the internal iliac, external iliac, and preaortic nodes, although only occasionally are they so large as to be palpable. Upper abdominal masses near the midline in a young man should suggest metastases from cancer of the testis; the primary growth may be minute and completely hidden in the substance of what appears to be a normal testicle.

NEUROLOGIC EXAMINATION

A careful neurologic survey may uncover sensory or motor impairment that will account for residual urine (neuropathic bladder) or incontinence. Since the bladder and its sphincter are innervated by the second to fourth sacral segments, much information can be gained by testing anal sphincter tone and the sensation of the perianal skin and by eliciting the Achilles tendon and bulbocavernosus reflexes. The bulbocavernosus reflex is elicited by placing a finger in the patient's rectum and squeezing the glans penis or clitoris or by jerking on an indwelling Foley catheter. The normal reflex is contraction of the anal sphincter and bulbocavernosus muscles in response to these maneuvers.

It is wise, particularly in children, to seek a dimple over the lumbosacral area. One should palpate the sacrum to be sure it is present and normally formed. Sacral agenesis or partial development is compatible with deficits of S2–4. If findings seem abnormal, x-ray examination is indicated.

REFERENCES

GENERAL

Braunstein GD: Gynecomastia. N Engl J Med 1993; 328:490.

Lemack GE, Poppas DP, Vaughan ED Jr: Urologic causes of gynecomastia: Approach to diagnosis and management. Urology 1995;45:313.

Leung AK: Gynecomastia. Am Fam Physician 1989;39 (4):215.

Neuman JF: Evaluation and treatment of gynecomastia. Am Fam Physician 1997;55:1835.

Spiro HM: An internist's approach to acute abdominal pain. Med Clin North Am 1993;77:963.

EXAMINATION OF THE KIDNEYS

Abdel-Razzak OM, Bagley DH: Clinical experience with flexible ureteropyeloscopy. J Urol 1992;148:1788.

Acino S, Resnick MI: Office urologic ultrasound. Urol Clin North Am 1988;15:577.

Ahn JH, Morey AF, McAninch JW: Workup and management of traumatic hematuria. Emerg Med Clin North Am 1998;16:145.

Bagley DH, Allen J: Flexible ureteropyeloscopy in the diagnosis of benign essential hematuria. J Urol 1990;143:549.

Bagley DH, Rivas D: Upper urinary tract filling defects: Flexible ureteroscopic diagnosis. J Urol 1990;143: 1196.

Choyke PL, Pollack HM: The role of MRI in diseases of the kidney. Radiol Clin North Am 1988;26:617.

Gross GW, Boal DK: Sonographic assessment of normal renal size in children with myelodysplasia. J Urol 1988;140:784.

Hennessy WT, Cromie WJ, Duckett JW: Congenital hemihypertrophy and associated abdominal lesions. Urology 1981;18:576.

Hodges CV, Barry JM: Non-urologic flank pain: A diagnostic approach. J Urol 1975;113:644.

Koop CE: Abdominal mass in the newborn infant. N Engl J Med 1973;289:569.

Mofenson HC, Greensher J: Transillumination of the abdomen in infants. Am J Dis Child 1968;115:428.

Perlman M, Williams J: Detection of renal anomalies by abdominal palpation in newborn infants. Br Med J 1976;3:347.

Restrepo NC, Carey PO: Evaluating hematuria in adults. Am Fam Physician 1989;40(2):149.

Saypol DC, Laudone VP: Congenital hemihypertrophy with adrenal carcinoma and medullary sponge kidney. Urology 1983;21:510.

Smith DR, Raney FL Jr: Radiculitis distress as a mimic of renal pain. J Urol 1976;116:269.

Williams MJ: Gynecomastia: Its incidence, recognition and host characterization in 447 autopsy cases. Am J Med 1963;34:103.

EXTERNAL GENITALIA IN MALES

Bemelmans BL et al: Penile sensory disorders in erectile dysfunction: Results of a comprehensive neuro-urophysiological diagnostic evaluation in 123 patients. J Urol 1991;146:777.

Conway GS et al: Importance of scrotal ultrasonography in gynaecomastia. Br Med J 1988;297:1176.

Donohue RE, Fauver HE: Unilateral absence of the vas deferens: A useful clinical sign. JAMA 1989;261: 1180. [See comments.]

Dubinsky TJ, Chen P, Maklad N: Color-flow and power Doppler imaging of the testes. World J Urol 1998;16:35.

Hall S, Oates RD: Unilateral absence of the scrotal vas deferens associated with contralateral mesonephric duct anomalies resulting in infertility: Laboratory, physical and radiographic findings, and therapeutic alternatives. J Urol 1993;150:1161.

Hanson P et al: Sacral reflex latencies in tethered cord syndrome. Am J Phys Med Rehab 1993;72(1):39.

Horstman WG: Scrotal imaging. Urol Clin North Am 1997;24:653.

Kaver I, Matzkin H, Braf ZF: Epididymo-orchitis: A retrospective study of 121 patients. J Fam Pract 1990;30:548.

Lavoisier P et al: Bulbocavernosus reflex: Its validity as a diagnostic test of neurogenic impotence. J Urol 1989;141:311.

Mineur P et al: Feminizing testicular Leydig cell tumor: Hormonal profile before and after unilateral orchidectomy. J Clin Endocrinol Metab 1987;64:686.

Rivkees SA et al: Accuracy and reproducibility of clinical measures of testicular volume. J Pediatr 1987; 110:914.

Sherrard J, Barlow D: Gonorrhoea in men: Clinical and diagnostic aspects. Genitourin Med 1996;72:422.

Vodusek DB, Janko M: The bulbocavernosus reflex: A single motor neuron study. Brain 1990;113(Part 3):813.

EXTERNAL GENITALIA IN FEMALES

Redman JF: Techniques of genital examination and bladder catheterization in female children. Urol Clin North Am 1990;17:1.

Redman JF, Bissada NK: How to make a good examination of the genitalia of young girls. Clin Pediatr 1976;15:907.

PROSTATE

Clarke HS Jr: Benign prostatic hyperplasia. Am J Med Sci 1997;314:239.

Goldstein MM, Messing EM: Prostate and bladder cancer screening. J Am Coll Surg 1998;186:63.

Kirby RS: The clinical assessment of benign prostatic hyperplasia. Cancer 1992;70(1 Suppl):284.

Nickel JC: The Pre and Post Massage Test (PPMT): A simple screen for prostatitis. Tech Urol 1997;3:38.

NEUROLOGIC EXAMINATION

Cardenas DD, Mayo ME, Turner LR: Lower urinary changes over time in suprasacral spinal cord injury. Paraplegia 1995;33:326.

Fernandes ET et al: Neurogenic bladder dysfunction in children: Review of pathophysiology. J Pediatr 1994;124:1.

Vodusek DB: Electromyogram, evoked sensory and motor potentials in neurourology. Neurophysiol Clin 1997;27:204.

5

Urologic Laboratory Examination

Karl J. Kreder, Jr., MD, & Richard D. Williams, MD

Examination of specimens of urine, blood, and genitourinary secretions or exudates commonly directs the subsequent urologic workup and frequently establishes a diagnosis. Since approximately 20% of patients who visit a primary physician's office have a urologic problem, it is important for the physician to have a broad knowledge of the laboratory methods available to test appropriate specimens. Judicious use of such tests permits rapid, accurate, and cost-effective determination of the probable diagnosis and the treatment needs of patients with urologic disease.

EXAMINATION OF URINE

Urinalysis is one of the most important and useful urologic tests available, yet all too often the necessary details are neglected and significant information is overlooked or misinterpreted. Reasons for inadequate urinalyses include: (1) improper collection, (2) failure to examine the specimen immediately, (3) incomplete examination (eg, many hospital laboratories do not perform a microscopic analysis unless it is specifically requested), (4) inexperience of the examiner, and (5) inadequate appreciation of the significance of the findings.

There is an extant controversy surrounding the necessity of routine urinalysis as a screen in asymptomatic individuals, those admitted to hospitals, or those undergoing elective surgery. Numerous studies appear to indicate that in these situations urinalysis is not cost-effective, ie, does not uncover more than 2.5% of conditions requiring treatment. Patients presenting with urinary tract symptoms or signs, however, should undergo urinalysis. Recent data also indicate that if macroscopic urinalysis (dip-strip) is normal, microscopic analysis is not necessary. If the patient has signs or symptoms suggestive of urologic disease, or the dipstick is positive for protein, heme, leukocyte esterase, or nitrite, a complete urinalysis, including microscopic examination of the sediment, should be completed.

Urine Collection

A. Timing of Collection: It is best to examine urine that has been properly obtained in the office. First-voided morning specimens are helpful for qualitative protein testing in patients with possible orthostatic proteinuria and for specific gravity assessment as a presumptive test of renal function in patients with minimal renal disease due to diabetes mellitus or sickle cell anemia or in those with suspected diabetes insipidus. Urine specimens that are obtained immediately after the patient has eaten or that have been left standing for a few hours become alkaline and thus may contain lysed red cells (erythrocytes), disintegrated casts, or rapidly multiplying bacteria; therefore, a freshly voided specimen obtained a few hours after the patient has eaten and examined within 1 h of voiding is most reliable. The patient's state of hydration may alter the concentration of urinary constituents. Timed urine collections may be required for definitive assessment of renal function or proteinuria.

B. Method of Collection: The importance of the method of urine collection cannot be overstated. Proper collection of the specimen is particularly important when patients have hematuria or proteinuria or are being evaluated for urinary tract infection. Examination of a urine specimen collected sequentially in several containers may help to identify the site of origin of hematuria or urinary tract infection (see pp. 55 and 57). Because urine specimens obtained at home are usually improperly collected and examination is delayed while they are delivered to the office or laboratory, such specimens are commonly useless. To gather consistent and meaningful urinalysis data, urine must be collected by a uniform method in the physician's office or laboratory. The specimen should be obtained before a genital or rectal examination in order to prevent contamination from the introitus or expressed prostatic secretions. Urine obtained from a collecting device, eg, a condom, chronic catheter, or intestinal conduit drainage bag, is *not* a proper specimen for urinalysis.

1. Men–It is usually simple to collect a clean-voided midstream urine sample from men. Routine instructions may be printed on a sheet given to the patient or placed on the lavatory wall. The procedure should include (1) retraction of the foreskin (a common source of contamination of the specimen) and cleansing of the meatus with benzalkonium chloride or hexachlorophene; (2) passing the first part of the stream (15–30 mL) without collection; (3) collecting the next portion (approximately 50–100 mL) in a sterile specimen container, which is capped immediately afterward; and (4) completely emptying the bladder into the toilet. A portion of the specimen is prepared immediately for both macroscopic and microscopic examination, and the rest is saved in the sterile container for subsequent culture if this proves necessary.

With this midstream clean-catch method, the likelihood that the specimen will be contaminated by meatal or urethral secretions is markedly decreased, although not completely eliminated. In adult males, it is rarely necessary to collect urine by catheterization unless urinary retention is present or assessment of residual urine is required.

2. Women–It is virtually impossible for a woman to obtain a satisfactory clean-voided midstream specimen without help. A voided specimen from an unprepped patient is not useful unless it is completely normal. The best method for collecting a clean-voided midstream specimen from a woman is as follows: (1) The patient is placed on the examining table in the lithotomy position. (2) The vulva and urethral meatus are cleansed with benzalkonium chloride or hexachlorophene. (3) The labia are separated. (4) The patient is instructed to initiate voiding into a container held close to the vulva. After she has passed the first 10–20 mL of urine, the next 50–100 mL is collected in a sterile container that is immediately capped. (5) The patient is allowed to complete emptying of the bladder. Because this technique requires considerable effort, it is acceptable to have the patient provide an initial specimen in a nonsterile container in the office lavatory. If results of urinalysis are normal, no further study is indicated; if abnormal, a urine specimen must be obtained by the more exacting technique. In either case, the specimen should be prepared for immediate examination.

If a satisfactory specimen cannot be obtained by the method described, assuming the necessity of examination has been assessed, one should not hesitate to obtain a specimen by catheterization, although suprapubic needle aspiration is the only sure way to obtain urine uncontaminated by urethrovaginal secretions or perineal organisms. Catheterization may be necessary to determine whether residual urine is present or to eliminate nonvaginal sources of hematuria. The possibility of introducing bladder infection by catheter is minimal when catheterization is performed carefully and should not prevent one from obtaining essential information. A satisfactory device with an 8F catheter attached to a centrifuge tube is available commercially.

3. Children–Obtaining a satisfactory urine specimen from a young child can be particularly challenging. Urine for analysis, other than bacterial cultures, can be obtained from males or females by covering the cleansed urethral meatus with a plastic bag; a urine specimen for culture may require catheterization or suprapubic needle aspiration. In girls, catheterization with a small catheter attached to a centrifuge tube is appropriate, but boys should *not* be routinely catheterized. It is often preferable in either sex to proceed with suprapubic needle aspiration. This is easier if the patient has been previously hydrated, so that the bladder is full. Suprapubic needle aspiration is performed as follows: (1) Cleanse the suprapubic area by sponging with alcohol. (2) With a small amount of local anesthetic, raise an intradermal wheal on the midline 1–2 cm above the pubis (the bladder lies just above the pubis in young children). (3) Attach a 10-mL syringe to a 22-gauge needle. Insert the needle perpendicularly through the abdominal wheal into the bladder wall, maintaining gentle suction with the syringe so that urine will be aspirated as soon as the bladder is entered.

Macroscopic Examination

Macroscopic examination of urine often provides a clue when diagnosis is difficult.

A. Color and Appearance: Urine is often colored owing to drugs: phenazopyridine (Pyridium) will turn the urine orange; rifampin will turn it yellow-orange; nitrofurantoin will turn it brown; and L-dopa, α-methyldopa, and metronidazole will turn it reddish-brown. Red urine does not always signify hematuria. A red discoloration unassociated with intact erythrocytes in the urine can result from betacyanin excretion after beet ingestion, phenolphthalein in laxatives, ingestion of vegetable dyes, concentrated urate excretion, myoglobinuria due to significant muscle trauma, or hemoglobinuria following hemolysis. In addition, *Serratia marcescens* bacteria can cause the "red diaper" syndrome. However, whenever red urine is seen, hematuria must be ruled out by microscopic analysis. Cloudy urine is commonly thought to represent pyuria, but more often the cloudiness is due to large amounts of amorphous phosphates, which disappear with the addition of acid, or urates, which dissolve with the use of alkali. The odor of urine is rarely clinically significant, except that a pungent odor may indicate that the specimen has been standing too long to be diagnostically useful.

B. Specific Gravity: The specific gravity of urine (normal, 1.003–1.030) is often important for diagnostic purposes: that of patients with significant intracranial trauma may be low owing to a lack of antidiuretic hormone (ADH, vasopressin); that of patients with primary diabetes insipidus is less than 1.010 even after overnight dehydration; that of patients with extensive acute renal tubular damage is consistently 1.010 (similar to the specific gravity of plasma); and a low specific gravity can be an early sign of renal damage from conditions such as sickle cell anemia. Urine specific gravity is the simplest time-honored test for evaluating hydration in postoperative patients. The specific gravity of urine may affect the results of other urine tests: in dilute urine, a pregnancy test may be falsely negative; in concentrated urine, protein may be falsely positive on dip-strips yet unconfirmed on quantitative tests. The specific gravity of urine may be falsely elevated by the presence of glucose, protein, artificial plasma expanders, or intravenous contrast agents.

The specific gravity of urine can be tested easily in the physician's office by a hydrometer or a refractometer. Both devices require occasional monitoring for precise calibration, and the specific gravity must be corrected to a standard temperature. Occasionally, a urine osmolality determination is required to confirm office specific gravity findings. Studies of specific-gravity reagent strips (method based on ionic alteration of a polyelectrolyte solution) have shown the method to be rapid, reliable, and unaffected by elevated amounts of glucose or contrast medium; however, alkaline pH may falsely lower the result (0.005/pH unit > 7.0) (Prodella, Dorizzi, and Rigalin, 1988). In the routine office setting, these strips are as reliable as either the hydrometer or refractometer methods (Bradley, Schumann, and Ward, 1984).

C. Chemical Tests: Chemically impregnated reagent strips that permit simultaneous rapid performance of a battery of chemical tests have replaced the specific individual tests. In general, these strips are accurate and have simplified routine urinalysis greatly. However, they must be monitored routinely by appropriate standardized quality-control reagents (Bradley, Schumann, and Ward, 1984), and more sophisticated chemical tests are occasionally required to confirm results and to maintain laboratory accreditation. The dip-strips are reliable only when not outdated and when used with *room temperature* urine.

1. pH—The pH of urine is important in a few specific clinical situations. Patients with uric acid stones rarely have a urinary pH over 6.5 (uric acid is soluble in alkaline urine). Patients with calcium stones, nephrocalcinosis, or both, may have renal tubular acidosis and will be unable to acidify urine below pH 6.0. With urinary tract infections caused by urea-splitting organisms (most commonly *Proteus* species), the urinary pH tends to be over 7.0. It should be reemphasized that urine obtained within 2 h of a large meal or left standing at room temperature for several hours tends to be alkaline. The indicator paper in most dip-strips is quite accurate; however, confirmation by a pH meter is occasionally required.

2. Protein—Dip-strips containing bromphenol blue can be used to determine the presence of > 10 mg/dL protein in urine, but persistent proteinuria detected in this manner requires quantitative protein testing for confirmation. The dip-strip measures primarily albumin and is not sensitive to Bence-Jones proteins (immunoglobulins). Concentrated urine may give a false-positive result, as will urine containing numerous white blood cells (leukocytes) or vaginal secretions replete with epithelial cells. Orthostatic proteinuria can be demonstrated by detecting elevated protein levels in a urine specimen obtained after the patient has been in the upright position for several hours, whereas normal levels are found in a specimen obtained in the early morning before ambulation. Prolonged fever and excessive physical exertion are also common causes of transient proteinuria.

Persistently elevated protein levels in the urine (> 150 mg/24 h) may indicate significant disease, eg, glomerulopathy or cancer. Therefore, specific quantitative protein tests on a timed urine collection, electrophoretic studies of the urine, or both, are required to determine the specific type of protein that is present. Ginsberg et al (1983) found that they could accurately assess proteinuria by determining the protein-creatinine ratio in an early-morning or late-afternoon single-voided urine specimen. They found that the normal ratio is 0.2 mg or less of protein per milligram of creatinine and that a ratio of 3.5 or more represents significant proteinuria (more than 1 g of protein excreted every 24 h). Results obtained by this method had an excellent correlation with the results of quantitative protein tests on 24-h urine specimens. This method of assessing proteinuria may obviate the need for the time-consuming and often inaccurate (due to incomplete collection) protein tests on 24-h urine collections.

3. Glucose—The glucose oxidase-peroxidase tests used in dip-strips are quite accurate and specific for urinary glucose. False-positive results may be obtained when patients have ingested large doses of aspirin, ascorbic acid, or cephalosporins. An occasional patient has a blood glucose level below 180 mg/dL and yet has significant glucosuria; this indicates a low renal threshold of glucose excretion. Most patients with a positive reading have diabetes mellitus, however, which may result in specific urinary tract manifestations such as renal papillary necrosis, recurrent urinary tract infections, neurovesical dysfunction, or impotence.

4. Hemoglobin—The dip-strip test for hemoglobin is not specific for erythrocytes and should be used only to *screen* for hematuria, with microscopic analysis of the urinary sediment used for confirmation. Free hemoglobin or myoglobin in the urine may give a positive reading; ascorbic acid in the urine can inhibit the dip-strip reaction and give a false-negative result. Note that dilute urine (< 1.008) will lyse erythrocytes and thus provide a positive dip-strip reading for hemoglobin but no visible erythrocytes on microscopic analysis (Wyker, 1991).

5. Bacteria and leukocytes–Test strips to determine the number of bacteria (nitrite) or leukocytes (leukocyte esterase) as predictors of bacteriuria are as accurate as microscopic sediment analysis in studies using quantitative urine cultures as the standard. The nitrite reductase test depends on the conversion of nitrate to nitrite. Many of the bacteria responsible for urinary tract infections, particularly enterobacteria, are capable of reducing nitrate to nitrite and therefore detectable by this test. When the nitrite test is positive, it suggests the presence of greater than 100,000 organisms/mL; however, several factors can lead to false-negative results. The nitrite test is positive only for coagulase-splitting bacteria and thus when used alone is only 40–60% accurate. Urine must be in the bladder for a sufficient time prior to sampling for the reduction of nitrate to occur (> 4 h); therefore, this test is most likely to be positive when first-voided morning urine is tested. A false-negative test will also result if the bacteria present do not contain nitrate reductase or if dietary nitrate is absent. A false-negative nitrate study may occur in a patient taking vitamin C. The leukocyte esterase test is a widely used chemical test that depends on the presence of esterase in granulocytic leukocytes. The leukocyte esterase test is an indication of pyuria and will remain positive even after the leukocytes have degenerated. The test accurately identifies patients with 10–12 leukocytes per high-power field in a centrifuged specimen. While this test is a good indicator of pyuria, it does not necessarily detect bacteriuria. Therefore, it is often combined with the nitrate test to detect both bacteriuria and inflammation to maximize the chances of predicting urinary tract infection. Used together, the 2 tests are equally as predictive as the microscopic analysis. A false-negative leukocyte esterase study can be caused by glucosuria, or by phenazopyridine hydrochloride (Pyridium), nitrofurantoin, vitamin C, or rifampin in the urine.

Microscopic Examination

Microscopic examination of the urinary sediment is an essential part of all urinalyses in the presence of urinary tract symptoms or an abnormal macroscopic analysis. To be most accurate, the microscopic sediment examination should be done personally by an experienced physician or technician. Early-morning urine is the best specimen if it can be examined within a few minutes of collection; however, this is rarely possible when the specimen is obtained at home, and for this reason, collection of a specimen for immediate examination in the office or hospital is the most useful method. In most cases, the sediment can be prepared as follows: (1) Centrifuge a 10-mL specimen at 2000 rpm for 5 min. (2) Decant the supernatant. (3) Resuspend the sediment in the remaining 1 mL of urine by tapping the tube gently against a counter top. (4) Place 1 drop of the mixture on a microscope slide, cover with a coverslip, and examine first under a low-power (× 10) and then under a high-power (× 40) lens. For maximal contrast of the elements in the sediment, the microscope diaphragm should be nearly closed to prevent overillumination. Significant elements (particularly bacteria) are more easily seen if the slide is stained with methylene blue, but staining is not essential. Figure 5–1 shows typical findings in the urinary sediment.

A. Staining: Staining with methylene blue (available commercially) may be helpful in microscopic examination of urinary sediment.

The urinary sediment is prepared as follows: (1) Place a drop of the centrifuged sediment on a glass slide and fix it slowly with heat from a laboratory burner or let it air dry. (2) Cool the slide and cover it with methylene blue for 10–20 s. (3) Rinse with tap water and let air dry or use with mild heat. Do not blot. (4) Examine the slide under oil immersion (with × 100 lens) without a coverslip.

The slide can be stained with Gram's stain (Table 5–1) instead of methylene blue, but this is more complex and time-consuming to perform, and the only advantage over staining with methylene blue is that *Neisseria gonorrhoeae* (gram-negative intracellular diplococci) can be more readily identified.

B. Interpretation

1. Bacteria–The significance of bacteria in the urinary sediment is discussed in the section that follows on bacteriuria.

2. Leukocytes–Just as the presence of bacteria in the sediment is not an absolute indication of infection, neither is the finding of pyuria. The method used to collect the specimen and the hydration status of the patient can alter the significance of the findings. In the sediment from clean-voided midstream specimens from men and those obtained by suprapubic aspiration or catheterization in women, a finding of more than 5–8 leukocytes per high-power field is generally considered abnormal (pyuria). If the patient has symptoms of a urinary tract infection as well as pyuria and bacteriuria, one is justified in making a diagnosis of infection and initiating empiric therapy. However, in a study of female patients with symptoms of urinary tract infection (Komaroff, 1984), 61% of those with pyuria had no bacterial growth from bladder urine obtained by catheterization or suprapubic aspiration. This underscores the unreliability of urinalysis alone for diagnosing urinary tract infections and further emphasizes the need for confirmation by bacterial cultures.

Renal tuberculosis can cause "sterile" acid-pyuria and should be considered in any patient with persistent pyuria and negative results on routine bacterial cultures. Specific staining of the urinary sediment for acid-fast bacteria (Ziehl-Neelsen stain) can be diagnostic; however, results will be positive from the sediment of spot specimens in only approximately 50%

Cells	Casts	Crystals	Other

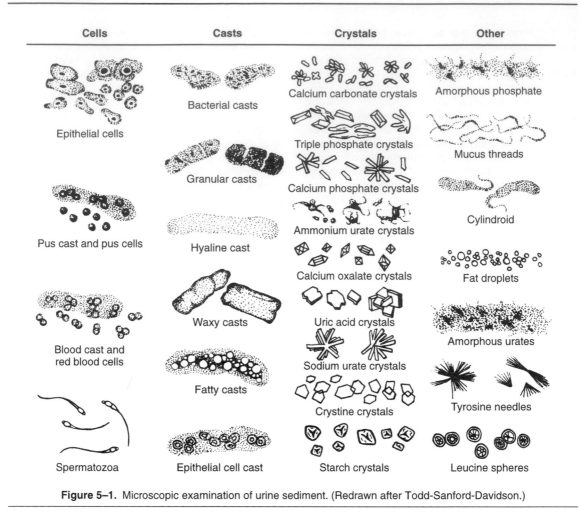

Figure 5–1. Microscopic examination of urine sediment. (Redrawn after Todd-Sanford-Davidson.)

of patients with renal tuberculosis, whereas they are positive in the sediment of 24-h specimens in 70–80% of such cases. *Mycobacterium smegmatis,* a commensal organism, may be present in the urine (particularly in uncircumcised men) and can give false-positive results on acid-fast stains.

Urolithiasis can also cause pyuria. In patients with persistent pyuria, the physician should consider ob-

taining at least a plain x-ray of the abdomen and possibly an intravenous urogram to determine whether urolithiasis is present. Similarly, a retained foreign body such as a self-induced bladder object or a forgotten internal ureteral stent can cause pyuria. A plain x-ray (KUB film) of the abdomen should reveal the offender.

Previous studies suggested that "glitter cells" (leukocytes with visible brownian movement of cytoplasmic granules) in the urinary sediment were pathognomonic of pyelonephritis; however, evidence has shown that these cells are not limited to patients with pyelonephritis.

3. Erythrocytes–The presence of even a few erythrocytes in the urine (hematuria) is abnormal and requires further investigation. Although gross hematuria is more alarming to the patient, microscopic hematuria is no less significant. Infrequent causes of hematuria include strenuous exercise (long-distance running), vaginal bleeding, and inflammation of organs near or directly adjoining the urinary tract, eg, diverticulitis or appendicitis. Hematuria associated

Table 5–1. Gram's staining method (Hucker modification).

1. Fix smear by heat.
2. Cover with crystal violet for 1 min.
3. Wash with water. Do not blot.
4. Cover with Gram's iodine for 1 min.
5. Wash with water. Do not blot.
6. Decolorize for 10–30 s with gentle agitation in acetone (30 mL) and alcohol (70 mL).
7. Wash with water. Do not blot.
8. Cover for 10–30 s with safranin (2.5% solution in 95% alcohol).
9. Wash with water and let dry.

with cystitis or urethritis generally clears after treatment. Persistent hematuria in an otherwise asymptomatic patient of either sex and any age signifies disease and is an indication for further testing.

In patients with microscopic hematuria, a 3-container method for collection of urine can provide information on the site of origin of erythrocytes. The method is as follows: (1) Give the patient 3 containers, labeled 1, 2, and 3 (or initial, mid, and terminal). (2) Instruct the patient to urinate and to collect the initial portion of the urine stream (10–15 mL) in the first container, the middle portion (30–40 mL) in the second, and the final portion (5–10 mL) in the third. (3) Using methods described previously, centrifuge the 3 specimens individually, prepare slides of the urinary sediment (with or without staining), and examine the slides microscopically. If erythrocytes predominate in the initial portion of the specimen, they are usually from the anterior urethra; those in the terminal portion are generally from the bladder neck or posterior urethra; and the presence of equal numbers of erythrocytes in all 3 containers usually indicates a source above the bladder neck (bladder, ureters, or kidneys). It is important to collect the urine before physical examination (particularly before rectal examination in men) to avoid misleading results.

The 3-container test may not be necessary in patients with gross hematuria, since the patients can usually tell the physician which portion of the stream contains the darkest urine (ie, the most erythrocytes). A specific dysmorphic erythrocyte configuration that can be detected with phase-contrast microscopy or by particle analyzer study of the urinary sediment and is highly indicative of active glomerular disease (Figure 5–2) has been described by Fairley and Birch (1982) and by Stamey and Kindrachuk (1985). This dysmorphism is thought to be a result of extreme changes in osmolality and the high concentration of urinary chemical constituents affecting erythrocytes during passage through the kidney tubules. An examiner experienced in viewing erythrocyte morphology can also detect these dysmorphic cells on routine microscopy if the light is diffracted appropriately. This finding represents a significant advance in routine urinalysis and should help define the origin of hematuria in patients with an elusive cause of bleeding.

Erythrocyte casts are discussed in a subsequent section.

4. Epithelial cells–Squamous epithelial cells in the urinary sediment indicate contamination of the specimen from the distal urethra in males and from the introitus in females; no other significance should

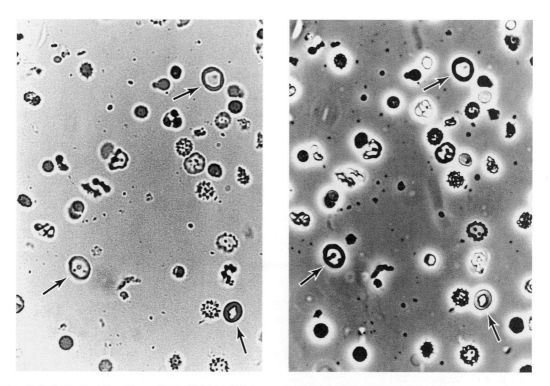

Figure 5–2. Left: Dysmorphic erythrocytes in urine (arrows), viewed under light microscopy (magnification × 400). **Right:** Dysmorphic erythrocytes in urine (identical field), viewed under phase-contrast microscopy. (Reproduced, with permission, from Stamey TA, Kindrachuk RW: *Urinary Sediment and Urinalysis: A Practical Guide for the Health Science Professional.* Saunders, 1985.)

be placed on them. It is not uncommon to find transitional epithelial cells in the normal urinary sediment; however, if they are present in large numbers or clumps and are abnormal histologically (including large nuclei, multiple nucleoli, and an increased ratio of nucleus to cytoplasm), they are indicative of a malignant process affecting the urothelium (Figure 5–3). Although staining the sediment with methylene blue may aid in visualizing the cells, the findings must be confirmed by an experienced cytopathologist.

5. Casts–Casts are formed in the distal tubules and collecting ducts and, for the most part, are not seen in normal urinary sediment; therefore, they commonly signify intrinsic renal disease.

Although **leukocyte casts** have been considered suggestive of pyelonephritis, they are not an absolute indicator and should not be used as the sole criterion for diagnosis. Leukocyte casts must be distinguished from **epithelial cell casts,** because the latter have little significance when present in small numbers. The distinction can be made easily if a small amount of acetic acid is added under the coverslip to enhance nuclear detail. (Note that casts tend to congregate near the edges of the coverslip.) Epithelial cell or leukocyte casts in large numbers signify underlying intrinsic renal disease requiring further diagnostic workup. In renal transplant recipients, an increase in the number of epithelial cells or casts from the renal tubules may be an early indication of acute graft rejection.

Erythrocyte casts are pathognomonic of underlying glomerulitis or vasculitis.

Hyaline casts probably represent a mixture of mucus and globulin congealed in the tubules; in small numbers, they are not significant. Hyaline casts are commonly seen in urine specimens taken after exercise and in concentrated or highly acidic urine specimens. As mentioned previously, casts are rarely seen in alkaline urine and are therefore not usually present in urine specimens that have been left standing or in specimens from patients unable to acidify urine (eg, those with advanced stages of chronic renal failure).

Granular casts most commonly represent disintegrated epithelial cells, leukocytes, or protein; they usually indicate intrinsic renal tubular disease.

6. Other findings–The finding of crystals in

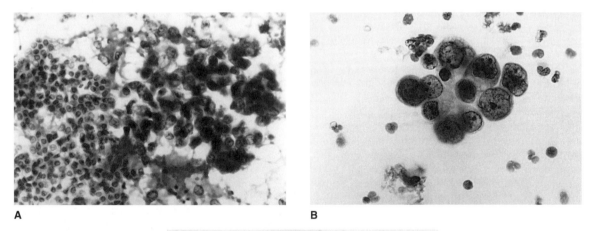

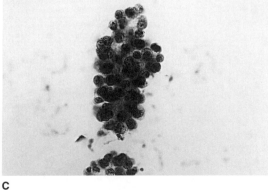

Figure 5–3. Papanicolaou-stained bladder cytology specimens. **A:** Normal cells (left) and malignant cells (right). **B:** High-power view of malignant cells. **C:** Papillary cluster of malignant cells. (Courtesy of Larry Kluskens, MD, Cytopathology Laboratory, University of Iowa.)

urine can be helpful in some instances, but the mere presence of crystals does not indicate disease. Crystals form in normal urine below room temperature. Cystine, leucine, tyrosine, cholesterol, bilirubin, hematoidin, and sulfonamide crystals are abnormal findings of varying importance. Several types of crystals that may be found on microscopic examination of urinary sediment are shown in Figure 5–1.

Recently, the use of protease inhibition for treatment of human immunodeficiency virus (HIV) has resulted in urolithiasis due to indinavir crystal formation in urine. The characteristic crystals are flat, rectangular plates, often in a fan or star-burst pattern (Gagnon, Tsoukas, and Watters, 1998; Kopp et al, 1997).

The presence of trichomonads or yeast cells in the stained or unstained smear of sediment from a properly obtained urine specimen establishes a diagnosis and the need for treatment.

Artifacts present in the urine sediment can be difficult to differentiate from real abnormalities. Dirt and small pieces of vegetable fiber or hair are frequently found, but the most common artifacts are starch granules from examination gloves.

Bacteriuria

A. Microscopic Examination: A presumptive diagnosis of bacterial infection may be made on the basis of results of microscopic examination of the urinary sediment. The significance of bacteria in the urinary sediment depends in part on the method used to collect the specimen, the specific gravity of the specimen, and whether the slide was stained. If several bacteria per high-power field are found in a urine specimen obtained by suprapubic aspiration or catheterization in a woman or in a properly obtained clean-voided midstream specimen from a man, a provisional diagnosis of bacterial infection can be made and empiric treatment started. The findings should be confirmed by bacterial culture. Finding several bacteria per high-power field in a voided specimen from a woman is of little significance. If the specific gravity of the urine specimen is low, the bacterial count may be low owing to dilution; if the specific gravity is high, the converse is true. It is easier to distinguish and count bacteria and to differentiate leukocytes from transitional epithelial cells when slides are stained with methylene blue (see earlier section).

B. Determining the Site of Origin of Infection: If the patient has a urinary tract infection but the site of the infection is not known, tests for antibody-coated bacteria may be performed. Although past studies have indicated that the presence of antibody-coated bacteria in the urine pointed to the kidney as the site of infection, antibody-coated bacteria may also be found in the urine of patients with neurogenic bladder, prostatitis, and chronic or recurrent cystitis. The test may be useful, however, in locating the site of origin of recurrent bacteriuria (particularly in women) if specimens are collected separately from the bladder and both ureters.

Another method for determining the site of origin of bacteriuria and pyuria is discussed subsequently in the section on examination of urethral discharge.

C. Bacterial Cultures: The presumptive diagnosis of bacterial infection based on microscopic examination of the urinary sediment should be confirmed by culture.

1. Indications and interpretation–Cultures can be used to estimate the number of bacteria in the urine (quantitative cultures), to identify the exact organism present, and to predict which drugs will be effective in treating the infection. Cultures are particularly important in patients with recurrent or persistent infections, renal insufficiency, or drug allergies.

The number of bacteria present in the urine (colony count) is influenced by the method used to collect the urine specimen, the patient's hydration status, and whether the patient has been taking antimicrobial drugs. These factors and the patient's symptoms must be considered in determining whether a urinary tract infection is present. The concept that urinary tract infection is present only when the urine specimen contains 10^5 or more bacteria per milliliter is not an absolute rule; a lower count does not exclude the possibility of an infection, particularly in a symptomatic patient. For example, a symptomatic patient with a urine specific gravity of 1.015 and a colony count of less than 10^5/mL in a clean-voided specimen may have a significant infection; a count of 10^5/mL in a specimen obtained by catheterization or an even lower count in a specimen obtained by suprapubic aspiration indicates significant bacteriuria. Cultures with growth of multiple organisms usually signify contamination, which may be due to an improper collection method or improper laboratory technique. The presence of a few organisms in a specimen with a low specific gravity is more significant than the same finding in a specimen with a high specific gravity, because the former is more dilute. The physician must take into account all of these factors when interpreting the results of bacterial cultures.

It is not always necessary to identify the specific organism causing the infection, particularly in "routine" lower urinary tract infections; however, identification of the causative organism may be important in patients with recurrent or persistent symptoms and signs of urinary tract infection. Some bacteria (eg, neisseriae, brucellae, mycobacteria, anaerobes), fungi, and yeasts will not grow with common culture methods, and thus special culture techniques are required.

Identifying the drugs to which the bacteria are sensitive may or may not be necessary. *Escherichia coli,* which causes 85% of "routine" urinary tract infections, is known to be sensitive to numerous oral antimicrobial drugs. However, in patients with septicemia, renal insufficiency, diabetes mellitus, or suspected enterococcal, *Proteus,* or *Pseudomonas* infections, it is important to determine the antibiotic sensitivity of the organism and the drug concentration necessary for efficacious treatment. Monitoring antibiotic levels in blood and urine during treatment may be indicated, especially in severely ill patients and those receiving highly toxic drugs. These measurements can be done by most hospital laboratories.

2. Rapid tests for bacteriuria–In general, seriously ill or hospitalized patients with urinary tract infections should have cultures processed by an accredited bacteriology laboratory. However, for "routine" infections encountered in office practice, there are many satisfactory, cost-effective testing methods.

Rapid methods to screen for bacteria include growth-independent systems and growth-dependent systems. Several growth-dependent systems are available. One measures the turbidity of urine incubated in a broth medium for several hours. Positive results can be determined in as short a time period as 4 h; however, 12 h of growth is required before a test sample can be regarded as negative. Another growth-dependent system is based on the measurement of electrical conductance; however, this test has a high false-positive rate. A single screening test uses the leukocyte esterase test and the nitrite test. The leukocyte esterase test is designed to detect pyuria, while the nitrate reductase test depends on the presence of bacteria in the urine that can reduce nitrate to nitrite. To maximize the probability of predicting urinary tract infection, these 2 tests have been combined in a single strip in which either or both may be positive.

One growth-independent screening test is an automated system of microscopy with acridine-orange staining. This system is very sensitive and predictive for a urinary tract infection, but it has a high false-negative rate and is costly. Another test traps leukocytes and bacteria in a filter. A dye is then applied to the filter, and a color change is indicative of a urinary tract infection. This system is very rapid; however, the filter is prone to clogging, and pigmented urine may interfere with the colorimetric end point. Particles in the urine (both bacteria and leukocytes) can be counted by measuring electrical impedance, although the test is less accurate when counting bacteria.

Reliable culture methods involve use of small strips or glass slides coated with eosin–methylene blue agar on one side and nutrient agar on the other. The strips or slides are dipped in the urine specimen and then incubated for 24 h. Although these methods are easy to use, their disadvantages are that (1) not all bacteria will grow under these conditions, and (2) the accuracy of colony counts is debatable.

Perhaps preferable for the physician's office (but still subject to some of the same limitations) is use of a divided plastic culture plate with blood agar on one side and deoxycholate agar on the other. A known amount of urine is inoculated onto the agar on each side of the plate, and colony counts are determined at 24–48 h. The numbers of bacteria in 1 mL of the original urine specimen can be determined by multiplying the number of colonies by the volume (in milliliters) and dilution (if any) of the inoculum. If antibiotic sensitivity testing is also desired, an additional culture plate can be inoculated and small antibiotic-impregnated disks placed on the agar. Zones of growth inhibition seen around the disks at 12–24 h indicate sensitivity. These methods are satisfactory for most office situations, although some organisms (see earlier section) may require specific media or conditions for growth.

3. Cultures for tuberculosis–Urine smears stained for acid-fast bacilli (Ziehl-Neelsen stain performed by the laboratory) may provide evidence to support the diagnosis of renal tuberculosis. However, regardless of the result of the smear, multiple urine cultures should be performed if renal tuberculosis is suspected, both to confirm the presence of *Mycobacterium* and to determine its species. Numerous atypical mycobacteria have been found to cause renal tuberculosis. Since they are not always sensitive to the commonly used antituberculous drugs, sensitivity testing may also be indicated. Because the procedures for urine culture for mycobacteria vary from one laboratory to another, the physician should consult the laboratory beforehand. Mycobacteria grow slowly; thus, culture results may require 6–8 weeks or longer.

Other Urine Tests

Many other tests of urine can be helpful in determining the presence of urologic disease.

A. Urothelial Cancer Tests

1. Urine cytology–The evaluation of voided or bladder wash (barbotage) urine for bladder urothelial cancer cells has been quite successful for higher-grade (2–3) transitional cell cancers. Lower-grade tumors less commonly shed abnormal cells. Cystoscopy remains the standard diagnostic test for initial diagnosis and surveillance of bladder cancer. However, a number of new tests have been developed to improve the noninvasive diagnosis of bladder cancer.

2. Bladder tumor antigen test–The bladder tumor antigen test (BTA; Bard Diagnostic Sciences, Inc, Redmond, WA) is a latex agglutination assay for the qualitative detection of bladder tumor antigen in the urine. This antigen is composed of basement membrane complexes that have been isolated and characterized from patients with bladder cancer. The bladder tumor antigen test may be performed rapidly on a voided urine specimen and requires minimal technical expertise (Sarosdy et al, 1995).

3. Bladder tumor antigen *stat* test–The BTA *stat* test (Bard Diagnostic Sciences) is a single-step immunochromatographic assay for bladder tumor-associated antigens in voided urine. The tumor-associated antigen detected by the BTA *stat* test has been identified as a human complement factor of protein (hCFHrp) that is similar in composition, structure, and function to human complement factor H (hCFH). The BTA *stat* test detects this bladder tumor antigen in approximately 5 min after a few drops of voided urine are placed into the test container (Sarosdy et al, 1997).

4. Nuclear matrix protein 22–The nuclear matrix protein 22 test (NMP22; Matritech, Inc, Newton, MA) is an immunoassay that measures nuclear matrix protein 22. Normal subjects will have low levels of NMP22 in the urine, whereas patients with active transitional cell carcinoma may have high levels of urinary NMP22. The test is currently performed by the manufacturer on the results of 3 voids, which are averaged in 1 sample (Soloway et al, 1996).

5. AuraTek FDP–Bladder tumor cells normally produce vascular endothelial growth factor, which increases the permeability of microvasculature leading to leakage of plasma proteins, including plasminogen, fibrinogen, and other clotting factors. These clotting factors rapidly convert fibrinogen into fibrin and fibrinogen degradation products. The AuraTek FDP test (PerImmune, Inc, Rockville, MD) is an immunoassay device designed for the qualitative measurement of fibrin/fibrinogen degradation products in the urine. The test is designed as an in-office test that is performed on a urine sample with a dipstick (Schmetter et al, 1997).

6. QUANTICYT System–The QUANTICYT System is a computer-based cytologic image analysis system. This system evaluates 50 randomly selected images containing 100–500 nuclei for DNA content and nuclear shape (van der Poel et al, 1996).

The characteristics of these bladder cancer tests are compared in Table 5–2.

B. Hormonal Studies: Tests for abnormalities in adrenal hormone secretion are important in the workup of patients with suspected adrenal tumors. Pheochromocytoma and neuroblastoma can be detected by measuring the excretion of vanillylmandelic acid (VMA). However, urinary levels of metanephrine, epinephrine, and norepinephrine are more sensitive indicators, particularly in cases of pheochromocytoma. While high levels of aldosterone in urine usually indicate an aldosterone-secreting tumor, drug interference may cause false-positive or false-negative results. Other adrenocortical tumors may be detected by their production of elevated levels of urinary 17-ketosteroids, although more specific urinary steroid tests are now available. In the past, determinations of urinary gonadotropin levels were helpful in the staging and follow-up of patients with testicular tumors or gestational trophoblastic tumors, but studies of the serum markers alpha-fetoprotein and the beta-subunit of human chorionic gonadotropin (hCG) have supplanted urinary studies in most of these patients (see Examination of Blood, Serum, & Plasma, following).

C. Studies of Stone Constituents: Patients with recurrent urolithiasis may have an underlying abnormality of excretion of calcium, uric acid, oxalate, magnesium, or citrate. Samples of 24-h urine collections can be tested to determine abnormally high levels of each. A few patients may have elevated cystine levels in urine. The nitroprusside test, a simple *qualitative* screening test for cystine, may indicate the need for quantifying cystine levels in timed urine collections. Whenever a stone is recovered, a formal stone analysis is recommended.

D. Miscellaneous Studies: Tests of urinary levels of lactate dehydrogenase, carcinoembryonic antigen, and other tumor markers (see Chapters 21 and 24) are not specific and thus are not generally helpful. The measurement of urinary levels of hydroxyproline has been described as a useful test for determining both the presence of bone metastases and the efficacy of treatment in patients with advanced prostatic adenocarcinoma. In patients with suspected fistulas of the urinary tract and bowel (eg, cancer of the colon, diverticulitis, regional ileitis), discoloration of the urine after ingestion of a poorly absorbed dye such as phenol red will confirm the diagnosis. In an equally satisfactory test for fistulas, the patient is instructed to ingest gelatin capsules filled with granulated charcoal and to submit a urine sample several days later. Examination of the centrifuged urinary sediment will reveal the typical black granules if a fistula is present.

Table 5–2. Comparison of different urine tests for transitional cell carcinoma of bladder.

Test	Sensitivity (%)	Specificity (%)	Positive Predictive Value (%)	Negative Predictive Value(%)
BTA	40	95	51	93
BTA *stat*	57	68	70	56
NMP22[a]	70	76	76	58
AuraTek FDP	68	80	59	35
QUANTICYT	59	93	76	76
Cytology (barbotage)	58	100	100	77
Cytology (voided)	59	100	100	78

[a] Used after transurethral resection of bladder tumor to predict recurrence.

EXAMINATION OF URETHRAL DISCHARGE & VAGINAL EXUDATE

Urethral Discharge

Examination of urethral discharge in males can be particularly helpful in establishing a diagnosis. The following procedure (as outlined by Stamey and others; see Stamey, 1980), although exacting, provides proper specimens for determining the site of origin of bacteriuria or pyuria. Four sterile containers are labeled VB_1, VB_2, EPS, and VB_3 (VB = voided bladder urine; EPS = expressed prostatic secretions). The patient is instructed to retract the foreskin and cleanse the meatus with benzalkonium chloride or hexachlorophene and to collect the urine specimens, capping the containers immediately afterward. The initial 10–15 mL of urine is collected in container VB_1 and the subsequent 15–30 mL in container VB_2. The prostate is then massaged, and secretions are collected in container EPS. The patient voids a final time, collecting the specimen in container VB_3. An aliquot of each specimen is tested for nitrite and leukocyte esterase and then centrifuged and the sediment prepared for microscopic examination as described previously. A separate aliquot of each VB specimen and the EPS specimen are saved for subsequent culture if necessary. The presence of leukocytes or bacteria (or both) only in VB_1 indicates anterior urethritis; if present in all 3 VB specimens, they may indicate cystitis or upper urinary tract infection; if present in EPS or VB_3 only, they indicate a prostatic source of infection. Quantitative cultures can be similarly interpreted. Patients with positive results should be treated with appropriate antimicrobial drugs.

If the patient presents with the thick yellowish discharge typical of *N gonorrhoeae* infection, the discharge should be stained with Gram's stain and examined for gram-negative intracellular diplococci. It is important to remember that commensal bacteria in smegma may produce false-positive results. Nevertheless, treatment of patients with positive results should be started immediately and not delayed until the results of confirmatory cultures are available. A spot test for *N gonorrhoeae* (Gonodecten) appears to be useful (Felman and William, 1982), but its accuracy is not absolute; therefore, confirmation of results by conventional culture of the exudate is still recommended.

If the patient presents with clear or whitish urethral discharge, a smear of the discharge obtained by milking the urethra or from VB_1 should be stained with methylene blue or Gram's stain and examined microscopically. The presence of trichomonads, yeast cells, or bacteria in properly collected specimens indicates disease requiring treatment.

In cases of acute epididymitis, urinalysis and urine culture are often helpful in establishing the cause.

Berger et al (1978) demonstrated that epididymitis is most commonly caused by *Chlamydia* species in young men and by *E coli* in men over 35 years of age. Culturing chlamydiae is time-consuming and expensive. Although a rapid immunofluorescence method of identifying *Chlamydia* is available, it is usually best to proceed with therapy based on the age of the patient and guided by clinical results.

The diagnosis of any sexually transmitted disease should raise the question of acquired immunodeficiency syndrome (AIDS). A study by Hart (1991) demonstrated that many patients who presented to a sexually transmitted disease clinic did not request to be tested for HIV infection. Had the clinical staff not provided education and urged HIV testing for all patients, 44% of patients diagnosed with HIV would have been missed.

Vaginal Exudate

Examination of the vaginal introitus is mandatory in evaluating symptoms involving the lower urinary tract in females. The underlying cause of vaginitis is often a viral, yeast, or protozoal infection or the presence of a foreign body (eg, retained tampon), and a simple physical examination may be all that is required for diagnosis.

Vaginal secretions obtained by use of a swab can be examined either stained or unstained. A drop of saline is added to a drop of specimen on a glass slide, mixed thoroughly, and covered with a coverslip. Examination under a low- or high-power lens may reveal yeast cells or trichomonads, thus suggesting appropriate therapy. Since bacteria are always present in the vagina, they generally are not significant findings in a wet smear. Culture of vaginal secretions may help to establish the cause of recurrent bacteriuria.

RENAL FUNCTION TESTS

If urologic disease is suspected, results of renal function tests may provide clues to the diagnosis, aid in determining which diagnostic studies should be performed or avoided, and assist in the choice of therapeutic alternatives.

Urine Specific Gravity

As noted previously, specific gravity is a simple and reproducible test of renal function. With diminished renal function, the ability of the kidneys to concentrate urine lessens progressively until the specific gravity of urine reaches 1.006–1.010. However, the ability to dilute urine tends to be maintained until renal damage is extreme. Even in uremia, although the concentrating power of the kidneys is limited to a specific gravity of 1.010, dilution power in the specific gravity range of 1.002–1.004 may still be found. Determination of urine osmolality is undoubtedly a more meaningful measurement of renal function, but determination of specific gravity lends itself to office diagnosis.

Serum Creatinine

Creatinine, the end product of the metabolism of creatine in skeletal muscle, is normally excreted by the kidneys. Because daily creatinine production is amazingly constant, the serum level is a direct reflection of renal function. Serum creatinine levels remain within the normal range (0.8–1.2 mg/dL in adults; 0.4–0.8 mg/dL in young children) until approximately 50% of renal function has been lost. Unlike most other excretory products, the serum creatinine level generally is not influenced by dietary intake or hydration status.

Endogenous Creatinine Clearance

Because creatinine production is stable and creatinine is filtered through the glomerulus (although a small amount is probably secreted), its renal clearance is essentially equal to the glomerular filtration rate. The endogenous creatinine clearance test has thus become the most accurate and reliable measure of renal function available without resorting to infusion of exogenous substances such as inulin or radionuclides. Determination of creatinine clearance requires only the collection of a timed (usually 24-h) urine specimen and a serum specimen. The clearance is calculated as follows:

$$\text{Clearance} = UV/P$$

where: **U = creatinine in urine (in mg/dL)**
P = creatinine in plasma (in mg/dL)
V = mL of urine excreted (per minute or 24 h)

The resulting clearance is expressed in milliliters per minute, with 90–110 mL/min considered normal.

Because muscle mass differs among individuals, further standardization has been achieved by using the following formula:

$$UV/P = 1.73 \text{ m}^2/\text{Estimated surface area} = \text{Corrected clearance}$$

A corrected clearance level of 70–140 mL/min is considered normal.

Although creatinine is highly reliable as an estimate of renal function, values may be falsely low, particularly if only part of the urine is collected over the timed period or if a serum specimen is not collected concurrently.

Blood Urea Nitrogen

Urea is the primary metabolite of protein catabolism and is excreted entirely by the kidneys. The blood urea nitrogen (BUN) level is therefore related to the glomerular filtration rate. Unlike creatinine, however, BUN is influenced by dietary protein intake, hydration status, and gastrointestinal bleeding. Approximately two-thirds of renal function must be lost before a significant rise in blood urea nitrogen level becomes evident. For these reasons, an elevated blood urea nitrogen level is less specific for renal insufficiency than an elevated serum creatinine level. However, the blood urea nitrogen-creatinine (BUN-Cr) ratio can provide specific diagnostic information. It is normally 10:1; in dehydrated patients and those with bilateral urinary obstruction or urinary extravasation, the ratio may range from 20:1 to 40:1; patients with advanced hepatic insufficiency and overhydrated patients may exhibit a lower than normal BUN level and BUN-Cr ratio. Patients with renal insufficiency may develop extremely high blood urea nitrogen levels that can be partially controlled by a decrease in dietary protein.

EXAMINATION OF BLOOD, SERUM, & PLASMA

Some of the serum and blood tests of diagnostic usefulness in urology were discussed previously. The following are also applicable to urologic disease.

Complete Blood Count

Normochromic normocytic anemia is often seen with chronic renal insufficiency. Chronic blood loss from microscopic hematuria is usually not sufficient to cause anemia, although gross hematuria certainly can be. A specific increase in the number of erythrocytes, as manifested by elevated hemoglobin and hematocrit levels (erythrocytosis, not polycythemia), may be indicative of a paraneoplastic syndrome associated with renal cell cancer. The leukocyte count is usually nonspecific, although marked elevations may indicate an underlying leukemia that may be the cause of urologic symptoms. In such cases, further testing is indicated to determine the specific diagnosis before any urologic surgery.

Blood Clotting Studies

Clotting studies are generally not necessary unless an insidious disorder such as von Willebrand disease, hepatic disease, or a sensitivity to ingested salicylates is suspected in a patient with unexplained hematuria. The determination of prothrombin time and bleeding time (and perhaps partial thromboplastin time) is usually sufficient. A platelet count is important in patients receiving chemotherapy and those who have received extensive radiation therapy.

Electrolyte Studies

Serum sodium and potassium determinations may be indicated in patients taking diuretics or digitalis preparations and in patients who have just undergone transurethral prostatectomy. Serum calcium determinations are useful in patients with calcium urolithiasis. Elevated calcium levels are occasionally indicative of a paraneoplastic syndrome in patients with renal cell cancer. Serum albumin levels should be measured simultaneously with calcium levels to adequately assess the significance of the latter.

Prostate Cancer Markers

Prostate-specific antigen (PSA) is an extremely important prostate cancer marker. PSA is prostate-specific but not cancer-specific. Serum elevation greater than 4.0 ng/mL is correlated with prostatic cancer; however, serum levels vary with prostate volume, inflammation, and amount of cancer within the gland. PSA has become useful as a screening tool and is most useful as a marker of effective treatment (falls to zero following removal of organ-confined cancer) and early recurrence (antedates other clinical evidence of tumor by 6 months or more). Recently, the percentage of free PSA (ratio of unbound to total PSA) in the serum has been approved for use in diagnosing prostate cancer. Studies show that when the percentage of free PSA is < 10%, approximately 60% of men will have prostate cancer, whereas if the percentage of free PSA is > 25%, only 10% will have it (Catalona et al, 1995).

Hormonal Studies

Serum parathyroid hormone studies are useful in determining the presence of a parathyroid adenoma in patients with urolithiasis and an elevated serum calcium level. Measurement of parathyroid hormone is not reliable, however, as a sole screening test for parathyroid adenoma and should not be used routinely in all patients with urolithiasis. Serum renin levels may be elevated in patients with renal hypertension, although many conditions can cause false-positive results. Studies of adrenal steroid hormones (eg, aldosterone, cortisol, epinephrine, norepinephrine) are useful in determining adrenal function or the presence of adrenal tumors. Determinations of serum levels of the beta-subunit of hCG and of alpha-fetoprotein are indispensable in staging and in treatment follow-up for testicular tumors. One of these tumor markers is usually elevated in up to 85% of patients with nonseminomatous testicular tumors and can predict the recrudescence of tumor several months before disease is clinically evident. Serum testosterone studies can help to establish the cause of impotence or infertility.

Other Studies

The finding of elevated fasting plasma glucose levels in patients with urologic disease can establish the diagnosis of diabetes mellitus and thus indicate a possible cause of renal insufficiency, neurovesical dysfunction, impotence, or recurrent urinary tract infection. Serum uric acid levels are often elevated in patients with uric acid stones. Elevated serum complement levels may be diagnostic of underlying glomerulopathies.

Table 5–3. Laboratory values that *do not* change with age.

Hepatic function tests
  Serum bilirubin
  AST
  ALT
  GGTP
Coagulation tests
Biochemical tests
  Serum electrolytes
  Total protein
  Calcium
  Phosphorus
  Serum folate
Arterial blood tests
  pH
  $Paco_2$
Renal function tests
  Serum creatinine
Thyroid function tests
  T_4
Complete blood count
  Hematocrit
  Hemoglobin
  Erythrocyte indices
  Platelet count

AST = aspartate aminotransferase; ALT = alanine aminotransferase; GGTP = gamma-glutamyltransferase

Table 5–4. Laboratory values that *do* change with age.

Value	Degree of Change
Alkaline phosphatase	Increases by 20% between third and eighth decades
Biochemical tests	
Serum albumin	Slight decline
Uric acid	Slight increase
Total cholesterol	Increases by 30–40 mg/dL by age 55 in women and age 60 in men
HDL cholesterol	Increases by 30% in men; decreases 50% in women
Triglycerides	Increases by 30% in men and 50% in women
Serum B_{12}	Slight decrease
Serum magnesium	Decreases by 15% between third and eighth decades
Pao_2	Decreases by 25% between third and eighth decades
Creatinine clearance	Decreases by 10 mL/min/1.73 sq m/decade
Thyroid function tests	
T_3	Possible slight decrease
TSH	Possible slight increase
Glucose tolerance tests	
Fasting blood sugar	Minimal increase (within normal range)
1-Hour postprandial blood sugar	Increases by 10 mg/dL/decade after age 30
2-Hour postprandial blood sugar	Increases up to 100 plus age after age 40
Leukocyte count	Decreases

HDL = high-density lipoprotein; TSH = thyroid-stimulating hormone.

Urologic diseases are rarely confined solely to urologic organs and may cause or result from diseases in other organ systems.

LABORATORY VALUES IN ELDERLY PATIENTS

To accurately diagnose and treat geriatric patients, physicians must have an understanding of the effect of aging on "normal" laboratory values. Clearly, some laboratory values change as patients age, others stay the same, and the effects of aging on some are as yet unknown. Laboratory values that do not change with increasing age include complete blood count, serum electrolytes, and hepatic function tests, among others (Table 5–3). Laboratory values that change as patients age include creatinine clearance, alkaline phosphatase, uric acid, and cholesterol (Table 5–4).

Other factors that may make laboratory interpretation more difficult include atypical disease presentation, multiple concurrent diseases, and prescription and nonprescription drug use.

REFERENCES

Abuelo JG: Proteinuria: Diagnostic principles and procedures. Ann Intern Med 1983;98:186.

Adams U: Evaluation of Ames Multistix-SG for urine specific gravity versus refractometer specific gravity. Am J Clin Pathol 1983;80:871.

Baum N, Dichoso CC, Carlton CE Jr: Blood urea nitrogen and serum creatinine: Physiology and interpretations. Urology 1975;5:583.

Berger RE et al: Chlamydia trachomatis as a cause of acute "idiopathic" epididymitis. N Engl J Med 1978;298:301.

Bolann BJ, Sandberg S, Digranes A: Implications of probability analysis for interpreting results of leukocyte esterase and nitrite test strips. Clin Chem 1989;35:1663.

Bradley M, Schumann GB, Ward PCJ: Examination of urine. In: Henry JB (editor): *Clinical Diagnosis and Management by Laboratory Methods,* 17th ed., Saunders, 1984.

Brody LH, Salladay JR, Armbruster K: Urinalysis and the urinary sediment. Med Clin North Am 1971;55:243.

Carlton CE Jr, Scardino PT: Initial evaluation. In: Harrison IH et al (editors): *Campbell's Urology,* 5th ed., vol 1, p. 276. Saunders, 1986.

Catalona WJ et al: Evaluation of percentage of free serum PSA to improve specificity of prostate cancer screening. JAMA 1995;274:1214.

Cavalieri TA, Chopra A, Bryman PN: When outside the norm is normal: Interpreting lab data in the aged. Geriatrics 1992;47:66.

Coudron PE et al: Detection of *Chlamydia trachomatis* in general specimens by the Microtrak direct specimen test. Am J Clin Pathol 1986;85:89.

deCaestecker MP et al: Localisation of haematuria by red cell analysers and phase contrast microscopy. Nephron 1989;52:170.

Diamond JR, McLaughlin ML: Urinary parameters to assess renal function. Clin Lab Med 1988;8:493.

Emanuel B, Aronson N: Neonatal hematuria. Am J Dis Child 1974;128:204.

Fairley KF, Birch DF: Hematuria: A simple method for identifying glomerular bleeding. Kidney Int 1982;21:105.

Fang LS: Urinalysis in the diagnosis of urinary tract infections. Clin Lab Med 1988;8:567.

Felman YM, William DC: New 3-minute in vitro diagnostic test for gonorrhea in the male without use of conventional culture or Gram stain. Urology 1982;19:252.

Friedman SA, Gladstone JL: The effects of hydration and bladder incubation time on urine colony counts. J Urol 1971;105:428.

Gagnon RF, Tsoukas CM, Watters AK: Light microscopy of indinavir urinary crystals. Ann Intern Med 1998;128:321.

Galambos JT, Hemdon EG Jr, Reynolds GH: Specific gravity determination: Fact or fancy. N Engl J Med 1964;270:506.

Gavan TL: In vitro antimicrobial susceptibility testing: Clinical implications and limitations. Med Clin North Am 1974;58:493.

Gillenwater JY et al: Home urine cultures by the dipstrip method: Results in 289 cultures. Pediatrics 1976;58:508.

Ginsberg JM et al: Use of single voided urine samples to estimate quantitative proteinuria. N Engl J Med 1983;309:1543.

Gleckman R: A critical review of the antibody-coated bacteria test. J Urol 1979;122:770.

Gleckman R, Crowley M: Epididymitis as cause of antibody-coated bacteria in urine. Urology 1979;14:241.

Hallander HO et al: Evaluation of rapid methods for the detection of bacteriuria (screening) in primary health care. Acta Pathol Microbiol Immunol Scand (Sect B) 1986;94:39.

Hardy JD, Fumell PM, Brumfitt W: Comparison of sterile bag, clean catch and suprapubic aspiration in the diagnosis of urinary infection in early childhood. Br J Urol 1976;48:279.

Hart G: Factors associated with requesting and refusing human immunodeficiency virus antibody testing. Med J Aust 1991;155:586.

Hubbell FA et al: Routine admission laboratory testing for general medical patients. Med Care 1988;26:619.

Kampmann J et al: Rapid evaluation of creatinine clearance. Acta Med Scand 1974;196:517.

Kass EH: Asymptomatic infections of the urinary tract. Trans Assoc Am Physicians 1956;69:56.

Kassirer JP, Harrington JT: Laboratory evaluation of renal function. In: Schrier RW, Gottschalk CW (editors): *Diseases of the Kidney,* 46th ed. Little, Brown, 1988.

Khanna OP, Son DL: Screening for urinary tract infection using Bac-T-Screen bacteriuria device. Urology 1986;27:424.

Komaroff AL: Acute dysuria in women. N Engl J Med 1984;310:368.

Kopp JB et al: Crystalluria and urinary tract abnormalities associated with indinavir. Ann Intern Med 1997; 127:119.

Kunin CM, DeGroot JE: Self-screening for significant bacteriuria: Evaluation of dip-strip combination nitrite/culture test. JAMA 1975;231:1349.

Kunin CM, DeGroot JE: Sensitivity of a nitrite indicator strip method in detecting bacteriuria in preschool girls. Pediatrics 1977;60:244.

Labovits ED et al: "Benign" hematuria with focal glomerulitis in adults. Ann Intern Med 1972;77:723.

Lawrence VA, Gafni A, Gross M: The unproven utility of the preoperative urinalysis: Economic evaluation. J Clin Epidemiol 1989;42:1185.

Littlewood JM, Jacobs SI, Ramsden CH: Comparison between microscopical examination of unstained deposits of urine and quantitative culture. Arch Dis Child 1977;52:894.

Lohr JA et al: Making a presumptive diagnosis of urinary tract infection by using a urinalysis performed in an on-site laboratory. J Pediatr 1993;122:22.

Madaio MP, Harrington JT: The diagnosis of acute glomerulonephritis. N Engl J Med 1983;309:1299.

McLin PH, Tavel FR: Urine culture and direct drug disc sensitivity testing: A rapid simple method for use in the office. Clin Med (Dec) 1971;78:16.

Merritt JL, Keys TF: Limitations of the antibody-coated bacteria test in patients with neurogenic bladder. JAMA 1982;247:1723.

Messing EM et al: Urinary tract cancers found by home-screening with hematuria dipsticks in healthy men over 50 years of age. Cancer 1989;64:2361.

Mills SJ et al: Screening for bacteriuria in urological patients using reagent strips. Br J Urol 1992;70:314.

Morgan MG, McKenzie H: Controversies in the laboratory diagnosis of community-acquired urinary tract infection. Eur J Clin Microbiol Infect Dis 1993;12:491.

Nanji AA, Adam W, Campbell DJ: Routine microscopic examination of the urine sediment: Should we continue? Arch Pathol Lab Med 1984;108:399.

Nettleman MD et al: Cost-effectiveness of culturing for Chlamydia trachomatis: A study in a clinic for sexually transmitted diseases. Ann Intern Med 1986;105:189.

Pels RJ et al: Dipstick urinalysis screening of asymptomatic adults for urinary tract disorders. 2. Bacteriuria. JAMA 1989;262:1221.

Prodella M, Dorizzi RM, Rigalin F: Relative density of urine: Methods and clinical significance. CRC Crit Rev Lab Sci 1988;26:195.

Sanford JP et al: Evaluation of the "positive" urine culture: An approach to the differentiation of significant bacteria from contaminants. Am J Med 1956;20:88.

Sarosdy MF et al: Results of a multicenter trial using the BTA test to monitor for and diagnose recurrent bladder cancer. J Urol 1995;154:379.

Sarosdy MF et al: Improved detection of recurrent bladder cancer using the Bard BTA *stat* test. Urology 1997;50:349.

Schmetter BS et al: A multicenter trial evaluation of the fibrin/fibrinogen degradation products test for detection and monitoring of bladder cancer. J Urol 1997; 158:801.

Soloway MS et al: Use of a new tumor marker, urinary NMP22, in the detection of occult or rapidly recurring transitional cell carcinoma of the urinary tract following surgical treatment. J Urol 1996;156:363.

Stamey TA: Diagnosis, localization, and classification of urinary infections. In: *Pathogenesis and Treatment of Urinary Tract Infections.* Williams & Wilkins, 1980.

Stamey TA, Kindrachuk RW: *Urinary Sediment and Urinalysis: A Practical Guide for the Health Science Professional.* Saunders, 1985.

Stamm WE et al: Diagnosis of coliform infection in acutely dysuric women. N Engl J Med 1982;307:463.

Unni Mooppan MM et al: Use of urinary hydroxyproline excretion as a tumor marker in diagnosis and follow-up of prostatic carcinoma. The Prostate 1983;4:397.

van der Poel HG et al: QUANTICYT: Karyometric analysis of bladder washing for patients with superficial bladder cancer. Urology 1996;48:357.

Wright DN, Saxon B, Matsen JM: Use of the Bac-T-Screen to predict bacteriuria from urine specimens held at room temperature. J Clin Microbiol 1986;24: 214.

Wyatt RJ, McRoberts JW, Holland NH: Hematuria in childhood: Significance and management. J Urol 1977;117:366.

Wyker AW: Standard diagnostic considerations. In: Gillenwater JY et al (editors): *Adult and Pediatric Urology,* 2nd ed. Year Book Medical Publishers, 1991.

Radiology of the Urinary Tract

6

Hedvig Hricak, MD, PhD, & William Okuno, MD

The field of diagnostic radiology has undergone momentous changes in the last decade with the development of sophisticated digital cross-sectional techniques. Uroradiologic procedures have benefited from these advances, and imaging of the urinary tract has become more precise, with new procedures offering a great selection of options. For example, ultrasonography, computed tomography (CT), and magnetic resonance imaging (MRI) permit higher soft-tissue contrast resolution than conventional radiography and represent significant advances in almost all areas of the discipline. They also have produced new algorithms for how to proceed with diagnostic imaging studies. The optimal choice of procedure, however, depends greatly on the equipment and professional talent available. As a result, uroradiology is an exciting, continuously advancing branch of imaging, indispensable in the diagnosis and treatment of patients with urologic disorders.

RADIOGRAPHY

X-rays are electromagnetic waves with photon energies that typically fall between those of gamma rays and ultraviolet radiation in the electromagnetic spectrum. Radiography makes use of the fact that all substances and tissues differ in their ability to absorb x-rays. A radiopaque contrast medium is frequently employed to enhance soft-tissue contrast resolution and thus make radiographs more informative.

Although newer imaging techniques are replacing radiography for diagnosis of some urologic problems, radiography remains essential for many urologic disorders; therefore, the urologist should be familiar with current x-ray equipment and uroradiologic techniques. The basic types of uroradiologic studies are plain (conventional) abdominal films, intravenous urograms, cystourethrograms, urethrograms, and angiograms. These studies are described separately in sections that follow.

Basic Equipment & Techniques

A. Equipment:

1. Radiography fluoroscopy–The basic requirements for radiography and fluoroscopy are a high-voltage electric generator, an x-ray tube, a collimating device, an x-ray detector, and a display device.

Many x-ray units contain both radiographic and fluoroscopic capabilities. These units combined with an electronic image intensifier and a television system are essential in a modern diagnostic radiology department. Today, more radiology departments are becoming completely "filmless" as digital recording, displaying, and archiving of images are rapidly replacing film-based techniques.

2. Image intensification–Image intensifiers electronically augment the ordinary dim fluoroscopic image. Image intensifiers are coupled to television cameras so that the intensified pictures can be recorded and relayed to television monitors conveniently placed for viewing, either in the x-ray room or elsewhere in the department.

3. Image recording–In addition to conventional recording of an x-ray image using film and intensifying screens, the image intensifier can be used to capture dynamic and static images by optically coupling the intensifier to a camera. A 35-mm cine camera can be used to obtain real-time images but at a cost of greatly increased patient radiation exposure in comparison to conventional fluoroscopy. In an alternative and more widely used method, the video signal from the television camera can be recorded and played back for real-time imaging. Conventional spot films can be replaced by use of 105-mm cameras coupled to the intensifier. These cameras reduce patient radiation exposure by a factor of 5 or so in comparison to conventional radiographic spot films, and images can be acquired at a rate of 4 per s or faster.

B. Patient Preparation: It is no longer considered necessary for patients to be dehydrated in preparation for intravenous urography (IVU). Indeed, dehydration is to be avoided in infants, debilitated and elderly patients, and patients with diabetes mellitus, renal failure, multiple myeloma, or hyperuricemia.

It is controversial whether preliminary bowel cleansing is beneficial. There are many ways to obtain good bowel preparation, and the choice may be made according to individual preference.

C. Urographic Contrast Media: Radiographic contrast agents are water-soluble, iodinated compounds that are radiopaque. The extracellular distribution of these contrast agents depends on many factors. This differential distribution of the contrast media results in improved contrast resolution and conspicuity of various structures.

These contrast agents can be administered by several routes, including intravascularly, and can be used to study many organ systems. Significant advances in water-soluble contrast media have been achieved with the introduction of low-osmolality (nonionic) organic iodine-containing compounds. When compared with conventional, high-osmolality agents, these nonionic agents significantly decrease the incidence of minor, moderate, and severe side effects. It is unclear, however, whether they reduce the mortality associated with the use of contrast media. The major obstacle to the universal use of nonionic agents is their higher cost.

D. Adverse Reactions to Urographic Contrast Media: All procedures using intravascular contrast media carry a small but definite risk of adverse reactions. The overall incidence of adverse reactions is about 5%.

Most reactions are minor, eg, nausea, vomiting, hives, rash, or flushing, and usually require no treatment other than reassurance. Cardiopulmonary and anaphylactoid reactions can occur with little or no warning, however, and can be life-threatening or fatal. In a large meta-analysis, the incidence of death due to intravascular injection of contrast media was 0.9 deaths per 100,000 injections. There are no reliable methods for pretesting patients for possible adverse reactions; therefore, the risks and benefits of using intravascular urographic contrast media should be carefully evaluated for each patient before the procedure is initiated.

The nonionic contrast media have produced fewer adverse reactions than the higher-osmolality ionic intravascular contrast agents now in general use. Although more expensive than ionic agents, these new nonionic agents are being used increasingly, particularly in patients with previous serious reactions to conventional ionic contrast agents or in patients with a strong history of allergies. In some departments they are used exclusively.

Treatment of adverse reactions involves the use of antihistamines, epinephrine, vascular volume expanders, and cardiopulmonary drugs as well as ancillary procedures indicated by the nature and severity of the reaction.

In some cases, imaging techniques that do not require contrast media are inadequate, and examination using intravascular contrast media is absolutely critical even if the patient has a history of reaction to such media. Such patients are given nonionic contrast agents and pretreated with corticosteroids, H_1-blockers, and sometimes H_2-blockers in an effort to prevent recurrence of the untoward response. This preventive treatment is not always successful, and the decision about the urgency of performing the procedure becomes critical.

Advantages & Disadvantages

Radiography produces anatomic images of almost any body part. Costs of equipment and examinations are moderate compared with those of some cross-sectional imaging systems. Space requirements for ordinary radiographic equipment are not excessive, and sophisticated portable equipment is available for use in hospital wards, operating rooms, and intensive care units. Because there are a great many specialists trained in radiography, its use is not confined to large medical centers. The major disadvantages of radiographic imaging are the use of ionizing radiation and a relatively modest soft-tissue contrast resolution. The evaluation of the urinary tract almost always requires opacification by iodine contrast media.

1. PLAIN FILM OF THE ABDOMEN (Figures 6–1 through 6–3)

A plain film of the abdomen, frequently called a KUB (kidney-ureter-bladder) film, is the simplest uroradiologic study and the first performed in any radiographic examination of the abdomen or the urinary tract. It is generally the preliminary radiograph in more extended radiologic examinations of the urinary tract, such as intravenous urography or angiography. It is usually taken with the patient supine, but when indicated, it may be taken with the patient in other positions. It may demonstrate abnormalities of bones and the presence of calcifications or large soft-tissue masses.

Because kidney outlines usually can be seen on the plain film of the abdomen, the size, number, shape, and position of the kidneys can be determined. These characteristics constitute useful urologic information. For example, the finding on a plain film of symmetrically shrunken rather than enlarged kidneys in a patient with unexplained acute renal failure is a useful indicator, suggesting that the cause of the renal failure is medical rather than surgically remediable bilateral urinary tract obstruction.

The size of normal kidneys varies widely, not only between like individuals but also with age, sex, and body stature. The long diameter (the length) of the kidney is the most widely used and most convenient radiographic measurement. The average adult kidney

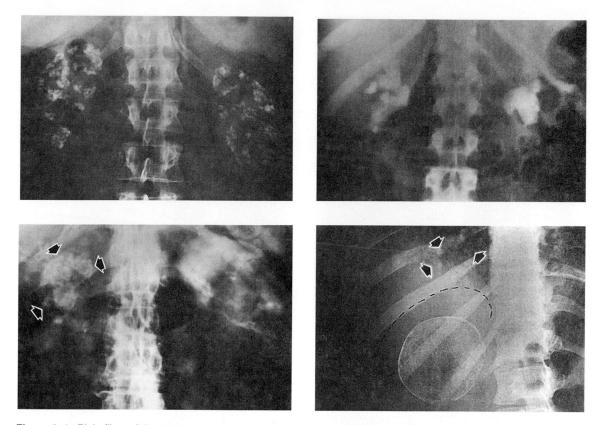

Figure 6–1. Plain films of the abdomen with abnormal radiopacities. **Upper left:** Bilateral nephrocalcinosis. Young adult male with renal tubular acidosis. **Upper right:** Bilateral staghorn calculi. 37-year-old woman with chronic pyelonephritis and history of previous right staghorn pyelolithotomy. **Lower left:** Renal tuberculosis. Shrunken, autonephrectomized and calcified right tuberculous kidney (arrows). 74-year-old man with history of renal and thoracolumbar spinal tuberculosis. **Lower right:** Papillary adenocarcinoma of right kidney. Remarkable tumor surface calcifications. Multiple pulmonary metastases (arrows) from the renal cancer. 22-year-old woman with painless soft tissue mass in the neck.

is about 12–14 cm long, and the left kidney is ordinarily slightly longer than the right one. In children older than 2 years of age, the length of a normal kidney is approximately equal to the distance from the top of the first to the bottom of the fourth lumbar vertebral body. In adults, the length of a normal kidney is approximately 3–4.5 times the height of the second lumbar vertebra.

The pattern of calcification in the urinary tract (Figures 6–1 and 6–2) is an important finding that may help to identify specific kidney diseases (eg, calcifications occasionally can be seen in kidney cancer, or the search for the primary disease elsewhere can be initiated when nephrocalcinosis is detected).

2. UROGRAPHY
(Figures 6–4 through 6–10)

The collecting structures of the kidneys, ureters, and bladder can be demonstrated radiologically with contrast media by the following methods.

Intravenous Urography

The IVU, also known as excretory urography (Eu) (Figure 6–4), and formerly called intravenous pyelography (IVP), is most commonly used. An IVU can demonstrate a wide variety of urinary tract lesions (Figures 6–5 and 6–6), is simple to perform, and is well tolerated by most patients.

Sonography, CT, and MRI are now used instead of urography in many cases. Nevertheless, urography remains the imaging study commonly used for demonstrating small lesions in the urinary tract (eg, papillary necrosis, medullary sponge kidney, uroepithelial tumors, pyeloureteritis cystica).

A. Standard Technique: Following a prelimi-

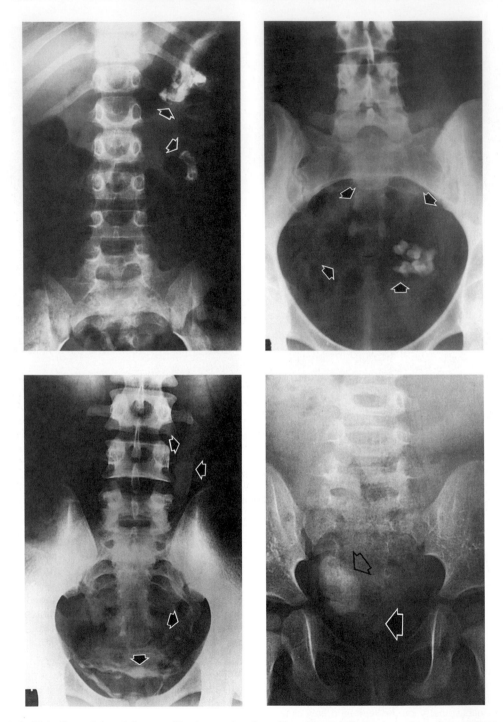

Figure 6–2. Plain films of the abdomen with abnormal radiopacities. **Upper left:** Benign retroperitoneal teratoma with bone formations. 9-year-old asthmatic girl with asymptomatic infradiaphragmatic calcifications (arrows) noted on routine chest film. **Upper right:** Benign ovarian cystic teratoma with teeth. Rounded cyst contains radiolucent fat (arrows) and a nest of well-formed teeth. 22-year-old woman with left pelvic mass. **Lower left:** Schistosomiasis calcification (arrows) in bladder and left ureter. 19-year-old male native of Aden with weight loss and hematuria. **Lower right:** Large vaginolith (open arrow) and small, barely visible bladder calculus (solid arrow). 4-year-old girl with common urogenital sinus.

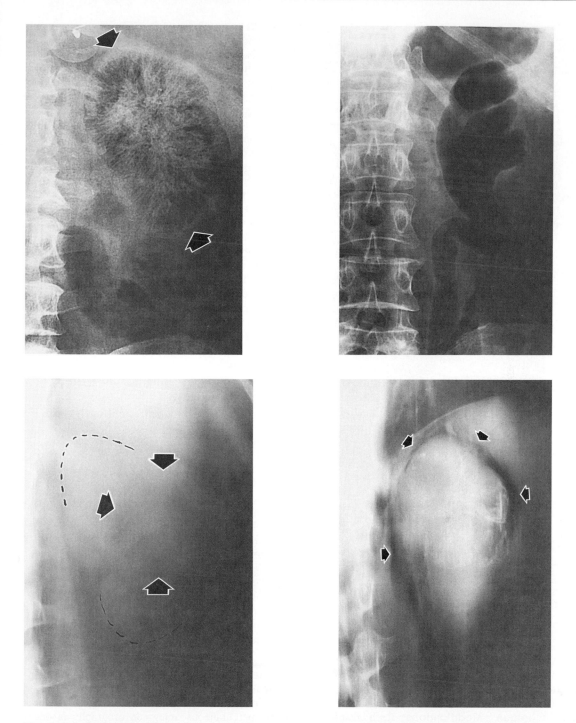

Figure 6–3. Plain films of the abdomen with abnormal radiolucencies. **Upper left:** Emphysematous pyelonephritis. Interstitial striated pattern of radiolucent gas throughout the entire left kidney. Similar changes were present in the right kidney. 58-year-old diabetic man with pyuria and septic shock. **Upper right:** Gas pyelogram. No interstitial gas, but gas fills dilated left kidney calices, pelvis, and ureter. 50-year-old diabetic woman with sepsis and left upper urinary tract infection due to gas-forming microorganisms. **Lower left:** Renal angiomyolipoma. Plain film tomogram shows left kidney mass containing radiolucent fat (arrows). 69-year-old woman with weight loss and left flank pain. **Lower right:** Calcified renal *Echinococcus* cysts. Retroperitoneal gas insufflation study, tomogram, adult male. Note how radiolucent gas (arrows) has dissected in the retroperitoneum about the minimally calcified cysts in the upper pole of the kidney.

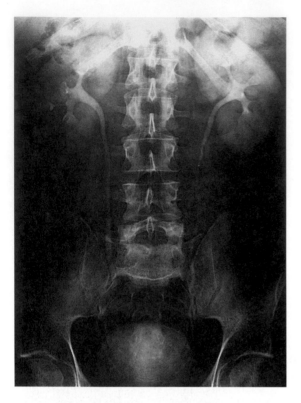

Figure 6–4. Normal excretory urogram. High-volume contrast medium study. The kidneys are normal in shape, size, and position; the calices and pelves are normal. The ureters are well shown because of the diuresis effect of the high volume of contrast medium. The bladder is normal. Healthy young adult male potential kidney donor.

nary plain film of the abdomen, radiographs of the abdomen are taken at timed intervals after the intravenous injection of a suitable iodine-containing contrast medium. Such substances are promptly excreted by normal kidneys, almost entirely by glomerular filtration.

The volume and speed of injection of the radiographic contrast medium (rapid bolus, slow infusion, etc), as well as the number and type of films taken following injection, vary depending on the institution at which the studies are performed and the patient's age, physical condition, and clinical problem.

B. Technique Modifications: Radiographic tomography, x-ray imaging of a selected plane in the body, permits recognition of kidney structures that otherwise are obscured on standard radiograms by extrarenal shadows, eg, those due to bone or feces (Figure 6–7). **Image-intensified fluoroscopy** and videotape recording permit real-time study of urinary tract dynamics. **"Immediate" films,** which are taken immediately after the rapid (bolus) injection of contrast medium, almost always show a dense nephro-

gram and permit better visualization of renal outlines. **Abdominal (ureteral) compression devices** that temporarily obstruct the upper urinary tract during excretory urography dramatically improve the filling of renal collecting structures. **"Delayed" films,** which are taken later on the same day or on the day after the contrast medium is administered, often contribute useful urologic information. **"Upright" films,** taken with the patient standing or partially erect, reveal the degree of mobility and drainage of the kidneys and, if taken immediately after the patient has voided (**"postvoiding" film**), show any residual urine in the bladder. In the past, a modified excretory urologic technique called **rapid-sequence (hypertensive) IVU** was used to evaluate suspected renovascular hypertension. In this method, a bolus injection of contrast medium was followed by rapid imaging in the first few minutes after the injection to look for signs of renal artery stenosis, eg, a small affected kidney with delayed contrast excretion and a progressively dense nephrogram. Today, more sensitive, noninvasive techniques such as **magnetic resonance angiography** (MRA), **CT angiography** (CTA), or **captopril-sensitized radionuclide renography** are used.

Retrograde Urograms

Retrograde urography is a moderately invasive procedure that requires cystoscopy and the placement of catheters in the ureters. A radiopaque contrast medium is introduced into the ureters or renal collecting structures through the ureteral catheters (Figures 6–8 through 6–10), and radiographs of the abdomen are taken. This study, which is more difficult to perform than an excretory urogram, must be performed by a urologist or experienced interventional uroradiologist. Some type of local or general anesthesia must be used, and the procedure occasionally causes later morbidity or urinary tract infection.

Retrograde urograms may be necessary if excretory urograms are unsatisfactory, if the patient has a history of adverse reaction to intravenous contrast media, or if other methods of imaging are unavailable or inappropriate.

Percutaneous Antegrade Urograms

Outlining the renal collecting structures and ureters by percutaneous antegrade urography is occasionally done when urinary tract imaging is necessary but excretory or retrograde urography has failed or is contraindicated, or when there is a nephrostomy tube in place and delineation of the collecting system of the upper urinary tract is desired. The contrast medium is introduced either through nephrostomy tubes, if these are present (nephrostogram), or by direct injection into the renal collecting structures via a percutaneous puncture through the patient's back.

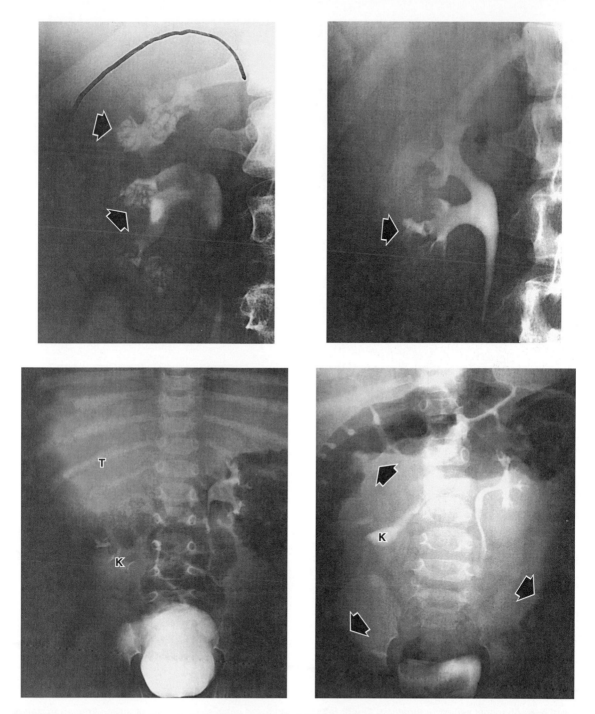

Figure 6–5. Abnormal excretory urograms. **Upper left:** Medullary sponge kidney. Pronounced medullary tubular ectasia (arrows) of entire right kidney. Similar findings in upper pole pyramids of left kidney. Small medullary calculi were present in some areas of tubular ectasia in both kidneys. 34-year-old woman with repeated bouts of chills, fever, and left flank pain. **Upper right:** Renal tuberculosis. Irregular cavitation of lower pole pyramid (arrow). 22-year-old woman with positive urine culture for tuberculosis. **Lower left:** Adrenal neuroblastoma. Diffuse small calcifications in a large right upper quadrant mass (T) depressing the right kidney (K). 12-year-old girl with proptosis of the right eye and an abdominal tumor. **Lower right:** Wilms tumor. Huge tumor of right kidney filling the entire abdomen (arrows), displacing bowel, and deforming collecting structures of the right kidney (K). Left kidney normal. 21-month-old girl with large abdominal mass.

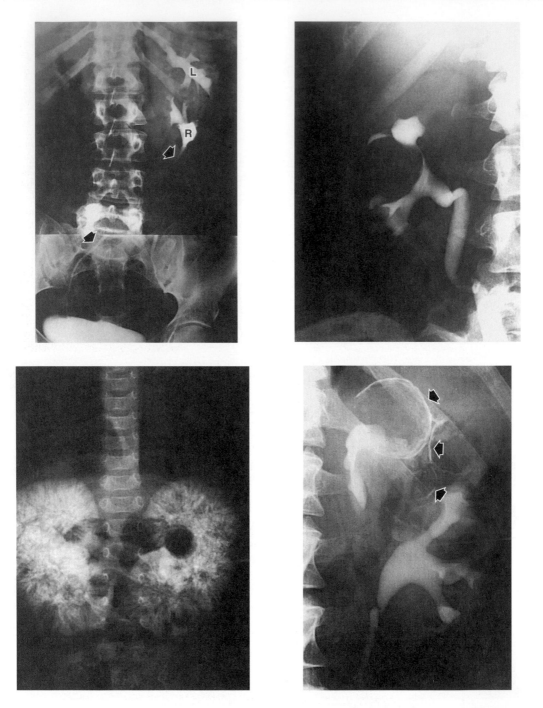

Figure 6–6. Abnormal excretory urograms. **Upper left:** Crossed fused ectopia. Composite of 2 films from an excretory urogram shows ectopic right kidney (R) fused to left kidney (L). Right ureter (arrows) crosses midline and enters normally into right side of bladder. Healthy 31-year-old female potential kidney donor. **Upper right:** Renal artery aneurysm. Right kidney collecting structures draped around a central mass. 41-year-old woman with hypertension and right abdominal bruit. **Lower right:** Infantile polycystic kidney disease. Very large kidneys with radiopaque spoke pattern radiating out to cortex. 26 h after administration of intravenous contrast medium. 4-month-old girl with bilateral abdominal masses. **Lower right:** Renal cell carcinoma. Unusual circular and curvilinear eggshell calcifications (arrows) in the tumor, which is compressing the infundibulum to deform upper pole calices. 39-year-old man with history of unroofing of left kidney cyst 3 years earlier.

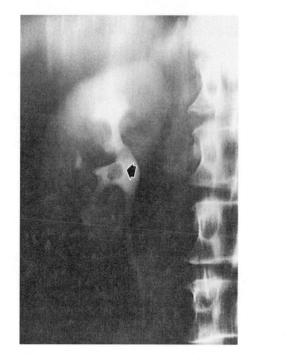
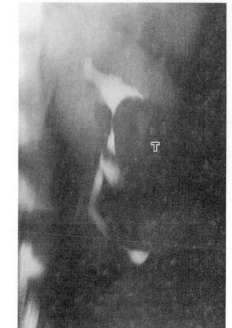
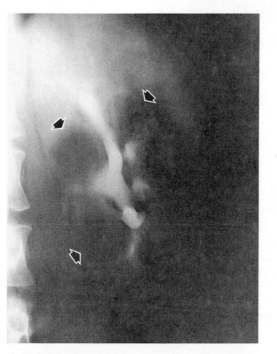

Figure 6–7. Radiographic tomography. Tomography is used to image a plane in the body. The technique is particularly useful in uroradiology, often permitting demonstration of lesions otherwise hidden by overlying soft tissues or obscuring bowel shadows. **Upper left:** Transitional cell carcinoma. The tumor in the pelvis (arrow) is clearly shown free of obscuring gas shadows present on the nontomographic films. 56-year-old man with history of renal calculi. **Upper right:** Renal cell carcinoma (T). Displacement of mid-kidney collecting structures and a nephrogram defect are seen free of obscuring splenic flexure fecal shadows that were present on the nontomographic films. 44-year-old woman with fever, weight loss, anemia, and history of contralateral nephrectomy for carcinoma 15 years earlier. **Bottom:** Adult polycystic kidney disease. The tomographic plane of the left kidney is outside the level of the bowel and shows to more advantage the numerous radiolucent cysts (arrows). Similar appearance in right kidney. 29-year-old man with family history of "cysts in the kidneys."

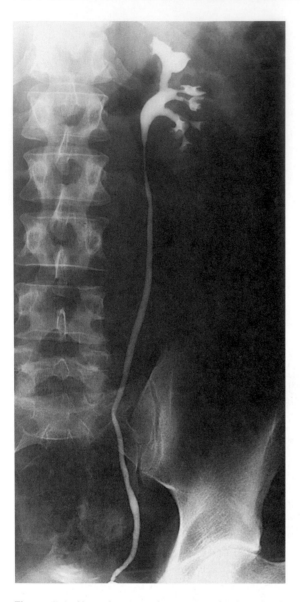

Figure 6–8. Normal retrograde urogram. Intrarenal collecting structures, pelvis, and ureter are normal. Adult male with microscopic hematuria and previous technically unsatisfactory excretory urogram.

Percutaneous Retrograde Urograms

Percutaneous retrograde urograms of the upper urinary tract are made by retrograde injection of contrast medium through the opening of a skin ureterostomy or pyelostomy (skin ureterogram, skin urogram) or through the ostium of an interposed conduit, usually a segment of small bowel (loopogram).

3. CYSTOGRAPHY & VOIDING CYSTOURETHROGRAPHY (Figures 6–11 through 6–14)

Although the urinary bladder can be visualized during excretory urography, direct instillation of contrast media into the urinary bladder (cystography) is required for a more thorough examination in patients with suspected bladder disease. The contrast medium is usually instilled via a transurethral catheter, but, when necessary, it can be administered via percutaneous suprapubic bladder puncture. Radiographs of the filled bladder can be taken using standard overhead x-ray tube equipment, or films can be taken during direct, image-intensified fluoroscopy. Voiding cystourethrograms are radiographs of the bladder and urethra obtained during micturition.

In addition to their use in imaging the bladder and urethra, cystography and cystourethrography are important radiologic techniques for detecting vesicoureteral reflux and are the bases of several radiographic methods used in the workup of patients with urinary stress incontinence. Recently, CT cystography (CT of the pelvis after the instillation of dilute contrast medium into the bladder) has been shown useful in the evaluation of bladder tumors and for the detection of bladder rupture.

4. URETHROGRAPHY (Figures 6–14 through 6–17)

The urethra can be imaged radiographically by retrograde injection of radiopaque fluid or in antegrade fashion with voiding cystourethrography. An antegrade urethrogram can also be obtained by taking radiographs as the patient voids at the termination of excretory urography, when the bladder is filled with contrast medium. The antegrade technique is required when lesions of the posterior urethra, eg, posterior urethral valves, are suspected; the retrograde technique is more useful for examining the anterior (penile) urethra.

5. VASOGRAPHY (Figure 6–18)

Vasoseminal vesiculography is most often used in the investigation of male sterility. The radiopaque contrast medium is introduced into the ductal system by direct injection into an ejaculatory duct following panendoscopy or, more commonly, by injection into the vas deferens after it has been surgically exposed through a small incision in the scrotal neck.

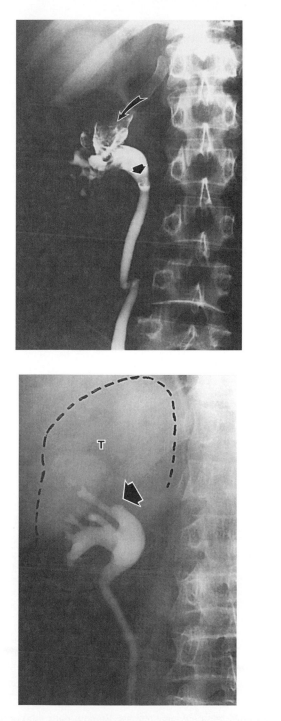

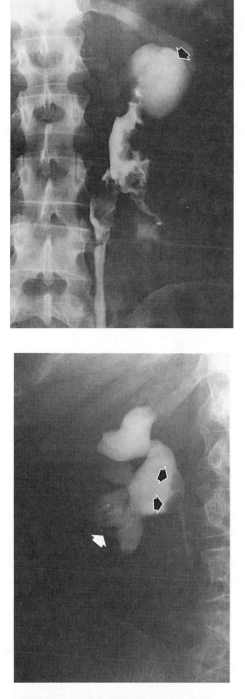

Figure 6–9. Abnormal retrograde urograms and nephrostograms; lower ureters not shown. **Upper left:** Transitional cell carcinoma. Severe deformity with filling defects in right upper pole calices (curved arrow) and blood clots in lower calices and at ureteropelvic junction (straight arrow). 65-year-old man with gross hematuria and right flank pain. **Upper right:** Squamous cell carcinoma. Marked irregular filling defects involving calices, pelvis, and proximal ureter, with communicating abscess cavity in upper pole (arrow). Kidney also showed squamous metaplasia and contained calculi. 51-year-old woman with 2-week history of left flank cellulitis and tenderness. **Lower left:** Renal cell carcinoma. Right upper pole mass (T) with amputation of superior calices and infundibulum (arrow). 76-year-old man with pulmonary metastases. **Lower right:** Fungus balls. Nephrostogram revealing 2 filling defects (arrows) in renal pelvis. Copious fungal matter aspirated through nephrostomy catheter. 65-year-old diabetic woman who had undergone left nephrectomy, with percutaneous nephrostomy catheter (white arrow) for obstruction of right kidney.

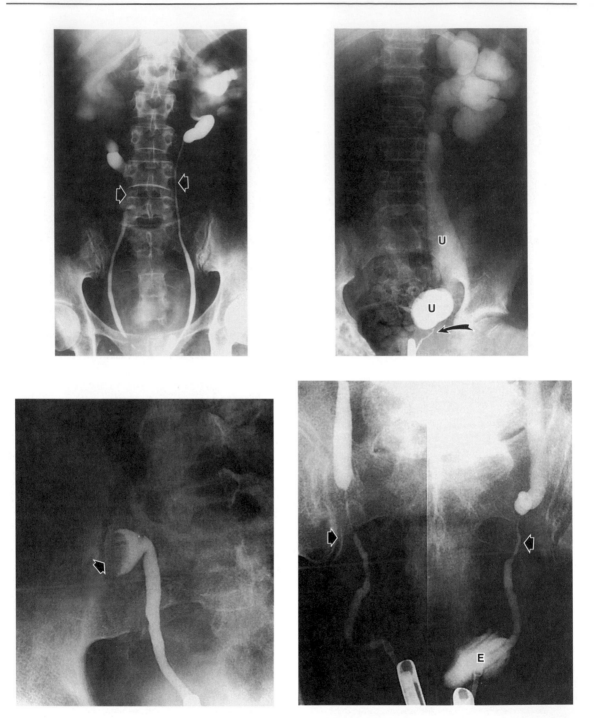

Figure 6–10. Abnormal retrograde urograms. **Upper left:** Idiopathic retroperitoneal fibrosis. Smooth narrowing of both mid ureters (arrows), with bilateral proximal ureterectasis and hydronephrosis. 51-year-old woman with no urinary tract symptoms. **Upper right:** Functional ureteral obstruction. Obstruction was due to congenitally abnormal muscle arrangements in the affected very distal ureter (curved arrow). Pronounced hydronephrosis and dilatation of ureter (U) proximal to the short segment of abnormal ureter. 13-year-old boy with repeated urinary tract infections. **Lower left:** Transitional cell carcinoma of the ureter. No contrast medium has passed beyond the large, bulky, right ureteral tumor (arrow). The ureteral widening below the tumor is distinctive and is sometimes referred to as the "champagne glass" sign (in this instance, the glass is tipped on its side). 76-year-old man with nonfunctioning right kidney. **Lower right:** Ureteral constrictions secondary to extension of carcinoma of the colon. Bilateral distal ureteral narrowings (arrows) with upper tract obstruction. Composite of separate retrograde urograms. E = unintended extravasation about tip of left ureteral catheter. 76-year-old man with cancer of the sigmoid colon.

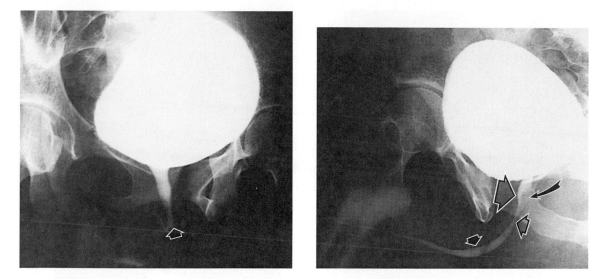

Figure 6–11. Normal voiding cystourethrograms. **Left:** Normal female bladder and urethra. Arrow indicates urethral meatus. 22-year-old woman with voiding symptoms. **Right:** Normal male penile urethra. Large open arrow = prostatic urethra; small open arrow = membranous urethra; closed arrow = penile urethra; curved arrow = verumontanum. 27-year-old man with vague right lower abdominal and testicular pain.

6. LYMPHANGIOGRAPHY (Figure 6–19)

Lymphangiography is performed by injecting an oily contrast medium through a cannula into a lymphatic vessel in the foot to produce radiopacification of the inguinal, pelvic, and retroperitoneal lymphatic system. This procedure has been largely replaced by CT and MRI. In some centers, however, lymphangiography is still performed to stage lymphomas, especially Hodgkin's disease, and testicular cancers when CT is equivocal or negative for lymphadenopathy.

7. ANGIOGRAPHY

Conventional angiography visualizes blood vessels by the use of radiopaque contrast media. Angiographic study of the urinary tract is almost exclusively used to visualize renal vessels. Although angiography is an established imaging technique with proven value and an acceptable incidence of complications and morbidity, it is moderately invasive and relatively expensive. Increasing use of ultrasonography, CT, and MRI has resulted in a marked decrease in the use of angiography for diagnosis of urologic problems.

Aortorenal & Selective Renal Arteriography (Figure 6–20)

Arteriographic studies of the kidneys are performed almost exclusively by percutaneous needle puncture and catheterization of the common femoral arteries or, much less often, the axillary arteries. Rapid serial radiograms are obtained during and after bolus injection of suitable radiopaque contrast medium into the aorta at the level of the renal arteries (aortorenal arteriogram, "flush" abdominal aortogram) or into one of the renal arteries (selective renal arteriogram). A reduced amount and concentration of contrast media can be injected when digital angiography is performed.

Renal angiography remains the gold standard for the diagnosis of renovascular hypertension. If renal artery stenosis is discovered at the time of angiography, treatment with endoluminal balloon angioplasty and, if necessary, stenting can be performed. Angiography of potential renal donors has largely been replaced by the less-invasive CTA and MRA.

Although cross-sectional imaging techniques are the primary modalities for the evaluation of renal masses, angiography still has a role in a minority of these cases. In patients with spontaneous renal hemorrhage, angiography may be useful in detecting an underlying hypervascular oncocytoma or renal cell carcinoma. Most of these patients, however, undergo follow-up cross-sectional imaging, mostly with CT and to a lesser extent MRI rather than angiography, to detect an underlying lesion. When nephron-sparing surgery is desirable in a patient with a renal mass, angiography provides a precise road map of the renal vessels to assist in surgical planning. In some patients with renal cell carcinoma, preoperative renal angiography and embolization are performed to decrease the amount of intraoperative blood loss.

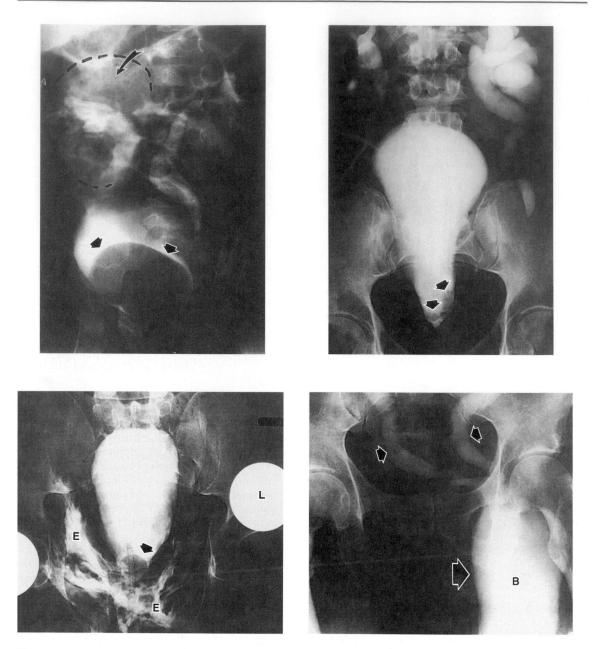

Figure 6–12. Abnormal cystograms: retrograde cystograms or "cystograms" as part of excretory urogram studies. **Upper left:** Ectopic ureterocele. Giant ureterocele (straight arrows) to hydronephrotic, nonfunctioning upper portion (curved arrow) of duplex right kidney. 9-month-old-girl with urinary tract infections. **Upper right:** Pelvic lipomatosis. Pear-shaped bladder and increased radiolucency of the pelvic soft tissues secondary to pelvic lipomatosis of severity sufficient to produce obstructive dilatation of the upper urinary tracts. Filling defects (arrows) at bladder base due to cystitis glandularis. 62-year-old man with intermittent left flank pain. **Lower left:** Rupture of the membranous urethra. Pear-shaped bladder secondary to extraperitoneal extravasation (E) and perivesical hematoma. Arrow = inflated balloon of Foley catheter. 41-year-old man with renal transplant, after a motor vehicle accident that resulted in pelvic bone fractures, separation of the sacroiliac joints, and dislocation of the left (L) but not the right hip prosthesis (patient has bilateral hip prostheses). **Lower right:** Bladder hernia. Bilateral obstructive ureterectasis (small arrows) secondary to remarkable herniation of the entire bladder (large arrow, B) into the inguinal region, 5'5", 225-pound, 53-year-old man with panniculus reaching to mid thigh, complaining of difficulty voiding.

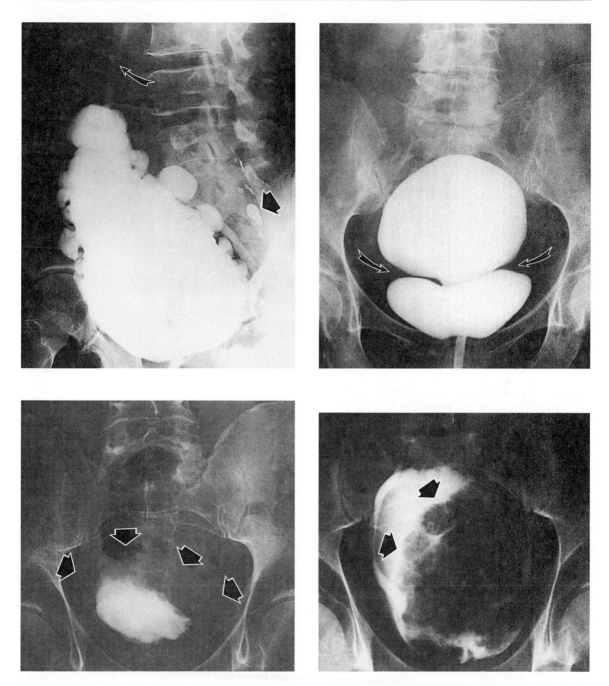

Figure 6–13. Abnormal cystograms: retrograde cystograms or "cystograms" as part of excretory urogram studies. **Upper left:** Neurogenic bladder. This neurogenic bladder has a "Christmas-tree" shape, with gross trabeculation and many diverticula. Residual myelographic contrast medium in spinal canal (straight arrow). Right vesicoureteral reflux (curved arrow). 70-year-old man with urinary incontinence. **Upper right:** Congenital "hourglass" bladder. Transverse concentric muscular band (arrows) separates upper and lower bladder segments, both of which contracted and emptied simultaneously and completely with voiding. 66-year-old woman with urinary stress incontinence. **Lower left:** Hodgkin's disease of bladder. Global thickening of the bladder wall (arrows), more apparent on the left. 54-year-old man with generalized Hodgkin's disease. **Lower right:** Papillary transitional cell bladder carcinoma. Huge (12 cm) cauliflowerlike bladder mass (arrows) filling almost the entire bladder. "Cystogram" film of an excretory urogram in a 40-year-old man with recurrent bladder tumor.

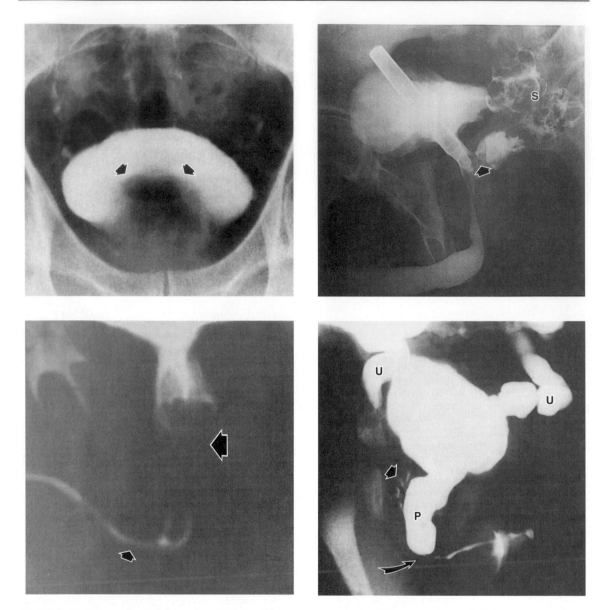

Figure 6–14. Abnormal prostate and posterior urethra: cystograms and urethrograms. **Upper left:** Benign prostatic hyperplasia. Gross enlargement of prostate gland producing marked elevation (arrows) of the bladder base. The bladder shows small diverticula and slight trabeculation. Excretory urogram (cystogram) in a 65-year-old man with history of obstructive voiding symptoms. **Upper right:** Foreign body (eyeliner pencil cover) lodged in bladder and prostatic urethra, with urethrorectal fistula. Radiopaque medium enters rectum and sigmoid colon (S) through fistula (arrow) from prostatic urethra. Retrograde urethrogram in a 43-year-old transsexual man. **Lower left:** Rhabdomyosarcoma of prostate. Lobulated filling defects (large arrow) encroaching on widened prostatic urethra. Voiding cystourethrogram in a 5-year-old boy with voiding difficulties. Small arrow = penile urethra. **Lower right:** Posterior urethral valves. Marked dilatation and elongation of prostatic urethra (P), with reflux into prostatic ducts (straight arrow) secondary to posterior urethral valves (curved arrow) with bilateral vesicoureteral reflux into dilated ureters (U). Voiding cystourethrogram in a 10-day-old boy.

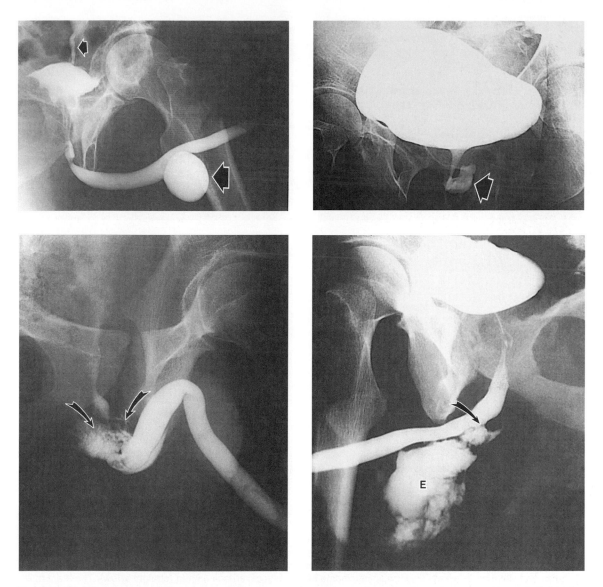

Figure 6–15. Abnormal anterior urethras: voiding cystourethrograms and retrograde urethrograms. **Upper left:** Voiding cystourethrogram in a 78-year-old man with a history of urethral diverticulum of unknown etiology. 4-cm anterior urethral diverticulum (large arrow) and left vesicoureteral reflux (small arrow). **Upper right:** Urethral diverticulum in a woman. Large irregular diverticulum (arrow). Voiding cystourethrogram in a 51-year-old woman with voiding difficulties and suspected urethral stricture. **Lower left:** Ruptured urethra. Extravasation of contrast medium around the bulbous urethra (arrows). Retrograde urethrogram in a 16-year-old boy in whom blunt perineal trauma was followed by bloody urethral discharge and inability to void. **Lower right:** Urethroscrotal fistula. Extravasation (E) into extraurethral tissues from fistula in bulbous urethra (arrow). Retrograde urethrogram in a 26-year-old man after end-to-end urethroplasty for stricture.

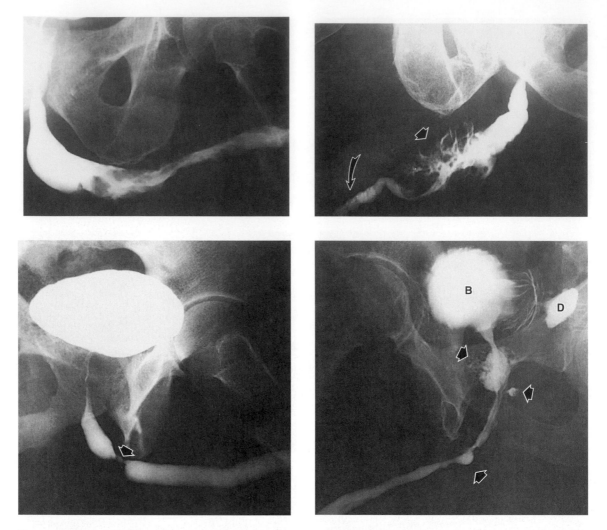

Figure 6–16. Abnormal anterior urethras: retrograde urethrograms. **Upper left:** Urethral carcinoma. Gross irregularities with filling defects involving most of penile urethra. Poorly differentiated carcinoma of anterior urethra in a 59-year-old man with obstructive voiding symptoms and inguinal adenopathy. **Upper right:** Urethral carcinoma. Filling of irregular sinus tracts and channels in a large epidermoid carcinoma of the bulbocavernous urethra (straight arrow). There are multiple thin transverse strictures of the penile urethra (curved arrow). 75-year-old man with obstructive voiding symptoms and 30-year history of urethral strictures requiring dilatations. **Lower left:** Focal urethral stricture (arrow). Middle-aged man with obstructive voiding symptoms who denied any previous urethritis. **Lower right:** Urethral strictures. Multiple strictures in the bulbocavernous urethra (lower arrow) with reflux into Cowper's gland (middle arrow) and prostatic ducts (upper arrow). B = bladder; D = bladder diverticulum. 62-year-old man with 25-year history of urethral strictures requiring frequent dilatations.

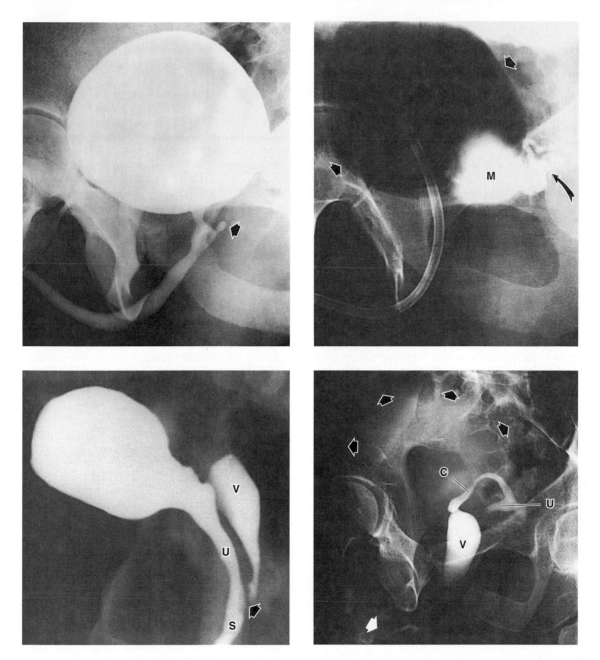

Figure 6–17. Congenital genitourinary anomalies: voiding cystograms and retrograde urethrograms. **Upper left:** Utricle. Midline outpouching (arrow) from verumontanum between orifices of ejaculatory ducts, representing müllerian duct cyst. **Upper right:** Gas cystogram combined with injection of utricle, oblique view. M = grossly dilated utricle (müllerian duct cyst); straight arrows = bladder distended with air; curved arrow = coincident partial filling of left seminal vesicle and vas deferens. 34-year-old man with urgency, frequency, and suspected retrograde ejaculation. **Lower left:** Common urogenital sinus. Vagina (V) and urethra (U) join (at arrow) into a common urogenital sinus (S). Voiding cystourethrogram in a 3-week-old female pseudohermaphrodite with ambiguous genitalia and congenital adrenal hyperplasia. **Lower right:** Male pseudohermaphrodite. Bladder is distended with urine (black arrows). Retrograde urethrogram via hypospadiac meatus has fortuitously and selectively filled with contrast medium an extensive müllerian duct remnant consisting of vagina (V), cervix and cervical canal (C), and retroverted uterus (U). Residual contrast medium in hypoplastic anterior urethra (white arrow). 27-year-old man with small external genitalia, hypospadias, and perineal pain.

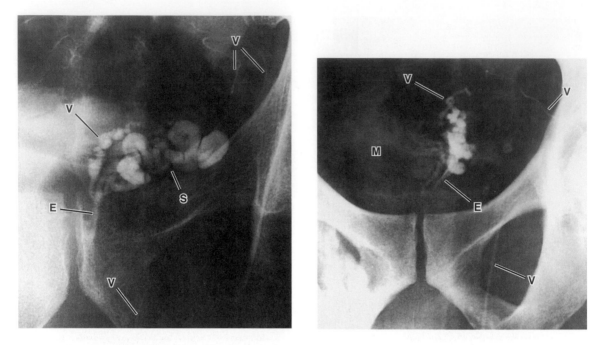

Figure 6–18. Vasoseminal vesiculography (vasography). **Left:** Normal left vasoseminal vesiculogram. V = vas deferens; S = seminal vesicle; E = ejaculatory duct. 40-year-old man with hypospermia. **Right:** Seminal vesiculitis. Bilateral vasogram. Mass (M) produced by the swollen, nonfilling right seminal vesicle has displaced both ejaculatory ducts (E) toward the left and indented the medial aspect of the proximal left seminal vesicle and vas deferens (V). 33-year-old man with painful ejaculations after repair of right varicocele.

Inferior Venacavography & Selective Renal Venography (Figures 6–21 and 6–22)

The common femoral veins are the usual site for catheterization and injection of contrast medium to visualize the inferior vena cava and renal veins.

Inferior venacavography (Figure 6–21) is useful to demonstrate extension of thrombus or tumor from renal veins into the vena cava. Renal vein tumors or thrombi that do not extend into the vena cava are not evident on inferior venacavograms but can be visualized by selective renal venography (Figure 6–22).

Sonography, CT scanning, and MRI are being used increasingly for visualization of abnormalities in the inferior vena cava and main renal veins, and inferior venacavography is much less commonly used today than just a few years ago. In fact, MRI and venography are equally sensitive in detecting venous tumors or thrombi, and MRI has effectively replaced venography for staging of renal cell carcinoma.

Miscellaneous Urologic Angiography (Figure 6–23)

Although angiography has little or no value in examination of the ureter, bladder, adrenals, and prostate, angiograms of these structures may be indicated in particular clinical situations, in which case the studies are usually "tailored" to the clinical problem. In this era of multiple cross-sectional methods, these procedures are rarely used.

Corpus cavernosograms are made by direct injection of suitable contrast material into the corpora cavernosa of the penis. They can be useful in examining for Peyronie's disease, impotence, priapism, and traumatic penile lesions, but these also are not commonly performed.

SONOGRAPHY (Figures 6–24 through 6–29)

Basic Principles

Sound is the propagation of a cyclic vibratory motion through a deformable medium. A wave frequency of one cycle/second (cps) is called a hertz (Hz). Sound frequencies greater than 20 kHz are beyond the range of human hearing and are called **ultrasound.** Medical sonography uses ultrasound to produce body images. The frequencies commonly used in medical sonography are between 3.5 and 10 MHz.

Ultrasound waves for imaging are generated by transducers, devices that convert electrical energy to

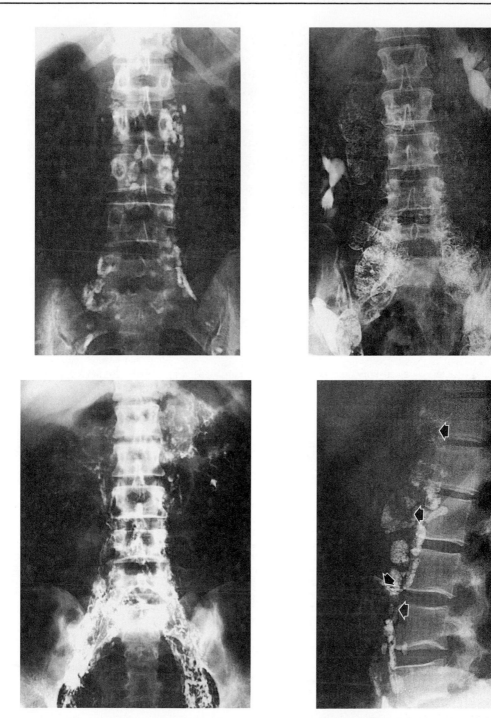

Figure 6–19. Lymphangiography. **Upper left:** Normal abdominal lymphangiogram. Lymph nodes appear normal. 15-year-old girl with fevers of unknown etiology. **Upper right:** Hodgkin's disease. Kidneys and ureters displaced by grossly involved abdominal and pelvic lymph nodes. 52-year-old woman with stage IV Hodgkin's disease. **Lower left:** Filariasis. Remarkable pattern of dilated, tortuous pelvic, abdominal, and renal lymphatics representing development of an extensive network of collateral channels secondary to obstruction of normal pathways. 42-year-old native of Okinawa with 12-year history of chyluria. **Lower right:** Metastatic testicular choriocarcinoma. Enlarged thoracolumbar lymph nodes partially replaced by metastatic tumor (arrows). 26-year-old man with enlarged left supraclavicular node after orchiectomy for choriocarcinoma.

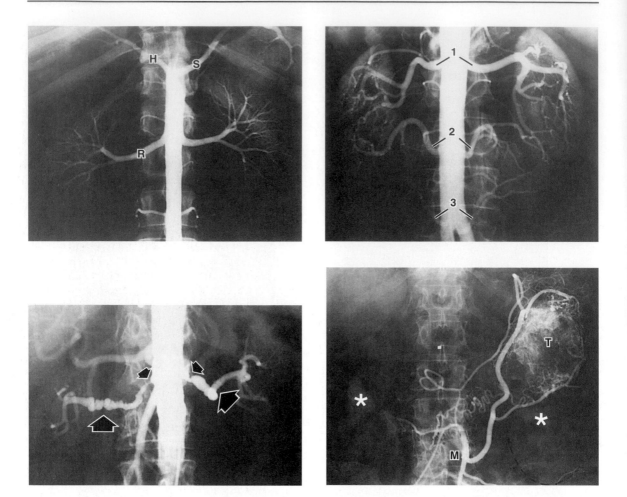

Figure 6–20. Angiography: aortorenal arteriography. **Upper left:** Normal abdominal aortogram. The aortic catheter is hidden by the opacified normal aorta. Right (R) and left renal arteries and branches are well shown, as are the splenic (S) and hepatic (H) arteries arising from the celiac axis. The superior mesenteric artery is superimposed over the aortic silhouette and is not visible on this study. 28-year-old healthy female potential kidney donor. **Upper right:** Multiple renal arteries. Horseshoe kidney with 3 renal arteries on each side, the 2 lowermost (3) supplying the renal isthmus. 42-year-old man with recurrent calculous disease, after left pyelolithotomy. **Lower left:** Bilateral renal artery stenoses. Typical angiographic appearance and location of stenoses caused by atherosclerosis (small arrows) and fibromuscular dysplasia (large arrows). 58-year-old woman with abdominal bruits and a 16-year history of hypertension. **Lower right:** Vascular parasitism by kidney cancer. Selective inferior mesenteric arteriogram (M) demonstrating large blood supply to a hypervascular adenocarcinoma (T) of the upper pole. Asterisk = renal pelvis. 69-year-old woman with polycythemia.

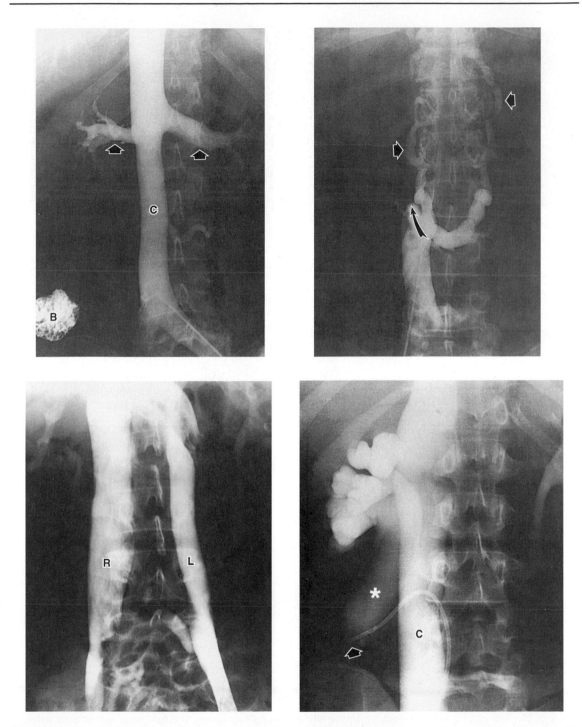

Figure 6–21. Angiography: inferior venacavography. **Upper left:** Normal inferior vena cava (C). Unusual retrograde filling of morphologically normal renal veins (arrows) from antegrade injection into the inferior vena cava is probably due to reduced venous outflow from the kidneys with the patient in Valsalva maneuver. B = retained contrast material in the cecum from previous barium enema examination. Woman with arteriolar nephrosclerosis and renal failure. **Upper right:** Inferior vena cava obstruction. Complete block of the vena cava (curved arrow) by extension from right renal vein of tumor thrombus from a right renal carcinoma. Note cephalad blood return via the paralumbar veins (straight arrows). 60-year-old man with gross hematuria. **Lower left:** Double inferior vena cava (R, L). Persistent left supracardinal vein anomaly. 23-year-old man after orchiectomy for testicular teratocarcinoma. **Lower right:** Retrocaval ureter. Hydronephrosis and proximal ureterectasis secondary to congenitally abnormal course of the right ureter behind the inferior vena cava (C). Catheter is in the right ureter, with its tip (arrow) at the lower curve of the redundant, dilated proximal ureter (asterisk). 17-year-old girl with history of pyelonephritis.

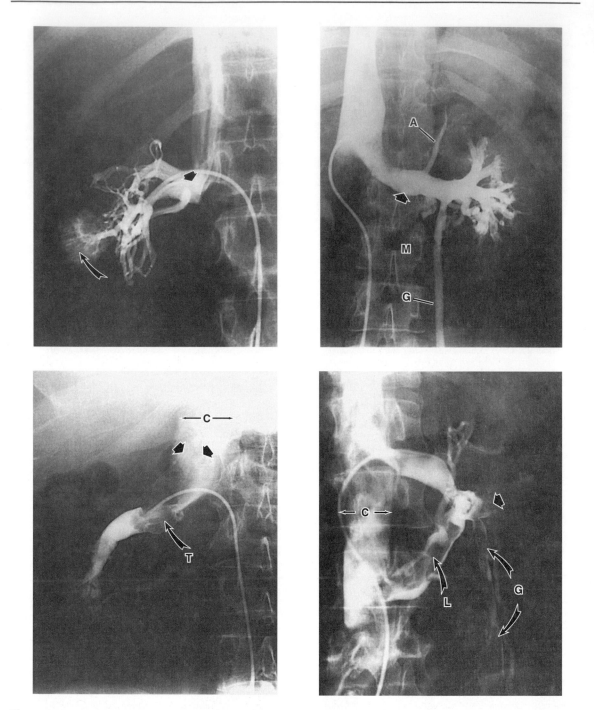

Figure 6–22. Angiography: renal venography. **Upper left:** Normal right renal vein. The right renal vein (straight arrow) is short and, unlike the left renal vein, does not receive the adrenal or gonadal vein; these veins empty directly into the inferior vena cava. Curved arrow = segmental intravasation of contrast medium from inadvertent wedging of the catheter tip in a small vein during injection. 19-year-old man with glomerulonephritis and nephrotic syndrome. **Upper right:** Normal left renal vein. On the left side, the adrenal (A) and gonadal (G) veins enter the renal vein (arrow). M = radiographic localization marker. Young woman with proteinuria. **Lower left:** Tumor thrombus. Straight arrows = upper margin of filling defect of the renal vein tumor thrombus (T) that extends into the vena cava (C). 68-year-old man with gross hematuria from adenocarcinoma of the right kidney. **Lower right:** Circumaortic left renal vein thrombosis. The catheter is in the patent upper limb of the venous anomaly. There is thrombosis of the intrarenal vein (straight arrow), with extension of thrombus into the lower limb (L) of the circumaortic renal vein and into the gonadal vein (G). C = inferior vena cava. 54-year-old man with nephrotic syndrome and edema of the legs and scrotum.

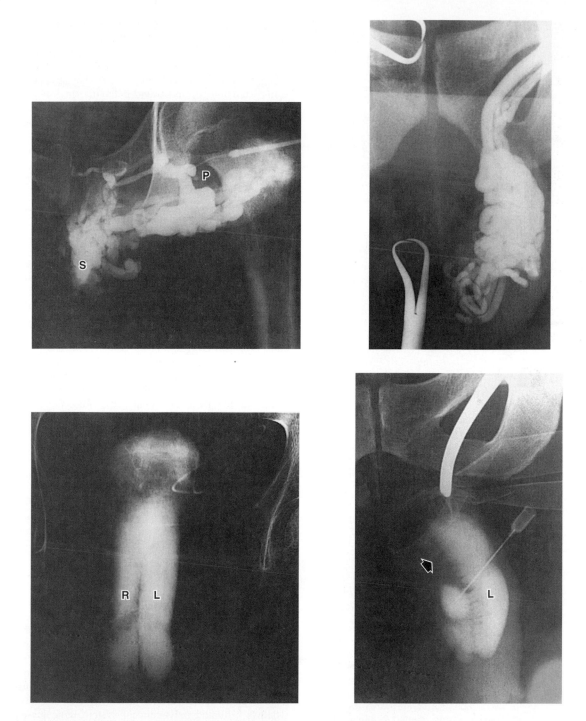

Figure 6–23. Angiography: miscellaneous urovenography. **Upper left:** Penoscrotal varices. Penile venography. Many tortuous veins in the penis (P) and scrotum (S). 14-year-old boy with long-standing penile and scrotal varicosities and numerous scrotal phleboliths. **Upper right:** Varicocele. Gonadal venography. Dilated, tortuous varicosities of the pampiniform plexus in the left scrotum. 31-year-old man with recurrence of scrotal pain after varicocele ligation. **Lower left:** Normal corpora cavernosogram. Injection of contrast medium into the left corpus (L), with normal (albeit slightly less) filling of the right corpus (R). 57-year-old man with impotence. **Lower right:** Penile fibrosis. Corpora cavernosogram. Injection of right corpus produces no filling of the proximal right corpus (arrow); there is normal filling of the left corpus (L). 33-year-old man with "crooked penis" following unsuccessful penile prosthesis operation.

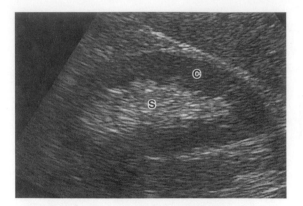

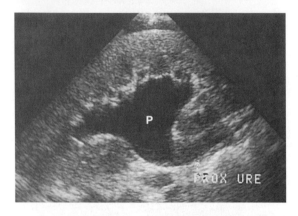

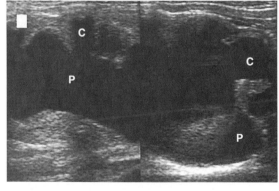

Figure 6–24. Sonography of the kidney. **Upper:** Normal kidney. Renal cortex (C), normal renal sinus echoes (S). **Middle:** Moderate hydronephrosis and hydroureter; dilated renal pelvis (P). Dilated proximal ureter (prox ure). **Lower:** Severe hydronephrosis of the transplanted kidney, compound sagittal scans, dilated clubbed calices (C), dilated renal pelvis (P).

sound energy and vice versa. These transducers are special piezoelectric crystals that emit ultrasound waves when they are deformed by an electrical voltage and, conversely, generate an electrical potential when struck by reflected sound waves. Thus, they act as both sound transmitters and sound detectors. In imaging, repeated bursts of ultrasound from the transducer are transmitted through tissues. Between transmissions, the transducer acts as a sound receiver.

In general concept, medical sonography resembles naval submarine sonar. Unlike radiographs, ultrasound images are reflection images formed when part of the sound that was emitted by the transducer bounces back from tissue interfaces to the transducer. These reflected sounds vary in intensity and time according to the nature and location of the tissues from which they are reflected.

The sound reflected by stationary tissues forms the data set for anatomic gray-scale images. The sound reflected by moving structures (eg, flowing blood in a vessel) has an altered frequency due to the Doppler effect. By determining the Doppler shift, vascular flow direction and velocity can be encoded graphically (spectral Doppler) or by color (color Doppler). A more sensitive method of detecting flow, called power mode Doppler, has recently been developed. To show flow, this technique displays the integrated power of the Doppler signal rather than the mean Doppler frequency shift. Unlike conventional color flow Doppler, the direction or velocity of flow is not displayed in the power mode.

The reflected sound energies received by the transducer are converted into electrical signals that are amplified, digitized, and stored in a computer. The information is converted by the computer into analog images and viewed directly on a cathode ray tube screen in real time; permanently recorded on hard copy, film, or videotape; or both.

Clinical Applications

The widespread use of ultrasonography has had a profound impact on urologic imaging. Ultrasound is now commonly used for the evaluation of the kidney, urinary bladder, prostate, testis, and penis.

In the evaluation of the kidney, ultrasound is useful for assessing renal growth in patients with vesicoureteral reflux. It is also helpful in triaging patients with renal failure. For example, small echogenic kidneys suggest renal parenchymal (medical) disease, whereas a dilated pelvocaliceal system indicates an obstructive, and potentially reversible, cause of renal failure.

Renal ultrasound, alone or in combination with other cross-sectional techniques, is indispensable for the detection and characterization of renal masses. Ultrasound is an effective method to distinguish benign cortical cysts from potentially malignant solid renal lesions. Since the most common renal mass detected on IVU is a simple cortical cyst, ultrasound is

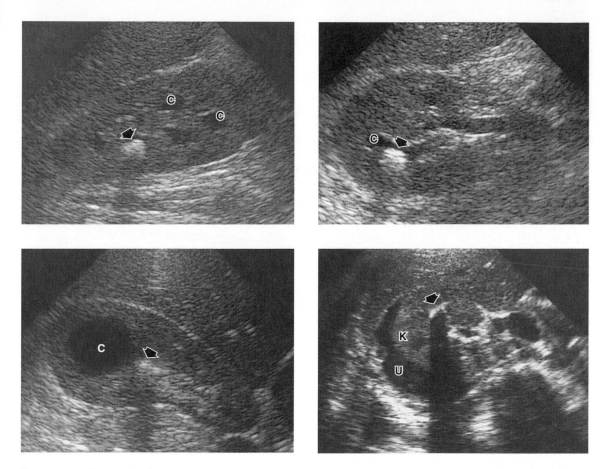

Figure 6–25. Renal calculi and the consequence of obstruction as detected by sonography. Longitudinal (**upper left**) and transverse (**upper right**) scans of the right kidney showing calicectasis (C) and renal calculus (arrow). **Lower left:** Renal calculus (arrow) at the infundibulum causing dilatation of the upper pole calyx (C). **Lower right:** Acute obstruction of the right kidney (K) with spontaneous urine (U) extravasation into the perirenal space. Renal calculus (arrow).

a cost-effective method to confirm this diagnosis, but when there is a suggestion of a solid mass on IVU, directly proceeding to CT is recommended. Ultrasound may also be used to follow up mildly complicated cysts detected on CT, eg, hyperdense cysts or cysts with thin septations.

The differential diagnosis for echogenic renal masses includes stones, angiomyolipomas, renal cell carcinomas, and, less commonly, abscesses and hematomas. All echogenic renal masses should be correlated with clinical history and, if necessary, confirmed with another imaging modality or follow-up ultrasound. Thin-section CT showing fat within the renal lesion characterizes it as a benign angiomyolipoma, and no further investigation is required. Echogenic lesions smaller than 1 cm are more difficult to characterize by CT owing to partial volume averaging; in the correct clinical setting, follow-up ultrasound rather than immediate CT may be more useful.

Doppler sonography is essential for the evaluation of complications following renal transplant. It can detect renal vein thrombosis, renal artery stenosis, ureteral obstruction prior to the development of hydronephrosis, arteriovenous fistulas, and pseudoaneurysms. Perinephric fluid collections following renal transplantation or extracorporeal shockwave lithotripsy are reliably detected by ultrasound.

Developments in other imaging modalities have decreased the use of ultrasound in several clinical scenarios. Most patients with suspected renovascular hypertension are evaluated with CTA, MRA, or radionuclide renography rather than Doppler ultrasonography. Unenhanced helical CT is now the initial procedure of choice for the evaluation of the patient with acute flank pain and suspected urolithiasis. In addition to rapidly and sensitively detecting renal stones without the need for intravenous contrast medium, helical CT also has the potential for identifying other causes of flank pain such as appendicitis

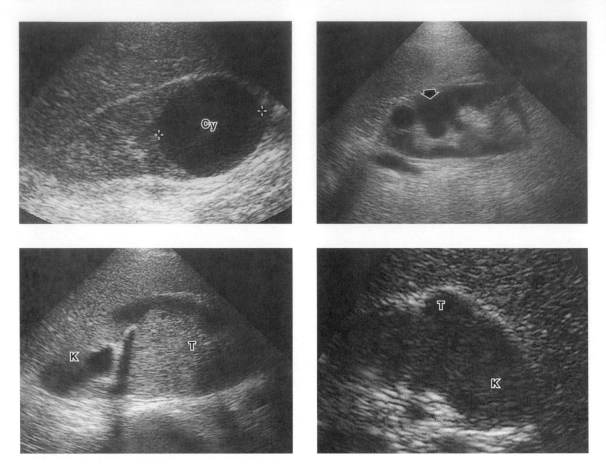

Figure 6–26. Sonography of renal neoplasms. **Upper left:** Simple renal cyst (Cy) demonstrating sharp interface toward the renal parenchyma, no internal echoes, and increase through transmission. **Upper right:** Complex renal cyst (arrow) with lobulated margins and thick wall. **Lower left:** Solid renal tumor (T) demonstrating homogeneous higher echogenicity than the adjacent renal parenchyma (K). **Lower right:** Small renal tumor (T) in the right kidney (K) the echogenicity of which is similar to that of the remaining renal parenchyma. The diagnosis is established by localized bulge in the outline.

and diverticulitis. In the past, some advocated KUB and ultrasound for the evaluation of hematuria, but recent studies indicate that IVU, CT, or both are the preferred modalities to evaluate this common clinical problem.

Applications of bladder sonography include assessment of bladder volume and bladder wall thickness and detection of bladder calculi and tumors. The suprapubic, transabdominal approach is most commonly used. The transurethral approach during cystoscopy has been recommended for tumor detection and staging.

Ultrasound examination of the testis has become an extension of the physical examination. The superficial location of the testis allows the use of a high-frequency transducer (5–10 MHz), which produces excellent spatial resolution. The addition of color Doppler sonography provides simultaneous real-time display of morphology and the temporospatial characteristics of blood flow. Normal intratesticular arterial blood flow is consistently detected with power or color Doppler. Sonography is highly accurate in differentiating intratesticular from extratesticular disease and in the detection of intratesticular pathology. Doppler ultrasound is commonly used to evaluate acute conditions of the scrotum. It can distinguish between inflammatory processes, inguinal hernias, and acute testicular torsion. In addition, epididymitis not responding to antibiotics within 2 weeks should be investigated further with scrotal ultrasonography.

Advantages & Disadvantages

The main advantages of ultrasound are that it is easy to perform, causes little or no patient discomfort, is noninvasive, does not use ionizing radiation, is relatively inexpensive, and is widely available.

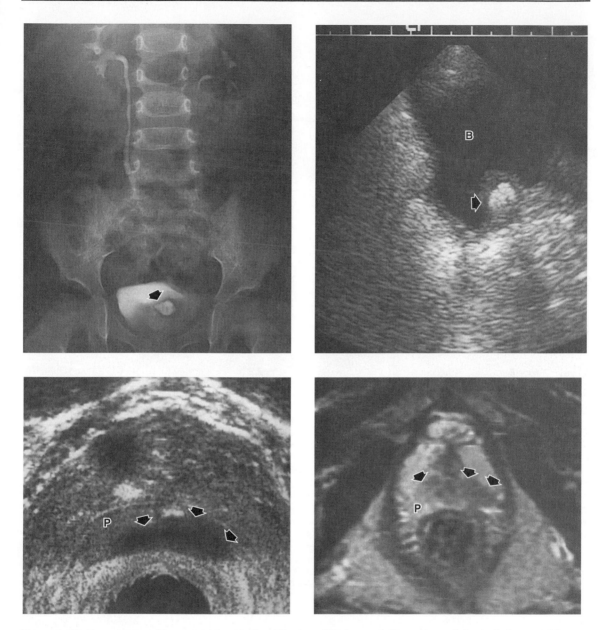

Figure 6–27. Sonography with comparative studies. Film from IVP (**upper left**) and transabdominal ultrasound (**upper right**) of the urinary bladder in a patient with duplication of the left kidney, ectopic ureterocele, and a calculus (arrow) within it. Urinary bladder (B). Transrectal ultrasound (**lower left**) and T2-weighted MR image (**lower right**) in a patient with prostate carcinoma (small arrows). On ultrasound, the tumor is hypoechoic as compared with the adjacent peripheral zone (P), and on MRI the tumor is of lower signal intensity than the adjacent peripheral zone (P). Tumor volume appears larger on MRI than it does on ultrasound.

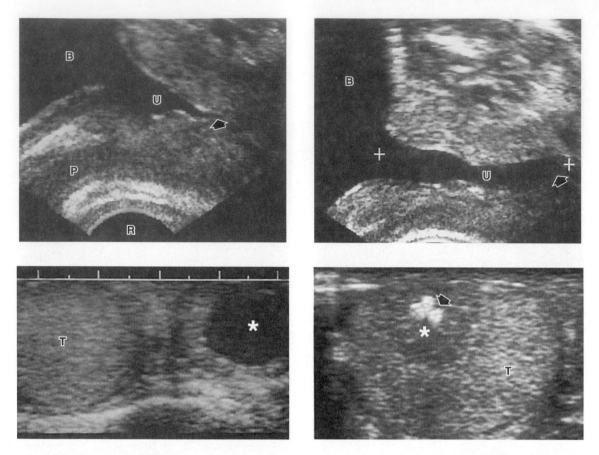

Figure 6–28. The use of transrectal ultrasound in the evaluation of the prostatic urethra. **Upper left:** Sonographic appearance of the prostatic urethra (U) following transurethral resection as seen on transrectal ultrasound in the sagittal plane of scanning. Urinary bladder (B). The urethra (U) is dilated to the level of the verumontanum (arrow). Peripheral zone (P), rectum (R). **Upper right:** The prostatic urethra (U) is dilated to the level to the membranous urethra (arrow). Urinary bladder (B). The cursors are placed to measure the length of the prostatic urethra. **Lower left and lower right:** Examples of testicular cancer. **Lower left:** The right testis (T) is normal. There is a hypoechoic lesion within the left testis (asterisk). At surgery, it was a seminoma. **Lower right:** The lesion (asterisk) within the right testis is hypoechoic with a hyperechogenic focus (arrow). Embryonal carcinoma was present at surgery. Surrounding normal testicular tissue (T).

Disadvantages include a relatively low signal-to-noise level, tissue nonspecificity, lack of contrast media, a small field of view, and dependence on the operator's skill and the patient's physique.

COMPUTED TOMOGRAPHY SCANNING (Figures 6–30 through 6–36)

Basic Principles

In conventional radiography, a broad beam of x-rays passes through the patient to produce an image on a detector, the x-ray film. In CT scanning, a thin, collimated beam of x-rays is passed through the patient and absorbed by a linear array of solid-state or gas detectors. CT scans give remarkable definition of body anatomy.

When scanning, the interconnected x-ray source and detector system are rapidly rotated in the gantry around the recumbent patient, the detectors recording a number of transmitted x-rays during the scan period. Digital computers assemble and integrate the collected x-ray transmission data to reconstruct a cross-sectional image (tomogram) that is displayed directly on a television screen. The image can be photographed, stored in digital form for later retrieval, or both.

Spiral CT uses a slip-ring gantry, which can rotate continuously using sliding contacts or brushes. The patient lies on a table moving at a constant speed

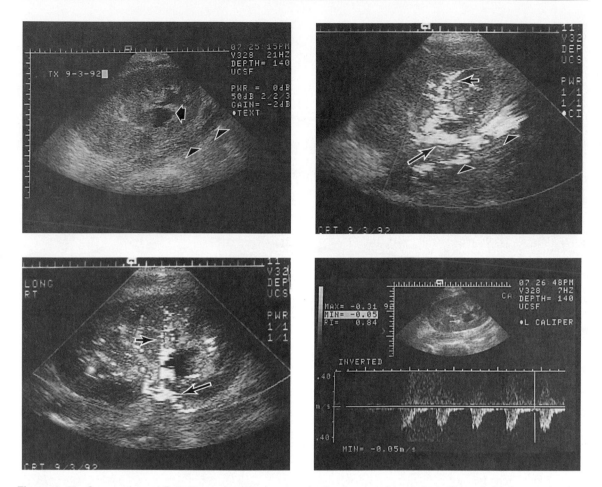

Figure 6–29. Gray-scale and Doppler sonography: acute rejection in a renal transplant. **Upper left:** Gray-scale ultrasound image of transplant kidney shows loss of corticomedullary differentiation. A small fluid collection is seen within the renal pelvis (arrow). Native external iliac vessels are seen as tubular hypoechoic structures (arrowheads). **Upper right and lower left:** Color Doppler images demonstrate flow within the native external iliac artery (arrowheads), the transplant renal artery (long arrow), and the interlobar arteries (short arrow). **Lower right:** Spectral Doppler analysis reveals an elevated resistive index of 0.84. These findings are compatible with but not specific for acute rejection.

through the continuously rotating gantry. This allows for volume acquisition of an image data set obtained in a helical spatial distribution. A helical exposure covering 30 cm of tissue can be obtained during a single 30-s breath-hold. Similar coverage using conventional CT scanners would require 2.5–4 min. In addition to increased scanning speed, spiral CT technology affords the ability to image during peak contrast levels, improved image reconstruction, and the ability to perform CT angiography.

Clinical Applications

CT examination can be applied to any kidney problem, but it is most commonly used in the evaluation of acute flank pain, hematuria, renal infection (search for abscess) and renal trauma, and in the characterization and staging of renal neoplasm. CT

evaluation of renal anatomy and pathology generally requires intravenous injection of iodinated contrast media. Noncontrast scans are needed, however, when renal or perirenal calcification, hemorrhage, or urine extravasation are suspected, since scans obtained after the administration of contrast media may mask these abnormalities. Thus, performance of both noncontrast and contrast-enhanced scans allows more complete evaluation of the urinary tract.

Contrast media may be administered either as a rapid intravenous bolus or by infusion techniques. The bolus technique is preferred for assessment of renal anatomy or measurement of aortorenal transit time. Infusion methods may facilitate evaluation of inferior vena cava patency. Using a bolus injection and rapid sequence scanning, renal arterial opacification is followed immediately by enhancement of the

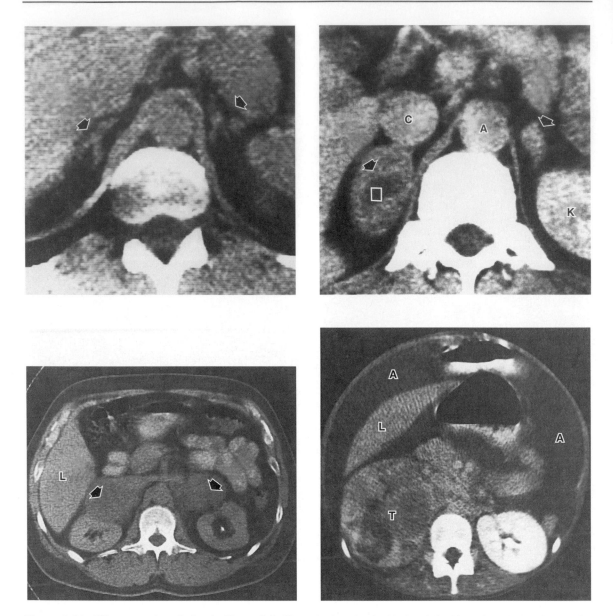

Figure 6–30. CT scans: adrenal glands. **Upper left:** Normal adrenals. At this level, in this patient, both adrenals (arrows) have an inverted Y shape. 34-year-old man with extra-adrenal pheochromocytoma. **Upper right:** Bilateral pheochromocytomas (arrows). Larger tumor on the right has a lower attenuation center (cursor). A = aorta, C = inferior vena cava, K = left kidney. 33-year-old man with multiple endocrine adenomatosis syndrome, after parathyroid adenoma and parathyroid carcinoma, with family history of medullary carcinoma. **Lower left:** Bilateral adrenal lymphoma. Enlarged adrenal glands (arrows) anterior to normal kidneys. L = liver. 53-year-old man with abdominal pain and histiocytic lymphoma of the central nervous system. **Lower right:** Carcinoma of the right adrenal. Scan through normal left kidney and large cystic and necrotic retrohepatic adrenal tumor (T). A = ascites, L = liver. 17-year-old girl with right abdominal mass and ascites.

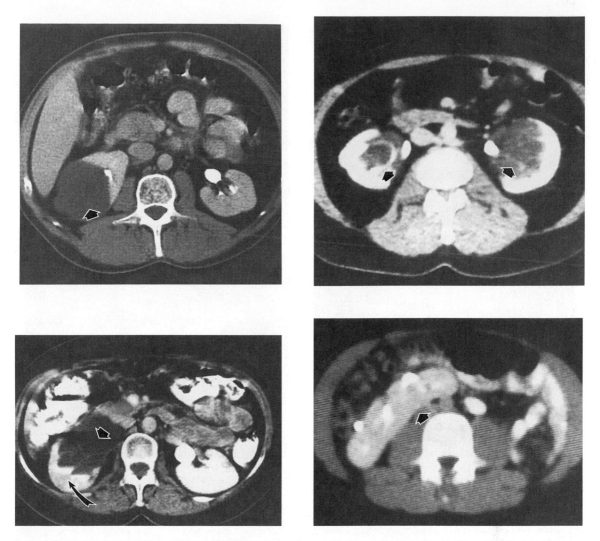

Figure 6–31. CT scans: kidneys. **Upper left:** Simple renal cyst. Cyst (arrow) has a CT number close to that of water. 49-year-old man with flank pain. **Upper right:** Bilateral peripelvic cysts (arrows). 52-year-old man with right flank mass found on routine physical examination. **Lower left:** Hydronephrosis. Dilated right renal pelvis (straight arrow) with layering of excreted contrast medium in distended calices (curved arrow). 54-year-old woman with obstructed distal right ureter from ovarian carcinoma. **Lower right:** Crossed fused renal ectopia (arrow). 14-year-old asymptomatic boy with abdominal mass palpated on school medical examination.

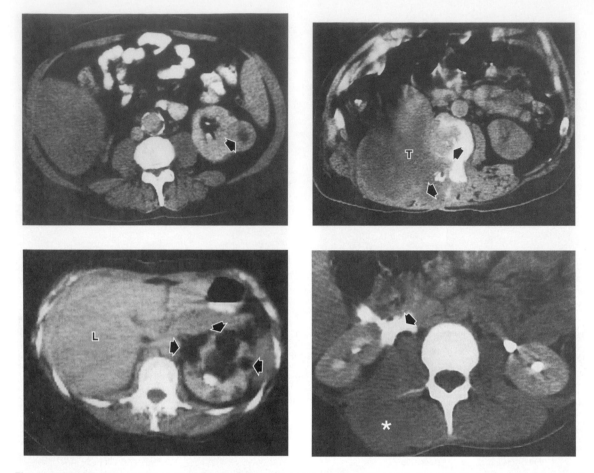

Figure 6–32. CT scans: kidneys. **Upper left:** Renal cell carcinoma. The left renal tumor (arrow) shows central necrosis. Note calcification in the arteriosclerotic abdominal aorta. 61-year-old man with previous right nephrectomy for renal carcinoma. **Upper right:** Recurrent renal adenocarcinoma. Massive recurrence in right renal fossa (T), with extensive invasion of posterior soft tissues and destruction of vertebral bodies (arrows). 51-year-old man after right nephrectomy for carcinoma. **Lower left:** Renal angiomyolipomas. Multiple low-attenuation mass lesions in the left kidney (arrows) with negative CT numbers compatible with fat. L = liver. 35-year-old woman with multiple bilateral renal hamartomas. **Lower right:** Right renal pelvic laceration. Enhanced CT scan through the kidneys showing extravasation of radiopaque material (arrow). Hemorrhage into the psoas and back muscles has enlarged their image (asterisk). 22-year-old man with laceration of the right renal pelvis due to a stab wound.

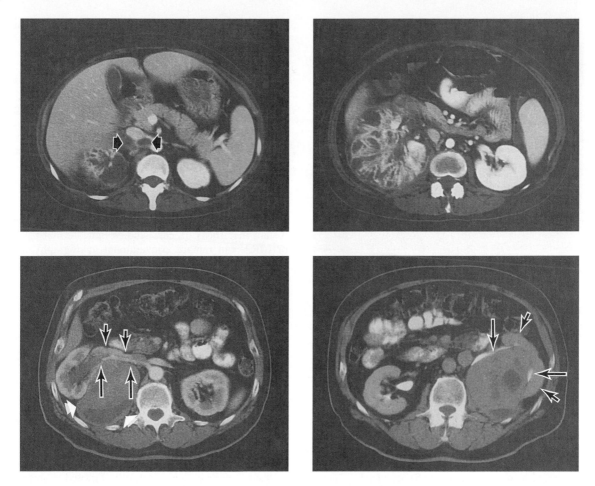

Figure 6–33. Spiral CT kidney. **Upper left:** 42-year-old woman with severe right pyelonephritis. An image through the upper pole of the right kidney shows low-density fluid collections between residual strands of enhancing renal parenchyma. Low-density inflammatory lymph nodes (arrows) displace the inferior vena cava anteriorly. **Upper right:** An image through the mid pole of the right kidney in the same patient reveals an enlarged kidney with marked destruction and striation of the renal parenchyma. Note the multiple low-density fluid collections. **Lower left:** Exophytic renal cell carcinoma. An image through the mid pole of the right kidney shows an apparent extrinsic mass (arrowhead) displacing the kidney laterally. The renal artery (long arrows) and renal vein (short arrows) are draped over the mass anteriorly. The renal vein is free of thrombus. **Lower right:** A lower image in the same patient reveals that the mass arises from the kidney. The renal parenchyma (short arrows) and contrast-containing collecting system (long arrows) are splayed by the mass.

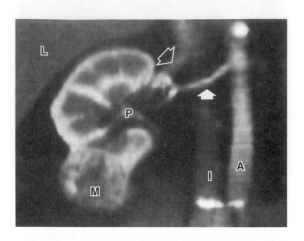

Figure 6–34. CT and CTA for staging renal cell carcinoma. This maximum intensity projection image from a renal CTA shows a 5-cm mass (M) in the lower pole of the right kidney which is localized to the cortex. The renal pelvis (P), artery (arrow), and vein (open arrow) are uninvolved. A = aorta, L = liver, I = inferior vena cava.

renal cortex. A nephrogram phase with medullary enhancement is reached within 60 s. Excretion of contrast material into the collecting structures can be expected within 2–3 min after initiation of contrast administration.

Although ureteral tumors can be detected by CT, the role of CT in the evaluation of the ureters is mostly in tumor staging and diagnosis of the cause and level of obstruction. As described in a previous section, helical CT without oral or intravenous contrast is the preferred imaging modality for patients with renal colic or suspected urolithiasis (Figure 6–35).

In the evaluation of the urinary bladder, CT is used primarily in staging bladder tumors and in diagnosing bladder rupture following trauma. Performing the CT after filling the bladder with dilute contrast medium (CT cystography) improves the sensitivity of this modality for detecting tumors and bladder rupture. For prostate diseases, CT is used for detection of lymphadenopathy and to evaluate prostatic abscesses. CT is used for detection of the abdominal location of suspected undescended testes, for staging of testicular tumors, and in the search for nodal or distant metastasis. Recent studies indicate that CTA or MRA can replace conventional angiography for the evaluation of potential renal donors.

Advantages & Disadvantages

The main advantages of CT include a wide field of view, the ability to detect subtle differences in the x-ray attenuation properties of various tissues, good spatial resolution, demonstration of cross-sectional images, and operator independence. These features contribute to the detailed demonstration of anatomy in all parts of the body and are particularly useful in the evaluation of the retroperitoneum. CT scanners presently in clinical use provide spatial resolution of 0.5–1 mm. Although CT is not as operator-dependent as ultrasound, much of the diagnostic information available from CT scans depends on patterns of contrast enhancement, and a carefully tailored examination is essential. Limitations of CT include restriction to the transaxial plane for direct imaging, tissue non-

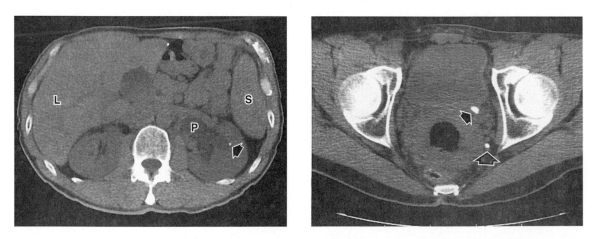

Figure 6–35. Helical CT without oral or intravenous contrast in a 42-year-old man with left flank pain. **Left:** CT image through the kidneys shows enlargement of the left kidney compared with the right, left pelvicalicectasis (P), and a stone in the mid pole of the left kidney (arrow). L = liver, S = spleen. **Right:** CT image through the base of the bladder shows an 8-mm stone (arrow) at the left ureterovesical junction with associated edema involving the left hemitrigone. Posterior to the ureteral stone is a 5-mm phlebolith (open arrow) within a pelvic vein.

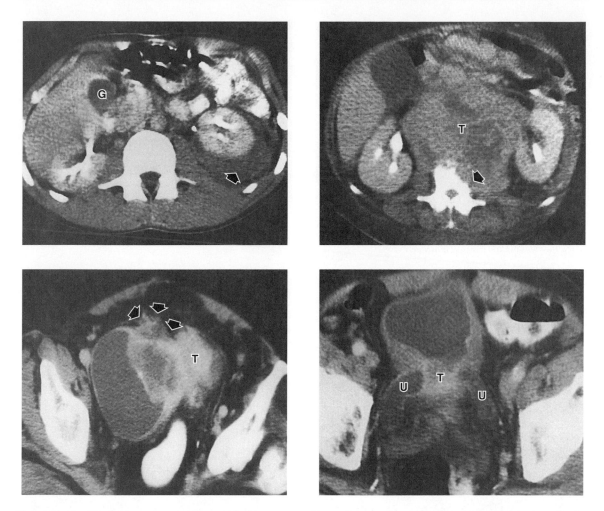

Figure 6–36. CT scans: retroperitoneum, bladder, prostate. **Upper left:** Perirenal hematoma. Hematoma (arrow) displaces the left kidney anteriorly. G = gallbladder. 16-year-old boy with acute glomerulonephritis; low-grade fever and left flank pain following left renal biopsy. **Upper right:** Retroperitoneal metastatic seminoma. Huge retroperitoneal mass of metastatic nodes (T) destroying vertebral body (arrow), obliterating outlines of central abdominal and retroperitoneal structures, and displacing kidneys laterally and bowel anteriorly. 46-year-old man with metastatic anaplastic testicular seminoma. **Lower left:** CT scan, transitional cell carcinoma of the urinary bladder with tumor (T) extension into the bladder diverticulum. There is tumor extension into the perivesical fat (arrows). **Lower right:** CT scan, transitional cell carcinoma of the urinary bladder with bilateral ureteral obstruction. Tumor (T), dilated ureters (U).

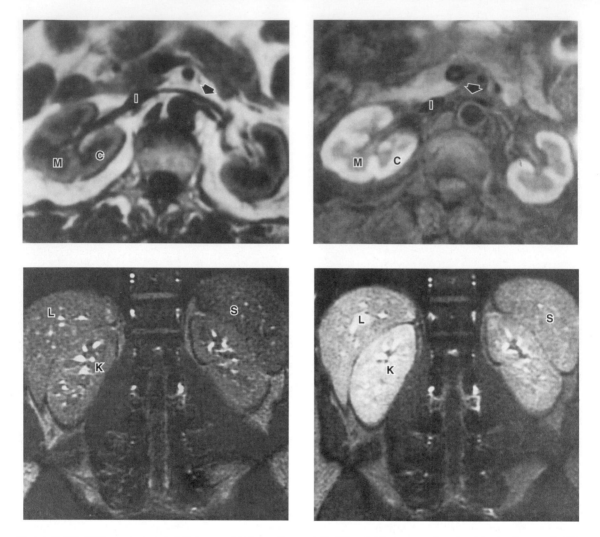

Figure 6–37. MRI appearance of the normal kidney. **Upper left:** T1-weighted conventional spin-echo image showing detailed anatomy of the kidney with differentiation between higher signal intensity cortex (C) and lower signal intensity medulla (M). Left renal vein (arrow), inferior vena cava (I). **Upper right:** T1-weighted spin-echo image using fat saturation technique. Because the fat signal has been suppressed, the computer automatically adjusts the gray scale of the signal intensity rendering even better contrast between higher signal intensity cortex (C) and lower signal intensity medulla (M). **Lower left and lower right:** Images of the normal kidney using GRASS (gradient recall acquisition steady state) technique. Gradient echo technique images are obtained while patient is holding his breath. **Lower left:** Noncontrast scan. **Lower right:** Scan obtained following gadolinium-DTPA injection of the contrast medium. The scan was obtained during the nephrogram phase showing uniform enhancement of both kidneys (K). There has been enhancement of the liver (L) and spleen (S).

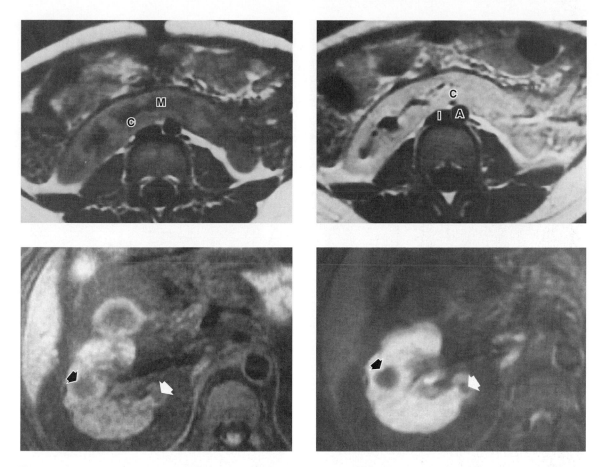

Figure 6–38. MR images (**upper left**) and horseshoe kidney (**upper right**). **Upper left:** Nonenhanced T1-weighted image; m, medulla; c, renal cortex. **Upper right:** Gadolinium-DTPA-enhanced T1-weighted image. Following injection of the contrast medium, there is uniform enhancement of the renal cortex (C). The addition of the contrast enhancement shows that the part of the kidney in front of the aorta (A) and the inferior vena cava (I) is functioning renal parenchyma. **Lower left and lower right:** T1-weighted fat saturation images of the renal cysts without and with contrast media. On a noncontrast scan (**lower left**), both the lateral (black arrow) and the medial (white arrow) renal cysts are seen, but the contrast between renal cysts and the adjacent renal parenchyma is better appreciated on the gadolinium-enhanced image (**lower right**).

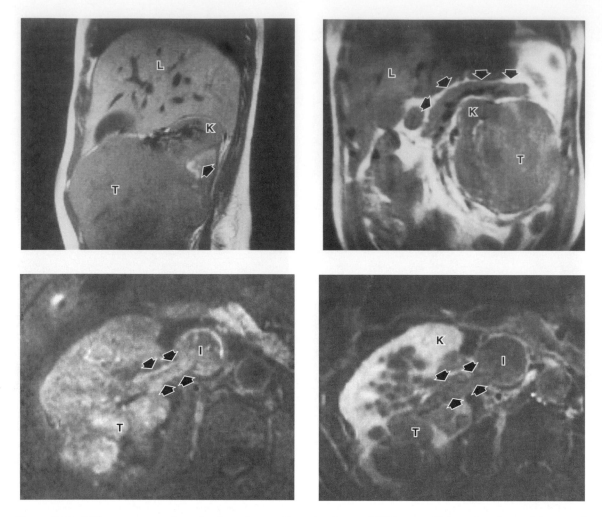

Figure 6–39. MRI appearance of renal cell carcinoma. The advantages of MRI are multiplanar imaging and the use of contrast media for better tumor characterization. **Upper left:** Sagittal T1-weighted image demonstrating a large renal cell carcinoma (T) arising from the inferior pole of the right kidney (K). Tumor extension in the posterior perirenal space (arrow). Liver (L). **Upper right:** Coronal image of a large renal cell carcinoma (T) replacing almost entire parenchyma of the left kidney (K). Superior displacement of the pancreas (arrows). Liver (L). **Lower left and lower right:** Fat saturation images before and after injection of the contrast medium. Heterogeneous tumor (**lower right**) in the posterior part of the right kidney shows heterogeneous enhancement following injection of gadolinium. The tumor is extending into the renal vein (arrows) and to the inferior vena cava (I).

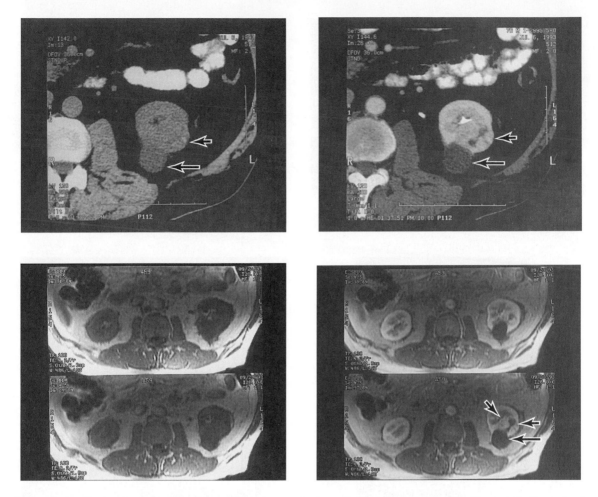

Figure 6–40. Pre- and postcontrast CT and MRI of a renal cell carcinoma adjacent to a cyst. **Upper left:** Precontrast CT image through the left kidney reveals a prominent posterior bulge (long arrow), which proved to be a cyst, and a subtle posterolateral convex contour deformity, which contains tiny calcifications (short arrow). **Upper right:** Postcontrast CT image reveals a nonenhancing cyst posteriorly (long arrow). The posterolateral contour deformity is caused by an enhancing renal cell carcinoma (short arrow) with a central low-density fluid collection. **Lower left:** Precontrast T1-weighted image shows similar intensities for the cyst, tumor, and normal renal parenchyma. **Lower right:** Postcontrast T1-weighted image. The cyst (long arrow) is nonenhancing. The margins of the enhancing renal cell carcinoma (short arrows) are seen. The central fluid collection does not enhance.

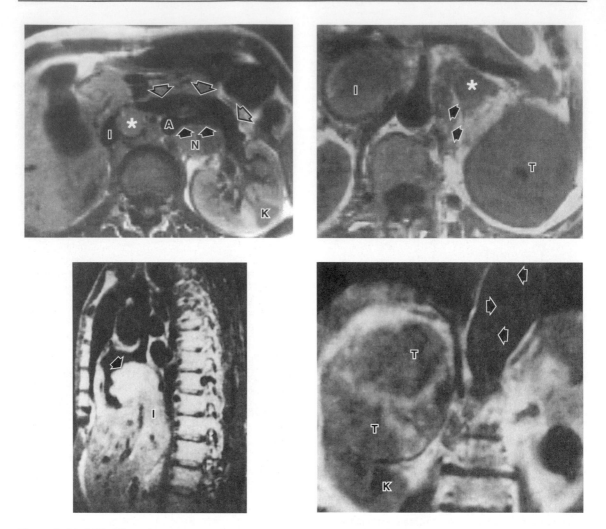

Figure 6–41. MRI ability to locally stage renal cell carcinoma. **Upper left:** Demonstration of adenopathy, T1-weighted MR image. The left para-aortic lymph nodes (N) are elevating the left renal artery (solid arrows), and there are also large nodes (asterisk) in the aortic caval window. The differentiation between the medium-signal-intensity nodes and the low signal intensity of the vessels (open arrows) is well seen. A, aorta. K, kidney. **Upper right:** Renal cell carcinoma (T) of the left kidney. Inferior vena cava (I) with tumor extension to the left adrenal gland (asterisk) and into the inferior vena cava (I). Enlarged nodes (arrows). **Lower left:** Sagittal image demonstrating a large tumor thrombus in the inferior vena cava (I) with tumor extending into the right atrium (arrow). **Lower right:** Large renal cell carcinoma (T) from the right kidney (K). Incidental finding is aortic dissection (small arrows). The patient died shortly after imaging from ruptured aortic dissection.

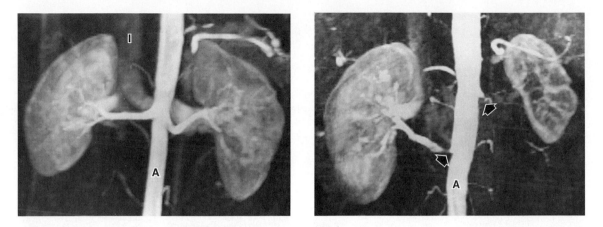

Figure 6–42. Gadolinium-enhanced renal MRA. **Left:** Maximum intensity projection (MIP) image from a renal MRA in a 22-year-old potential renal donor. The renal arteries are normal. **Right:** MIP image from a renal MRA in a 56-year-old man with suspected renovascular hypertension shows an atrophic left kidney with an occluded left renal artery (arrow) and a severely stenotic right renal artery (open arrow). The collateral capsular renal vessels are not seen. A = aorta, I = inferior vena cava.

specificity, low soft-tissue contrast resolution, and the need for contrast media, both oral and intravenous. Even with careful use of contrast media, tissue contrast is sometimes unsatisfactory.

MAGNETIC RESONANCE IMAGING
(Figures 6–37 through 6–46)

Basic Principles

Clinical MRI has its basis in the nuclear properties of the hydrogen atoms in the body. The nucleus of a hydrogen atom has the nuclear property of spin, with the result that the nucleus behaves like a tiny magnet.

Ordinarily, the spin axes of the hydrogen nuclei in the body are randomly oriented. However, if the nuclei are placed in a strong magnetic field (like that produced in MR imagers by large magnets housed in suitable gantries), they precess (wobble like a spinning top) around the lines of magnetic force.

If these hydrogen nuclei in the magnetic field are additionally stimulated by very short pulses of radio waves of appropriate frequency, they absorb energy and invert their orientation with respect to the magnetic field, ie, they are elevated to a state of higher energy. Once the short radiofrequency pulse terminates, the hydrogen nuclei return at various rates to their original (low-energy) orientation within the magnetic field, emitting energy in the form of radio waves of the same frequency as the one absorbed in the process. This phenomenon is called **nuclear magnetic resonance.** The emitted energies from the resonating hydrogen nuclei are collected and are transformed with various computer programs into cross-sectional images.

MR tomographic images are reflections of the hydrogen densities in the various body tissues, modified importantly by the differing physical, cellular, and chemical microenvironments and any flow (fluid) characteristics of the tissues. The energy signals emitted from nuclei under MR investigation contain no innate information defining their origin. In MRI, that information is obtained by the use of gradient magnetic coils that vary the magnetic field within the main magnet in space, thereby changing the nature of the emitted MR signals from the different body regions to permit exact localization of the hydrogen nuclei emitting the signals.

There are biologically important nuclei other than hydrogen nuclei that are MR-sensitive, including those of phosphorus, sodium, and potassium, but these more complex nuclei have lower inherent sensitivities to MRI and occur in lower physiologic concentrations than hydrogen. Notwithstanding these inherent limitations, imaging of these nuclei for tissue typing and mapping and as biologic tracers (MR spectroscopy) is undergoing intense research and development.

Clinical Applications

MRI has been applied in imaging the kidney, retroperitoneum, urinary bladder, prostate, testis, and penis. Applications for nonenhanced MR in renal imaging include demonstration of congenital anomalies, diagnosis of renal vein thrombosis, and staging of renal cell carcinoma. MR angiography, which does not require intravenous contrast media, is useful in evaluating renal transplant vessels, renal vein tumor or thrombosis, and renal artery stenosis.

The use of contrast media in MRI of the kidney has

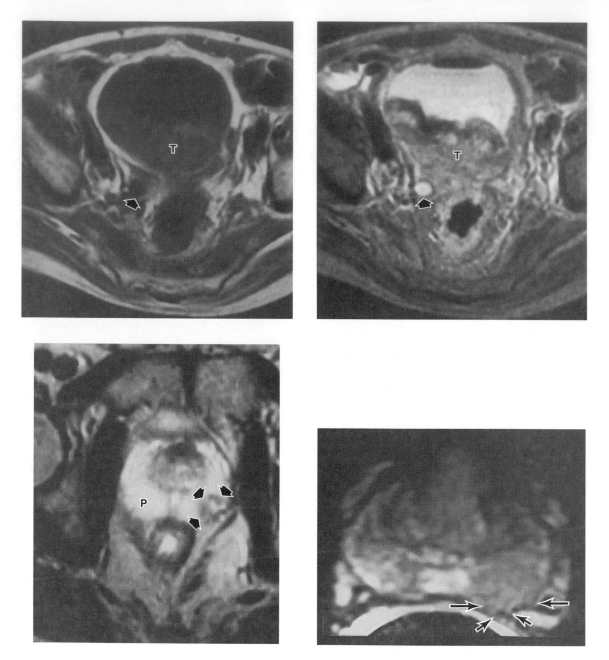

Figure 6–43. MRI examination of the pelvis. The upper images are examples of the ability of MRI to demonstrate a bladder tumor and show its extent. **Upper left:** T1-weighted. **Upper right:** T2-weighted transaxial image. The large tumor (T) at the bladder base shows perivesical extension. Also seen is a dilated right ureter (arrow). **Lower left:** Example of prostate carcinoma as seen on a T2-weighted image. The prostate carcinoma (small arrows) demonstrates lower signal intensity as compared with the adjacent higher signal intensity peripheral zone (P). **Lower right:** T2-weighted image; an example of extracapsular extension of prostatic carcinoma (Jewett stage C disease). Low-signal tumor is seen within the left peripheral zone. There is breach of the prostatic capsule (between long arrows) with extension of tumor beyond the capsule to involve the neurovascular bundle (short arrows).

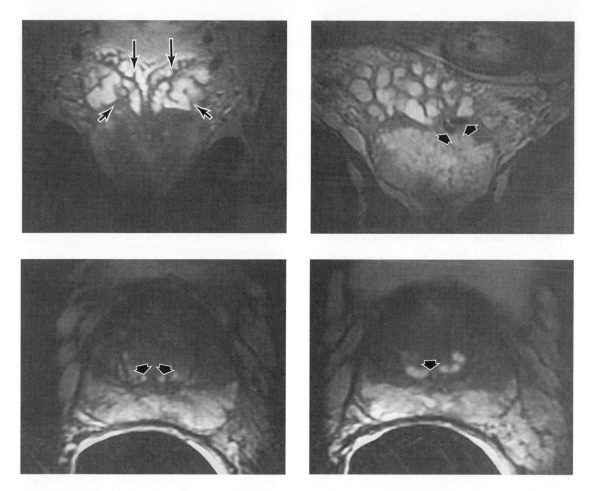

Figure 6–44. MRI of seminal vesicles, ductus deferens, and ejaculatory ducts. **Upper left:** T2-weighted image, normal seminal vesicles, and ductus deferens, and ejaculatory ducts. The ampullae of the ductus deferens (long arrows) are normally of high signal intensity on T2-weighted images and are immediately medial to the seminal vesicles (short arrows). The seminal vesicles are also of high signal intensity and are draped over the prostate gland. **Upper right:** Seminal vesicle and ductus deferens calculi. Coronal T2-weighted images show low-signal calculi within the proximal ductus deferens and medial aspect of the seminal vesicle on the left side (arrows). The patient had a history of prostatitis, prostatic pain, and hemorrhagic ejaculate. **Lower left:** Axial T2-weighted image through the prostate. The peripheral zone is of normal high signal intensity. The normal ejaculatory ducts (arrows) are identified as two small foci of high signal intensity within the lower-signal central zone. **Lower right:** Axial T2-weighted image through the prostate reveals a low-signal-intensity calculus (arrow) within the right ejaculatory duct (same patient as in upper right image).

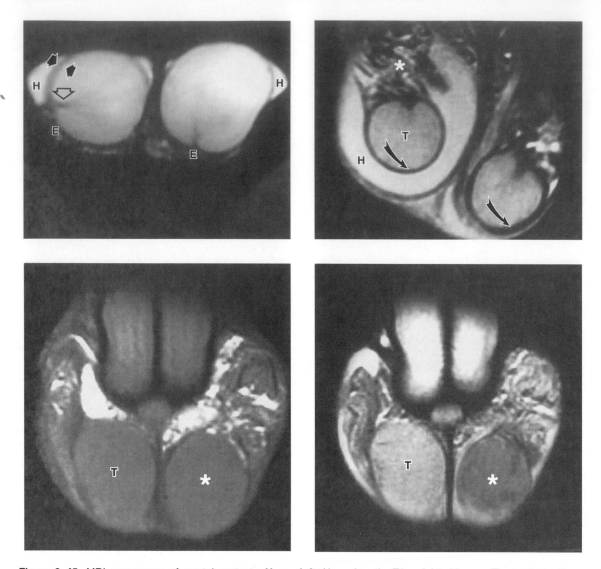

Figure 6–45. MRI appearance of scrotal contents. **Upper left:** Normal testis, T2-weighted image. The testicular tissue is of homogeneous high signal intensity. The tunica albuginea (arrows) demonstrates low signal intensity as does the mediastinum testis (open arrowhead). A small amount of fluid—hydrocele (H). Epididymis (E) is of low signal intensity. **Upper right:** Hydrocele of the right scrotum (T2-weighted image). Hydrocele (H) demonstrates high signal intensity. Testis (T). Tunica albuginea (curved black arrows). Varicocele (asterisk). **Lower left and lower right:** Images of a testicular tumor. On the proton density image (**lower left**), the signal intensity from both testicles is similar. On the T2-weighted image (**lower right**), testicular tumor (asterisk) demonstrates lower signal intensity as compared with the higher signal intensity of the normal testicular tissue (T).

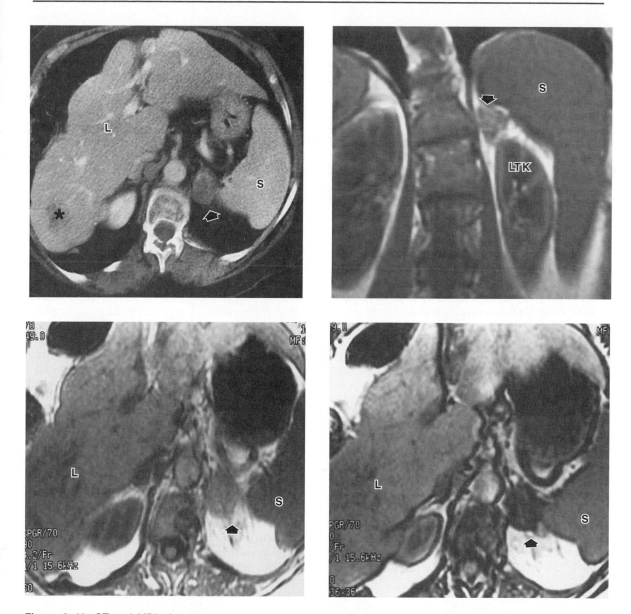

Figure 6–46. CT and MRI of an adrenal adenoma. **Upper left:** Contrast-enhanced CT through the left adrenal gland shows a 3-cm mass (arrow). Since the CT was performed after the administration of contrast, the x-ray attenuation of this lesion, 35 Hounsfield units, was indeterminate for adenoma, and MRI was performed. The hypodense lesion (asterisk) in the liver (L) is a metastasis from this patient's known colon cancer. Spleen, (S). **Upper right:** A coronal T1-weighted image shows the left adrenal lesion (arrow) above the left kidney (LTK). Spleen, (S). **Lower left:** An in-phase gradient echo image shows a left adrenal lesion (arrow), which has a signal intensity brighter than that of the adjacent spleen (S). Liver, (L). **Lower right:** On the opposed-phase gradient echo image, the adrenal lesion (arrow) has decreased in signal intensity and now appears darker than the spleen (S). This signal loss on opposed-phase images is characteristic of adrenal adenomas. Liver, (L).

broadened the clinical application of this technique. Using bolus injection, gadolinium, and rapid sequence imaging, both anatomy and function of the kidney can be assessed. Gadolinium, similar to iodine contrast media, is an extracellular contrast agent primarily excreted by glomerular filtration. Unlike iodine contrast media, however, gadolinium has shown good renal tolerance in patients with preexisting renal failure. Whereas iodine contrast agents uniformly enhance the tissue density on x-ray or CT images, the effect of gadolinium on MR tissue signal intensity depends on its concentration. This relationship between signal intensity and concentration is nonlinear. At lower concentrations gadolinium causes an increase in signal intensity (predominantly due to shortening of the T1 relaxation time), whereas at higher concentrations there is a decrease in signal intensity (due to intervening shortening of the T2 relaxation time).

The use of gadolinium has extended the application of MRI to the evaluation of renal obstruction (when other studies are inconclusive) and the detection and characterization of renal tumors. Although MRI is capable of imaging blood vessels without contrast media, the rapid injection of gadolinium followed by rapid imaging can also be used for this purpose. This gadolinium-enhanced MRA is useful for assessing renal artery stenosis and for evaluating potential renal donors (Figure 6–42).

In evaluation of the urinary bladder, MRI is used primarily to stage bladder tumors and to differentiate between benign bladder wall hypertrophy and infiltrating malignant neoplasm. In imaging the prostate gland, MRI has stirred much interest because multiplanar imaging and very good tissue contrast allow an excellent display of anatomy and intraprostatic pathology. MRI is used in the evaluation of congenital anomalies and in the staging of prostate carcinoma. MRI of the testis is appropriate only when other imaging studies (eg, ultrasonography) are inconclusive and is applicable to the evaluation of undescended testis, trauma, epididymoorchitis, and tumors.

A modification of the MRI technique, called gradient echo imaging, can detect microscopic amounts of fat within lesions (Figure 6–46). This technique is commonly used to characterize adrenal masses. Adrenal masses containing fat are either adrenal adenomas or myelolipomas, so the CT or MRI demonstration of fat in an adrenal lesion characterizes it as a benign lesion, even in the oncologic patient.

In a technique called MR urography, heavily fluid-weighted MR images are obtained to produce urogramlike pictures without the need for contrast media. This technique is sensitive in the detection of ureterohydronephrosis and is particularly useful in patients in whom contrast material is contraindicated, such as patients with prior contrast reactions or renal failure. It is still under investigation for the detection and staging of urothelial tumors.

Advantages and Disadvantages

Advantages of MRI include direct imaging in any plane desired (although the 3 orthogonal planes—transverse, sagittal, and coronal—are most commonly used), a large field of view, excellent soft-tissue contrast, imaging without exposure to ionizing radiation, and operator independence. It can also image blood vessels and the urinary tract without contrast material. MR scanning, however, is not without drawbacks. The scanning time is relatively slow (often leading to images that are marred by motion), and image clarity is often inferior compared with CT. Although no deleterious effects of clinical MRI have been identified to date, a patient undergoing an MRI examination is subject to ECG changes, temporary anisotropy, heat generation, and claustrophobia. None of these effects has been shown to be important during clinical scanning. There are also contraindications to MRI. Absolute contraindications include the presence of (1) intracranial aneurysm clips, unless the referring physician is certain that the clip is made of a nonferromagnetic material (such as titanium); (2) intra-orbital metal fragments; and (3) any electrically, magnetically, or mechanically activated implants (including cardiac pacemakers, biostimulators, neurostimulators, cochlear implants, and hearing aids). Relative contraindications such as pregnancy should always be viewed in the light of risk versus benefit of the examination.

COMPARISON OF IMAGING METHODS (Figures 6–47 through 6–50)

Radiography, sonography, CT scanning, and MRI all have advantages and disadvantages. As new imaging methods have been developed, changes have occurred in both the frequency used and applications of each type of imaging. For example, increased familiarity with and confidence in sonography and CT scanning have resulted in a decrease in the use of some long-established conventional uroradiologic studies, eg, excretory urography, retrograde urography, and lymphography; adrenal and renal angiograms are not being performed anymore for strictly diagnostic purposes. MRI is also producing dramatic changes in medical and urologic diagnosis.

Several factors are involved in these changes: (1) the increased effectiveness of newer imaging methods over older ones for some aspects of urodiagnosis; (2) the availability of equipment, trained technical personnel to operate it, and physicians to interpret the results; (3) increased awareness of the hazards of ionizing radiation; and (4) the desire to avoid using invasive diagnostic procedures if possible.

Because so many different types of imaging are available, each with different costs, risks, and areas of effectiveness, it may be difficult for the clinician

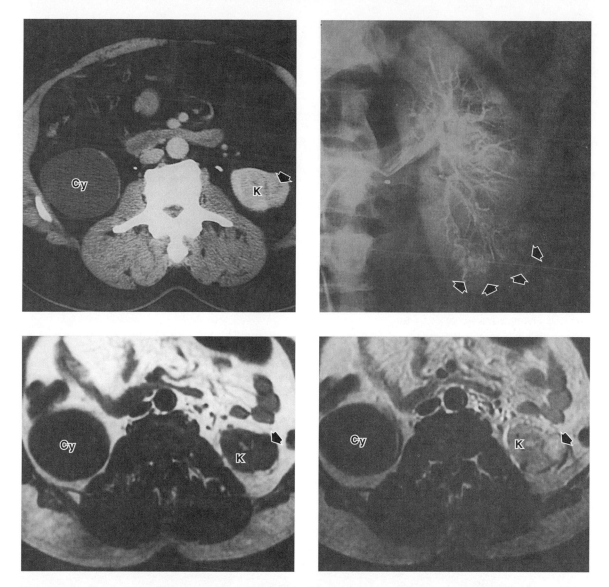

Figure 6–47. Comparison of imaging methods in the evaluation of renal cell carcinoma. **Upper left:** CT scan showing a renal cyst (Cy) in the right kidney. There is bulging (arrow) in the contour of the left kidney (K), but it is difficult to discern if the lesion represents a neoplasm. **Upper right:** Angiogram showing small vascular lesions in the inferior pole of the left kidney (arrows). **Lower left and lower right:** MRI scans. **Lower left:** T1-weighted noncontrast scan. **Lower right:** T1-weighted postcontrast scan. The renal cyst (Cy) in the right kidney does not show any enhancement. The lesion (arrow) in the left kidney (K) shows marked enhancement, indicating that it is solid in nature. In this example, the contrast-enhanced MRI is superior to CT in the detection and characterization of the left renal mass.

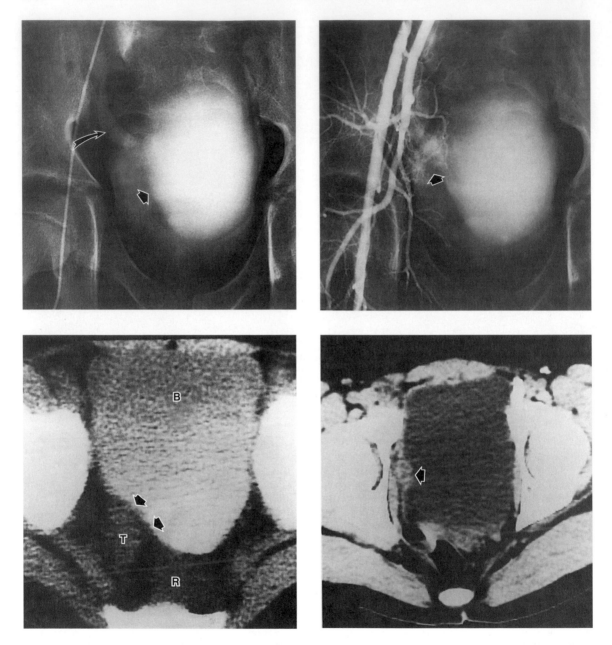

Figure 6–48. Comparison of imaging methods: metastatic extra-adrenal familial pheochromocytoma. 10-year-old boy with hypertension and seizures precipitated by abdominal palpation. Family history of multiple extra-adrenal pheochromocytomas in the mother. **Upper left:** Excretory urogram. The right ureter is dilated and elevated (curved arrow), with the right posterior portion of the bladder displaced toward the left (straight arrow). The urographic diagnosis is possible extra-adrenal paravesical pheochromocytoma. **Upper right:** Right femoral arteriogram. Tumor stain (arrow) in right paravesical location. The angiographic diagnosis is extra-adrenal paravesical pheochromocytoma. **Lower left:** CT scan. Transverse tomogram through bladder (B) shows the tumor (T) indenting the bladder (arrows). R = rectum. **Lower right:** CT scan. Transverse tomogram through bladder. Recurrence of symptoms following removal of the right paravesical pheochromocytoma prompted another CT study, which shows recurrent tumor (arrow) in the bladder wall. Each imaging study complemented or supplemented the previous one. None, however, diagnosed the small liver metastases discovered at surgery.

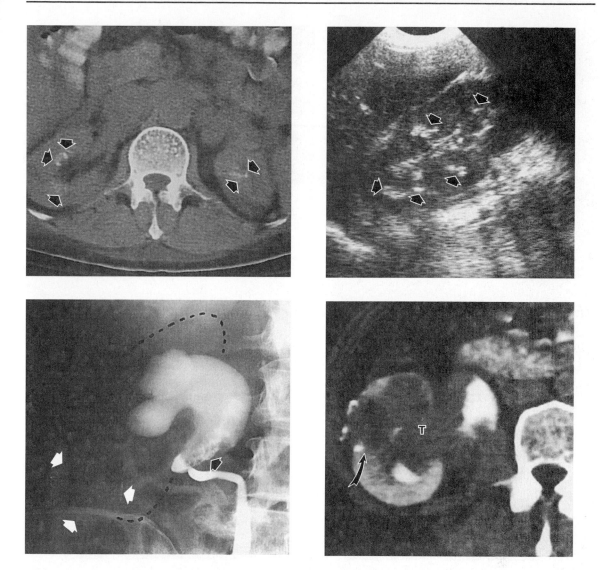

Figure 6–49. Comparison of imaging methods. **Upper left** is an example of a nonenhanced CT, and **upper right** is an ultrasound study in the demonstration of renal calcifications. Fine calcifications in the medullary region indicate medullary nephrocalcinosis. They are of high density on CT (arrows) and are shown as echogenic foci (arrows) on an ultrasound scan. **Lower left and lower right:** Example of images of a transitional cell carcinoma and the calcified renal cyst. Retrograde urogram (**lower left**) shows filling defects due to tumor in the renal pelvis (black arrow) at ureteropelvic junction, and also seen are the calcifications in a lower pole mass (white arrows). Note that the infundibulum and calices of the lower pole failed to opacify in this 45-year-old woman with hematuria. On the CT scan (**lower right**) the cystic nature of the calcified renal mass (curved arrow) is well demonstrated and the CT scan shows better the extent of the tumor (T), which involves the entire lower pole of the kidney and extends into the dilated renal pelvis.

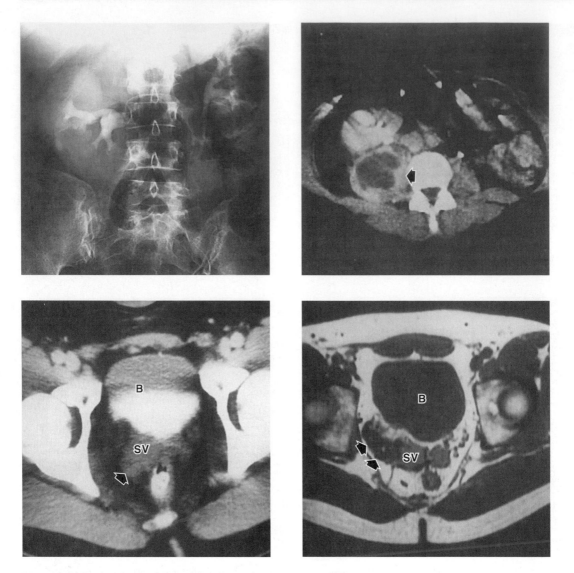

Figure 6–50. Comparison of imaging methods. **Upper left and upper right:** Psoas abscess. Excretory urogram (**upper left**) reveals abnormal orientation of the right kidney and an enlarged psoas muscle. On the CT scan (**upper right**) in the same patient, the psoas abscess (arrow) is well seen. The CT scan is exceptionally helpful for imaging retroperitoneal structures. The abscess was drained percutaneously under CT control. **Lower left and lower right:** Demonstration of an arterial venous malformation to the seminal vesicles. On the CT scan (**lower left**), the right seminal vesicle (SV) is enlarged, but the nature of the enlargement (arrow) is difficult to discern. On an MRI scan (**lower right**), the enlarged vessels (arrows) are demonstrated as the flowing blood within the vessel lacks signal intensity in contrast to the medium signal intensity of the seminal vesicles (SV). Urinary bladder (B).

to decide which method will yield the most information with the least cost and risk. A particular study may be critical in one diagnostic situation but useless in another. For example, sonography, CT scanning, and MRI are usually ineffective in demonstrating small uroepithelial tumors, and an excretory urogram is the study of choice for such lesions. Sonography is an excellent noninvasive, relatively inexpensive method for differentiating simple cysts from other mass lesions in the kidney but is much less effective in imaging the retroperitoneum than is CT scanning. Sonography also relies considerably on the skill of the operator. CT scanning produces excellent images and is currently the preferred imaging method for the examination of the retroperitoneum. MRI rivals CT scanning in imaging capability for some structures, eg, the kidney, but has surpassed CT in imaging the pelvis. With advances in equipment and speed of scanning and the introduction of contrast media, the use of MRI in urology can only be extended further.

The patient and the clinician both benefit from careful consultation with the radiologist to ensure that the methods of imaging chosen are of value in diagnosis and treatment planning and do not duplicate or merely confirm established findings, with loss of time and additional expense.

REFERENCES

GENERAL

Baum S (editor): *Abrams' Angiography and Interventional Radiology,* 4th ed. Little, Brown, 1997.

Bushberg JT et al: *The Essential Physics of Medical Imaging.* Williams & Wilkins, 1994.

Davidson AJ, Hartman DS: *Radiology of the Kidney and Urinary Tract,* 2nd ed. Saunders, 1994.

Dunnick NR et al: *Textbook of Uroradiology,* 2nd ed. Williams & Wilkins, 1997.

Lee JKT et al: *Computed Body Tomography with MRI Correlation,* 3rd ed. Lippincott-Raven, 1998.

Pollack HM: *Clinical Urography.* Saunders, 1990.

Taylor A Jr, Nally JV: Clinical applications of renal scintigraphy. AJR 1995;164:31.

CONTRAST AGENTS

Caro JJ, Trindade E, McGregor M: The risks of death and of severe nonfatal reactions with high- vs low-osmolality contrast media: A meta-analysis. AJR 1991; 156:825.

Cohan RH, Ellis, JH: Iodinated contrast material in uroradiology. Choice of agent and management of complications. Urol Clin North Am 1997;24:471.

Katzberg RW: Urography into the 21st century: New contrast media, renal handling, imaging characteristics, and nephrotoxicity. Radiology 1997;204:297.

Weissleder R: Can gadolinium be safely given in renal failure? AJR 1996;167:278.

Wittbrodt ET, Spinler, SA: Prevention of anaphylactoid reactions in high-risk patients receiving radiographic contrast media. Ann Pharmacother 1994;28:236.

RADIOGRAPHY

Berlin JW et al: Voiding cystourethrography after radical prostatectomy: Normal findings and correlation between contrast extravasation and anastomotic strictures. AJR 1994;162:87.

Bircan MK, Sahin H, Korkmaz K: Diagnosis of urethral strictures: Is retrograde urethrography still necessary? Int Urol Nephrol 1996;28:801.

Boisclair C et al: Treatment of renal angioplasty failure by percutaneous renal artery stenting with Palmaz stents: Midterm technical and clinical results. AJR 1997;168:245.

Bradley AJ, Taylor PM: Does bowel preparation improve the quality of intravenous urography? Br J Radiol 1996;69:906.

Ditchfield MR et al: Voiding cystourethrography in boys: Does the presence of the catheter obscure the diagnosis of posterior urethral valves? AJR 1995;164: 1233.

Dyer R et al: The segmental nephrogram. AJR 1985; 145:321.

Goessl C et al: Is routine excretory urography necessary at first diagnosis of bladder cancer? J Urol 1997;157:480.

Harding M et al: Does lymphangiography have any role in the management of early non-seminomatous germ cell tumours? Clin Radiol 1990;41:392.

Kadner W: Nephrotomography as a routine part of the excretory urogram. AJR 1995;165:491.

Kass DA, Hricak H, Davidson AJ: Renal malignancies with normal excretory urograms. AJR 1983;141:731.

Kayigil O, Atahan O, Metin A: Dynamic infusion cavernosometry and cavernosography in diagnosing and classifying venoocclusive dysfunction. Int Urol Nephrol 1995;275:615.

Kuchta SG, Manco LG, Evans JA: Prominent iliopsoas muscles producing a gourd-shaped deformity of the bladder. J Urol 1982;127:1188.

Lebowitz RL et al: International system of radiographic grading of vesicoureteric reflux: International Reflux Study in Children. Pediatr Radiol 1985;15:105.

Marks LB et al: Role of lymphangiography in staging testicular seminoma. Urology 1991;38:264.

Mussurakis S, Sprigg A, Steiner M: Patterns of integration and clinical value of voiding cystourethrography in the work-up of urinary tract infection in children. Eur Urol 1995;28:165.

Patriquin HB, O'Regan S: Medullary sponge kidney in childhood. AJR 1985;145:315.

Sandler CM, Corriere JN Jr: Urethrography in the diagnosis of acute urethral injuries. Urol Clin North Am 1989;16:283.

Schuster GA, Nazos D, Lewis GA: Preparation of outpatients for excretory urography: Is bowel preparation with laxatives and dietary restrictions necessary? AJR 1995;164:1425.

Smith RC, McClennan BL: Voiding cystourethrography. JAMA 1996;275:1876.

Thornbury JR, Stanley JC, Fryback DG: Hypertensive urogram: A nondiscriminatory test for renal vascular hypertension. AJR 1982;138:43.

Wasserman NF et al: Ureteral pseudodiverticula: Frequent association with uroepithelial malignancy. AJR 1991;157:69.

Zeitlin SI et al: Is intravenous urography indicated in a young adult with hematuria? Urology 1996;48:365.

ULTRASOUND

Benson CB, Doubilet PM, Richie JP: Sonography of the male genital tract. AJR 1989;153:705.

Cronan JJ, Tublin ME: Role of the resistive index in the evaluation of acute renal obstruction. AJR 1995;164:377.

Dacher JN et al: Power Doppler sonographic pattern of acute pyelonephritis in children: Comparison with CT. AJR 1996;166:1451.

Grantham JG et al: Testicular neoplasms: 29 tumors studied by high-resolution US. Radiology 1985;157:775.

Habboub HK, Abu-Yousef MM, Williams RD: Accuracy of color Doppler sonography in assessing venous thrombus extension in renal cell carcinoma. AJR 1997;168:267.

Hamm B: Differential diagnosis of scrotal masses by ultrasound. Eur Radiol 1997;7:668.

Hricak H et al: Renal parenchymal disease: Sonographic-histologic correlation. Radiology 1982;144:141.

Kaude JV et al: Renal morphology and function immediately after extracorporeal shockwave lithotripsy. AJR 1985;145:305.

Mallek R et al: Distinction between obstructive and nonobstructive hydronephrosis: Value of diuresis duplex Doppler sonography. AJR 1996;166:113.

Meacham RB, Townsend RR, Drose JA: Ejaculatory duct obstruction: Diagnosis and treatment with transrectal sonography. AJR 1995;165:1463.

Migaleddu V et al: Imaging of renal hydatid cysts. AJR 1997;169:1339.

Mokulis JA et al: Should renal ultrasound be performed in the patient with microscopic hematuria and a normal excretory urogram? J Urol 1995;154:1300.

Siegel CL et al: Angiomyolipoma and renal cell carcinoma: US differentiation. Radiology 1996;198:789.

Steinhardt GF, Slovis TL, Perlmutter AD: Simple renal cysts in infancy. Radiology 1985;155:349.

COMPUTED TOMOGRAPHY

Choi SH, Anllo V: Left renal vein "nutcracker" phenomenon. Urology 1982;20:549.

Cochran ST et al: Helical CT angiography for examination of living renal donors. AJR 1997;168:1569.

Curry NS: Atypical cystic renal masses. Abdom Imaging 1998;23:230.

Degesys GE et al: Retroperitoneal fibrosis: Use of CT in distinguishing among possible causes. AJR 1986;146:57.

Fielding JR et al: Spiral CT in the evaluation of flank pain: Overall accuracy and feature analysis. J Comput Assist Tomogr 1997;21:635.

Katz DS, Lane MJ, Sommer FG: Unenhanced helical CT of ureteral stones: Incidence of associated urinary tract findings. AJR 1996;166:1319.

Perlman ES et al: CT urography in the evaluation of urinary tract disease. J Comput Assist Tomogr 1996;20:620.

Sivit CJ, Cutting JP, Eichelberger MR: CT diagnosis and localization of rupture of the bladder in children with blunt abdominal trauma: Significance of contrast material extravasation in the pelvis. AJR 1995;164:1243.

Smith RC et al: Acute ureteral obstruction: Value of secondary signs of helical unenhanced CT. AJR 1996;167:1109.

Szolar DH, Kammerhuber FH: Adrenal adenomas and nonadenomas: Assessment of washout at delayed contrast-enhanced CT. Radiology 1998;207:369.

Urban BA et al: CT appearance of transitional cell carcinoma of the renal pelvis: Part 1. Early-stage disease. AJR 1997;169:157.

Urban BA et al: CT appearance of transitional cell carcinoma of the renal pelvis: Part 2. Advanced-stage disease. AJR 1997;169:163.

Vining DJ et al: CT cystoscopy: An innovation in bladder imaging. AJR 1996;166:409.

Vinnicombe SJ et al: Normal pelvic lymph nodes: Evaluation with CT after bipedal lymphangiography. Radiology 1995;194:349.

Weyman PJ, McClennan BL, Lee JKT: Computed tomography of calcified renal masses. AJR 1982;138:1095.

Zeman RK et al: Helical CT of renal masses: The value of delayed scans. AJR 1996;167:771.

Zeman RK et al: Helical (spiral) CT of the abdomen. AJR 1993;160:719.

MAGNETIC RESONANCE IMAGING

Bakker J et al: Renal artery stenosis and accessory renal arteries: Accuracy of detection and visualization with gadolinium-enhanced breath-hold MR angiography. Radiology 1998;207:497.

Buzzas GR et al: Use of gadolinium-enhanced, ultrafast, three-dimensional, spoiled gradient-echo magnetic resonance angiography in the preoperative evaluation of living renal allograft donors. Transplantation 1997;64:1734.

De Cobelli F et al: Renal artery stenosis: Evaluation with breath-hold, three-dimensional, dynamic, gadolinium-enhanced versus three-dimensional, phase-contrast MR angiography. Radiology 1997;205:689.

Fisher MR, Hricak H, Crooks LE: Urinary bladder MR imaging. 1. Normal and benign conditions. Radiology 1985;157:467.

Fisher MR, Hricak H, Tanagho EA: Urinary bladder MR imaging. 2. Neoplasm. Radiology 1985;157:471.

Grenier N et al: Diagnosis of renovascular hypertension: Feasibility of captopril-sensitized dynamic MR imaging and comparison with captopril scintigraphy. AJR 1996;166:835.

Hussain S et al: MR urography. Magn Reson Imaging Clin North Am 1997;5:95.

Ikonen S et al: Magnetic resonance imaging of clinically localized prostatic cancer. J Urol 1998;159:915.

Kaji Y et al: Localizing prostate cancer in the presence

of postbiopsy changes on MR images: Role of proton MR spectroscopic imaging. Radiology 1998;206:785.

Low RN et al: Potential renal transplant donors: Evaluation with gadolinium-enhanced MR angiography and MR urography. Radiology 1998;207:165.

Mattrey RF: Magnetic resonance imaging of the scrotum. Semin Ultrasound CT MR 1991;12:95.

Regan F et al: MR urography using HASTE imaging in the assessment of ureteric obstruction. AJR 1996;167:1115.

Ros PR et al: Diagnosis of renal artery stenosis: Feasibility of combining MR angiography, MR renography, and gadopentetate-based measurements of glomerular filtration rate. AJR 1995;165:1447.

Schiebler ML et al: Efficacy of prostate-specific antigen and magnetic resonance imaging in staging stage C adenocarcinoma of the prostate. Invest Radiol 1992;27:575.

Tang Y et al: The value of MR urography that uses HASTE sequences to reveal urinary tract disorders. AJR 1996;167:1497.

COMPARISON OF VARIOUS IMAGING METHODS

Berman JM et al: Sonographic evaluation of acute intrascrotal pathology. AJR 1996;166:857.

Bosniak MA: The current radiologic approach to renal cysts. Radiology 1986;158:1.

Curry NS: Small renal masses (lesions smaller than 3 cm): Imaging evaluation and management. AJR 1995;164:355.

Einstein DM et al: Evaluation of renal masses detected by excretory urography: Cost-effectiveness of sonography versus CT. AJR 1995;164:371.

Friedland GW, Chang P: The role of imaging in the management of the impalpable undescended testis. AJR 1988;151:1107.

Griebling TL, Williams RD: Staging of incidentally detected prostate cancer: Role of repeat resection, prostate-specific antigen, needle biopsy, and imaging. Semin Urol Oncol 1996;14:156.

Hoeffel C et al: Spontaneous unilateral adrenal hemorrhage: Computerized tomography and magnetic resonance imaging findings in 8 cases. J Urol 1995;154:1647.

Hricak H: Noninvasive imaging for staging of prostate cancer: Magnetic resonance imaging, computed tomography, and ultrasound. NCI Monogr 1988;7:31.

Hricak et al: Prostate carcinoma: Staging by clinical assessment, CT, and MR imaging. Radiology 1987;162:325.

James JM, Testa HJ: Imaging techniques in the diagnosis of urinary tract infection. Curr Opin Nephrol Hypertens 1994;3:660.

Kallman DA et al: Renal vein and inferior vena cava tumor thrombus in renal cell carcinoma: CT, US, MRI, and venacavography. J Comput Assist Tomogr 1992;16:240.

Kloos RT et al: Incidentally discovered adrenal masses. Endocr Rev 1995;16:460.

Lemaitre L et al: Renal angiomyolipoma: Growth followed up with CT and/or US. Radiology 1995;197:598.

McCarthy P, Pollack HM: Imaging of patients with stage D prostatic carcinoma. Urol Clin North Am 1991;18:35.

McNicholas MM et al: An imaging algorithm for the differential diagnosis of adrenal adenomas and metastases. AJR 1995;165:1453.

McSherry SA et al: Preoperative prediction of pathological tumor volume and stage in clinically localized prostate cancer: Comparison of digital rectal examination, transrectal ultrasonography and magnetic resonance imaging. J Urol 1991;146:85.

Mindell HJ: Do all homogeneously echogenic renal lesions that are smaller than 1.5 cm and are seen incidentally on sonograms lesions presumed to be angiomyolipomas require CT to confirm fat content of such lesions? AJR 1996;167:1590.

Parivar F et al: Detection of locally recurrent prostate cancer after cryosurgery: Evaluation by transrectal ultrasound, magnetic resonance imaging, and three-dimensional proton magnetic resonance spectroscopy. Urology 1996;48:594.

Postlethwaite RJ, Wilson B: Ultrasonography vs cystourethrography to exclude vesicoureteric reflux in babies. Lancet 1997;350:1567.

Rifkin MD et al: Comparison of magnetic resonance imaging and ultrasonography in staging early prostate cancer. Results of a multi-institutional cooperative trial. N Engl J Med 1990;323:621.

Sanchez-Chapado M et al: Comparison of digital rectal examination, transrectal ultrasonography, and multicoil magnetic resonance imaging for preoperative evaluation of prostate cancer. Eur Urol 1997;32:140.

Serra AD et al: Inconclusive clinical and ultrasound evaluation of the scrotum: Impact of magnetic resonance imaging on patient management and cost. Urology 1998;51:1018.

Smith RC et al: Acute flank pain: Comparison of non-contrast-enhanced CT and intravenous urography. Radiology 1995;194:789.

Thurnher S et al: Imaging the testis: Comparison between MR imaging and US. Radiology 1988;167:631.

Valji K: What is the radiologist's current role in the diagnosis and treatment of sexual impotence in men? AJR 1994;163:217.

Yoder IC, Papanicolaou N: Imaging the urethra in men and women. Urol Radiol 1992;14:24.

Zagoria RJ: With the high cost of nonionic contrast media, it has been suggested that we use a plain abdominal radiograph (KUB) and renal sonography to evaluate patients with hematuria. AJR 1995;165:1297.

Zagoria RJ, Bechtold RE, Dyer RB: Staging of renal adenocarcinoma: Role of various imaging procedures. AJR 1995;164:363.

7

Vascular Interventional Radiology

Allan I. Bloom, MD, Shelley R. Marder, MD, & Roy L. Gordon, MD

Interventional uroradiologic procedures can be divided into 2 major groups: vascular and percutaneous nonvascular. Percutaneous nonvascular interventional procedures are discussed elsewhere in this volume. The intravascular route is used, as the therapy of choice, for the embolization of arteriovenous fistulas or malformations and for bleeding sites. Transcatheter embolization is used for tumor embolization, for the ablation of renal function, and for the treatment of testicular vein and ovarian vein varices. Balloon angioplasty and stenting of stenotic renal arteries are endovascular techniques frequently used for the treatment of ischemic nephropathy and secondary hypertension. Occasionally, fibrinolytic agents are delivered via an endovascular catheter to occluded renal arteries. In this chapter we will review these intravascular interventions.

TRANSCATHETER EMBOLIZATION

Renal Arteriovenous Fistulas & Malformations

Transcatheter embolization is the treatment of choice for renal arteriovenous fistulas (AVFs), which may be congenital, spontaneous, or acquired. Iatrogenic AVFs are the type most commonly treated by transcatheter embolization. These occur as a complication of such procedures as percutaneous renal biopsy, nephrostomy placement, and pyelolithotomy (Phadke et al, 1997). Trauma or surgery can also result in AVFs (Reilly, Shapiro, and Haskal, 1996). AVF in the transplant kidney is successfully managed by embolization (Perrini et al, 1998). The classic angiographic finding of spontaneous or acquired AVF is a feeding artery with an early draining vein. Ancillary findings include pseudoaneurysm and extravasation of contrast material. Congenital AVFs (arteriovenous malformations) consist of a group of multiple coiled communicating vessels that may be associated with enlarged feeding arteries and draining veins.

The modes of clinical presentation include hematuria, retroperitoneal or intraperitoneal hemorrhage, congestive heart failure, and cardiomegaly. Hypertension can result from ischemia secondary to venous shunting of blood away from the affected area. A bruit may be heard on physical examination. Duplex Doppler ultrasound is the most useful diagnostic study, performed before angiographic intervention.

Successful intervention requires the angiographic identification, selective catheterization, and embolization of the feeding artery (Figure 7–1A, B). Using a transfemoral approach, an abdominal aortogram is performed to identify the arterial supply to the bleeding kidney. In the case of a renal transplant, an initial pelvic angiogram is performed in a steep oblique projection. The artery supplying the bleeding site is selectively catheterized. A 3F coaxial microcatheter is then used for subselective catheterization and embolization of the feeding artery. The use of a microcatheter permits accurate placement of the embolic material. Microcoils are used for the occlusion of iatrogenic AVFs because they can be deployed precisely, thereby minimizing the loss of renal parenchyma due to resultant ischemia (Figure 7–2A–C).

The procedure is usually performed without significant complications. Rarely, inadvertent nontarget embolization or thrombosis of the renal artery can occur.

Bleeding Sites

Transcatheter embolization plays a key role in the management of hemorrhage in the urinary tract originating in the kidney, ureter, bladder, and pelvis (Agolini et al, 1997). Acute life-threatening hemorrhage can occur as a consequence of trauma, instrumentation, and tumors. Chronic intractable hemorrhage is associated with radiation cystitis, tumors, prostatectomy, and infiltrative disorders. Hemodynamically stable patients undergo a noninvasive diagnostic study such as contrast-enhanced computed tomography (CT) before embolization.

Pelvic fractures resulting in life-threatening hemorrhage require embolization for control, if resuscitation and external pelvic fixation have been ineffective. Embolization has been shown to be 100%

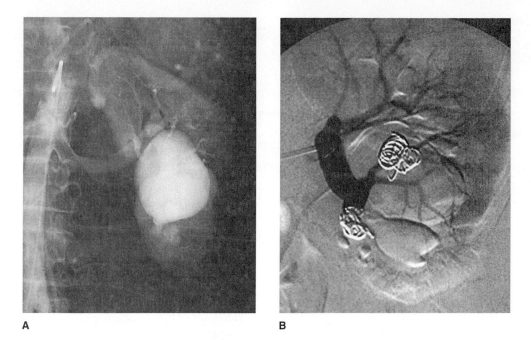

A B

Figure 7–1. Transcatheter embolization of a large arteriovenous malformation (AVM) in a 64-year-old woman who presented with hematuria. **A:** A conventional film midstream aortogram. An enlarged left renal artery is seen. There is a large serpiginous AVM arising from the lower pole renal artery branch with aneurysmal dilatation of the draining renal vein. **B:** Selective left renal digital subtraction arteriogram following coil embolization shows cessation of flow in the AVM. Coils have been placed in the terminal portion of the lower pole artery and within the AVM. Embolization resulted in resolution of the hematuria.

effective at arresting hemorrhage (Agolini et al, 1997). Using a transfemoral approach, a nonselective pelvic arteriogram is performed before selective catheterization and embolization of the hypogastric arteries. Because of contralateral crossover blood supply, pelvic lesions are treated by bilateral embolization. Gelfoam pledgets are frequently used because they can be deployed rapidly, are immediately effective if the patient has a normal coagulation profile, and produce temporary vascular occlusion. Gelfoam sponge is easily cut into pieces appropriate to the caliber of the vessel to be embolized. Coils may be used with, or instead of, Gelfoam. However, they may hamper future access to the hypogastric artery in the event of rebleeding. Small embolic materials such as Gelfoam powder or Ivalon particles are not used to treat hemorrhage from pelvic trauma because they produce peripheral occlusion of small vessels, thereby risking ischemia of nontarget organs.

Complications specific to pelvic embolization are extremely uncommon. Nontarget embolization is rare.

Tumors

Renal Cell Carcinoma: Primary renal cell carcinoma (RCC) is treated by surgical excision. In some cases, preoperative occlusive embolization of the re-

nal artery is used as an adjunct to surgery. Embolization reduces intraoperative hemorrhage and permits immediate ligation of the renal vein. It is used in patients with very large tumors and or tumors supplied by many parasitized vessels. Embolization accentuates cleavage planes and therefore facilitates nephrectomy (Wallace et al, 1981). It is performed several hours to several days before surgery.

Palliation of nonresectable disease that causes pain and hematuria can be achieved by transcatheter embolization (Park et al, 1994; Saitoh et al, 1997). Patients with bilateral RCC, and those with RCC in a single kidney, can undergo subselective embolization as an alternative to surgery, thereby sparing normal parenchyma. Occasionally, embolization of RCC metastases to bone is performed before surgical resection (Sun and Lang, 1998) to decrease intraoperative blood loss. Computed tomography or magnetic resonance imaging is used for tumor evaluation before and after intervention.

A transfemoral aortogram and selective arteriogram are performed to determine the blood supply to the kidney and tumor. An occlusive balloon catheter may be placed within the vessel and inflated before embolization to prevent reflux of embolic material and inadvertent nontarget embolization. However, many physicians use a simple selective

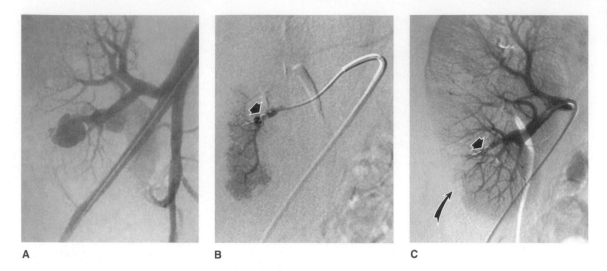

A   **B**   **C**

Figure 7–2. Transcatheter embolization of a postbiopsy arteriovenous fistula (AVF) in a 14-year-old boy with hypertension and previous renal transplantation. A bruit was heard on examination. **A:** Pelvic digital subtraction arteriogram (DSA) shows an AVF arising from a lower pole branch artery. There is aneurysmal dilatation of the draining vein. **B:** DSA shows that the renal artery has been selectively catheterized, and a 3F coaxial catheter is positioned peripherally within the lower pole branch artery supplying the AVF. Several microcoils have been placed (arrow), and no flow is seen in the AVF. **C:** Completion DSA of the main renal artery shows absent flow in the AVF (straight arrow) with minimal devascularization of lower pole parenchyma (curved arrow).

catheter. Gelfoam pledgets are used for preoperative embolization (Figure 7–3A, B). Coils are not used, because they can be dislodged during surgery when the kidney is manipulated. Absolute ethanol is the preferred embolic material for ablative palliative embolization of nonresectable tumor. Bone metastases are embolized by positioning a microcatheter in the vessel(s) supplying the tumor and injecting polyvinyl alcohol until maximal obliteration of the angiographic tumor stain is achieved.

Tumor embolization is a safe procedure. Complications such as puncture-site hematoma and inadvertent nontarget embolization occur in less than 2% of patients. Almost all patients, however, experience the postembolization syndrome, which consists of severe pain, nausea and vomiting, fever, and leukocytosis. Postembolization syndrome is probably caused by tissue necrosis that results from successful embolization. Transient ileus, transient hypertension, sepsis and reversible renal failure have also been described. This syndrome occurs within a few hours of the procedure and may last for several days. Its occurrence should not delay surgical intervention. Tissue swelling and tissue gas formation are seen on imaging studies. The severity of postembolization syndrome is related to the quantity of infarcted tissue. Analgesics and antibiotics are used for treatment. Administration of steroids and antibiotics before embolization may reduce its severity (Meglin, 1997).

Angiomyolipoma: Selective embolization has proved to be an effective method of controlling hemorrhage from benign renal lesions while preserving normal parenchyma. This technique has been used in the treatment of active bleeding from angiomyolipoma (Lee et al, 1998) and for the elective prevention of hemorrhage, especially if the tumors are multiple or bilateral, as in patients with tuberous sclerosis (Soulen et al, 1994; Han et al, 1997). The procedure is effective in decreasing tumor size and in preventing or treating hemorrhage in 85–90% of patients. Computed tomography can clearly identify the fat component of the tumor and is therefore used for diagnosis before intervention and for follow-up.

The technique for embolization is similar to that described for RCC. Using a transfemoral approach, angiography is used to define the arterial supply to the kidney and tumor. The feeding vessels are then selectively catheterized using a coaxial microcatheter. The tumor volume is estimated, and an equal amount of absolute ethanol admixed with iodized oil is carefully injected until the flow ceases. Ethanol is easy to handle, is inexpensive, and produces permanent occlusion of the vascular bed. Iodized oil is radiopaque and therefore is useful for visualizing the flow of the embolic material during the embolization. It remains within the tumor thereby allowing measurement of tumor response on follow-up CT. An occlusion balloon is reserved for more proximal embolization in a main renal artery when the risk of nontarget embolization is greatest.

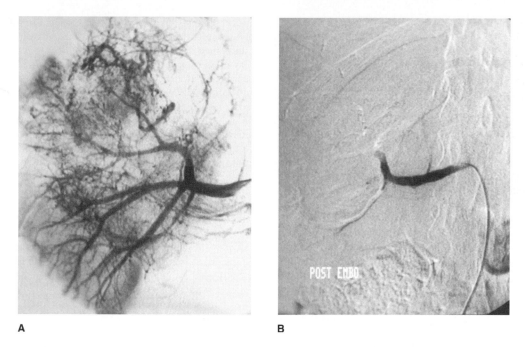

A   B

Figure 7–3. Preoperative embolization of a large right renal cell carcinoma in a 28-year-old female patient. **A:** Digital subtraction arteriogram (DSA) of the right renal artery shows a large hypervascular mass involving most of the right kidney. There is tumor thrombus within the renal vein. **B:** Completion DSA of the right renal artery after Gelfoam embolization shows complete cessation of flow within the tumor and kidney. Contrast is seen within the main renal artery only.

The reported complications are similar to those seen after RCC embolization. Recurrence of tumor hemorrhage occurs in approximately 10–15% of patients and is treated by repeat embolization.

Ablation of Renal Function: Total renal infarction using transcatheter embolization may be indicated in certain circumstances, eg, abolition of urine production to assist in healing or palliation of terminal patients with urinary fistulae; prevention of excessive proteinuria; and management of uncontrollable hypertension. For patients with end-stage renal disease and intractable hypertension or nephrotic syndrome, the advantages of ablation must be weighed against the loss of production of vitamin D_3 and erythropoietic factors and, occasionally, the loss of the ability to eliminate some water. Total renal ablation must be achieved so that perfusion of surviving parenchyma via pericapsular branches cannot occur. The embolic agent must perfuse the entire renal substance but must be safe if it passes through the kidney into the venous circulation. The technique is applicable in adults and children and in both native and allograft kidneys. Renal ablation appears to be a safe procedure and is successful in most patients (Borge et al, 1992; Golwyn et al, 1997).

Initially, a midstream aortogram is performed to identify the arterial supply to the kidneys. This is followed by renal artery catheterization and selective arteriography. An occlusion balloon catheter is placed in the vessel, and contrast is injected to measure the volume of embolic agent needed to fill the vascular tree of the kidney. Absolute ethanol is the embolic agent of choice for the reasons mentioned above. An equal volume is carefully injected with the balloon inflated to prevent reflux to nontarget regions. The contents are then aspirated, and an angiogram is performed to assess flow. The procedure is repeated as many times as necessary to completely occlude all blood flow.

Postembolization syndrome of several days' duration occurs in all patients and is managed with antibiotics and analgesics. Inadvertent embolization of the adrenal artery and other visceral vessels is a rare but serious complication that can be avoided by using the occlusion balloon technique. Systemic toxicity from ethanol injection is not a clinical problem. Morbidity and mortality from the procedure is less than that from surgical nephrectomy (Golwyn et al, 1997).

Embolization of Primary Varicocele: The subject of varicocele and male infertility is discussed in detail in Chapter 46. The basis for intervention is the presence of a varicocele on physical examination; most varicoceles are left-sided. Several reports have suggested a positive association between improvement of seminal parameters and pregnancy. Surgery and percutaneous transvenous embolization appear to be equally effective (Shlansky-Goldberg et al, 1997).

However, advantages of the percutaneous route include greater patient comfort, ease of bilateral treatment, and reduced recovery time.

The procedure is performed with conscious intravenous sedation and local anesthesia. The transjugular venous approach is preferred by many physicians, although the procedure can be performed transfemorally. Direct ultrasound guidance is used to gain access to the jugular vein; a catheter is then guided fluoroscopically into the left gonadal vein. The left gonadal vein usually drains into the left renal vein, whereas the right gonadal vein usually drains directly into the inferior vena cava. The patient is placed in reverse Trendelenburg position, and left gonadal venography is performed. A positive venogram demonstrates incompetence with filling of collateral vessels. Embolization is achieved by placing coils within the gonadal vein, commencing at the region of the inguinal ligament and continuing cranially toward the renal vein, until the gonadal vein and collateral vessels have been occluded. If a right-sided varicocele is also present, the right gonadal vein is then interrogated and embolized.

The recurrence rate of varicocele after embolization is approximately 4%. Minor complications include contrast extravasation from perforation of the vein, nontarget embolization, venospasm, and hematoma. Rarely, cardiac arrhythmia and contrast allergy can occur.

Embolization of Ovarian Vein Varices (Pelvic Congestion Syndrome): Pelvic congestion syndrome in women is a recognized cause of chronic pelvic pain that has been associated with lumboovarian vein varices. Dyspareunia may be a poor prognostic indicator (Capasso et al, 1997). Symptoms are often worse with fatigue, before menstruation, and in the upright position. Occasionally, vulval and thigh varicosities are present on examination. The cause is probably multifactorial. The diagnosis is confirmed with duplex Doppler ultrasound that is also used for postintervention follow-up. Transvenous embolization has produced durable relief of symptoms in most patients (> 70%), with most responses occurring within 2 weeks of treatment. Using a transfemoral approach, the ovarian vein is catheterized, and embolic agents such as coils or synthetic glue are deployed in the vessel at the level of the pelvic inlet.

Reported complications are similar to those for varicocele embolization. The procedure does not appear to have a deleterious effect on fertility.

RENAL ARTERY ANGIOPLASTY & STENTING

Ischemic nephropathy due to atherosclerotic vascular disease (ASVD) and renal artery stenosis is a leading cause of progressive renal failure. Renal artery stenosis is the most common cause of secondary hypertension. Surgical revascularization is an established method of treatment, with reported success rates of > 70% (Steinbach et al, 1997). In recent years, percutaneous transluminal angioplasty (PTA) and stent placement have become a viable alternative to surgery. Percutaneous transluminal angioplasty is the treatment of choice in the management of fibromuscular dysplasia, which occurs in a subset of hypertensive patients. The technique involves the use of an inflatable balloon catheter that is positioned endoluminally across the stenosis and then inflated (angioplasty).

Several diagnostic imaging modalities are used for patient selection and for post-procedure follow-up, including captopril radioisotope assay, duplex Doppler ultrasound, CT angiography, magnetic resonance angiography, and arteriography. Discussion of the advantages and disadvantages of these techniques is beyond the scope of this chapter.

Renal artery stenosis is described as ostial, nonostial, or branch vessel stenosis. An ostial lesion is located within 3 mm of the aortic lumen and is typical of ASVD. In fibromuscular dysplasia, nonostial and branch vessel lesions are more typically seen. The initial technical success rate of PTA varies. It may be as low as 35% for some ASVD ostial lesions, but in most studies the overall rate approximates 95–100%. Percutaneous transluminal angioplasty results in stabilization or improvement of renal function in > 80% of patients with ischemic nephropathy (Greco and Breyer, 1997) and leads to durable improvement or cure in 63–70% of patients with hypertension (Bonelli et al, 1995). The best results following PTA have been achieved in hypertensive patients with fibromuscular dysplasia, in whom improvement or cure is achieved in approximately 90% (Tegtmeyer et al, 1991).

Stent placement has traditionally been reserved for immediate failure or complication of PTA, such as elastic recoil or intimal dissection, for residual stenoses of > 30%, for early restenosis, and for ostial lesions that are difficult to treat by PTA alone. Renal artery stenting results in stabilization or improvement of renal function in 38% and 27% of patients, respectively, and in durable improvement or cure of hypertension in 56% and 10% of patients, respectively (Palmaz, 1998). Percutaneous transluminal angioplasty and stenting have also been used successfully to treat renal allograft artery stenosis (Sierre et al, 1998). Primary patency rates vary after stenting. In a review of the literature, the average restenosis rate was approximately 16% after a mean follow-up period of 10.9 months (Palmaz, 1998). However, the rate increased to 20–30% with longer follow-up. Secondary patency may be achieved in > 90% of patients (Blum et al, 1997).

Usually, the transfemoral approach is used, although a transaxillary approach may be required. Ini-

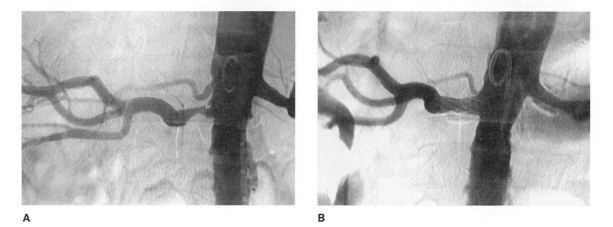

A   B

Figure 7–4. Renal artery stenting in an 80-year-old woman with labile hypertension and right renal artery stenosis due to atherosclerotic vascular disease. Her hypertension was poorly controlled on 3 antihypertensive medications. **A:** A midstream aortogram at the level of the renal arteries demonstrates a high-grade ostial right renal artery stenosis. **B:** Repeat midstream aortogram after placement of a 20-mm-long Palmaz stent, dilated to 6 mm. A widely patent renal artery is seen. The stent protrudes slightly into the aortic lumen. The patient's hypertension improved after the procedure.

tially, a midstream aortogram is performed to identify the renal arteries, followed by a selective injection to evaluate the morphologic features and location of the stenosis, the diameter of the vessel, and the percentage of stenosis. In the presence of altered renal function with elevated creatinine levels, alternatives to iodinated contrast agents include gadolinium and carbon dioxide gas. Indicators of a significant stenosis include a reduction of cross-sectional diameter of 50%, post-stenotic dilatation, collateral vessels to the affected kidney and a transtenotic systolic pressure gradient of > 20 mm Hg across the lesion. Before intervention, the patient is heparinized, and a vasodilating agent such as nitroglycerine is administered via the arterial catheter. Initially, the lesion is crossed with a guidewire. If a high-grade stenosis is present, predilatation with a small balloon may be necessary before definitive angioplasty or stent placement. An outer guiding catheter or sheath is used to facilitate contrast injection during the procedure and to improve catheter stability. Continuous fluoroscopic guidance and "vascular roadmapping" are also used to ensure precision. Frequently, a small tear in the vessel intima is seen after PTA. We prefer to use the Palmaz balloon expandable stent, as it can be accurately deployed. The stent is mounted on a balloon catheter before insertion. The minimal recommended vessel diameter for stenting is 6 mm. A 10- to 20-mm-long stent is used, and approximately 1–2 mm should protrude into the aortic lumen when ostial lesions are treated (Figure 7–4A, B).

Success of the procedure is defined by < 30% residual stenosis and by the resolution of a significant transtenotic pressure gradient. After the procedure, the patient is placed on antiplatelet medication,

such as aspirin or dipyridamole and is carefully followed up by clinical evaluation and repeat imaging.

The reported complication rate after PTA and stenting varies considerably but ranges from 3 to 10% for experienced operators. Complications include puncture-site hematoma, femoral artery pseudoaneurysm, contrast nephropathy, cholesterol embolization, stent malpositioning, and injury to the renal artery such as dissection, thrombosis, and rupture. Rarely, procedure-related deaths have occurred.

CATHETER-DIRECTED FIBRINOLYSIS

Catheter-directed fibrinolysis has been used extensively in the peripheral vasculature but with only limited success in the management of native renal artery or aortorenal bypass graft thrombosis. Small studies and individual case reports have suggested a possible role in the treatment of recent renal artery occlusion before PTA (Boyer et al, 1994; Morris et al, 1998) and for the treatment of acute renal artery thromboembolic disease.

The diagnosis is made by noninvasive imaging, such as duplex Doppler ultrasound or magnetic resonance or CT angiography, and is then confirmed by intrarterial angiography, at which time fibrinolytic therapy is begun. A diagnostic arteriogram is performed from a transfemoral approach, after which an infusion catheter or wire is embedded within the thrombosed segment. Urokinase is the most frequently used fibrinolytic agent. Several infusion protocols exist including initial "pulse spray" or bolus and low- to high-dose continuous infusion. Our preferred technique is continuous intermediate dose infusion of 150,000 U of urokinase per h in addition to systemic heparinization to prevent pericatheter thrombosis. Prophylactic antibiotics are administered. The patient is monitored for puncture-site and systemic bleeding in the intensive care or step-down unit throughout the infusion therapy. A repeat arteriogram is performed 12–24 h after the initiation of therapy. When recanalization has been achieved, an underlying stenotic lesion is usually identified, at which time PTA or stenting is performed.

Complications include puncture-site and systemic hemorrhage and infection. Bleeding may be severe enough to require transfusion or discontinue the infusion. The incidence of complications is related to the duration of therapy and to the dose administered. True allergic reactions to urokinase are rare. Shaking chills can occur, but the patient usually responds to intravenous meperidine.

REFERENCES

Agolini SF et al: Arterial embolization is a rapid and effective technique for controlling pelvic fracture hemorrhage. J Trauma 1997;43:395.

Blum U et al: Treatment of ostial renal artery stenoses with vascular endoprostheses after unsuccessful balloon angioplasty. N Engl J Med 1997;336:459.

Bonelli FS et al: Renal artery angioplasty: Technical results and clinical outcome in 320 patients. Mayo Clin Proc 1995;70:1041.

Borge MA et al: Percutaneous renal ablation in children with end-stage renal disease. J Vasc Interv Radiol 1992;3:467.

Boyer L et al: Percutaneous recanalization of recent renal artery occlusions: Report of 10 cases. Cardiovasc Interv Radiol 1994;17:258.

Capasso P et al: Treatment of symptomatic pelvic varices by ovarian vein embolization. Cardiovasc Interv Radiol 1997;20:107.

Golwyn DH Jr et al: Percutaneous transcatheter renal ablation with absolute ethanol for uncontrolled hypertension or nephrotic syndrome: Results in 11 patients with end-stage renal disease. J Vasc Interv Radiol 1997;8:527.

Greco BA, Breyer JA. Atherosclerotic ischemic renal disease. Am J Kidney Dis 1997;29:167.

Han YM et al: Renal angiomyolipoma: Selective arterial embolization—effectiveness and changes in angiomyogenic components in long-term follow-up. Radiology 1997;204:65.

Lee W et al: Renal angiomyolipoma: Embolotherapy with a mixture of alcohol and iodized oil. J Vasc Interv Radiol 1998;9:255.

Meglin AJ. Renal embolization. In: Sandhu J, Meglin AJ, Trerotola SO (editors): *SCVIR Syllabus,* vol. 7. *Thoracic and Visceral Nonvascular Interventions/Genitourinary Interventions.* Society of Cardiovascular and Interventional Radiology, 1997.

Morris CS et al: Treatment of acute aortorenal bypass graft thrombosis by means of primary stent placement and adjunctive thrombolysis. J Vasc Interv Radiol 1998;9:961.

Palmaz JC. The current status of vascular intervention in ischemic nephropathy. J Vasc Interv Radiol 1998; 9:539.

Park JH et al: Transcatheter arterial embolization of unresectable renal cell carcinoma with a mixture of ethanol and iodized oil. Cardiovasc Interv Radiol 1994;17:323.

Perrini S et al: Transcatheter embolization of biopsy related vascular injury in the transplanted kidney: Immediate and long-term outcome. J Vasc Interv Radiol 1998;9:1011.

Phadke RV et al: Iatrogenic renal vascular injuries and their radiological management. Clin Radiol 1997;52: 119.

Reilly KJ, Shapiro MB, Haskal ZJ: Angiographic embolization of a penetrating traumatic renal arteriovenous fistula. J Trauma 1996;41:763.

Saitoh H et al: Long term results of ethanol embolization of renal cell carcinoma. Radiat Med 1997;15:99.

Shlansky-Goldberg RD et al: Percutaneous varicocele embolization versus surgical ligation for the treatment of infertility: Changes in seminal parameters and pregnancy outcomes. J Vasc Interv Radiol 1997; 8:759.

Sierre SD et al: Treatment of recurrent transplant renal artery stenosis with metallic stents. J Vasc Interv Radiol 1998;9:639.

Soulen NC et al: Elective embolization for prevention of hemorrhage from renal angiomylipomas. J Vasc Interv Radiol 1994;5:587.

Steinbach F et al: Long-term survival after surgical revascularization for atherosclerotic renal artery disease. J Urol 1997;158:38.

Sun S, Lang EV. Bone metastases from renal cell carcinoma: Preoperative embolization. J Vasc Interv Radiol 1998;9:263.

Tegtmeyer CJ et al: Results and complications of angioplasty in fibromuscular disease. Circulation 1991;83 (Suppl. I)155.

Wallace SW et al: Embolization of renal carcinoma. Experience with 100 patients. Radiology 1981;138:563.

Percutaneous Endourology & Ureterorenoscopy

8

Joachim W. Thüroff, MD, & Christian P. Gilfrich, MD

In contrast to retrograde instrumentation such as ureterorenoscopy, which invades the urinary tract via the natural route of the urethra under endoscopic guidance, techniques of antegrade instrumentation involve access via a percutaneous puncture. This approach must respect the intrarenal anatomy just as in open surgical nephrotomy, and imaging techniques are essential to guide the procedure.

First, and most important, a puncture route must be established that will provide straightforward access to the target and safe, bloodless instrumentation. Thus, the location and direction of the puncture tract on the site of entry into the renal collecting system determine the success of all subsequent steps of radiologically and endoscopically controlled instrumentation. Visualization of the puncture needle and target and precise guidance to the target require the use of imaging techniques such as ultrasound, fluoroscopy, and, in selected cases, computed tomography (CT).

For percutaneous puncture, ultrasound is the imaging technique of choice. For subsequent procedures (eg, tract dilation, nephrostomy catheter placement), fluoroscopy is required. For intrarenal surgical procedures, endoscopy is superior to radiographic imaging techniques.

Contraindications to percutaneous kidney puncture are blood clotting anomalies due to coagulopathies or pharmacologic anticoagulation. Preparation and draping of the surgical field are required as for open surgery, and the same standards of asepsis must be followed. Local anesthesia only is sufficient for puncture of the kidney and small-bore tract dilation (6–12F) for antegrade insertion of a ureteral stent or nephrostomy catheter. Lidocaine hydrochloride 1% USP, 10 mL, can be given for infiltration of the skin and tissues along the intended route of puncture down to the renal capsule. During dilation of the tract, administration of a local anesthetic in lubricant (eg, lidocaine hydrochloride jelly 2%) serves the dual purpose of anesthetization and lubrication. Dilation of nephrostomy tracts up to 30F and extraction of small renal stones can be done under local anesthesia. However, extracorporeal shockwave lithotripsy

(ESWL) is the treatment of choice for most of these small stones.

Percutaneous nephrolithotomy (PNL) is still indicated for treatment of staghorn calculi and stones in caliceal diverticula, but the extent of intrarenal instrumentation for stone disintegration and extraction usually requires epidural or general anesthesia. Because puncture, tract dilation, and stone disintegration and removal are preferably performed as a one-stage procedure, the use of local anesthesia in PNL is limited.

IMAGING & PUNCTURE TECHNIQUES

Percutaneous puncture of the renal collecting system may be performed for diagnostic procedures (eg, antegrade pyelography, pressure/perfusion studies) or to establish access for therapeutic interventions such as percutaneous catheter placement or endoscopic procedures (Table 8–1). Regardless of indication, techniques for imaging and percutaneous puncture of the kidneys and retroperitoneum are identical.

Both ultrasonic scanning and fluoroscopy provide visualization and guidance for a safe, accurate percutaneous puncture, but ultrasound has definite advantages.

(1) No intravenous or retrograde administration of contrast dye.

(2) No radiation exposure.

(3) Continuous real-time control of puncture.

(4) Imaging of radiolucent, non-contrast-enhancing renal and extrarenal structures (eg, renal cyst, retroperitoneal tumor) for puncture.

(5) Imaging of all tissues along an intended nephrostomy tract (eg, bowel, lung).

(6) Imaging in numerous planes simply by shifting, tilting, and rotating the scanning head.

(7) Three-dimensional information during puncture: If the 2-dimensional image plane shows both the target and the puncture needle (which has to be directed and aligned accordingly), the position of the needle remains confined to the volume of the slice of the scan without lateral deviation of the needle into the third dimension.

Table 8–1. Indications for percutaneous puncture of the renal collecting system.

Diagnostic indications
  Antegrade pyelography
  Pressure/perfusion study (Whitaker test)
Therapeutic indications
  Nephrostomy catheter drainage
  Antegrade ureteral stenting
  Dilation of ureteral strictures
  Percutaneous endopyeloplasty
  Perfusion chemolysis of renal stones
  Percutaneous nephrolithotomy (PNL)
  Percutaneous resection and coagulation of urothelial
    tumors

Once the puncture needle has entered the renal collecting system, fluoroscopy is required for control and guidance of subsequent steps (eg, guide wire insertion, tract dilation, catheter insertion). In selected cases, insertion and placement of a nephrostomy catheter in a dilated renal system may be possible with ultrasonic control only. However, while the rigid puncture needle can be readily visualized and directed within the 2-dimensional ultrasonic scanning

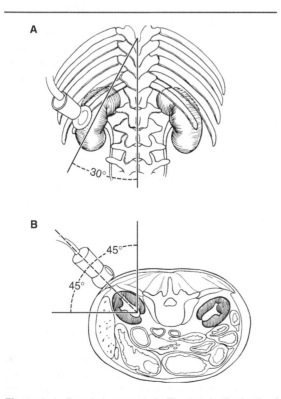

Figure 8–1. Renal ultrasound. **A:** The longitudinal axis of the kidney forms a 30-degree angle with the midline. **B:** The transverse axis of the kidney forms a 45-degree angle with both a horizontal and a vertical line.

plane, flexible instruments such as guide wires and catheters follow the anatomy of the renal collecting system and may deviate, therefore, from the scanning plane. Fluoroscopy provides a 2-dimensional image with complete integration of all information from the third (anterior-posterior) dimension, so that the entire length of radiopaque catheter, wires, and so on, can be visualized.

For percutaneous puncture of the renal collecting system, the patient should be placed on the fluoroscopy table in the prone position. Radiolucent bolsters may be placed under the abdomen to correct for lumbar lordosis and to support the kidney. A standard puncture site is in the posterior axillary line midway between the 12th rib and the ileal crest; this site ensures that later the patient does not lie on the nephrostomy catheter in the supine position. Ultrasonic scanning is performed below the 12th rib to obtain a median longitudinal scan through the kidney. For optimal coupling of the ultrasonic beam to the skin, sterile gel (eg, K-Y jelly) is applied to the skin at the scanning site. The position, rotation, and tilt of the scanning head, which determine the plane of ultrasonic scanning, must be oriented along the normal topography of the kidney. In the frontal view of an intravenous pyelogram (IVP), the long axis of the kidney usually follows the psoas muscle, forming about a 30-degree angle with the midline (Figure 8–1A). In the transverse view of a CT scan, the transverse axis of the kidney forms about a 45-degree angle with both a horizontal and a sagittal line (Figure 8–1B). The position and direction of the transducer should be oriented roughly to the following marks: below the 12th rib (if possible), cranial to the puncture site, with a 30-degree caudal-lateral rotation, and with a 45-degree lateral tilt of the scanning head. Fine adjustment of the position and direction of the scanning head must be made during imaging.

Factors that may influence the choice of scanning technique and puncture site include patient size; position and rotation of the kidney; anomalies of bony structures; positions of the colon, spleen, liver, and lung relative to the kidney; and the target of puncture (upper, middle, or lower calyx; caliceal diverticulum). Ultrasound can image all these structures, and the scanning head can be positioned to provide the best visualization and optimum puncture site for each patient. Thus, a puncture site as high as above the 11th rib may be chosen if the lung is not visualized in the puncture route. A different puncture site must be chosen if bowel gas or the liver or spleen is visualized within the intended nephrostomy route.

If puncture is performed for nephrostomy drainage of a dilated system or antegrade stent placement only, the site of entry into the collecting system is not as crucial as for endoscopic stone manipulation or other procedures. On principle, however, the route of puncture should always aim through a pyramid into a dorsal calyx; puncture into an infundibulum may result in bleeding from segmental and interlobar vessels in the renal sinus, and direct puncture of the renal pelvis renders dilation of the nephrostomy tract and insertion of catheters and instruments difficult, with increased risk of accidental catheter dislodgment after successful entry. Performance of PNL for complicated stones such as staghorn calculi or stones in caliceal diverticula requires careful planning and precise entry into the target area of the renal collecting system. For large, complete staghorn calculi, when PNL is to be performed for debulking the stone volume (followed by ESWL for disintegrating retained caliceal stones), puncture is usually performed through a lower dorsal calyx, a position from which the lower caliceal group, the renal pelvis, and part of the upper caliceal group can be reached easily with rigid instruments. However, for staghorn stones that can be completely removed by PNL alone (without ESWL), another route (eg, middle or upper calyx puncture) may be chosen. Stones in caliceal diverticula are better approached by direct puncture of the diverticulum than by puncture of the collecting system with endoscopic access to the diverticulum. In every case, peripheral puncture of the collecting system through a papilla allows maximal use of available space within the collecting system.

Once chosen, the target for access to the renal collecting system must be visualized ultrasonically. The cutaneous puncture site should be chosen in a virtual caudal extension of the perpendicular orientation (width) of the scanning plane. (Most transducers have a mark indicating the orientation of the scanning plane relative to the transducer head, or an attachment for a needle guide at this site.) Skin and fascia are incised with a No. 11 blade. At this time, the scanning head may be shifted over the incision to measure the exact distance between the incision and the target. A 16- to 18-gauge puncture needle (Figure 8–2) may then be inserted blindly through the incision and aimed in the direction previously determined by ultrasound. However, the needle should never be advanced blindly farther than through the abdominal fascia.

The scanning head is now placed in such a way that both the target and the puncture needle are visualized in the same scanning plane, and the needle is aligned so that its tip can be clearly seen. Time and patience may be necessary to align the direction of the needle and the position of the scanning head so that both the needle and the target can be seen simultaneously on the monitor. Vibrating the needle makes the tip more visible while the position of the scanning head is being adjusted. If the angle of puncture is too steep or too flat, the needle can be withdrawn into the subcutaneous fat and reinserted through the abdominal wall. The needle can be safely moved back and forth down to the renal capsule as often as necessary, but the renal parenchyma ideally should be punctured only once.

A needle guide can be used to direct the needle exactly within the ultrasonic scanning plane. This device

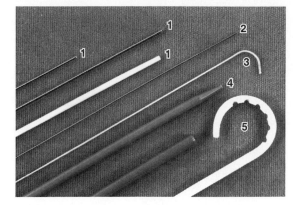

Figure 8–2. Universal nephrostomy set (Bard-Angiomed), containing (1) coaxial 17.5-gauge needle/6F catheter system with obturator; (2) fine needle (22 gauge); (3) 0.035-in stiff guidewire with floppy J-tip; (4) coaxial 10F dilator/12F introducer catheter system; and (5) 10F pigtail nephrostomy catheter.

usually has a slot or duct configuration and must be sterilized and attached to the transducer head. With some needle guides, the angle of puncture relative to the longitudinal axis of the scanning plane (depth) is also fixed and may be indicated on the monitor by an electronically generated beam. If a steeper or flatter angle of puncture is desired, the entire scanning head and attached needle guide must be tilted, and the choice of puncture site is therefore limited. Another drawback of this device is that it does not allow for independent adjustment of the puncture and scanning direction if the needle deviates from its intended direction after being advanced through the skin. This frequently occurs in patients with scars from previous operations and becomes more of a problem the farther the target is from the cutaneous puncture site. Freehand puncture with individual adjustment of puncture and scanning direction is preferable in these cases.

Movement of the kidney during respiration may complicate puncture if the target is small and is visible on the monitor only during a specific respiratory phase. If the direction of the needle and the position of the target are aligned and both are clearly seen on the monitor, the needle is advanced through the renal capsule during the appropriate phase of respiration (Figure 8–3). In this phase, the kidney is usually pushed to some extent by the puncture needle, so that visualization of needle and target may be momentarily impaired. However, as soon as the tip of the needle has penetrated the fibrous renal capsule, it is seen even more clearly as it is advanced through the renal parenchyma, which has a low echogenicity, and into a dilated calyx, the renal pelvis, or a renal cyst, all of which are free of internal echoes. If both the tip of the needle and the target are visualized clearly at the

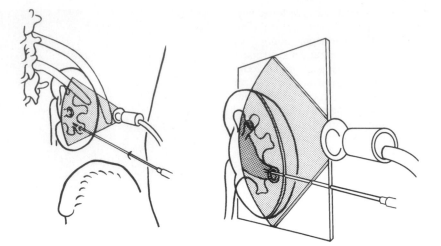

Figure 8–3. Ultrasonically guided puncture of a dorsal lower calyx. Needle must be in the scanning plane to be visualized.

same spot on the scanning plane, the needle is in the desired space.

A stone may be felt by the needle tip, or its movement may be observed on the monitor. Antegrade injection of a small amount of contrast dye for fluoroscopy outlines the renal collecting system after successful puncture. However, if the collecting system has not been successfully punctured at the first attempt, contrast dye may fill the interlobar veins, which form a basketlike structure around the calyx, or may extravasate. In rare cases in which contrast dye is injected into the adventitia of the renal collecting system, extravasation may assume the configuration of the collecting system, mimicking successful puncture. Care must be taken to inject the least amount of dye necessary so that further fluoroscopic and ultrasonic orientation will not be hindered. A larger amount of dye injected outside the collecting system may compress the calyx to be entered and render puncture more difficult. At this stage, the position of the needle tip should be checked by repeated sonography and the findings compared with the fluoroscopic appearance. If the position of the needle tip on ultrasound is close to its destination (ascertained by a small vibratory movement), the needle should be retracted a few millimeters only and readvanced at the appropriate angle and tilt. Once the collecting system is entered (Figure 8–4A), fluoroscopy alone is used to guide the subsequent steps of the procedure.

If fluoroscopy is used instead of ultrasound for guiding renal puncture, a fine-needle (20–22 gauge) puncture technique may be used. Intravenous or retrograde administration of contrast dye is needed. With retrograde injection, a ureteral balloon occlusion catheter can be inserted and blocked in the ureteropelvic junction to cause slight distention of

the renal collecting system; this facilitates puncture of a nondilated system. First, a 16- to 18-gauge needle is inserted through the abdominal wall only, and a longer fine needle is inserted coaxially through the larger needle (Figure 8–4B). This technique improves control of the fine needle. As soon as the fine needle has entered the collecting system, the larger needle can be advanced over the fine needle, which

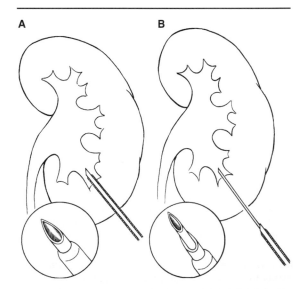

Figure 8–4. Percutaneous puncture techniques. **A:** Ultrasonically guided technique: puncture with a 16- to 18-gauge coaxial needle/catheter system. **B:** Fluoroscopically guided technique: coaxial fine-needle puncture through a larger needle/catheter system.

serves as a guide. After withdrawal of the fine needle, a regular guide wire can be inserted through the large needle into the collecting system.

Urine aspirated from the collecting system should be cultured, especially if there is suspicion of a urinary tract infection.

ANTEGRADE PYELOGRAPHY & PRESSURE/PERFUSION STUDIES

Renal puncture is rarely indicated for diagnostic antegrade pyelography only, because less invasive radiographic techniques are available (eg, intravenous pyelography with tomograms, ultrasound, CT, magnetic resonance imaging, retrograde pyelography). However, obtaining a radiograph after antegrade injection of contrast dye should be an integral part of every percutaneous puncture for any indication. Before contrast dye is injected, urine must be aspirated to decompress an obstructed collecting system. The contrast dye should be diluted to 20–30% for better visualization of details; antegrade pyelography then provides images of the collecting system with about the same resolution of detail as retrograde pyelography.

Antegrade pyelography is also performed in conjunction with a percutaneous pressure/perfusion study (Whitaker test) to assess pyeloureteral resistance. Percutaneous urodynamic studies of the dilated upper urinary tract are indicated only in the 10–30% of cases in which noninvasive radioisotope studies (diuresis renogram; see Chapter 10) fail to differentiate an obstructed from a nonobstructed dilated system (more likely in cases of ureterovesical obstruction than in pelvic-ureteral obstruction, in which diuresis renograms are reliable).

The Whitaker test provides simultaneous measurements of intrapelvic and intravesical pressures during antegrade perfusion, with flow rates of 5, 10, 15, and 20 mL/min. Puncture of the renal collecting system is performed with a coaxial needle/catheter system with an outer 6F catheter for the renal pressure/perfusion study; thus, puncture and catheter insertion can be done as a one-step procedure. Perfusion is started with flow rates of 5–10 mL/min until a steady-state equilibrium of pressure readings is reached and the entire upper urinary tract is opacified (Figure 8–5). Pressure readings may be obtained intermittently, from the perfusion catheter via a 3-way stopcock, or continuously, if a double-lumen nephrostomy catheter or 2 separate catheters for perfusion and pressure measurement are used. Continuous recordings during perfusion from a single-lumen perfusion catheter via a T connection yield erroneous pressure readings (the smaller the lumen of the nephrostomy catheter and the higher the perfusion rate, the higher the pressure reading), unless the resistance of the entire system was previously calibrated for each rate of perfusion. In order to obtain accurate pressure read-

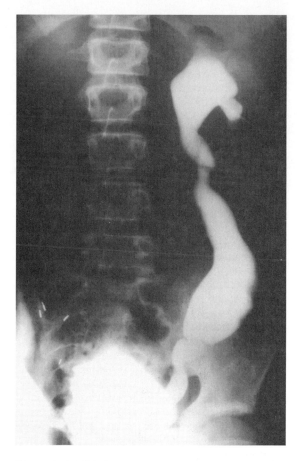

Figure 8–5. Whitaker test in a dilated upper tract after vesicoureteral reimplantation (prune belly syndrome). Antegrade perfusion with 10 mL/min results in a vesicopelvic pressure gradient of 10 cm of water, with unobstructed flow.

ings, the positions of the intrapelvic and intravesical pressure manometers must be adjusted to the level of the renal pelvis and bladder, respectively. At a flow rate of 10 mL/min, differential pressures (renal pelvic pressure minus bladder pressure) below 13 cm water are normal, between 14 and 22 cm water suggest mild obstruction, and above 22 cm water suggest moderate to severe obstruction. At flow rates of 15 mL/min and 20 mL/min, upper limits of normal pressure are 18 cm and 21 cm water, respectively.

PERCUTANEOUS CATHETER PLACEMENT

Percutaneous nephrostomy catheter placement for drainage and decompression of the upper urinary tract is indicated if retrograde ureteral catheterization is not advisable (eg, in sepsis secondary to ureteral obstruction) or proves to be impossible (eg, impassable ureteral obstruction due to stone, tumor, or stricture). Nephrostomy catheters also may be used for diagnostic purposes (Whitaker test) or therapeutic procedures (chemolysis of stones). After percutaneous endourologic procedures, a nephrostomy catheter is usually left indwelling for a few days. To convert a nephrostomy catheter diversion into an internal stent drainage, antegrade ureteral stenting through the nephrostomy tract may be attempted even in cases in which previous attempts at retrograde stenting have failed. The antegrade approach to stenting can be expected to be successful if failure of retrograde stenting was not related to mere mechanical ureteral obstruction but rather to ureteral tortuosity, false passage (ureterovaginal fistula, urinoma after open surgery), or inability to identify the orifice endoscopically (ureteroileal anastomosis).

In percutaneous puncture for catheter placement, the diameter of tract dilation depends on the size of the catheter to be inserted. For diagnostic procedures such as pressure/perfusion studies (Whitaker test), a 6F catheter is sufficient. Catheters of this size can be placed in a one-step procedure of puncture if coaxial needle/catheter systems are used (Figure 8–2). For therapeutic interventions such as nephrostomy drainage or antegrade ureteral stenting, softer, larger catheters must be inserted, and puncture tract dilation is necessary before catheter insertion. For dilation of a puncture tract, a 0.035- or 0.038-in guidewire must be inserted into the collecting system, either directly through the puncture needle or through the outer catheter of a coaxial needle/catheter system. Curved-tip (J) guidewires are less likely to cause damage to the mucosa of the renal pelvis than are straight guide wires. One of the most common problems of tract dilation is kinking of the guidewire during insertion of fascial dilators; therefore, guidewires with a floppy tip and a stiff proximal section (Lunderquist wire) are preferable over floppy guidewires. If the tip of the guidewire cannot be advanced into the renal pelvis because it is trapped in a dilated calyx with a narrow infundibulum or because an obstructing stone hinders passage, the outer catheter of a coaxial needle/catheter system can be used to manipulate the guide wire into the collecting system (Figure 8–6A), or angiographic catheters with different curved-tip configurations may be inserted over the guide wire for this purpose. Once the guidewire is in the correct position (upper calyx, renal pelvis, upper ureter), radiopaque fascial dilators can be inserted under fluoroscopic control with rotating movement of the dilator during advancement. If flexible plastic fascial dilators are used, sequential insertion of dilators of increasing size (usually in 2F steps) is necessary. If stiff metal or Kevlar dilators are used, dilation from 6F to 10–12F is possible in a one-step procedure.

After tract dilation, relatively stiff nephrostomy catheters (eg, polyethylene catheters) can be introduced easily over the guidewire. However, if softer catheters (eg, silicone or polyurethane) are to be inserted, use of an introducer catheter is helpful. An introducer catheter is also helpful for antegrade ureteral stenting and for insertion of nephrostomy catheters with various self-retaining configurations of the tip (eg, pigtail). These catheters can be stretched into a straight configuration while being inserted through the introducer catheter and over a guidewire; the tip resumes its original configuration due to the memory function of the material once the guidewire is withdrawn. The introducer catheter can be inserted with the last fascial dilator in a one-step procedure if a coaxial dilator/introducer catheter system is used (Figures 8–6B and C). The use of an introducer catheter provides universal access to the renal collecting system for placement of all types of catheters (nephrostomy catheters [Figure 8–6D], ureteral stents, balloon dilation catheters) and safety and working wires for different systems of large-bore nephrostomy tract dilation required for insertion of endoscopic instruments.

Nephrostomy catheters should be soft to avoid discomfort and irritation of the renal pelvis and should have a self-retaining mechanism or should be placed with enough slack to prevent dislodgment from the collecting system during movement of the kidney. Standard nephrostomy catheters are Malecot catheters, pigtail catheters, and loop catheters. Loop catheters have a very effective retaining mechanism; it may cause serious complications, however, if the catheter is accidentally pulled out of the kidney.

Antegrade ureteral stenting can be done through an introducer catheter using either open- or closed-tip stents. Catheters with open-tip configuration are advanced with a pusher catheter over a guidewire, which must be inserted through the introducer sheath down the ureter and into the bladder as a first step. Catheters with closed-tip configuration are advanced by pushing the indwelling wire. In either technique, a thread should be pulled through one of the proximal side holes of the catheter so that the catheter can be pulled back into the renal pelvis if it is advanced too far. The thread must be pulled out before the guidewire is withdrawn so that the pusher catheter can still hold the double-J stent in place.

An introducer catheter may also be used for insertion of a 7F balloon dilation catheter over a guidewire into the ureter to dilate ureteral strictures to 12–18F with balloon pressures of up to 15 atm. After successful dilation, an 8–10F stent is usually left indwelling for several weeks. This technique is most successful in ureteral strictures that are a complication of recent surgery for benign disorders, except ureteropelvic obstruction. Long-standing strictures or strictures due to tumor compression of the ureter, radiation damage, or ischemic ureteral necrosis after radical pelvic surgery are not likely to respond favorably to balloon dilation. Long-term results of ureteral balloon dilation cannot be determined from pub-

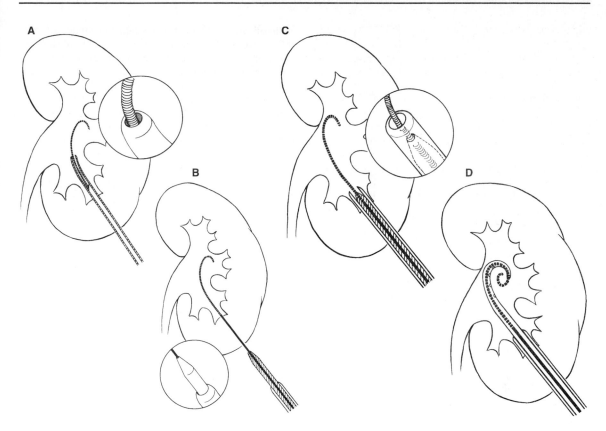

Figure 8–6. Small-bore tract dilation and nephrostomy catheter insertion. **A:** J-guidewire inserted through the needle-catheter system and advanced with assistance of the catheter into the renal pelvis. **B:** Insertion of a coaxial dilator/introducer catheter system over the guidewire. Stiff proximal section of the guidewire prevents extrarenal kinking. **C:** After the dilator has entered the collecting system, the introducer catheter is advanced over its tip. **D:** Pigtail nephrostomy catheter is inserted into the renal pelvis over the guidewire and through the introducer catheter.

lished data, either because the periods of follow-up were too short or because balloon dilations were repeated periodically.

PERFUSION-CHEMOLYSIS OF RENAL STONES

Nephrostomy catheters may be used for perfusion of the renal collecting system with chemolytic agents for dissolution of renal stones. In principle, uric acid, cystine, struvite, or apatite stones are amenable to chemolysis. However, the success of ESWL and the possibility of oral chemolysis (for uric acid stones) have limited the use of percutaneous chemolysis to adjunctive treatment of residual stones after open surgery, PNL, or ESWL. Primary percutaneous chemolysis may still be indicated in patients who are poor anesthetic risks, since anesthesia is required for several alternative procedures. Benefits of percutaneous chemolysis must be weighed against disadvantages and possible risks, eg, prolonged hospitaliza-

tion for dissolution of large stones (cystine, struvite, or apatite stones) and possible complications of treating infection stones (sepsis, hypermagnesemia).

To limit risks, perfusion chemolysis should always be performed with a double-catheter system for irrigation and simultaneous continuous drainage. This is achieved by using either 2 separately or coaxially inserted nephrostomy catheters (Figure 8–7A) or a ureteral catheter in conjunction with a nephrostomy catheter (Figure 8–7B). To ensure effective flow around the stone, the irrigation catheter must be placed close to the stone. Lack of continuous, complete drainage of the perfusate with increased intrapelvic pressures above 30 cm water may lead to pyelotubular and pyelovenous reflux of chemolytic agents and, possibly, infected urine, resulting in hypermagnesemia (perfusion with hemiacidrin or Suby's solution G or M) and sepsis. Irrigation should be started only in the absence of urinary tract infection or if infection is under control. Irrigation must first be tested with saline at the lowest possible height above kidney level to achieve a flow rate of

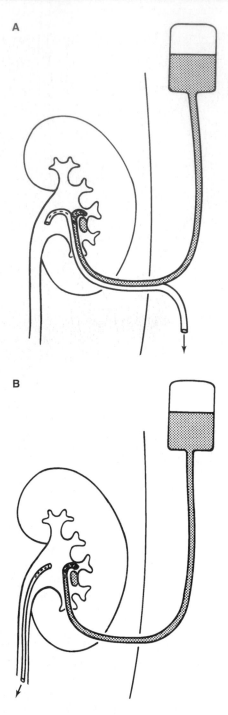

Figure 8–7. Catheter placement for perfusion chemolysis of renal stones. **A:** Perfusion and drainage of the irrigating fluid through 2 nephrostomy catheters. **B:** Perfusion through nephrostomy catheter, and drainage of the irrigant through ureteral catheter.

100–120 mL/h. Discomfort, pain, or leakage of perfusate may indicate inappropriate drainage of the irrigant, and patients should be instructed to interrupt the irrigation themselves in such instances.

Uric acid stones can be dissolved by sodium or potassium bicarbonate solution; cystine stones with D-penicillamine, acetylcysteine, or tromethamine-E solution; and struvite and apatite stones with Suby's solution G or M or hemiacidrin (Renacidin; not FDA-approved for renal irrigation). Patients must be monitored for developing urinary tract infection or fever, and serum creatinine, phosphorus (hemiacidrin-perfusion), and magnesium levels (perfusion with hemiacidrin, Suby's solution G or M) must be obtained every other day.

The time necessary for complete stone dissolution depends on the composition and size of the stone and may vary from a few days (uric acid stones) to several weeks (cystine or struvite stones).

ENDOSCOPIC INTRARENAL INSTRUMENTATION

Nephroscopes are endoscopic instruments with sheaths of 15–26F that are inserted percutaneously through a nephrostomy tract. Standard rigid instruments are available in sizes 24–26F; these have telescopes with offset eyepieces (Figure 8–8 Left). Rigid instruments such as graspers and ultrasound probes can be inserted through a central working channel (Figure 8–8 Right). Flexible fiberoptic nephroscopes may be used as well. These have a deflecting mechanism for the tip that allows inspection of otherwise difficult-to-reach calyces. A smaller working channel allows insertion of flexible instruments such as stone baskets, wire graspers, and electrohydraulic or laser probes. However, instrumentation through flexible nephroscopes is limited by the size and flexibility of working instruments such as stone forceps, and flexible endoscopes do not offer the optical quality and durability of rigid nephroscopes.

Nephroscopy is rarely indicated for diagnostic purposes only; in most cases, it is performed for percutaneous lithotripsy and extraction of renal stones (PNL). However, ESWL has gradually replaced PNL for treatment of renal stones and is now used in more than 90% of cases. PNL is still indicated in cases for which ESWL is not the primary choice of treatment. Such cases include urinary obstruction not caused by the stone itself, large-volume stones, and stones that cannot be positioned within the focus of the shock wave apparatus. Nephroscopes also may be used for direct-vision internal incision of ureteropelvic stenosis and for palliative treatment of urothelial cancer of the upper urinary tract.

Insertion of a nephroscope into the renal collecting system requires dilation of the puncture tract to 24–30F. Different systems of dilators can be em-

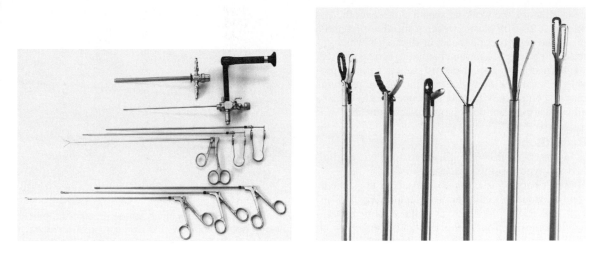

Figure 8–8. Rigid nephroscope. **Left:** A continuous-flow sheath, telescope with offset eyepiece for central access to a straight working channel, and rigid forceps and graspers. **Right:** Graspers and forceps for percutaneous endoscopic stone extraction.

ployed, all of which are introduced over a working wire. A safety wire should be inserted parallel to the working wire and advanced into an upper calyx or the upper ureter to guide the way back into the collecting system in case the dilator and working wire become dislodged accidentally. Insertion of an introducer catheter during small-bore tract dilation to 10–12F facilitates parallel insertion of safety and working wires. The central metal catheter of a coaxial metal dilator system (Figure 8–9 Left), the central plastic catheter for insertion of sequential plastic dilators, or a balloon dilator catheter can be inserted over the working wire. Balloon dilator catheters of 9F size can dilate a nephrostomy tract to a diameter of 30F under pressure up to 10–12 atm in a one-step procedure. This may prove difficult or impossible if perirenal scar tissue from previous surgery prevents complete expansion of the balloon over its entire length. Sequential plastic dilators allow stepwise dilation of the tract under fluoroscopic control; however, on withdrawal for insertion of the next larger dilator, compression of the tract is lost intermittently and bleeding occurs into the collecting system, sometimes hindering subsequent endoscopy. Coaxial metal dilators (Figure 8–9 Right) (each dilator slides over the next smaller one) allow stepwise tract dilation even in the presence of severe scarring with continuous nephrostomy tract compression for improved hemostasis.

With any dilation technique, the last step is insertion of a working sheath, which may be either the 24–26F metal working sheath of the nephroscope or a larger plastic sheath. With the balloon dilation technique, the working sheath must be introduced over a plastic dilator; with use of serial plastic or coaxial

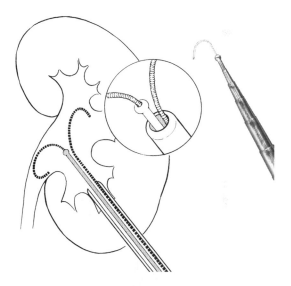

Figure 8–9. Large-bore tract dilation for nephroscopy. **Left:** Insertion of the central catheter of the Alken dilator system over a working wire through an introducer catheter (see also Figure 8–7). An introducer catheter allows parallel insertion of a safety wire into the collecting system. **Right:** Alken coaxial metal dilators for sequential tract dilation without loss of tract compression. Final step is coaxial insertion of a plastic working sheath or the metal nephroscope sheath.

metal dilators, the working sheath slides over the last dilator. A 28–30F plastic working sheath is preferable to a metal nephroscope sheath in all cases in which extensive, prolonged instrumentation is anticipated (eg, staghorn stones). Larger plastic sheaths not only provide better irrigation with lower intrapelvic pressures than do continuous-flow nephroscope sheaths but also allow easier extraction of large stone fragments.

Renal Stones

In the era of ESWL, indications for PNL are limited to 4 types of stone disease:

(1) Urinary obstruction not caused by the stone itself (eg, stone in a caliceal diverticulum [Figure 8–10 Left and Right], stone in association with ureteropelvic stenosis). These stones could be broken up by ESWL, but gravel would not pass spontaneously.

(2) Large-volume stones (> 3 cm, stone surface > 500 mm^2) (Figure 8–11 Left and Right) (eg, staghorn stones). These stones can be treated by several sessions of ESWL, but only about 30% become stone free. However, problems associated with passing large quantities of gravel (eg, ureteral obstruction, pain, fever, sepsis) can be prevented by first percutaneously debulking the stone and then performing ESWL for endoscopically inaccessible stones.

(3) Stones that cannot be positioned within the focus of the shock wave apparatus (eg, stones in kidneys with abnormal position due to anomalies of the urinary tract or skeleton, stones in transplanted kidneys).

(4) PNL may be of benefit for lower-pole caliceal calculi even under the 2–3 cm range. The overall stone-free rate for these stones with ESWL is only about 60%.

Large-volume staghorn stones are a much more common indication for PNL than stones that can be extracted in toto. Small stones can be extracted with a variety of rigid forceps and graspers (Figure 8–8

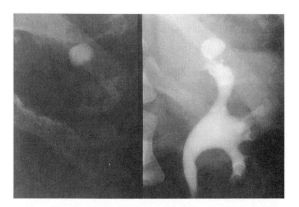

Figure 8–10. Stone in upper caliceal diverticulum requiring percutaneous nephrolithotomy. **Left:** Plain abdominal radiograph. **Right:** Intravenous pyelogram.

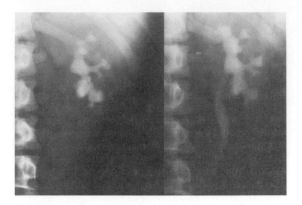

Figure 8–11. Staghorn stone requiring combined percutaneous nephrolithotomy and extracorporeal shockwave lithotripsy. **Left:** Plain abdominal radiograph. **Right:** Intravenous pyelogram.

Right). Stones may be retrieved from difficult-to-reach calyces with flexible wire baskets and graspers inserted through flexible nephroscopes. Large stones must be disintegrated using mechanical, ultrasonic, electrohydraulic, or laser energy. Strong nutcracker-type forceps (visual lithotrite, stone punch; derived from instruments for transurethral bladder stone disintegration) can be used only in a spacious renal pelvis. Hollow ultrasonic probes allow for controllable, systematic stone disintegration under continuous suction for removal of sand and smaller fragments. Electrohydraulic probes are more powerful than ultrasonic probes and may be used through flexible nephroscopes but do not provide continuous suction and are associated with a higher risk of scattering stone fragments into inaccessible calyces and of damaging the mucosa of the renal pelvis. However, with electrohydraulic probes and the holmium:YAG laser, disintegration of hard or large stones is faster.

For soft stones, continuous disintegration and evacuation of fragments with ultrasound probes is most time-efficient. Hard stones should be broken up into the largest possible fragments that can be extracted through the working sheath. The ureteropelvic portion of a staghorn stone should be left in place until the procedure is nearly completed, as it will act like a plug in a drain to prevent the loss of fragments into the ureter. An antegradely or retrogradely positioned ureteral balloon occlusion catheter might serve the same purpose; however, the extra procedure of retrograde ureteral catheterization is rarely indicated.

Normal saline should be used as the irrigation fluid except in the case of electrohydraulic lithotripsy, in which 1/6 normal saline is more appropriate. However, even with the low-pressure system provided by a large plastic working sheath, considerable amounts of irrigation fluid may be absorbed if small veins are opened and intrarenal manipulation is prolonged. This may cause transurethral resection (TUR) syndrome with use of hypotonic fluids. Intraoperative administration of diuretics (eg, mannitol, 12.5 g) is advisable and also has proved effective in preventing intrarenal reflux. If there is suspicion of extravasation, contrast dye must be injected and a diagnostic radiograph obtained. On completion of the procedure, a plain film should be obtained and a nephrostomy catheter placed. A Foley catheter with a 5-mL balloon may be inserted through a fenestrated trocar or the plastic working sheath, which then is withdrawn and cut lengthwise for removal from the Foley catheter. Malecot catheters or straight polyethylene catheters (eg, chest tubes) may be used as well and should be secured to the skin with sutures. A final nephrostogram documents appropriate position of the catheter.

Nephrostomy catheters may be removed after 1–4 days, the interval depending on the amount and duration of instrumentation and related persistence of hematuria. If ESWL is to be performed, it can be done 1–4 days after the percutaneous procedure. The nephrostomy catheter should be left in place during and after ESWL to provide drainage for urine and stone gravel and to allow for a second endoscopic procedure if some of the stone fragments do not pass spontaneously after ESWL.

Ureteropelvic Stenosis

With the advent of PNL and ureterorenoscopy, other endosurgical techniques have been developed that are similar to procedures used in the lower urinary tract. Direct-vision internal incision of ureteropelvic stenosis (pyelolysis, endopyelotomy, endopyeloplasty) seems to be a natural outgrowth of endoscopic techniques in the upper urinary tract. Compared with the retrograde techniques of endopyelotomy (incision with a cold knife, Acucise catheter, Greenwald electrode, or laser) and the endoballoon rupture, the antegrade technique offers the advantage of an incision under direct vision. The cold-knife incision must be extended into the perirenal fat and is stented for 4–6 weeks to allow for healing, according to the principle of Davis' intubated ureterotomy.

Success rates of antegrade endopyelotomy of up to 65–95% are reported for primary cases and up to 89% for secondary cases after failed open-surgical pyeloplasty.

The success rates for retrograde endopyelotomy with fewer patients and less follow-up than in antegrade endopyelotomy range between 79% and 94%, for the Acucise endopyelotomy between 73% and 81%. The candidates for best endoscopic (antegrade and retrograde) outcome are those with less than grade II hydronephrosis and good renal function.

In most reports on endopyelotomy, the criteria of success differ from those of open pyeloplasty; relief of subjective symptoms is given priority over results

of imaging studies such as decompression of a dilated collecting system on intravenous pyelography or renal ultrasound. Inadequate results after endopyelotomy may be related to a crossing vessel or to redundancy of the renal pelvis, which would be resected during open pyeloplasty. According to the law of Laplace, wall tension of a renal pelvis is, at the same intrapelvic pressures, higher in a more dilated collecting system with a larger diameter than in a less dilated system with a smaller diameter. A raised wall tension supposedly represents a more important pathogenetic factor for developing progressive dilatation than do elevated intrapelvic pressures due to anatomic obstruction of outflow. Secondary open pyeloplasty after failed endopyelotomy may be a more tedious operation with less satisfactory results in cases with extensive periureteral scarring due to extravasation of urine after endopyelotomy than primary open pyeloplasty.

Renal Pelvis Tumor

Another technique of endoscopic surgery in the upper urinary tract is use of electroresection, electrocoagulation, electrovaporization, and neodymium:YAG laser coagulation for treatment of urothelial tumors of the renal pelvis. However, with the limited reports of treatment of upper urinary tract urothelial cancer endoscopically, recurrence rates are yet to be compared with those of standard surgical treatment.

Ensuring a strict follow-up, percutaneous management of transitional cell carcinoma of the collecting system may be an alternative to nephroureterectomy for patients with grade I disease and for palliative treatment.

PERCUTANEOUS ASPIRATION & BIOPSY

Percutaneous puncture of cystic or solid lesions of the kidney and the adjacent retroperitoneum is usually performed for diagnostic purposes, in some cases in combination with therapeutic intentions such as drainage of fluid collections or obliteration of renal cysts (Tables 8–2 and 8–3). Because most of these lesions are radiolucent and are not enhanced with intravenously administered contrast dye, they cannot be visualized by fluoroscopy. Thus, ultrasound or CT is the imaging technique of choice to depict these lesions and guide percutaneous puncture. The technique of ultrasonically guided puncture is the same whether the target is the renal collecting system or a cystic or solid renal or extrarenal lesion. Depending on the purpose of the puncture, the size and configuration of puncture needles may vary. For cytologic aspiration, a fine-needle (20–22 gauge) aspiration technique is used that is comparable to fine-needle aspiration biopsy of the prostate. There is no evidence that one type of needle is preferable to the others. For aspiration and evacuation of renal cysts or

Table 8–2. Indications for puncture of renal and retroperitoneal lesions.

Diagnostic indications
Fluid aspiration
Fluid chemistry
Bacteriology and sensitivity
Cytology
Radiography with percutaneously injected contrast dye
Histology (core biopsy)
Therapeutic indications
Catheter drainage
Urinoma, lymphocele
Abscess, hematoma
Fluid evacuation and injection of sclerosing agent
Simple renal cyst

extrarenal fluid collections (urinoma, lymphocele), the same coaxial needle/catheter system can be used as for percutaneous puncture of the renal collecting system. A small catheter (6–10F) is placed for a few days to ensure complete drainage of fluid. When fluids of high viscosity (abscess, hematoma) are to be drained, large-bore catheters (14–20F) must be inserted, necessitating dilation of the percutaneous tract. Percutaneous renal biopsy for histologic diagnosis and classification of renal disease is performed with 14- to 16-gauge needles (eg, Franklin-Silverman, Tru-Cut) at the lower pole of the kidney.

Renal Cysts

Renal cysts are found in about 50% of autopsy specimens in persons over the age of 50 years and are a frequent accidental finding on ultrasound or CT studies. On ultrasound examination, a simple benign cyst will appear as a smooth-walled, echo-free spherical lesion, which may occur at any location within the kidney: it may protrude exophytically from the kidney, or be located in the renal parenchyma or re-

Table 8–3. Differential diagnosis of renal and retroperitoneal lesions.

Renal cystic lesion
Benign cyst
Hydrocalix
Abscess
Hematoma
Cystic tumor
Tumor in cyst
Retroperitoneal fluid collection
Urinoma
Lymphocele
Hematoma
Abscess
Cystic tumor
Solid renal and retroperitoneal lesions
Benign tumor
Malignant primary tumor
Metastatic tumor

nal sinus and compress the renal collecting system. Septations in a cyst and multilocular cysts may be difficult to differentiate from tumors on ultrasound, and CT may become necessary; however, only a few cases require diagnostic percutaneous puncture. Indications for diagnostic puncture of a cystic lesion are an irregular, thick wall and internal echoes on ultrasound examination, density numbers on CT higher than those of serous fluid, and hematuria. Puncture for therapeutic procedures (evacuation of fluid and instillation of a sclerosing agent) is indicated only if, due to its size or location, the cyst causes compression and urinary obstruction of a caliceal infundibulum or the ureter, or discomfort and pain.

Various tests may be performed on aspirated fluid. No one test is pathognomonic except cytologic findings of malignant cells. However, neoplasms within a cyst are exceedingly rare, and cystic degeneration of a renal neoplasm can usually be easily identified by ultrasound and CT. Benign cysts contain clear, straw-colored fluid with low fat and protein content and lactic acid dehydrogenase (LDH) levels of less than 250 mIU/mL. Cancer is suspected if the fluid is bloody or murky and has a high content of fat, protein, and LDH. After aspiration of 20–30% of the cystic fluid, the same amount of 60% contrast dye is injected, and diagnostic radiographs are obtained in the prone, supine, upright, decubitus, and Trendelenburg positions. If necessary, another 20–30% of the cystic fluid may be replaced by air for obtaining double-contrast radiographs.

For therapeutic obliteration of cysts, sclerosing agents such as Pantopaque or 95% ethanol can be injected after complete evacuation of the cystic fluid. A volume of 10–100 mL of 95% ethanol, approximating 10–20% of the original volume of cystic fluid, is injected into the cyst and should be drained after 30 min.

Retroperitoneal Fluid Collections

Low-viscosity retroperitoneal fluid collections (urinoma, lymphocele) are usually a complication of surgical procedures. However, urinoma may also be caused by exogenous trauma or by fornix rupture due to acute ureteral obstruction. Percutaneous techniques of catheter drainage eliminate the need for open surgical revision in most cases.

Insertion of a small (6–10F) catheter (with numerous side holes) is usually sufficient. Adjunctive procedures are performed to ensure sealing of the fluid leak and obliteration of the cystic lesion. In cases of urinoma, the upper urinary tract must also be drained by a ureteral catheter or percutaneous nephrostomy catheter until drainage from the urinoma stops. Lymphoceles that develop following pelvic or retroperitoneal lymphadenectomy or renal transplantation often undergo spontaneous regression and usually do not require puncture and drainage. However, large lymphoceles developing after retroperitoneal lymphadenectomy may cause pain and even ureteral obstruction (Figure 8–12). Patients should be treated with parenteral nutrition and abdominal compression by bandaging, but if lymph drainage after percutaneous puncture and catheter placement persists for more than 1 week, surgical intervention with intraperitoneal marsupialization of the lymphocele and ligation or electrocoagulation of lymphatic vessels is indicated.

High-viscosity fluid collections (hematoma, abscess) usually require large-bore (14–20F) percutaneous catheters for sufficient drainage. Perirenal hematomas are most frequently caused by surgical or exogenous trauma and rarely develop spontaneously in the presence of a bleeding disorder or due to rupture of a renal tumor. Indications for percutaneous drainage are rare, as most small hematomas resolve spontaneously and should be followed by ultrasound or CT only. A hematoma that increases in size requires surgical intervention rather than percutaneous drainage. Secondary infection of a hematoma may be an indication for percutaneous drainage.

A perirenal abscess is mostly a complication of open surgery; hematogenic renal abscess (renal carbuncle) is less frequent. Indications for puncture and drainage should be based on CT finding of a unifocal process that can be effectively and safely drained percutaneously. Multifocal renal abscess formation is not amenable to percutaneous drainage.

Renal & Retroperitoneal Tumors

Percutaneous aspiration biopsy of renal and retroperitoneal tumors is indicated if less invasive radiographic studies are inconclusive and if cytologic findings may have an impact on further medical or surgical therapy (Figure 8–13). If curative treatment by open surgery seems to be feasible, aspiration biopsy is generally not indicated. If the identity of a renal lesion is questionable or if conservative, organ-sparing surgery is technically feasible, surgical excision of the lesion with intraoperative frozen sections is preferable over percutaneous aspiration biopsy. However, aspiration biopsy may be indicated to avoid radical nephrectomy of a possibly benign lesion. In multifocal or possibly metastatic lesions, cytologic evaluation can be crucial for planning surgical or medical therapy, and in these cases, aspiration biopsy is usually indicated. Interpretation of cytologic findings is limited by a 10–25% incidence of false-negative findings and the difficulty in discriminating normal renal tubular cells from low-grade renal cell cancer. As a rare complication, tumor seeding in the puncture tract has been described. The aspirate is immediately spread on glass slides. For standard Papanicolaou stains, alcohol fixation must be used.

Renal Biopsy

Renal biopsy for diagnosis and classification of medical renal disease can be performed percutaneously or by open surgery. Because specimens, rather than aspirates, are needed for diagnostic histologic study, large-bore (14–16 gauge) Franklin-Silverman or Tru-Cut needles are used. Ultrasonic or fluoroscopic guidance is preferable to blind renal puncture. However, even with puncture aimed precisely at the dorsal aspect of the lower pole of the kidney, where accidental injury to large vessels is less likely, bleeding is to be expected because of the vascularity of the parenchyma and is the major complication of this procedure (about 5% of cases, with a mortality rate of 0.1%). Hematoma can usually be followed conservatively by ultrasound or CT, but transvascular embolization, open surgical revision, and even nephrectomy have been required following diagnostic renal biopsy. Therefore, open surgical biopsy rather than percutaneous biopsy is indicated in patients with solitary kidneys or uncontrolled hypertension.

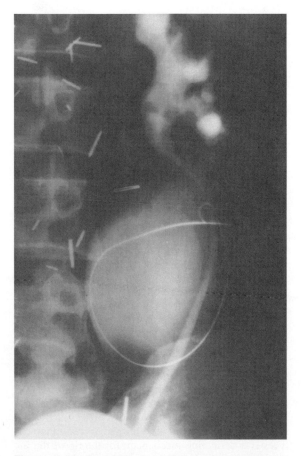

Figure 8–12. Percutaneous drainage of a lymphocele causing ureteral displacement and compression.

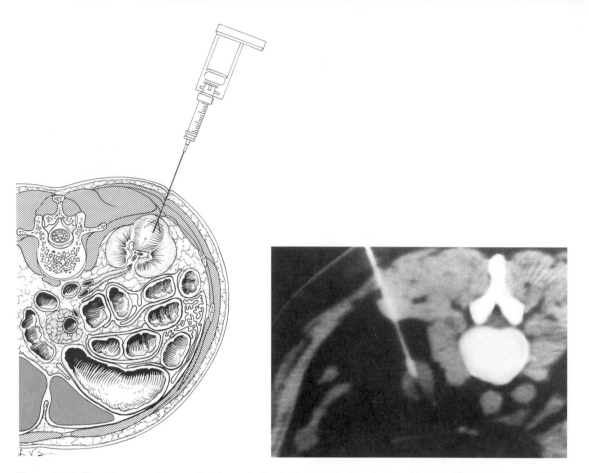

Figure 8–13. Percutaneous fine-needle biopsy. **Left:** Aspiration biopsy of a renal lesion. **Right:** Guidance with computed tomography scanning for fine-needle aspiration biopsy of an exophytic renal cell carcinoma.

URETERORENOSCOPY

Ureterorenoscopy (URS) is endoscopy of the ureter up to the renal pelvis for both diagnostic evaluation and therapeutic intervention (Table 8–4). Treatment of ureteral stones is the most frequent indication for therapeutic ureterorenoscopy; other indications are endoscopic treatment of ureteral strictures or ureteral tumors.

Table 8–4. Indications for ureterorenoscopy.

Diagnostic indications
  Lesions of ureter or renal pelvis
  Hematuria from upper tract
Therapeutic indications
  Ureteral stone treatment
  Direct vision internal ureterotomy of ureteral strictures
  Endoscopic resection and coagulation of ureteral tumors

Ureterorenoscopes (Figure 8–14) are endoscopes for retrograde insertion into the ureter; however, they also may be used in an antegrade fashion via a percutaneously established nephrostomy tract. Rigid ureterorenoscopes are available in sizes 6.9–12.6F, and semirigid fiberoptic ureterorenoscopes and flexible ureterorenoscopes may be found in sizes 6.2–9.3F. The size of the instrument chosen depends on the diagnostic or therapeutic use. The smallest instruments, which allow easier and safer instrumentation, do not provide a working channel and are for diagnostic procedures only. Larger instruments, with a 3–6F working channel, can accept stone baskets, wire graspers, stone forceps, biopsy forceps, and ultrasonic, electrohydraulic, or laser probes for stone disintegration. Flexible ureterorenoscopes follow the topographic anatomy of the ureter more easily and facilitate inspection of middle and lower renal calyces if a deflecting mechanism for the tip of the instrument is provided. However, the use of instrumentation through flexible nephroscopes is limited by the

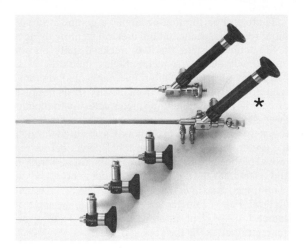

Figure 8–14. Ureterorenoscopes: Telescopes with center and offset eyepieces for use through a 12.5F working sheath. 10.5F ureterorenoscope with integrated sheath (asterisk).

visibility. If the urine has cleared, the chances of identifying a lesion that could not be detected on radiographic studies are small as well.

Ureteral Stones

Ureterorenoscopy is most frequently performed for treatment of ureteral stones, although more than 90% of ureteral stones can be treated by ESWL either in situ or after dislodgment of the ureteral stone into the renal pelvis using a ureteral catheter (push-back or flush-back procedures). For the remaining indications of ureteral stone treatment, ureterorenoscopy is used for extraction of stones, dislodgment of stones into the renal pelvis for subsequent ESWL, and intraureteral stone disintegration.

For extraction of distal ureteral stones that are unresponsive to ESWL, short rigid ureterorenoscopes and alligator forceps or Dormia baskets are most helpful. Impacted proximal ureteral stones that did not respond to in situ ESWL and could not be dislodged with a ureteral catheter usually can be repositioned into the renal pelvis under direct vision for

size and flexibility of working instruments such as stone forceps, and flexible ureterorenoscopes do not offer the optical quality and durability of rigid instruments.

Insertion of a ureterorenoscope into the ureteral orifice may be facilitated by dilation of the intramural ureter, either with sequential plastic dilators of increasing size, which are slid over a guidewire, or with a balloon dilator catheter (Figure 8–15). Dilation of the ureter is often unnecessary if a small (3–5F) ureteral catheter is inserted through the working channel of the ureterorenoscope into the ureter as a guide, and the ureterorenoscope is then rotated 180 degrees and introduced in an upside-down orientation (Figure 8–16). In this position, the ureteral catheter will spread the roof of the intramural ureter like a tent and the nose of the instrument will slide flat on the trigone into the orifice. The orifice and intramural ureter will thus be dilated only to the extent necessary for insertion of the instrument.

Diagnostic Ureterorenoscopy

Indications for diagnostic ureterorenoscopy are those rare lesions of the ureter or renal pelvis whose nature cannot be determined with less invasive diagnostic procedures such as retrograde pyelography, selective urinary cytology, CT, or magnetic resonance imaging. If a small ureterorenoscope without a working channel is used for a diagnostic procedure, a biopsy of a lesion cannot be obtained. If ureterorenoscopy is performed for evaluation of hematuria from the upper tract, the source of bleeding can rarely be identified during gross hematuria because of limited irrigation through ureterorenoscopes, resulting in poor

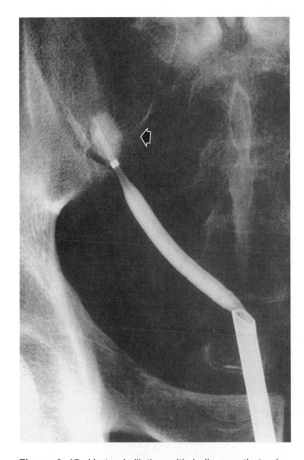

Figure 8–15. Ureteral dilation with balloon catheter before ureterorenoscopic removal of a distal ureteral stone (arrow).

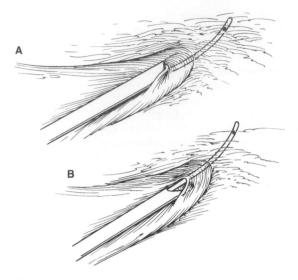

Figure 8–16. Ureterorenoscopy. **A:** Straightforward advancement of the instrument over a thin ureteral catheter can catch the mucosa of the orifice. **B:** With 180-degree upside-down rotation of the instrument, the ureteral catheter holds the orifice open like a tent.

subsequent ESWL using a small semirigid or rigid ureterorenoscope. If the stones are too large or impacted, intraureteral lithotripsy for stone disintegration may be necessary in a few cases.

To prevent the pushing back of stones or fragments into the renal pelvis during lithotripsy, a 3F wire basket can be used to hold the stone during disintegration or a 3F balloon catheter can be passed alongside the stone and be blocked proximally. Ultrasound probes allow safe stone disintegration under continuous suction, but they are not as effective as electrohydraulic and laser probes and can be used through rigid ureterorenoscopes only. Both electrohydraulic and laser probes can be used through rigid or flexible ureterorenoscopes. Laser probes for intraureteral lithotripsy have the smallest diameter (< 1F) and do not injure the mucosa of the ureter if used under direct vision. Several pulsed lasers such as the holmium:YAG laser, pulsed-dye laser, and Alexandrite laser are available for intraureteral lithotripsy. Electrohydraulic probes, which are available in sizes 1.6–5F, require less expensive equipment, but they bear the risk of ureteral damage if used inappropriately.

If ureteral perforation occurs as a complication of intraureteral instrumentation, ureteral stenting using a 6–8F double-J stent for 2–6 weeks usually allows healing without late sequelae. Stents should be used for a few days even after uncomplicated ureterorenoscopy to prevent pain from urinary stasis because of edema of the intramural ureter after instrumentation. Stents are easily introduced over a guidewire (open tip technique), which should be inserted through the ureterorenoscope into the renal pelvis before removal of the instrument. If there is ureteral perforation and a stent has been placed, the bladder should be on continuous drainage for a few days using a transurethral Foley catheter or a suprapubic cystotomy catheter to prevent urinoma formation from vesicoureteral reflux via the double-J stent.

Ureteral Strictures

Direct-vision internal ureterotomy of ureteral strictures is the ureterorenoscopic variant of percutaneous endopyeloplasty for ureteropelvic stenosis (see the section: Endoscopic Intrarenal Instrumentation, Ureteropelvic Stenosis). Cold-knife incision of the stenosis into the periureteral fat and stenting of the ureter for 4–6 weeks are the principles of Davis' intubated ureterotomy. Success rates depend on the extent of the stricture, its cause, and its duration.

Best results are obtained in ureteral strictures that are a complication of surgery for benign disorders if treatment is established early. However, long-term results of this technique as compared with open surgical repair remain to be determined. Long-standing strictures or strictures due to external ureteral compression, radiation damage, or ischemic ureteral necrosis after surgery are not satisfactorily treated by internal ureterotomy.

Ureteral Tumors

Endoscopic electroresection and laser coagulation of ureteral tumors are the ureterorenoscopic variants of percutaneous endoscopic treatment of renal pelvis tumors (see the section: Endoscopic Intrarenal Instrumentation, Renal Pelvis Tumor). While a rare, benign fibroepithelioma of the ureter is sufficiently treated by ureterorenoscopic techniques, the same precautions and limitations apply for endoscopic treatment of urothelial cancer of the ureter as listed previously for percutaneous endoscopic treatment of renal pelvis tumors. Recurrence rates remain to be determined as compared with standard surgical treatment, and indications need to be defined in regard to tumor location, multiplicity, staging, and grading.

REFERENCES

PERCUTANEOUS PUNCTURE & CATHETER PLACEMENT

Davidoff R, Bellman GC: Influence of technique of percutaneous tract creation on incidence of renal hemorrhage. J Urol 1997;157:1229.

Dyer RB, Assimos DG, Regan JD: Update on interventional uroradiology. Urol Clin North Am 1997;24: 623.

Goodwin WE, Casey WC, Woolf W: Percutaneous trocar (needle) nephrostomy in hydronephrosis. JAMA 1955;157:891.

Kaye KW, Goldberg ME: Applied anatomy of the kidney and ureter. Urol Clin North Am 1982;9:3.

Lau MWM et al: Urinary tract obstruction and nephrostomy drainage in pelvic malignant disease. Br J Urol 1995;76:565.

Pedersen JF: Percutaneous nephrostomy guided by ultrasound. J Urol 1974;112:157.

Seldinger SI: Catheter: Catheter replacement of the needle in percutaneous arteriography. Acta Radiol 1953; 39:368.

Smith AD, Badlani GH: Special use of retrograde percutaneous nephrostomy in endourology. J Endourol 1987;1:23.

Thüroff JW, Alken P: Ultrasound for renal puncture and fluoroscopy for tract dilatation and catheter placement: A combined approach. Endourology 1987;2:1.

Thüroff JW, Becht E: Urologists ultrasound. In: Lytton B et al (editors): *Advances in Urology,* vol. 1. Year Book Medical Publishers, 1988.

Watson G: Problems with double-J stents and nephrostomy tubes. J Endourol 1997;11:413.

ANTEGRADE PRESSURE/PERFUSION STUDIES

Ahlawat R, Basarge N: Objective evaluation of the outcome of endopyelotomy using Whitaker's test and diuretic renography. Br J Urol 1995;76:686.

Jones A et al: Compliance studies, pressure flow measurements and renal function assessment in patients with upper urinary tract dilatation. J Urol 1987;138:571.

Kashi SH, Irving HC, Sadek SA: Does the Whitaker test add to antegrade pyelography in the investigation of collecting system dilatation in renal allografts? Br J Radiol 1993;66:877.

Pagne S, Ramsay J: The effect of double-J-stents on renal pelvic dynamics in the pig. J Urol 1988;140:637.

Whitaker RH: Methods of assessing obstruction in dilated ureters. Br J Urol 1973;45:15.

Whitaker RH, Buxton-Thomas MS: A comparison of pressure flow studies and renography in equivocal upper urinary tract obstruction. J Urol 1984;131:446.

Woodburg P et al: Constant pressure perfusion: A method to determine obstruction in the upper urinary tract. J Urol 1989;142:632.

PERCUTANEOUS RENAL STONE TREATMENT

Alken P, Günther R, Thüroff J: Percutaneous nephrolithotomy: A routine procedure? Br J Urol [Suppl] 1983; 51:1.

Alken P et al: Extracorporeal shock wave lithotripsy (ESWL): Alternatives and adjuvant procedures. World J Urol 1985;3:48.

Callaway TW et al: Percutaneous nephrolithotomy in children. J Urol 1992;148:1067.

Carr LK et al: New stone formation: A comparison of extracorporeal shock wave lithotripsy and percutaneous nephrolithotomy. J Urol 1996;155:1565.

Cato AR, Tulloch AGS: Hypermagnesemia in a uremic patient during renal pelvis irrigation with renacidin. J Urol 1974;111:313.

el-Damanhoury H, Burger R, Hohenfellner R: Surgical aspects of urolithiasis in children. Pediatr Nephrol 1991;5:339.

Esuvaranathan K et al: Stones in horseshoe kidneys: Results of treatment by extracorporeal shock wave lithotripsy and endourology. J Urol 1991;146:1213.

Fernström I, Johansson B: Percutaneous pyelolithotomy: A new extraction technique. Scand J Urol Nephrol 1976;10:257.

Jones DJ, Wickham JE, Kellet MJ: Percutaneous nephrolithotomy for calculi in horseshoe kidneys. J Urol 1991;145:481.

Jones DJ et al: The changing practice of percutaneous stone surgery. Review of 1000 cases 1981–1988. Br J Urol 1990;66:1.

Kamihira O et al: Long-term stone recurrence rate after extracorporeal shock wave lithotripsy. J Urol 1996; 156:1267.

Kurzrock EA et al: Endoscopic management of pediatric urolithiasis. J Pediatr Surg 1996;31:1413.

Lingemann J et al: Comparison of results and morbidity of percutaneous nephrostolithotomy and extracorporeal shockwave lithotripsy. J Urol 1987;138:485.

McDougall E et al: Comparison of extracorporeal shockwave lithotripsy and percutaneous nephrolithotomy for the treatment of renal calculi in lower pole calices. J Endourol 1989;3:265.

Meretyk S et al: Complete staghorn calculi: Random prospective comparison between extracorporeal shock wave lithotripsy monotherapy and combined with percutaneous nephrolithotomy. J Urol 1997;157:780.

Minon Cifuentes J et al: Percutaneous nephrolithotomy in transplanted kidney. Urology 1991;38:232.

Motola JA, Smith AD: Therapeutic options for the management of upper tract calculi. Urol Clin North Am 1990;17:191.

Narasimham DL et al: Percutaneous nephrolithotomy through an intercostal approach. Acta Radiol 1991; 32:162.

Rao PN et al: Prediction of septicemia following endourological manipulation for stones in the upper urinary tract. J Urol 1991;146:955.

Saad F et al: Staghorn calculi treated by percutaneous nephrolithotomy: Risk factors for recurrence. Urology 1993;41:141.

Saxby MF et al: A case-control study of percutaneous nephrolithotomy versus extracorporeal shock wave lithotripsy. Br J Urol 1997;79:317.

Segura JW: Role of percutaneous procedures in the management of renal calculi. Urol Clin North Am 1990; 17:207.

Segura JW et al: Percutaneous removal of kidney stones: Review of 1000 cases. J Urol 1985;134:1077.

Smith JJ III, Hollowell JG, Roth RA: Multimodality treatment of complex renal calculi. J Urol 1990;143:891.

Suby HI, Albright F: Dissolution of phosphatic urinary calculi by the retrograde introduction of citrate solution containing magnesium. N Engl J Med 1943;228:81.

Teichmann JM et al: Holmium:YAG percutaneous nephrolithotomy: The laser incident angel matters. J Urol 1998;159:690.

Thüroff JW, Alken P: Stones in caliceal diverticula: Removal by percutaneous nephrolithotomy. In: Jonas U, Dabhoiwala NF, Debruyne FMJ (editors): *Endourology: New and Approved Techniques.* Springer-Verlag, 1988.

Wolf JS Jr, Clayman RV: Percutaneous nephrostolithotomy. What is its role in 1997? Urol Clin North Am 1997;24:43.

PERCUTANEOUS ENDOSCOPIC SURGERY

Aslan P, Preminger GM: Retrograde balloon cautery incision of ureteropelvic junction obstruction. Urol Clin North Am 1998;25:295.

Bierkens AF et al: Anterograde percutaneous treatment of ureterointestinal strictures following urinary diversion. Eur Urol 1996;30:363.

Clayman RV et al: Ureteronephroscopic endopyelotomy. J Urol 1990;144:246.

Danuser H et al: Endopyelotomy for primary ureteropelvic junction obstruction: Risk factors determine the success rate. J Urol 1998;159:56.

Davis DM: Intubated ureterotomy: A new operation for ureteral and ureteropelvic strictures. Surg Gynecol Obstet 1943;76:513.

Elliott DS et al: Long-term follow-up of endoscopically treated upper urinary tract transitional cell carcinoma. Urology 1996;47:819.

Figenshau RS, Clayman RV: Endourologic options for management of ureteropelvic junction obstruction in the pediatric patient. Urol Clin North Am 1998;25:199.

Gill HS, Liao JC: Pelvi-ureteric junction obstruction treated with Acucise retrograde endopyelotomy. Br J Urol 1998;82:8.

Goldfischer ER, Smith AD: Endopyelotomy revisited. Urology 1998;51:855.

Goldfischer ER et al: Techniques of endopyelotomy. Br J Urol 1998;82:1.

Gupta M et al: Open surgical exploration after failed endopyelotomy: A 12-year perspective. J Urol 1997;157:1613.

Hoenig DM et al: Impact of etiology of secondary ureteropelvic junction obstruction on outcome of endopyelotomy. J Endourol 1998;12:131.

Hulbert J, Hunter D, Castaneda-Zuniga W: Classification of and techniques for the reconstitution of acquired strictures in the region of the ureteropelvic junction. J Urol 1989;140:468.

Hulbert JC et al: Percutaneous intrarenal marsupialization of a perirenal cystic collection: Endocystolysis. J Urol 1988;139:1039.

Jabbour ME et al: Endopyelotomy after failed pyeloplasty: The long-term results. J Urol 1998;160:690.

Jarrett TW et al: Percutaneous management of transi-tional cell carcinoma of the renal collecting system: 9-year experience. J Urol 1995;154:1629.

Martinez-Pineiro JA et al: Endourological treatment of upper tract urothelial carcinomas: Analysis of a series of 59 tumors. J Urol 1996;156:377.

Meretyk I, Meretyk S, Clayman RV: Endopyelotomy: Comparison of ureteroscopic retrograde and antegrade percutaneous techniques. J Urol 1992;148:775.

Motola JA, Badlani GH, Smith AD: Results of 212 consecutive endopyelotomies: An 8-year followup. J Urol 1993;149:453.

Nadler RB et al: Acucise endopyelotomy: Assessment of long-term durability. J Urol 1996;156:1094.

Nakada SY, Clayman RV: Percutaneous electrovaporization of upper tract transitional cell carcinoma in patients with functionally solitary kidneys. Urology 1995;46:751.

Nakada SY et al: Retrospective analysis of the effect of crossing vessels on successful retrograde endopyelotomy outcomes using spiral computerized tomography angiography. J Urol 1998;159:62.

Ozgok IY et al: Intrarenal pressure following pyeloplasty or percutaneous surgery. Br J Urol 1991;67:251.

Patel A et al: Long-term outcome after percutaneous treatment of transitional cell carcinoma of the renal pelvis. J Urol 1996;155:868.

Segura JW: Antegrade endopyelotomy. Urol Clin North Am 1998;25:311.

Shalhav AL et al: Adult endopyelotomy: Impact of etiology and antegrade versus retrograde approach on outcome. J Urol 1998;160:685.

Shalhav AL et al: Endopyelotomy for high-insertion ureteropelvic junction obstruction. J Endourol 1998;12:127.

Van Cangh PJ, Nesa S: Endopyelotomy. Urol Clin North Am 1998;25:281.

Wolf JS: Retrograde acucise endopyelotomy. Urology 1998,51:859.

PERCUTANEOUS ASPIRATION & BIOPSY

Bodner L et al: The role of interventional radiology in the management of intra- and extra-peritoneal leakage in patients who have undergone continent urinary diversion. Cardiovasc Intervent Radiol 1997;20:274.

Bolton WK, Vaughan ED: A comparative study of open surgical and percutaneous renal biopsies. J Urol 1977;117:696.

Bush WH Jr, Burnett LL, Gibbons RP: Needle tract seeding of renal cell carcinoma. AJR 1977;129:725.

Coptcoat MJ, Ison KT, Wickham JE: Endoscopic tissue liquidization and surgical aspiration. J Endourol 1988;2:321.

Diaz-Buxo JA, Donadio JV Jr: Complications of percutaneous renal biopsy: An analysis of 1,000 consecutive biopsies. Clin Nephrol 1975;4:223.

Ferrucci JT et al: Malignant seeding of the tract after thin-needle aspiration biopsy. Radiology 1979;130:345.

Gibbons RP, Bush WH Jr, Burnett LL: Needle tract seeding following aspiration of renal cell carcinoma. J Urol 1977;118:865.

Herts BR, Baker ME: The current role of percutaneous biopsy in the evaluation of renal masses. Semin Urol Oncol 1995;13:254.

Kovalik EC et al: No change in complication rate using spring-loaded gun compared to traditional percutaneous renal allograft biopsy techniques. Clin Nephrol 1996;45:383.

Marwah DS, Korbet SM: Timing of complications in percutaneous renal biopsy: What is the optimal period of observation? Am J Kidney Dis 1996;28:47.

Sadi MV, Nardozza A, Gianotti J: Percutaneous drainage of retroperitoneal abscesses. J Endourol 1988;2:293.

Schmidt A, Baker R: Renal biopsy in children: Analysis of 61 cases of open wedge biopsy and comparison with percutaneous biopsy. J Urol 1976;116:79.

Wehle MJ, Grabstald H: Contraindications to needle aspiration of a solid renal mass: Tumor dissemination by renal needle aspiration. J Urol 1986;136:446.

STONE BASKETING, URETERORENOSCOPY

Aso Y et al: Treatment of staghorn calculi by fiberoptic transureteral nephrolithotripsy. J Urol 1990;144:17.

Berkoff WB, Meijer F: Percutaneous antegrade fiberoptic ureterorenoscopic treatment of ureteral calculi. J Urol 1990;144:628.

Clayman RV et al: Ureterorenoscopic endopyelotomy. J Urol 1990;144:246.

Conlin MJ, Marberger M, Bagley DH: Ureteroscopy, development and instrumentation. Urol Clin North Am 1997;24:25.

Denstedt J, Clayman R: Electrohydraulic lithotripsy of renal and ureteral calculi. J Urol 1990;143:13.

Dourmashkin RL: Cystoscopic treatment of stones in the ureter with special reference to large calculi: Based on a study of 1550 cases. J Urol 1945;54:245.

Dretler SP: Clinical experience with electromechanical impactor. J Urol 1993;150:1402.

Elashry OM et al: Flexible ureteroscopy: Washington University experience with the 9.3F and 7.5F flexible ureteroscopes. J Urol 1997;157:2074.

Erhard M, Salwen J, Bagley DH: Ureteroscopic removal of mid and proximal ureteral calculi. J Urol 1996;155:38.

Evans CP, Stoller ML: The fate of the iatrogenic retroperitoneal stone. J Urol 1993;150:827.

Gautier JR et al: Pulsed dye laser in the treatment of 325 calculi of the urinary tract. Eur Urol 1990;18:6.

Goldfischer ER, Gerber GS: Endoscopic management of ureteral strictures. J Urol 1997;157:770.

Gould DL: Holmium:YAG laser and its use in the treatment of urolithiasis: Our first 160 cases. J Endourol 1998;12:23.

Grasso M et al: Techniques in endoscopic lithotripsy using pulsed dye laser. Urology 1991;37:138.

Grocela AJ, Dretler SP: Intracorporeal lithotripsy. Urol Clin North Am 1997;24:13.

Higashihara E et al: Laser ureterolithotripsy with combined rigid and flexible ureterorenoscopy. J Urol 1990;143:273.

Hill DE et al: Ureteroscopy in children. J Urol 1990;144:481.

Kramolowski EV, Tucker RD, Nelson CMK: Management of benign ureteral strictures: Open surgical repair or endoscopic dilatation? J Urol 1989;141:285.

Morgentaler A, Bridge S, Dretler S: Management of the impacted ureteral calculus. J Urol 1990;143:263.

Morse RM, Resnick MI: Ureteral calculi: Natural history and treatment in an era of advanced technology. J Urol 1991;145:263.

Nakada SY et al: Long-term outcome of flexible ureterorenoscopy in the diagnosis and treatment of lateralizing essential hematuria. J Urol 1997;157:776.

Netto NR et al: Endourological management of ureteral strictures. J Urol 1990;144:631.

Netto NR et al: Ureteroscopic stone removal in the distal ureter. Why change? J Urol 1997;157:2081.

Puppo P et al: Flexible antegrade and retrograde nephroscopy: Review of 50 cases. Eur Urol 1990;17:193.

Rao PN et al: Prediction of septicemia following endourological manipulation for stones in the upper urinary tract. J Urol 1991;146:955.

Razvi HA et al: Intracorporeal lithotripsy with the holmium:YAG laser. J Urol 1996;156:912.

Santarosa RP, Hensle TW, Shabsigh R: Percutaneous transvesical ureteroscopy for removal of distal ureteral stone in reimplanted ureter. Urology 1993;42:313.

Segura JW: Ureteroscopy for lower ureteral stones. (Editorial.) Urology 1993;42:356.

Shroff S: The holmium:YAG laser for ureteric stones. Br J Urol 1996;78:836.

Singal RK, Denstedt JD: Contemporary management of ureteral stones. Urol Clin North Am 1997;24:59.

Singal RK et al: Holmium:YAG laser endoureterotomy for treatment of ureteral stricture. Urology 1997;50:875.

Thomas R et al: Safety and efficacy of pediatric ureteroscopy for management of calculous disease. J Urol 1993;149:1082.

Vijayan P: An aid to rigid ureteroscopy: Stone basket. Br J Urol 1991;68:215.

9 Laparoscopic Surgery

Howard N. Winfield, MD, FRCS, FACS

The application of laparoscopic techniques over the last decade has gained an important role in all surgical fields, including urology. If asked 10 years ago to write a manuscript on the state of laparoscopy as applied to urology, I would have been hard-pressed to come up with more than diagnostic "look-and-see" procedures. However, because of remarkable advances in video and fiberoptic technology, miniaturization of instrumentation, and the realization that minimally invasive surgical intervention may be as effective as open surgery, the era of laparoscopic surgery was truly born in the 1990s.

The intent of this chapter is to bring the reader from the beginnings of laparoscopy to the present year and then beyond. Basic laparoscopic techniques and equipment are discussed, and the more common urologic ablative and reconstructive procedures are described in detail.

HISTORY OF LAPAROSCOPIC SURGERY

It was in 1901 that G. Kelling of Germany first experienced the excitement of peering into the abdominal cavity of a dog by using a Nitze cystoscope. Nine years later, Jacobaeus applied this technique to the human abdomen. Thus, through the bold actions of these two independent investigators with the aid of a piece of urologic equipment, laparoscopy was born (Gunning, 1977). Initially, those predominantly interested in laparoscopy were the gynecologists and gastroenterologists, who slowly improved the techniques and instrumentation. The realization that filtered room air was a potential hazard for air embolus owing to its relative insolubility led Zollikofer to employ carbon dioxide (CO_2) as the insufflating gas (Zollikofer, 1924). In 1938, a medical internist from Budapest by the name of J. Veress was using a spring-loaded needle to puncture the thoracic cavity to create a pneumothorax in patients with tuberculosis (Veress, 1938). An unknown astute surgeon realized that this needle would be ideal for the initial blind puncture of the abdominal cavity. The Veress needle is still used today for the pneumoperitoneum.

Over the ensuing 30 years, there were considerable improvements in laparoscopic optics and instrumentation. In the 1960s and 1970s, Steptoe, Hulka, and Semm, well-known gynecologists, published extensively on laparoscopic surgical interventions and equipment and are considered pioneers of modern-day laparoscopy (Steptoe, 1967; Hulka et al, 1979; Semm, 1977). However, laparoscopy was being taught primarily as a diagnostic procedure, and very few gynecologists used it therapeutically.

In 1988, a clinical report from F. Dubois of France described the first laparoscopic cholecystectomy, and, through the extensive work of Reddick and Olsen, laparoscopic surgery spread throughout the United States during 1989 to the present time (Dubois et al, 1990; Reddick and Olsen, 1989).

Despite the fact that the Nitze cystoscope was the first instrument used for inspection of the peritoneal cavity, minimal interest in this form of minimally invasive surgery was shown by urologic surgeons until 1990. As of 1990, the peer-reviewed urologic literature describes laparoscopy's being applied for (1) the investigation of nonpalpable testes; (2) the evaluation of intersex disorders with occasional biopsy of gonads; and (3) the biopsy of abdominal or pelvic masses in rare situations (Cortesi et al, 1976; Lowe, Brock, and Kaplan, 1984; Das and Amar, 1988; Elder, 1989). More advanced forms of laparoscopy had been described as case reports by Wickham (1979), who performed a laparoscopic ureterolithotomy by a retroperitoneal flank approach. In 1985, Eshghi and colleagues used laparoscopy to monitor the percutaneous transabdominal removal of a staghorn calculus from a pelvic kidney (Eshghi, Roth, and Smith, 1985).

In early 1988, Winfield and Ryan began performing laparoscopic pelvic lymph node dissection (L-PLND), cystectomy, ureteral ligation, and other procedures using the porcine model to determine its potential role in urology (Winfield and Ryan, 1990). By late 1989, Schuessler and Vancaille took the bold step of performing an L-PLND for staging purposes in a patient with cancer of the prostate (Schuessler et al, 1991). Over the subsequent 12 months, there was a progressive trickle of laparoscopic procedures as applied to urology, with a significant increase in interest by urologic surgeons. As of the spring of 1992, approximately 24 centers had offered one or more laparoscopic training courses consisting of 1 or more days of hands-on experience using animal models. Over the ensuing 3 years, the vast majority of American urologists had taken a course or were being exposed to laparoscopic surgery in some form (See et al, 1993).

After the initial excitement and flurry of case reports, the science of laparoscopic surgery needed to be developed in the form of comparative studies against the "gold standard." There is no question that the use of laparoscopic surgery in urology is here to stay. Its current and predicted future role as applied to each urologist's practice is defined in this chapter.

BASIC LAPAROSCOPIC TECHNIQUES & EQUIPMENT

General Principles

Laparoscopic intervention is very different from open surgery and requires the surgeon to become familiar with a completely new set of instruments and equipment. This "techno-intensive" procedure requires that the surgeon become familiar with a wide variety of laparoscopic instruments, such as CO_2 insufflator, needles, trocars and sheaths, graspers, forceps, scissors, clip applicators, monopolar and bipolar coagulation probes and needles, and irrigation and suction devices, to name a few. The urologist has an advantage over other surgical specialists in that he or she is familiar with endoscopic and percutaneous surgery and should rapidly master the limited 2-dimensional visual field inherent to laparoscopic surgery. Similarly, the blunted tactile sensation of using long instruments to perform surgery is also not new to the endoscopic surgeon. With any new surgical procedure, it is important that the surgeon fully understand the indications and contraindications of the operation. To successfully perform laparoscopic surgery, 2 experienced surgeons should be capable of operating on the patient in tandem and in synchrony, while visualizing the procedure on a television monitor by use of a full-beam camera attached to the laparoscope. Finally, the nursing staff must be fully acquainted with the laparoscopic instrumentation and steps of the proposed procedure. A separate table with a laparotomy setup should be available in the operating room should emergencies develop. The arrangement of the equipment and surgical personnel should be planned in advance of all laparoscopic procedures.

Preoperative Patient Evaluation

To ensure optimal results and to increase the chances of successful laparoscopic intervention, it is critical that one attempt to choose the "ideal patient" early in one's experience. This patient should not have any of the relative or absolute contraindications for laparoscopic surgery and should have clear indications for the proposed procedure (Table 9–1). Patients who are more than 25 pounds over their ideal weight should be initially avoided, as well as patients who have had previous abdominal surgery. Umbilical or hiatal hernias may create problems, and these patients should be avoided as well. Once the surgeon has gained experience and confidence, more difficult and complicated cases may be attempted. Absolute contraindications to laparoscopy are self-evident, and alternative forms of treatment should be considered.

Once the correct patient is identified, he or she should be fully informed of the proposed laparoscopic procedure as well as alternative treatment options. Risks and benefits need to be spelled out in the informed consent form. In addition, the surgeon is obligated to inform the patient of his or her experience with this form of surgery, and if a more experienced laparoscopist will be assisting in the procedure, this person should be identified or introduced. The patient should also be made aware that should complications arise or the procedure not be technically possible, the traditional open incision would be used to complete the procedure.

Depending on the laparoscopic procedure to be performed, a modified bowel preparation as well as antibiotics may be required. Cross matching or type and screening for blood products is also dependent on the operation to be performed and the experience of the surgeon. These points are delineated in further detail below for each procedure.

Operating Room Preparation

Before the patient arrives in the operating room, the surgeons and nursing staff should arrange the equipment and instruments for the laparoscopic procedure. It may be helpful to prepare a checklist to be sure all equipment is present and functional. In addition, a brief summary for the nursing staff concerning patient positioning, expected laparoscopic equipment, and approach is extremely useful. In this way,

Table 9–1. Relative and absolute contraindications for laparoscopic surgery.

Relative	Absolute
Gross obesity	Generalized peritonitis
Hiatal hernia	Severe obstructive airways
Umbilical hernia	disease
Bowel obstruction	Coagulopathy—uncorrectable
Previous significant	Cardiac disease—inoperable
intraperitoneal surgery	Shock
Abdominal wall infection	Morbid obesity

delays, unexpected surprises, and frustrations, will be minimized.

Endoscopic telescopes should be checked to see that the lens system is intact. Camera chip and video units as well as television monitors should be correctly wired and assessed to be appropriately focused, white, and color-balanced. All operative instrumentation (graspers, scissors, trocars, clip applicators, etc) should be checked to be sure that working components move freely and that all screws and nuts are tightened. It is mandatory that all electrocautery instruments be carefully inspected to ensure that the insulation coating is intact and that all connecting cables are appropriate and fit tightly. Unfortunately, pinhole breaks in the instrument insulation may not be noticed, and the resultant high electrical power density may cause severe injury to surrounding viscera. Aspiration-irrigation systems need to be adequately primed and secured to prevent malfunction or leakage. The CO_2 insufflation system should be working properly and give an accurate measurement of intraperitoneal pressure. Finally, gas tanks should be checked for adequate pressure before insufflation is begun. It is suggested that a full backup tank be available in the operating theater should this be necessary.

The last potential problem that needs to be addressed is how to safely arrange the laparoscopic equipment around the patient so that there is still room for the surgeons, assistants, anesthesiology team, and nursing staff. Needless to say, the operating room can turn into a jungle if the spatial arrangements are not planned ahead of time. This arrangement should be jointly agreed upon by all participants listed above. The location of the television monitors, depending on whether a pelvic or renal procedure is being performed, needs to be considered before the arrival and positioning of the patient. Normally, the television monitors are positioned off each hip for pelvic procedures or off the shoulders for kidney cases. Each laparoscopic surgeon develops his or her own preferences, however, as described below. The optimal setup would be an operating room that had "power booms" with the television monitors and associated video transmitting equipment suspended from the ceiling (Figure 9–1). This arrangement would optimize room space and make the operating theater truly dedicated to state-of-the-art minimally invasive surgery.

Patient Positioning & Preparation

After general anesthesia is obtained, a Foley catheter is inserted into the bladder of all patients and put to straight drainage. An orogastric tube is placed for all upper abdominal procedures or when the operative time is expected to be lengthy. Although regional or local anesthesia is feasible for laparoscopic surgery, general anesthesia using agents other than inhaled nitrous gas is strongly advised. A poorly

anesthetized patient will strain at the time of trocar insertion, potentially resulting in bowel or vascular catastrophes. In addition, the CO_2 pneumoperitoneum will create diaphragmatic and peritoneal irritation, leading to considerable discomfort and shoulder tip pain in the awake patient. Although there is considerable controversy in the anesthesiology literature, it has been my experience that inhaled nitrous oxide routinely causes bowel distention which interferes with the laparoscopic intervention.

Having obtained suitable anesthesia, the patient's abdomen or flank is fully prepared and draped as one would do for a laparotomy. The genitals may be included in the preparation if a pelvic procedure is planned and access to these structures is necessary.

Creation of the Pneumoperitoneum

If transperitoneal surgery is planned, a pneumoperitoneum must be created. This may be achieved by either the closed (Veress needle) or open (Hassan cannula) technique. Both techniques are effective, and the laparoscopic surgeon should be comfortable with both. This part of the procedure is perhaps the most critical to the successful outcome of the laparoscopic intervention. A poorly positioned Veress needle or Hassan cannula may result in preperitoneal emphysema or visceral injury, requiring, in some cases, that the surgery be aborted. Therefore, time taken at this initial step of the procedure will pay dividends later on.

Veress Needle (Closed) Technique

Using a no. 15 scalpel blade, a tiny nick is made through the abdominal skin at a chosen location. Traditionally, the inferior crease of the umbilicus is the chosen site because the anterior abdominal wall is very thin at this level, with all fascial layers fusing. However, with experience, the Veress needle can be safely placed in the upper or lower quadrants of the abdomen, lateral to the rectus muscles. For renal or adrenal surgery, I routinely insert the Veress needle in the upper quadrant just below the costal margin.

My preferred technique of inserting the Veress needle into the peritoneal cavity is by careful steady pressure at the level of the previously made abdominal incision, feeling for 2 points of resistance: the fascial layers and the peritoneal membrane (Figure 9–2). Alternatively, the Veress needle may be placed by lifting up on the abdominal wall with two towel clips or by grasping the wall with the nondominant hand. These latter maneuvers may lift the anterior abdominal wall away from underlying loops of bowel. However, they may also result in lifting only subcutaneous fat and causing the needle to go a greater distance before penetrating the peritoneal membrane. In more corpulent individuals, the risk of inadequate needle positioning and preperitoneal emphysema is increased owing to these problems as well as to a lax

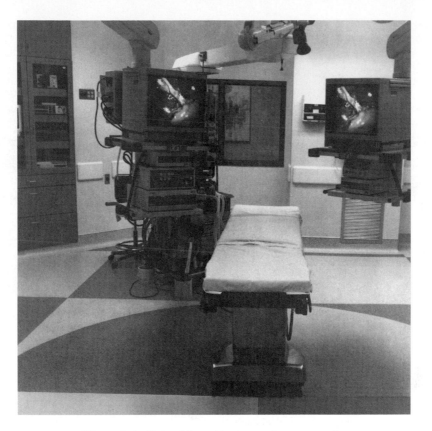

Figure 9–1. State-of-the-art laparoscopic surgery suite.

anterior peritoneal membrane that dips downward under pressure to touch the posterior peritoneal membrane (Figure 9–3).

There are a few tricks that have been learned by trial and error to overcome these problems in positioning the pneumoperitoneum needle. Should the peritoneal cavity not be satisfactorily entered from the inferior crease of the umbilicus, attempts from the superior crease are made. By aiming toward the sacral promontory from this supraumbilical approach, the needle should penetrate the peritoneal membrane just below the umbilicus, which is the point where all fascial layers are fused. Alternatively, other sites may be selected. Failing this, my approach is to employ the open laparoscopy approach by using a Hassan or similar blunt-tip trocar-sheath unit (Hassan, 1971).

An important test to determine correct positioning of the Veress needle is the saline drop test. Placing a drop of saline at the hub of the Veress needle, the surgeon lifts up on the abdominal wall. The negative intraperitoneal pressure should suck this drop downward. The second maneuver is the aspiration-injection technique. A Veress needle that is correctly positioned in the peritoneal cavity should not yield blood,

bowel contents, or other liquids and gases on aspiration. In addition, injection of 5 to 10 mL of saline should flow easily into the peritoneal cavity without return on reaspiration. As a final check of the position of the needle, the initial intraperitoneal pressure, as monitored on the insufflation machine, should begin at a low baseline pressure of < 7 mm Hg and gradually increase as the pneumoperitoneum progresses. Respiratory variations of intraperitoneal pressures should be apparent. A high initial intraperitoneal pressure and poor CO_2 flow suggest incorrect positioning. The needle may be inserted too far or tangled in omentum or in the preperitoneal fat. If not positioned correctly, the needle should be slowly withdrawn and the procedure repeated. The tendency of the laparoscopic neophyte is not to trust the abnormal readings and to continue insufflation, resulting in a massive extraperitoneal gas collection and an aborted procedure. A low intraperitoneal pressure is not a guarantee of correct needle positioning, as the bladder and bowel lumens may allow considerable gas instillation before detection. However, performing the aspiration-injection technique and other steps should eliminate this complication. Moving the needle in a circular maneuver or in and out in an attempt

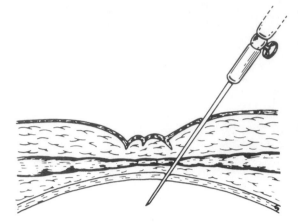

Figure 9–2. Insertion of the Veress needle into the peritoneal cavity.

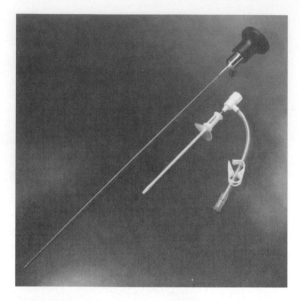

Figure 9–4. Surgineedle–2-mm introducer (Autosuture Co, Norwalk, CT).

to reach the peritoneal cavity is mentioned only to condemn this practice as a cause of complications.

In recent years, a number of devices have been marketed to diminish the risks of blind peritoneal puncture. One such device is the disposable Surgineedle–2-mm introducer. A 0-degree minilaparoscope can be inserted through this device to visualize loops of bowel to be certain that the peritoneal cavity has been entered (Figure 9–4).

Hassan Cannula (Open) Technique

If inserting the Veress needle does not gain access into the peritoneal cavity, the laparoscopic surgeon should not hesitate to use the open laparoscopic approach. In addition, in certain patients it may not be possible or advisable to create the pneumoperitoneum with the Veress needle or to blindly place the

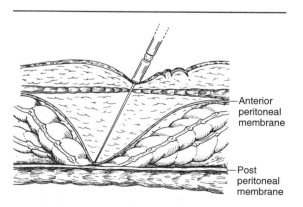

Figure 9–3. The Veress needle penetrating the lax anterior peritoneal membrane in an obese patient.

Anterior peritoneal membrane

Post peritoneal membrane

initial trocar-sheath units. These patients may be obese, may have certain congenital or acquired abdominal anomalies, or may have previously undergone multiple intraperitoneal surgical procedures. Because the risk of injuring underlying structures or viscera may be increased, it may be safer to use the open laparoscopy approach. This approach requires a specially designed unit first described by Hassan (Figure 9–5). The unit consists of a 10- or 11-mm sheath with a blunt tip obturator. In addition, there is a cone-shaped outer adjustable sleeve that occludes the larger abdominal wall opening. For placement, a 3-cm incision is made at a chosen site and deepened down to the peritoneal membrane, which is opened under direct vision. A finger is inserted to determine the presence of underlying adhesions or loops of bowel that may be tethered. Two stay stitches of 0-polypropylene are placed, one on either side of the fascial incision, and the Hassan cannula is inserted into the peritoneal cavity. The conical sleeve is cinched down against the fascia, and the polypropylene stitches are put on traction and fixed to the cannula handle to allow the formation of a tight seal. Gas insufflation then proceeds in a routine fashion.

Insufflation

Initial insufflation begins at 2 L/min and can be increased to maximum flow once the numerical readings on the insufflation machine are correct and the abdomen is becoming diffusely tympanic. The insufflator is a sophisticated valve mechanism that gates the flow of the pressurized gas from the tank into the patient's peritoneal cavity. High-flow insufflators are

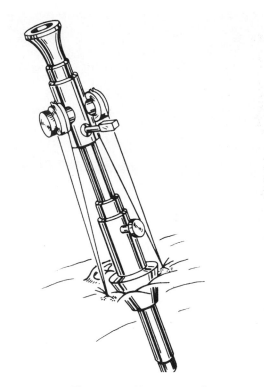

Figure 9–5. Hassan cannula.

now available that can deliver up to 15 L of CO_2 per min. The most important component of the insufflator is the analog or digital display for monitoring the patient's intraperitoneal pressure. This must accurately report the initial insufflation pressures (< 7 mm Hg) and demonstrate a smooth progression up to the preset maximum intraperitoneal pressure (15 mm in most adults; 10–15 mm in children). Deviation off this predicted course would suggest a problem and allow the operator to take action so as to prevent a complication. Once the intraperitoneal pressure reaches the preset pressure on the insufflator, the gas flow should automatically be closed off to prevent excessive pressures being reached. When the intraperitoneal pressure falls below the set level, the insufflator should automatically bring the pressure back up. This control mechanism allows laparoscopic surgery to be performed effectively and safely. The normal adult male requires 4–6 L of CO_2 to obtain an intraperitoneal pressure of 15 mm Hg. Discrepancy between the volume initially insufflated and the intraperitoneal pressure suggests problems that must be addressed. The total volume of gas used during a procedure is variable and probably reflects the length of the procedure and the skill of the laparoscopist.

Currently, CO_2 is the most frequently used gas for insufflation. Its relative solubility in blood diminishes the risk of gas embolus. It has been estimated that upward of 500 mL of CO_2 must be rapidly absorbed directly into the bloodstream to develop a CO_2 embolus. Carbon dioxide does not support combustion, so electrocautery and lasers can be used safely in its presence. However, CO_2 is a peritoneal irritant and may result in acid-base disorders during prolonged procedures. Carbon dioxide is converted to carbonic acid on the peritoneal surface and can result in postoperative discomfort. Shoulder pain postoperatively due to CO_2 diaphragmatic irritation is not uncommon. Absorption of CO_2 may result in a significant increase in arterial $PaCO_2$ if the anesthesiologist is not careful to increase the minute ventilatory rate. Subsequent acidosis may occur owing to conversion of CO_2 to carbonic acid (Glascock et al, 1996). The benefit-risk ratio of CO_2 is such that it is the insufflant of choice for most laparoscopic urologic procedures.

Nitrous oxide is, however, a good choice for short diagnostic or therapeutic procedures under local anesthesia when electrocautery or laser will not be used (El-Minawi et al, 1981). Unlike CO_2, it is not irritating to the diaphragm and peritoneal membrane. Other gases such as xenon, argon, and krypton have very desirable qualities as laparoscopic insufflants, but these qualities are outweighed by their high cost.

Insertion of Telescopic Trocar-Sheath Unit

The blind puncture of the initial 5- or 10-mm trocar-sheath unit into the peritoneal cavity may be the most dangerous and anxiety-provoking step in the laparoscopic procedure. However, there are a few key steps that may help to improve the safety of this maneuver. To obtain as firm an abdominal wall as possible, bring the initial intraperitoneal pressure up to 20 mm Hg. The site of first trocar placement is enlarged and deepened, and a small nick is made in the abdominal fascia. This facilitates the subsequent insertion of the initial trocar-sheath unit by allowing the tip of this instrument to insinuate with less force into the created pneumoperitoneum. Safety can also be improved by extending the index finger to act as a buffer on the abdominal wall from overly aggressive insertion of the trocar-sheath unit. Use of towel clips applied laterally to the umbilical incision is an optional safety measure to stabilize or elevate the abdominal wall and diminish the risk of intraperitoneal injury. The laparoscope is inserted, and the intraperitoneal contents should be inspected to rule out injury. Once the position of the telescopic sheath is ascertained, the intraperitoneal pressure is lowered to 15 mm Hg.

Equipment manufacturers have continued to develop instruments that are safer and more efficient. The Visi-Port (AutoSuture Co, Norwalk, CT) allows a laparoscope to be directly inserted into the cannula as a cutting blade is seen going through the abdominal wall layers (Figure 9–6). The InnerDyne system

(InnerDyne Inc, Sunnyvale, CA) creates a dilation of the entry site rather than a puncture (Figure 9–7). This theoretically should create less tissue trauma and a smaller defect when terminating the laparoscopic procedure.

Insertion of Working Trocar-Sheath Units

Depending on the uro-laparoscopic operation planned, anywhere from 1 to 5 working ports may be required. These working ports are each placed under laparoscopic television-video monitoring so that the tip of the trocar can be seen penetrating the peritoneal membrane and aimed in such a way to avoid underlying bowel. By shining the light of the laparoscope up against the anterior abdominal wall in a darkened operating room theater, abdominal wall vessels, specifically the superficial epigastric vessels, are illuminated and avoided. The inferior and superior epigastric vessels will not be seen as they are covered by the rectus abdominis muscle. However, in slender patients, the lateral border of this muscle may be transilluminated. The anatomic spatial arrangement of the working ports depends on the laparoscopic surgery planned.

Trocar-sheath units come in a variety of sizes varying from 3 to 15 mm. The most common sizes are 5 and 10 mm for adult surgery, whereas 3-mm (needlescopic) sheaths are now being used more frequently for pediatric and adult procedures (Figure 9–8).

To avoid inadvertent removal of the sheath from the peritoneal cavity during instrument exchanges, anchor the sheath to the skin by means of a 2-0 silk suture. Alternatively, various companies have gripping and locking devices that are available, but they add to the cost of instrumentation.

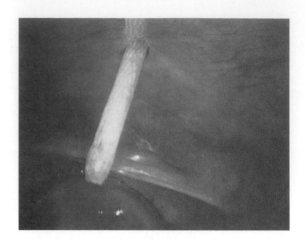

Figure 9–7. InnerDyne system (InnerDyne Inc, Sunnyvale, CA).

Retroperitoneoscopic (Extraperitoneal) Surgery

Laparoscopic surgery has traditionally been performed by a transperitoneal route. However, genitourinary organs and structures are in the retroperitoneum, and therefore many surgeons have advocated this route to minimally invasive surgery. Despite a number of investigators attempting this approach, it was not until 1992 that Gaur showed that distention of a balloon device placed directly within the retroperitoneum could rapidly and safely create a working space (Gaur, 1992). Modifications of this technique and instrumentation have progressed significantly since then and are now applied to almost all genitourinary laparoscopic procedures.

The basic technique involves a small incision down through the rectus fascia for the pelvis or lumbodorsal fascia in the flank. The preperitoneal space is digitally developed and then a balloon distention device is inserted into this space. A number of com-

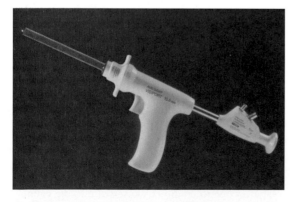

Figure 9–6. Visi-Port system (Autosuture Co, Norwalk, CT).

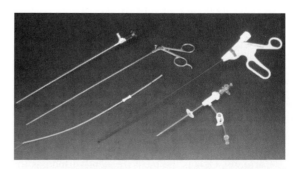

Figure 9–8. Needlescopic equipment and sheath (3 mm) (Autosuture Co, Norwalk, CT).

mercial distention devices are available that work well in creating the working space (Figure 9–9). However, one can also fashion a homemade device by using the finger of a surgical glove or finger cot of a transurethral resection drape (Figure 9–10). The distention device chosen is inflated with normal saline to 800–1000 mL in adults or 400–600 mL in children. A suitable working space is created, allowing subsequent insertion of working ports directly into the retroperitoneal space under laparoscopic or finger guidance. It is important to avoid tearing the peritoneal membrane or traversing this membrane with insertion of working ports. The initial port site is filled with a Hassan-type cannula so as to prevent CO_2 leakage. The retroperitoneal CO_2 insufflation is brought up to 12–15 mm Hg. Details of the retroperitoneal approach are discussed in greater detail for bladder suspension and nephrectomy (see below).

Laparoscope & Television-Video Units

The great advances in this technology have made laparoscopic surgery a reality. One cannot perform this "keyhole" type of surgery unless the laparoscope, video, and television units are functional and of good quality. As mentioned earlier, the modern-day laparoscope is an offshoot of the cystoscope, which is used on a daily basis in urology. Laparoscopes are constructed of a rod-lens system consisting of an objective lens, rod lenses, an eyepiece lens, and a fiberoptic cable.

The most common laparoscope used in adult procedures is 10 mm in diameter. For pediatric surgery, a 5- or 2-mm minilaparoscope is advised. The larger laparoscopes are capable of transmitting a greater amount of light and provide a slightly wider field of view and a higher-quality resolution than their smaller counterparts.

The laparoscopic optical system most commonly used is a 0- or 30-degree lens. The 30-degree lens system is now the camera of choice for procedures

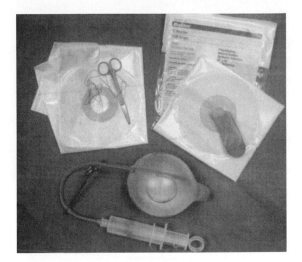

Figure 9–10. Finger cot of transurethral resection drape attached to a 22F red rubber catheter to create extraperitoneal space.

such as nephrectomy, adrenalectomy, and most pelvic laparoscopic procedures.

The television-video system consists of a camera chip, video unit, and preferably 2 television monitors. The optimal laparoscopic camera used today is a full-beam 3-chip CCD (charged coupled devices) unit that provides clarity of image and color spectrum. In addition to the laparoscope and television-video unit, a powerful laparoscopic xenon light source with automatic adjustments for variable light intensity is required to aid in visualization. Proper automatic control of light intensity allows for just the right amount of light output so as to afford increased depth of field and image clarity. Finally, documentation of each operation may be accomplished by videocassette recording or by use of a video printer.

Laparoscopic Instrumentation

With the explosion of interest in laparoscopic surgery, there has been a similar expansion in the types and varieties of laparoscopic instrumentation. The laparoscopic operating equipment can be subdivided into 7 major categories: (1) operative grasping and dissection instruments; (2) incisional instruments; (3) hemostatic and suturing instruments; (4) aspiration-irrigation systems; (5) retracting instruments; (6) morcellation and entrapment systems; and (7) miscellaneous equipment such as bowel or vascular stapling devices, laparoscopic ultrasound or Doppler probes, argon beam coagulators and harmonic scalpel, as well as a variety of other instruments (Figures 9–11 and 9–12). Many instruments are available in both disposable and nondisposable models, and one must evaluate the relative merits of

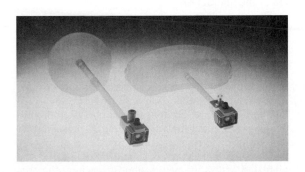

Figure 9–9. Trocar-mounted preperitoneal distention device (Origin Medsystems, Menlo Park, CA).

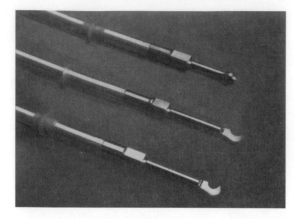

Figure 9–11. Harmonic scalpel (Ethicon Endo-Surgery Inc, Cincinnati, OH).

each, including price, maintenance, and quality. The diameter and length of laparoscopic instruments must be such that they can be passed through a laparoscopic port and reach the area of interest. Most standard instruments are 5 or 10 mm in diameter and 35 cm in length. Recently, mini-instruments (needlescopic) that are 2 mm in size are gaining increasing application for routine cases.

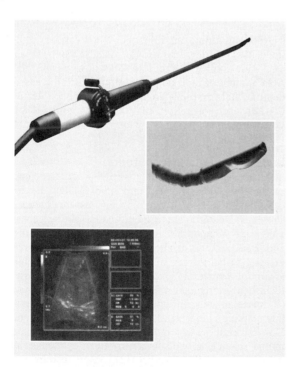

Figure 9–12. Laparoscopic 7.5-MHz ultrasound probe (B&K Medical Systems Inc, Marlborough, MA).

Exiting the Abdomen

After completion of a laparoscopic procedure it is essential to exit the peritoneal cavity in a safe and systematic fashion. All working ports are removed under vision. In this fashion, any unexpected bleeding from the abdominal wall that may occur can be detected and treated laparoscopically. In adults, all port sites 10 mm or larger are closed by using a 2-0 absorbable polydioxanone suture with a Carter-Thomason (Inlet Medical Inc, Eden Prairie, MN) port closure or similar device (Figure 9–13). These devices improve fascial closure, thus diminishing the risk of postoperative incisional hernia. In children, all port sites must be carefully closed. Before closure of the fascia of the last port site, all CO_2 is desufflated. A subcuticular running stitch of 4-0 polyglycolic acid is used on > 10-mm skin incisions and then Steri-Strips are applied. A Tegaderm dressing is applied over each skin incision.

LOWER GENITOURINARY PROCEDURES

Testis

A. Nonpalpable Testis

1. Diagnostic laparoscopy and Fowler-Stephens—As described previously, diagnostic laparoscopy for nonpalpable testes was one of the earliest applications of this technique in urology (Cortesi et al, 1976; Lowe, Brock, and Kaplan, 1984). In 1991, Bloom described the laparoscopic first stage of the Fowler-Stephens maneuver for high intra-abdominal testes. Using a Hulka clip, the testicular vessels were clipped in situ. Six months later, the testicle was brought down by an open surgical procedure into the scrotum, based on the vasal vasculature (Bloom, 1991).

2. Laparoscopic orchiopexy—Jordan and Winslow (1992) took this procedure one step further when they reported performing a complete laparoscopic orchiopexy of an intra-abdominal testis. Subsequently, other surgeons have refined this procedure, which is now considered the procedure of choice for intra-abdominal testes that are within 2.5 cm of the internal ring.

The procedure requires no more than 3 ports arranged in the lower abdomen of sizes varying from 3 to 10 mm. After identification of the salvageable testis, the gubernaculum is freed at the level of the internal ring and a triangular incision is made, freeing up the testicular vessels laterally and the vas inferiorly along the pelvic side wall (Figure 9–14). The intervening web of peritoneal tissue between the testicular vessels and the vas is carefully preserved. In this fashion, adequate length for the testis is obtained, such that the testis should be able to be manipulated across the pelvis, almost reaching the contralateral internal ring. Then a subdartos pouch is created and a 5- to 10-mm trocar-sheath unit is in-

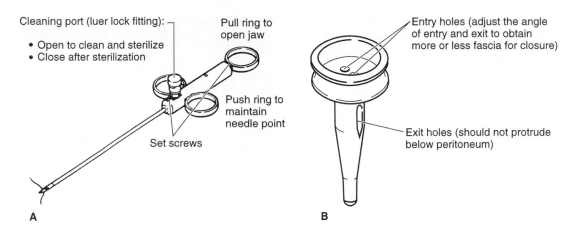

Cleaning port (luer lock fitting):
- Open to clean and sterilize
- Close after sterilization

Pull ring to open jaw

Push ring to maintain needle point

Set screws

Entry holes (adjust the angle of entry and exit to obtain more or less fascia for closure)

Exit holes (should not protrude below peritoneum)

A   B

Figure 9–13. Carter-Thomason device (Inlet Medical Inc, Eden Prairie, MN). **A:** Needle point suture passer. **B:** Fascial closure guide.

serted along the inguinal canal and punctures into the peritoneal cavity just medial to the obliterated umbilical ligament, always being certain the bladder is decompressed and not entered. The testis is carefully brought down to the subdartos pouch and secured at this level. The testicular vessels are inspected and further dissection of the cord may be performed if required. The defect at the point of dissection near the internal ring may be closed simply by clipping or suturing the peritoneal membrane, although this is often unnecessary.

3. Laparoscopic orchiectomy–Should the intra-abdominal testis be found to be atrophic, a laparoscopic orchiectomy is a simple procedure in experienced hands (Castilho et al, 1992).

B. Evaluation of Intersex Patients: Diagnostic laparoscopy is ideal when the anatomic gender of

the infant is uncertain. With the use of 3-mm minilaparoscopes and 2-mm needlescopic instruments, gonadal biopsies may be easily obtained with minimal trauma to the child (Yu et al, 1995).

C. Varicocele:

1. Laparoscopic varix ligation–Laparoscopic varix ligation is one of the simplest laparoscopic surgical procedures performed for the treatment of clinically significant varicocele. Although it was a popular operation in the early 1990s, it is rarely performed in light of data that indicate it to be more invasive and costly than the subinguinal (Marmar) or percutaneous embolization approaches (Thomas and Geisinger, 1990; Ivanissevich and Gregorini, 1918; Palomo, 1949; Marmar, DeBenedictis, and Praiss, 1985; Mitchell et al, 1985). However, it should be realized that not all medical institutions have a skilled interventional radiologist capable of performing these embolization procedures or a urologist capable of the results reported for the subinguinal microsurgical approach (Goldstein et al, 1992).

The greatest advantages of laparoscopic varix ligation seem to involve the following points: (1) an excellent approach for treatment of bilateral varices; (2) minimal postoperative pain; (3) very short convalescence period with resultant financial saving; (4) avoidance of injury to the vas deferens as may occur with the inguinal or subinguinal approaches; and (5) an option in the presence of a failed inguinal/subinguinal or percutaneous embolization approach or in patients who have had previous inguinal hernia repair (Donovan and Winfield, 1992).

a. Preoperative preparation–All patients are fully informed of the various surgical and radiologic options available to correct their varix. Benefits, risks, and complications are described as well as known statistics concerning pregnancy rates. Patients are not required to undergo any type of bowel prepa-

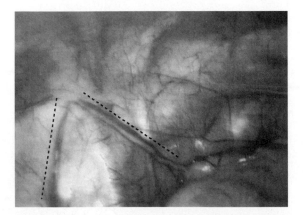

Figure 9–14. Left intra-abdominal testis. Dashed lines represent an incision into the posterior peritoneum for orchiopexy.

ration before surgery and are admitted to the "day-of-surgery" ambulatory center. All patients fast from the midnight before, and some patients receive a broad-spectrum cephalosporin administered empirically 1 h before surgery. Type and screen for blood products may be obtained early in one's experience but may be phased out of the preoperative preparation as one gains greater experience with laparoscopic varix ligation.

b. Technique of laparoscopic varix ligation– Under general anesthesia, the patient is shaved from just above the umbilicus to just below the pubic symphysis. The genitalia are prepared into the operative field to provide access to the testicles during the procedure. In some cases, tugging on the testicle allows the surgeon to be certain all testicular veins have been divided in the retroperitoneal space. A Foley catheter is inserted into the bladder and placed to dependent drainage. A nasogastric tube is inserted only if the anesthesiologist has had difficulty with induction or performing endotracheal intubation.

With the patient in a 10-degree Trendelenburg position, a small skin incision is made within the inferior crease of the umbilicus. The Veress needle is inserted into the peritoneal cavity as described earlier. Normally only 3 ports are necessary. The 5- or 10-degree laparoscope is brought in through a periumbilical port. Then one 3- or 5-mm port is placed in the left lower quadrant and suprapubic regions, respectively, for a unilateral left varicocele. If bilateral varicoceles are present, a port is placed in the right lower quadrant and the suprapubic port is eliminated.

The patient is now rotated laterally to elevate the affected side so that loops of intestine should migrate away from the operative field under the forces of gravity. The testicular vessels and vas deferens are usually easily seen lying just below the translucent posterior peritoneal membrane running to and from the internal inguinal ring (Figure 9–15). In some cases, the sigmoid colon may be adherent to the internal ring or over the testicular vessels. The position of the sigmoid colon probably represents an anatomic variant rather than adhesions due to inflammatory changes associated with diverticulitis. These adhesions are easily taken down by incising along the lateral peritoneal reflection.

The initial incision for a laparoscopic varix ligation should be through the posterior peritoneum, just lateral to the testicular vessels about 3 cm cephalad to the internal inguinal ring. This incision is made with curved scissors and then made into a **T** by incising medially toward the iliac vessels (Figure 9–16). Having gained access into the retroperitoneal space, the packet of testicular vessels is freed away from the psoas muscle by using a curved or straight 2- to 5-mm dissecting instrument. Then the testicular veins are separated away from the testicular artery and carefully clipped and transected. The testicular artery is usually in the posteromedial portion of the testicu-

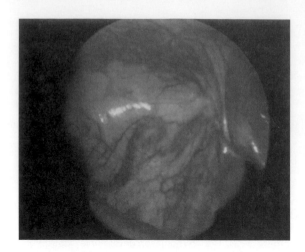

Figure 9–15. Left testicular vessels for laparoscopic varix ligation.

lar vascular bundle. However, as with all aspects of human anatomy, there are frequent variations, and, in fact, 2 testicular arteries have been found in some cases. Spasm of the artery may be relieved by dripping 1% lidocaine or papavarine solution onto the vessel. Alternatively, a laparoscopically designed "Doppler probe," which may be inserted through a 5-mm port, is helpful in locating the testicular artery. The surgeon stands on the contralateral side of the patient and maneuvers instruments through the ipsilateral and midline ports. The assistant is responsible for precise positioning of the laparoscope and stabilizing the ports as the surgeon moves instruments in and out of the peritoneal cavity.

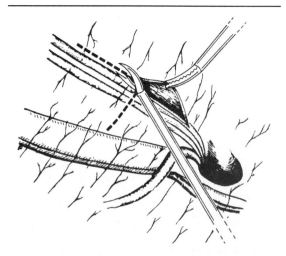

Figure 9–16. T-shaped incision made through the posterior peritoneum to gain access to testicular vessels.

At the termination of the procedure, the ipsilateral testicle is pulled to demonstrate that only the testicular artery remains intact in the region of the dissection. The vas should be seen exiting from the internal ring and remain intact. The surgeon should be cautioned to avoid wandering too far medially or laterally from the testicular bundle. Medially, the external iliac vessels may be encountered; laterally, the genitofemoral nerve fibers may be injured by electrocautery or traction. In fact, occasional patients complain of postoperative transient sensory numbness in the region of the anterior thigh. This complication usually resolves over the course of a few weeks.

After ensuring that hemostasis is satisfactory and no viscera have been injured, the laparoscope and trocar units are removed from the abdomen as described earlier for exiting the peritoneal cavity. The Foley catheter is removed during anesthetic reversal.

Typically, patients recover rapidly and are discharged later in the day. They are advised to return to full activity as tolerated with no time restrictions. Analgesic medication in the form of codeine or other narcotic is prescribed to be taken as needed for pain management. Semen analyses are evaluated at 6 and 12 months after surgery.

The application of laparoscopic varix ligation is not considered superior to the other options but is an alternative procedure. Laparoscopic varix ligation appears to result in an equal improvement in semen analysis and pregnancy rates compared with the other alternatives. The recurrence rate is lower than that with the open or radiologic approaches (Donovan, 1993).

D. Cancer of the Testis:

1. Laparoscopic retroperitoneal lymph node dissection—The management of cancer of the testis has changed dramatically over the last 25 years, primarily because of the advent of improved and highly effective chemotherapeutic regimens (Richie, 1990). As a result, the survival and cure rates for all forms of germ cell testis tumors are very high, even for advanced stages. Thus, the role of extensive retroperitoneal lymph node dissection (RPLND) for nonseminomatous germ cell tumors (NSGCT) has diminished, and modified anatomic templates are now being advocated (Donohue et al, 1990). By performing a modified nerve-sparing RPLND in correctly selected cases, the perioperative morbidity has diminished and preservation of antegrade ejaculation with improved fertility has been demonstrated (Richie, 1990).

For low-stage NSGCT (stage I) in association with negative tumor markers (alpha-fetoprotein and beta--human chorionic gonadotropin) and favorable histologic findings, close surveillance alone has been advocated as a management option. If surveillance is decided upon, a careful follow-up plan must be arranged, and patient compliance must be optimal (Young et al, 1991; Nicolai and Pizzocar, 1995). However, it should be noted that clinical relapse has

been reported in 25–30% of patients on surveillance protocols (Freedman et al, 1987; Hoskin et al, 1986). Fortunately, salvage combination chemotherapy has been reported to yield a > 90% cure rate (> 5 years disease-free) in this situation but still with a death rate of up to 10% in patients who may not respond to second-line treatment modalities (Skinner and Skinner, 1997).

Patients with Stage I or low-volume Stage II pure seminoma are effectively treated with postorchiectomy radiation therapy yielding 5-year survival rates of > 90% (Richie, 1997). Combination chemotherapy is generally indicated as primary treatment for clinical stages IIB, IIC, and III testis tumors, irrespective of the histologic findings. After combination chemotherapy for advanced testis cancer, residual tumor mass may be visualized on computerized tomography (CT scan), for which surgical intervention may be required to determine if viable malignant tissue remains. Such operations are normally very difficult owing to the desmoplastic reaction and loss of normal tissue planes as a result of the chemotherapy (Skinner and Skinner, 1997).

Within the current treatment strategies described above for patients with testis cancer, laparoscopic RPLND can offer a minimally invasive alternative for precise lymph node staging to determine metastatic disease in patients with clinical stage I NSGCT (Gerber et al, 1994; Janetschek et al, 1996; Klotz, 1994; Rassweiler, Seemann, and Henkel, 1996). Its role as a therapeutic surgical procedure, however, has not been clarified, in that all patients who have been found with positive lymph node tissue for metastases have received adjunctive combination chemotherapy. Furthermore, the role of RPLND in resection of post-chemotherapy residual abdominal masses visualized on CT scans is currently being examined (Rassweiler, Seemann, and Henkel, 1996; Janetschek et al, 1997).

Laparoscopic RPLND was first described as a case report by Rukstalis and Chodak (1992) and was quickly followed by further case reports. Laparoscopic RPLND is a technically advanced procedure, primarily owing to the difficulty with exposure of the midline retroperitoneal structures and the presence of the great vessels with their associated branches. Such laparoscopic procedures normally require considerably longer operative time, resulting in higher intraoperative surgical costs (Troxel and Winfield, 1994). At centers where laparoscopic RPLND has been successfully undertaken, these patients experience the usual benefits of minimally invasive surgery—less postoperative pain and narcotic use with shortened hospitalization and convalescence compared with open surgical intervention. The cosmetic appearance of the laparoscopic scars has been reported by patients to be superior to the usual extensive midline or thoracoabdominal incisions.

When considering laparoscopic RPLND for the

management of testis cancer, one must be certain that the end result will be equivalent to that of open surgery without surgically compromising the patient's chance for cure. This is the critical issue that needs to be addressed with all minimally invasive procedures but especially with testis tumors, since careful and detailed management should yield high cure rates with minimal morbidity. Anything less may potentially compromise the life of a patient in his most productive years. Table 9–2 lists my indications for performing laparoscopic RPLND. The ideal candidate would be a slender healthy man who has not had previous abdominal surgery and whose radical orchiectomy specimen contains a NSGCT. The testicular tumor markers should be negative, and CT scan of the abdomen, pelvis, and chest should not reveal radiologic evidence of metastatic disease (clinical stage I). The goal of laparoscopic RPLND is to replicate what would ordinarily be achieved with a modified RPLND template as described by Donohue et al (1990). Direct attempts to preserve sympathetic fibers are not made, but preaortic dissection directly below the inferior mesenteric artery is avoided.

a. Preoperative patient preparation–After obtaining informed consent, the patient undergoes a mechanical bowel preparation by imbibing 1 gallon of GoLytely (Braintree Laboratories, Braintree, MA) the afternoon before surgery and has only clear liquids until midnight. The patient is admitted into hospital the day of surgery. Broad-spectrum intravenous antibiotics are administered on call to the operating room. Pneumatic stockings are placed on the lower extremities.

b. Technique of laparoscopic RPLND–After general anesthesia is obtained by agents other than nitrous oxide, the patient is placed in the semiflank position (60 degrees) with the ipsilateral side elevated and the extremities well padded. An orogastric tube is inserted into the stomach, and appropriate venous or arterial lines (or both) are obtained.

Early in one's experience one might prefer to perform flexible cystoscopy with insertion of a 6F endhole ureteral catheter over a 0.038-in Amplatz superstiff guidewire into the ipsilateral renal unit. This is secured to a 16F Foley catheter inserted into the bladder. By manipulating the ureteral catheter, one can locate the ureter more quickly and potentially protect it during the node dissection. This approach is now used only in select cases where the patient is obese or has had previous retroperitoneal surgery.

Access into the peritoneal cavity may be by the Veress needle with insertion into the ipsilateral upper quadrant 2 finger-breadths below the costal margin in the midclavicular line. A pneumoperitoneum is created up to 20 mm Hg pressure, and a 10/11-mm laparoscopic port is inserted carefully at this location. A 10-mm 30-degree laparoscope is inserted and then 3 other 10/11-mm ports are inserted as shown in Figure 9–17. In some cases a fifth port is required suprapubically for retraction of bowel. All ports are secured in place using 2-0 silk suture, and then the pneumoperitoneal pressure is lowered to 15 mm Hg.

The template for the laparoscopic RPLND follows that described by Donohue et al (1990). This is a modified template that is bordered, for a right-sided dissection, by the ureter laterally, the right renal vessels superiorly, the anterior surface of the aorta medially, and the inferior mesenteric artery caudally on the aorta but extending below over the inferior vena cava and the right common iliac artery. On the left side, the borders include the left ureter laterally, the left renal vessels superiorly, and the precaval region medially. Caudally, the dissection stops at the inferior mesenteric artery over the aorta but continues lateral to the aorta and over the lateral aspect of the left common iliac artery.

Once the laparoscopic ports are placed, the table is rotated to bring the patient into almost the full-flank position with the involved side elevated. The laparoscope is placed through the periumbilical port and,

Table 9–2. Indications for laparoscopic retroperitoneal lymph node dissection.

- Clinical stage I nonseminomatous testis tumor
- Negative testis tumor markers
- Candidate otherwise considered for surveillance
- No absolute contraindications to laparoscopic surgery
- Individualized decision if patient has relative contraindications to laparoscopic surgery
- Residual isolated abdominal or pelvic mass following chemotherapy in the presence of negative testis tumor markers. These cases must be individualized and approached very cautiously.

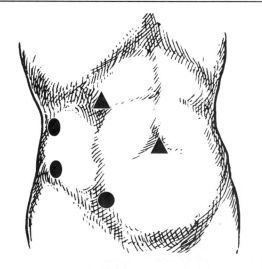

Figure 9–17. Port placement for right-sided retroperitoneal lymph node dissection.

using the midclavicular ports, the colon is mobilized medially by incising along the white line of Toldt. The mobilization is extended around the hepatic or splenic flexure such that the posterior peritoneum is incised along the inferior margin of the liver or spleen, respectively, toward the midline. This type of mobilization is important to allow adequate access to the dissection around the great vessels and the renal vessels in the interaortocaval region. Fortunately, gravity works well with the flank position to move loops of bowel out of the operative field. This becomes more problematic in obese patients.

Having gained access to the retroperitoneal space, one identifies the involved internal ring. The stump of the testicular vessels is dissected free, and it is hoped that the nonabsorbable suture placed at the time of the radical orchiectomy can be seen. The testicular vessels are then dissected cranially toward the inferior vena cava or left renal vein and aorta below the junction of the renal hilum. The proximal ureter must be carefully identified, because the testicular vessels pass over this structure. In addition, undue traction or manipulation of the testicular veins should be avoided to prevent avulsion at the level of the inferior vena cava or renal vein. The testicular vein(s) is doubly clipped at the junction of the inferior vena cava or left renal vein and the testicular artery close to the aorta. The testicular vascular remnants are delivered intact through a laparoscopic port.

The fibrolymphatic packages are now divided by using the templates described above for a right- or left-sided dissection and removed en bloc using a 10-mm laparoscopic spoon-shaped grasper through a 10/11-mm port and sent immediately for frozen section. Dissection in the interaortocaval region must proceed very cautiously owing to the variability of the network of small vascular branches off the great vessels. To adequately excise this nodal tissue, it is not uncommon to clip and transect 2 or 3 lumbar vessels. These are carefully secured with laparoscopic clips. The dissection should expose the paraspinous tissue, and if sympathetic fibers can be identified, they are spared so long as no lymphatic tissue in this region is spared (Figure 9–18). Hemostasis is carefully evaluated, and the laparoscopic ports are closed in the usual fashion.

During the laparoscopic node dissection, should pathologic interpretation of frozen sections demonstrate evidence of significant metastatic nodal disease, I would abort this approach and convert to open surgery to perform a more extensive and possibly curative RPLND. I have not yet been faced with this situation. Final pathologic evaluation would determine the need for adjunctive chemotherapy.

c.   Post-chemotherapy or -radiotherapy laparoscopic RPLND–Patients with initial clinical stage IIb, IIc, or III are usually advised to receive 3 or 4 courses of combination chemotherapy as primary initial treatment. If, after chemotherapy, there

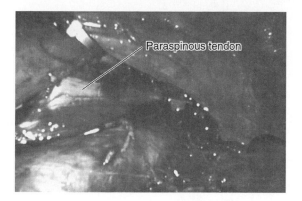

Figure 9–18. Exposure of paraspinous tissue during right-sided retroperitoneal lymph node dissection.

is evidence of residual or new tumor mass in the absence of elevated tumor markers, RPLND is recommended for diagnostic and therapeutic purposes. If the pathologic interpretation of the residual mass is carcinoma, the patient may require second-line chemotherapy. The finding of teratoma or residual necrotic tissue portends a more favorable prognosis for the patient.

It is known that RPLND in the post-chemotherapy or -radiotherapy setting is fraught with difficulty, whether performed in an open or laparoscopic fashion (Skinner and Skinner, 1997). Tissue planes are distorted and fixed with a desmoplastic reaction to major surrounding structures, specifically, the great vessels. However, the goal of these cases is to remove residual tumor mass seen on CT scan for histologic evaluation. Attempts to follow the usual template map or laparoscopically dissect above the renal hilar region are not easy and are rarely accomplished. Laparoscopic dissection in this setting must be approached cautiously.

d.   Postoperative care–The true benefits of a successful laparoscopic RPLND are realized the moment the patient reaches the recovery room. Although pain is present around the port sites, it generally diminishes within 24 h. None of my patients have required continuous intravenous narcotic pain medication postoperatively. Bowel function returns rapidly, with most patients tolerating oral fluids within 24 h of surgery. Discharge is usually within 2–4 days. Convalescence to full activity is reported to require between 10 and 20 days.

Only a limited number of centers have been able to report small studies of laparoscopic RPLND for nonseminomatous stage I testis tumors (Gerber et al, 1994; Janetschek et al, 1996; Klotz, 1994; Rassweiler, Seemann, and Henkel, 1996). As can be seen in Table 9–3, the cumulative operative times of these studies are lengthy for stage I NSGCT, varying from

Table 9–3. Summary of clinical studies for laparoscopic RPLND for NSGCT.

Study	No. Pts	Stage I	Stage II Post-chemo.	Mean OR Time (min) R	L	Both	Nodal Pathology	Complications	Postop. Days	Convalescence Days	Mean Follow-up and Recurrence	Success Rate
Rassweiler, Seemann, and Henkel, 1996	26	17	9	312	268		1/17 Embryonal 9/9 Necrosis	Delayed ureteral stenosis (1) Pulm. embolism (1) Retrograde ejaculation (1) Retrop hematoma (1) Lymphocele (1)	4.5		27 mo: pulmonary mets (2) Local relapse (0)	Stage I: 16/17 Post-chemo.: 2/9
Janetschek et al, 1996b	29	29	0	Initial 14 pts 558 Last 15 pts 354	348 240	480 306	8/29 Positive	Bleeding requiring laparotomy (1) Pressure sores (2) Lymphocele (1) Transient lymphedema (1) Retrograde ejaculation (0)	Initial 14 pts: 5.5 Last 15 pts: Pulmonary edema (1)	4	16 mo: no recurrences	28/29
Gerber et al, 1994	20	20	0			480	3/18 Positive	Gonadal vessel injury requiring laparotomy (2) Suncapsular myonecrosis (1) Injury to inferior mesenteric artery (1) Lymphocele (1) Trocar site bleeding (1) Retrograde ejaculation (0)	3	14	10 mo: pulmonary mets (2) Local relapse (0)	18/20
Klotz, 1994	4	4	0			All left	0/4 Positive	None reported	2–5	10		Stage 1: 3/4
Janetschek et al, 1997	27	0	27			252	1/27 Active tumor 11/27 Teratoma 15/27 Necrosis	Bleeding (1) Lymphascites (2) Lymphocele (1)	3.6			27/27

R, right RPLND; L, left RPLND.

240 to 558 min (mean 355 min), reflecting a steep learning curve but also the technical difficulty of this procedure. The cumulative success rate of all reported stage I cases is 93%, with node positivity occurring in 18%. There have been no reported cases of local recurrence or tumor seeding at the port site. Cumulative complications are 20–25%; most are not unique to laparoscopic surgery but are more accentuated owing to the minimally invasive access. To date, the sole comparative study, albeit retrospective, of laparoscopic versus open RPLND shows a clear benefit postoperatively for the laparoscopic approach. This study of Janetschek and colleagues (1997) demonstrates the longer operative time with laparoscopy but a marked reduction in time with practice.

Therefore, one can conclude that laparoscopic RPLND for stage I NSGCT is feasible in the hands of surgeons skilled with advanced laparoscopic techniques. Based on few studies laparoscopic RPLND following chemotherapy for residual abdominal lesions is fraught with difficulty and should be considered only in centers with advanced laparoscopic surgical experience.

Prostate
A. Laparoscopic Pelvic Lymph Node Dissection: The evaluation of pelvic lymph nodes for staging purposes for cancer of the prostate was previously the most frequent application of laparoscopic surgery performed by urologists. The first report in a peer-reviewed journal describing L-PLND was by Schuessler and colleagues (1991). Since then, many other authors have reported their experience with this procedure (Winfield et al, 1992; Parra, Andrus, and Boullier, 1992).

The importance of determining the presence or absence of metastatic lymph node involvement with cancer of the prostate, or any other urologic malignancy, is that this finding will most likely determine the extent of treatment and the feasibility of curative therapy (Whitmore, 1963). Radiologic evaluation of the pelvic lymph nodes by the use of abdominal and pelvic CT scan for detection of involved lymph nodes has been demonstrated to have an accuracy rate of only 65%; therefore, the routine use of this modality is not advocated (Benson et al, 1981). The use of ultrasound and magnetic resonance imaging for the detection of nodal metastases has also been found to be rather unreliable (Rifkin et al, 1990). Lymphangiography has been shown to have a high false-positive and false-negative rate (25–60%) for cancer of the prostate (Grossman et al, 1980; Smith, 1966; Castellino et al, 1973; Loening et al, 1977). Consequently, PLND has been shown to be the most accurate staging test to determine lymph node status for cancer of the prostate, as well as bladder, penile, and urethral tumors.

Recently, several authors have analyzed the utility of PLND. With the advent of prostate-specific antigen (PSA) as a screening tool, the frequency of detection of pelvic lymph node metastasis from prostate cancer has decreased. Factors that predict lymph node involvement include elevation of serum PSA, high Gleason score, and advanced clinical stage by digital rectal examination. According to Campbell and associates (1995), lymph node metastases were particularly uncommon in patients with nonpalpable tumors (1.5%), PSA values < 10 ng/dL (1.3%), and Gleason score < 6 (3.8%). Of the 245 patients studied, 179 (73.1%) presented with at least one of these favorable characteristics, and only 4 (2.2%) demonstrated lymph node involvement.

In a review of the medical records of 1632 patients who had undergone PLND, Bluestein and associates (1994) found that PSA provided the best predictive value of lymph node metastases and could be enhanced with the addition of Gleason score and clinical stage. Deeming 3% as an acceptable false-negative rate, they suggest that 61% of patients with stage T1a-T2b and 29% of patients with stage T1a-T2c could be spared the risk and expense of PLND. Partin et al (1994) published their retrospective analysis of patients who had undergone PLND and radical retropubic prostatectomy at Johns Hopkins University. To achieve a false-negative rate no greater than 3%, a review of Partin's data would suggest the need for PLND in the following: (1) patients with PSA between 0.0 and 10.0 ng/mL, whose clinical stage is T2a-T3a, and whose Gleason score is > 6; (2) patients with PSA between 10 and 20 ng/mL, whose clinical stage is T2a-T3a, and whose Gleason score is > 5; and (3) virtually all patients with PSA > 20 ng/mL. Until more precise noninvasive staging is available (ie, radioimmunodetection, positron emission), the PLND remains the definitive method of identifying prostate cancer metastasis to regional lymph nodes.

Why should one consider the laparoscopic approaches to PLND for staging cancer of the prostate? The advantages to the patient are decreased hospitalization and postoperative convalescence with staging effectiveness comparable to that of the open procedure (Winfield et al, 1992). Finally, from a cosmetic point of view, the 4 or 5 small (3- to 11-mm) abdominal puncture sites appear to be superior to the disfigurement of the midline incision from umbilicus to symphysis pubis.

1. Preoperative preparation–If only a laparoscopic PLND is planned, the patient is admitted on the day of surgery, having self-administered enemas and oral laxatives the day before. If immediate retropubic or perineal prostatectomy is planned should the nodes come back negative after frozen pathologic examination, a full bowel preparation is administered the night before when the patient is admitted into the hospital. All patients receive 1 dose of a broad-spectrum parenteral antibiotic 1 h before the procedure and are typed and screened for blood products before laparoscopic surgery is begun.

2. Laparoscopic PLND procedure—After induction of general anesthesia, a Foley catheter and orogastric tube are positioned in the bladder and stomach, respectively.

This procedure may be performed by either a transperitoneal or extraperitoneal approach. For the transperitoneal route, the pneumoperitoneum is created as described previously; the working port configuration is shown in Figure 9–19. In very corpulent patients in whom abundant fatty tissue hangs in the region of the obliterated umbilical ligaments, 4 working ports are placed, as shown in Figure 9–20. Alternatively, an extraperitoneal approach should be considered, because the intact peritoneal membrane effectively retracts back the loops of bowel from the pelvic region.

3. Transperitoneal route—The patient is now placed in a 30-degree Trendelenburg position with lateral rotation to allow loops of small bowel to migrate under gravity away from the iliac region of dissection. It is important to identify certain key landmarks, as shown in Figure 9–21. Familiarity with

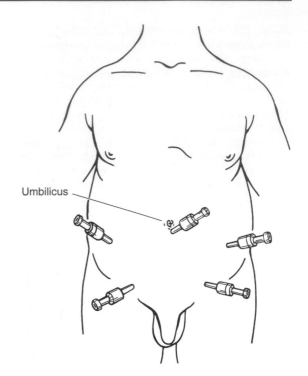

Figure 9–20. Horseshoe port placement for laparoscopic pelvic lymph node dissection in an obese patient.

these structures will aid in avoiding major surgical accidents. On the left side, it is often necessary to take down adhesions from the sigmoid colon by cutting along the white line of Toldt, whereas on the right side the cecum and appendiceal regions may be tethered down over the iliac region, requiring release.

The initial incision through the posterior peritoneal membrane begins just lateral to the obliterated umbilical ligament, high over the pubic bone, and is brought down just medial to the pulsating external iliac artery back toward the bifurcation of the common iliac artery, where the ureter may be identified. The vas deferens becomes apparent and is then coagulated or clipped and then transected. The external iliac vein is located and cleared of all fibrolymphatic tissue off its anterior and medial surfaces. This essentially creates the lateral border of the obturator lymph node packet. The tissue below the external iliac vein is swept off the pelvic side wall, which is then traced to its junction with the pubic bone. With the obliterated umbilical ligament retracted medially, a plane is created just lateral to form the medial border of the obturator nodal packet. At this point, the obturator nerve and associated vessels should be identified, and thus the inferior apex of the nodal tissue is created. Normally, there are no significant vessels in this apical tissue, and therefore electrocautery can be used to release it away from the pubic bone. The

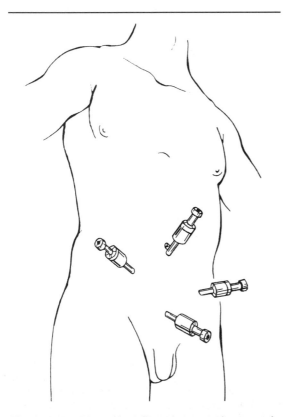

Figure 9–19. Diamond-configuration port placement for laparoscopic pelvic lymph node dissection or extraperitoneal bladder neck suspension.

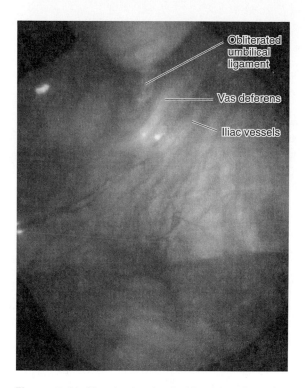

Figure 9–21. Key landmarks for laparoscopic pelvic lymph node dissection showing right obliterated umbilical ligament, testicular vessels, and internal ring with vas deferens.

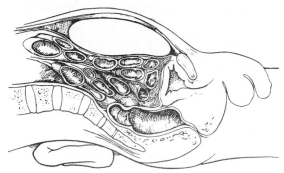

Figure 9–22. Balloon device inflated in the preperitoneal space for laparoscopic pelvic lymph node dissection or bladder suspension.

lymph node packet is then stripped proximally off the obturator nerve back toward the bifurcation of the iliac vessels.

The nodal packet is then removed through the 11-mm suprapubic port with spoon-shaped graspers. Frozen pathologic examination is always requested if immediate prostatectomy is being considered or if the dissected tissue is palpably hard and suggestive of malignancy. Hemostasis is ensured, and the abdomen is exited in the usual fashion.

4.   Extraperitoneal route–Should an extraperitoneal route be chosen, a 2-cm infraumbilical midline incision is made and deepened down through the rectus fascia. Stay sutures are placed in the fascia, and then a preperitoneal plane is digitally initiated such that the back of the pubic bone can be felt. The balloon inflation device is then inserted and inflated to 800–1000 mL of saline (Figure 9–22). After deflation and removal of the balloon, a Hassan-type cannula is inserted and secured with the stay sutures and the CO_2 is insufflated up to 15 mm Hg. A large working space should be developed with no significant bleeding apparent. In many cases, the pubic bone as well as the iliac vessels are fully exposed. Working ports are carefully inserted to complete a diamond-shape configuration directly into the created extraperitoneal

space. This can be done under laparoscopic vision or digital guidance. The key here is not to traverse the peritoneal membrane, which will then result in CO_2 flowing into the peritoneal cavity with subsequent collapse of the extraperitoneal space.

It should be remembered that the extraperitoneal route should not be considered if the patient has had previous lower abdominal surgery or inguinal hernia surgery, because the peritoneal membrane is likely to be easily torn, resulting in the scenario described above.

The dissection proceeds as described above directly onto the iliac vessels, which are often already exposed. The vas deferens is pushed cephalad with the peritoneal membrane and may not need to be transected. The boundaries of the dissection should be identical to that which would be performed in an open extraperitoneal approach.

Postoperatively, most patients are allowed to begin oral feeding the night of surgery. The Foley catheter is removed when the patient is alert and ambulating. Barring any problems, discharge is within 24 h of surgery, with return to full activity at 1 week.

Comparative studies of laparoscopic versus open PLND demonstrate similar intraoperative times with laparoscopy after the learning curve is overcome, thus reducing the costs. There is a marked benefit with laparoscopy in the postoperative period. The minilaparotomy approach advocated by Steiner and Marshall (1993) is a viable surgical alternative for those uncomfortable with laparoscopy. My current indications for performing L-PLND are listed in Table 9–4.

B.   Laparoscopic Mobilization of Seminal Vesicles: In anticipation of a radical perineal prostatectomy, it is possible to continue laparoscopic intervention after L-PLND so as to mobilize the seminal vesicles and transect the ampulla of the vas (Kavoussi et al, 1993b). Using the distal transected segment of the vas deferens as a guide, these struc-

Table 9–4. Indications for L-PLND in men with cancer of the prostate.

1. Clinical stage B2 to C (T2b to T4) regardless of the follow-up treatment under consideration
2. Stage A2 (T1b) and a Gleason score of ≥ 7
3. Elevated enzymatic assay for serum prostatic acid phosphatase in patients with a negative nuclear bone scan (stage D0)
4. Patients with a serum PSA of > 30 ng/mL (Hybritech assay)
5. Patients electing transperineal prostatectomy in whom a pelvic lymph node dissection is planned
6. Stage A1, A2, or B1 (T1a, T1b, T2a) disease in patients with moderately to poorly differentiated histologic subtypes (Gleason score of ≥ 7) who are considered to be candidates for definitive radiotherapy or surgery
7. Biopsy-proven persistent adenocarcinoma of prostate following full-course radiotherapy in patients being considered for salvage prostatectomy

tures are followed medially into the deep pelvis behind the bladder. The tips of the seminal vesicles as well as associated vessels are well within the operative field and easily dissected. The ampullae of the vas deferens are freed of fibrous surrounding tissues and then clipped and transected. Care to identify the artery to the tips of the seminal vesicles must be heeded as well as the close proximity of the distal ureter.

The predominant advantage of laparoscopic mobilization of the seminal vesicles is in conjunction with perineal prostatectomy, in which complete visualization and dissection of the tips of these structures is optimal. This technique is unnecessary if radical retropubic prostatectomy is planned.

C. Laparoscopic Prostatectomy: As an extension of laparoscopic mobilization of the seminal vesicles, select urologic surgeons have reached out to explore the possibility of performing a complete laparoscopic prostatectomy. The laparoscopic prostatectomy is feasible, albeit difficult, but the major obstacle has been the subsequent bladder neck tapering and urethrovesical reanastomosis (Schuessler et al, 1992). Although this procedure should be considered futuristic at the present time, it is anticipated that improved laparoscopic instrumentation and suturing devices augmented by transurethral guidance will allow this procedure to be performed with greater ease and reliability.

Penis and Urethra

A. Laparoscopic PLND–Extended: In rare situations where ilioinguinal node dissection is anticipated for staging and curative therapy for carcinoma of the urethra or penis, an extensive laparoscopic node dissection is feasible for evaluation of the internal, external, and common iliac lymph node chains (Assimos and Jarow, 1994).

Such dissections are best approached transperi-toneally, and a more extensive mobilization of the sigmoid colon and cecoappendiceal regions are required to provide a broader exposure of the operative field. Although greater lymphocele formation has been reported after extended PLND, this is less likely with the laparoscopic transperitoneal approach. Detection of positive iliac lymph nodes would alleviate the need for inguinal node dissection with its attendant morbidity.

B. Laparoscopic Penile Revascularization: Patients meeting the criteria for penile arterial bypass surgery for treatment of impotence may be candidates for laparoscopic penile revascularization. The most common donor vessel is the inferior epigastric artery, which normally requires a transverse or paramedial abdominal open incision. To diminish the incision size and postoperative morbidity, Winfield and colleagues described a laparoscopic approach to mobilize the inferior epigastric vessels. The artery is then carefully tunneled to the base of the penis, where it is anastomosed to the proximal dorsal penile artery or suitable recipient vessels using microsurgical techniques. Limited studies describing this technique have reported good results (Lund, Winfield, and Donovan, 1995; Trombetta et al, 1997).

Laparoscopic Ablative Bladder Surgery

A. Laparoscopic PLND–Extended: The treatment for invasive bladder cancer is PLND and radical cystoprostatectomy in men or anterior exenteration in women. In certain situations, the preoperative physical examination, cystoscopic inspection, and radiographic studies may suggest but not be diagnostic of pelvic lymphadenopathy. When the histologic finding is transitional cell cancer, and neoadjuvant combination chemotherapy is considered, a staging extended L-PLND may be warranted. Alternatively, L-PLND can be performed after chemotherapy to improve the restaging accuracy before embarking on radical exenterative surgery.

The preoperative management of the patient is identical to that described for prostate surgery. The limits of the extended dissection are the common iliac arteries cephalad, the genitofemoral nerve laterally, and the bladder medially; Cloquet's intraoperatively is critical. The dissection is more hazardous if preoperative chemotherapy or extensive radiotherapy has been administered, resulting in the loss of normal tissue planes.

B. Laparoscopic Cystectomy: Laparoscopic cystectomy is an advanced ablative laparoscopic procedure that has been performed primarily for benign disease such as pyocystis in patients who have preexisting urinary diversion (Parra et al, 1992). The endoscopic gastrointestinal anastomotic (endo-GIA) stapling device (Autosuture Co, Norwalk, CT) is instrumental in taking down the vascular pedicles.

C. Laparoscopic Bladder Diverticulectomy:

Bladder diverticuli that involve the lateral, dome, or anterior regions of the bladder are easily accessible to dissection and repair by laparoscopic techniques (Iselin et al, 1996). In fact, posterior diverticuli are suitably approached by using a laparoscopic route. The location of the ureter relative to the diverticula must be determined preoperatively, and placement of an end-hole ureteral stent is suggested. To date, my experience has involved a transperitoneal approach to the bladder and use of laparoscopic absorbable suture repair. Intraoperative use of flexible cystoscopy allows more rapid identification of the diverticula(e). Movement of the flexible scope and the bright light emanating from it allows the dissection to proceed directly over the diverticular region. Consideration of an extraperitoneal route is possible as well as the use of laparoscopic absorbable clips. Should the ureter be involved in the diverticulum, laparoscopic ureteral refluxing reimplantation may be feasible.

The urologist should also relieve any bladder neck outlet obstruction by the transurethral route before or after the laparoscopic intervention.

D. Combined Laparoscopic and Transurethral Ablation of Bladder Tumor: Patients with symptomatic invasive bladder tumors who are not considered suitable candidates for radical surgery or who refuse such aggressive therapy may be considered for deep transurethral laser ablation under transor extraperitoneal laparoscopic guidance with bowel protection. Furthermore, laser energy may be applied to the bladder serosal surface by way of the laparoscopic working port.

E. Urachal Anomalies: Anomalies of the urachus may be easily managed by laparoscopic intervention. Determination of the presence of malignancy should be assessed preoperatively, as this would necessitate partial or total cystectomy. The key to successful laparoscopic excision of urachal structures is correct port placement so as to gain optimal working maneuverability to the anterior abdominal wall. This may necessitate the ports' being placed far laterally (Fried-Siegal, Winfield, and Smith, 1994).

Laparoscopic Bladder Reconstructive Surgery

A. Bladder Neck Suspension: Numerous surgical procedures for the management of women with type I and II hypermobility stress urinary incontinence have been advocated, including transabdominal, transvaginal, or a combination of these approaches. The fact that no one procedure prevails indicates that the long-term efficacy and morbidity of each operation is not optimal. The literature, however, does contain prospective randomized clinical trials, as reported by Bergman and associates, showing that the 1-year cure rate is > 85% with Burch colposuspension compared with a cure rate of 72% with the vaginal Pereyra urethropexy (Bergman, Ballard, and Koonings, 1989). A long-term randomized prospective study comparing the Burch and Marshal-Marchetti-Krantz procedures indicates superior results with Burch, with persistent cure rates of 92% and 80% at 2 and 7 years, respectively (Colombo et al, 1994).

However, it is generally believed, although not definitively proved, that postoperative pain and hospitalization are greater after retropubic suspension. In an extensive review, Jarvis (1994) noted that the surgical and postoperative morbidity of the vaginal approach appears to be no less than that of the open retropubic operation.

To potentially diminish postoperative pain, hospitalization, and morbidity as well as maintain efficacy, the laparoscopic Burch-type urethropexy has gained increasing attention and favor since Vancaillie and Schuessler (1991) first described this minimally invasive approach.

1. Extraperitoneal laparoscopic bladder neck suspension–After initially using a transperitoneal approach to laparoscopic bladder neck suspension, it has become apparent that the extraperitoneal approach is simpler and more expeditious. A mechanical bowel preparation without oral antibiotics is suggested before the procedure. After general anesthesia is obtained, the patient is positioned in low lithotomy, and the abdomen and genitalia are prepared. An 18F Foley is placed into the bladder.

A midline incision is made approximately 4 cm below the umbilicus. The extraperitoneal space is created with the balloon inflation device as previously described for extraperitoneal L-PLND (Figure 9–22). A 10/11-mm Hassan cannula is secured, and the laparoscope guides 3 working ports directly into the extraperitoneal space. These ports vary in size from 5 to 10 mm and are placed in a diamond-shape configuration as described for L-PLND (Figure 9–19). Much of the dissection is often already accomplished after extraperitoneal balloon inflation. Care is exercised to clear fibrofatty tissue away from the periurethral–bladder neck region to improve exposure to the endopelvic fascia covering the anterior vaginal wall.

For a right-handed surgeon, the left lateral port and the suprapubic port are best for laparoscopic suture placement. A long strand (48 in) of 2-0 Gortex on a CV-2 tapered style needle is inserted into the working space, and then solid bites into the endopelvic fascia at the level of the bladder neck are obtained using the index finger of the operator's left hand or the assistant's hand in the vagina as a guide to correct placement. The suture is then transferred through Cooper's ligament, and the two ends are brought out through a 5- or 10-mm port. Extracorporeal knots are secured while the assistant lifts the bladder neck anteriorly by digital transvaginal upward pressure. Ideally, 2 stitches are placed on each side of the bladder neck (Figure 9–23). With this approach, the goal is to elevate the bladder neck suffi-

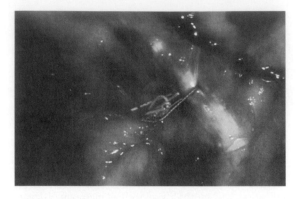

Figure 9–23. Laparoscopic sutures placed for bladder neck suspension through Cooper's ligament.

ciently in a sort of hammock position but not to overcorrect. Attempting to bring the vaginal endopelvic fascia directly in contact with Cooper's ligament will cause excessive tension and certain postoperative urinary retention. Cystoscopic examination is normally performed before CO_2 desufflation of the abdomen and removal of the laparoscopic port to examine the bladder wall and to visualize efflux of urine from the ureteric orifices. The Foley catheter is left in place overnight and, if necessary, intermittent catheterization is used if temporary urinary retention occurs.

Numerous other variations of the laparoscopic bladder neck suspension, as well as techniques to place and secure the sutures, have been advocated. Each laparoscopic surgeon seems to develop his or her method.

2. Intraperitoneal laparoscopic bladder neck suspension–Intraperitoneal laparoscopic bladder neck suspension is occasionally necessary when previous lower abdominal surgery has been performed and a suitable extraperitoneal space is not created. After establishment of pneumoperitoneum, 4 ports are placed in the diamond-shape configuration, and a vertical incision is made just medial to the left obliterated umbilical ligament aiming toward the pubic bone. The surgeon must be cognizant of the possibility of injury to the inferior epigastric vessels or perforation of the bladder, especially in women having undergone previous bladder or uterine surgery.

Having located the pubic bone and exposed the left Cooper's ligament, the dissection is carried medially to expose the symphysis pubis and region of the right pubic bone. Manipulating the Foley catheter allows identification of the urethra and bladder. Fibrofatty tissue is gently cleared in the region of the vesicourethral junction to expose the endopelvic fascia covering the anterior vaginal wall. There are often some unnamed blood vessels traversing through this area that require careful electrocoagulation. Placement of sutures through the endopelvic fascia at

the level of the bladder neck proceeds as described for the extraperitoneal approach.

Preliminary 1-year data from Burton (1994), who randomized 60 patients to open Burch versus laparoscopic colposuspension, suggests less favorable results with the latter. In contrast, a retrospective study by McDougall et al suggests comparable success at 2 years between the laparoscopic (71%) and Raz transvaginal (73%) approaches but reports less postoperative pain, analgesia requirement, and need for catheterization with laparoscopy (McDougall, Klutke, and Cornell, 1994). Clearly, long-term, larger randomized prospective studies must be performed to determine the appropriate role for the laparoscopic approach.

3. Laparoscopically assisted bladder sling urethropexy–The definitive treatment for intrinsic urethral sphincter dysfunction (type III stress urinary incontinence) is sling urethropexy. Attempts at using fascia later have met with mixed results (Narepalem, Kreder, and Winfield, 1995; Gilling et al, 1994). A laparoscopic "cutting" device to develop the plane between the urethra and the anterior vaginal wall is currently under investigation. Other authors are also gaining some experience with this technique in limited series.

B. Bladder Autoaugmentation and Augmentation: Laparoscopic seromyotomy or autoaugmentation of the bladder has been performed in both children and adults (Erlich and Gershman, 1993). The use of laser energy may improve the detrusor dissection. Attempts at bladder augmentation using the intestine or stomach has been technically hampered by the need for suturing. Laparoscopic gastrocystoplasty has been reported but clearly is in the early stages of development (Docimo et al, 1995). A laparoscopically assisted appendicovesicostomy (Mitrofanoff) has also been described (Jordan and Winslow, 1993b). It is believed that improved suturing devices such as the Endostitch (Autosuture Co) may make such technical feats easier.

C. Ileal Conduit Urinary Diversion: Although creation of an ileal conduit diversion by laparoscopic techniques has been reported in small studies, this advanced reconstructive endeavor may become easier with improved laparoscopic suturing and stapling devices (Kozminski and Partamian, 1992). This procedure has been done primarily in patients who require only urinary diversion, although Sanchez-de-Badajoz and colleagues (1993) have reported this technique in combination with laparoscopic cystectomy.

UPPER GENITOURINARY TRACT PROCEDURES

Ureter

A. Laparoscopic Ureterolysis: The surgical treatment for retroperitoneal fibrosis is ureterolysis, which requires an extensive abdominal incision. By employing laparoscopic techniques, this procedure with intraperitonealization and/or lateralization of the ureter is feasible (Kavoussi et al, 1992). Although considered an advanced procedure, it may be accomplished with the use of trocar-sheath units. Placement of an end-hole ureteral catheter over a 0.038-in Amplatz super-stiff guidewire allows the assistant to wiggle the stent and more rapidly identify the ureter. Alternatively, an infrared ureteral stent (Stryker Endoscopy, Santa Clara, CA) may assist in identifying the diseased ureter. Once the ureter is recognized, it is freed from the fibrotic process with care not to tear the ureter or compromise the blood supply. The ureter can be intraperitonealized by closing the medial and lateral cut edges of peritoneum behind it. Alternatively, it can be lateralized or wrapped with omentum using laparoscopic clips or sutures.

B. Laparoscopic Ureterectomy: Removal of the ureter can be performed as part of a nephroureterectomy procedure for transitional cell carcinoma (described below) or as a separate procedure for refluxing ureter with an associated nonfunctioning kidney, a pyoureter from a previous partial or simple nephrectomy, renal tuberculosis, or an ectopic ureterocele (Clayman, 1993). The distal ureter may be followed far down into the pelvis to its junction with the bladder. This may be aided by the preoperative placement of an end-hole stent and Amplatz super-stiff guidewire.

The intramural portion of the ureter may be excised using a Colling's knife, circumscribing the involved ureteric orifice and resecting out to the perivesical fat. Normally, only 1 or 2 laparoscopic sutures are required to close the bladder. Alternatively, the ureter can be stapled using an endo-GIA device at its junction with the ureter. The titanium staple line is normally not exposed to urine and is not a cause for stone formation.

C. Laparoscopic Ureterolithotomy: Laparoscopic ureterolithotomy is rarely required because of the high efficacy of endoscopic antegrade and retrograde stone techniques as well as extracorporeal shock wave lithotripsy. However, in those rare patients in whom stones cannot be removed by using endoscopic techniques, laparoscopic ureterolithotomy may be a less invasive approach than open surgery (Harewood, Webb, and Pope, 1994).

This procedure may be performed by an extraperitoneal or transperitoneal approach. Laparoscopic suturing may be required to close the ureterotomy after removal of the stone. Placement of a double-J catheter and drain is suggested postoperatively.

D. Other Ureteral Procedures: Isolated cases of laparoscopic ureteral reimplantation, ureteroureterostomy, and cutaneous ureterostomy have been reported. Much of the work for these procedures is still in the experimental phase (Reddy and Evans, 1994; Nezhat et al, 1992).

Alternative methods of tissue reconstruction using laser welding and fibrin glue may make such advanced procedures easier and more surgeon-friendly.

Kidney

A. Laparoscopic Renal Ablative Procedures: The first laparoscopic nephrectomy was performed in 1990 through the pioneering work of Clayman and colleagues (1991a). Since that date, numerous types of procedures have been performed laparoscopically for the full gamut of benign and malignant diseases of the upper urinary tract. In fact, the indications for laparoscopic surgery are greater today for upper urinary tract disease than for the lower tract.

1. Laparoscopic nephrectomy–Laparoscopic nephrectomy is primarily considered for benign renal disease but may be used for malignant disease of the kidney and ureter in select cases. The approach may be transperitoneal or retroperitoneal.

a. Preoperative preparation–After the correct patient is selected for this procedure, a full mechanical bowel preparation is administered. All patients receive a broad-spectrum parenteral antibiotic and are cross-matched for 2 units of packed red blood cells (erythrocytes).

Early in one's experience or in select cases, an end-hole ureteral catheter may be placed before embarking on the laparoscopic procedure. This may be placed with the use of the flexible cystoscope without the need for fluoroscopy. An Amplatz super-stiff guidewire is left in the ureteral catheter, and this unit is then fixed to a 16F Foley catheter placed in the bladder. The ureteral catheter–Amplatz wire unit may be helpful in locating the ureter intraoperatively.

2. Transperitoneal laparoscopic simple nephrectomy–General anesthesia is administered, and appropriate intravenous and arterial monitoring lines are established as deemed necessary by the anesthesiologist. Foley catheter and nasogastric tubes are mandatory. The patient is positioned at about 70 degrees flank and secured on an inflatable "bean bag," with the extremities well padded and secured.

In most patients, access to the peritoneal cavity is by use of the Veress needle through a puncture in the upper quadrant just lateral to the midclavicular line. The initial telescopic port is inserted at this level just below the costal margin. Normally, 2 additional ports are now placed at the superior crease of the umbilicus and just below the umbilicus in the midclavicular line. The laparoscope is moved to the umbilical port (Figure 9–24). The size and location of these ports is variable but generally will require one 12-mm port for insertion of the sac for kidney removal and subsequent extraction.

After the white line of Toldt is incised and the colon is rotated medially, a third working port may be placed in the midaxillary line for retraction. It is important to extend the incision around the hepatic or

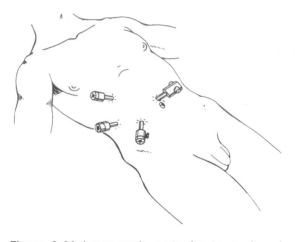

Figure 9–24. Laparoscopic ports for transperitoneal nephrectomy.

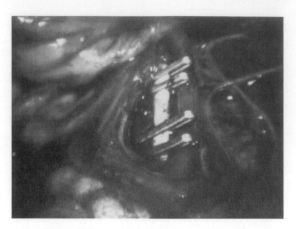

Figure 9–25. Laparoscopic clips (double) on renal artery.

splenic flexures to adequately mobilize the liver or spleen superomedial, which will improve access to the hilar and upper pole regions of the kidney. The location of the proximal ureter may be sought and then followed cranially, or, alternatively, dissection in the renal hilar region may be initiated immediately. Care must be taken in identifying the gonadal vessels as they cross the proximal ureter. In some cases these vessels should be clipped and transected, because they will compromise further ureteral dissection and may be avulsed from their associated great vessels. With the ureter identified, it is grasped with an endo-babcock or similar instrument and then traced upward toward the lower pole of the kidney and renal hilum.

Using a careful dissecting technique with straight and curved instruments, the renal artery(s) and vein(s) are individually cleared of surrounding fibrolymphatic and fatty tissue. At least 2 9-mm clips are placed on the proximal or "stay" side of these vessels and 1 or 2 on the distal or "go" side (Figure 9–25). It is strongly advised that the arterial vessels first be interrupted to prevent excessive venous pressure and undesirable bleeding. The main renal vein may require a laparoscopic endo-GIA staple to secure this vessel.

With the renal hilum transected, the lateral attachments of the kidney are released. Pulling inferiorly on the ureter, the upper pole of the kidney and upper medial portion of the kidney are dissected free; one should be careful of adrenal vessels or direct vascular branches off the inferior vena cava or aorta.

With the kidney fully mobilized, an impermeable sac (LapSac; Cook Urological Inc, Spencer, IN; or Endocatch; Autosuture Co), is placed down the 12-mm umbilical port into the peritoneal cavity (Figure 9–26). The laparoscope is moved to the upper mid-clavicular port, and then grasping instruments through the other ports are used to manipulate the kidney into the sac. The neck of the sac is brought out through the umbilical port site, and then the kidney may be morcellated within the sac using an electric tissue morcellator (Cook Urological Inc) or more simply digitally fragmented with the aid of ring forceps. This process is monitored laparoscopically to be certain the sac is not perforated. Keeping steady upward tension, the sac is delivered out of the abdomen, and the morcellated specimen is delivered to the pathologist. Alternatively, if the kidney is small, the periumbilical incision can be extended 1 or 2 cm farther to allow the kidney to be delivered intact. This approach is strongly suggested if laparoscopic nephrectomy is being considered for renal cancer.

The periumbilical incision may be closed at this point or the 12-mm port reestablished, and then a final laparoscopic inspection for hemostasis and visceral integrity is completed. Sheaths are removed as described previously for exiting the abdomen.

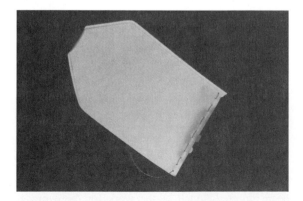

Figure 9–26. LapSac entrapment device (Cook Urological Inc, Spencer, IN).

3. Extraperitoneal laparoscopic simple nephrectomy–An extraperitoneal approach is preferred by many laparoscopic surgeons in reaching the kidney, because it is more direct and does not require mobilizing bowel or dealing directly with liver or spleen. Many of the potential risks of injuring intraperitoneal viscera are reduced, if not eliminated. Drawbacks to this approach are the loss of familiar anatomic landmarks, limited or reduced working space, and the potential for increased CO_2 absorption compared with the transperitoneal route (Glascock et al, 1996). It has been my policy to use the extraperitoneal route for laparoscopic nephrectomy in cases where the kidney is relatively small (as for renovascular hypertension) and there has not been previous retroperitoneal renal surgery or perinephric infection. I still prefer the transperitoneal approach in the presence of an enlarged polycystic kidney, recurrent pyelonephritis or xanthogranulomatous disease, or renal cell carcinoma.

As with the transperitoneal route, insertion of an end-hole ureteral catheter is optional. The patient is positioned in full flank and secured to the bean bag with care that the extremities are well padded.

A 2-cm transverse incision is made over Petit's triangle (inferior lumbar triangle) and deepened down to the lumbodorsal fascia. This fascia is incised, and then stay sutures are placed on each fascial edge. The finger is inserted into the retroperitoneal space and initiates the space. Feeling the back of the 12th rib and the back of the posterior iliac crest assures the operator that the correct space has been entered. No attempt is made to incise Gerota's fascia at this point in the procedure. An inflation balloon device is inserted, and the retroperitoneal working space is created as described for laparoscopic bladder neck suspension and laparoscopic PLND. A Hassan-type cannula is then inserted and secured to the 2 fascial stay sutures. Carbon dioxide is then insufflated up to 15 mm Hg.

On insertion of the laparoscope, the neophyte to the retroperitoneal space may be confronted with abundant pararenal fat and no landmarks. Working ports are placed just off the tip of the 12th rib at about the midaxillary line and a second port just above the iliac crest. These ports should be placed directly into the retroperitoneal space under laparoscopic or digital control and should not traverse the peritoneal membrane. If an opening in the peritoneal membrane does occur, it should be opened further to allow the CO_2 to equalize between both compartments and not cause compression of the retroperitoneal space.

Gerota's fascia is incised to locate the lateral aspect of the kidney. The kidney is freed laterally as well as toward the polar regions. At this point in the procedure it is advisable to place a third working port in the anterior axillary line directly opposite the initial entry site over Petit's triangle. Thus, the location of the laparoscopic ports take a diamond-shape configuration (Figure 9–27). This third working port in the anterior axillary line is important for retracting the kidney medially to allow access to the posterior and hilar regions of the kidney. The beauty of the retroperitoneal approach is improved access to the renal artery before having to deal with the renal vein. After securing the main renal artery or branches as described for the transperitoneal route, the renal vein and branches can be approached either anteriorly or posteriorly. Having secured the renal hilum, the remainder of the procedure involves mobilizing the kidney and transecting the ureter. In many cases the kidney is brought out directly through the flank incision, which can be enlarged slightly, or the laparoscopic sac technique can be used. Using a sac is more difficult owing to limited working space. After he-

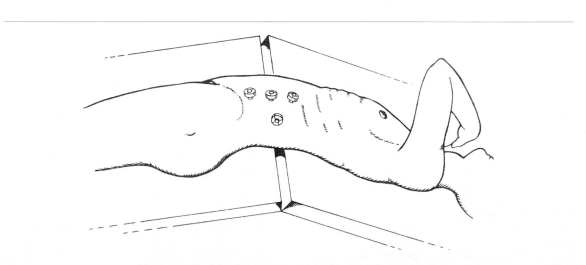

Figure 9–27. Port placement for extraperitoneal renal surgery.

mostasis is ensured, the laparoscopic ports are closed as described previously.

4. Laparoscopic radical nephrectomy–My preference is to perform laparoscopic radical nephrectomy by a transperitoneal route. However, a number of authors are very comfortable with the retroperitoneal approach (Gill et al, 1998c; Rassweiler et al, 1998). The key difference in performing a laparoscopic radical nephrectomy is intact preservation of Gerota's fascia with en bloc resection of the kidney. Upper pole renal cell tumors also require en bloc resection of the ipsilateral adrenal gland. I also prefer to limit laparoscopic radical nephrectomy to smaller tumors (≤ 8 cm) not involving the central hilar regions of the kidney or with obvious radiologic evidence of renal vein or inferior vena caval tumor involvement. Clinical data indicate comparable pathologic results with the laparoscopic approach compared with open radical nephrectomy, whereas the postoperative and convalescent period is markedly improved with laparoscopic nephrectomy (McDougall, Clayman, and Elashry, 1996; Caddedu et al, 1998). It is suggested that the resected kidney be placed in an entrapment sac before removal from the peritoneal cavity. Controversy has been raised about the intact removal of the kidney, which would require enlarging the incision, versus morcellation of the bagged kidney, which would obliterate tumor margins. My preference is to manually maneuver the bagged intact kidney through a 4- to 5-cm incision.

5. Laparoscopic cryosurgery for renal cell carcinoma–Very few centers have used laparoscopic cryosurgery as a curative alternative to the management of renal cell carcinoma. The laparoscopic ultrasound probe is mandatory to visualize the progressing "ice ball." Peripheral renal tumors < 4 cm in size are reasonable choices for this ablative technique (Gill et al, 1998a).

6. Laparoscopic live donor nephrectomy–To date, only a few centers worldwide have performed the advanced laparoscopic procedure, live donor nephrectomy. Initial cases, as pioneered by Kavoussi and colleagues, demonstrated excellent results with comparable renal graft function to open live donor nephrectomy (Ratner et al, 1997; Flowers et al, 1997). Most centers, including my own, use a transperitoneal approach and remove the kidney intact through an enlarged 5- to 7-cm midline or lower abdominal lateral incision. Warm ischemic time has averaged 2–5 min. As an incision will be required to remove the intact kidney, our approach has been to use hand-assisted laparoscopic surgery with the use of the PneumoSleeve (Dexterity Inc, Blue Bell, PA). Early results from Baltimore centers where the procedure was initiated indicate equivalent early graft survival with the open donor procedure, while complications are not excessive.

7. Postoperative Management–In most cases of laparoscopic nephrectomy, oral feeding can be initiated on the first postoperative day, and ambulation is encouraged the evening of surgery. Two doses of parenteral antibiotics are administered, but this is an empiric practice. In most cases, a full diet and hospital activity are achieved by the second or third postoperative day, and discharge closely follows. My patients have resumed full activity within 2 weeks of laparoscopic surgery.

8. Results–Contemporary comparative studies of laparoscopic versus open nephrectomy for benign and malignant tumors show that the procedure is feasible and has been done at many centers worldwide. Although the intraoperative surgical times are longer than those with the open approach, the patient benefits significantly in the postoperative period with respect to length of hospitalization, need for analgesic control, and return to normal daily activities.

9. Laparoscopic nephroureterectomy–As an extension of nephrectomy, laparoscopic nephroureterectomy was first described by Clayman et al (1991b). This operation, performed primarily for transitional cell carcinoma of the upper collecting system, is similar to laparoscopic nephrectomy in that it may be approached transperitoneally or by the retroperitoneal route. However, it is also necessary to excise the distal ureter and cuff of surrounding bladder.

Our approach to the distal ureter has been the following. The patient is positioned in dorsolithotomy, and a glide wire (Terumo) is cystoscopically inserted up the involved ureter. A glide wire is chosen to minimize conduction of the electric current along the guidewire. Using a Colling's knife set at 50W pure cut, the ureteric orifice is encircled transurethrally up to the level of the ureterovesical junction where fat becomes visible. Then using a roller electrode, the entire ureteral os and tunnel as well as a 2-cm perimeter are electrocauterized. At the termination, a 6F end-hole ureteral catheter is advanced over the glide wire up to the renal pelvis and left to straight drainage. Recent modifications of this technique using needlescopic instruments have been described by Soble et al (1998). The patient is then positioned as for a laparoscopic nephrectomy. A fifth or sixth laparoscopic port may be required for dissection of the distal ureter. Some authors have described the use of hand-assisted laparoscopy with the PneumoSleeve (Dexterity, Inc) to make the procedure faster and allow rapid en bloc removal of the nephroureteral specimen (Wolfe, Tehltgen, and Merion, 1998). It has been my policy to close the bladder opening using laparoscopic absorbable sutures. Other authors report closure of the bladder with a GIA stapler (Autosuture Co) without subsequent stone formation (Kerbl et al, 1993).

The postoperative course is normally similar to that described previously, and the Foley catheter should be left indwelling for 10 days and removed after a satisfactory cystogram is obtained. Sizeable studies of laparoscopic nephroureterectomy demonstrate long operative times but a marked improvement in postoperative course compared with the open approach (Keeley and Tolley, 1998; McDougall, Clayman, and Elashry, 1995). As mentioned previously, the use of the PneumoSleeve (Dexterity, Inc) may make this procedure faster but with the benefits of minimally invasive surgery.

Laparoscopic nephroureterectomy may also be considered for benign disease such as renal tuberculosis with pyoureteronephrosis or nonfunctioning hydroureteronephrotic kidneys. Excision of a bladder cuff in such situations is not necessary (Doehn et al, 1998).

10. Laparoscopic renal cyst decortication–Laparoscopic renal cyst decortication is ideal for those patients who have a benign simple renal cyst that causes significant flank or back pain. The other major indication for laparoscopic decortication is compression of the renal pelvis or infundibulocalyceal system, resulting in poor drainage of urine and possible stone formation or compromised renal function. Some authors have recommended laparoscopic decortication of multiple cysts in patients presenting with polycystic kidney disease (Elashry et al, 1996). Although improvement of renal function is not expected with such procedures, the laparoscopic approach does offer these patients a considerable lessening of pain without having to undergo maximally invasive surgery.

It has been my policy to percutaneously decompress the cyst(s) in patients complaining of significant pain from simple solitary cysts. Patients in whom the pain returns as the cyst fluid reaccumulates will benefit from definitive decortication. As a word of caution, a large calyceal diverticulum with tiny infundibular connection to the renal pelvis may be mistaken for a simple renal cyst. This entity should be considered preoperatively.

a. Preoperative evaluation–The usual preoperative criteria for laparoscopy should be considered for this procedure. Radiologic imaging based on renal ultrasound, CT scan, or cyst puncture with cytologic and biochemical tests of the fluid should not be suggestive of malignancy. In most cases these tests are accurate, but unfortunately in < 1% of cases, a renal cell carcinoma may be found within the wall of a "simple cyst." Therefore, every attempt should be made to determine the clinical status of the symptomatic cyst. A CT scan is strongly advised to clearly identify the location of the cyst. Cysts located posteriorly or laterally are preferably approached by a retroperitoneal laparoscopic route, whereas anterior or perihilar cysts are approached transperitoneally.

b. Technique–The laparoscopic approach to patients with a renal cyst is similar to that described for retroperitoneal or transperitoneal nephrectomy. However, in most cases, only 3 ports are required. In most cases, the cyst is easily visualized bulging off

the contour of the kidney. Overlying fibrofatty tissue is carefully peeled off the cyst wall and generally transmits a bluish hue that is clearly different from surrounding parenchyma (Figure 9–28). It has been my policy to insert a 5-mm laparoscopic aspiration needle into the cyst to be absolutely sure the landmarks are correct. Fluid obtained should be straw-colored and clear and should be sent for cytologic and biochemical analysis.

The cyst wall is then carefully excised using electrocautery or a harmonic scalpel. The edges of the cyst are fulgurated and the specimen sent for pathologic examination. The base of the cyst is carefully inspected. Any lesion suggestive of malignancy is biopsied and sent for frozen pathologic evaluation. Malignancy discovered at this point would require an immediate open nephrectomy to prevent further tumor spillage.

After malignancy is ruled out, surrounding perirenal fat or omentum may be mobilized into the confines of the cyst cavity and sutured or stapled to the edges. A drain is not normally placed. The ports are removed as described earlier, and the skin is handled in the usual fashion.

In cases of perihilar or multiple renal cysts, it has been my policy to perform flexible cystoscopy and insert an end-hole ureteral catheter. After excision of the outer cyst wall, methylene blue may be injected through the ureteral catheter to be certain the collecting system has not been entered. Should this be the case, the opening is laparoscopically repaired and a double-J catheter is inserted.

The patient is started on fluids the evening of surgery and may be discharged from hospital the following day.

c. Results–The experience of a number of authors has been uniformly good in laparoscopically managing symptomatic renal cysts (Denis et al, 1998; Hoenig et al, 1997). However, cases must be chosen carefully to be certain the indications for treatment are correct.

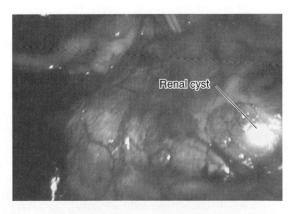

Figure 9–28. Bluish hue of a renal cyst.

11. Laparoscopic partial nephrectomy–Laparoscopic partial nephrectomy is an advanced procedure that may be indicated for the removal of a small segment of the upper or lower pole region of the kidney (Jordan and Winslow, 1993a; Winfield et al, 1995). I have seen this in conjunction with a poorly functioning, atrophic segment of a duplicated collecting system (Winfield et al, 1995). Alternatively, the procedure has been used for excision of the lower calyceal portion of the kidney harboring recurrent calculi and minimal surrounding cortex. Many of these patients have undergone many previous attempts to render them stone- and infection-free, resulting in considerable surrounding fibrotic tissue. In rare cases, laparoscopic partial nephrectomy has been undertaken for excision of small renal tumors that are located close to or beyond the renal cortex. In such cases, frozen biopsies must be taken from the surgical margins. The threshold for conversion to open surgery in such cases must be low.

Although arteriogram or spiral CT is not always required for open partial nephrectomy, it is strongly suggested for the laparoscopic approach. In addition, specialized laparoscopic equipment should be available, primarily to aid in hemostasis. The harmonic scalpel (Ethicon Endo-Surgery Inc, Cincinnati, OH), argon beam coagulator, and laparoscopic Satinsky vascular clamps or bulldog clamps (MicroFrance Co, Montreal, Canada) are of great use in controlling the bleeding expected with partial nephrectomy. The 10-mm laparoscopic 7.5-MHz ultrasound probe with color Doppler vascular component may also be helpful in locating the area and depth of renal pathology.

a. Technique–The laparoscopic exposure to the kidney may be transperitoneal or retroperitoneal, depending on the location of the pathologic lesion. It is reasonable to cystoscopically insert a 6F end-hole ureteral catheter before beginning the procedure. This is used to inject methylene blue during the procedure, if necessary, and to allow conversion to a double-J catheter at termination. It is usual to use 3 or 4 laparoscopic ports.

Mobilization of the renal hilum with dissection of the renal arterial branches is suggested if a sizeable segment of the kidney is to be excised. With this preparation, a laparoscopic vascular or bulldog clamp may be quickly applied should bleeding be significant. An electrocautery hook is used, followed closely by the 5- or 10-mm laparoscopic argon beam coagulator probe to excise the diseased segment of kidney in a controlled fashion. If and when the collecting system is entered, the raw surface may be extensively coagulated with the argon beam. If the opening is small, this coagulation may be sufficient, whereas larger openings may require a few laparoscopic sutures. Perirenal fat or surrounding renal capsule should be secured over the raw parenchyma.

It is best to convert the end-hole catheter to a double-J catheter. This may be done simply by inserting a guidewire through the end-hole catheter and then removing the catheter. A double-J catheter is then back-loaded over the guidewire and introduced via the pusher. Choosing a longer double-J stent and carefully estimating the location of the ureteral orifice should prevent one from advancing the stent too far into the ureter. Alternatively, fluoroscopy can be used if available.

A 1/2-in Penrose drain is introduced through a posterior 10-mm trocar-sheath unit, and then laparoscopic hernia staples are used to reperitonealize the colon if a transperitoneal route was used. Ports and skin are managed as described previously.

Postoperatively, most patients follow a course similar to that described for laparoscopic nephrectomy and are started on fluids the first postoperative day. Drainage has been minimal, and in most cases the drain may be advanced on the second or third postoperative day. A retrograde pyelogram is performed on day 14, and the double-J stent may be removed if no extravasation is present.

12. Renal biopsy–Renal biopsy is an important diagnostic test for determining the renal pathological condition associated with severe proteinuria or unexplained renal disease. Normally, this procedure is performed by percutaneous biopsy.

When percutaneous renal biopsy is not feasible or safe, a laparoscopic approach can be undertaken with excellent results. The kidney should be approached by a retroperitoneal route, and biopsies can be easily obtained using laparoscopic scissors. Hemostasis is controlled with simple electrocautery or argon beam coagulation (Gimenez et al, 1998).

B. Laparoscopic Renal Reconstructive Procedures:

1. Laparoscopic pyeloplasty–Ureteropelvic junction (UPJ) obstruction is a well-known urologic disease that can be treated by different surgical approaches. While open dismembered pyeloplasty has been the gold standard, less invasive techniques have been developed, including antegrade or retrograde endoscopic incision (endopyelotomy) of the narrowed UPJ. Antegrade endopyelotomy was developed in the 1980s as an alternative to open pyeloplasty (Wickham and Kellett, 1983; Badlani, Eshghi, and Smith, 1986). Overall success rates are reported to be around 85% (ranging from 78 to 89%), with slightly better results in secondary UPJ obstruction (Badlani, Eshghi, and Smith, 1986; Motola, Badlani, and Smith, 1993; Kletscher et al, 1995; Danuser et al, 1998; Thomas, Monga, and Klein, 1996). Endopyelotomy may also be accomplished via a retrograde ureteroscopic approach with success rates of around 80% (Thomas, Monga, and Klein, 1996; Conlin and Bagley, 1998). The Acucise ureteral cutting balloon device (Applied Medical, Laguna Hills, CA) offers yet another alternative, with reported success rates of 68–87% (Nadler et al, 1996; Gelet et al, 1997).

Laparoscopic pyeloplasty has now been described

by authors in several centers where advanced laparoscopy is performed. This procedure mirrors the gold standard except for the surgical access. Success rates in limited studies rival those of open pyeloplasty (Brooks et al, 1995). Concomitant stones can be removed during the repair (Moore et al, 1997). The procedure is particularly suited for those patients with a large, redundant renal pelvis, or a prominent crossing vessel, because these patients may have lower success rates with endopyelotomy. In fact, Van Cangh et al (1994) have reported a successful result in only 66% of patients with high-grade hydronephrosis and in 42% of patients with a crossing vessel. In patients with both characteristics, the success rate of endopyelotomy may be as low as 39% (Van Cangh et al, 1994).

Preoperative evaluation should include a lasix diuretic renal scan. In recent years the use of helical CT scanning with 3-dimensional reconstruction has yielded outstanding vascular anatomy in the region of the UPJ. The use of endoluminal sonographic imaging (Bagley, Kiu, and Goldberg, 1996) has also been considered in select cases. These radiologic modalities aid in determining the optimal treatment approach for each patient.

Laparoscopic pyeloplasty may be performed by the transperitoneal or retroperitoneal approach. The advantages of the transperitoneal approach are the familiarity of the anatomic landmarks and the larger operating space (especially important for large kidneys or masses), making intracorporeal suturing somewhat easier. The disadvantages are the violation of the peritoneum with its attendant risks to intraperitoneal structures, the increased risk of ileus with mobilization of the colon (minimal in my experience), increased risk of incisional hernia, and the risks of intraperitoneal urine extravasation. My preference is the transperitoneal route.

a. Patient preparation–Preoperative consultation must include a discussion of alternative approaches and the possibility of conversion to open surgery. The patient is given a simple mechanical bowel preparation. Broad-spectrum intravenous antibiotics are administered preoperatively. An open-end ureteral catheter is placed at the beginning of the procedure by using the flexible cystoscope, with fluoroscopic guidance if needed. A Foley catheter is also placed, and both are secured. The ureteral catheter is included in the sterile field for intraoperative access.

b. Surgical technique–The patient is placed in a full flank position, as for laparoscopic nephrectomy. A nasogastric or orogastric tube is recommended. Standard skin preparation and draping are performed. Initial access may be gained by Veress needle placement or the Hassan technique at the umbilicus or at a subcostal location in the midclavicular line, and pneumoperitoneum is obtained as described previously. An umbilical port and 2 midclavicular

ports are used. An optional lateral port may be placed in the midaxillary line to assist with retraction if necessary. By using primarily 10/11-mm ports, maximum versatility with the instruments is preserved, although smaller ports are recommended.

After inspection of the peritoneal cavity, the colon is mobilized medially to expose the kidney. The lower pole of the kidney is identified, and the ureter is exposed and isolated at this level. The ureter can then be followed up to the renal pelvis, where the UPJ is identified (Figure 9–29). Lower pole crossing vessels may be found in up to 40% of these cases (Sampaio and Favorito, 1993) and should be identified at this point (Figure 9–30). The preoperative radiographic images may have already clarified this anatomy. The previously placed ureteral catheter is helpful for identifying the ureter. For additional assistance, an Amplatz stiff guidewire can be passed through the ureteral catheter and the catheter can be wiggled by the assistant.

c. Dismembered pyeloplasty–A stay suture of 4-0 polyglactin (vicryl) is placed in the medial aspect of the ureter just below the area to be excised. The ends of the suture are cut and held together with a clip for use in retracting the ureter. The ureter is then divided below the UPJ obstruction. The ureter can be spatulated along the lateral edge, as would be done in an open pyeloplasty. The renal pelvis is opened above the UPJ, and the narrowed segment is excised and removed from the operative field. At this point the renal pelvis is transposed to the opposite side of any crossing vessels. A large, redundant pelvis can be excised and tailored.

The sutured anastomosis—admittedly the most difficult portion of this procedure—is prepared. The first 4-0 polyglactin suture is placed through the apex of the ureteral spatulation and the most dependent

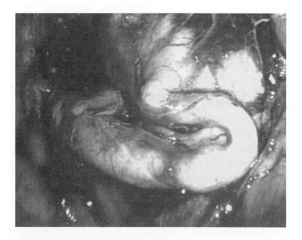

Figure 9–29. Kinking ureteropelvic junction anatomy for laparoscopic pyeloplasty.

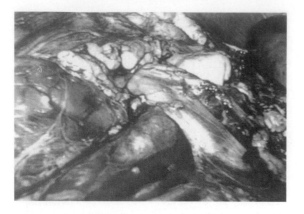

Figure 9–30. Crossing vessel at ureteropelvic junction causing obstruction.

portion of the renal pelvis. The ureteral stay suture is used to ensure that the ureter lies in the proper orientation. Additional interrupted sutures are placed along the back wall first. When the anastomosis is partially completed, the ureteral guidewire is manipulated into the renal pelvis. The open-end ureteral catheter is replaced with a 7F double-J stent of appropriate length. The ureteropelvic anastomosis is completed with the interrupted sutures. The remainder of the pyelotomy can be closed with running sutures.

With the anastomosis complete, the colon is repositioned over the kidney and (optionally) tacked to the lateral abdominal wall with hernia staples. This maneuver theoretically recreates the retroperitoneal space. A small passive drain is placed through the most lateral port site into the retroperitoneum. The ports are removed and the incisions closed in standard fashion.

d. Alternative surgical techniques–It is important that the laparoscopic surgeon be familiar with alternative approaches to the repair of the UPJ. Using the flap techniques such as Y-V-plasty and Culp (or Scardino) pyeloplasty, a flap of renal pelvis wall is mobilized down across the UPJ to expand the lumen of the ureter. These approaches are ideal for high UPJ insertion with nondilated renal pelvis or where the area of narrowing at the UPJ is lengthy. Because of the difficulty of suturing in a dismembered anastomosis or flap technique, the Fenger-plasty has been advocated by some authors (Janetschek et al, 1996a). The Fenger-plasty is accomplished by making a longitudinal incision across the UPJ and closing it transversely. Each of these nondismembered techniques has the advantage of leaving the renal pelvis and ureter in continuity so that the technical aspect of suturing is more manageable.

e. Alternative anastomotic techniques–Alternative methods of anastomotic closure have been

investigated and are now reported more frequently. The greatest advance has come from the use of the automated suturing device (Endostitch; Autosuture Co). This device passes a short needle with swaged-on suture between opposing jaws, thus eliminating the time-consuming task of grasping and positioning a free needle with laparoscopic instruments. This enables the surgeon to place and tie a suture in one-third the time required for free needle suturing (Adams et al, 1995). In one study, operative time was reduced by 2.1 h with the introduction of this instrument (Moore et al, 1997). However, the jaws of the Endostitch are large when compared with the size of the ureteral anastomosis to be accomplished. I prefer to suture the ureter with a free needle and close the pyelotomy with the Endostitch device.

Another group has reported the use of a few fixation sutures along with fibrin glue to complete the anastomosis and make a watertight seal (Eden et al, 1997). The use of small, nonperforating titanium clips has been reported in an animal model to facilitate reconstruction of the urinary tract (McDougall et al, 1997). All of these techniques are introduced to decrease the time required for the most tedious portion of this procedure while preserving optimal results.

f. Postoperative care–Patients are advanced quickly to a regular diet, and pain is controlled with oral or intravenous analgesics (or both). The drain is removed in 2–4 days, and the ureteral double-J stent is removed in 4 weeks in the office with the use of a flexible cystoscope.

g. Results–Laparoscopic pyeloplasty offers the possibility of success rates equivalent to those of open dismembered pyeloplasty, combined with the benefits of minimally invasive surgery and a shorter recovery period. The procedure has been demonstrated in a few centers to be safe and feasible. Furthermore, improvements in technology and alterations in technique have contributed to decreased operating time. There is evidence that some prognostic factors reduce the likelihood of success of endoscopic incision and stenting. For these patients, it is reasonable to consider laparoscopic pyeloplasty as a definitive procedure with a high rate of success.

2. Laparoscopic nephropexy–Nephroptosis is characterized by a downward displacement of the kidney by more than 3 vertical bodies when the patient moves from a supine to an erect position (Moss, 1997). Although rare, it often presents in very slender adult females and may result in significant flank pain and a palpable mass. In rare cases it may cause intermittent hematuria and hypertension. After excluding all other causes of flank pain by history and radiologic and provocative testing, fixation of the kidney (nephropexy) may be considered. This procedure has been accomplished laparoscopically by both the retroperitoneal and the transperitoneal approach (Fornara, Doehn, and Jocham, 1997). Freeing up the lateral and upper portion of the kidney, laparoscopic sutures are placed through the renal capsule and secured to the fascia of the psoas or quadratis lumborum muscle as far cephalad within the retroperitoneum as possible. To tie the knots well, an extracorporeal knot may be required or secured with the lapra Ty suture clip applier (Ethicon Endo-Surgery Inc). Normally, only 3–6 sutures are sufficient to secure the kidney well.

ADRENAL GLANDS

1. Laparoscopic adrenalectomy–Laparoscopic adrenalectomy was first reported by Gagner and colleagues in 1992 and has gained attention worldwide over the ensuing years. Initial studies indicate marked benefits to the patient in the postoperative period (Gagner, Lacroix, and Bolte, 1992; Sardi and McKinnon, 1993; Susuki et al, 1993). To date this technique has shown great promise in the treatment of metabolically active adrenal tumors, such as aldosteronomas, pheochromocytomas, and Cushing disease. It has also been considered for solitary metastatic disease to the adrenal gland, which is often associated with renal cell carcinoma. The use of laparoscopic techniques for adrenal lesions in excess of 8 cm or for primary adrenal carcinoma is discouraged.

a. Preoperative preparation–As with all other laparoscopic techniques, patients are informed of all treatment options as well as potential risks and complications. A mechanical bowel preparation with GoLytely (Braintree Laboratories) the previous afternoon is recommended. All patients require a Foley catheter inserted into the bladder, and an orogastric tube is mandatory because a distended stomach will compromise exposure of the adrenal gland.

b. Surgical technique–My preference for laparoscopic adrenalectomy has been the transperitoneal route. However, other authors have approached the adrenal gland by the retroperitoneal (flank) route or even the posterior lumbar (prone) route with excellent results (Ono et al, 1996; Baba et al, 1997).

For the transperitoneal route, patients are placed in full flank position after general anesthesia has been obtained. Access into the peritoneal cavity is by the Veress needle or Hassan cannula open technique into the respective abdominal upper quadrant in the midclavicular line, and a pneumoperitoneum is created with CO_2 up to 15 mm Hg. Four 10/11-mm laparoscopic ports are arranged subcostal in the respective upper abdominal quadrant, as shown in Figure 9–31. It has been a goal to decrease the port sizes; Gill and colleagues (1998b) have presented data on the use of miniports and instrumentation for laparoscopic adrenalectomy.

On the left side, a T-shaped incision is made to mobilize the splenic flexure inferomedially and the

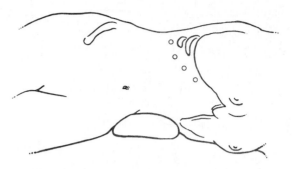

Figure 9–31. Placement of ports for right laparoscopic adrenalectomy.

spleen superomedially (Figure 9–32). It is important to fully mobilize the spleen so that it literally falls over onto itself by gravitational pull alone. After creating a working space in the retroperitoneum to access the adrenal gland, the inferior and superior borders of the gland are identified and dissected. Misidentification of the tail of the pancreas for the adrenal gland can be avoided by not dissecting medial to the splenic vessels and by recognizing the nongolden color of the pancreas. Once the dissection of the adrenal gland progresses medially, the left adrenal vein(s) should be identified and then doubly clipped and transected (Figure 9–33). Liberal use of the electrocautery hook has been helpful in this delicate dissection, and avoidance of direct manipulation of the adrenal capsule prevents troublesome bleeding. If available, the 7.5-MHz laparoscopic ultrasound probe with deflecting transducer tip capabilities (B&K Medical Systems, Inc, Marlborough, MA) may aid in the localization of the adrenal gland among the often abundant periadrenal and renal fat.

For the right laparoscopic adrenalectomy, port size and location are similarly placed in the right upper quadrant. The T-shaped incision now allows inferomedial retraction of the hepatic flexure, and the liver is mobilized superomedially (Figure 9–32). As with the spleen on the left side, it is important to fully retract the liver upward by incising the triangular ligaments. Identification of the inferior vena cava allows access to the large right adrenal vein emanating off the posterolateral aspect of this great vessel. When the adrenal vein is short and fat and there is concern that 2 clips cannot be safely placed on the caval side, the endo-GIA stapling device is used. It is also not uncommon for there to be large adrenal vessels emanating from the renal vein and artery.

The adrenal gland is then manipulated into a 4 × 6-in LapSac (Cook Urological Inc) or similar entrapment device and removed via the lateral 10-mm laparoscopic port site. On rare occasions, it is necessary to slightly enlarge this opening to accommodate the adrenal tissue.

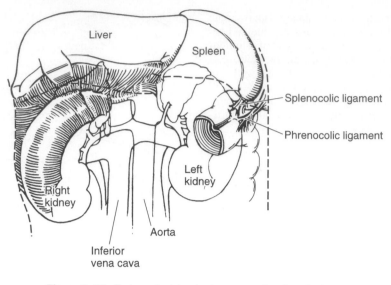

Figure 9–32. T-shape incision for laparoscopic adrenalectomy.

All ports are closed with the Carter-Thomason port closure device (Inlet Medical Inc) using 2-0 polydioxanone suture for the fascia and 4-0 dexon (polyglycolic acid) for the skin.

Although operative times with laparoscopy are longer than those with open surgery, a retrospective comparison of laparoscopic to open adrenalectomy demonstrates clear advantages of the minimally invasive approach in the postoperative period. Once the learning curve of laparoscopic adrenalectomy is overcome, the surgical times become comparable (Winfield et al, 1998).

Despite the apparent minimal invasiveness of laparoscopic adrenalectomy, its availability should not encourage expansion of the accepted indications for removal of nonfunctioning adrenal masses (Mugiya et al, 1996). It has been my policy to offer laparoscopic adrenalectomy as a treatment option for incidentally discovered, nonfunctioning adrenal masses > 3 cm or for those demonstrating measurable growth on serial CT scans or magnetic resonance images. Tumors > 6 cm and those highly suggestive of primary adrenal carcinoma are believed to be best handled by an open surgical approach. Adrenal lesions < 6 cm that are suspected of harboring metastatic disease from renal cell carcinoma are easily managed by laparoscopy. The dissection planes, however, are not as well defined owing to the uncontrolled growth pattern of the carcinoma. This, of course, would be accentuated by primary adrenal carcinomatous lesions > 6 cm. The chances of cure would be low without en bloc resection, which would be very difficult with a laparoscopic approach.

As outlined in reports from centers throughout the world, many other laparoscopic approaches have been advocated for adrenalectomy that involves direct lateral retroperitoneal and posterior retroperitoneal routes. Baba and colleagues (1997) compared the efficacy of retroperitoneoscopic adrenalectomy by a posterior lumbar approach with that obtained by a lateral flank approach or the transperitoneal route. It was found that adrenalectomy by the retroperitoneoscopic posterior lumbar approach was accomplished more rapidly than the alternative endoscopic routes, and there appeared to be little risk of injury to intraperitoneal organs. They did caution that the retroperitoneal working space is smaller, causing limited mobility of instruments. Undoubtedly, this could present more of a problem in patients of larger body weight in whom retroperitoneal fat would be more abundant. Each procedure has its advantages

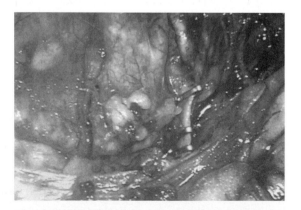

Figure 9–33. Clipping of the left adrenal vein.

and disadvantages as well as its unique complications (Ono et al, 1996; Baba et al, 1997). By a retroperitoneal approach, injury to the epigastric vessels or spleen would not be expected, whereas pneumothorax, severe hemorrhaging, and technical difficulties in accessing and dissecting the adrenal gland that are due to the limited working space have been reported with the retroperitoneal approach, requiring open conversion.

LYMPHOCELE

Lymphocele formation associated with extrapelvic surgery or following renal transplantation may result in significant complications. The definitive management of a lymphocele may prevent lower extremity edema, deep vein thrombosis, and renal graft loss. Treatment modalities have included fine-needle aspiration, percutaneous drainage, and open surgical internal drainage (Bischof et al, 1998).

The transperitoneal laparoscopic approach to decompression of lymphoceles has been shown to be highly successful while allowing the rapid recovery of the patient compared with open surgical intervention (Melvin et al, 1997).

Critical to the success of this procedure is correct localization of the ureter relative to the lymphocele. This can be aided by placement of an end-hole ureteral catheter preoperatively as well as previous spiral CT scanning with reformatting. It is not unusual for the ureter to course directly in the field of the planned peritoneal window.

After the ureter is identified, a peritoneal window is excised from the lymphocele cavity such that the space is obliterated by omentum. The use of the laparoscopic ultrasound probe may also be helpful in the rapid localization of small lymphoceles located deep in the pelvis.

COMPLICATIONS OF LAPAROSCOPIC SURGERY

If one reviews the general laparoscopic literature before 1989, it would appear that rates of major (0.6%) and minor (4%) complications are low and that complications occur relatively infrequently (Mintz, 1977; Cuschieri, 1980). However, one must be careful to note that these data are based primarily on diagnostic "look-and-see" laparoscopy. As demonstrated by multicenter studies of more advanced laparoscopic urologic procedures, complications do occur (Kavoussi et al, 1993a; Gill et al, 1995). There is no question that there is a steep learning curve with laparoscopic surgery and that many initial complications would have been avoided or are more appropriately managed today. On the other hand, as one gains greater experience and confidence, more complicated cases will be undertaken. J. Wickham said in 1991, "The complications of surgery are the complications of surgery." One cannot expect to perform major laparoscopic procedures in large numbers without having complications. Surgeons who boast that they have not had complications are probably saying one of 2 things: They do not do the surgery very often, or they do not know (or are lying about) what is happening to their patients.

A complete description of all the complications and management approaches is beyond the scope of this chapter. What is important to mention is that a standardized approach to performing the basic steps of laparoscopic surgery should be followed in every case (Table 9–5). By preparing one's operating room and personnel thoroughly, as well as having a clear plan of what is to be performed laparoscopically, complications will be minimized. Finally, correct patient selection is crucial in safely performing laparoscopic surgery.

THE FUTURE OF LAPAROSCOPIC SURGERY IN UROLOGY

It is clear that laparoscopic surgery is here to stay in the specialty of urology. This is reflected by the number of urologists who have sought training in this minimally invasive form of surgery. Indeed, major

Table 9–5. Standardization of laparoscopic surgery.

Adequate laparoscopic training and supervision
Organized operating room and a reliable surgical nursing team
Comprehensive understanding of laparoscopic equipment and instrumentation
Properly maintained equipment
Correct patient selection
Preoperative preparation and informed consent
Careful patient positioning
Placement of Foley catheter and other tubes
Entering the abdomen
  Establish and assess pneumoperitoneum or retropneumoperitoneum (Veress needle or open laparoscopic approach).
  Monitor CO_2 pressures being insufflated.
  Control placement of all trocar-sheath units. Inspect underlying viscera.
  Secure all ports in place to prevent slippage.
  Verbally communicate with anesthesiologist.
Exiting the abdomen
  Inspect for visceral integrity at termination of procedure.
  Inspect for hemorrhaging by lowering intraperitoneal or retroperitoneal pressure to 5 mm Hg.
  Laparoscopically visualize working port removal for abdominal wall bleeding.
  Close 10-mm (or larger) working port puncture sites with 2-0 absorbable suture in adults under laparoscopic guidance. Close all ports in children.
  Desufflate all CO_2 from last port and remove. Close last port site with 2-0 suture.
  Cover skin incisions with SteriStrips.

academic and urologic residency programs have attending staff dedicated to minimally invasive surgery. Advertisements offering positions in private urologic practice encourage residency or fellowship training in laparoscopy.

Despite the initial enthusiasm for laparoscopic surgery in the early 1990s, it has not, unfortunately, become a major portion of most urologists' practices. This can be explained by the fact that laparoscopic surgery is not easy to perform and there is a definite learning curve, steep at times. The simpler procedures such as laparoscopic varix ligation and laparoscopic PLND are now less commonly performed. As mentioned previously, with the advent of PSA testing and increased public awareness, prostate cancer is usually detected at an earlier stage, when laparoscopic PLND is unnecessary. Laparoscopic varix ligation is as invasive as the inguinal or subinguinal approach and more costly. Therefore, the indications for laparoscopic surgery have moved to more advanced bladder, renal, and adrenal surgery, which require greater experience and skill.

Equipment companies continue to develop better and more user-friendly laparoscopic instruments and devices. This is clearly reflected in the stapling and suturing instrumentation. Alternative imaging equipment, such as laparoscopic color ultrasound or Doppler probes, allows the laparoscopic surgeon to overcome the tactile deficiencies.

To overcome the human fatigue factor, robotics has played an increasingly important role in laparoscopic surgery. Robotics has been championed by Kavoussi and colleagues (1995) at Johns Hopkins University in conjunction with Computer Motion (Goleta, CA). The AESOP allows the surgeon to attach the laparoscope to the robotic arm and then actively maneuver the robot by means of a foot or hand switch or through the use of voice activation. Thus, the laparoscopic surgeon regains complete control over the operative visual field without having to translate the movements to a first or second assistant. The incorporation of robots into the operating theater now allows a consultant surgeon to teleoperate and/or telementor from a remote site. Thus, the consultant surgeon may now be able to actively move the robot arm via toggle switches from another location within the hospital, city, or country, thereby moving the laparoscope or other instrument in an appropriate fashion. Such long-distance robotic-aided laparoscopic procedures have been accomplished (Janetschek et al, 1998).

The goal of robotic surgery, telesurgery, and telementoring is to make laparoscopic surgery easier and more accessible to the novice. In addition, such endeavors allow mainstream laparoscopic surgery to be brought to more remote and distant medical centers throughout the world.

Finally, to help overcome the learning curve of laparoscopic surgery, the use of virtual reality programs has been considered by a number of centers. Such computer-supported programs allow the trainee to adapt to the equipment, the optics, and the usual anatomic parameters before embarking on the human model (Coleman, Nduka, and Darzi, 1994).

As has been discussed in this chapter, laparoscopic surgery has been considered for almost all types of genitourinary pathology. Julius Caesar said many years ago, "If it is possible, it has been done. If it is impossible, it will be done." However, just because it can be done does not necessarily mean it is better or safer for our patients. As intelligent surgeons we must continue to prospectively compare laparoscopic procedures with the traditional approaches of treatment so as to gain the optimal results for our patients. Only in this way will laparoscopic urologic intervention find its rightful role in the management of genitourinary pathology.

Finally, although laparoscopic surgery may not always be easy, it is critically important that we support and encourage individuals interested in this form of surgery. There are now many general surgeons who are extremely adept at laparoscopic interventions around and on the kidney and adrenal glands. Laparoscopic donor nephrectomy is being performed in many centers solely by general or transplant surgeons. Needless to say, if they are capable of laparoscopically removing a kidney for the purpose of transplantation, there is very little reason to believe that they could not also remove a diseased kidney should a urologic surgeon not be capable of doing such minimally invasive surgery. It is critical that we protect our "surgical turf" by maintaining clear foresight about the necessity to train laparoscopic surgeons.

In the interim, however, we should be proud of our creativity and leading role in this new form of minimally invasive surgery and should encourage our engineering colleagues to continue to develop these wonderful new instruments. The future for urology is bright, and we must continue to stay on the leading edge of this technology.

REFERENCES

Adams JB et al: New laparoscopic suturing device: Initial clinical experience. Urology 1995;46:242.

Assimos, Jarow JP: Role of laparoscopic pelvic lymph node dissection in the management of patients with penile cancer and inguinal adenopathy. J Endourol 1994;8:365.

Baba S et al: A posterior lumbar approach for retroperitoneoscopic adrenalectomy: Assessment of surgical efficacy. Urology 1997;50:19.

Badlani G, Eshghi M, Smith AD: Percutaneous surgery for ureteropelvic junction obstruction (endopyelotomy): Technique and early results. J Urol 1986;135: 26.

Bagley DM, Kiu JB, Goldberg B: Endoluminal sonographic imaging of the ureteropelvic junction. J Endourol 1996;10:105.

Benson KH et al: The value of computerized tomography in evaluation of pelvic lymph nodes. J Urol 1981; 126:63.

Bergman A, Ballard CA, Koonings PP: Comparison of three different surgical procedures for genuine stress incontinence: Prospective randomized study. Am J Obstet Gynecol 1989;160:1102.

Bischof G et al: Management of lymphocele after kidney transplantation. Transplant Int 1998;11:277.

Bloom DA: Two-step orchiopexy with pelvioscopic clip ligation of the spermatic vessels. J Urol 1991;145: 1030.

Bluestein DL et al: Eliminating the need for bilateral pelvic lymphadenectomy in select patients with prostate cancer. J Urol 1994;151:1315.

Brooks JD et al: Comparison of open and endourologic approaches to the obstructed ureteropelvic junction. Urology 1995;46:791.

Burton G: A randomized comparison of laparoscopic and open colposuspension. Neurourol Urodyn 1994; 13:497.

Caddedu JA et al: Laparoscopic nephrectomy for renal cell cancer: Evaluation of efficacy and safety: A multicenter experience. Urology 1998;52:773.

Campbell SC et al: Open pelvic lymph dissection for prostate cancer: A reassessment. Urology 1995;46: 352.

Castellino RA et al: Lymphangiography in prostatic carcinoma: Preliminary observations. JAMA 1973;223: 877.

Castilho LN et al: Laparoscopic pediatric orchiectomy. J Endourol 1992;6:155.

Clayman RV: Laparoscopic ureteral surgery. In: Clayman RV, McDougall EM (editors): *Laparoscopic Urology.* Quality Medical Publishing, 1993.

Clayman RV et al: Laparoscopic nephrectomy. N Engl J Med 1991a;324:1370.

Clayman RV et al: Laparoscopic nephroureterectomy: initial clinical case report. Lap Surg 1991b;1:343.

Coleman J, Nduka CC, Darzi A: Virtual reality and laparoscopic surgery. Br J Surg 1994;81:1709.

Colombo M et al: Burch colposuspension versus modified Marshall-Marchetti-Krantz urethropexy for primary genuine stress urinary incontinence: A prospective, randomized clinical trial. Am J Obstet Gynecol 1994;171:1573.

Conlin MJ, Bagley DH: Ureteroscopic endopyelotomy at a single setting. J Urol 1998;159:727.

Cortesi N et al: Diagnosis of bilateral abdominal cryptorchidism by laparoscopy. Endoscopy 1976;8:33.

Cuschieri A: Laparoscopy in general surgery and gastroenterology. Br J Hosp Med 1980;24:252.

Danuser H et al: Endopyelotomy for primary ureteropelvic junction obstruction: Risk factors determine the success rate. J Urol 1998;159:56.

Das S, Amar AD: The impact of laparoscopy on modern urologic practice. Urol Clin North Am 1988;15:537.

Denis E et al: Laparoscopic surgical treatment of simple cysts of the kidney. Prog Urol 1998;8:195.

Docimo SG et al: Laparoscopic bladder augmentation using stomach. Urology 1995;46:565.

Doehn C et al: Comparison of laparoscopic and open nephroureterectomy for benign disease. J Urol 1998; 159:732.

Donohue JP et al: Nerve-sparing retroperitoneal lymphadenectomy with preservation of ejaculation. J Urol 1990;144:287.

Donovan JF Jr: Laparoscopic varix ligation. Atlas Urol Clin North Am 1993;1:15.

Donovan JF Jr, Winfield HN: Laparoscopic varix ligation. J Urol 1992;147:77.

Dubois F et al: Coelioscopic cholecystectomy. Preliminary report of 35 cases. Ann Surg 1990;211:60.

Eden CG et al: Extraperitoneal laparoscopic dismembered fibrin-glued pyeloplasty: Medium-term results. Br J Urol 1997;80:382.

Elashry OM et al: Laparoscopy for adult polycystic kidney disease: A promising alternative. Am J Kidney Dis 1996;27:224.

Elder JS: Laparoscopy and Fowler-Stephens orchiopexy in the management of the impalpable testis. Urol Clin North Am 1989;16:399.

El-Minawi MF et al: Physiologic changes during CO_2 and N_2O pneumoperitoneum in diagnostic laparoscopy; A comparative study. J Reprod Med 1981;26: 338.

Erlich RM, Gershman A. Laparoscopic seromyotomy (autoaugmentation) for non-neurogenic bladder in a child: Initial case report. Urology 1993;42:175.

Eshghi AM, Roth JS, Smith AD: Percutaneous transperitoneal approach to a pelvic kidney for endourological removal of staghorn calculus. J Urol 1985; 134:525.

Flowers JL et al: Comparison of open and laparoscopic live donor nephrectomy. Ann Surg 1997;226:489.

Fornara P, Doehn C, Jocham D: Laparoscopic nephropexy: 3-year experience. J Urol 1997;158:1679.

Freedman LS et al: Histopathology in the prediction of relapse of patients with Stage I testicular teratoma treated by orchiectomy alone. Lancet 1987;2:294.

Fried-Siegal J, Winfield HN, Smith AD: Laparoscopic excision of urachal cyst. J Urol 1994;151:1631.

Gagner M, Lacroix A, Bolte E: Laparoscopic adrenalectomy in Cushing's syndrome and pheochromocytoma. N Engl J Med 1992;327:1033.

Gaur DD: Laparoscopic operative retroperitoneoscopy. J Urol 1992;148:1137.

Gelet A et al: Endopyelotomy with the Acucise cutting

balloon device: Early clinical experience. Eur Urol 1997;31:389.

Gerber GS et al: Laparoscopic retroperitoneal lymphadenectomy: Multi-institutional analysis. J Urol 1994;152:1188.

Gill IS et al: Complications of laparoscopic nephrectomy in 185 patients: A multi-institutional review. J Urol 1995;154:479.

Gill IS et al: Laparoscopic renal cryoablation: Initial clinical series. Urology 1998a;52:543.

Gill IS et al: Needlescopic adrenalectomy—the initial series: Comparison with conventional laparoscopic adrenalectomy. Urology 1998b;52:180.

Gill IS et al: Retroperitoneal laparoscopic nephrectomy. Urol Clin North Am 1998c;25:343.

Gilling PJ et al: Laparoscopic extraperitoneal approaches to female urinary incontinence: The colposuspension and pubovaginal sling. J Urol 1994;151:344A.

Gimenez LF et al: Laparoscopic renal biopsy. Kidney Int 1998;54:525.

Glascock JM et al: Carbon dioxide homeostasis during lymphadenectomy: A real-time intraoperative comparison. J Endourol 1996;10:319.

Goldstein M et al: Microsurgical inguinal varicocelectomy with delivery of the testis: An artery and lymphatic sparing technique. J Urol 1992;148:1808.

Grossman IC et al: Staging pelvic lymphadenectomy for carcinoma of the prostate: Review of 91 cases. J Urol 1980;124:632.

Gunning JE: History of laparoscopy. In: Phillips JM (editor): *Laparoscopy.* Williams & Wilkins, 1977.

Harewood LM, Webb DR, Pope AJ: Laparoscopic ureterolithotomy: The results of an initial series, and an evaluation of its role in the management of ureteric calculi. Br J Urol 1994;74:170.

Hassan HM: Modified instrument and method for laparoscopy. Am J Obstet Gynec 1971;110:886.

Hoenig DM et al: Laparoscopic ablation of peripelvic renal cysts. J Urol 1997;158:1345.

Hoskin P et al: Prognostic factors in Stage I non-seminomatous germ cell testicular tumors managed by orchiectomy and surveillance: Implications for adjuvant chemotherapy. J Clin Oncol 1986;4:1031.

Hulka JF et al: Laparoscopic sterilization with the spring clip: Instrumentation development and current clinical experience. Am J Obstet Gynecol 1979;135:1016.

Iselin CE et al: Sequential laparoscopic bladder diverticulectomy and transurethral resection of the prostate. J Endourol 1996;10:545.

Ivanissevich O, Gregorini H: A new operation for the cure of the varicocele. Semana Med 1918;61:17.

Janetschek G, Bartsch G, Kavoussi LR: Transcontinental interactive laparoscopic telesurgery between the United States and Europe. J Urol 1998;160:1413.

Janetschek G et al: Laparoscopic and retroperitoneoscopic repair of ureteropelvic junction obstruction. Urology 1996a;47:311.

Janetschek G et al: Retroperitoneal lymphadenectomy after chemotherapy for low-volume Stage II nonseminomatous testicular tumor: Laparoscopy versus open surgery. J Endourol 1997;11:S131.

Janetschek G et al: Retroperitoneal lymphadenectomy for clinical Stage I non-seminomatous testicular tumor: Laparoscopy versus open surgery and impact of learning curve. J Urol 1996b;156:89.

Jarvis GL: Surgery for genuine stress incontinence. Br J Obstet Gynaecol 1994;101:371.

Jordan GH, Winslow BH: Laparoendoscopic surgical management of the abdominal/transinguinal undescended testicle. J Endourol 1992;6:159.

Jordan GH, Winslow BH: Laparoendoscopic upper pole partial nephrectomy with ureterectomy. J Urol 1993a;150:940.

Jordan GH, Winslow BH: Laparoscopically assisted continent catheterizable cutaneous appendicovesicostomy. J Endourol 1993b;7:517.

Kavoussi LR et al: Comparison of robotic versus human laparoscopic camera control. J Urol 1995;154:2134.

Kavoussi LR et al: Complications of laparoscopic pelvic lymph node dissection. J Urol 1993a;149:322.

Kavoussi LR et al: Laparoscopic approach to the seminal vesicles. J Urol 1993b;150:417.

Kavoussi LR et al: Laparoscopic ureterolysis. J Urol 1992;147:426.

Keeley FX Jr, Tolley DA: Laparoscopic nephroureterectomy: Making management of upper tract transitional cell carcinoma entirely minimally invasive. J Endourol 1998;12:139.

Kerbl K et al: Laparoscopic stapled bladder closure: Laboratory and clinical experience. J Urol 1993;149:1437.

Kletscher BA et al: Percutaneous antegrade endopyelotomy: Review of 50 consecutive cases. J Urol 1995;153:701.

Klotz L: Laparoscopic retroperitoneal lymphadenectomy for high-risk Stage I non-seminomatous germ cell tumor: Report of four cases. Urology 1994;43:752.

Kozminski M, Partamian KO: Case report of laparoscopic ileal loop conduit. J Endourol 1992;6:147.

Loening SA et al: A comparison between lymphangiography and pelvic lymph node dissection in the staging of prostatic cancer. J Urol 1977;117:752.

Lowe DH, Brock WA, Kaplan GW: Laparoscopy for localization of nonpalpable testes. J Urol 1984;131:728.

Lund GO, Winfield HN, Donovan JF: Laparoscopically assisted penile revascularization for vasculogenic impotence. J Urol 1995;153:1123.

Marmar JL, DeBenedictis TJ, Praiss D: The management of varicoceles by microdissection of the spermatic cord at the external inguinal ring. Fertil Steril 1985;43:583.

McDougall E et al: The use of titanium staples for laparoscopic reconstructive surgery: Uretero-ureterostomy in a porcine model. J Endourol 1997;11:S53.

McDougall EM, Clayman RV, Elashry O: Laparoscopic nephroureterectomy for upper tract transitional cell cancer: The Washington University experience. J Urol 1995;154:975.

McDougall EM, Clayman RV, Elashry OM: Laparoscopic radical nephrectomy for renal tumor: The Washington University experience. J Urol 1996;155:1180.

McDougall EM, Klutke CG, Cornell T: Comparison of transvaginal versus laparoscopic bladder neck suspension for stress urinary incontinence. Urology 1994;45:641.

Melvin WS et al: The laparoscopic management of post-transplant lymphocele. A critical review. Surg Endosc 1997;11:245.

Mintz M: Risks and prophylaxis in laparoscopy: A survey of 100,000 cases. J Reprod Med 1977;18:269.

Mitchell SE et al: Long-term results of outpatient balloon embolotherapy in 300 varicoceles. Radiology 1985;157:90.

Moore RG et al: Laparoscopic pyeloplasty: Experience with the initial 30 cases. J Urol 1997;157:459.

Moss SW: Floating kidneys: A century of nephroptosis and nephropexy. J Urol 1997;158:699.

Motola JA, Badlani GH, Smith AD: Results of 212 consecutive endopyelotomies: An 8-year follow-up. J Urol 1993;149:453.

Mugiya S et al: Laparoscopic adrenalectomy for nonfunctioning adrenal tumors. J Endourol 1996;10:539.

Nadler RB et al: Acucise endopyelotomy: Assessment of long-term durability. J Urol 1996;156:1094.

Narepalem N, Kreder KJ, Winfield HN: Laparoscopic urethral sling for the treatment of intrinsic urethral weakness (Type III stress urinary incontinence). Tech Urol 1995;2:1.

Nezhat C et al: Laparoscopic ureteroureterostomy. J Endourol 1992;6:143.

Nicolai N, Pizzocar G: Ten year follow-up of a surveillance study in clinical Stage I non-seminomatous germ cell tumors of the testis (NSGCTT). J Urol 1995;153:245A.

Ono Y et al: Laparoscopic adrenalectomy via the retroperitoneal approach: First five cases. J Endourol 1996;10:361.

Palomo A: Radical cure of varicocele by a new technique: Preliminary report. J Urol 1949;61:604.

Parra RO, Andrus C, Boullier J: Staging laparoscopic pelvic lymph node dissection: Comparison of results with open pelvic lymphadenectomy. J Urol 1992;147:875.

Parra RO et al: Laparoscopic cystectomy: Initial report on a new treatment for the retained bladder. J Urol 1992;148:1140.

Partin AW et al: The use of prostate specific antigen, clinical stage and Gleason score to predict pathological stage in men with localized prostate cancer. (Letter.) J Urol 1994;152:172.

Rassweiler J et al: Laparoscopic nephrectomy: the experience of the laparoscopy working group of the German Urologic Association. J Urol 1998;160:18.

Rassweiler JJ, Seemann O, Henkel TO: Laparoscopic retroperitoneal lymph node dissection for non-seminomatous germ cell tumors: Indications and limitations. J Urol 1996;156:1108.

Ratner LE et al: Laparoscopic assisted live donor nephrectomy: A comparison with the open approach. Transplantation 1997;63:229.

Reddick EJ, Olsen DO: Laparoscopic laser cholecystectomy. A comparison with mini-lap cholecystectomy. Surg Endosc 1989;3:131.

Reddy PK, Evans RM: Laparoscopic ureteroneocystostomy. J Urol 1994;152:2057.

Richie JP: Modified retroperitoneal lymphadenectomy for clinical state I testicular cancer. J Urol 1990;144:1160.

Richie JP: Neoplasms of the testis. In: Walsh PC et al (editors): *Campbell's Urology,* 7th ed. Saunders, 1997.

Rifkin MD et al: Comparison of magnetic resonance imaging and ultrasonography in staging early prostate cancer. N Engl J Med 1990;323:621.

Rukstalis DB, Chodak GW: Laparoscopic retroperitoneal lymph node dissection in a patient with Stage I testicular carcinoma. J Urol 1992;148:1907.

Sampaio FJB, Favorito LA: Ureteropelvic junction stenosis: Vascular anatomical background for endopyelotomy. J Urol 1993;150:1787.

Sanchez-de-Badajoz et al: Laparoscopic cystectomy. J Endourol 1993;7:S227.

Sardi A, McKinnon W: Laparoscopic adrenalectomy for primary aldosteronism. (Letter.) JAMA 1993;269:989.

Schuessler WW et al: Laparoscopic radical prostatectomy: Initial case report. J Urol 1992;147:246A.

Schuessler WW et al: Transperitoneal endosurgical lymphadenectomy in patients with localized prostate cancer. J Urol 1991;145:988.

See WA et al: Laparoscopic surgical training: Effectiveness and impact on urologic surgical practice patterns. J Urol 1993;149:1054.

Semm K: *Atlas of Gynecologic Laparoscopy and Hysteroscopy.* Saunders, 1977.

Skinner EC, Skinner DG: Surgery of Testicular Neoplasms. In: Walsh PC et al (editors): *Campbell's Urology,* 7th ed. Saunders, 1997.

Smith MJV: The lymphatics of the prostate. Invest Urol 1966;3:439.

Soble JJ, Sung GY, Gill IS: A new technique of excising the distal ureter and bladder cuff during laparoscopic nephroureterectomy. J Endourol 1998;12:S235.

Steiner MS, Marshall FF: Mini-laparotomy staging pelvic lymphadenectomy (mini laparotomy): Alternative to standard and laparoscopic pelvic lymphadenectomy. Urology 1993;41:201.

Steptoe PC: *Laparoscopy in Gynaecology.* E & S Livingstone Ltd, 1967.

Suzuki K et al: Laparoscopic adrenalectomy: Clinical experience with 12 cases. J Urol 1993;150:1099.

Thomas AJ Jr, Geisinger MA: Current management of varicoceles. Urol Clin North Am 1990;17:893.

Thomas R, Monga M, Klein EW: Ureteroscopic retrograde endopyelotomy for management of ureteropelvic junction obstruction. J Endourol 1996;10:141.

Thompson PI, Nixon J, Harvey VJ: Disease relapse in patients with Stage I non-seminomatous germ cell tumor of the testis on active surveillance. J Clin Oncol 1988;6:1597.

Trombetta C et al: Laparoscopically assisted penile revascularization for vasculogenic impotence: 2 additional cases. J Urol 1997;158:1783.

Troxel SA, Winfield HN: Comparative financial analysis of laparoscopic versus open pelvic lymph node dissection for men with cancer of the prostate. J Urol 1994;151:675.

Vancaillie TG, Schuessler WW: Laparoscopic bladder neck suspension. J Laparoendosc Surg 1991;1:169.

Van Cangh PJ et al: Long-term results and late recurrence after endoureteropyeloplasty: A critical analysis of prognostic factors. J Urol 1994;151:934.

Veress J: Ein neues Instrument zur Ausfuhrung von

Brust-oder Bauchpunktionen und Pneumothoraxbe-handlung. Deutsche Med Wchnschr 1938;64:1480.

Whitmore WF Jr: The rationale and results of ablative surgery for prostatic cancer. Cancer 1963;16:119.

Wickham JEA: The surgical treatment of renal lithiasis. In: *Urinary Calculous Disease.* Churchill Living-stone, 1979.

Wickham JEA, Kellett MJ: Percutaneous pyelolysis. Eur Urol 1983;9:122.

Winfield HN, Ryan KJ: Experimental laparoscopic surgery: Potential clinical applications in urology. J Endourol 1990;4:37.

Winfield HN et al: Laparoscopic adrenalectomy: The preferred choice? A comparison to open adrenalec-tomy. J Urol 1998;160:325.

Winfield HN et al: Laparoscopic partial nephrectomy: Initial experience and comparison to the open surgi-cal approach. J Urol 1995;153:1409.

Winfield HN et al: Laparoscopic pelvic lymph node dis-section for genitourinary malignancies: Indications, techniques, and results. J Endourol 1992;6:103.

Wolfe JS, Tehltgen MB, Merion RM: Hand-assisted lap-aroscopic live donor nephrectomy. Urology 1998; 52:885.

Young BJ et al: Compliance with follow-up of patients treated for non-seminomatous testicular cancer. Br J Cancer 1991;64:606.

Yu TJ et al: Use of laparoscopy in intersex patients. J Urol 1995;154:1193.

Zollikofer R: Zur Laparoskopie. Schweiz Med Wchn-schr 1924;54:264.

Radionuclide Imaging

10

Barry A. Kogan, MD, Robert S. Hattner, MD, & Jeffrey A. Cooper, MD

Radioisotopic imaging of the genitourinary tract permits anatomic and functional evaluations without disturbance of physiologic processes. These studies have benefited from numerous technical advances in radiopharmaceuticals, scintillation cameras, and computer processing. Currently, the most common studies emphasize the physiologic properties of radiopharmaceuticals and, consequently, allow for dynamic, functional evaluations of the organ being studied.

Radiopharmaceuticals

Imaging radiopharmaceuticals are moieties with specific physiologic properties allowing them to trace normal and abnormal processes. They are labeled with a readily available radionuclide that can be easily imaged, most commonly technetium-99m. Because extremely small molar quantities of radionuclide can provide a photon flux adequate for imaging, radiopharmaceuticals rarely disturb the physiologic processes of the organs being investigated. These radioisotopes are safe and noninvasive, with radiation exposure being in most instances considerably less than in standard radiographic or fluoroscopic procedures. Owing to the tiny quantities used, allergic reactions are virtually unknown and the potential toxicity of contrast media is avoided. In most instances, the radiopharmaceutical is delivered intravenously and the agent enters the target organ physiologically. Thus, nuclear medicine images are not as much anatomic as they are functional—the concentration of the pharmaceutical being proportionate to the amount of function as much as to the anatomy of the organ being investigated.

Scintillation Camera

The amount of radiopharmaceutical present within a given organ is monitored externally by a scintillation camera. The camera has a central crystal, a collimator, and a photomultiplier. The crystal, made of thallium-drifted sodium iodide, is generally circular and optically clear. It is 20–50 cm in diameter and 6–12 mm thick. A photon interacting in the crystal causes a quantitative release of visible-light photons proportionate to the energy of the incident photon. The collimator usually has parallel channels of dense radiation-absorbing material, usually lead, which are applied to the crystal in such a way that only photons with a path parallel to the long axis of the channel are permitted to reach the crystal and react with it. By doing this, the 3-dimensional distribution of radiopharmaceutical is converted into a 2-dimensional projection of the activity. The photomultiplier is attached to the back of the crystal on the side opposite the collimator. This device detects visible-light photons released from the crystal and uses an electronic algebraic scheme to determine the spatial location of the incident photon. As each incident photon is examined independently, the scintillation camera samples the source distribution at random and can be used to sample the distribution of radioactivity over short time intervals. This produces a quantitative cinematic data set that can be subjected to computer analysis. The data are also mapped onto film by conversion of the electron pulses to light flashes for subsequent photography.

Most gamma cameras built today are capable of single photon emission computed tomography (SPECT). With SPECT, the camera rotates in a circular or elliptical arc around the patient and obtains a series of images from multiple angles. These images are reconstructed by a computer into transaxial, coronal, or sagittal slices comparable to the images obtained with magnetic resonance imaging. The advantages of performing tomography are marked contrast enhancement and the elimination of overlapping radioactivity, resulting in improved sensitivity.

Computer Analysis

The analog signals from the scintillation camera are digitized and stored in the computer memory. In most instances, they are subsequently transferred to a peripheral storage device, for example, a magnetic disk. A standard mini- or microcomputer is then programmed to direct the acquisition, analysis, and display of data. The acquisition program is flexible and allows for specification of the precision of spatial sampling, the temporal resolution, the study length, and the total amount of data to be collected. In renal cortical imaging, for instance, the data are collected based on the total number of counts for each image. In contrast, for diuretic renography, the data are collected in a series of images each of the same duration, independent of the number of counts per image. Analysis programs allow study of a particular region of interest and will also compute and display activity in a quantitative manner (eg, as a function of time). This type of analysis is used extensively for diuretic renography. Finally, the display program can provide graphs, images, and tables that can be photographed for the clinician's use. Other analysis programs use the linear systems theory to solve multiple differential equations and analyze raw data to look at the rate of disappearance of radioisotopes from various body pools. This type of computer analysis is used for calculations of the glomerular filtration rate (GFR) with Tc-99m diethylenetriaminepentaacetic acid (^{99m}Tc-DTPA) or of effective renal plasma flow with Tc-99m mercaptoacetyltriglycine (^{99m}Tc-MAG-3).

Computer processing is particularly important for SPECT. The program controls the acquisition of images by directing the camera to move the appropriate angular steps, obtaining images for the acquisition time at each angle and controlling the number of angles imaged. The computer program then performs image reconstruction, usually by filtered back projection. Coronal or sagittal images or a series of oblique images parallel to any desired plane can be obtained. The computer can also read volume-rendered or surface-mapped images.

As in most investigations, communication between clinician and nuclear medicine specialist is essential, because the choice of radioisotope, imaging technique, and computer analysis should be adapted and adjusted to the particular problem.

KIDNEY

Nuclear medicine studies of the kidney are extremely valuable for noninvasive evaluation of renal function and anatomy. In some instances, these are the only studies capable of delineating the anatomy.

Function

When quantifying renal function, either glomerular or tubular function can be measured. Glomerular function has traditionally been assessed by the GFR and tubular function by renal blood flow (RBF). Any substance that is freely filtered by the glomerulus but is not reabsorbed or secreted by the tubular or collecting duct cells can be used to quantify the GFR. The polysaccharide inulin meets these criteria and has been the classic agent used for this purpose. It remains the "gold standard" by which other agents are

judged. GFR can be expressed in the following equation:

$$\frac{[\text{Inulin}]_{\text{urine}} \times \text{Volume}_{\text{urine}}}{[\text{Inulin}]_{\text{plasma}}}$$

Unfortunately, accurate measurement of inulin clearance is complex, time-consuming, and expensive, making it impractical for clinical use. Labeling inulin with a radioisotope allows for easier quantification of concentrations. ^{14}C-inulin is available for these purposes, but it requires special handling and is not useful in the clinical setting. The most commonly used alternatives are ^{125}I-iothalamate, chromium-51 ethylenediaminetetraacetic acid (^{51}Cr-EDTA), and ^{99m}Tc-DTPA. All are excreted in a manner similar to that of inulin and are easier to handle and measure. ^{51}Cr-EDTA and ^{125}I-iothalamate clearances correlate well with inulin clearance, but accurate measurements require collection of multiple serum or urine samples or both. ^{99m}Tc-DTPA has the advantage of providing excellent renal images as well, allowing simultaneous imaging and clearance measurements. Clearances can be measured in the same way as with ^{51}Cr-EDTA, or a close estimate can be obtained by quantitative analysis of scintillation counts obtained on gamma camera imaging in adults (Gates, 1982, 1983). An important advantage of this technique is the ease with which simultaneous split renal function studies can be obtained. This is of considerable practical benefit. However, the technique may not produce accurate results of total renal function in children, particularly in those with decreased renal function (Chandhoke et al, 1990).

RBF is measured by determining the clearance of a substance that is eliminated completely from blood in one pass through the kidney. Para-aminohippuric acid (PAH) meets this criterion, and its clearance has been the traditional reference standard for measurement of RBF. As with inulin, it is not easy to measure PAH clearance, nor is it easy to radiolabel PAH. However, ^{131}I-hippuran is widely available and is almost completely extracted from renal blood in one pass; hence, it provides accurate measurements of RBF. It is also used for renal imaging; however, ^{123}I-hippuran, although considerably more expensive, has better imaging qualities and is used more commonly in Europe (O'Reilly et al, 1977). Its clearance also correlates well with PAH clearances. ^{99m}Tc-MAG-3 has similar physiologic properties and is much less expensive; hence, it has largely replaced hippuran for this purpose in the United States (Russell et al, 1988; Bagni et al, 1990). The absolute uptake of Tc-99m dimercaptosuccinic acid (^{99m}Tc-DMSA) can also be used for this purpose, but, again, its measurement is not straightforward (Daly et al, 1979).

The easy assessment of renal function is invaluable in urology. Furthermore, the ability to quantify individual renal function noninvasively allows for comparison of renal health before, during, and after treatment for a number of urologic diseases (eg, vesicoureteral reflux or ureteropelvic junction obstruction). This is perhaps the principal advantage of nuclear medicine techniques over all other imaging modalities. In fact, they constitute the only noninvasive method of determining relative renal function.

Imaging

Two basic types of renal imaging are possible: (1) cortical imaging, with agents that are bound to renal parenchymal cells, and (2) imaging of the transit of GFR or RBF agents that are excreted in the urine. Some agents are known to do both (eg, Tc-99m glucoheptonate).

^{99m}Tc-DMSA is used most commonly for cortical imaging. A dose of 75 µCi/kg, but not less than 0.3 mCi, is given intravenously. Although a small amount is excreted in the urine, at least 50% is bound to renal proximal tubular cells within 4 h. Images taken thereafter show details of the renal parenchyma. This is particularly useful when looking for segmental abnormalities of the kidney (eg, renal scarring, tumors, or evidence of trauma).

^{99m}Tc-DTPA (200 µCi/kg, but not less than 2 mCi) and ^{99m}Tc-MAG-3 (100 µCi/kg, but not less than 1 mCi) are the agents most often used for "excretory" imaging, since large amounts of these are excreted rapidly in the urine. ^{99m}Tc-MAG-3 has mostly replaced ^{131}I-hippuran because of its similar physiologic properties along with vastly better imaging and radiation dosimetry (Russell et al, 1988; Bagni et al, 1990). Image resolution is much less satisfactory than with traditional uroradiographic studies (eg, excretory urograms), and these agents are therefore not used for examining details of the collecting system. Although nuclear medicine techniques provide crude anatomic information (enough, for instance, to delineate the level of upper tract obstruction) (Koff et al, 1984), their principal advantage is quantification of amounts of radioisotope entering and leaving the collecting system, allowing for dynamic, functional, and anatomic imaging simultaneously.

As noted previously, each agent has somewhat different physiologic properties, causing their functional and anatomic capabilities to vary. The choice of agent can greatly affect the information obtained, and it is therefore preferable to tailor the study to the clinical problem under evaluation. This will be demonstrated by looking more closely at the clinical applications in which radioisotopes are most helpful.

UPPER URINARY TRACT OBSTRUCTION

Traditionally, a dilated upper urinary tract has been assumed to be obstructed, but this is not always the case (eg, following pyeloplasty, the collecting system may remain dilated but may not be obstructed). Sonography or excretory urography can delineate the anatomy but in many cases will not determine the degree of obstruction. Nuclear medicine studies are helpful, as they quantify the amount of radioisotope entering and leaving the collecting system. These studies are dynamic in that quantification is done sequentially and, when indicated, after diuresis (O'Reilly et al, 1978; Koff, Thrall, and Keyes, 1979).

In evaluating obstruction, radionuclide renography should be performed according to recommended standards (Mandell et al, 1997a). ^{99m}Tc-MAG-3 is the desired tracer, although ^{99m}Tc-DTPA is acceptable. The patient should be hydrated, preferably intravenously, before undergoing imaging. Urine output should be monitored and additional hydration given for patients with inadequate urine flow. Patients who are young, incontinent, or those with reflux, abnormal bladders, or with suspected lower tract obstruction should be catheterized. After injection of the radioisotope, a series of images is obtained, with the duration of imaging held constant. The amount of emptying of the system can be visually determined by observing the decrease in activity in the kidney over time. With computerized techniques, a region of interest is selected over the kidney (or in the case of ureteral dilation, over the distal ureter) and the number of counts at any given time quantified. The number of counts can be expressed as a function of time and a time-activity curve generated (see Figure 38–12). In the dilated system, which does not drain readily, a diuretic (usually furosemide, 1 mg/kg) is given when the collecting system is full of radioisotope. In patients with poor renal function, doses of 2–4 mg/kg may be required to induce adequate diuresis. After administration of the diuretic, the unobstructed system will drain and the number of counts over the kidney will decrease. In the obstructed system, however, the amount of radioisotope will stay constant or even increase (Figure 10–1).

In some instances, the diagnosis of obstruction is clear-cut. However, in most cases, the obstruction is partial, and the surgeon must determine when operative intervention is appropriate. A number of investigators have documented the usefulness of diuretic renography in these circumstances (Kass, Majd, and Belman, 1985). However, there is no definitive criterion, and the final decision remains a clinical one. The shape of the time-activity curve is a measure of the severity of the obstruction, and a number of authors have attempted to use the slope of the curve or the time until 50% of the isotope has drained to judge this. A problem with this technique is that each case must be individualized, as the rapidity of drainage is determined not only by the degree of obstruction but also by the size and compliance of the collecting system, as well as by the urinary output provoked by the diuretic. In fact, when a kidney has been damaged

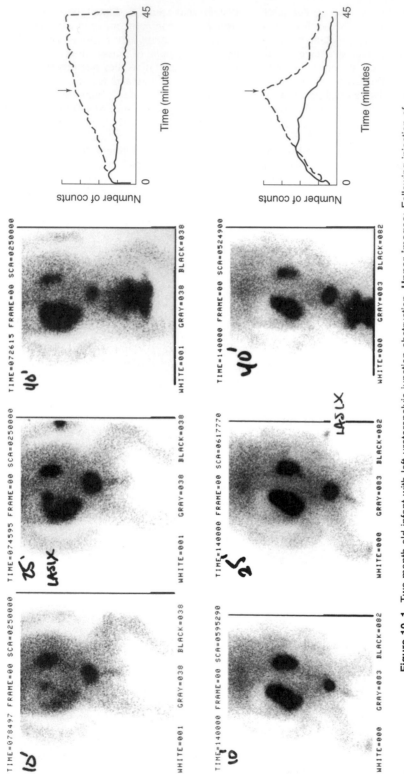

Figure 10–1. Two-month-old infant with left ureteropelvic junction obstruction. **Upper images:** Following injection of ^{99m}Tc-diethylenetriaminepentaacetic acid, the left kidney is seen to be large and hydronephrotic with a rim of cortex (10 min). After the administration of furosemide (25 min), the left renal pelvis fills with increasing amounts of radioisotope (40 min). **Upper graph:** Computer-generated time-activity curves demonstrate normal uptake and "washout" of the right kidney and progressive increase in counts over the left kidney. The arrow marks the administration of furosemide. **Lower images:** Following successful pyeloplasty, there is still hydronephrosis, but after administration of furosemide, the amount of radioisotope in the left collecting system decreases (arrows). **Lower graph:** The same findings are displayed graphically. Note the excellent "washout" of the dilated left kidney.

significantly by obstruction, it may respond poorly to the diuretic; the dilated system may not fill sufficiently to induce drainage. The time-activity curve must be interpreted cautiously in these patients, as limited or delayed "washout" of radioisotope may be falsely interpreted as an indication of obstruction. Modifications are being developed to make the scan more sensitive and specific (English et al, 1987). However, because of individual variations, the clinician must be involved actively in interpretation of these studies (Maizels et al, 1986). A standardized protocol involving hydration and bladder drainage has made diuretic renography the only noninvasive technique useful for documenting the degree of obstruction (Conway and Maizels, 1992; Mandell, 1997a). In patients in whom function is too poor, diagnosis of obstruction is better made by other means, usually pressure-flow studies.

In practice, these studies are useful in following patients with long-term hydronephrosis. Examples are newborns with antenatally diagnosed hydronephrosis, children with posterior urethral valves, and patients after surgery for a ureteropelvic junction obstruction or vesicoureteral reflux (Koff et al, 1981; Bayne and Shapiro, 1985).

CHRONIC PYELONEPHRITIS IN CHILDREN

Evaluation of renal damage from urinary infections has traditionally been done with excretory urography. The classic abnormalities include small kidneys, thinned parenchyma, and blunted calyces, with thinning of the parenchyma primarily overlying the calyces. These changes, although pathognomonic, are not always seen, partly because it is difficult to obtain a high-quality excretory urogram during childhood when careful follow-up of renal growth is most important, since vesicoureteral reflux with associated pyelonephritis is a major cause of renal damage. The difficulties with excretory urography are multifactorial. (1) Young children have diminished renal function, even when compared on a per kilogram basis with adults. (2) Bowel preparation is not used, as it may cause excessive dehydration. (3) Crying causes swallowing of air and markedly increases bowel gas. (4) Abnormally positioned kidneys may be hidden by bony structures. (5) The use of oblique films and tomography is limited by attempts to keep exposure to radiation to a minimum. Similarly, sonography has considerable limitations when evaluating renal injury (Benador et al, 1994).

Nuclear medicine obviates many of these problems. ^{99m}Tc-DTPA or ^{99m}Tc-MAG-3 scans can be used, but are suboptimal (Piepsz et al, 1992). Only the images obtained in the first several minutes are valuable because thereafter the radioisotope is excreted in the urine and the images are primarily of the collecting system. A better alternative is an agent

that images the renal cortex primarily, the optimal one being ^{99m}Tc-DMSA (Kogan et al, 1983; Mandell et al, 1997b). By binding directly to renal proximal tubular cells, these agents provide excellent delineation of parenchymal anatomy. Because the binding is prolonged and the half-life of the ^{99m}Tc is 6 h, images can be obtained in different positions to visualize specific lesions more completely. When necessary, 24-h images can be obtained to reduce the background further and to allow any radioisotope in the urine to be excreted, giving further definition to the renal parenchymal images.

These studies are particularly beneficial in chronic pyelonephritis (Figure 10–2). First, they are not affected by bowel gas, bony structures, or any of the other problems associated with excretory urography. Furthermore, they appear to be more sensitive than excretory urography or sonography, even when a high-quality study is available (McLorie et al, 1989). This sensitivity results in part from failure of the injured renal parenchyma to bind the radiopharmaceutical immediately after being damaged, whereas on excretory urography or sonography, the size and shape of the kidney do not change until the injured area is replaced by collagen and the collagen contracts, distorting the calyces and thinning the cortex.

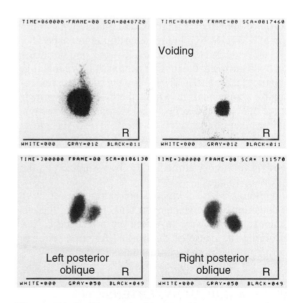

Figure 10–2. Six-month-old girl with recurrent urinary tract infection. **Top:** Posterior images from a nuclear cystogram, performed by injecting ^{99m}Tc-diethylenetriaminepentaacetic acid into a urethral catheter and filling the bladder with saline. Images are also obtained during voiding. Right vesicoureteral reflux is demonstrated during both filling and voiding. **Bottom:** Left posterior oblique and right posterior oblique images from a ^{99m}Tc-dimercaptosuccinic acid scan in the same patient clearly delineate right renal scarring.

Clinically, renal cortical scans are invaluable shortly after an episode of pyelonephritis in order to document the amount of renal damage. This information is important in planning therapy and particularly useful in evaluating the results of treatment (eg, in determining the progression of scarring in children followed medically for vesicoureteral reflux; Stoller and Kogan, 1986).

RENAL TRANSPLANTATION

After renal transplantation, the kidney must be monitored continuously. Numerous disease processes can lead to graft dysfunction (eg, acute tubular necrosis, acute rejection, cytomegalovirus infection, acute pyelonephritis, cyclosporine toxicity, aminoglycoside toxicity, and recurrence of the original renal disease). Measurement of serum creatinine is the most common clinical determination of renal function, but changes are slow and this measurement is relatively insensitive to small changes in function. Nuclear medicine studies are highly sensitive and provide quantitative information with low risk (Hattner and Engelstad, 1984). Many different techniques have been investigated and a number of good results published, but the recent availability of ^{99m}Tc-MAG-3, with its excellent physical and imaging qualities, has made it the isotope of choice at this time (Taylor, Ziffer, and Eshima, 1990). Perhaps the most common protocol involves a combination of quantitative analysis and qualitative evaluation of ^{99m}Tc-MAG-3 kinetics. Although nonspecific, this study permits repeated evaluations and comparison even during acute tubular necrosis. This capability is particularly beneficial in following patients after cadaveric transplants, in whom there is a higher incidence of acute tubular necrosis. Major vascular abnormalities can be identified on the ^{99m}Tc-MAG-3 flow study (ie, monitoring the radionuclide on its first transit through the bloodstream and kidney), and urinary extravasation or dysfunction can be visualized on the follow-up images.

Although MAG-3 kinetics are extremely sensitive in detecting subtle changes in renal function, the clinician must be aware that they are nonspecific. Determining the cause of diminished function requires correlation with other clinical data.

RENOVASCULAR HYPERTENSION

In typical renovascular hypertension, there is decreased blood flow and diminished uptake and delayed excretion of radioisotope over the involved area, the renal mass is smaller, and there is compensatory hypertrophy of uninvolved areas (Figure 10–3). This is best demonstrated by agents that correlate with RBF (eg, ^{99m}Tc-MAG-3). ^{99m}Tc-DMSA also has been shown to be valuable, especially in de-

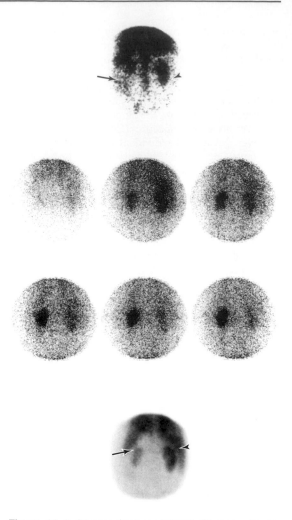

Figure 10–3. Images from a 65-year-old man with severe hypertension. **Top:** Posterior image from a ^{99m}Tc-diethylenetriaminepentaacetic acid (DTPA) blood flow study after captopril. The aorta is clearly seen, as is the right kidney (arrowhead). The blood flow to the left kidney is delayed (arrow). **Middle:** On a ^{131}I-hippuran study done immediately following, there is not only slow uptake but delayed excretion. Images were obtained at 4-min intervals. **Bottom:** A delayed ^{99m}Tc-DTPA image shows the small left kidney (arrow) and the larger, possibly hypertrophied, right kidney (arrowhead).

lineating segmental vascular disease (Stringer et al, 1984; Rosen, Treves, and Ingelfinger, 1985).

Unfortunately, the classic findings are not often seen. However, nuclear scans can be enhanced when used with captopril. This particular technique is based upon interfering with the physiologic autoregulation that occurs in a kidney with renal artery stenosis. In a typical kidney with renal artery stenosis, the kidney maintains perfusion and function by constriction of the post-glomerular arterioles. This constriction occurs through an angiotensin-mediated mechanism. An angiotensin-converting enzyme inhibitor, such as captopril, will interfere with this regulatory mechanism causing reduced filtration. After a baseline scan showing normal blood flow, prolonged cortical uptake after captopril is highly specific for renal artery stenosis. Captopril-enhanced renal scanning with ^{99m}Tc-MAG-3 has been reported to be approximately 85% sensitive and 90% specific for the detection of renal artery stenosis. However, it must be kept in mind that a large percentage of the population has anatomic findings of renal artery stenosis in the absence of significant hypertension. Of importance, though, is the fact that captopril-enhanced renal scanning is more than 95% accurate for predicting which patients have physiologically significant renal artery stenosis that will respond to surgical revascularization (Taylor and Martin, 1991; Roccatello et al, 1992; Mittal et al, 1996).

FUNCTIONAL RENAL MASS QUANTIFICATION

One of the most important problems in clinical urology and nephrology is the quantification of renal mass. Excretory urography provides some information on renal size and amount of contrast excretion, but this correlates only loosely with function. Similarly, sonography can evaluate renal size and character (ie, echogenicity) but also is not functional. On the other hand, radioisotopes, by virtue of their physiology, provide functional information; the amount of uptake of radioisotope is proportionate to the amount of function. Excretory agents can be used for this purpose but are not optimal because many kidneys being evaluated are abnormal in shape and position

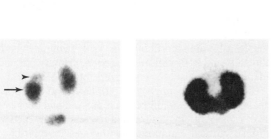

Figure 10–4. Dimercaptosuccinic acid renal cortical scans. **Left:** Posterior images from a 3-month-old girl with left duplication and ureterocele. The dilated upper pole (arrowhead) has 12% of the total renal function compared with the lower pole (arrow), which has 32%. Enough function remained so that heminephroureterectomy was deemed inappropriate. **Right:** Posterior images from a 1-week-old female with a horseshoe kidney, right duplication, and ureterocele arising from the upper pole segment. This scan delineates the renal anatomy better than any other study.

and have dilated collecting systems or vesicoureteral reflux. Cortical agents (eg, ^{99m}Tc-DMSA) are superior in these instances (Gordon, 1987) (Figure 10–4).

In practice, these studies are useful in evaluating unilateral renal pathology. In order to decide whether a significantly damaged kidney should be removed, it is crucial to know what percentage of renal function the kidney contributes. Radioisotopic imaging is the only currently available study that can provide this information noninvasively.

SPACE-OCCUPYING RENAL LESIONS

Renal cortical agents are capable of delineating mass lesions within the kidney, particularly those larger than 1–2 cm. Because of numerous technologic advances in recent years, ultrasonography, computed tomography (CT) scanning, and magnetic resonance imaging (MRI) can provide similar information while also evaluating associated renal and extrarenal findings. Hence, nuclear medicine studies are not the investigation of choice in patients with renal infarctions, tumors, or lesions due to trauma. However, in unusual circumstances or when some of the studies mentioned are unavailable, renal cortical agents can provide extremely useful information (eg, delineating the degree of segmental renal damage from trauma or differentiating a hypertrophied column of Bertin from a renal tumor). A high-quality ^{99m}Tc-DMSA scan can clearly differentiate functional from nonfunctional renal tissue.

BLADDER

Radioisotopic imaging of the bladder is useful primarily for detecting vesicoureteral reflux. This application was first discussed by Winter (1959). Refinements in widefield gamma camera imaging and new radioisotopes have made this technique highly sensitive and useful, especially in children (Conway et al, 1972; Merrick, Uttley, and Wild, 1977).

A catheter is placed in the bladder, and the bladder is filled with normal saline to which 1 mCi of ^{99m}Tc-DTPA has been added. The cooperative child is placed upright on a portable toilet or bedpan. Once the bladder is distended, the catheter is removed and the child voids. Gamma camera imaging is performed from behind and is continuous during both filling and voiding. The images obtained often demonstrate reflux (see Figure 10–2). Very mild degrees of reflux can also be identified by computer analysis of radioactivity over the kidneys. The test can be combined with a simple cystometrogram to obtain more information and to increase accuracy (Nasrallah et al, 1978).

The major advantage of radioisotopic cystography is its high sensitivity with relatively limited radiation exposure, approximately 1/100th that obtained from conventional voiding cystourethrography. Because image resolution is relatively poor, fine anatomic detail is not seen as well as with traditional radiography, and this procedure is not useful as the initial study of the lower urinary tract in males, for whom visualization of the urethra is important. It is also of questionable usefulness as the first study in females with urinary tract infection because the spine is not visualized, a ureterocele may not be seen, and visualization of bladder wall thickening and trabeculation is not possible. It is, however, an ideal test for follow-up studies of children with vesicoureteral reflux either after ureteral reimplantation or during expectant management for spontaneous resolution. In these children, the quality of image resolution is not important but limited exposure to radiation is, particularly when many studies must be performed.

A variation of this technique (indirect radionuclide cystography) was developed to avoid catheterization (Conway and Kruglik, 1976). For indirect radionuclide cystography, the child undergoes a renal scan and voids the excreted tracer during dynamic imaging of the ureters and kidneys. If able to live up to its promise, this study would be very useful. However, besides requiring patient cooperation, the indirect method cannot be used to detect the 20% of reflux that occurs only during bladder filling, measure the volume of the bladder at the time of reflux, measure the volume of urine refluxed, or calculate the residual volume. In addition, this test has a higher radiation dose and, because it requires a very cooperative, toilet-trained child, its use is precluded in many children who are being evaluated for reflux. Even among successful studies, indirect radionuclide cystography misses about half of all grades of reflux (Majd, Kass, and Belman, 1985). Overall, this is a study that does not live up to its promise. If a parent or patient insists on avoiding catheterization, renal cortical imaging with ^{99m}Tc-DMSA is more likely to provide clinically useful information.

TESTIS

The primary benefit of radionuclide imaging of the testis is in differentiating degrees of testicular vascularity. Angiography is performed with a bolus injection of ^{99m}Tc sodium pertechnetate (200 µCi/kg but not less than 2 mCi) and imaging at 5-s intervals during its first pass through the groin area. Approximately 10 min later, blood pool images are obtained, as concentration of this agent correlates reasonably well with vascularity. Areas of increased vascularity appear denser than normal, and avascular tissues appear as a filling defect.

This study is used primarily to differentiate testicular torsion from epididymitis. The latter classically appears as an area of hypervascularity and the former as avascular (Figure 10–5). A number of reports have

suggested that this technique is both sensitive and specific (Falkowski and Firlit, 1980; Blacklock et al, 1983).

Unfortunately, there are some limitations. First, because torsion must be diagnosed and treated immediately, a nuclear medicine technician must be available on short notice 24 h a day. Furthermore, false-negative and false-positive results do occur (Stoller, Kogan, and Hricak, 1985). Late torsion may appear as a hypervascular area due to an inflammatory response, and intermittent torsion can also demonstrate hypervascularity, resulting in delayed diagnosis and correction. A large hydrocele and even gross purulence can result in a large filling defect, simulating torsion (Wilkins et al, 1985). In summary, radioisotopic studies of the scrotum can be helpful in the differential diagnosis of acute scrotal pain, but the diagnosis is made primarily on clinical grounds and the scan should be used only as an adjunct.

ADRENAL SCINTIGRAPHY

Adrenal Cortex

The adrenal cortex uses blood cholesterol as the primary substrate for steroid synthesis, in contrast to other organs, which synthesize cholesterol de novo from acetate. Hence, radiolabeled derivatives of cholesterol are taken up by the adrenal and can be imaged 3–5 days after injection (Lieberman et al, 1971). The best agent for this purpose is 7-iodomethyl-19-norcholesterol labeled with ^{131}I (NP59) (Sarkar et al, 1975). These scans are useful in both Cushing syndrome and Conn syndrome (Beierwaltes, 1984).

In Cushing syndrome, it is important to distinguish between a primary adrenal source of corticosteroids and a paraneoplastic or pituitary source. Often biochemical and other radiographic tests can help, but NP59 can distinguish the origin when it is unclear (Figure 10–6). Either a pituitary or paraneoplastic source of adrenocorticotropin will stimulate both adrenals, and both will be imaged. A primary adrenal adenoma will also be visualized, but the increased corticosteroids suppress the pituitary, and the contralateral adrenal therefore is suppressed and does not take up NP59. In contrast, a metabolically active adrenal cortical carcinoma synthesizes its own cholesterol and corticosteroids and consequently suppresses both adrenals. In these cases, neither adrenal is visualized.

In Conn syndrome, primary hyperaldosteronism is demonstrated by biochemical studies. It is then important therapeutically to distinguish between bilateral adrenal hyperplasia and a unilateral adenoma. This can be done by suppressing both adrenals with dexamethasone and imaging with NP59. The scan images any autonomously functioning tissue, either the unilateral adenoma or the bilateral hyperplastic glands. The appropriate surgical approach can then be planned.

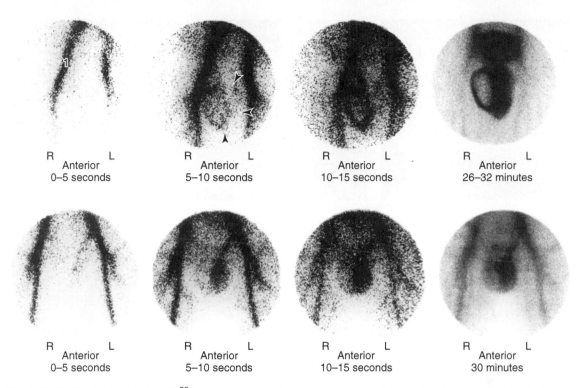

R	L
Anterior	
0–5 seconds	

R	L
Anterior	
5–10 seconds	

R	L
Anterior	
10–15 seconds	

R	L
Anterior	
26–32 minutes	

R	L
Anterior	
0–5 seconds	

R	L
Anterior	
5–10 seconds	

R	L
Anterior	
10–15 seconds	

R	L
Anterior	
30 minutes	

Figure 10–5. Scrotal scanning with ^{99m}Tc-sodium pertechnetate. **Top:** This adolescent had proven right testicular torsion. Early scans of the pelvis show both iliac arteries (1) and increased flow around the right testis (arrowheads). However, later pictures, especially the 30-min delayed film, demonstrate a clear photopenic area involving the right testis. **Bottom:** In contrast, this young man with left epididymo-orchitis has obviously increased blood flow to the entire left scrotum. In this instance, the delayed film demonstrates the increased flow to the entire testis. (Courtesy of MCC Ling.)

In the United States, high-resolution CT scanning has largely supplanted the adrenal cortical scan. However, when CT scanning is equivocal, cortical scanning with NP59 remains very useful.

Adrenal Medulla

In somewhat the same manner as cholesterol in the adrenal cortex, meta-iodobenzylguanidine (MIBG) is taken up by adrenergic neurons. It can be radiolabeled with iodine and used to image the adrenal medulla and other endocrinologically active adrenergic tissues, in particular pheochromocytoma and neuroblastomas (Sisson et al, 1981; Munkner, 1985; Hattner et al, 1984a, b).

^{123}I-MIBG is 85–90% sensitive and virtually 100% specific for localizing pheochromocytomas (Sisson et al, 1984) (Figure 10–7). This ability is particularly helpful in extra-adrenal pheochromocytomas when CT scanning is unrevealing or when symptoms and signs of pheochromocytoma persist after resection, indicating multiple neoplasms. Because the incidence of this condition may be as high as 10%, some surgeons perform routine preoperative MIBG scans. ^{123}I-MIBG is also helpful in screening the family members of patients with type 2 multiple endocrine neoplasia, in whom a high incidence of pheochromocytoma or adrenal medullary hyperplasia is seen. In a few cases, large doses of ^{131}I-MIBG have been used therapeutically in patients with otherwise untreatable metastatic malignant pheochromocytoma (Sisson et al, 1984).

In patients with neuroblastoma, ^{123}I-MIBG is almost 100% sensitive and specific. This level is crucial for staging and subsequently defining the optimal therapy. Imaging with MIBG has uncovered numerous soft-tissue and bony metastases not found by any other means. Consequently, it has considerable promise as a means of delivering high doses of radiation directly to metastatic neuroblastoma. Trials of ^{131}I-MIBG radiotherapy are now under way in patients with otherwise unresponsive stage IV tumors.

SKELETAL SCINTIGRAPHY

Bone scans obtained with conventional bone-seeking radiopharmaceuticals such as ^{99m}Tc-methylenediphosphonate (MDP) occupy a unique place in the staging of cancer patients. Nowhere is this more true than in urogenital cancers, particularly carcinoma of the prostate (McNeil, 1984) (Figure 10–8).

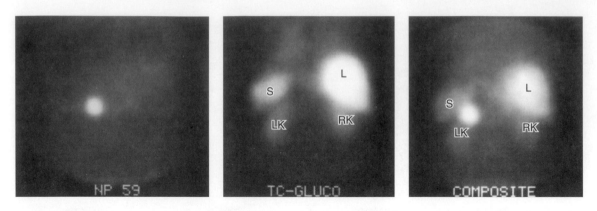

Figure 10–6. In this 45-year-old woman with Cushing syndrome, computed tomography scanning suggested a left adrenal mass, but biochemical studies were unclear as to the primary pathology. **Left:** An NP59 scan shows very strong uptake in the abdomen. **Center:** A ^{99m}Tc-glucoheptinate scan was performed to localize the uptake in relation to the liver (L), spleen (S), right kidney (RK), and left kidney (LK). **Right:** A composite of both scans shows that the uptake is clearly unilateral and in the left adrenal. A left adrenal adenoma was removed, and the patient was cured.

MDP and similar compounds are chemisorbed to the surface of bone crystals, intercalating into crystal imperfections. The relative localization of a radiopharmaceutical is equal to the product of its extraction efficiency, blood flow, and blood concentration. Since blood concentration after intravenous injection is equal throughout the body and since MDP has a very high extraction efficiency, it follows that the bone scan correlates mostly with the vascularity of the skeleton. The response of bone to a variety of insults is limited but nearly always includes increased blood flow; hence, bony lesions are seen as foci of increased radioisotope in scans. Although bone scans are nonspecific for any solitary abnormality, a high degree of specificity may be obtained from imaging the entire skeleton. The spatial distribution and appearance of

metastatic disease is usually distinct from osteoarthritis and Paget disease of bone, and in many cases the definitive diagnosis can be made. When questionable, correlation with plain radiographs or bone biopsy is required. Overall, the sensitivity of bone scans in skeletal metastasis for prostate cancer exceeds 95%, making it important in the evaluation and follow-up of patients with this disease.

SCINTIGRAPHIC DETECTION OF OCCULT INFLAMMATION

Gallium-67 (^{67}Ga) was investigated originally as a tumor-imaging agent. However, it has been found to be more useful in the detection of acute and chronic in-

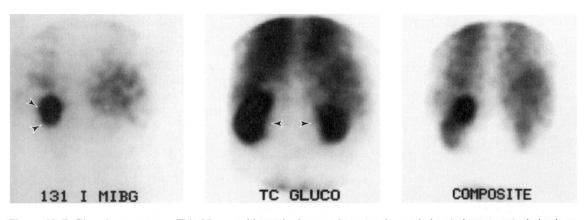

Figure 10–7. Pheochromocytoma. This 35-year-old man had severe hypertension and elevated serum catecholamines. **Left:** A ^{131}I-meta-iodobenzylguanidine scan shows marked uptake in the left abdomen. **Center:** A ^{99m}Tc-glucoheptinate scan was done to help localize the lesion. The kidneys are clearly seen. **Right:** A composite view shows the lesion in the left adrenal. With surgical excision of a left adrenal pheochromocytoma, the patient was cured.

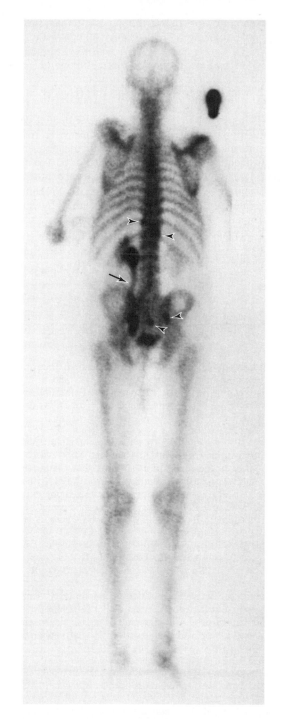

Figure 10–8. An 83-year-old man with carcinoma of the prostate. A ^{99m}Tc-methylenediphosphonate bone scan shows metastasis in the sacrum and at T10 and T11 (arrowheads). Since some radioisotope is excreted in the urine, the obstructed left ureter is also well delineated (arrow).

flammation (Halpern and Hagan, 1980). The exact mechanism of localization of ^{67}Ga in inflammatory foci is disputed. Because it resembles ferric iron, it probably binds to iron-binding molecules of microorganisms (siderophores) and to lactoferrin, an iron-binding protein abundant in neutrophils. For unknown reasons, ^{67}Ga is also accumulated by macrophages. Since any or all of these cells are found at the site of inflammatory processes, ^{67}Ga is an excellent compound for finding inflammation.

Gallium scans are hampered by nonspecific colonic activity, which reduces their imaging capabilities significantly. Nonetheless, they can serve to direct further diagnostic workup in cases of occult inflammation (eg, suspected perinephric abscess, interstitial nephritis, or pelvic abscess). They can also be used to confirm suspicious or nondiagnostic findings seen on other studies.

Indium-111- or ^{99m}Tc-labeled granulocytes are prepared by labeling of the patient's own white blood cells (leukocytes). These cells are then reinjected into the patient. Although the labeled granulocytes are distributed throughout the body, areas of high concentration are easily imaged with a gamma camera. In contrast to ^{67}Ga, there is minimal colonic binding. These scans are therefore very sensitive and specific for acute suppurative infections (Coleman, 1982). Unfortunately, these labeled granulocytes are not as accurate for finding chronic inflammatory conditions. Because the radiolabeling is generally performed out of hospital by a community radiopharmacy, these scans are relatively expensive and usually available only during regular working hours, a distinct disadvantage, since this particular study is often needed urgently. Nonetheless, in selected cases these scans can be extremely useful.

TUMOR IMAGING

General

In the early 1970s, it became possible to create large quantities of pure antibodies in a relatively inexpensive way. Monoclonal antibodies are made by immunizing a mouse with a specific antigen, then hybridizing the mouse's spleen cells with murine myeloma cells and subsequently growing these hybridomas within other mice. A continuous supply of pure antibodies can be created. These antibodies can be developed against a variety of antigens and are used primarily for in vitro immunoassays.

By choosing a tumor-specific antigen, it is theoretically possible to radiolabel the monoclonal antibodies to the tumor in question. In practice, monoclonal antibodies highly specific for prostatic, renal cell carcinoma, and others, have been produced. Cancer-specific radiopharmaceuticals have been used to image these neoplasms with moderate success, and it is hoped that in the future this technique will permit radioimmunotherapy, so that radioisotopes can be directed only against the neoplasm, allowing for high-dose radiation therapy to the tumor yet limiting toxicity to normal tissues (Larson, Carrasquillo, and Reynolds, 1984).

Prostate Cancer

One very successful radiolabeled monoclonal antibody for the imaging of prostate cancer is ^{111}In-capromab pendetide. Capromab is a murine monoclonal antibody against the prostate-specific membrane antigen found on the surface of prostate cancer cells. The tracer is injected intravenously, and imaging is performed immediately to assess blood pool distribution. Reimaging is performed again 4–7 days after injection. The two sets of images are compared to identify regions of capromab uptake unrelated to blood pool localization. Among untreated patients with a definitive diagnosis of prostate cancer who are at high risk for pelvic lymph node metastases, capromab imaging is 75% sensitive, in contrast to CT and MRI, which are only 20% sensitive. Similarly, based on pathology and long-term follow-up, capromab is 90% specific, again in contrast to CT or MRI, which are only 30% specific (Hinkle et al, 1998).

Among patients with prostate cancer treated with radical prostatectomy, but with a positive or rising prostate-specific antigen, capromab imaging correctly identifies the site of recurrence in 60% of patients (Kahn et al, 1998a). Again, this is in contrast to CT scanning, which is only 20% sensitive. Prognostically, patients undergoing salvage pelvic radiation therapy after a failed radical prostatectomy are most likely to respond if their capromab scan is either negative or with limited uptake in the prostatic bed (Kahn et al, 1998b).

REFERENCES

Bagni B et al: ^{99m}Tc-MAG-3 versus ^{131}I-orthoiodohippurate in the routine determination of effective renal plasma flow. J Nucl Med Allied Sci 1990;34:67.

Bayne DP, Shapiro CE: Diuretic radionuclide urography: Functional assessment following pyeloplasty. J Urol 1985;134:344.

Beierwaltes WH: The adrenals. In: Harbert J, DaRocha AFG (editors): *Textbook of Nuclear Medicine,* vol. 2: *Clinical Applications,* 2nd ed., p. 56. Lea & Febiger, 1984.

Benador D et al: Cortical scintigraphy in the evaluation of renal parenchymal changes in children with pyelonephritis. J Pediatr 1994;125:334.

Blacklock ARE et al: Radionuclide imaging in scrotal swellings. Br J Urol 1983;55:749.

Chandhoke PS et al: Monitoring renal function in children with urologic abnormalities. J Urol 1990;144:601.

Coleman RE: Radiolabeled leukocytes. In: Freeman LM, Weissman H (editors): *Nuclear Medicine Annual 1982.* Raven Press, 1982.

Conway JJ, Kruglik GD: Effectiveness of direct and indirect radionuclide cystography in detecting vesicoureteral reflux. J Nucl Med 1976;17:81.

Conway JJ, Maizels M: The "well tempered" diuretic renogram: A standard method to examine the asymptomatic neonate with hydronephrosis or hydroureteronephrosis. J Nucl Med 1992;33:2047.

Conway JJ et al: Detection of vesicoureteral reflux with radionuclide cystography: A comparison study with roentgenographic cystography. Am J Roentgenol Radium Ther Nucl Med 1972;115:720.

Daly MJ et al: Differential renal function using technetium-99m dimercaptosuccinic acid (DMSA): In vitro correlation. J Nucl Med 1979;20:63.

English PJ et al: Modified method of diuresis renography for the assessment of equivocal pelviureteric junction obstruction. Br J Urol 1987;59:10.

Falkowski WS, Firlit CF: Testicular torsion: The role of radioisotopic scanning. J Urol 1980;124:886.

Gates GF: Glomerular filtration rate: Estimation from fractional renal accumulation of ^{99m}Tc-DTPA (stannous). AJR 1982;138:565.

Gates GF: Split renal function testing using Tc-99m DTPA: A rapid technique for determining differential glomerular filtration. Clin Nucl Med 1983;8:400.

Gordon I: Indications for ^{99m}technetium dimercaptosuccinic acid scan in children. J Urol 1987;137:464.

Halpern S, Hagan P: Gallium-67 citrate imaging in neoplastic and inflammatory disease. In: Freeman LM, Weissman H (editors): *Nuclear Medicine Annual 1980.* Raven Press, 1980.

Hattner RS, Engelstad BE: Radionuclide evaluation of renal transplants. In: Freeman LM, Weissman HS (editors): *Nuclear Medicine Annual 1984.* Raven Press, 1984.

Hattner RS et al: Localization of m-iodo (^{131}I) benzylguanidine in neuroblastoma. AJR 1984;143:373.

Hattner RS et al: Scintigraphic detection of pheochromocytomas using m-iodo (^{131}I) benzylguanidine. Noninvasive Med Imaging 1984;1:105.

Hinkle GH et al: Multicenter radioimmunoscintigraphy evaluation of patients with prostate carcinoma using indium-111 capromab pendetide. Cancer 1998;83:739.

Kahn D et al: 111-Indium capromab pendetide in the evaluation of patients with residual or recurrent prostate cancer after radical prostatectomy. J Urol 1998a;159:2041.

Kahn D et al: Radioimmunoscintigraphy with In-111-labeled capromab pendetide predicts prostate cancer response to salvage radiotherapy after failed radical prostatectomy. J Clin Oncol 1998b;16:284.

Kass EJ, Majd M, Belman AB: Comparison of the diuretic renogram and the pressure perfusion study in children. J Urol 1985;134:92.

Koff SA, Thrall JH, Keyes JW Jr: Diuretic radionuclide urography: A noninvasive method for evaluating nephroureteral dilatation. J Urol 1979;122:451.

Koff SA et al: Diuretic radionuclide localization of upper urinary tract obstruction. J Urol 1984;132:513.

Koff SA et al: Early postoperative assessment of the functional patency of ureterovesical junction following ureteroneocystostomy. J Urol 1981;125:554.

Kogan BA et al: ^{99m}Tc-DMSA scanning to diagnose pyelonephritic scarring in children. Urology 1983;21:641.

Larson SM, Carrasquillo JA, Reynolds JC: Radioimmunodetection and radioimmunotherapy. Cancer Invest 1984;2:363.

Lieberman LM et al: Diagnosis of adrenal disease by visualization of human adrenal glands with ^{131}I-19-iodo-cholesterol. N Engl J Med 1971;285:1387.

Maizels M et al: Troubleshooting the diuretic renogram. Urology 1986;28:355.

Majd M, Kass EJ, Belman AB: Radionuclide cystography in children: Comparison of direct (retrograde) and indirect (intravenous) techniques. Ann Radiol 1995;28:322.

Mandell GA et al: Procedure guideline for diuretic renography in children. J Nucl Med 1997a;38:1647.

Mandell GA et al: Procedure guideline for renal cortical scintigraphy in children. J Nucl Med 1997b;38:1644.

McLorie GA et al: ^{99m}Technetium-dimercaptosuccinic acid renal scanning and excretory urography in the diagnosis of renal scans in children. J Urol 1989;142:790.

McNeil BJ: Value of bone scanning in neoplastic disease. Semin Nucl Med 1984;14:277.

Merrick MV, Uttley WS, Wild R: A comparison of two techniques of detecting vesicoureteric reflux. Br J Radiol 1977;50:792.

Mittal BR et al: Role of captopril renography in the diagnosis of renovascular hypertension. Am J Kidney Dis 1996;28:209.

Munkner T: ^{131}I-meta-iodobenzylguanidine scintigraphy of neuroblastomas. Semin Nucl Med 1985;15:154.

Nasrallah PF et al: Quantitative nuclear cystogram: Aid in determining spontaneous resolution of vesicoureteral reflux. Urology 1978;12:654.

O'Reilly PH et al: Diuresis renography in equivocal urinary tract obstruction. Br J Urol 1978;50:76.

O'Reilly PH et al: ^{123}-Iodine: A new isotope for functional renal scanning. Br J Urol 1977;49:15.

Piepsz A et al: Replacing ^{99m}Tc-DMSA for renal imaging? Nucl Med Commun 1992;13:494.

Roccatello D et al: Prospective study on captopril renography in hypertensive patients. Am J Nephrol 1992;12:406.

Rosen PR, Treves S, Ingelfinger J: Hypertension in children: Increased efficacy of technetium Tc-99m succimer in screening for renal disease. Am J Dis Child 1985;139:173.

Russell CD et al: Quantitation of renal function with ^{99m}Tc-MAG-3. J Nucl Med 1988;29:1931.

Sarkar JD et al: A new and superior adrenal scanning agent: Np-59. J Nucl Med 1975;16:1038.

Sisson JC et al: Radiopharmaceutical treatment of malignant pheochromocytoma. J Nucl Med 1984;25:197.

Sisson JC et al: Scintigraphic localization of pheochromocytoma. N Engl J Med 1981;305:12.

Stoller ML, Kogan BA: Sensitivity of ^{99m}technetium-dimercaptosuccinic acid for diagnosis of chronic pyelonephritis: Clinical and theoretical considerations. J Urol 1986;135:977.

Stoller, ML, Kogan BA, Hricak H: Spermatic cord torsion: Diagnostic limitations. Pediatrics 1985;76:929.

Stringer DA et al: Comparison of aortography, renal vein renin sampling, radionuclide scans, ultrasound and IVU in the investigation of childhood renovascular hypertension. Br J Radiol 1984;57:111.

Taylor A Jr, Martin LG: The utility of ^{99m}Tc-MAG-3 in captopril renography. Am J Hypertens 1991;4(12–part 2):731s.

Taylor A Jr, Ziffer JA, Eshima D: Comparison of ^{99m}Tc-MAG-3 and ^{99m}Tc-DTPA in renal transplant patients with impaired renal function. Clin Nucl Med 1990;15:371.

Wilkins SA Jr et al: Acute appendicitis presenting as acute left scrotal pain: Diagnostic considerations. Urology 1985;25:634.

Winter CC: A new test for vesicoureteral reflux: An external technique using radioisotopes. J Urol 1959;81:105.

11

Retrograde Instrumentation of the Urinary Tract

Marshall L. Stoller, MD

The ability to manipulate the urinary tract without the need for an open surgical incision differentiates urology from other disciplines. Such intervention may be required for diagnostic or therapeutic purposes (or both). Understanding the various catheters, guidewires, stents, endoscopes, and associated instrumentation is key in helping physicians accomplish their desired tasks. Manipulation of the urinary tract should be performed in a gentle fashion; instruments need not be forced. An understanding of anatomy and alternative instrumentation should allow physicians to accomplish their tasks with finesse. The patient should understand the proposed procedure and potential complications. For example, the attempt to place a retrograde ureteral catheter to drain an infected kidney may ultimately lead to a percutaneous nephrostomy if the surgeon is unable to achieve retrograde drainage. Knowing when to stop is as important as knowing when to start.

Many procedures are performed at the bedside or in a cystoscopy suite under local anesthesia. A patient who is comfortable, informed, and assured will more likely cooperate and tolerate the procedure. A physician who is familiar with the proposed instrumentation and understands its limitations and alternatives will win the patient's confidence.

Manipulation of the urinary tract can result in significant injury. Anticipated prolonged procedures should be covered with appropriate antibiotics directed by preoperative urine cultures and sensitivities. Generous use of a water-soluble lubricant and low-pressure irrigation decreases the likelihood of significant iatrogenic infections. Patient positioning is as important as proper choice of instrumentation. Pressure points must be identified and adequately padded, especially when the patient is placed in the dorsal lithotomy position. Additionally, the legs should be secured in their stirrups to prevent accidental injury, such as might result from a leg hitting the surgeon after an unexpected obturator reflex during endoelectric surgery.

URETHRAL CATHETERIZATION

Urethral catheterization is the most frequent retrograde manipulation performed on the urinary tract. Catheters are placed to drain the bladder during and after surgical procedures requiring anesthetics, to assess urinary output in critically ill patients, to collect reliable urine specimens, for urodynamic evaluation, for radiographic studies (eg, cystograms), and to assess residual urine. Such catheters can be left indwelling with a self-retaining balloon, as is done with a Foley catheter. An in-and-out procedure to drain a bladder does not require a self-retaining device. Adequate lubrication and sufficient frequency to keep the bladder at reasonable volumes are critical and must be emphasized to the patient performing self-intermittent catheterization; sterility is secondary. In contrast, when a catheter is left indwelling it is important to use sterile technique.

Technique of Catheterization

A. In Men: The penis should be positioned pointing toward the umbilicus to decrease the acute angulation as the catheter traverses the bulbar urethra. On most occasions, the catheter passes without difficulty. When difficulties arise, a careful history relating to previous urologic manipulations is critical. Strictures are not infrequent. Soon after endourologic surgery, urethral strictures can be found, initially at the meatus and 1–2 months postoperatively at the bladder neck. History of a straddle injury may suggest a bulbar urethral stricture. Adequate lubrication injected into the urethra and instruction of the patient to relax his pelvic floor eases the passage beyond the striated rhabdosphincter. A large-caliber catheter of approximately 18F should be used. Narrow, stiff, small catheters have greater potential of creating false passages and possible perforation. Coudé (elbowed) tipped catheters frequently help negotiate a high bladder neck, as seen with benign prostatic hyperplasia. With self-retaining Foley catheters, complete advancement until the elbowed valve is at the meatus or until the urine returns is important. Inflating the balloon prematurely (while it is in the urethra) may result in severe pain and possible urethral rupture. This must be emphasized to ancillary nursing personnel dealing with demented patients unable to communicate effectively, because under such circumstances, urethral rupture may present only after severe infection is evident.

B. In Women: It may be difficult to identify the meatus, especially in patients with hypospadias. Lateral traction on the labia and a vaginal speculum may be needed. With adequate instruction and a mirror to visualize the meatus, women can learn to catheterize themselves. For repeat catheterizations, a finger inserted into the vagina can help to guide the catheter.

C. Difficult Placement and Removal: When a urethral catheter cannot be placed, filiforms and followers may be used with caution; the narrow filiform leaders are stiff and can easily puncture the urethra. Gentle advancement should stop when resistance is encountered, and the initial filiform should be left in place. A second and third filiform, and possibly additional ones, should be placed next to the previously placed catheters in hopes that the existing catheter occupies false passages or tortuous kinks. Eventually, one of the filiforms should pass and coil into the bladder. A female screw mount can be secured to the end of the filiform and used to progressively dilate the narrowed urethra. After adequate dilatation, an open-tipped Councill catheter can be placed over the filiform and into the bladder. If at any stage a problem or resistance is encountered, the procedure should be aborted and a suprapubic cystostomy should be performed to achieve adequate drainage.

Indwelling catheters should be secured to a closed gravity drainage system. For long-term requirements in males, the catheter should be secured to the abdominal wall to decrease the likelihood of stricture formation. Meatal care is needed to ensure adequate egress of urethral secretions.

Difficulty is much less common when removing indwelling urethral catheters, which are usually balloon retaining types. Inspection of the valve frequently reveals any problem. One may attempt to cut proximal to the valve in hopes of evacuating the balloon contents, but this is not always successful. Other options include transperineal or transabdominal puncture, injection of an organic agent such as ether through the balloon port (with a full bladder to prevent chemical cystitis) to dissolve the balloon wall. Occasionally, a narrow endoscope must be placed next to the catheter in the urethra and an unintended retaining suture cut after an open surgical procedure. Another complication of urethral catheters is incrustation, especially when a catheter is left indwelling for a long time.

Catheter Design

Catheters differ in size, shape, type of material, number of lumens, and type of retaining mechanism (Figure 11–1). Standard sizes of external catheter diameters and most endoscopic instruments are given according to Charriére's French scale (units of 0.33 mm = 1 French [F] or 1 Charriére [Charr]). Thus, 3F equals 1 mm in diameter and 30F equals 10 mm in diameter.

The choice of catheter size is dependent on the patient and the purpose. Large-caliber catheters are used to evacuate potential blood clots. Other catheters are used to stabilize grafts after open urethroplasties, for stenting after endoscopic incisions of strictures, for support of external ureteral catheters, or to assess urinary output. Triple-lumen catheters (one port for balloon inflation and deflation, and one each for inflow and outflow) have smaller lumens than 2-way catheters. Other catheter variables include balloon size and construction materials; smaller catheters have smaller balloons. Large balloons (eg, 30 mL) can be inflated well over 50 mL to decrease the likelihood of the balloon migrating into the prostatic fossa, especially after transurethral resection of the prostate, and can be used as traction devices against the bladder neck in hopes of controlling hemorrhage from the prostatic fossa.

The rigidity of the catheter, the ratio between internal and external diameters, and the biocompatibility depend on the material with which the catheter is made. The standard latex catheter can result in severe reactions in patients with latex allergies, most commonly those with myelomeningoceles. Silicone varieties are good alternatives in such situations. Mucosal irritation is decreased when catheters with a low coefficient of friction are used. Hydromers are placed onto catheters to allow for transient coating, creating an interface between biologic tissues and the foreign catheter; this interface lasts for only approximately 5 days. Permanent hydrogel coatings last the life of the catheter. Decreasing the coefficient of friction of these catheters brings about a decrease in mucosal irritation and better biocompatibility. Catheters with a longer lasting interface result in decreased incrustation.

URETHROSCOPY

To identify and aid in treating urethral pathology, endoscopic inspection via a urethroscope with a 0-degree lens is helpful. Stricture disease can be identified or confirmed after radiographic studies. Strictures are characterized by circumferential narrowing. Sequential dilation of urethral strictures by inserting catheters of increasing size exerts shear and tear forces to the mucosa and is likely to produce extended scarring. Thus, stricture recurrence is common if periodic urethral dilation is terminated. Balloon dilation of a stricture with 7–9F balloon dilators (which can be passed over guidewires and inflated up to 30F with pressures of up to 15 atm) does not exert shear force, but the long-term results are poor. Limited circumferential strictures can be incised under

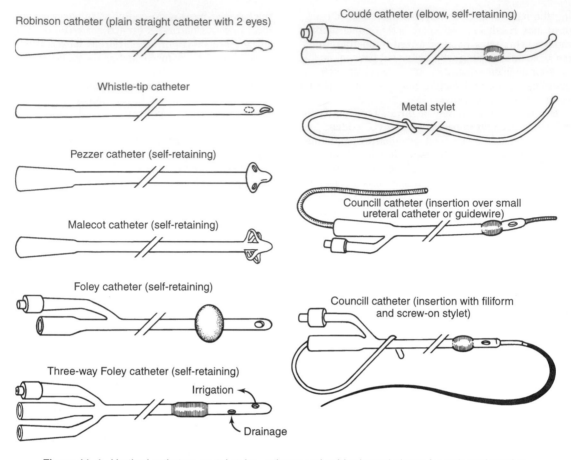

Robinson catheter (plain straight catheter with 2 eyes)

Whistle-tip catheter

Pezzer catheter (self-retaining)

Malecot catheter (self-retaining)

Foley catheter (self-retaining)

Three-way Foley catheter (self-retaining)

Irrigation

Drainage

Coudé catheter (elbow, self-retaining)

Metal stylet

Councill catheter (insertion over small ureteral catheter or guidewire)

Councill catheter (insertion with filiform and screw-on stylet)

Figure 11–1. Urethral catheters, metal stylet, catheter and guidewire techniques for catheter insertion.

direct vision with a cold knife. The incision is usually made at the 12 o'clock position, adequate to allow passage of the urethroscope. The bladder then can be evacuated and adequate irrigation used if further incision results in hemorrhage. It is difficult to identify the true limits of a stricture solely by vision.

A urethral diverticulum can be confirmed with urethroscopy. If it has been identified, a catheter can be placed through the neck of the diverticulum to help identify it during definitive open surgical repair. Urethroscopy can be used to inject dye into rare retained müllerian duct cysts, to identify and extract foreign bodies or rare calculi, and to access biopsy-suspicious lesions. Urethroscopy allows endoscopic access to treat urethral condylomata.

CYSTOSCOPY

Endoscopic inspection of the lower urinary tract requires irrigation, illumination (fiberoptics), and optics. The optics and illumination are offset by the irrigating and working port. To optimize a complete examination, the rigid endoscope should be rotated, and 0-, 30-, 70-, and 120-degree lenses may be required. Suprapubic pressure facilitates inspection of the bladder dome, which frequently has an air bubble. A systematic approach is required when evaluating the urethra, prostate, bladder walls, dome and neck, and ureteral orifices (including location, number, shape, and character of efflux). The bladder should be evaluated at different levels of filling. It is only after full distention of the bladder that characteristic glomerulations and ecchymoses are seen in interstitial cystitis. Rectal examination with the endoscope in place is informative, especially in assessing prostate size and length of prostatic urethra.

Choice of irrigant during endoscopic manipulation is important. There are conductive and nonconductive irrigants. Conductive irrigants, which include saline and lactated Ringer's solution, would be inappropriate during endoelectric surgery. Nonconductive irrigants include water and glycine. Water has a theoretic advantage of increasing visibility, and because it is hypotonic, it can lyse tumor cells. If the potential exists for increased intravascular absorption, isoosmotic or other nonhemolyzing agents are preferred to hypotonic solutions.

Rigid endoscopy results in discomfort, which can be minimized with 1% lidocaine per urethra as a local anesthetic. Flexible endoscopes that decrease patient discomfort and allow for instrumentation in the supine rather than the routine dorsal lithotomy position are becoming more popular. They are now used routinely in an office setting, especially for hematuria/tumor surveillance and double-J stent retrieval. Videoendoscopy with flexible scopes allows patients to visualize normal and abnormal anatomy and thus helps them understand their pathology. Videoendoscopy reduces fluid contact to the urologist and can help reduce cervical neck disease. Such scopes have smaller irrigating ports that decrease maximal irrigation and they do not have a working sheath. As a result, changing lenses, assessing residual urine, and repeat evacuation of irrigant cannot be completed without entirely removing the endoscope. Rigid endoscopy allows for a greater variety of instrumentation, better optics, and increased durability.

Instrumentation similar to that used to evaluate the urethra and bladder can be used to inspect continent urinary reservoirs or conventional ileal loops. A Robinson or a Foley catheter placed prior to the endoscope gives the operator a visual landmark and an exit port for irrigation to keep the procedure at a low pressure. Alternatively, the Foley balloon can be inflated and the catheter plugged to transiently expand the intestinal segment in hopes of helping to identify landmarks or pathologic lesions. Endoscopic inspection allows for identification of calculi, foreign bodies, mucous plugs, and eroded Marlex collars and also has the potential for intubation of ureterointestinal anastomoses.

URETERAL CATHETERIZATION

Ureteral catheterization is required in performing retrograde pyelography, collecting urine for cytologic examination or appropriate cultures, performing brush biopsies (Figure 11–2), and placing a ureteral catheter for stone pushback procedures or for localization during lithotripsy. Other procedures that often require ureteral catheterization include fluoroscopically controlled stone basket manipulations (Figure 11–3), draining an obstructed kidney due to either intrinsic or extrinsic compressions, and placement of an internal double-J catheter. Finding the ureteral orifice can be difficult. Long-term indwelling Foley catheters, infection, history of a psoas hitch and ureteral reimplantation, or renal transplantation can hinder identification of the ureteral orifice. One must first try to identify the interureteric ridge and then look for a jet of efflux. Varying bladder volumes can facilitate localizing

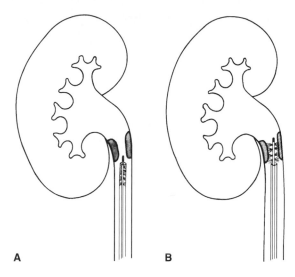

Figure 11–2. Brushing of a proximal ureteral lesion. **A:** Insertion of the brush covered by a catheter. **B:** Advancement of the brush through the lesion.

ureteral orifices. Intravenous methylene blue may be helpful once it is excreted out of the ureteral orifice (it usually takes longer than anticipated). Once the orifice is identified, catheters usually are placed uneventfully. However, in the setting of benign prostatic hyperplasia with J-hooking of the distal ureter, previous retroperitoneal surgery, reimplantation of the ureter, decreased lower extremity mobility or other skeletal abnormalities, or edema or kinking secondary to long-standing impacted ureteral calculi, catheterization procedures can be difficult or impossible. An Albiron bridge may help direct catheters and guidewires.

There are many configurations of catheter tips (Figure 11–4). Acorn or cone-tipped catheters are excellent for routine retrograde pyelography. Care should be taken to eliminate air in the catheter before injection to avoid confusing air with a filling defect. Fluoroscopy helps determine the appropriate volume of radiocontrast material to decrease the likelihood of pyelolymphatic or pyelovenous reflux or forniceal rupture. The average collecting system holds 7–9 mL of contrast material. If performed under local anesthesia, overdistension is recognized by severe ipsilateral flank pain. With low-pressure injections, there is no systemic absorption of contrast material. A coudé-tipped catheter allows for dramatic mobility of the tip of the catheter by merely twisting it; there is no need for exaggerated motion of the endoscope. This is helpful in orifices that are difficult to identify because of edema or tumor infiltration.

To bypass severe angulations, passage of a guidewire must first be attempted. Straight guidewires can be made floppy if they have removable cores, and

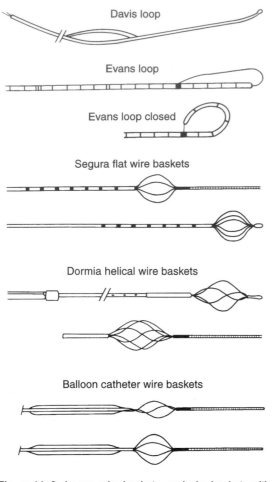

Figure 11–3. Loops, wire baskets, and wire baskets with balloon catheters for extraction of ureteral stones.

frequently this allows easy passage. At times, hydrophilic coudé-tipped torque guidewires are helpful. If the orifice can be engaged with the tip of the guidewire but the guidewire cannot be advanced, the tip of the endoscope should be pivoted toward the contralateral orifice while the guidewire is advanced through the endoscope just enough to keep the guidewire engaged in the orifice. The guidewire should then be advanced against the back wall of the bladder, effectively changing the vector force so that the wire can be advanced through a severe J deformity (Figure 11–5). With the guidewire advanced, an exchange catheter can be advanced over the guidewire for injection of contrast material, to be exchanged later for another guidewire or an open-ended catheter. A coudé-tipped guidewire or floppy-tipped guidewire (with a removable core guide) can be advanced through such exchange catheters to facilitate bypassing stones or severe kinks. A push-pull maneuver (pulling the exchange catheter while pushing

the guidewire) frequently straightens the ureter as a result of resistance from the exchange catheter, allowing advancement of the guidewire. To increase resistance, an occlusion balloon ureteral catheter can be inflated and with gentle traction can help straighten a kinked or tortuous ureter. Additional helpful maneuvers include deep exhalation, thus elevating the diaphragm, external cephalad pressure by an assistant, or Trendelenburg patient positioning. Impacted ureteral calculi can be advanced back into the renal pelvis with mechanical force applied from the catheter or via hydrostatic pressure.

Double-J catheters are used to facilitate internal drainage due to obstruction from ureteral angulation and internal or external ureteral compression; they are also used to help decrease the likelihood of sepsis or obstruction in the presence of steinstrasse after extracorporeal shock-wave lithotripsy. Double-J stents increase the internal lumen of the ureter. This increase may be used to one's advantage after attempts at ureteroscopy have been unsuccessful because of a narrow ureter. Placing a double-J catheter and postponing the ureteroscopy for a few days significantly decreases the difficulty of the procedure. Double-J stents disrupt normal ureteral peristalsis.

Double-J catheters can be placed over a guidewire or with a closed leading end. With proper placement of the proximal end into the renal pelvis, the J should project in the lateral position when seen on fluoroscopy or x-ray. Projecting in an anterior-posterior position suggests a proximal ureteral location. Proximal J stent placement can be confirmed by renal ultrasonography during placement in pregnant patients. If it is too long, the distal end in the bladder can result in severe irritative voiding symptoms; if too short, it is more likely to advance inadvertently beyond the ureteral orifice into the ureter. In such situations, drainage cannot be ensured, and thus the catheter must be extracted with a ureteroscope or snared with a ureteral stone basket. Patients must be informed that such stents have been placed. Frequently, they will not feel the stent. However, if the stent is left in place for long periods, the likelihood of incrustations, with potentially poor drainage and difficult extraction, is increased. It is unclear whether double-J stents facilitate drainage because of drainage around the catheter or via the numerous side holes communicating with the internal lumen. New helically ridged double-J ureteral stents likely enhance ureteral stone passage through unidirectional ratchetlike motion over the external ridges during respiratory and body wall motion. Additional potential complications include distal migration into the bladder, distal migration beyond the bladder neck (resulting in total urinary incontinence), and flank pain during micturition secondary to reflux. The catheter can be removed with cold cup forceps via a flexible or rigid cystoscope or by pulling a string that has been attached to the distal end of the catheter and

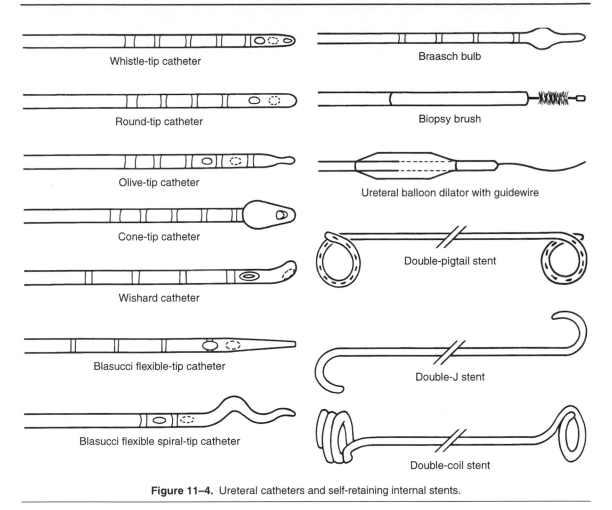

Figure 11–4. Ureteral catheters and self-retaining internal stents.

left exiting through the meatus. Although double-J catheters have potential complications, they can help ensure internal urinary drainage.

Balloon dilators can be used to ease passage of ureteroscopes (rigid or flexible; see chapter on ureteroscopy) and extract intact large calculi. Balloons are routinely passed over a guidewire. Woven balloons have a tight, unfolded outer surface that shortens in longitudinal length when inflated. In contrast, nonwoven varieties are folded and may be difficult to pass after initial inflation and deflation; however, they do not shorten in length with inflation. Balloons inflated alongside distal ureteral calculi can result in balloon perforation or extrusion of the calculus outside the ureteral lumen. Balloon inflation is best achieved with ratcheted or torqued syringe aids directed with pressure gauges.

Retrograde endopyelotomy is an alternative to open surgical repair and percutaneous antegrade approaches. After documentation of the exact location of the ureteropelvic junction obstruction under fluo-

roscopic control, a 150-cm superstiff Linderquist guidewire is advanced into the renal pelvis. The endoscope is removed and the retrograde endopyelotomy device is advanced over the guidewire under fluoroscopic control (such devices are approximately 9F in size). After the incising wire is directed laterally, the balloon is inflated during cautery. Successful results are seen in approximately 80% of patients. An internal endopyelotomy double-J stent, 14F at the proximal end, straddling the ureteropelvic junction, and tapered to 6–8F as it enters and coils in the bladder, or a routine 7F double-J ureteral stent is then placed over the stiff guidewire and left in place for 6 weeks. Placing a standard double-J catheter before this procedure dilates the ureter and eases passage of the balloon cutting device (Acucise) and the endopyelotomy double-J catheter.

A large selection of endoscopic baskets are available to entrap and remove material including calculi, sloughed papillae, bulky tumors, fungal bezoars, and other foreign bodies. Baskets are designed with and

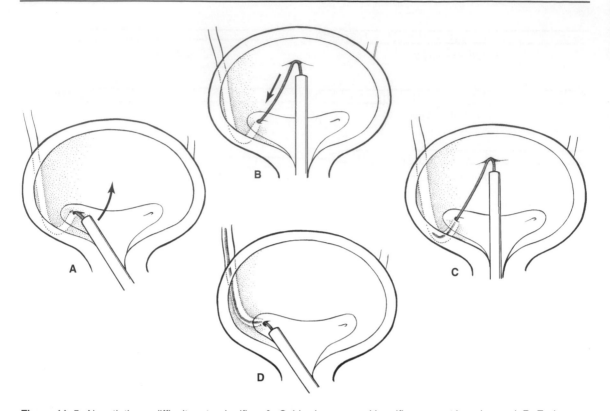

Figure 11–5. Negotiating a difficult ureteral orifice. **A:** Guidewire engaged in orifice, cannot be advanced. **B:** Endoscope is rotated toward contralateral orifice. Guidewire remains engaged in orifice. **C:** Guidewire is advanced against bladder wall. **D:** Guidewire negotiated beyond angulation.

without filiform leaders and can be advanced on their own or, more commonly, through the working ports of flexible and rigid ureteroscopes. Round wire baskets can be torqued to help entrap the target material. A few (2–3) wired baskets are used for large material, while numerous (4–6) wired baskets are used for small or numerous objects. Flat wired baskets can engage stones effectively. If twisted, however, the wire can fold and transform into a knifelike edge. Once the basket is engaged, one should ensure that the endothelium is not entrapped. Gentle traction helps extract these foreign materials. Engaged baskets may be difficult to disengage. Occasionally, one must cut the handle and place a ureteroscope alongside the basket to facilitate stone and basket extraction. Nitinol baskets have rounded tops and decrease potential endothelial trauma.

TRANSURETHRAL SURGERY

Resectoscopes are endoscopes with sheaths of 10–30F (Figure 11–6) designed for transurethral surgery; they allow urologists to excise, fulgurate, or vaporize tissue from the lower genitourinary tract.

Applying an alternating current at high frequencies decreases muscular contractions and allows for cutting and coagulation properties. A pure sine wave is optimal for cutting, whereas dampened oscillating waveforms are best for coagulation. It is possible to combine the 2 waves to allow for simultaneous cutting and coagulation. A ground plate, as an indifferent electrode, usually applied over the hip, is required. The cutting current results in rapid vaporization of tissue, allowing the cutting loop to move easily through tissue with minimal resistance, and separates the chip, enabling easy flow into the bladder. Rapid succession of cutting sweeps allows rapid surgical excision. In contrast, a coagulation current results in less rapid vaporization and thus decreased separation of tissue from the cutting current. If a resectoscope does not cut tissue, the operator should check for a broken resecting loop, a broken or disconnected cable or generator, or a conductive irrigant (as with saline) that diffuses the current.

Before endoelectric surgery, the urethra should be calibrated with sounds to ensure ease in placing the resectoscope. Urethral sounds and probes come in numerous varieties (Figure 11–7). An Otis urethrotome can be used to incise the urethra at the 12 o'clock posi-

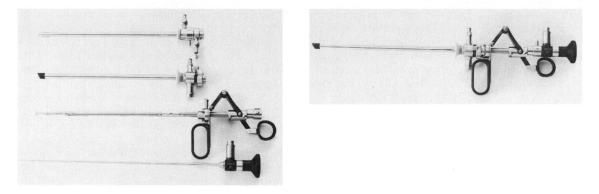

Figure 11–6. Transurethral resectoscope. **Left:** Continuous-flow sheath, standard sheath, working element with cutting loop, telescope. **Right:** Instrument assembled.

tion, thereby decreasing the potential for stricture disease in narrow urethras. Generous use of a water-soluble lubricant is indicated. Before placement of the resectoscope, the loop should be inspected for defects and for appropriate engagement to ensure complete re-

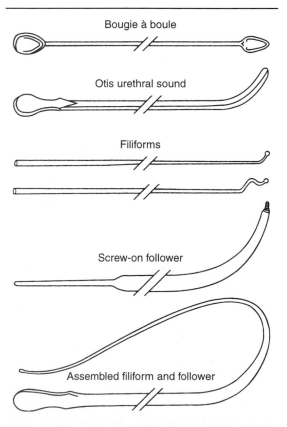

Figure 11–7. Urethral probes and sounds.

traction into the sheath, thereby allowing resected tissue to flow easily into the bladder. A spare loop should be available to decrease the time needed for replacement if need be. The endoscope can be placed under direct vision, especially if the patient has not recently been cystoscoped. Alternatively, a Timberlake obturator allows for blind placement of the resectoscope sheath. Timberlake obturators can be placed under direct vision. Most endoscopes require the operator to intermittently remove the working element to allow evacuation of bladder contents. Other endoscopes have an additional channel for continuous operation. An alternative is a percutaneous suprapubic drainage catheter, which allows for continuous flow. Orientation with identification of landmarks, such as the verumontanum and the ureteral orifices, before resection dramatically decreases the potential for complications. Bladder lesions are best resected with minimal bladder distention to decrease the likelihood of perforation. A Bugbee electrode can be used for point coagulation of bleeding points or pathologic lesions. A rollerball can be used to coagulate large areas. Transurethral resection can be used to resect an obstructing prostate gland, to drain prostatic abscesses, or to unroof the ejaculatory duct in select infertility patients.

Transurethral resection of the prostate (TURP) is a time-tested procedure for resecting prostatic tissue and decreasing symptoms of urinary obstruction. In experienced hands, this can be done with minimal complications. New, alternative procedures are being investigated, especially with patients who are poor anesthetic risks, whose life expectancy is limited, or who are averse to TURP. Those with small glands or with bladder neck contractures have been treated by transurethral incision of the prostate from a point just distal to the ureteral orifices to the verumontanum. Transcystoscopic urethroplasty, also known as prostatic balloon dilatation, dilates the prostatic urethra under visual and fluoroscopic control. Intraurethral coils can be placed in high-risk patients to avoid permanent catheter drainage. Thermotherapy requires 6–10 treatments delivering temperatures of 41–44 °C for 60 min. Results of such new methods of treatment are limited, and long-term comparison with the more traditional TURP is lacking. Obstructing median lobes are unsuited for such newer techniques.

Transurethral laser ablation of the prostate gland has been described as a method for the management of prostatic enlargement. The beam of neodymium:YAG laser is deflected at 90 degrees using a specially designed probe, which is positioned in the prostatic urethra through a standard cystoscope. Sequential evaporation and coagulation of obstructing prostatic tissue may then be undertaken, with significantly less bleeding than usually results from conventional electrocautery resection. The major disadvantage of this procedure in comparison with standard resection techniques is that an immediate clearance of tissue is not obtained and that a complete histologic examination of the prostate is unavailable. The denatured prostatic tissue is instead allowed to slough and pass in the urinary stream over ensuing weeks. Initial enthusiasm for this technique has been replaced with caution owing to delayed symptom improvement and irritating symptoms as tissue is sloughed. More recently, holmium:YAG laser techniques allow enucleation of prostatic tissue into the bladder. Long-term studies are required to compare this technique with TURP.

There are various cutting techniques for resecting an obstructing prostate gland during TURP. All require good vision, a comfortable operator, identification of the surgical capsule, and established goals that are met before starting additional stages of the procedure. Pulsatile arterial bleeders should be coagulated first and venous hemorrhage next. Occasionally, arterial bleeders cannot be coagulated without additional resection of tissue. An Ellik bulb or piston syringe should be available to evacuate resected tissue. At the conclusion of the procedure, one should ensure adequate resection and hemostasis, and perform an inspection for forgotten chips of tissue and possible injuries. A Foley catheter should be placed into the bladder and irrigated to confirm unobstructed flow and adequate hemostasis. If an undermined trigone is suspected, a coudé-tipped catheter, a finger in the rectum, or a stylet inserted into the catheter can help in proper placement. The Foley balloon should be inflated 20 mL plus 1 mL for each gram of resected tissue. Gentle traction on the catheter can aid hemostasis.

Video cameras can be attached to the optical eyepiece while transurethral surgery is performed. Use of the camera can reduce the risk of cervical disc disease and distance the surgeon from blood products. It is an excellent resource to improve the teaching of endoscopic surgery. Additionally, still pictures taken with 35-mm film can document disease progression.

Acute complications include intra- or extraperi-toneal rupture of the bladder, rectal perforation, incontinence, incision of a ureteral orifice with possible reflux or stricture, hemorrhage, gas explosion (especially during resection of a bladder lesion at the dome in the presence of accumulated gas), epididymitis, sepsis, and transurethral resection syndrome. The transurethral resection syndrome is characterized by delusional hyponatremia resulting in possible confusion, congestive heart failure, or pulmonary edema. It is secondary to a large amount of fluid being absorbed, usually through a perforation of a low-pressure system such as the venous sinusoids. If perforations are noted, especially into a sinus, the height of the irrigating solution should be lowered, hemostasis achieved, and the procedure brought to a rapid conclusion. Other complications include impotence (with excessive coagulation) and urethral stricture disease. After an adequate transurethral resection of the prostate, retrograde ejaculation almost always occurs.

LOWER TRACT CALCULI

Most bladder calculi originating from the upper tract pass spontaneously through the urethra. In contrast, bladder calculi resulting from outlet obstruction may require endoscopic extraction. Many of these calculi can be washed out or extracted with the aid of various forceps or a resectoscope loop. Calculi too large to pass through an endoscopic sheath first require fragmentation. Visual lithotrites with crushing jaws or a punch type mechanism are effective. Introduction of these bulky devices is potentially dangerous. A distended bladder facilitates effective engagements of the stone without injuring the bladder wall. Twisting the lithotrite before crushing ensures that the bladder wall is free from the instrument.

Other methods available to fragment bladder calculi include ultrasonic, electrohydraulic, and pneumatic lithotrites. Ultrasonic lithotrites use vibratory energy delivered via a rigid metal transducer. An offset endoscopic lens is required. Gentle pressure of the transducer against the stone facilitates fragmentation; excessive pressure can erode or perforate the bladder wall. A hollow core with suction extracts the fragments. Electrohydraulic lithotripsy generates a spark-gap, resulting in a shock wave. It is delivered at the end of a flexible catheter and can be applied as single or repetitive shocks. Fragmentation can be performed with normal saline. Initially, it was performed with 1/6–1/7 normal saline (6 mL of 23.4% concentrated saline added to 1 L of distilled water). A rheostat can adjust the power output. A high setting can result in the stone caroming to various locations in the bladder; lower settings result in suboptimal fragmentation. To optimize fragmentation, the tip of the lithotrite should be a few millimeters away from the stone. To protect the endoscopic optics, the endoscope should be kept at a distance. Shock waves fragment brittle material, such as the stone or a lens. Biologic tissues are elastic and are unharmed as long as the spark-gap does not touch them. Air-driven, jack-hammer-like devices (rigid and flexible) can be used for stone fragmentation. The photothermal mechanism of holmium lasers is effective in fragmenting very large bladder stones. Uric acid calculi produce small amounts of cyanide gas when fragmented with holmium lasers; the clinical significance is unknown. Pneumatic lithotrites are now becoming popular. They are effective, with minimal tissue trauma, use reusable probes, and are powered by compressed gas. Initial start-up costs are significantly less than those for laser systems.

ADVANCED INSTRUMENTATION

Lasers

Lasers (light amplification by stimulated emission of radiation) have recently been used through flexible and rigid endoscopes. Carbon dioxide and argon lasers result in tissue penetration that is inadequate for the needs of urology. Neodymium:YAG lasers give adequate tissue coagulation and are useful for various lesions. The holmium:YAG system is excellent for stone fragmentation and tissue ablation and is now the most popular system in use. Disadvantages are the lack of adequate tissue for histopathologic evaluation and the initial cost of machinery.

Ultrasonography

Ultrasound has found increased application to the lower genitourinary tract. It results in minimal discomfort; gives a 3-dimensional appreciation of the shape, size, and volume of organs and disease; and can provide direct intervention. Various transducers are available; high-megahertz transducers are required for superficial structures (for example, scrotal structures) to assess testicular disease (including tumors and torsion), while low-megahertz transducers are reserved for deep structures (for example, guiding percutaneous access for kidneys and bladders). Intervening tissue can significantly reduce image quality.

Transrectal ultrasound is valuable in evaluating the prostate to determine size and confirm digital information on the presence and stage of a suspected malignant tumor. Because of the low incidence of detecting malignancies (1.6–7%), mass screening programs are not cost-effective. Direct needle biopsies, with automatic biopsy mechanisms, are quick, well-tolerated, and result in reliable tissue cores and less pain than traditional needles (such as Tru-Cut) directed under digital palpation. Percutaneous drainage tubes, radioactive seed implants, and temperature coils used for cryosurgery of the prostate can be placed safely under transrectal ultrasonic guidance. Transrectal ultrasonography can yield unreliable images that often are misinterpreted by the novice. Pitfalls include faulty instrument settings, poor coupling caused by feces or gas, and unrecognized artifacts resulting from reverberation, deflection, shadowing, or enhancement.

Suprapubic ultrasonography can help to assess prostate anatomy, especially size and intravesical extension. It can help to evaluate the bladder for residual urine and for calculi that are questionable on plain abdominal radiographs. (Changing the patient's position can shift the position of a calculus.) Distal ureteral stones can be identified, especially when visualized through a full bladder used as an acoustic window. Double-J stents, incrustations, diverticula, and large malignant lesions can be identified. The procedure also can direct placement of suprapubic

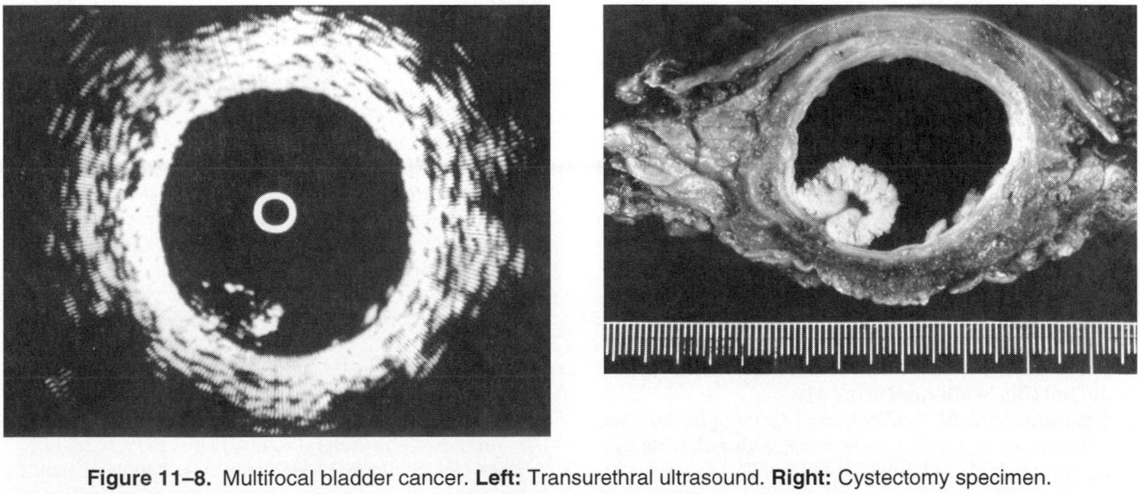

Figure 11–8. Multifocal bladder cancer. **Left:** Transurethral ultrasound. **Right:** Cystectomy specimen.

cystostomy drainage catheters and often can avert overlying bowel, especially in patients who have had lower abdominal surgery.

Additional applications include endocavitary, color, Doppler, and dynamic ultrasonography. Endocavitary ultrasound, which includes transvaginal, transurethral (Figure 11–8), and transcystoscopic techniques, can delineate vaginal, urethral, and blad-

der disease. Endoureteral ultrasound can help in the identification of crossing vessels, preferably before an endopyelotomy. Color and Doppler ultrasound can assess blood flow as related to erectile dysfunction. Dynamic ultrasound can supplement urodynamic findings. Ultrasound applied to the lower genitourinary tract causes minimal discomfort and provides valuable information.

REFERENCES

URETHRAL CATHETERIZATION CYSTOSCOPY

Berci G: Instrumentation 1: Rigid endoscopes. In: Berci G (editor): *Endoscopy.* Appleton-Century-Crofts, 1976.

Berci G: Instrumentation 2: Flexible fiber endoscopes. In: Berci G (editor): *Endoscopy.* Appleton-Century-Crofts, 1976.

Berci G et al: Permanent film records. In: Berci G (editor): *Endoscopy.* Appleton-Century-Crofts, 1976.

Bloom DA, McGuire EJ, Lapides J: A brief history of urethral catheterization. J Urol 1994;151:317.

Brechtelsbauer DA: Care with an indwelling urinary catheter: Tips for avoiding problems in independent and institutionalized patients. Postgrad Med 1992;92:127.

Brocklehurst JC: The management of indwelling catheters. Br J Urol 1978;50:102.

Choong S et al: A prospective, randomized, double-blind study comparing lignocaine gel and plain lubricating gel in relieving pain during flexible cystoscopy. Br J Urol 1997;80:69.

Clayman RV, Reddy P, Lange PH: Flexible fiberoptic and rigid-rod lens endoscopy of the lower urinary tract: A prospective controlled comparison. J Urol 1984;131:715.

Cox CE, Hinman F Jr: Experiments with induced bacteriuria, vesical emptying and bacterial growth on the mechanism of bladder defense to infection. J Urol 1961;86:739.

Desautels RE, Chibaro EA, Lang JR: Maintenance of sterility in urinary drainage bags. Surg Gynecol Obstet 1981;154:838.

Fuselier HA Jr, Mason C: Liquid sterilization versus high level disinfection in the urologic office. Urology 1997;50:337.

Koss EH, Schneiderman JJ: Entry of bacteria in urinary tracts of patients with in-lying catheter. N Engl J Med 1957;256:556.

Lapides J et al: Clean, intermittent self-catheterization in the treatment of urinary tract disease. J Urol 1972;107:458.

Madsen FA, Bruskewitz RC: Cystoscopy in the evaluation of benign prostatic hyperplasia. World J Urol 1995;13:14.

Nanninga JB: Care of the catheter-dependent patient. Urol Clin North Am 1980;7:41.

Simonato A, Galli S, Carmignani G: Simple, safe and inexpensive retrieval of JJ stents with a flexible cystoscope. Br J Urol 1998;81:490.

Williams JC et al: Deflation techniques for faulty Foley catheter balloons: Presentation of a cystoscopic technique. Tech Urol 1996;2:174.

TRANSRECTAL & TRANSURETHRAL ULTRASOUND

Carpentier PJ, Schroder FH: Transrectal ultrasonography in the follow-up of prostatic carcinoma patients: A new prognostic parameter? J Urol 1984;131:903.

Hernandez AD, Smith JA Jr: Transrectal ultrasonography for the early detection and staging of prostate cancer. Urol Clin North Am 1990;17:45.

Nash PA et al: Sono-urethrography in the evaluation of anterior urethral strictures. J Urol 1995;154:72.

Rickards D: Transrectal ultrasound 1992. Br J Urol 1992;69:449.

URETERAL CATHETERIZATION

Bigongiari LR: Transluminal dilatation of ureteral strictures. In: Lang EK (editor): *Percutaneous and Interventional Urology and Radiology.* Springer-Verlag, 1986.

Elyaderani MK, Kandzari SJ: Ureteral stent insertion and brush biopsy. In: Elyaderani MK et al (editors): *Invasive Uroradiology: A Manual of Diagnostic and Therapeutic Techniques.* Heath, 1984.

Finney RP: Double-J and diversion stents. Urol Clin North Am 1982;9:89.

Fritzche PJ: Antegrade and retrograde ureteral stenting. In: Lang EK (editor): *Percutaneous and Interventional Urology and Radiology.* Springer-Verlag, 1986.

Gibbons RP et al: Experience with indwelling ureteral stent catheters. J Urol 1976;115:22.

Goldstein AG, Conger KB: Perforation of the ureter during retrograde pyelography. J Urol 1965;94:658.

Huffman JL, Bagley DH, Lyon ES: Ureteral catheterization, retrograde ureteropyelography and self retaining ureteral stents. In: Bagley DH, Huffman JL, Lyon ES (editors): *Urologic Endoscopy: A Manual and Atlas.* Little, Brown, 1985.

Irby PI et al: Long term followup of ventriculoureteral shunts for the treatment of hydrocephalus. Urology 1993;42:193.

Mardis HK, Hepperlen TW, Kammandel H: Double pigtail ureteral stent. Urology 1979;14:23.

Oswalt GC Jr, Bueschen AJ, Lloyd IK: Upward migration of indwelling ureteral stents. J Urol 1979;122:249.

Phan CN, Stoller ML: Helically ridged ureteral stent facilitates the passage of stone fragments in an experimental porcine model. Br J Urol 1993;72:17.

Ramsay JWA et al: The effects of double J stenting on unobstructed ureters: An experimental and clinical study. Br J Urol 1985;57:630.

STONE BASKETING, URETERORENOSCOPY

Abdelsayed M, Onal E, Wax SH: Avulsion of the ureter caused by stone basket manipulation. J Urol 1977; 118:868.

Aslan P, Malloy B, Preminger GM: Access to the distal ureter after failure of direct visual ureteroscopy. Br J Urol 1998;82:290.

Dourmashkin RL: Cystoscopic treatment of stones in the ureter with special reference to large calculi: Based on a study of 1550 cases. J Urol 1945;54:245.

Fabrizio MD, Behari A, Bagley DH: Ureteroscopic management of intrarenal calculi. J Urol 1998;159:1139.

Hofmann R, Hartung R: Laser-induced shock-wave lithotripsy of ureteric calculi. World J Urol 1989;7: 142.

Kandzari SJ, Elyaderani MK: Retrograde extraction, chemolysis, and intraoperative ultrasonographic localization of urinary calculi. In: Elyaderani MK et al (editors): *Invasive Uroradiology: A Manual of Diagnostic and Therapeutic Techniques.* Heath, 1984.

Low RK, Stoller ML: Endoscopic mapping of renal papillae for Randall's plaques in patients with urinary stone disease. J Urol 1997;158:2062.

Perez-Castro Ellendt E, Martinez-Pineiro JA: Ureteral and renal endoscopy: A new approach. Eur Urol 1982; 8:117.

Rutner AB: Ureteral balloon dilatation and stone basketing. Urology 1985;23(5 Spec No.):44.

Rutner AB, Fucilla IS: An improved helical stone basket. J Urol 1976;116:784.

Schwartz BA, Wise HA II: Endourologic techniques for the bladder and urethra. Urol Clin North Am 1982;9: 165.

Shihata AA, Greene JE: Ureteric stone extraction by a new double-balloon catheter: An experimental study. J Urol 1983;129:616.

Stoller ML et al: Endoscopic management of upper tract urothelial tumors. Tech Urol 1997;3:1.

Wolf JS Jr, Carroll PR, Stoller ML: Cost-effectiveness v patient preference in the choice of treatment for distal ureteral calculi: A literature-based decision analysis. J Endourol 1995;9:243.

CYTOLOGY, BIOPSY HISTOLOGY

Barry JM et al: The influence of retrograde contrast medium on urinary cytodiagnosis: A preliminary report. J Urol 1978;119:633.

Crawford ED et al: Prevention of urinary tract infection and sepsis following transrectal prostatic biopsy. J Urol 1982;127:449.

Dodd LG et al: Endoscopic brush cytology of the upper urinary tract. Evaluation of its efficacy and potential limitations in diagnosis. Acta Cytol 1997;41:377.

Epsoti PL: Cytologic malignancy grading for prostatic carcinoma for transurethral aspiration biopsy. Scand J Urol Nephrol 1971;5:199.

Epstein NA: Prostatic biopsy: A morphologic correlation of aspiration cytology with needle biopsy histology. Cancer 1976;38:2078.

Franzen S et al: Cytological diagnosis of prostatic tumors by transrectal aspiration biopsy: A preliminary report. Br J Urol 1960;32:193.

Gill WB, Lu C, Bibbo M: Retrograde brush biopsy of the ureter and renal pelvis. Urol Clin North Am 1979; 6:573.

Lieberman RP, Cummins KB, Leslie SW: Sheathed catheter system for fluoroscopically guided retrograde catheterization, and brush and forceps biopsy of the upper urinary tract. J Urol 1984;131:450.

Rife CC, Farrow GM, Utz DC: Urine cytology of transitional cell neoplasm. Urol Clin North Am 1979;6: 599.

ENDOSCOPY

Hopkins HH: The modern urological endoscope. In: *A Handbook of Urological Endoscopy.* Churchill Livingstone, 1978.

Merkle EM et al: Virtual cystoscopy based on helical CT scan datasets: Perspectives and limitations. Br J Radiol 1998;71:262.

Nicholson P: Problems encountered by early endoscopists. Urology 1982;19:114.

Reuter MA, Reuter HJ: The development of the cystoscope. J Urol 1998;159:638.

LITHOTRIPSY

Bapat SS: Endoscopic removal of bladder stones in adults. Br J Urol 1977;49:527.

Bigelow HJ: Lithotripsy by a single operation. Am J Med Sci 1978;75:117.

Reuter HJ: Electronic lithotripsy: Transurethral treatment of bladder stones in 50 cases. J Urol 1970; 104:834.

Vassar GJ, Teichman JM, Glickman RD: Holmium:YAG lithotripsy efficiency varies with energy density. J Urol 1998;160:471.

12

Urinary Obstruction & Stasis

Emil A. Tanagho, MD

Because of their damaging effect on renal function, obstruction and stasis of urinary flow are among the most important of urologic disorders. Either leads eventually to hydronephrosis, a peculiar type of atrophy of the kidney that may terminate in renal insufficiency or, if unilateral, complete destruction of the organ. Furthermore, obstruction leads to infection, which causes additional damage to the organs involved.

Classification

Obstruction may be classified according to cause (congenital or acquired), duration (acute or chronic), degree (partial or complete), and level (upper or lower urinary tract).

Etiology

Congenital anomalies, more common in the urinary tract than in any other organ system, are generally obstructive. In adult life, many types of acquired obstruction can occur.

A. Congenital: The common sites of congenital narrowing are the external meatus in boys (meatal stenosis) or just inside the external urinary meatus in girls, the distal urethra (stenosis), posterior urethral valves, ectopic ureters, ureteroceles, and the ureterovesical and ureteropelvic junctions. Another congenital cause of urinary stasis is damage to sacral roots 2–4 as seen in spina bifida and myelomeningocele. Vesicoureteral reflux causes both vesical and renal stasis (see Chapter 13).

B. Acquired: Acquired obstructions are numerous and may be primary in the urinary tract or secondary to retroperitoneal lesions that invade or compress the urinary passages. Among the common causes are (1) urethral stricture secondary to infection or injury; (2) benign prostatic hyperplasia or cancer of the prostate; (3) vesical tumor involving the bladder neck or one or both ureteral orifices; (4) local extension of cancer of the prostate or cervix into the base of the bladder, occluding the ureters; (5) compression of the ureters at the pelvic brim by metastatic nodes from cancer of the prostate or

cervix; (6) ureteral stone; (7) retroperitoneal fibrosis or malignant tumor; and (8) pregnancy.

Neurogenic dysfunction affects principally the bladder. The upper tracts are damaged secondarily by ureterovesical obstruction or reflux and, often, complicating infection. Severe constipation, especially in children, can cause bilateral hydroureteronephrosis from compression of the lower ureters.

Elongation and kinking of the ureter secondary to vesicoureteral reflux commonly lead to ureteropelvic obstruction and hydronephrosis. Unless a voiding cystourethrogram is obtained in children with this lesion, the primary cause may be missed and improper treatment given.

Pathogenesis & Pathology

Obstruction and neuropathic vesical dysfunction have the same effects on the urinary tract. These changes can best be understood by considering (1) the effects on the lower tract (distal to the bladder neck) of severe external urinary meatal stricture and (2) the effects on the mid tract (bladder) and upper tract (ureter and kidney) of benign prostatic hyperplasia.

A. Lower Tract (eg, Urethral Stricture): Hydrostatic pressure proximal to the obstruction causes dilation of the urethra. The wall of the urethra may become thin, and a diverticulum may form. If the urine becomes infected, urinary extravasation may occur, and periurethral abscess can result. The prostatic ducts may become widely dilated.

B. Mid Tract (eg, Prostatic Hyperplasia): In the earlier stages (compensatory phase), the muscle wall of the bladder becomes hypertrophied and thickened. With decompensation, it becomes less contractile and, therefore, weakened.

1. Stage of compensation–In order to balance the increasing urethral resistance, the bladder musculature hypertrophies. Its thickness may double or triple. Complete emptying of the bladder is thus made possible.

Hypertrophied muscle may be seen microscopically. With secondary infection, the effects of infection are often superimposed. There may be edema of the submucosa, which may be infiltrated with plasma cells, lymphocytes, and polymorphonuclear cells.

At cystoscopy, surgery, or autopsy, the following evidence of this compensation may be visible (Figure 12–1):

a. Trabeculation of the bladder wall–The wall of the distended bladder is normally quite smooth. With hypertrophy, individual muscle bundles become taut and give a coarsely interwoven appearance to the mucosal surface. The trigonal muscle and the interureteric ridge, which normally are only slightly raised above the surrounding tissues, respond to obstruction by hypertrophy of their smooth musculature. The ridge then becomes prominent. This trigonal hypertrophy causes increased resistance to urine flow in the intravesical ureteral segments owing to accentuated downward pull on them. It is this mechanism that causes relative functional obstruction of the ureterovesical junctions, leading to back pressure on the kidney and hydroureteronephrosis. The obstruction increases in the presence of significant residual urine, which further stretches the ureterotrigonal complex. (A urethral catheter relieves the obstruction somewhat by eliminating the trigonal stretch. Definitive prostatectomy leads to permanent release of

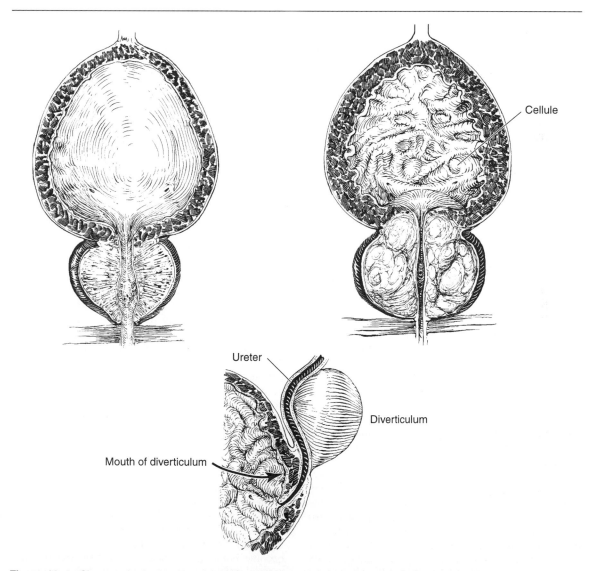

Figure 12–1. Changes in the bladder developing from obstruction. **Upper left:** Normal bladder and prostate. **Upper right:** Obstructing prostate causing trabeculation, cellule formation, and hypertrophy of the interureteric ridge. **Bottom:** Marked trabeculation (hypertrophy) of the vesical musculature; diverticulum displacing left ureter.

stretch and gradual softening of trigonal hypertrophy with relief of the obstruction.)

b. Cellules–Normal intravesical pressure is about 30 cm of water at the beginning of micturition. Pressures 2–4 times as great may be reached by the trabeculated (hypertrophied) bladder in its attempt to force urine past the obstruction. This pressure tends to push mucosa between the superficial muscle bundles, causing the formation of small pockets, or cellules (Figure 12–1).

c. Diverticula–If cellules force their way entirely through the musculature of the bladder wall, they become saccules, then actual diverticula, which may be embedded in perivesical fat or covered by peritoneum, depending on their location. Diverticula have no muscle wall and are therefore unable to expel their contents into the bladder efficiently even after the primary obstruction has been removed. When secondary infection occurs, it is difficult to eradicate; surgical removal of the diverticula may be required. If a diverticulum pushes through the bladder wall on the anterior surface of the ureter, the ureterovesical junction will become incompetent (see Chapter 13).

d. Mucosa–In the presence of acute infection, the mucosa may be reddened and edematous. This may lead to temporary vesicoureteral reflux in the presence of a "borderline" junction. The chronically inflamed membrane may be thinned and pale. In the absence of infection, the mucosa appears normal.

2. Stage of decompensation–The compensatory power of the bladder musculature varies greatly. One patient with prostatic enlargement may have only mild symptoms of prostatism but a large obstructing gland that can be palpated rectally and observed cystoscopically; another may suffer acute retention and yet have a gland of normal size on rectal palpation and what appears to be only a mild obstruction cystoscopically.

In the face of progressive urethral obstruction, possibly aggravated by prostatic infection with edema or by congestion from lack of intercourse, decompensation of the detrusor may occur, resulting in the presence of residual urine after voiding. The amount may range up to 500 mL or more.

C. Upper Tract:

1. Ureter–In the early stages of obstruction, intravesical pressure is normal while the bladder fills and is increased only during voiding. The pressure is not transmitted to the ureters and renal pelves because of the competence of the ureterovesical "valves." (A true valve is not present; the ureterotrigonal unit, by virtue of its intrinsic structure, resists the retrograde flow of urine.) However, owing to trigonal hypertrophy (see the section Trabeculation of the bladder wall) and to the resultant increase in resistance to urine flow across the terminal ureter, there is progressive back pressure on the ureter and kidney, resulting in ureteral dilatation and hydronephrosis. Later, with the phase of decompensation accompanied by residual urine, there

is an added stretch effect on the already hypertrophied trigone that increases appreciably the resistance to flow at the lower end of the ureter and induces further hydroureteronephrosis. With decompensation of the ureterotrigonal complex, the valvelike action may be lost, vesicoureteral reflux occurs, and the increased intravesical pressure is transmitted directly to the renal pelvis, aggravating the degree of hydroureteronephrosis.

Secondary to the back pressure resulting from reflux or from obstruction by the hypertrophied and stretched trigone or by a ureteral stone, the ureteral musculature thickens in its attempt to push the urine downward by increased peristaltic activity (stage of compensation). This causes elongation and some tortuosity of the ureter (Figure 12–2). At times, this change becomes marked, and bands of fibrous tissue develop. On contraction, the bands further angulate the ureter, causing secondary ureteral obstruction. Under these circumstances, removal of the obstruction below may not prevent the kidney from undergoing progressive obstruction due to the secondary ureteral obstruction.

Finally, because of increasing pressure, the ureteral wall becomes attenuated and therefore loses its contractile power (stage of decompensation). Dilatation may be so extreme that the ureter resembles a loop of bowel (Figures 12–3 and 13–8, upper right).

2. Kidney–The pressure within the renal pelvis is normally close to zero. When this pressure increases because of obstruction or reflux, the pelvis and calyces dilate. The degree of hydronephrosis that develops depends on the duration, degree, and site of the obstruction (Figure 12–4). The higher the obstruction, the greater the effect on the kidney. If the renal pelvis is entirely intrarenal and the obstruction is at the ureteropelvic junction, all the pressure will be exerted on the parenchyma. If the renal pelvis is extrarenal, only part of the pressure produced by a ureteropelvic stenosis is exerted on the parenchyma; this is because the extrarenal renal pelvis is embedded in fat and dilates more readily, thus "decompressing" the calyces (Figure 12–2).

In the earlier stages, the pelvic musculature undergoes compensatory hypertrophy in its effort to force urine past the obstruction. Later, however, the muscle becomes stretched and atonic (and decompensated).

The progression of hydronephrotic atrophy is as follows:

(1) The earliest changes in the development of hydronephrosis are seen in the calyces. The end of a normal calyx (as seen on a urogram, Figure 6–4) is concave because of the papilla that projects into it; with increase in intrapelvic pressure, the fornices become blunt and rounded. With persistence of increased intrapelvic pressure, the papilla becomes flattened, then convex (clubbed) as a result of compression enhanced by ischemic atrophy (Figure 12–5).

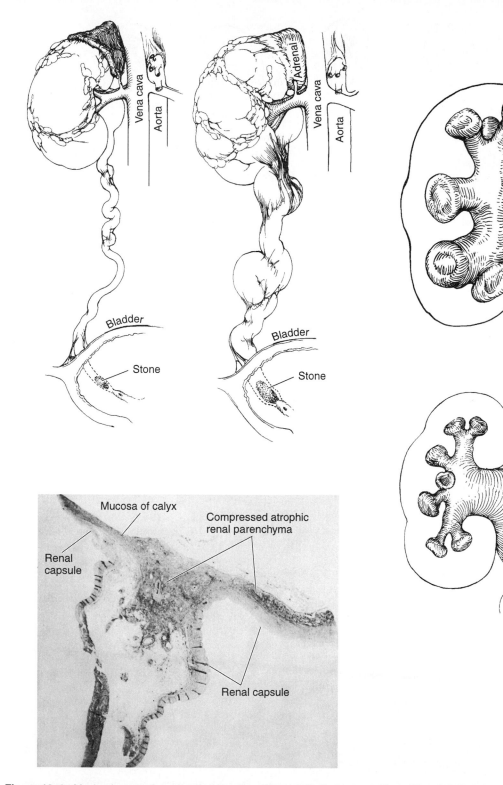

Figure 12–2. Mechanisms and results of obstruction. **Upper left:** Early stage. Elongation and dilatation of ureter due to mild obstruction. **Upper center:** Later stage. Further dilatation and elongation with kinking of the ureter; fibrous bands cause further kinking. **Lower left:** Photomicrograph of advanced hydronephrosis. Thin layer of renal parenchyma covered by fibrous capsule. **Upper right:** Intrarenal pelvis. Obstruction transmits all back pressure to parenchyma. **Lower right:** Extrarenal pelvis, when obstructed, allows some of the increased pressure to be dissipated by the pelvis.

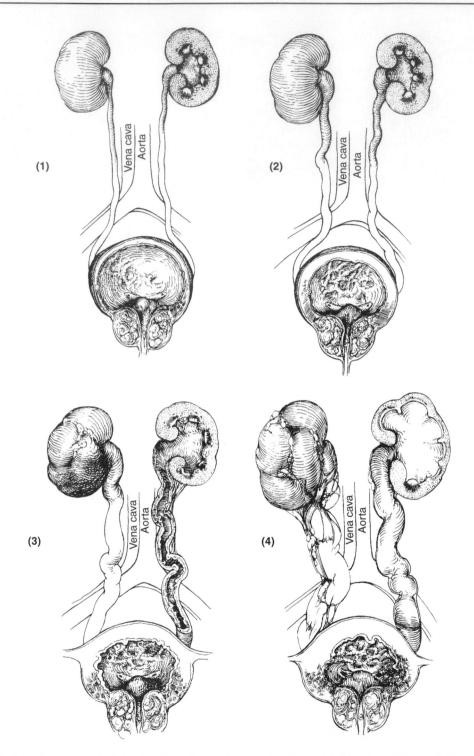

Figure 12–3. Pathogenesis of bilateral hydronephrosis. Progressive changes in bladder, ureters, and kidneys from obstruction of an enlarged prostate: thickening of bladder wall, dilatation and elongation of ureters, and hydronephrosis.

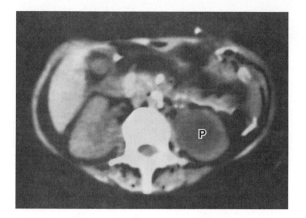

Figure 12–4. Hydronephrotic left renal pelvis. Low-density mass (P) in left renal sinus had attenuation value similar to that of water, suggesting the correct diagnosis. Unless intravenous contrast material is used, differentiation from peripelvic cyst may be difficult.

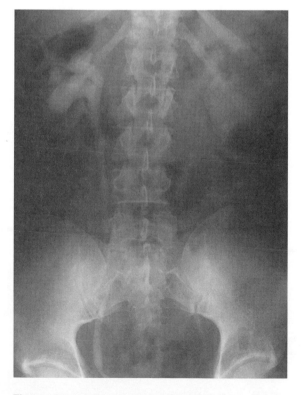

Figure 12–5. Lower right ureteral obstruction. Mild-to-moderate dilatation of the collecting system with rounded blunting of the calyces.

The parenchyma between the calyces is affected to a lesser extent. The changes in the renal parenchyma are due to (1) compression atrophy from increase in intrapelvic pressure (more accentuated with intrarenal pelves) and (2) ischemic atrophy from hemodynamic changes, mainly manifested in arcuate vessels that run at the base of the pyramids parallel to the kidney outline and are more vulnerable to compression between the renal capsule and the centrally increasing intrapelvic pressure.

This spotty atrophy is caused by the nature of the blood supply of the kidney. The arterioles are "end arteries"; therefore, ischemia is most marked in the areas farthest from the interlobular arteries. As the back pressure increases, hydronephrosis progresses, with the cells nearest the main arteries exhibiting the greatest resistance.

This increased pressure is transmitted up the tubules. The tubules become dilated, and their cells atrophy from ischemia.

It should be pointed out that a few instances of dilated renal pelves and calyces are not due to the presence of obstruction. Rarely, the renal cavities are congenitally capacious and thus simulate hydronephrosis. More commonly, hydronephrosis may occur in childhood owing to the back pressure associated with vesicoureteral reflux. If the valvular incompetence resolves (and this is common), some degree of the hydronephrotic changes may persist. These persisting changes may cause the physician to suspect the presence of obstruction, which may lead to unnecessary surgery. An isotope renogram or the Whitaker test (**see p 131**) can be performed to determine whether organic obstruction is present.

(2) Only in unilateral hydronephrosis are the advanced stages of hydronephrotic atrophy seen. Eventually the kidney is completely destroyed and appears as a thin-walled sac filled with clear fluid (water and electrolytes) or pus (Figure 12–6).

If obstruction is unilateral, the increased intrarenal pressure causes some suppression of renal function on that side. The closer the intrapelvic pressure approaches the glomerular filtration pressure (6–12 mm Hg), the less urine can be secreted. Glomerular filtration rate and renal plasma flow are reduced, concentrating power is gradually lost, and the urea-creatinine concentration ratio of urine from the hydronephrotic kidney is lower than that of urine from the normal kidney.

Hydronephrotic atrophy is an unusual type of pathologic change. Other secretory organs (eg, the submaxillary gland) cease secreting when their ducts are obstructed. This causes primary (disuse) atrophy. The completely obstructed kidney, however, continues to secrete urine. (If this were not so, hydronephrosis could not occur, since it depends on increased intrarenal pressure.) As urine is excreted into the renal pelvis, fluid and, particularly, soluble substances are reabsorbed, through either the tubules or

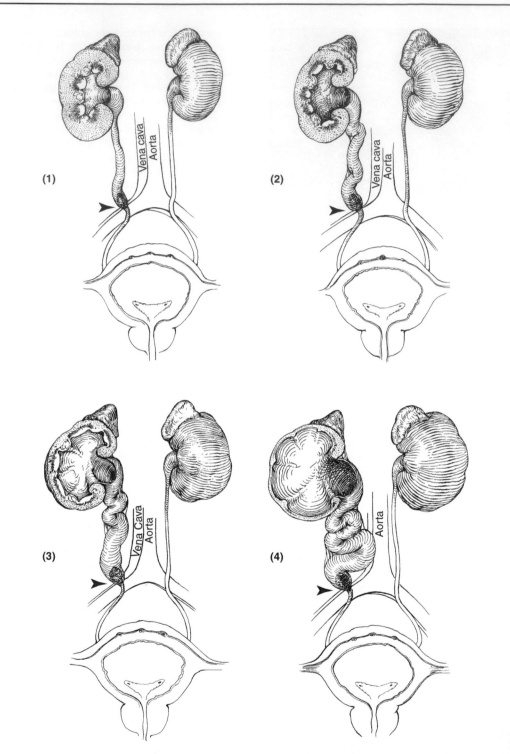

Figure 12–6. Pathogenesis of unilateral hydronephrosis. Progressive changes in ureter and kidney secondary to obstructing calculus (arrows). As the right kidney undergoes gradual destruction, the left kidney gradually enlarges (compensatory hypertrophy).

the lymphatics. This has been demonstrated by injecting phenolsulfonphthalein (PSP) into the obstructed renal pelvis. It disappears (is reabsorbed) in a few hours and is excreted by the other kidney. If the intrapelvic pressure in the hydronephrotic kidney rapidly increases to a level approaching filtration pressure (resulting in cessation of filtration), a safety mechanism is activated that produces a break in the surface lining of the collecting structure at the weakest point—the fornices. This leads to escape and extravasation of urine from the renal pelvis into the parenchymal interstitium (pyelointerstitial backflow). The extravasated fluid is absorbed by the renal lymphatics, and the pressure in the renal pelvis drops, allowing further filtration of urine. This explains the process by which the markedly hydronephrotic kidney continues to function. Further evidence of the occurrence of extravasation and reabsorption is that the markedly hydronephrotic kidney does not contain urine in the true sense; only water and a few salts are present.

Functional impairment in unilateral hydronephrosis, as measured by PSP tests or excretory urograms, is greater and increases faster than that seen in bilateral hydronephrotic kidneys showing comparable damage on urography. As unilateral hydronephrosis progresses, the normal kidney undergoes compensatory hypertrophy (particularly in children) of its nephrons (renal counterbalance), thereby assuming the function of the diseased kidney in order to maintain normal total renal function. For this reason, successful anatomic repair of the ureteral obstruction of such a kidney may fail to improve its powers of waste elimination.

If both kidneys are equally hydronephrotic, a strong stimulus is continually being exerted on both to maintain maximum function. This is also true of a hydronephrotic solitary kidney. Consequently, the return of function in these kidneys after repair of their obstructions is at times remarkable.

Experimental studies have shown recovery of function after release of complete obstruction of up to 4 weeks' duration. In 2 well-documented human cases, function was recovered after obstruction of 56 and 69 days. However, irreversible loss of function can begin as early as 7 days, as evidenced by dilatation and necrosis of the proximal tubules, which progressively increase with time.

The extent of recovery after partial obstruction is difficult to determine preoperatively. Renal scanning with DMSA (dimercaptosuccinic acid) is most helpful. Temporary drainage, especially by nephrostomy, followed by tests to assess renal function is the best measure.

Physiologic Explanation of Symptoms of Bladder Neck Obstruction

The following hypothesis has been proposed to explain the syndrome known as "prostatism," which occurs with progressive vesical obstruction:

The bladder, like the heart, is a hollow muscular organ that receives fluid and forcefully expels it. And, like the heart, it reacts to an increasing work load by going through the successive phases of compensation and finally decompensation.

Normally, contraction of the detrusor muscle and the trigone pulls the bladder neck open and forms a funnel through which the urine is expelled. The intravesical pressure generated in this instance varies between 20 and 40 cm of water; this force further widens the bladder neck.

With bladder neck obstruction, hypertrophy of the vesical musculature develops, allowing the intravesical voiding pressure to rise to 50–100 cm or more of water in order to overcome the increased outlet resistance. Despite this, the encroaching prostate appears to interfere with the mechanisms that ordinarily open the internal orifice. Also, the contraction phase may not last long enough for all of the urine to be expelled; "exhaustion" of the muscle occurs prematurely. The refractory phase then sets in, and the detrusor is temporarily unable to respond to further stimuli. A few minutes later, voiding may be initiated again and completed.

A. Compensation Phase:

1. Stage of irritability–In the earliest stages of obstruction of the bladder neck, the vesical musculature begins to hypertrophy. The force and size of the urinary stream remain normal because the balance is maintained between the expelling power of the bladder and urethral resistance. During this phase, however, the bladder appears to be hypersensitive. As the bladder is distended, the need to void is felt. In patients with a normal bladder, these early urges can be inhibited, and the bladder relaxes and distends to receive more urine. However, in patients with a hypertrophied detrusor, the contraction of the detrusor is so strong that it virtually goes into spasm, producing the symptoms of an irritable bladder. The earliest symptoms of bladder neck obstruction, therefore, are urgency (even to the point of incontinence) and frequency, both day and night.

2. Stage of compensation–As the obstruction increases, further hypertrophy of the muscle fibers of the bladder occurs, and the power to empty the bladder completely is thereby maintained. During this period, in addition to urgency and frequency, the patient notices hesitancy in initiating urination while the bladder develops contractions strong enough to overcome resistance at the bladder neck. The obstruction causes some loss in the force and size of the urinary stream, and the stream becomes slower as vesical emptying nears completion (exhaustion of the detrusor as it nears the end of the contraction phase).

B. Decompensation Phase: If vesical tone becomes impaired or if urethral resistance exceeds detrusor power, some degree of decompensation (imbalance) occurs. The contraction phase of the vesical muscle becomes too short to completely expel the contents of the bladder, and some urine remains in the bladder (residual urine).

1. Acute decompensation–The tone of the compensated vesical muscle can be temporarily embarrassed by rapid filling of the bladder (high fluid intake) or by overstretching of the detrusor (postponement of urination though the urge is felt). This may cause increased difficulty of urination, with marked hesitancy and the need for straining to initiate urination; a very weak and small stream; and termination of the stream before the bladder completely empties (residual urine). Acute and sudden complete urinary retention may also occur.

2. Chronic decompensation–As the degree of obstruction increases, a progressive imbalance between the power of the bladder musculature and urethral resistance develops. Therefore, it becomes increasingly difficult to expel all the urine during the contraction phase of the detrusor. The symptoms of obstruction become more marked. The amount of residual urine gradually increases, and this diminishes the functional capacity of the bladder. Progressive frequency of urination is noted. On occasion, as the bladder decompensates, it becomes overstretched and attenuated. It may contain 1000–3000 mL of urine. It loses its power of contraction, and overflow (paradoxic) incontinence results.

Clinical Findings

A. Symptoms:

1. Lower and mid tract (urethra and bladder)–Symptoms of obstruction of the lower and mid tract are typified by the symptoms of urethral stricture, benign prostatic hyperplasia, neurogenic bladder, and tumor of the bladder involving the vesical neck. The principal symptoms are hesitancy in starting urination, lessened force and size of the stream, and terminal dribbling; hematuria, which may be partial, initially, with stricture or total with prostatic obstruction or vesical tumor; and burning on urination, cloudy urine (due to complicating infection), and occasionally acute urinary retention.

2. Upper tract (ureter and kidney)–Symptoms of obstruction of the upper tract are typified by the symptoms of ureteral stricture or ureteral or renal stone. The principal complaints are pain in the flank radiating along the course of the ureter, gross total hematuria (from stone), gastrointestinal symptoms, chills, fever, burning on urination, and cloudy urine with onset of infection, which is the common sequel to obstruction or vesicoureteral reflux. Nausea, vomiting, loss of weight and strength, and pallor are due to uremia secondary to bilateral hydronephrosis. A history of vesicoureteral reflux in childhood may be significant. Obstruction of the upper tract may be silent even when uremia supervenes.

B. Signs:

1. Lower and mid tract–Palpation of the urethra may reveal induration about a stricture. Rectal examination may show atony of the anal sphincter (damage to the sacral nerve roots) or benign or malignant enlargement of the prostate. Vesical distention may be found.

Although observation of the force and caliber of the urinary stream affords a rough estimate of maximum flow rate, the rate can be measured accurately with a urine flowmeter or, even more simply, by the following technique: Have the patient begin to void. When observed maximum flow has been reached, interpose a container to collect the urine and simultaneously start a stopwatch. After exactly 5 s, remove the container. The flow rate in milliliters per second can easily be calculated. The normal urine flow rate is 20–25 mL/s in males and 25–30 mL/s in females. Any flow rate under 15 mL/s should be regarded with suspicion. A flow rate under 10 mL/s is indicative of obstruction or weak detrusor function. Flow rates associated with an atonic neurogenic (neuropathic) bladder (diminished detrusor power), or with urethral stricture or prostatic obstruction (increased urethral resistance) may be as low as 3–5 mL/s. A cystometrogram can differentiate between these 2 causes of impaired flow rate. After definitive treatment of the cause, the flow rate should return to normal.

In the presence of a vesical diverticulum or vesicoureteral reflux, although detrusor power is normal, the urinary stream may be impaired because of the diffusion of intravesical pressure into the diverticulum and vesicoureteral junction as well as the urethra. Excision of the diverticulum or repair of the vesicoureteral junctions leads to efficient expulsion of urine via the urethra.

2. Upper tract–An enlarged kidney may be discovered by palpation or percussion. Renal tenderness may be elicited if infection is present. Cancer of the cervix may be noted; it may invade the base of the bladder and occlude one or both ureteral orifices, or its metastases to the iliac lymph nodes may compress the ureters. A large pelvic mass (tumor, pregnancy) can displace and compress the ureters. Children with advanced urinary tract obstruction (usually due to posterior urethral valves) may develop ascites. Rupture of the renal fornices allows leakage of urine retroperitoneally; with rupture of the bladder, urine may pass into the peritoneal cavity through a tear in the peritoneum.

C. Laboratory Findings: Anemia may be found secondary to chronic infection or in advanced bilateral hydronephrosis (stage of uremia). Leukocytosis is to be expected in the acute stage of infection. Little if any elevation of the white blood count accompanies the chronic stage.

Large amounts of protein are usually not found in the obstructive uropathies. Casts are not common from hydronephrotic kidneys. Microscopic hematuria may indicate renal or vesical infection, tumor, or stone. Pus cells and bacteria may or may not be present.

In the presence of unilateral hydronephrosis, results of the PSP test are normal because of the contralateral renal hypertrophy. Suppression of PSP excretion indicates bilateral renal damage, residual urine (vesical or bilateral ureterorenal), or vesicoureteral reflux.

In the presence of significant bilateral hydronephrosis, urine flow through the renal tubules is slowed. Thus, urea is significantly reabsorbed but creatinine is not. Blood chemistry therefore reveals a urea-creatinine ratio well above the normal 10:1.

D. X-Ray Findings (Figure 12–7): A plain film of the abdomen may show enlargement of renal shadows, calcific bodies suggesting ureteral or renal stone, or tumor metastases to the bones of the spine or pelvis. Metastases in the spine may be the cause of spinal cord damage (neuropathic bladder); if they are osteoblastic, they are almost certainly from cancer of the prostate.

Excretory urograms reveal almost the entire story unless renal function is severely impaired. They are more informative when obstruction is present because the radiopaque material is retained. These urograms demonstrate the degree of dilatation of the pelves, calyces, and ureters. The point of ureteral stenosis is revealed. Segmental dilatation of the lower end of a ureter implies the possibility of vesicoureteral reflux (Figure 12–7), which can be revealed by cystography. The cystogram may show trabeculation as an irregularity of the vesical outline and may show diverticula. Vesical tumors, nonopaque stones, and large intravesical prostatic lobes may cause radiolucent shadows. A film taken immediately after voiding will show residual urine. Few tests that are as simple and inexpensive give the physician so much information.

Retrograde cystography shows changes of the bladder wall caused by distal obstruction (trabeculation, diverticula) or demonstrates the obstructive lesion itself (enlarged prostate, posterior urethral valves, cancer of the bladder). If the ureterovesical valves are incompetent, ureteropyelograms are obtained by reflux.

Retrograde urograms may show better detail than the excretory type, but care must be taken not to overdistend the passages with too much opaque fluid; small hydronephroses can be made to look quite large. The degree of ureteral or ureterovesical obstruction can be judged by the degree of delay of drainage of the radiopaque fluid instilled.

Computed tomography scanning and sonography can also help determine the extent of dilatation and parenchymal atrophy.

E. Isotope Scanning: (See Chapter 10.) In the presence of obstruction, the radioisotope renogram may show depression of both the vascular and secretory phases and a rising rather than a falling excretory phase due to retention of the radiopaque urine in the renal pelvis.

The ^{131}I activity recorded on the gamma camera will show that the isotope is poorly taken up, slowly transported through the parenchyma, and accumulated in the renal pelvis.

F. Instrumental Examination: Exploration of the urethra with a catheter or other instrument is a valuable diagnostic measure. Passage may be blocked by a stricture or tumor. Spasm of the external sphincter may make passage difficult. Passage of the catheter immediately after voiding allows estimation of the amount of residual urine in the bladder. Residual urine is common in bladder neck obstruction (enlarged prostate), cystocele, and neurogenic (neuropathic) bladder. Residual urine is usually absent with urethral stricture, even though the urinary stream may be markedly impaired.

Measurement of vesical tone by means of cystometry is helpful in diagnosing neurogenic bladder and in differentiating between bladder neck obstruction and vesical atony.

Inspection of the urethra and bladder by means of cystoscopy and panendoscopy may reveal the primary obstructive agent. Catheters may be passed to the renal pelves and urine specimens obtained. The function of each kidney may be measured (PSP test), and retrograde ureteropyelograms can be obtained.

G. Interventional Uroradiology: If there is doubt about the presence of true obstruction, either the Whitaker test (**see p 131**) or an isotope renogram can be done. However, Whitaker and Buxton-Thomas (1984) have shown that neither test is without error.

Differential Diagnosis

A thorough examination usually leaves no doubt about the diagnosis. The differential diagnosis under these circumstances is rarely difficult. If seemingly simple infection does not respond to medical therapy or if infection recurs, obstruction, a foreign body, or vesicoureteral reflux is the probable cause, and complete study of the urinary tract is indicated.

Complications

Stagnation of urine leads to infection, which then may spread throughout the entire urinary system. Once established, infection is difficult and at times impossible to eradicate even after the obstruction has been relieved.

Often the invading organisms are urea-splitting (*Proteus,* staphylococci), which causes the urine to become alkaline. Calcium salts precipitate and form bladder or kidney stones more easily in alkaline urine.

If both kidneys are affected, the result may be renal insufficiency. Secondary infection increases renal damage.

Pyonephrosis is the end stage of a severely infected and obstructed kidney. The kidney is functionless and filled with thick pus. At times, a plain film

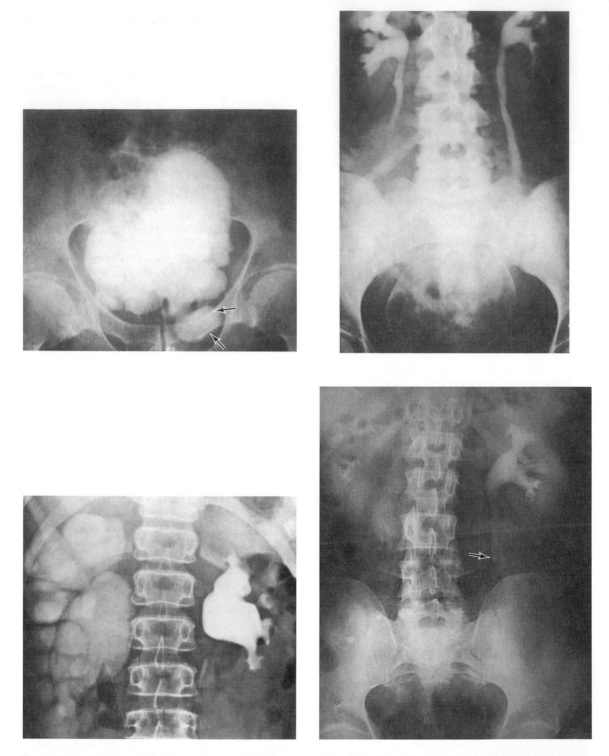

Figure 12–7. Changes in bladder, ureters, and kidneys caused by obstruction. **Upper left:** Cystogram showing benign prostatic enlargement and multiple diverticula. Arrows point to femoral hernia that probably developed as a result of straining to urinate. **Upper right:** Pregnancy. Significant dilatation and elongation of upper right ureter due to compression at the pelvic line. Left side normal. **Lower left:** Excretory urogram, 70 min after injection. Advanced right hydronephrosis secondary to ureteropelvic obstruction. Mild ureteropelvic obstruction on left. **Lower right:** Stone in left ureter (at arrow) with mild hydronephrosis.

of the abdomen may show an air urogram caused by gas liberated by infecting organisms.

Treatment

A. Relief of Obstruction: Treatment of the main causes of obstruction and stasis (benign prostatic hyperplasia, cancer of the prostate, neurogenic bladder, ureteral stone, posterior urethral valves, and ureteral stenosis) is described in detail elsewhere in this book.

1. Lower tract obstruction (distal to the bladder)–With patients in whom secondary renal or ureterovesical damage (reflux in the latter) is minimal or nonexistent, correction of the obstruction is sufficient. If significant reflux is demonstrated and does not subside spontaneously after relief of obstruction, surgical repair may be needed. Repair becomes imperative if there is considerable hydronephrosis in addition to reflux. Preliminary drainage of the bladder by an indwelling catheter or other means of diversion (eg, loop ureterostomy) is indicated in order to preserve and improve renal function. If, after a few months of drainage, reflux persists, the incompetent ureterovesical junction should be surgically repaired.

2. Upper tract obstruction (above the bladder)–If tortuous, kinked, dilated, or atonic ureters have developed secondary to lower tract obstruction (so that they are themselves obstructive), vesical drainage will not protect the kidneys from further damage; the urine proximal to the obstruction must be diverted by nephrostomy or ureterostomy. The kidneys then may regain some function. Over a period of many months, the ureter may become less tortuous and less dilated; its obstructive areas may open up. If radiopaque material instilled into the nephrostomy tube passes readily to the bladder, it may be possible to remove the nephrostomy tube. If obstruction or reflux persists, surgical repair is indicated. Permanent urinary diversion (eg, ureteroileal conduit) may be necessary.

If one kidney has been irreversibly damaged, as measured by kidney function tests, urography, sonography, computed tomography scan, or scintigraphy, nephrectomy may be necessary.

B. Eradication of Infection: Once the obstruction is removed, every effort should be made to eradicate infection. If the infection has been severe and prolonged, antibiotics may fail to sterilize the urinary tract.

Prognosis

No simple statement can be made about the prognosis in this group of patients. The outcome depends on the cause, site, degree, and duration of the obstruction. The prognosis is also definitely influenced by complicating infection, particularly if the infection has been present for a long time.

If renal function is fair to good, if the obstruction or other causes of stasis can be corrected, and if complicating infection can therefore be eradicated, the prognosis is generally excellent.

REFERENCES

Abrams P: Objective evaluation of bladder outlet obstruction. Br J Urol 1995;76(Suppl 1):11.

Bauer SB, Joseph DB: Management of the obstructed urinary tract associated with neurogenic bladder dysfunction. Urol Clin North Am 1990;17:395.

Belman AB, King LR: Vesicostomy: Useful means of reversible urinary diversion in selected infants. Urology 1973;1:208.

Bloom DA, Lebowitz RL, Bauer SB: Correlation of cystographic bladder morphology and neuroanatomy in boys with posterior urethral valves. Pediatr Radiol 1997;27:553.

Blyth B, Snyder HM, Duckett JW: Antenatal diagnosis and subsequent management of hydronephrosis. J Urol 1993;149:693.

Bomalaski MD, Hirschl RB, Bloom DA: Vesicoureteral reflux and ureteropelvic junction obstruction: Association, treatment options and outcome. J Urol 1997;157:969.

Bratt CG et al: Long-term followup of maximum concentrating ability and glomerular filtration rate in adult obstructed kidneys after pyeloplasty. J Urol 1988;140:273.

Cardenas DD, Mayo ME, Turner LR: Lower urinary changes over time in suprasacral spinal cord injury. Paraplegia 1995;33:326.

Carr LK, Webster GD: Bladder outlet obstruction in women. Urol Clin North Am 1996;23:385.

Cartwright PC et al: Managing apparent ureteropelvic junction obstruction in the newborn. J Urol 1992;148:1224.

Clark WR, Malek RS: Ureteropelvic junction obstruction. I. Observations on the classic type in adults. J Urol 1987;138:276.

Cockett AT et al: Indications for treatment of benign prostatic hyperplasia: The American Urological Association Study. Cancer 1992;70(Suppl 1):280.

Colodny AH: Antenatal diagnosis and management of urinary abnormalities. Pediatr Clin North Am 1987;34:1365.

DeMaeyer P et al: Clinical study of technetium dimercaptosuccinic acid uptake in obstructed kidneys: Comparison with creatinine clearance. J Urol 1982;128:8.

Devine CJ Jr, Devine PC: Urethral strictures. (Editorial.) J Urol 1980;123:506.

Dinneen MD, Duffy PG: Posterior urethral valves. Br J Urol 1996;78:275.

Dowling KJ et al: Ureteropelvic junction obstruction: The effect of pyeloplasty on renal function. J Urol 1988;140:1227.

Emmott RC, Tanagho EA: Ureteral obstruction due to fecal

impaction in patient with colonic loop urinary diversion. Urology 1980;15:496.

Ewalt DH, Bauer SB: Pediatric neurourology. Urol Clin North Am 1996;23:501.

Fourcroy JL, Azoury B, Miller HC: Bilateral ureteral obstruction as a complication of vascular graft surgery. Urology 1980;15:556.

Gillenwater JY et al: Renal function after release of chronic unilateral hydronephrosis in man. Kidney Int 1975;7:179.

Hanna MK, Jeffs RD: Primary obstructive megaureter in children. Urology 1975;6:419.

Hines JE: Symptom indices in bladder outlet obstruction. Br J Urol 1996;77:494.

Hinman F Jr, Oppenheimer RO, Katz IL: Accelerated obstruction at ureteropelvic junction in adults. J Urol 1983; 129:812.

Hollowell JG et al: Coexisting ureteropelvic junction obstruction and vesicoureteral reflux: Diagnostic and therapeutic implications. J Urol 1989;142:490.

Hutch JA, Tanagho EA: Etiology of non-occlusive ureteral dilatation. J Urol 1965;93:177.

Hydronephrosis, renal obstruction, and renography. (Editorial.) Lancet 1987;1:1301.

Jepsen JV, Bruskewitz RC: Comprehensive patient evaluation for benign prostatic hyperplasia. Urology 1998;51 (4A Suppl):13.

Johnston JH et al: Pelvic hydronephrosis in children: A review of 219 personal cases. J Urol 1977;117:97.

Jones DA, Holden D, George NJ: Mechanism of upper tract dilatation in patients with thick walled bladders, chronic retention of urine and associated hydroureteronephrosis. J Urol 1988;140:326.

Jones DA et al: Compliance studies, pressure flow measurements and renal function assessment in patients with upper urinary tract dilatation. J Urol 1987;138:571.

Keating MA et al: Changing concepts in management of primary obstructive megaureter. J Urol 1989;142:636.

Koff SA: Pathophysiology of ureteropelvic junction obstruction: Clinical and experimental observations. Urol Clin North Am 1990;17:263.

Koff SA, Thrall JH, Keyes JW Jr: Diuretic radionuclide methods for investigating hydroureteronephrosis. Eur Urol 1982;8:82.

Lee WJ et al: Treatment of ureteropelvic strictures with percutaneous pyelotomy: Experience in 62 patients. AJR 1988;151:515.

Levin RM et al: Genetic and cellular characteristics of bladder outlet obstruction. Urol Clin North Am 1995;22:263.

Lipitz S et al: Fetal urine analysis for the assessment of renal function in obstructive uropathy. Am J Obstet Gynec 1993;168:174.

Maizels M, Zaontz MR, Firlit CF: Role of in-office ultrasonography in screening infants and children for urinary obstruction. Urol Clin North Am 1990;17:429.

Maizels M et al: Grading nephroureteral dilatation detected in the first year of life: Correlation with obstruction. J Urol 1992;148:609; discussion 615.

Mandell J et al: Prenatal diagnosis of the megacystis-megaureter association. J Urol 1992;148:1487.

McGrath MA, Estroff J, Lebowitz RL: The coexistence of obstruction at the ureteropelvic and ureterovesical junctions. AJR 1987;149:403.

Montagnino B: Posterior urethral valves: Pathophysiology and clinical implications. ANNA J 1994;21:26.

Nguyen HT, Kogan BA: Upper urinary tract obstruction: Experimental and clinical aspects. Br J Urol 1998;81 (Suppl 2):13.

O'Reilly PH: Functional outcome of pyeloplasty for ureteropelvic junction obstruction: Prospective study in 30 consecutive cases. J Urol 1989;142:273.

Perlmutter AD, Kroovand RL, Lai Y-W: Management of ureteropelvic obstruction in first year of life. J Urol 1980;123:535.

Peters CA, Bauer SB: Evaluation and management of urinary incontinence after surgery for posterior urethral valves. Urol Clin North Am 1990;17:379.

Peters CA et al: The response of the fetal kidney to obstruction. J Urol 1992;148:503.

Platt JF et al: Duplex Doppler US of the kidney: Differentiation of obstructive from nonobstructive dilatation. Radiology 1989;171:515.

Reinberg Y, Gonzalez R: Upper urinary tract obstruction in children: Current controversies in diagnosis. Pediatr Clin North Am 1987;34:1291.

Rink RC, Mitchell ME: Physiology of lower urinary tract obstruction. Urol Clin North Am 1990;17:329.

Ross JH, Kay R: Ureteropelvic junction obstruction in anomalous kidneys. Urol Clin North Am 1998;25:219.

Sacks SH et al: Late renal failure due to prostatic outflow obstruction: A preventable disease. Br Med J 1989;298:156.

Sarmina I, Resnick MI: Obstructive uropathy in patients with benign prostatic hyperplasia. J Urol 1989;141:866.

Semelka RC et al: Obstructive nephropathy: Evaluation with dynamic Gd-DTPA-enhanced MR imaging. Radiology 1990;175:797.

Skinner DG, Lieskovsky G, Boyd S: Continent urinary diversion. J Urol 1989;141:1323.

Smart WR: Chapter 55. In: Campbell MF, Harrison JH (editors): Urology, 3rd ed. Saunders, 1970.

Staskin DR: Hydroureteronephrosis after spinal cord injury: Effects of lower urinary tract dysfunction on upper tract anatomy. Urol Clin North Am 1991;18:309.

Styles RA et al: Long-term monitoring of bladder pressure in chronic retention of urine: The relationship between detrusor activity and upper tract dilatation. J Urol 1988; 140:330.

Tanagho EA: Congenitally obstructed bladders: Fate after defunctionalization. J Urol 1974;111:102.

Tanagho EA: The pathogenesis and management of megaureter. In: Johnson JH, Goodwin WF (editors): Excerpta Medica in Paediatric Urology. North Holland, 1974.

Tanagho EA, Meyers FH: Trigonal hypertrophy: A cause of ureteral obstruction. J Urol 1965;93:678.

Tanagho EA, Smith DR, Guthrie TH: Pathophysiology of functional ureteral obstruction. J Urol 1970;104:73.

Walther PC, Parsons CL, Schmidt JD: Direct vision internal urethrotomy in management of urethral strictures. J Urol 1980;123:497.

Wein AJ: Bladder outlet obstruction—an overview. Adv Exp Med Biol 1995;385:3, 75.

Whitaker RH, Buxton-Thomas M: A comparison of pressure flow studies and renography in equivocal upper urinary tract obstruction. J Urol 1984;131:446.

Witherow RO, Whitaker RH: The predictive accuracy of antegrade pressure flow studies in equivocal upper tract obstruction. Br J Urol 1982;53:496.

Vesicoureteral Reflux

13

Emil A. Tanagho, MD

Under normal circumstances, the ureterovesical junction allows urine to enter the bladder but prevents urine from regurgitating into the ureter, particularly at the time of voiding. In this way, the kidney is protected from high pressure in the bladder and from contamination by infected vesical urine. When this valve is incompetent, the chance for development of urinary infection is significantly enhanced, and pyelonephritis is inevitable. With few exceptions, pyelonephritis—acute, chronic, or healed—is secondary to vesicoureteral reflux.

ANATOMY OF THE URETEROVESICAL JUNCTION

An understanding of the causes of vesicoureteral reflux requires a knowledge of the anatomy of the ureterovesical valve. Anatomic studies performed by Hutch (1972) and by Tanagho and Pugh (1963) (Figure 13–1) are incorporated into the following discussion.

Mesodermal Component
The mesodermal component, which arises from the wolffian duct, is made up of 2 parts that are innervated by the sympathetic nervous system:

A. The Ureter and the Superficial Trigone: The smooth musculature of the renal calyces, pelvis, and extravesical ureter is composed of helically oriented fibers that allow for peristaltic activity. As these fibers approach the vesical wall, they are reoriented into the longitudinal plane. The ureter passes obliquely through the vesical wall; the intravesical ureteral segment is thus composed of longitudinal muscle fibers only and therefore cannot undergo peristalsis. As these smooth-muscle fibers approach the ureteral orifice, those that form the roof of the ureter swing to either side to join those that form its floor. They then spread out and join equivalent muscle bundles from the other ureter and also continue caudally, thus forming the superficial trigone. The trigone passes over the neck of the bladder, ending at the verumontanum in the male

and just inside the external urethral orifice in the female. Thus, the ureterotrigonal complex is one structure. Above the ureteral orifice, it is tubular; below that point, it is flat.

B. Waldeyer's Sheath and the Deep Trigone: Beginning at a point about 2–3 cm above the bladder, an external layer of longitudinal smooth muscle surrounds the ureter. This muscular sheath passes through the vesical wall, to which it is connected by a few detrusor fibers. As it enters the vesical lumen, its roof fibers diverge to join its floor fibers, which then spread out, joining muscle bundles from the contralateral ureter and forming the deep trigone, which ends at the bladder neck.

Endodermal Component
The vesical detrusor muscle bundles are intertwined and run in various directions. As they converge on the internal orifice of the bladder, however, they tend to become oriented into 3 layers:

A. Internal Longitudinal Layer: The internal longitudinal layer continues into the urethra submucosally and ends just inside the external meatus in the female and at the caudal end of the prostate in the male.

B. Middle Circular Layer: The middle circular layer is thickest anteriorly and stops at the vesical neck.

C. Outer Longitudinal Layer: The muscle bundles of the outer longitudinal layer take a circular and spiral course about the external surface of the female urethra and are incorporated within the peripheral prostatic tissue in the male. They constitute the true vesicourethral sphincter.

The vesical detrusor muscle is innervated by the parasympathetic nerves (S_2–S_4).

PHYSIOLOGY OF THE URETEROVESICAL JUNCTION

Although many investigators had suspected that normal trigonal tone tended to occlude the intravesi-

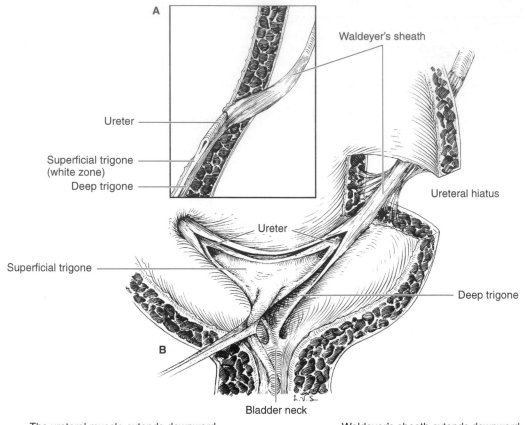

Figure 13–1. Normal ureterotrigonal complex. **A:** Side view of ureterovesical junction. Waldeyer's muscular sheath invests the juxtavesical ureter and continues downward as the deep trigone, which extends to the bladder neck. The ureteral musculature becomes the superficial trigone, which extends to the verumontanum in the male and stops just short of the external meatus in the female. **B:** Waldeyer's sheath is connected by a few fibers to the detrusor muscle in the ureteral hiatus. This muscular sheath, inferior to the ureteral orifices, becomes the deep trigone. The musculature of the ureters continues downward as the superficial trigone. (Redrawn and modified, with permission, from Tanagho EA, Pugh RCB: The anatomy and function of the ureterovesical junction. Br J Urol 1963;35:151.)

cal ureter, it remained for Tanagho et al (1965) to prove it. Using nonrefluxing dogs, they demonstrated the following:

(1) Interruption of the continuity of the trigone resulted in reflux. An incision was made in the trigone 3 mm below the ureteral orifice, resulting in an upward and lateral migration of the ureteral orifice with shortening of the intravesical ureter. Reflux was demonstrable. After the incision healed, reflux ceased.

(2) Unilateral lumbar sympathectomy resulted in paralysis of the ipsilateral trigone. This led to lateral and superior migration of the ureteral orifice and reflux.

(3) Electrical stimulation of the trigone caused the ureteral orifice to move caudally, thus lengthening the intravesical ureter. This maneuver caused a marked rise in resistance to flow through the ureterovesical junction. Ureteral efflux of urine ceased. Intravenous injection of epinephrine caused the same reaction. On the other hand, isoproterenol caused the degree of occlusion to drop below normal. If the trigone was incised, however, electrical stimulation of the trigone or the administration of epinephrine failed to increase ureteral occlusive pressure.

(4) During gradual filling of the bladder, intravesical pressure increased only slightly, whereas pressure within the intravesical ureter rose progressively—owing, apparently, to increasing trigonal stretch. A few seconds before the expected sharp rise in intravesical pressure generated for voiding, the closure pressure in the intravesical ureter rose sharply and was maintained for 20 s after detrusor contraction had ceased. This experiment demonstrated that

ureterovesical competence is independent of detrusor action and is governed by the tone of the trigone, which contracts vigorously just before voiding, thus helping to open and funnel the vesical neck. At the same time, significant pull is placed on the intravesical ureter, so that it is occluded during the period when intravesical pressure is high. During the voiding phase, there is naturally no efflux of ureteral urine.

One may liken this function to the phenomenon of the Chinese thimble: The harder the finger (trigone) pulls, the tighter the thimble (intravesical ureter) becomes. Conversely, a deficient pull may lead to incomplete closure of the ureterovesical junction.

It was concluded from these experiments that normal ureterotrigonal tone prevents vesicoureteral reflux. Electrical or pharmacologic stimulation of the trigone caused increased occlusive pressure in the intravesical ureter and increased resistance to flow down the ureter, whereas incision or paralysis of the trigone led to reflux. The theory that ureterovesical competence was maintained by intravesical pressure compressing the intravesical ureter against its backing of detrusor muscle was thereby disproved.

Biopsy of the trigone (and the intravesical ureter) in patients with primary reflux revealed marked deficiency in the development of its smooth muscle (Figure 13–2). Electrical stimulation of such a trigone caused only a minor contraction of the ureterotrigonal complex. This work led to the conclusion that the common cause of reflux, particularly in children, is congenital attenuation of the ureterotrigonal musculature.

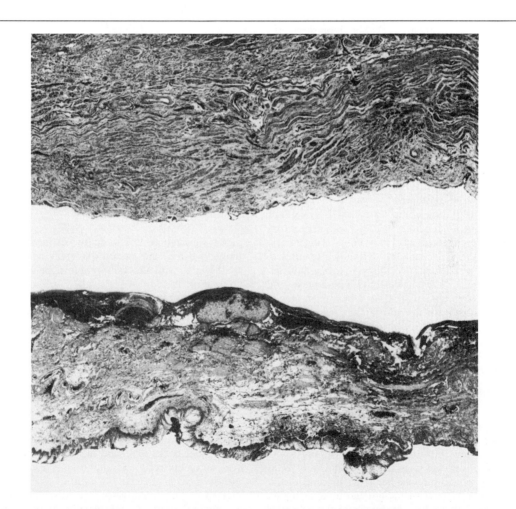

Figure 13–2. Histology of the trigone in primary reflux. **Top:** Normal trigone demonstrating wealth of closely packed smooth-muscle fibers. **Bottom:** The congenitally attenuated trigonal muscle that accompanies vesicoureteral reflux. Note absence of inflammatory cells. (Reproduced, with permission, from Tanagho EA et al: Primary vesicoureteral reflux: Experimental studies of its etiology. J Urol 1965;93:165.)

VESICOURETERAL REFLUX

CAUSES

The major cause of vesicoureteral reflux is attenuation of the trigone and its contiguous intravesical ureteral musculature. Any condition that shortens the intravesical ureter may also lead to reflux, but this is less common. Familial vesicoureteral reflux has been observed by a number of authors. It appears to be a genetic trait.

Congenital Causes

A. Trigonal Weakness (Primary Reflux): Trigonal weakness is by far the most common cause of ureteral reflux. It is most often seen in young girls, though it occurs occasionally also in boys. Reflux in adults—usually women—probably represents the same congenital defect. Weakness of one side of the trigone leads to a decrease in the occlusive pressure in the ipsilateral intravesical ureter. Diffuse ureterotrigonal weakness causes bilateral reflux.

It is postulated that ureteral trigonal weakness is related to the development of the ureteral bud on the mesonephric duct. It is known that the ureter acquires its musculature from its cranial end caudally, so that if a segment is muscularly deficient, it is deficient in its most caudal part. It is also postulated that if the ureter is too close to the urogenital sinus on the mesonephric duct, it will join the latter relatively early in embryonic life, before acquiring adequate mesenchymal tissue around itself to be differentiated later into proper trigonal musculature as well as lower ureter. This embryologic hypothesis explains all the known features of refluxing ureters: their muscular weakness, their lateral placement on the bladder base with a very short submucosal segment, and their usual association with weak ureteral musculature and gaping ureteral orifices (which, in severe cases, ensures a golf-hole endoscopic appearance at their junction with the bladder wall). It also explains why, in duplicated systems, if there is only one refluxing unit, it is the upper orifice (which originated closer to the urogenital sinus on the mesonephric duct and thus has the least muscular development).

In the normal state, the intravesical ureterotrigonal muscle tone exerts a downward pull, whereas the extravesical ureter tends to pull cephalad (Figure 13–3). If trigonal development is deficient, not only is its occlusive power diminished but the ureteral orifice tends to migrate upward toward the ureteral hiatus. The degree of this retraction relates to the degree of incompetence of the junction (Figure 13–4). If the ureteral orifice lies over the ureteral hiatus in the bladder wall (so-called golf-hole orifice), it is com-

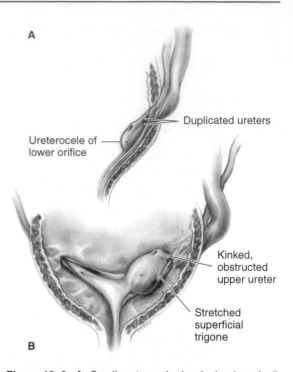

A

Duplicated ureters

Ureterocele of lower orifice

Kinked, obstructed upper ureter

Stretched superficial trigone

B

Figure 13–3. A: Small ureterocele developing in a duplicated system (where it always involves a lower ureteral orifice). **B:** Expansion of submucosal segment leads to lifting and angulation of ipsilateral lower pole ureteral orifice. Duplicated system ureteroceles are rarely so small. (Diagrammatic representation.) (Reproduced, with permission, from Tanagho EA: Ureteroceles: Embryogenesis, pathogenesis and management. J Cont Educ Urol [Feb] 1979;18:13.)

pletely incompetent. The degree of incompetence is judged by the findings on excretory urography and cystography and the cystoscopic appearance of the ureteral orifices.

B. Ureteral Abnormalities:

1. Complete ureteral duplication (Figure 13–5)–The intravesical portion of the ureter to the upper renal segment is usually of normal length, whereas that of the ureter to the lower pole is abnormally short; this orifice is commonly incompetent. However, Stephens (1957) demonstrated that the musculature of the superiorly placed orifice is attenuated, which further contributes to its weakness.

2. Ectopic ureteral orifice–A single ureter or one of a pair may open well down on the trigone, at the vesical neck, or in the urethra. In this instance, vesicoureteral reflux is the rule. This observation makes it clear that the length of the intravesical ureter is not the sole factor in reflux. Such intravesical ureteral segments are usually devoid of smooth muscle. Thus, they have no occlusive force.

3. Ureterocele–A ureterocele involving a single ureter rarely allows reflux, but this lesion usually in-

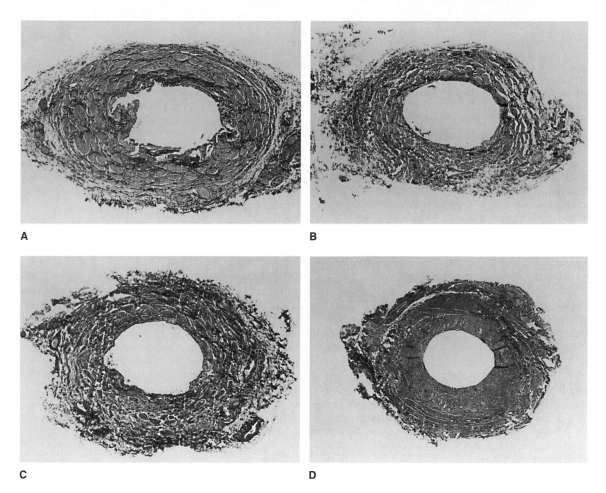

Figure 13–4. Histology of the various grades of submucosal muscular weakness of the ureteral orifice. (See also Figure 13–9.) **A:** Normal. Minimal deficiency. (Cone orifice.) **B:** More marked muscular weakness. (Stadium orifice.) **C:** Marked muscular deficiency. (Horseshoe orifice.) **D:** Extreme muscular deficiency. Only a few muscle fibers can be seen; the rest is collagen tissue.

volves the ureter that drains the upper pole of a duplicated kidney. Because the ureteral orifice is obstructed, the intramural ureter becomes dilated. This increases the diameter of the ureteral hiatus, further shortening the intravesical segment of the other ureter, which therefore may become incompetent. Resection of the ureterocele usually causes its ureter to reflux freely as well.

Vesical Trabeculation

Occasionally, a heavily trabeculated bladder may be associated with reflux. The causes include spastic neurogenic bladder and severe obstruction distal to the bladder. These lesions, however, are associated with trigonal hypertrophy as well; the resultant extra pull on the ureterotrigonal muscle tends to protect the junction from incompetence. In a few such cases,

however, the vesical mucosa may protrude through the ureteral hiatus just above the ureter to form a diverticulum, or saccule (Figure 13–6). The resulting dilatation of the hiatus shortens the intravesical segment; reflux may then occur.

Edema of the Vesical Wall Secondary to Cystitis

As noted previously, valves vary in their degrees of incompetence. A "borderline" junction may not allow reflux when the urine is sterile, but valvular function may be impaired when cystitis causes associated edema involving the trigone and intravesical ureter. In addition, the abnormally high voiding pressure may lead to reflux, in which case secondary pyelonephritis may ensue. After cure of the infection, cystography again reveals no reflux. It is believed

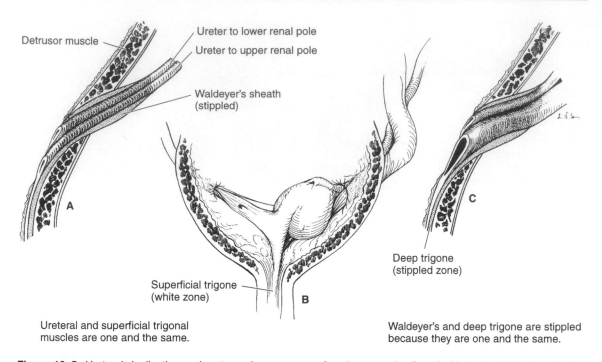

Figure 13–5. Ureteral duplication and ureterocele as causes of vesicoureteral reflux. **A:** Ureteral duplication showing juxtavesical and intravesical ureters encased in common sheath (Waldeyer's). The superior ureter, which always drains the lower renal pole, has a shorter intravesical segment; in addition, it is somewhat devoid of muscle. It therefore tends to allow reflux. **B:** Duplication with ureterocele that always involves caudal ureter, which drains upper renal pole. Pinpoint orifice is obstructive, causing hydroureteronephrosis. Resulting wide dilatation of ureter and ureteral hiatus shortens the intravesical segment of the other ureter, often causing it to reflux. **C:** Resection of ureterocele allows reflux into that ureter.

that a completely normal junction will not decompensate even under these circumstances.

It has been shown that pyelonephritis of pregnancy is associated with vesicoureteral reflux. Many patients give a history of urinary tract infections during childhood. The implication is that they "outgrew" reflux at puberty, but if bacteriuria becomes established during pregnancy, their "borderline" valves may become incompetent. This condition may be aggravated by the hormones of pregnancy, which may contribute to a further loss of tone of the ureterotrigonal complex. After delivery, reflux is usually no longer demonstrable (Hutch and Amar, 1972).

Eagle-Barrett (Prune Belly) Syndrome

The Eagle-Barrett syndrome is a relatively rare condition in which there is failure of normal development of the abdominal muscles and the smooth muscle of the ureters and bladder. Bilateral cryptorchidism is the rule. At times, talipes equinovarus and hip dislocation are also noted. Because the smooth muscle of the ureterotrigonal complex is deficient, reflux is to be expected; advanced hydroureteronephrosis is therefore found.

Iatrogenic Causes

Certain operative procedures may lead to either temporary or permanent ureteral regurgitation.

A. Prostatectomy: With any type of prostatectomy, the continuity of the superficial trigone is interrupted at the vesical neck. If the proximal trigone moves upward, temporary reflux may occur. This mechanism may account for the high fever (and even bacteremia) that is sometimes observed when the catheter is finally removed. Fortunately, in 2–3 weeks the trigone again becomes anchored and reflux ceases.

Preexisting trigonal hypertrophy (due to prostatic obstruction) helps to compensate for the effect of trigonal interruption; thus, reflux may never occur.

B. Wedge Resection of the Posterior Vesical Neck: Wedge resection of the posterior vesical neck, often ill-advised when performed in conjunction with plastic revision of the vesical neck for supposed vesical neck stenosis or dysfunction, may also upset trigonal continuity and allow reflux.

C. Ureteral Meatotomy: Extensive ureteral meatotomy may be followed by reflux. Fortunately, however, limited incision of the roof of the intravesical ureter divides few muscle fibers, since the fibers

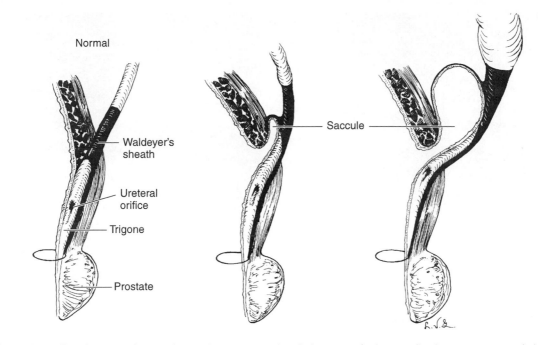

Figure 13–6. Development of ureteral saccule, seen occasionally in cases of primary reflux but more commonly in obstructed or neurogenic bladders with marked trabeculation. Note that the vesical mucosa herniates through the ureteral hiatus, pulling the ureteral orifice upward with it. The orifice may ultimately open in the saccule rather than in the bladder.

have left the roof to join muscle fibers on the floor. Wide resection for treatment of vesical cancer is often followed by ureteral reflux.

D. Resection of Ureterocele: If the ureteral hiatus is widely dilated, this procedure is often followed by reflux.

Contracted Bladder

A bladder that is contracted secondary to interstitial cystitis, tuberculosis, radiotherapy, carcinoma, or schistosomiasis may be associated with ureteral reflux.

COMPLICATIONS

Vesicoureteral reflux damages the kidney through one or both of 2 mechanisms: (1) pyelonephritis and (2) hydroureteronephrosis.

Pyelonephritis

Vesicoureteral reflux is one of the common contributing factors leading to the development of cystitis, particularly in females. When reflux is present, bacteria reach the kidney and the urinary tract cannot empty itself completely, so infection is perpetuated. Pyelonephritis is discussed in more detail in Chapter 14.

Hydroureteronephrosis
(See also Chapter 12)

Dilation of the ureter, renal pelvis, and calyces is usually observed in association with reflux (Figure 13–7), sometimes to an extreme degree (Figure 13–8). In males, because they have a relatively long segment of sterile urethra, such changes are often seen in the absence of infection. Sterile reflux is less damaging than infected reflux.

There are 3 reasons for the dilatation:

(1) Increased work load: The ureter is meant to transport the urine secreted by the kidney to the bladder only once. In the presence of reflux, variable amounts of urine go back and forth, and the work load may be doubled, quadrupled, or increased 10-fold or even more. Eventually, the ureter is not able to transport the increased volume of urine, and stasis and dilatation result.

(2) High hydrostatic pressure: The ureter is protected from the high pressures of the urinary bladder by a competent ureterovesical junction. If there is free reflux, the high intravesical pressure is directly transmitted to the ureteral and pelvic walls, which results in marked stretching and dilation.

(3) Weak ureteral musculature: In reflux, the ureteral wall is invariably deficient in musculature to some degree. The more severe the reflux, the more apparent the muscular deficiency. Some cases show

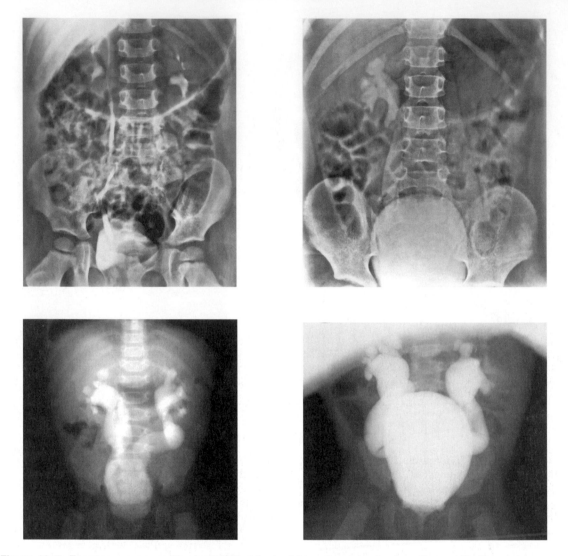

Figure 13–7. Excretory urogram with changes that imply right vesicoureteral reflux. **Upper left:** Excretory urogram showing normal right urogram and a ureter that is mildly dilated and remains full through its entire length. The ureteral change implies reflux. **Upper right:** Cystogram demonstrates the reflux. Note, now, the degree of dilatation of the ureter, pelvis, and calyces. **Lower left:** Excretory urogram shows bilateral hydroureteronephrosis with pyelonephritic scarring. These findings imply the presence of reflux. **Lower right:** Voiding cystourethrogram. Free reflux bilaterally.

more massive dilatation than others. The properly muscularized ureter is better able to resist and compensate for overwork and hydrostatic pressure than the muscularly deficient ureter. The latter tends to undergo further dilatation once it is subjected to any increased intraluminal pressure.

Whether sterile reflux is harmful is the subject of controversy. My colleagues and I believe there is conclusive evidence that severe sterile reflux can lead to parenchymal damage. Pyelointerstitial backflow or pyelotubular backflow under the high pressures of reflux (not infrequently seen during cystographic studies) leads to extravasation of urine in the interstitium

of the kidney. The presence of urine in any interstitium will result in a marked inflammatory response with cellular infiltration, resulting finally in fibrosis and scarring. On a long-term basis, this can lead to parenchymal changes indistinguishable from pyelonephritic scarring caused by inflammation due to bacterial infection. This damage may be termed **reflux nephropathy.** If severe, it will produce parenchymal damage serious enough to lead to end-stage kidney disease.

Ransley's studies (1976) indicate that intrarenal reflux is more likely to occur in the presence of flat, concave, or compound papillae, because their collecting

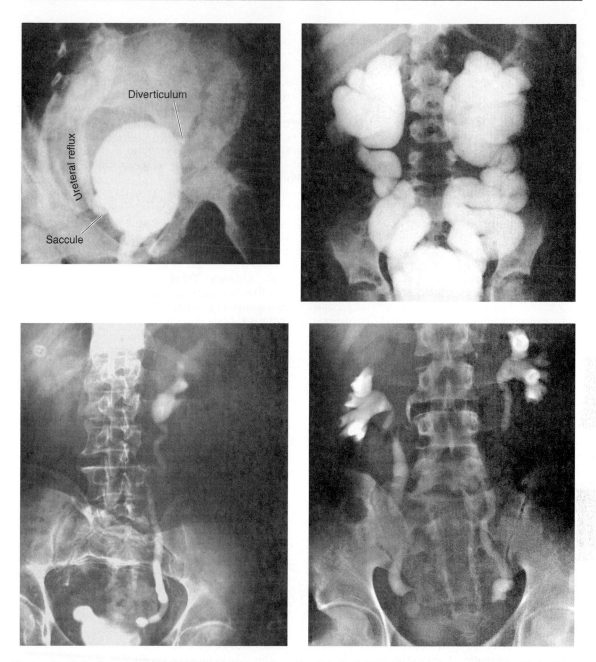

Figure 13–8. Cystograms revealing vesicoureteral reflux. **Upper left:** Saccule at right ureterovesical junction. **Upper right:** Meningomyelocele. Reflux with severe bilateral hydroureteronephrosis; serum creatinine, 0.6 mg/dL; phenolsulfonphthalein excretion, 5% in 1 h. **Lower left:** Post-prostatectomy patient with reflux on left and bilateral saccules. **Lower right:** Ten-year-old boy with meningomyelocele. Bladder has been emptied. Impairment of drainage at ureterovesical junctions is demonstrated. (Courtesy of JA Hutch.)

ducts tend to open with an increase in intrapelvic pressure and reflux. Papillae prone to reflux are more commonly seen in the polar segments of the kidney. Normal papillae might also permit intrarenal reflux if flattened as a result of the changes due to reflux.

Intravesical pressure is transmitted through the incompetent ureteral orifice. This back pressure is quite high at the time of voiding. Furthermore, the ureteropelvic and ureterovesical junctions are less distensible than the rest of the ureter. Either junction may have trouble passing the normal amount of secreted urine plus the refluxed urine; functional obstruction may result. A common cause of ureteropelvic and uretero-vesical "obstruction" is vesicoureteral reflux. Such changes indicate the need for cystography.

INCIDENCE

Vesicoureteral reflux occurs in 50% of children with urinary tract infection but in only 8% of adults with bacteriuria. This discrepancy is explained by the fact that girls usually have pyelonephritis, whereas women usually have cystitis only. Bacteriuria does not always imply pyelonephritis.

The fairly competent (borderline) valve refluxes only during an acute attack of cystitis. Since cystography is performed in such cases only after the infection has been eradicated, the incidence of reflux found on cystography is abnormally low. On the other hand, reflux is demonstrable in 85% of patients whose excretory urograms reveal significant changes typical of healed pyelonephritis.

When infection associated with reflux occurs during the first few weeks of life, many patients are septic and uremic. Most are boys with posterior urethral valves. After age 6 months, the female-male ratio of infection with reflux is 10:1.

CLINICAL FINDINGS

A history compatible with acute pyelonephritis implies the presence of vesicoureteral reflux. This is most commonly seen in females, particularly young girls. Persistence of recurrent "cystitis" should suggest the possibility of reflux. Such patients often have asymptomatic low-grade pyelonephritis.

Symptoms Related to Reflux

A. Symptomatic Pyelonephritis: The usual symptoms in adults are chills and high fever, renal pain, nausea and vomiting, and symptoms of cystitis. In children, only fever, vague abdominal pains, and sometimes diarrhea are apt to occur.

B. Asymptomatic Pyelonephritis: The patient may have no symptoms whatsoever. The incidental findings of pyuria and bacteriuria may be the only clues. This fact points up the need for a screening urinalysis in all children.

C. Symptoms of Cystitis Only: In cases of symptoms of cystitis only, bacteriuria is resistant to antimicrobial drugs, or infection quickly recurs following treatment. These patients may have reflux with asymptomatic chronic pyelonephritis.

D. Renal Pain on Voiding: Surprisingly, renal pain on voiding is a rare complaint in patients with vesicoureteral reflux.

E. Uremia: The last stage of bilateral reflux is uremia due to destruction of the renal parenchyma by hydronephrosis or pyelonephritis (or both). The patient often adjusts to renal insufficiency and may appear quite healthy. Many renal transplants are performed in patients whose kidneys have deteriorated secondarily to reflux and accompanying infection. Early diagnosis, based on careful urinalysis, would have led to the proper diagnosis in childhood. Progressive pyelonephritis is, with few exceptions, preventable.

F. Hypertension: In the later stages of atrophic pyelonephritis, a significant incidence of hypertension is observed.

Symptoms Related to the Underlying Disease

The clinical picture is often dominated by the signs and symptoms of the primary disease.

A. Urinary Tract Obstruction: Young girls may have hesitancy in initiating the urinary stream and an impaired or intermittent stream secondary to spasm of the periurethral striated muscle (see Distal Urethral Stenosis in Chapter 41). In males, the urinary stream may be slow as a result of posterior urethral valves (infants) or prostatic enlargement (men over age 50).

B. Spinal Cord Disease: The patient may have a serious neurogenic disease such as paraplegia, quadriplegia, multiple sclerosis, or meningomyelocele. Symptoms may be limited to those of neurogenic bladder: incontinence of urine, urinary retention or large residual volume, and vesical urgency.

Physical Findings

During an attack of acute pyelonephritis, renal tenderness may be noted. Its absence, however, does not rule out chronic renal infection. Palpation and percussion of the suprapubic area may reveal a distended bladder secondary to obstruction or neurogenic disease. The finding of a hard midline mass deep in the pelvis in a male infant is apt to represent a markedly thickened bladder caused by posterior urethral valves. Examination may reveal a neurologic deficit compatible with a paretic bladder.

Laboratory Findings

The most common complication of reflux, particularly in females, is infection. Bacteriuria without pyuria is not uncommon. In males, the urine may be sterile because of the long, sterile urethra.

The serum creatinine may be elevated in the advanced stage of renal damage, but it may be normal even when the degree of reflux and hydronephrosis is marked (Figure 13–8, upper right).

X-Ray Findings

The plain film may reveal evidence of spina bifida, meningomyelocele, or absence of the sacrum and thus point to a neurologic deficit. Even in vesicoureteral reflux, excretory urograms may be normal, but usually one or more of the following clues to the presence of reflux is noted (Figure 13–7): (1) a persistently dilated lower ureter, (2) areas of dilatation in the ureter, (3) ureter visualized throughout its entire length, (4) presence of hydroureteronephrosis with a narrow juxtavesical ureteral segment, (5) changes of healed pyelonephritis (caliceal clubbing with narrowed infundibula or cortical thinning). A normal intravenous urogram does not rule out reflux.

The presence of ureteral duplication suggests the possibility of reflux into the lower pole of the kidney. In this case, hydronephrosis or changes compatible with pyelonephritic scarring may be seen. Abnormality of the upper segment of a duplicated system can be caused by the presence of an ectopic ureteral orifice with reflux or by obstruction secondary to a ureterocele.

Reflux is diagnosed by demonstration of its existence with one of the following techniques: simple or delayed cystography, voiding cystourethrography, or voiding cinefluoroscopy. Radionuclide scanning can be used: 1 mCi of ^{99m}Tc is instilled into the bladder along with sterile saline solution, and the gamma camera will reveal ureteral reflux (see Chapter 10).

Reflux can be demonstrated by a technique using indigotindisulfonate sodium (indigo carmine), a blue dye. The bladder is filled with sterile water containing 5 mL of indigo carmine per 100 mL, after which the patient voids and the bladder is thoroughly flushed out with sterile water. The ureteral orifices are then viewed cystoscopically for blue-tinged efflux. This technique has the advantage that no ionizing radiation is used, and its efficiency is equal to that of voiding cystourethrography. In general, reflux demonstrable only with voiding implies a more competent valve than does reflux that occurs at low pressures. As has been pointed out, failure to demonstrate reflux on one study does not rule out intermittent reflux.

The voiding phase of the cystogram may reveal changes compatible with distal urethral stenosis with secondary spasm of the voluntary periurethral muscles in girls (Figure 39–1) or changes diagnostic of posterior urethral valves in young boys.

Instrumental Examination

A. Urethral Calibration: In females, urethral calibration using bougies à boule should be done. Distal urethral stenosis is almost routinely found in young girls suffering from urinary infection. Dilation of the ring of stenosis is an important step in improving the hydrodynamics of voiding: lowering intravesical voiding pressure and eliminating the presence of residual vesical urine (see Chapter 41). Less commonly, urethral stenosis is discovered in women and should be treated.

B. Cystoscopy: Most young girls with reflux have smooth-walled or only slightly trabeculated bladders. Chronic cystitis, ureteral duplication, or ureterocele may be evident. An orifice may be ec-

topic and be found at the bladder neck or even in the urethra. As the bladder is filled, a small diverticulum may form on the roof of the ureteral orifice (Figure 13–6). These findings imply the possibility of reflux. The major contribution of cystoscopy is to allow study of the morphologic characteristics of the ureteral orifice and its position in relation to the vesical neck (Figure 13–9).

1. Morphology–The orifice of a normal ureter has the appearance of a volcanic cone. That of a slightly weaker valve looks like a football stadium; an even weaker one has the appearance of a horseshoe with its open end pointing toward the vesical neck. The completely incompetent junction has a golf-hole orifice that lies over the ureteral hiatus.

2. Position–By and large, the more defective the appearance of the ureteral orifice, the farther from the vesical neck it lies. The degree of lateralization of the orifice reflects the degree of ureterotrigonal deficiency.

DIFFERENTIAL DIAGNOSIS

Functional (nonocclusive) vesicoureteral obstruction may cause changes similar to those suggesting the presence of reflux on excretory urography. Multiple cystograms fail to show reflux. Tanagho, Smith, and Guthrie (1970) showed that this congenital obstruction is due to an abundance of circularly oriented smooth-muscle fibers in the ureteral musculature at this point. Its action is sphincteric.

Significant obstruction distal to the vesical neck leads to hypertrophy of both the detrusor and trigonal muscles. The latter exert an exaggerated pull on the intravesical ureter and thus cause functional obstruction (Tanagho and Meyers, 1965). Hydroureteronephrosis is therefore to be expected; vesicoureteral reflux is uncommon.

Other lesions that may cause hydroureteronephrosis without reflux include low ureteral stone, occlusion of the ureter by cervical or prostatic cancer, urinary tract tuberculosis, and schistosomiasis.

TREATMENT

It is impossible to give a concise and definitive discourse on the treatment of vesicoureteral reflux because of the many factors involved and because there is no unanimity of opinion among urologists on this subject. In general, probably more than half of the cases of primary reflux that occur in children can be controlled by nonsurgical means; the rest require some form of operative procedure. Adults with reflux usually require vesicoureteroplasty.

Medical Treatment

A. Indications: A child with primary reflux (at-

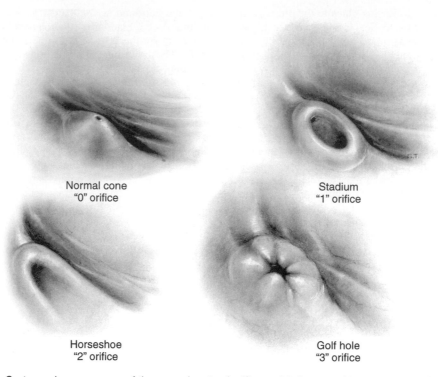

Normal cone
"0" orifice

Stadium
"1" orifice

Horseshoe
"2" orifice

Golf hole
"3" orifice

Figure 13–9. Cystoscopic appearance of the normal ureteral orifice and 3 degrees of incompetence of the ureterovesical junction. (See also Figure 13–4.) (Reproduced, with permission, from Lyon RP, Marshall SK, Tanagho EA: The ureteral orifice: Its configuration and competency. J Urol 1969;102:504.)

tenuated trigone) who has fairly normal upper tracts on urographic study and whose ureterovesical valves appear fair to good on cystoscopy has an excellent chance of "outgrowing" the defect, particularly if cystograms show only transient or "high-pressure" reflux. A boy with posterior urethral valves may cease to have reflux once these valves are destroyed.

In a woman who occasionally develops acute pyelonephritis following intercourse but whose urine quickly clears on antimicrobial therapy, reflux will probably be controlled if she takes steps to prevent vesical infections (see Acute Cystitis, **p 252**). This is particularly true if reflux cannot be demonstrated cystographically when her urine is sterile. The maintenance of sterile urine allows her "borderline" valve to remain competent.

B. Methods of Treatment: Dilation of the ring of distal urethral stenosis in young girls or of posterior urethral valves in boys usually gives excellent results, reducing intravesical voiding pressure and abolishing vesical residual urine and reflux.

Urinary infection should be definitively treated with antimicrobial drugs, after which chronic suppressive therapy should be continued for 6 months or more.

Triple voiding is the least effective method of treating reflux. Since vesicoureteral reflux prevents the urinary tract from emptying itself completely, thus destroying the vesical defense mechanism, triple voiding once a day is helpful if the child is old enough to be trained. When reflux is present, the bladder empties itself on voiding, but some urine ascends to the kidneys and then returns to the bladder. Voiding again a few minutes later pushes less urine into the ureters. A third voiding usually completely empties the urinary tract. This allows the patient's own natural resistance to operate to a maximum degree.

Children with reflux often have thin-walled bladders and do not perceive the normal urge to void when the bladder is full. Further detrusor tone is lost with overfilling, increasing the likelihood of residual urine. Such children should "void by the clock" every 3–4 h whether they have the urge or not. Vesical residual urine may then be minimized.

Infant girls with markedly dilated upper urinary tracts may be tided over by means of an indwelling urethral catheter. Over a period of months, ureteral dilatation and elongation may regress; renal function is protected. At a convenient and strategic time, more definitive therapy can be accomplished.

C. Evaluation of Success of Medical Treatment: Urinalysis should be done at least once a month for a year or more. Maintenance of sterile urine is an encouraging sign. Cystograms should be repeated every 4–6 months. Excretory urography or nuclear renal scan should be performed at 6 and 12 months to be sure that renal deterioration does not occur. About half of children with reflux are cured by medical treatment.

Surgical Treatment

A. Indications: Reflux caused by the following abnormalities will not disappear spontaneously: (1) ectopic ureteral orifice, (2) ureteral duplication, (3) ureterocele associated with ureteral duplication and reflux into the uninvolved ureter, (4) golf-hole ureteral orifice, and (5) low-pressure reflux with significant hydroureteronephrosis.

Surgery is indicated (1) if it is not possible to keep the urine sterile and reflux persists; (2) if acute pyelonephritis recurs despite a strict medical regimen and chronic suppressive antimicrobial therapy; or (3) if increased renal damage is demonstrated by serial excretory urograms.

B. Types of Surgical Treatment: In cases of markedly impaired kidney function and massively dilated ureters, preliminary urinary diversion may be required to improve renal function and to allow dilated ureters to regain tone, after which definitive relief of obstruction (eg, posterior urethral valves) and ureterovesicoplasty can be performed at the optimum time. Some patients with irreversible lesions causing reflux (eg, meningomyelocele) or badly damaged and atonic ureters may require permanent diversion of the urine (ie, ureteroileocutaneous anastomosis).

1. Temporary urinary diversion–If refluxed urine drains freely into the bladder, cystostomy (or an indwelling urethral catheter in girls) may prove helpful. If the ureters are dilated and kinked, a low redundant loop can be brought to the skin. The ureter is opened at this point and urine collected into an ileostomy bag. Later, the loop and the section of ureter distal to it can be resected and the ureter proximal to the loop reimplanted into the bladder. Nephrostomy may be necessary if there is no ureteral redundancy.

2. Permanent urinary diversion–If it is felt that successful ureterovesicoplasty cannot be accomplished, a Bricker type of diversion is indicated. If renal function is poor and the ureters are widely dilated and atonic, ureterocutaneous diversion may be the procedure of choice.

3. Other surgical procedures–

a. If reflux is unilateral, with the affected kidney badly damaged and the other kidney normal, nephrectomy is indicated.

b. If one renal pole of a duplicated system is essentially functionless, heminephrectomy with removal of its entire ureter should be done. If there is moderate hydronephrosis of one renal pole with duplication, an alternative is anastomosis of the dilated ureter or

pelvis to the normal ureter or pelvis. The remainder of the dilated refluxing ureter should be removed.

c. In unilateral reflux, anastomosis of the lower end of the refluxing ureter into the side of its normal mate (transureteroureterostomy) has a few proponents.

4. Definitive repair of ureterovesical junction (ureterovesicoplasty)–

a. Principles of repair (Tanagho, 1970)–

1. Resect the lower 2–3 cm of the ureter in which the muscle is underdeveloped.

2. Free up enough extravesical ureter so that an intravesical segment 2.5 cm long can be formed.

3. Place the intravesical ureter in a submucosal position.

4. Suture the wall of the new ureteral orifice to the cut edge of the trigonal muscle.

b. Types of operation–The following procedures satisfy the preceding principles and have been successful in a high percentage of cases: suprahiatal repair, increasing the length of intravesical ureter above the level of the ureteral hiatus (Paquin, 1959; Politano and Leadbetter, 1958); infrahiatal repair, the advancement procedures of Hutch (1963) and Glenn and Anderson (1967); combined supra- and infrahiatal repair, which is the most attractive; and transtrigonal repair (Cohen, 1975).

If the ureters are unduly tortuous, the redundant portions must be resected. If they are widely dilated, the lower ends must be tailored to a more normal size.

c. Results of ureterovesicoplasty–About 93% of patients no longer show reflux after ureterovesicoplasty. About 3% develop ureterovesical stenosis that requires reoperation. At least 75% have and maintain sterile urine without antimicrobial drugs 3–6 months after surgery. Many patients in whom bacteriuria persists have cystitis only. This has been demonstrated by the finding that renal urine specimens collected by ureteral catheters are sterile. Febrile attacks cease. Considering that only the most severe and advanced cases are submitted to surgical repair, these are impressive results, and they exceed by far the cure rates reported when only antimicrobial drugs are used (10–15%). This operation is rightly considered one of the most significant accomplishments of modern urology.

PROGNOSIS

In patients with reflux who are judged to have fairly competent valves, conservative therapy as outlined previously is highly successful in the cure of the reflux and therefore of infection.

Patients with very incompetent ureterovesical valves subjected to surgical repair also have an excellent prognosis. A few children, however, have such badly damaged urinary tracts when finally submitted to diagnostic procedures that little help other than permanent urinary diversion can be offered.

REFERENCES

Ahmed S, Boucaut HA: Vesicoureteral reflux in complete ureteral duplication: Surgical options. J Urol 1988;140:1092.

Alon U, Berant M, Pery M: Intravenous pyelography in children with urinary tract infection and vesicoureteral reflux. Pediatrics 1989;83:332.

Ambrose SS et al: Observations on small kidney associated with vesicoureteral reflux. J Urol 1980;123:349.

Arap S, Abrao EG, Menezes de Goes G: Treatment and prevention of complications after extravesical antireflux technique. Eur Urol 1981;7:263.

Arap S et al: The extra-vesical antireflux plasty: Statistical analysis. Urol Int 1971;26:241.

Askari A, Belman AB: Vesicoureteral reflux in black girls. J Urol 1982;127:747.

Atwell JD, Allen NH: The interrelationship between pararauretric diverticula, vesicoureteric reflux and duplication of the pelvicaliceal collecting system: A family study. Br J Urol 1980;52:269.

Atwell JD, Cox PA: Growth of the kidney following unilateral antireflux surgery. Eur Urol 1981;7:257.

Bailey RR, Rolleston GL: Vesicoureteric reflux and reflux nephropathy: The Christchurch contribution. N Z Med J 1997;110:266.

Bakshandeh K, Lynne C, Carrion H: Vesicoureteral reflux and end stage renal disease. J Urol 1976;116:557.

Bauer SB, Colodny AH, Retik AB: The management of vesicoureteral reflux in children with myelodysplasia. J Urol 1982;128:102.

Belman AB: Vesicoureteral reflux. Pediatr Clin North Am 1997;44:1171.

Ben-Ami T et al: Vesicoureteral reflux in boys: Review of 196 cases. Radiology 1989;183:681.

Birmingham Reflux Study Group. Operative versus nonoperative treatment of severe vesicoureteric reflux in children: Five years' observation. Br Med J Clin Res 1987;295:237.

Bisset GS III, Strife JL, Dunbar JS: Urography and voiding cystourethrography: Findings in girls with urinary tract infection. AJR 1987;148:479.

Bjorgvinsson E, Jajd M, Eggli KD: Diagnosis of acute pyelonephritis in children: Comparison of sonography and 99mTc-DMSA scintigraphy. AJR 1991;157:539.

Blake NS, O'Connell E: Endoscopic correction of vesicoureteric reflux by subureteric Teflon injection: Follow-up ultrasound and voiding cystography. Br J Radiol 1989;62:443.

Bomalaski MD, Hirschl RB, Bloom DA: Vesicoureteral reflux and ureteropelvic junction obstruction: Association, treatment options and outcome. J Urol 1997; 157:969.

Bourne HH et al: Intrarenal reflux and renal damage. J Urol 1976;115:304.

Casale AJ: Early ureteral surgery for posterior urethral valves. Urol Clin North Am 1990;17:361.

Chisholm GD et al: DMSA scan and the prediction of recovery in obstructive uropathy. Eur Urol 1982;8: 227.

Cohen SJ: Ureterocystoneostomie: Eine neue antireflux Technik. [Ureterocystoneostomy: A new technique for reflux prevention.] Aktuelle Urologie 1975;6:1.

DeKlerk DP, Reiner WG, Jeffs RD: Vesicoureteral reflux and ureteropelvic junction obstruction: Late oc-

currence of ureteropelvic obstruction after successful ureteroneocystostomy. J Urol 1979;121:816.

Devriendt K et al: Vesico-ureteral reflux: A genetic condition? Eur J Pediatr 1998;157:265.

Duckett JW, Bellinger MF: A plea for standardized grading of vesicoureteral reflux. Eur Urol 1982;8:74.

Duckett JW Jr: Ureterovesical junction and acquired vesicoureteral reflux. J Urol 1982;127:249.

Elo J et al: Character of urinary tract infections and pyelonephritic renal scarring after antireflux surgery. J Urol 1982;129:343.

Garin EH, Campos A, Homsy Y: Primary vesicoureteral reflux: Review of current concepts. Pediatr Nephrol 1998;12:249.

Glenn JF, Anderson EE: Distal tunnel ureteral reimplantation. J Urol 1967;97:623.

Griffiths DJ, Scholtmeijer RJ: Vesicoureteral reflux and lower urinary tract dysfunction: Evidence for 2 different reflux/dysfunction complexes. J Urol 1987;137: 240.

Hawtry CE et al: Ureterovesical reflux in an adolescent and adult population. J Urol 1983;130:1067.

Hellström M et al: Voiding cystourethrography as a predictor of reflux nephropathy in children with urinary-tract infection. AJR 1989;152:801.

Hendren WH: Complications of megaureter repair in children. J Urol 1975;113:228.

Hendren WH: Reoperation for the failed ureteral reimplantation. J Urol 1974;111:403.

Holland NH et al: Relation of urinary tract infection and vesicoureteral reflux to scars: Follow-up of thirty-eight patients. J Pediatr 1990;116:S65.

Huland H et al: Vesicoureteral reflux in end stage renal disease. J Urol 1979;121:10.

Hutch JA: The mesodermal component: Its embryology, anatomy, physiology and role in prevention of vesicoureteral reflux. J Urol 1972;108:406.

Hutch JA: Ureteric advancement operation: Anatomy, technique, and early results. J Urol 1963;89:180.

Hutch JA, Amar AD: *Vesicoureteral Reflux and Pyelonephritis.* Appleton-Century-Crofts, 1972.

Jequier S, Jequier JC: Reliability of voiding cystourethrography to detect reflux. AJR 1989;153:807.

Jodal U et al: Infection pattern in children with vesicoureteral reflux randomly allocated to operation or long-term antibacterial prophylaxis: The International Reflux Study in Children. J Urol 1992;148:1650.

Johnston JH: Vesicoureteric reflux with urethral valves. Br J Urol 1979;51:100.

Kallen RJ: Paleonephrology and reflux nephropathy: From the "big bang" to end-stage renal disease. Am J Dis Child 1991;145:860.

Koff SA: Relationship between dysfunctional voiding and reflux. J Urol 1992;148:1703.

Koff SA, Murtagh DS: The uninhibited bladder in children: Effect of treatment of recurrence of urinary infection and on vesicoureteral reflux resolution. J Urol 1983;130:1138.

Leadbetter GW Jr: Skin ureterostomy with subsequent ureteral reconstruction. J Urol 1972;107:462.

Lenaghan D et al: The natural history of reflux and long-term effects of reflux on the kidney. J Urol 1976;115: 728.

Lerner GR, Fleischmann LE, Perlmutter AD: Reflux nephropathy. Pediatr Clin North Am 1987;34:747.

Lewy PR, Belman AB: Familial occurrence of nonobstructive, noninfectious vesicoureteral reflux with renal scarring. J Pediatr 1975;86:851.

Lyon RP: Treatment of vesicoureteral reflux: Point system based on 20 years of experience. Urology 1980; 16:38.

Lyon RP, Marshall SK, Scott MP: Treatment of vesicoureteral reflux: Point system based on 20 years of experience. Trans Am Assoc Genitourin Surg 1979; 71:146.

Lyon RP, Marshall SK, Tanagho EA: The ureteral orifice: Its configuration and competency. J Urol 1969; 102:504.

Malek RS et al: Vesicoureteral reflux in the adult. 3. Surgical correction: Risks and benefits. J Urol 1983; 130:882.

Mulcahy JJ, Kelalis PP: Non-operative treatment of vesicoureteral reflux. J Urol 1978;120:336.

Mundy AR et al: Improvement in renal function following ureteric reimplantation for vesicoureteric reflux. Br J Urol 1982;53:542.

Noe HN et al: The transmission of vesicouretal reflux from parent to child. J Urol 1992;148:1869.

O'Donnell B: Management of urinary tract infection and vesicoureteric reflux in children. 2. The case for surgery. Br Med J 1990;300:1393.

Paltiel HJ, Lebowitz RL: Neonatal hydronephrosis due to primary vesicoureteral reflux: Trends in diagnosis and treatment. Radiology 1989;170:787.

Paquin AJ Jr: Ureterovesical anastomosis: The description and evaluation of a technique. J Urol 1959;82: 573.

Parrott TS, Woodard JR: Reflux in opposite ureter after successful correction of unilateral vesicoureteral reflux. Urology 1976;7:276.

Politano VA, Leadbetter WF: An operative technique for correction of vesicoureteral reflux. J Urol 1958; 79:932.

Ransley PG: The renal papilla and intrarenal reflux. In: Williams PI, Chisholm GD (editors): *Scientific Foundations of Urology.* Year Book, 1976.

Ransley PG: Vesicoureteral reflux: Continuous surgical dilemma. Urology 1978;12:246.

Roberts JA: Experimental pyelonephritis in the monkey. 4. Vesicoureteral reflux and bacteria. Invest Urol 1976;14:198.

Rolleston GL, Maling TMJ, Hodson CJ: Intrarenal reflux and the scarred kidney. Arch Dis Child 1974;49:531.

Rose JS, Glassberg KI, Waterhouse K: Intrarenal reflux and its relationship to renal scarring. J Urol 1975; 113;400.

Salvatierra O Jr, Kountz SL, Belzer FO: Primary vesicoureteral reflux and end-stage renal disease. JAMA 1973;226:1454.

Salvatierra O Jr, Tanagho EA: Reflux as a cause of end stage kidney disease: Report of 32 cases. J Urol 1977; 117:441.

Savage JM et al: Five year prospective study of plasma renin activity and blood pressure in patients with long-standing reflux nephropathy. Arch Dis Child 1987;62:678.

Seruca H: Vesicoureteral reflux and voiding dysfunction: A prospective study. J Urol 1989;142:494.

Shimada K et al: Renal growth and progression of reflux nephropathy in children with vesicoureteral reflux. J Urol 1988;140:1097.

Skoog SJ, Belman AB, Majd M: A nonsurgical approach to the management of primary vesicoureteral reflux. J Urol 1987;138:941.

Smith JW: Prognosis in pyelonephritis: Promise or progress? Am J Med Sci 1989;297:53.

Soulen MC, Fishman EK, Goldman SM: Sequelae of acute renal infections: CT evaluation. Radiology 1989;173:423.

Stephens FD: Treatment of megaloureters by multiple micturition. Aust N Z J Surg 1957;27:130.

Stickler GB et al: Primary interstitial nephritis with reflux: A cause of hypertension. Am J Dis Child 1971; 122:144.

Strand WR, Sesterhenn I, Rushton HG: Role of superoxide dismutase in the pathogenesis of pyelonephritis: Immunological localization of superoxide dismutase in human renal tissues. J Urol 1989;142:616.

Sty JR et al: Imaging in acute renal infection in children. AJR 1987;148:471.

Tanagho EA: The pathogenesis and management of megaureter. In: Johnston JH, Goodwin WE (editors): *Reviews in Paediatric Urology.* North Holland, 1974.

Tanagho EA: Surgical revision of the incompetent ureterovesical junction: A critical analysis of techniques and requirements. Br J Urol 1970;42:410.

Tanagho EA: Ureteral tailoring. J Urol 1971;106:194.

Tanagho EA, Guthrie TH, Lyon RP: The intravesical ureter in primary reflux. J Urol 1969;101:824.

Tanagho EA, Jonas U: Reduced bladder capacity: Cause of ureterovesical reflux. Urology 1974;4:421.

Tanagho EA, Meyers FH: Trigonal hypertrophy: A cause of ureteral obstruction. J Urol 1965;93:678.

Tanagho EA, Pugh RCB: The anatomy and function of the ureterovesical junction. Br J Urol 1963;35:151.

Tanagho EA, Smith DR, Guthrie TH: Pathophysiology of functional ureteral obstruction. J Urol 1970;104:73.

Tanagho EA et al: Primary vesicoureteral reflux: Experimental studies of its etiology. J Urol 1965;93:165.

Van den Abbeele AD et al: Vesicoureteral reflux in asymptomatic siblings of patients with known reflux: Radionuclide cystography. Pediatrics 1987;79:147.

Verber IG, Strudley MR, Meller ST: 99mTc dimercaptosuccinic acid (DMSA) scan as first investigation of urinary tract infection. Arch Dis Child 1988;63:1320.

Wacksman J, Anderson EE, Glenn JF: Management of vesicoureteral reflux. J Urol 1978;119:814.

Walker RD: Renal functional changes associated with vesicoureteral reflux. Urol Clin North Am 1990;17: 307.

Walker RD III et al: Renal growth and scarring in kidneys with reflux and concentrating defect. J Urol 1983;129:784.

Warren JW, Muncie HL Jr, Hall-Craggs M: Acute pyelonephritis associated with bacteriuria during long-term catheterization: A prospective clinicopathological study. J Infect Dis 1988;158:1341.

Weiss RA: Update on childhood urinary tract infections and reflux. Semin Nephrol 1998;18:264.

Weiss RM, Biancani P: Characteristics of normal and refluxing ureterovesical junctions. J Urol 1983;129:858.

Whitaker RH: Reflux induced pelvi-ureteric obstruction. Br J Urol 1976;48:555.

Whitaker RH, Flower CDR: Ureters that show both reflux and obstruction. Br J Urol 1979;51:471.

White RH: Management of urinary tract infection and vesicoureteric reflux in children. 1. Operative treatment has no advantage over medical management. Br Med J 1990;300:1391.

White RH: Vesicoureteric reflux and renal scarring. Arch Dis Child 1989;64:407.

Williams DI: The natural history of reflux. Urol Int 1971;26:350.

Woodard JR, Rushton HG: Reflux uropathy. Pediatr Clin North Am 1987;34:1349.

Woodard JR, Zucker I: Current management of the dilated urinary tract in prune belly syndrome. Urol Clin North Am 1990;17:407.

Zel G, Retik AB: Familial vesicoureteral reflux. Urology 1973;2:249.

Bacterial Infections of the Genitourinary Tract

14

Simon N. McRae, MD, & Linda M. Dairiki Shortliffe, MD

Urinary tract infections (UTIs) caused by pathogenic bacteria are a significant source of morbidity and mortality in modern medicine, despite the widespread use of antibiotics. Although most cases are susceptible to a variety of antibiotic agents and respond quickly to short-term therapy, fulminant infections with resistant organisms are difficult to treat and require a multimodal therapeutic approach. Even then, they yield a significant mortality rate.

Progress in the management of bacterial UTIs has come about with the development of new antibiotic agents that have excellent activity against the usual uropathogens while simultaneously having fewer adverse effects on the patients. In many cases, oral forms of these antibiotics have made it possible to treat some infections on an outpatient basis that previously had required parenteral therapy. Better understanding of the pathogenesis of UTIs has also led to better patient management, particularly in allowing the physician to tailor therapy to specific infectious processes and thereby reduce adverse therapeutic outcomes.

Fortunately, the organisms responsible for UTIs are still quite predictable. Most UTIs are caused by aerobic gram-negative rods, especially *Escherichia coli*. Certain gram-positive cocci (eg, enterococci) also cause UTIs with some frequency. Some organisms that require special techniques of identification can also become infectious, especially in the lower genitourinary tract (eg, *Chlamydia trachomatis, Ureaplasma urealyticum, Gardnerella vaginalis*). Gram-positive rods and anaerobic bacteria are rarely implicated in UTIs. Table 14–1 gives a complete list of microorganisms that can cause genitourinary infections.

CLASSIFICATION

Urinary tract infections can be classified according to their natural history. In general, they can be thought of as either first infections or recurrent infections. The term chronic should not be applied to most UTIs, mainly because the duration of infection is in-

correctly reflected by the term. Stamey (1980) subclassified recurrent infections into 3 types: unresolved bacteriuria, bacterial persistence, and reinfection.

First infection typically refers to infection in a nonhospitalized patient without structural or functional abnormalities of the urinary tract. These infections can also be considered isolated infections if they are separated from other infections by at least 6 months. Young and middle-aged women commonly get this type of infection. As many as 30% of all women in their 30s will have a first or isolated infection.

Unresolved bacteriuria implies inadequate therapy of a diagnosed UTI. Cultures taken during treatment will differentiate these infections from the other types of recurrence, namely, persistence and reinfection; the culture shows that the original infecting pathogen has not been eradicated by therapy. The most common cause of unresolved bacteriuria is antibiotic resistance to the selected agent. Antibiotic resistance is more prevalent in patients who have undergone recent antibiotic therapy, especially with penicillins or sulfonamides, which commonly produce resistance in fecal bacteria. Unresolved bacteriuria may also be due to azotemia and papillary necrosis, in which adequate levels of antibiotic in the urine are not achieved. Occasionally, giant staghorn calculi can present a mass of bacterial growth that is too great for bacterial inhibition, leading to unresolved bacteriuria.

When sterilization of the urine has been documented, an organism may cause recurrence of infection if it is sequestered from adequate concentrations of antibiotic. In this case, the bacteria are considered to be persistent. Abnormalities that may underlie bacterial persistence are listed in Table 14–2.

Reinfection is the most common cause of recurrent infections. Reinfection implies a new infection with new pathogens, typically via the fecal-perineal-urethral route, after a variable period of sterility from a previous infection. Biologic susceptibility factors probably play a significant role in the predisposition

Table 14–1. Bacteria causing genitourinary tract infections.

Gram-positive cocci	Gram-negative rods	Other pathogens
Staphylococcus aureus	Citrobacter	Chlamydiae (Chlamydia trachomatis)
Staphylococcus epidermidis	Escherichia coli	Myocoplasmas (Ureaplasma urealyticum)
Staphylococcus saprophyticus	Enterobacter sp.	
Streptococcus, group D	Gardnerella vaginalis	
Streptococcus faecalis	Klebsiella sp.	
Streptococcus bovis	Morganella morganii	
Streptococcus, group B	Proteus sp. (P mirabilis)	
	Providencia stuartii	
Gram-negative cocci	Pseudomonas aeruginosa	
Neisseria gonorrhoeae	Serratia sp.	

to reinfections, and their identification may help improve management.

Generally, bacterial persistence is differentiated from bacterial reinfection by identification of the infecting organisms. With bacterial persistence, the same bacterial species are usually isolated. With reinfection, periodic infections can be caused by a variety of bacteria.

PATHOGENESIS OF URINARY TRACT INFECTIONS

Bacterial pathogenesis in the urinary tract depends on a number of factors, chief of which are the virulence characteristics of the bacteria themselves and the host's ability to protect itself against infection. The interplay between these 2 forces determines not only the pathogenic potential but also the potential to cause renal damage.

There are 4 possible modes of bacterial entry into the urinary tract:

(1) Ascending infection from the urethra is clearly the most prevalent cause of UTIs in both men and women. In women, because of a shortened urethra and a tendency for rectal bacteria to colonize the perineum and vaginal vestibule, susceptibility to ascending infection is higher. This may explain why sexual intercourse is a major precipitating factor of UTI in women (Nicolle et al, 1982). The antibacterial properties of prostatic secretions may offer men additional protection from this mode of entry.

(2) Hematogenous spread of infection into the urinary tract is much less common in adults but may be important in neonates. Tuberculosis spreads in this way, as do the bacteria (primarily staphylococcal) that sometimes produce renal and perirenal abscesses.

(3) Lymphatogenous spread is probably very rare. Indeed, whether bacteria can actually travel through rectal and colonic lymphatics to infect the urinary tract has not been clearly established, and there is little evidence that lymphatic routes play any role in most UTIs.

(4) Direct extension of infection from neighboring organs may occur in certain circumstances. Intraperitoneal abscesses, especially those associated with inflammatory bowel disease and severe pelvic inflammatory disease, may cause infection through this route. Additionally, extension of bacteria through vesicointestinal and vesicovaginal fistulas can lead to UTI.

Table 14–2. Correctable urologic abnormalities that cause bacterial persistence.

Infection stones
Chronic bacterial prostatitis
Unilateral infected atrophic kidneys
Ureteral duplication and ectopic ureters
Foreign bodies
Urethral diverticula
Unilateral medullary sponge kidneys
Infected ureteral stumps following nephrectomy
Infected urachal cysts
Infected communicating renal calyceal cysts
Papillary necrosis
Paravesical abscess with fistula to bladder

Bacterial Virulence Factors

About 90% of simple UTIs are caused by *E coli*. The ability of a few of the more than 150 strains of *E coli* to colonize the perineum and urethra and migrate into the urinary tract relies on certain virulence properties found in those strains (mostly O1, O2, O4, O6, O18, and O75) that enable them to adhere to epithelium and urothelium. Other virulence properties allow for progression of infection in situ, including the ability to resist bactericidal activity and the ability to produce hemolysin.

Bacterial adherence to vaginal and urothelial cells is mediated by bacterial fimbriae or pili. These are long, proteinaceous, hairlike appendages that extend off the bacterial cell surface. Adherence of the bacterium to a cell is dependent on the interaction between the pili and certain sugar sequences in the form of glycolipids or glycoproteins found on the host cell surface.

Pili are classified according to their ability to cause hemagglutination and the ability of certain sugars to block this process. Type 1 pili agglutinate guinea pig erythrocytes. Because this agglutination is inhibited by the sugar D-mannose, strains with this type are said to exhibit mannose-sensitive hemagglutination. P pili agglutinate human (not guinea pig) erythrocytes in a fashion not inhibited by D-mannose. Strains with this type exhibit mannose-resistant hemagglutination. P pili bind specifically to glycolipid receptors on uroepithelium that are also found on P-blood group antigens. These glycolipid receptors can be found on renal tubular cells as well as on uroepithelium.

The importance of bacterial adherence in determining the severity of infection has been demonstrated. Kallenius et al (1981) studied 97 children with UTI and compared them with 82 control subjects. They found that P pili were expressed by 91% of E coli strains causing pyelonephritis, 19% of strains causing cystitis, 14% of strains causing asymptomatic bacteriuria, and only 7% of fecal E coli isolates from healthy control subjects. Similar findings have been reported in adult women with acute nonobstructive pyelonephritis (Jacobson et al, 1985). The association of P piliated E coli and pyelonephritis may not be as strong in patients with abnormal urinary tracts, however. Girls with gross vesicoureteral reflux (VUR) had recurrent infections that were minimally associated with strains of E coli expressing P pili (Lomberg et al, 1983).

Most E coli isolates causing UTI possess both type 1 pili and P pili. However, phase variation may occur during UTI (Schaeffer, 1997). Phase variation refers to the phenomenon wherein bacteria can alternate between piliated and nonpiliated forms depending on their microenvironment. Indeed, the presence or absence of pili has biologic implications for the infectivity of bacteria. Although type 1 pili may be advantageous to the bacteria for adhering to bladder mucosa, and P pili may be advantageous for attachment to upper tract epithelial surfaces, both may be detrimental when bacteria come into contact with the neutrophils, as they could facilitate phagocytosis.

Host Susceptibility Factors

An important factor in the establishment of ascending infection in women is the receptivity of vaginal epithelial cells to bacterial colonization. Several studies have shown that infectious strains of E coli adhere more readily in vitro to vaginal epithelial cells from women with recurrent UTIs than to cells from healthy control subjects (Fowler and Stamey, 1977; Schaeffer, Jones, and Dunn, 1981).

Susceptible women may have increased adherence of E coli to their epithelial cells for 2 reasons. They may simply have more binding sites for bacterial ad-

hesins, in the form of glycolipid or glycoprotein receptors, on their cell surfaces. Or possibly, they may be what are called nonsecretors. The mucosal secretion of soluble compounds that can bind to the same receptors that bind bacterial adhesins may provide competitive inhibition of bacterial adherence and colonization. Women who lack this secretion, then, would be less able to inhibit the attachment of pathogenic E coli to their vaginal epithelium. Blood group antigens may constitute the soluble compounds responsible for decreasing the availability of receptor sites for bacterial adherence. Sheinfeld et al (1989) determined that Lewis antigens within the blood group phenotype differed between susceptible women and control subjects. Lewis antigens act as fucosyltransferases and may affect the ability of certain oligosaccharides on the cell surface to "cover up" bacterial adhesin receptor sites (Navas et al, 1993).

The normal flora of the periurethral area forms a defense against the colonization of pathogenic bacteria. Alterations in this environment, resulting from shifts in local pH or estrogen levels or the use of antimicrobial agents, may alter the makeup of the protective flora and also the ability of pathogenic bacteria to colonize. Not much else is known about urethral defense mechanisms, although bacterial adherence, periurethral gland secretions, and urine flow all probably play an important role.

In males, the prostate plays an important role in antimicrobial defense. Zinc has been identified as a component of prostatic fluid that carries potent bactericidal properties (Fair, Couch, and Wehner, 1976). Men with chronic bacterial prostatitis exhibit absent or reduced amounts of zinc in their prostatic fluid; they are also most likely to suffer recurrent infections of the urine.

The most important defense of the bladder against bacterial colonization is the prompt and efficient emptying of urine. Patients with neurogenic bladder dysfunction, or those who are otherwise unable to empty their bladder effectively, are much more susceptible to bladder infections. The ability of bacteria to adhere to the bladder wall may be affected by surface mucins, urinary antibodies, urinary osmolality, and pH, and alterations in any of these factors may predispose to bacterial colonization.

The presence or absence of VUR, the quality of ureteral peristalsis, and the relative susceptibility of the renal medulla to infection are all factors that influence the establishment of bacterial infection in the upper tracts. These factors are greatly influenced by ureteral obstruction, renal scarring, and poor renal blood flow.

DIAGNOSIS

Diagnosis of infections in the urinary tract relies primarily on urinalysis and urine culture. Localization techniques can supplement information obtained from urinalysis and culture when the source of infection is presumed to lie outside the bladder, as with the prostate and kidneys.

Urine Collection

The reliability of results obtained from the collection of any urine specimen can be greatly influenced by the method of collection. The method least likely to introduce contaminants from urethra, skin, or introitus into the specimen is suprapubic needle aspiration of the bladder. Although this practice is commonly used in infants and in patients with spinal cord injury, it is rarely used in healthy adults unless the problem of contamination is being specifically addressed.

In men, voided urine specimens are generally adequate for diagnostic purposes. No cleaning is required for circumcised men; uncircumcised men should retract their foreskin and wash the glans with soap and water before giving the specimen. The urine collection can then be segmented according to the purposes of the investigation. The first 10 mL of urine represents a urethral specimen. The midstream urine represents a bladder specimen. If prostatitis is suspected, expressed prostatic secretions can be collected, followed by another 10 mL of urine to reveal any additional prostatic fluid. In men who can void spontaneously, catheterization is not indicated.

In females, contamination of voided urine is more common. Introital bacteria and vaginal flora can easily come into contact with the urinary stream and affect the results of urinalysis and culture. For this reason, women should be more fastidious about urine collection. They should carefully spread the labia and wash the introitus and periurethral area before collecting a midstream urine specimen. If a specimen cannot be obtained without contamination, as evidenced by vaginal flora or epithelial cells on urinalysis, then the patient should be catheterized and a midcatheterized specimen collected. Unfortunately, single catheterization does carry a risk of introducing infection, and for this reason it may be prudent to treat patients requiring catheterization with 1 or 2 doses of antibiotics after the specimen is collected.

Urinalysis

Microscopic examination of urine sediment often allows presumptive diagnosis of UTIs. Once a urine specimen has been centrifuged, most of the urine is poured off and the sediment is resuspended in a few drops of residual urine. This suspension is transferred to a glass slide, placed under a coverslip, and examined at high power for the presence of white blood cells (leukocytes), red blood cells (erythrocytes), microorganisms, epithelial cells, and crystals. Only when the bacterial counts are greater than 100,000 colony-forming units per milliliter can bacteriuria usually be detected microscopically (Jenkins, Fenn,

and Matsen, 1986). Pyuria is more easily detected. Three or more fresh leukocytes per high-power field suggest infection and are rarely found in normal, nonbacteriuric patients (Stamm et al, 1981). The presence of pyuria in voided urine samples has a reported sensitivity of 80–95% and specificity of 50–76% for UTI (Stamm et al, 1982; Schultz et al, 1984; Wigton et al, 1985). Microscopic hematuria occurs in about one-half of all patients with acute cystitis (Wigton et al, 1985).

Chemical screening of urine for markers of infection may provide some useful clinical information, although it is less sensitive than microscopic urinalysis for detecting UTIs. Bacteria can reduce nitrates in the urine to nitrites, which are then detectable biochemically as indirect evidence of bacterial presence. Activated leukocytes secrete leukocyte esterase, which, similarly, can be exploited as indirect evidence of immune response to infection. These 2 markers have a sensitivity ranging from 56% to 92% (Lachs et al, 1992), and they are rarely positive in the absence of infection. For this reason, they are used primarily as a screening tool for asymptomatic patients (Pezzlo, 1988).

Urine Culture

Quantitative urine culture confirms the presence of pathogenic bacteria in urine specimens and allows for their identification. Generally, once the specimen is collected in a sterile container, it should be processed onto culture medium quickly. If a delay is foreseen, the specimen can be refrigerated for up to 24 h before plating. Small samples of 0.1 mL or less are spread onto plates containing nutrient agars. After several hours of growth, each rod or group of cocci will form an identifiable colony on the surface of the medium. The colonies can then be counted, and bacterial growth can be quantified as colony-forming units per milliliter (CFU/mL). The threshold for significant bacteriuria was originally defined as 100,000 CFU/mL to exclude patients with bacterial contamination from the introitus or foreskin; nevertheless, 20% of positive results were attributed to contamination (Kass, 1960). Subsequently, however, it was found that women often have significant bacterial infections with growth of only 100 to 10,000 CFU/mL on culture medium; in symptomatic patients, then, depending on the circumstances, more than 100 CFU/mL could be considered significant (Stamm and Hooton, 1993).

Upper Urinary Tract Localization Studies

Stamey and Pfau (1963) introduced a technique for localization of infection in the bacteriuric patient to an upper or lower tract source and to the right or left side. First, a bladder specimen is collected. The bladder is then irrigated thoroughly with sterile saline solution. Under cystoscopic guidance, ureteral catheters are passed into the bladder. Control specimens of bladder urine are obtained through the catheters. The catheters are passed simultaneously into each ureteral orifice. An initial ureteral sample is taken on each side, and then the catheters are passed up to the renal pelvis, where serial cultures are collected. Examples of quantitative results for various sources of infection are given in Table 14–3 (Stamey, 1980). This approach reveals that about one-half of bacteriuric patients have bladder infections only, and one-half have renal bacteriuria (Stamey, Govan, and Palmer, 1965).

ANTIBIOTIC AGENTS

The goal of antibacterial therapy is the complete elimination of bacterial growth in the urine. If growth of bacteria in the urine is only suppressed to lower counts and not eradicated, then the infection is considered unresolved and the treatment unsuccessful. Often, documentation of complete resolution of infection is necessary to determine whether subsequent episodes of bacteriuria are recurrent or unresolved infections.

Choice of Antibiotic

The urinary concentration of antibiotic is much more important than serum concentration in the treatment of UTIs. Most antibiotics are excreted by the kidney and appear in the urine at higher concentrations than they do in serum or tissue. As a result, doses sufficient to produce bactericidal urinary levels are often a fraction of the usual systemic dose. Table 14–4 gives the typical doses as well as the serum and urine concentrations for the drugs commonly used in UTIs. Table 14–5 lists the common microorganisms found in UTI and the antibiotics that reliably treat each of them.

Trimethoprim-Sulfamethoxazole: Trimethoprim combined with sulfamethoxazole (TMP-SMX) interferes with the bacterial metabolism of folate. TMP-SMX has activity against most of the common uropathogens, with the exception of *Enterococcus* and *Pseudomonas* species. It is one of the most widely used drugs for the treatment of UTIs because of its efficacy and low cost. However, adverse drug reactions, especially to the sulfa component, are not rare. These include hypersensitivity reactions, rashes, gastrointestinal (GI) upset, and photosensitivity. Patients with glucose-6-phosphate dehydrogenase deficiency, folate deficiency, or acquired immunodeficiency syndrome (AIDS) can experience hematologic toxicity. Use of the drug can significantly prolong the prothrombin time in patients taking warfarin. Preg-

Table 14–3. Localization patterns for patients with bacteriuria from various sources.

Source	Bacteria/mL	Organism	Diagnosis
Patient P.G.			Lower tract
CB	69,000,000	*Proteus mirabilis*	source
WB	94	*P mirabilis*	
LK_1	0	None	
RK_1	0	None	
LK_2	0	None	
RK_2	0	None	
LK_3	0	None	
RK_3	0	None	
Patient S.I.			Unilateral renal
CB	1,260,000	*Escherichia coli*	source
WB	3720	*E coli*	
LK_1	394,000	*E coli*	
RK_1	91	*E coli*	
LK_2	228,000	*E coli*	
RK_2	2	*E coli*	
LK_3	33,400	*E coli*	
RK_3	0	*None*	
Paitent L.P.			Bilateral renal
CB	> 100,000	*E coli*	source
WB	50,000	*E coli*	
LK_1	> 100,000	*E coli*	
RK_1	> 100,000	*E coli*	
LK_2	> 100,000	*E coli*	
RK_2	> 100,000	*E coli*	
LK_3	> 100,000	*E coli*	
RK_3	> 100,000	*E coli*	

CB = catheterized bladder specimen; WB = washed bladder specimen; LK_{1-3} = serial left kidney specimens; RK_{1-3} = serial right kidney specimens.
Source: Adapted from Stamey TA: *Pathogenesis and Treatment of Urinary Tract Infections.* Williams & Wilkins, 1980.

Table 14–4. Serum and urinary antimicrobial levels in adults.

Antibiotic	Dose[1]	Route	Peak Serum Level (μg/mL)	Mean Urine Level (μg/mL)
Ampicillin	250 every 6 h	Oral	3	350
Carbenicillin	764 every 6 h	Oral	11–17	1000
Cephalexin	250 every 6 h	Oral	9	800
Ciprofloxacin	500 every 12 h	Oral	2.3	200
Colistin	75 every 12 h	Intramuscular	1.8	34
Gentamicin	1 mg/kg every 8 h	Intramuscular	4	125
Kanamycin	500 every 12 h	Intramuscular	18	750
Nalidixic Acid	1000 every 6 h	Oral	34	75
Nitrofurantoin	100 every 6 h	Oral	< 2	150
Norfloxacin	400 every 12 h	Oral	1.5	170
Penicillin G	500 every 6 h	Oral	1	300
Tetracycline	250 every 6 h	Oral	2–3	500
TMP-SMX	160/800 every 12 h	Oral	1.7/32	150/400
Trimethoprim	100 μg every 12 h	Oral	1	92

[1] Milligrams unless indicated otherwise.
TMP-SMX = trimethoprim plus sulfamethoxazole.
Adapted from: Stamey TA: Pathogenesis & treatment of Urinary Tract Infections, Williams & Wilkins, 1980.

nant women should avoid TMP-SMX because of fetal hepatotoxicity. TMP alone may be just as efficacious as the combination and may carry fewer side effects (Harbord and Grueneberg, 1981).

Fluoroquinolones: The fluoroquinolones inhibit bacterial DNA gyrase, an enzyme necessary for DNA replication. They have a broad spectrum of activity, especially against the gram-negative enterics (including *Pseudomonas* species). Although activity against staphylococci is also good, the fluoroquinolones in general have marginal activity against streptococcal species. They are ineffective against most anaerobic bacteria, which means they do not significantly interfere with the fecal flora. Common adverse reactions include mild GI effects, dizziness, and lightheadedness. Currently, these drugs are not indicated for use in children or in pregnant or nursing women because of animal studies showing damage to developing cartilage (Christ, Lehnert, and Ulbrich, 1988).

Nitrofurantoin: Nitrofurantoin works by inhibiting a number of bacterial enzyme pathways. It has good activity against most gram-negative enterics, except for *Pseudomonas* and *Proteus* species. It has activity against staphylococci and enterococci. Nitrofurantoin is rapidly cleared by the kidneys and never achieves significant serum levels. As such, it is not suitable for treatment of renal parenchymal or other complicated infections. Patients taking nitrofurantoin may experience GI upset and, more seriously, peripheral polyneuropathy. Patients with impaired renal function, or those otherwise predisposed to neuropathies (ie, those with diabetes or vitamin B_{12} deficiencies) should avoid using this agent. Additionally, with long-term use, pulmonary hypersensitivity reactions may develop, leading to interstitial changes. However, nitrofurantoin has minimal effects outside

the urinary tract and has been used effectively in prophylactic regimens for long periods. The development of acquired bacterial resistance is infrequent.

Aminoglycosides: The aminoglycosides inhibit protein synthesis by inactivating bacterial ribosomes. They cover most gram-negative pathogens, including *Pseudomonas* spp. When combined with ampicillin, they provide a synergistic effect against enterococci. An aminoglycoside, combined with ampicillin, is the first line of therapy in patients with febrile UTIs requiring intravenous antibiotics. They have well-recognized nephrotoxicity and should be used with caution in patients with impaired renal function. Serum levels can adequately predict potential for renal damage and should generally be checked in all patients receiving sustained therapy. Aminoglycosides also have potential ototoxicity, affecting the vestibular and auditory apparatuses.

Cephalosporins: The cephalosporins inhibit bacterial cell wall synthesis, similar to the other beta-lactam antibiotics. They generally have good activity against most uropathogens, but there are differences between generations. First-generation cephalosporins have increased activity against gram-positive organisms but also cover *E coli, Proteus mirabilis,* and *Klebsiella* species. Second-generation agents add higher activity against anaerobes, as well as more reliable coverage of *Haemophilus influenzae.* The third-generation cephalosporins have broader and more reliable gram-negative coverage in general, including activity against *Pseudomonas* spp. Hypersensitivity reactions can occur, but they are much less common than those with penicillins. Pseudomembranous colitis has also resulted from cephalosporin use. The oral agents can cause some GI upset.

Penicillins: First-generation penicillins are not effective enough against gram-negative organisms to

Table 14–5. Choices of drugs for bacteria commonly encountered in genitourinary infections.

Bacteria	Oral Therapy	Parenteral Therapy
Gram-positive cocci		
Staphylococcus aureus	Nafcillin, nitrofurantoin, ciprofloxacin	Nafcillin, vancomycin
Staphylococcus epidermidis	Ampicillin, nitrofurantoin, ciprofloxacin	Ampicillin, penicillin G
Staphylococcus saprophyticus	Ampicillin, nitrofurantoin, ciprofloxacin	Ampicillin, penicillin G
Streptococcus, group D		
S faecalis (enterococci)	Ampicillin, nitrofurantoin	Ampicillin plus gentamicin
S bovis	Penicillin G, ampicillin	Ampicillin, vancomycin
Streptococcus, group B	Ampicillin, cephalosporin	Ampicillin, cephalosporin
Gram-negative cocci		
Neisseria gonorrhoeae	Ciprofloxacin plus doxycycline	Ceftriaxone
Gram-negative rods		
Escherichia coli	TMP-SMX, ciprofloxacin, nitrofurantoin	Gentamicin
Enterobacter sp.	TMP-SMX, ciprofloxacin, nitrofurantoin	Gentamicin plus piperacillin
Gardnerella vaginalis	Metronidazole, ampicillin	Metronidazole
Klebsiella sp.	TMP-SMX, ciprofloxacin	Gentamicin plus cephalosporin
Proteus sp.	Ampicillin, TMP-SMX, ciprofloxacin	Ampicillin, gentamicin
Pseudomonas aeruginosa	Carbenicillin, tetracycline, ciprofloxacin	Gentamicin plus piperacillin
Serratia sp.	TMP-SMX, carbenicillin	TMP-SMX, amikacin
Other pathogens		
Chlamydiae	Tetracycline, erythromycin	Tetracycline, erythromycin
Mycoplasmas, ureaplasmas	Tetracycline, erythromycin	Tetracycline, erythromycin
Obligate anaerobes	Metronidazole, clindamycin	Metronidazole, clindamycin

TMP-SMX = trimethoprim plus sulfamethoxazole.

be useful in most UTIs. The aminopenicillins, however, including ampicillin and amoxicillin, have been used in the treatment of UTIs. They have good activity against enterococci and staphylococci, as well as *E coli* and *P mirabilis.* However, they are frequently associated with the emergence of resistance, which limits their practical utility (Hooton and Stamm, 1991). β-Lactamase inhibitors like clavulanic acid help overcome this resistance, but they also add expense. The antipseudomonal penicillins provide better coverage of gram-negative organisms while maintaining effectiveness against gram-positive organisms. Again, however, their expense limits their usefulness to more resistant, nosocomially acquired infections. All penicillins carry the risk of hypersensitivity, whether immediate or delayed. They can also cause GI upset, and ampicillin is especially prone to cause diarrhea. Pseudomembranous colitis can be related to the use of penicillins.

ANTIBIOTIC PROPHYLAXIS FOR ENDOURO- LOGIC PROCEDURES

Endourologic procedures are considered clean-contaminated in the operative wound classification system. As such, prophylaxis is strongly recommended only for those patients with prostheses, those

at risk for endocarditis, or those at high risk for complications from infection because of significant co-morbidity (diabetes, immunocompromise, age). Despite these general recommendations, the issue of systemic antibiotic prophylaxis in patients who do not have these specific risks and who are undergoing endourologic procedures remains controversial.

Outpatient diagnostic cystoscopy is safe and well tolerated, with an infection risk similar to that of straight catheterization. Manson (1988) performed a prospective, randomized trial comparing the use of antimicrobial prophylaxis and placebo in 138 patients undergoing outpatient cystoscopy. On follow-up urine cultures, he found no difference in the rate of culture positivity between the 2 groups. Other studies have shown the overall infection rate without prophylaxis to be from 1% to 4%. The risk for women, however, may be higher. Bhatia et al (1992) studied 362 women undergoing urethral instrumentation in a randomized trial and found significant infection rates in women treated with placebo compared with those receiving antibiotic prophylaxis.

UTIs identified on preprocedure culture need to be eradicated before the procedure is started. Failure to do this can result in bacteremia in as many as 50% of cases. Equally mandatory is the approach to patients with risk of endocarditis (prosthetic valves or valvular heart disease) undergoing genitourinary manipulation. For any transurethral manipulation (including catheterization, cystoscopy, and urethral dilation), broad-spectrum antibiotic coverage should be given. Generally, this consists of ampicillin and gentamicin given intramuscularly 30 min before the procedure, followed by an oral dose of amoxicillin 6 h later. For patients allergic to penicillin, vancomycin should be given intravenously in combination with gentamicin 1 h before the procedure. This regimen can be repeated once 8 h later.

The incidence of bacteriuria following transurethral resection of the prostate (TURP) varies widely; reports have ranged from 6% to 64%. Several studies have addressed the role of prophylactic antibiotics for this procedure, including their timing, dosing, and duration. In studies in which antibiotics were given preoperatively and then continued postoperatively until either the catheter was removed or 5 days to 3 weeks had passed, the post-TURP incidence of infection decreased to a range of 0–12%. Some studies have examined single-dose antibiotic prophylaxis given at the time of surgery. These studies generally show a significantly lower incidence of bacteriuria in treated patients compared with control subjects. Scholz and colleagues (1998) gave ceftriaxone, 1 g intravenously, at induction of anesthesia and observed a reduction in the incidence of bacteriuria from 26% to 9%. Other studies have compared the use of single-dose antibiotics with longer perioperative courses and found no difference between these 2 approaches (Janknegt, 1992). However, Duclos, Larrouturou, and Sarkis (1992) observed a significant benefit to giving patients a second dose of antibiotics at the time the catheter was removed. They suggested that antibiotics at the time of catheter removal are more important in preventing bacteriuria than are those at the time of operation.

In otherwise asymptomatic patients who do not have a preoperative urine culture available, 6–12% should be considered to have unsuspected bacteriuria at any given time. As a result, as many as 67% of these patients who undergo genitourinary manipulation could go on to develop bacteremia if not treated prophylactically. They should be treated with appropriate antibiotics in the preoperative period, and treatment should be continued for at least 24 h postoperatively.

Any patient with an indwelling catheter for longer than 24–48 h preoperatively is presumably infected and should achieve sterile urine cultures before undergoing TURP. In addition to antibiotics with broad coverage against gram-negative organisms, eradication of bacteria may be aided at times by removal of the indwelling catheter and conversion to clean intermittent catheterization.

Transrectal ultrasound–guided prostate biopsies carry a significant risk of infection. Asymptomatic bacteriuria, UTI, fever and urosepsis can all occur following biopsy. With the advent of smaller-caliber biopsy needles and the spring-loaded biopsy gun, infection rates with fever of > 38 °C are 1–6%, quite a bit lower than the 14–37% seen previously. A review of modern studies investigating the use of short-course (1- to 2-dose) quinolone prophylaxis demonstrated febrile infection rates of 0.8–20%. Studies that used longer treatments, for up to 4 days, showed 0–0.8% infection rates. Given the expense and morbidity involved with febrile infections, antibiotic prophylaxis is recommended for transrectal prostate biopsies. Fluoroquinolones are generally used for 24–48 h, but duration of therapy is still controversial.

Urosepsis can result from shock wave lithotripsy (SWL) when bacteria are released from calculi as they are fragmented. This complication is rare, with an incidence of 0.1–1.5%. It is postulated that shock waves may induce microtrauma by propelling stone fragments into ureteral or renal tissue. This tissue trauma could allow entry of released bacteria into the bloodstream. Pyelonephritis and cystitis may also result from SWL therapy and incur significant added cost in terms of patient morbidity, treatment, and lost wages.

For these reasons, patients with infection stones, those with a history of recurrent or current bacteriuria, immunocompromised patients, and those undergoing endourologic manipulation before SWL all require preprocedure antibiotics to minimize the risk of these complications. The role of antibiotics for low-risk patients without evidence of infection is controversial. In a meta-analysis of all the published studies on this topic, Pearle and Roehrborn (1997) found that, in randomized controlled trials, 2% of prophylactically treated patients and 7% of untreated patients developed a UTI after SWL. With an overall relative risk of 0.45 (95% confidence interval of 0.22–0.93), this suggested that antibiotic prophylaxis was effective in preventing post-SWL UTIs. They concluded that the cost of treating the 5.7% of patients who would probably develop a UTI without prophylaxis and the occasional resulting sepsis warrants the use of routine prophylaxis.

KIDNEY INFECTIONS

Acute Pyelonephritis

Etiology & Pathogenesis: Acute pyelonephritis is bacterial infection causing inflammation of the parenchyma and pelvis of the kidney. The bacteriology of this disease resembles that of most UTIs. *E coli* predominates, accounting for 80% of cases. Other gram-negative enteric organisms, such as *Klebsiella, Proteus, Pseudomonas, Serratia, Enterobacter,* and *Citrobacter* spp., are cultured less frequently from infected patients. Enterococci and *Staphylococcus aureus* are occasional pathogens.

Pathogens usually ascend from the lower urinary

tract to establish renal infection. Evidence for this fecal-perineal-urethral progression of bacteria comes from studies that document the clonality of urinary and fecal isolates in cases of uncomplicated pyelonephritis in women (Mitsumori et al, 1997). Once bacteria have reached the bladder, ascent to the upper tracts can depend on a number of conditions. The presence of VUR provides bacterial entry to the ureter and puts patients at significantly increased risk for acute pyelonephritis. Particular microbial virulence factors can also influence the establishment of renal infection. Of the adhesins, P fimbriae, which dominate the fecal flora in one-third of normal healthy women (Mitsumori et al, 1997), show the most clear-cut association with acute pyelonephritis (Johnson, 1991). Impaired ureteral peristalsis may also predispose to upper tract infection.

When hematogenous spread of infection does occur, it is often associated with staphylococcal bacteremia. In this setting, renal abscesses are also more common, and the clinical course is fulminant.

Clinical Features: The abrupt onset of fever, chills, and unilateral or bilateral flank pain constitutes the classic presentation of acute pyelonephritis. Lower urinary tract symptoms, including dysuria, frequency, and urgency, are also common. Nausea, vomiting, and malaise often accompany the more specific signs. Variations in presentation do occur, however. Patients occasionally complain of diffuse abdominal pain that, when accompanied by nausea, vomiting, and diarrhea, can lead the clinician to suspect a GI illness. Similarly, children often do not localize pain to their flanks and instead complain of nonspecific abdominal discomfort. In patients with compromised immune systems, acute pyelonephritis may be relatively asymptomatic.

On physical examination, the patient generally appears ill. Measurement of the vital signs usually reveals tachycardia as well as a fever ranging from 101 to 104 °F. Palpation or percussion over the costovertebral angle on the affected side causes pain. The patient sometimes has a paralytic ileus as well, which manifests as abdominal distention, tenderness, and a quiet intestine.

Diagnosis: A complete blood count regularly shows significant leukocytosis, with a shift toward neutrophils and immature forms. The urinalysis typically shows numerous leukocytes as well, accompanied by bacteria, protein, and varying numbers of erythrocytes. Large neutrophils containing cytoplasmic granules in a state of Brownian motion are called glitter cells. Along with leukocyte casts, their presence in the urinary sediment is suggestive of acute pyelonephritis, but not diagnostic. Urine culture is always positive and typically yields heavy growth of the pathogenic bacteria (> 100,000 CFU/mL). In the presence of ureteral obstruction, however, bacterial growth and activity of the urinary sediment may be diminished. Blood cultures are warranted, as bacteremia coexists in about one-third of patients (Behr et al, 1996).

Diagnostic imaging techniques in the management of acute pyelonephritis have improved significantly in the past decade. Previously, intravenous urography (IVU) was the standard imaging modality. In only 25–30% of cases, however, did this study show abnormalities (Little, McPherson, and Wardener, 1965; Silver et al, 1976). General or focal renal enlargement is seen in about 20% of patients and is caused by interstitial inflammation and edema. During the nephrogram phase, cortical striations may be seen (Davidson and Talner, 1973; Silver et al, 1976; Teplick et al, 1978). Congestion in renal tubules caused by edema, along with local vasoconstriction, could delay excretion of contrast material, resulting in a diminished nephrogram and pyelogram. In addition, bacterial endotoxin-mediated effects on ureteral peristalsis might cause a dilated ureter in some cases, in the absence of any mechanical obstruction (Kass et al, 1976; Silver et al, 1976; Teplick et al, 1978).

More recently, computed tomography (CT), radionuclide studies, and power Doppler ultrasonography have been useful for patients with unclear or complicated clinical pictures. Acute bacterial infection causes constriction of peripheral arterioles and reduces perfusion to affected segments of renal parenchyma. The perfusion deficits can be picked up on contrast-enhanced CT images as focal, multifocal, or diffuse areas of reduced signal density (Figure 14–1). Radionuclide study with the ^{99m}Tc-dimercaptosuccinic acid scan probably has a sensitivity similar to that of contrast-enhanced CT in detecting perfusion defects from pyelonephritis (Talner, Davidson, and Lebowitz, 1994). Power Doppler ultrasonogra-

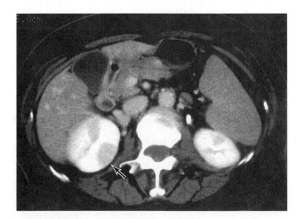

Figure 14–1. Acute pyelonephritis. Contrast-enhanced computed tomography scan shows an enlarged right kidney with wedge-shaped areas of decreased contrast enhancement (arrow). Local vasoconstriction brought about by bacterial infection has reduced blood flow to these renal segments.

phy extends the dynamic range of the Doppler scale down to the noise threshold, allowing assessment of local vascularity and blood volume (Breidahl et al, 1996; Rubin et al, 1994). It is therefore capable of detecting vasoconstriction caused by bacterial infection. A recent study showed that this technique is nearly as sensitive as CT in diagnosing acute pyelonephritis (Sakarya et al, 1998).

For patients with acute pyelonephritis, the biggest concern is missing the diagnosis of urinary tract obstruction. Ultrasonography can reliably exclude this possibility, but it is poor at demonstrating inflammation (Talner, Davidson, and Lebowitz, 1994). Indeed, 70% of patients with acute pyelonephritis may have normal kidneys on ultrasound, with the most common finding in the remainder being renal enlargement (Bailey et al, 1996). Although the assessment of urinary tract obstruction is important in the seriously ill patient, some authors suggest that ultrasound might not be necessary in patients who are not toxic or in those who are responding well to therapy (Johnson et al, 1992).

Management: Treatment strategy depends primarily on whether the patient is ill enough to require hospitalization. In any case, empiric antibiotic therapy directed against the most common pathogens should be started. For adults being treated as outpatients, the fluoroquinolones or TMP-SMX are generally efficacious and well tolerated. After using the sensitivity results to make any necessary adjustments, therapy should be continued for 10–14 days. In patients with a more toxic appearance, hospitalization with bed rest, intravenous fluids, and parenteral antibiotics may be required. Traditionally, an aminoglycoside combined with ampicillin, to provide effective coverage of both enterococci and *Pseudomonas* spp., have been employed. Recently, however, increasing resistance to ampicillin has prompted a switch to TMP-SMX combined with an aminoglycoside or, alternatively, fluoroquinolones or parenteral third-generation cephalosporins as monotherapy (Johnson et al, 1991).

Fever may persist for several days in patients with acute pyelonephritis despite initiation of appropriate therapy. Behr et al (1996) observed an average duration of 39 h of fever in these patients, with 26% still being febrile after 48 h. If fever persists beyond 72 h, or if the urine does not become sterile after initiation of antibiotics, then complications such as abscess, obstruction, or urinary tract abnormality needs to be ruled out with either ultrasound or CT (Soulen et al, 1989). Any complicating factor should be dealt with quickly to minimize potential renal damage.

If bacteremia is present, parenteral therapy should continue for 7–10 days. If the blood cultures are negative, parenteral therapy can stop after 3–5 days. In both cases, oral antibiotic therapy should follow for 10–14 days. Patients should get repeat urine culture 4–6 weeks after therapy to document eradication of infection. Some patients may require follow-up radiologic examination depending on their age, urologic evaluation, or treatment response. Such examination might consist of voiding cystourethrography, cystoscopy, or bacterial localization studies.

Complications: When treated adequately, uncomplicated pyelonephritis in adult patients usually resolves without leaving renal scars or any permanent damage. In children, in whom renal development is not complete, acute pyelonephritis can produce scarring and permanently diminish renal function. The most serious complication in adults is septicemia with shock. Renal abscess requiring drainage may also develop.

Emphysematous Pyelonephritis

Etiology & Pathogenesis: Emphysematous pyelonephritis is a necrotizing renal infection characterized by gas within the renal parenchyma or perinephric tissue. In larger studies, 80–90% of patients have diabetes; and of the nondiabetics, urinary tract obstruction from either calculi or papillary necrosis is present in all (Michaeli, 1984; Shokeir et al, 1997; Chen et al, 1997). It is postulated that impaired host response due either to systemic disease (diabetes) or local factors (obstruction) allows bacteria to utilize necrotic tissue to ferment glucose and produce carbon dioxide gas. By far the most frequently isolated organism is *E coli,* with *Klebsiella* also seen (Michaeli, 1984; Ahlering et al, 1985). Ten percent of cases are polymicrobial. Only one case of anaerobic infection has been reported (Levy and Schwinger, 1953), and *Clostridium* spp. have never been isolated (Michaeli, 1984).

Clinical Findings: Typically, patients present with severe acute pyelonephritis that fails initial management with parenteral antibiotics. A classic triad of fever, flank pain, and vomiting has been described (Schainuck, Fouty, and Cutler, 1968). If gas extends into the collecting system, pneumaturia may be present. Urine cultures are generally positive. Blood cultures are positive in 30–100% of cases (Chen et al, 1997; Shokeir et al, 1997; Wan et al, 1998).

The diagnosis is made following radiographic investigation. A plain abdominal radiograph often shows mottled gas shadows over the affected kidney. In some cases, a crescent of gas over the superior pole can be made out. As the illness progresses, gas can track out into the retroperitoneum. A noncontrast CT scan is very sensitive for the presence of gas (Figure 14–2); it can also describe the extent of infection as well as any concurrent obstruction. Ultrasonography demonstrates obstruction well, but it is much less sensitive than CT at picking up renal gas (Shokeir et al, 1997). Because these patients usually have abnormal renal function, their risk of contrast nephropathy is high and IVU or contrast-enhanced CT should be avoided.

Several prognostic factors have been identified for

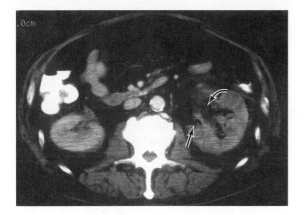

Figure 14–2. Emphysematous pyelonephritis. Computed tomography scan without intravenous contrast enhancement shows gas formation in the left renal parenchyma (straight arrow), extending into the collecting system (curved arrow).

patients with emphysematous pyelonephritis (Wan et al, 1998). Elevated serum creatinine, severe thrombocytopenia (probably a marker of disseminated intravascular coagulation), and hematuria were all associated with poor outcome. The type of emphysematous pyelonephritis was also significant. Type I emphysematous pyelonephritis consists of renal necrosis with either absence of fluid content on CT or presence of a mottled gas pattern. Type II is characterized by renal or perirenal fluid in association with a bubbly gas pattern or the presence of air in the collecting system. Type I patients generally had a worse clinical prognosis (Wan et al, 1998).

Management: Patients should be given fluids and broad-spectrum antibiotics intravenously. Prompt control of blood glucose should be achieved. Ureteral obstruction should be relieved quickly. Beyond these measures, treatment of emphysematous pyelonephritis is controversial. Klein et al (1986) reviewed 66 cases from the literature and found a mortality of 71% among medically treated patients, 29% among surgically treated patients, and 38% overall. Citing the high mortality of medical therapy, several authors have advocated aggressive early surgical intervention, consisting of total nephrectomy (Freiha, Messing, and Gross, 1979; Michaeli, 1984; Ahlering et al, 1986). Attempts at renal sparing through partial nephrectomy have been unsuccessful at retaining renal function or decreasing morbidity (Freiha, Messing, and Gross, 1979).

More recently, investigators have attempted percutaneous drainage combined with medical therapy in treating emphysematous pyelonephritis (Hall, Choa, and Wells, 1988). Chen et al (1997) reported their experience with 25 patients over 10 years. They treated 20 patients successfully with percutaneous

drainage alone. The duration of therapy averaged 3–4 weeks, with interval CT scans to check for resolution of disease. Three patients eventually underwent nephrectomy because of nonfunctioning kidneys or staghorn calculi, and the other 2 patients died. Their overall success rate was 92%, with an 80% nephron-sparing rate. They found that drained kidneys could preserve meaningful excretory function. For patients without perfusion on follow-up renal scan, they recommended nephrectomy.

Chronic Pyelonephritis

Etiology & Pathogenesis: Chronic pyelonephritis refers to a process of renal scarification and atrophy resulting in renal insufficiency. It should more aptly be termed pyelonephritic scarring. While the sequelae of chronic pyelonephritis are easily discernible pathologically and on imaging studies, the pathogenic mechanisms themselves are more obscure. Repeated bacterial infections cause renal insufficiency, it seems, only in the presence of some underlying urinary tract abnormality of either structure or function. Acute uncomplicated UTIs do not commonly lead to renal scarring and progressive renal disease, at least in adults. Factors such as diabetes, calculi, analgesic nephropathy, and obstructive nephropathy in the presence of repeated UTIs, however, can lead to renal loss of function. Huland and Busch (1982) analyzed 42 patients with end-stage renal disease as a result of chronic pyelonephritis. They found that all 42 patients had some complicating defect, such as those mentioned above, in addition to a history of UTIs. Murray and Goldberg (1975) evaluated 101 patients with end-stage renal disease from chronic pyelonephritis and concluded that UTI is rarely the sole cause of chronic renal insufficiency in adults. Indeed, they readily identified some other structural-anatomic cause in 89% of their patients. The point is this: Underlying abnormality of urinary tract structure or function, and not recurrent infection alone, is primarily responsible for chronic pyelonephritis.

In children, the most important association in the development of renal scarring is that between VUR and UTI. This association is often referred to as **reflux nephropathy.** Immature, developing kidneys are much more susceptible to damage brought on by bacterial infection alone than are mature kidneys. As such, the susceptibility to renal scarring is age-related. It appears that new scars seldom develop in children with reflux after 4 years old, but established scars can progress beyond this age (Cardiff-Oxford Bacteriuria Study Group, 1978). The severity of renal scarring brought on by reflux nephropathy seems to relate directly to the grade of VUR in children with repeat UTIs. Experimental studies suggest that those children with intrarenal reflux of infected urine, as a result of altered papillary morphology, are at the highest risk for permanent damage (Ransley and Ridson, 1979).

Clinical Features: In the absence of acute infection, patients with pyelonephritic scarring are asymptomatic. In those patients whose renal function has been significantly impaired by chronic pyelonephritis, symptoms of hypertension and renal failure may be present. There are also no specific physical findings for chronic pyelonephritis alone, save for those brought on by renal insufficiency. In general, the condition is usually discovered incidentally.

Diagnosis: Urinalysis can show pyuria and bacteriuria in the presence of active infection, but it may equally show no signs of infection. If renal impairment has advanced to the stage of glomerular involvement, proteinuria is present. Urine cultures are positive only in the presence of bacteriuria. Serum creatinine and urea nitrogen reflect the severity of renal impairment.

Plain radiography of the abdomen might show that the kidneys have an irregular outline and are small. The IVU typically shows small, atrophic kidneys, which demonstrate impaired excretion of contrast material. Focal, coarse renal scarring often overlies clubbed calyces, especially at the renal poles. If the atrophy is only unilateral, compensatory hypertrophy may be seen on the contralateral side. Urolithiasis may be present, and the ureters may be dilated, signifying chronic obstruction or reflux.

If VUR is present, a voiding cystourethrogram will show the abnormality and allow assessment of its severity.

Management: Unfortunately, the renal damage incurred by chronic pyelonephritis is irreversible. By identifying and correcting any underlying structural abnormalities, as well as by preventing recurrence of UTIs, the clinician may be able to save the patient from any further renal damage. The long-term use of continuous prophylactic antibiotic therapy is often required, especially in children, to keep the urine sterile. In certain cases, management with low-dose antibiotics alone may be sufficient, until the VUR has resolved on its own. If medical management fails to prevent reinfection in the face of VUR, surgical intervention may be necessary to prevent chronic pyelonephritis from developing.

In those patients with structural causes of urinary obstruction, surgery is generally needed to correct the defect. Similarly, any stones (especially infected ones) require removal. Close follow-up and prompt attention to eradication of any urinary infection are crucial in preserving renal function. Nephrectomy may be necessary in patients with unilateral atrophic kidneys who have renin-mediated hypertension or in patients with large infected stone burdens whose renal function on that side is poor.

Renal Abscess

Etiology & Pathogenesis: Widespread antibiotic use has greatly changed the pathogenesis of renal abscesses. In the past, most abscesses arose from hematogenous spread of bacteria, mostly staphylococci. Because infected skin lesions were a predisposing factor, those with diabetes mellitus, those undergoing hemodialysis, or those using intravenous drugs were at higher risk. Over the past quarter century, however, the nature of the illness has changed. Gram-positive abscess formation still occurs but is less prevalent today. Aerobic gram-negative organisms commonly found in other UTIs now predominate. Additionally, the most common mechanism for inoculation of the kidney now appears to be through an ascending, not a hematogenous, route. Patients with previous infections or those with renal calculi are particularly susceptible. Some investigators have noted the increased frequency of renal abscess formation in patients with VUR (Timmons and Perlmutter, 1976). Similarly, Anderson and McAninch (1980) found that patients with UTIs complicated by stasis, calculi, pregnancy, neurogenic bladder, and diabetes were more prone to abscess formation.

The location of the abscess within the renal parenchyma relates to the pathogenesis of the illness. Abscesses that form in the renal cortex (carbuncles) probably arise from hematogenous spread. Corticomedullary abscesses, in contrast, are more often caused by coliform bacteria in conjunction with some other underlying urinary tract abnormality.

Clinical Features: Fever, chills, and flank pain are the typical presenting signs. Nausea, vomiting, and malaise are common. If the abscess-forming bacteria arose from a lower tract source, or if the abscess communicates with the collecting system, then cystitislike symptoms may also be present. Patients usually have costovertebral angle tenderness and may also have abdominal tenderness. The physical findings in general, however, are rather nonspecific.

The complete blood count discloses a pronounced leukocytosis, with a shift toward neutrophils and immature forms. Blood cultures usually indicate bacteremia. Urinalysis may show pyuria and bacteriuria. The absence of these findings, however, is not uncommon, especially in cortical abscesses, which less frequently connect with the pyelocalyceal system. Similarly, urine culture may be misleading. No growth, or growth of an organism distinct from that forming the abscess, may occur in cortical abscesses. Urine studies are more revealing in cases of corticomedullary abscess.

Diagnosis: Because the clinical presentation and laboratory findings are nonspecific, imaging studies are crucial in the diagnosis of renal abscess. CT, with and without contrast enhancement, is the diagnostic procedure of choice. Early on, CT shows renal enlargement and focal areas of hypoattenuation (Figure 14–3). Once the abscess has matured to a discrete liquefied collection of pus, an inflammatory wall surrounds the mass. With its increased vascularity, this wall enhances with contrast material, producing a "ring" sign. Aspiration of the abscess under CT guid-

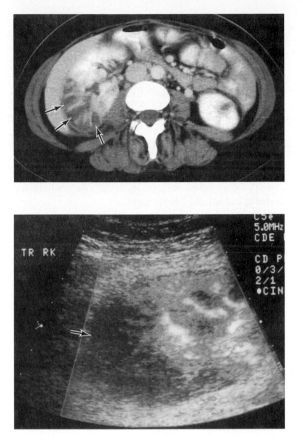

Figure 14–3. Renal abscess. **Top:** Contrast-enhanced computed tomography scan shows dramatic renal enlargement, with a large mottled mass posteriorly. Areas of low density (arrows) represent parenchymal liquefaction. **Bottom:** Renal ultrasound shows a large hypoechoic mass (arrow) at the pole of the affected kidney.

ance can assist in diagnosis and identification of the infecting organism. Ultrasound is also effective in detecting renal abscesses, as well as in guiding aspiration. A hypoechoic density, with increased through-transmission, is generally found at the abscess site. Edema in the surrounding renal tissue usually accompanies the density in the early stages; subsequently, the interface of abscess and surrounding parenchyma becomes more well-defined. Depending on the amount of tissue debris within the abscess cavity, the internal echotexture of the mass can vary. With ultrasound, abscess is frequently difficult to differentiate from renal neoplasm, as the two often have similar ultrasound characteristics.

Management: Appropriate antibiotic therapy constitutes the first step in therapy. When a staphylococcal abscess is suspected as a result of hematogenous spread, a penicillinase-resistant penicillin is the antibiotic of choice. Vancomycin or a cephalosporin can be substituted in cases of penicillin hypersensi-

tivity. Renal abscesses that are associated with more typical urinary pathogens can be effectively treated with aminoglycosides or third-generation cephalosporins.

Although surgical drainage had been recommended in the past, several studies have shown that intravenous antibiotics begun early enough may be sufficient management (Hoverman et al, 1980; Levin et al, 1984). If no favorable clinical response is apparent after 48 h of antibiotic treatment, however, percutaneous CT- or ultrasound-guided aspiration and drainage should be employed. Follow-up imaging is necessary to document resolution of the abscess. If the abscess still does not resolve, then open surgical drainage becomes the definitive treatment.

Perinephric Abscess

Etiology & Pathogenesis: Perinephric abscesses are collections of purulent material within the perinephric space, which lies between the kidney and Gerota's fascia. If the abscess extends beyond Gerota's fascia, it becomes **paranephric.** Renal abscesses can rupture out into the perinephric space, and this probably represents the primary way in which perinephric abscesses develop. As a result, the bacteriology resembles that of renal abscesses. Ascending aerobic gram-negative enteric infection (especially *E coli*) is more common than staphylococcal infection from hematogenous spread. Factors that predispose patients to development of renal abscess, such as urinary stasis or obstruction, calculi, neurogenic bladder, and diabetes, also predispose patients to perinephric abscesses.

Clinical Features: Fever, flank pain, and lower urinary tract symptoms are the most common complaints. These symptoms will often have been present for more than a week before presentation. Patients may also complain of abdominal pain or, if the abscess abuts the diaphragm, pleuritic chest pains. On physical examination, patients usually have tenderness over the costovertebral angle. A flank mass, with overlying skin erythema, may be present in 47% of patients (Saiki, Vaziri, and Barton, 1982). Patients may also have tenderness, guarding, and a palpable mass on abdominal examination. The diaphragm on the affected side may be elevated or fixed, and the patient may have an associated pleural effusion.

Diagnosis: Most patients have an elevated leukocyte count. Urinalysis is normal in about 25% of patients on admission. Otherwise, it generally shows pyuria and proteinuria, with hematuria being rare. Urine cultures identify the pathogenic organism in only one-third of cases, and blood cultures are positive in only about 40% of cases. Percutaneous aspiration of the abscess contents under ultrasound or CT guidance allows for absolute identification of the infecting organism.

CT is the most sensitive tool for diagnosing perinephric abscesses. CT can define the full extent of tissue involvement and demonstrate the mass effects caused by the abscess and any urinary obstruction or calculi that may be associated with it. Characteristically, CT will show a soft tissue mass that has a central area of low attenuation. A ring sign may be present, representing an inflammatory shell that enhances with contrast administration. CT may also show thickening of Gerota's fascia and stranding in the perinephric fat, as well as obliteration of surrounding soft tissue planes. Ultrasound is a useful imaging modality as well, but it is less sensitive than CT and cannot show the anatomic detail or associated findings nearly as well. The internal echopatterns of abscess cavities can vary widely on ultrasound, depending on the amount of tissue debris contained within them. Ultrasound is most convenient for percutaneous aspiration of abscesses and is often suitable for diagnosis.

Intravenous urography and plain abdominal films are less reliable tests in the patient with perinephric abscess. They do not show any abnormality at all in about 20% of cases (Thorley, Jones, and Sanford, 1974). When they do show abnormalities, they are generally nonspecific. Findings may include decreased excretion on the affected side, renal displacement, calyceal stretching or calyectasis, abnormal or obliterated renal outline, and renal calculi. Radionuclide studies are also less useful, playing only a minor role in diagnosis. With radiolabeled leukocytes, a day or two is required to allow accumulation of radioactivity in the abscess. When the test is suggestive of some disease, it often cannot be used to discriminate perinephric abscess from other forms of renal disease.

Management: Antibiotic therapy combined with abscess drainage is the mainstay of therapy. Until the results of culture and sensitivity tests taken from the abscess itself have returned, antibiotic therapy should be directed against the most likely organisms. The same drugs used to treat pyelonephritis would be appropriate in treating renal and perinephric abscesses. If blood cultures are negative and the patient responds to initial treatment, parenteral therapy can be converted to appropriate oral therapy after 3–5 days. Oral therapy should continue until full resolution both clinically and on repeat imaging studies. This usually takes several weeks. If bacteremia is present, parenteral therapy should last for 7–10 days before converting to oral therapy.

Drainage by placement of an appropriate percutaneous catheter under CT or ultrasound guidance is effective in certain patients (Finn, Palestrant, and De-Wolf, 1982; Fernandez, Miles, and Buck, 1985). If the abscess cavities are large, however, and filled with thick purulent material, then some authors suggest open surgical drainage, and possibly even nephrectomy if the kidney is nonfunctioning (Haaga and Weinstein, 1980). Also, if the patient's clinical course worsens or does not improve following percutaneous drainage and administration of appropriate antibiotics, open drainage should be performed.

Pyonephrosis & Infected Hydronephrosis

Infected hydronephrosis and pyonephrosis refer to the early and late stages of bacterial infection in a hydronephrotic, obstructed kidney. With pyonephrosis, suppurative destruction of the renal parenchyma results in significant loss of renal function and poses a threat to the patient's life. Patients with this condition usually present in extremis, with high fever, chills, and flank pain. Their past medical histories are often significant for calculi, UTIs, or previous urologic surgery. On urine culture, the bacterial pathogen can usually be isolated, except in those cases where the ureter is completely obstructed.

Ultrasound is helpful in establishing the diagnosis of pyonephrosis. It will show a dilated collecting system with dependent echoes suggestive of the accumulation of purulent sediment (Figure 14–4). These fluid-debris levels typically shift with changes in patient position. On the other hand, if the patient has only infected hydronephrosis, the collecting system will not show any internal echotexture.

Rapid treatment of pyonephrosis is essential. This consists of broad-spectrum parenteral antibiotic therapy combined with relief of obstruction and drainage of purulent material. Drainage can either be approached transurethrally, with a ureteral drainage catheter, or percutaneously via a nephrostomy tube.

Xanthogranulomatous Pyelonephritis

Etiology & Pathogenesis: Xanthogranulomatous pyelonephritis is an unusual form of chronic bacterial infection of the kidney that most often affects middle-aged and older women. The infection is severe and can cause widespread renal destruction.

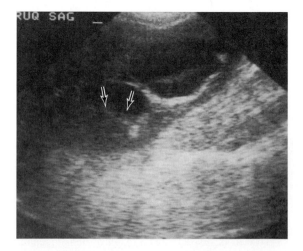

Figure 14–4. Pyonephrosis. Renal ultrasound shows a dilated pelvis with a discrete fluid-debris level indicative of pus in the collecting system.

The involved kidney is almost always hydronephrotic and obstructed, and the association with urolithiasis is high (Parsons et al, 1983). Although the etiology is obscure, it is likely that urinary obstruction followed by infection leads to accumulation of foamy lipid-laden macrophages (xanthoma cells). These xanthoma cells distribute around calyces and areas of parenchymal abscess and are associated with a granulomatous process that eventually obliterates the renal parenchyma. Because of their histologic characteristics, xanthoma cells may be confused with those seen in renal clear cell carcinoma. The most common organisms isolated from tissue cultures are *P mirabilis* and *E coli* (Tolia et al, 1981; Chuang et al, 1992; Eastham, Ahlering, and Skinner, 1994). On pathologic examination, the kidney typically shows yellow nodules of inflammatory tissue next to areas of parenchymal abscess. The inflammatory process can extend beyond the kidney, into the perinephric fat and retroperitoneum.

Clinical Features: Xanthogranulomatous pyelonephritis has been termed a great imitator owing to its variable presentation of clinical signs and symptoms. Intermittent flank pain and fever or chills are the most frequent symptoms, seen in 70–90% and 45–70% of patients, respectively; on physical examination, a palpable flank mass is present in 11–48% of patients (Malek and Elder, 1978; Chuang et al, 1992; Eastham, Ahlering, and Skinner, 1994). Patients may also present with symptoms attributable to involvement of adjacent tissues and organs in the inflammatory process. Draining flank sinuses have been described, as well as fistulas to bowel and joint spaces (Parsons et al, 1986; Eastham, Ahlering, and Skinner, 1994).

Diagnosis: Urine cultures are positive in about two-thirds of affected patients. Urinalysis shows protein and leukocytes. Tissue aspiration and culture are most effective in isolating the offending organism. Blood tests often reveal leukocytosis and anemia (Chuang et al, 1992; Eastham, Ahlering, and Skinner, 1994). Abnormal liver function tests are found in 50–80% of patients and may be due to a reactive hepatitis (Malek and Elder, 1978; Chuang et al, 1992; Eastham, Ahlering, and Skinner, 1994).

CT is the imaging modality of choice and can suggest the diagnosis preoperatively in up to 90% of cases (Eastham, Ahlering, and Skinner, 1994; Claes et al, 1987). It usually demonstrates areas of decreased signal intensity within the kidney, representing parenchymal infiltration by xanthoma cells, calyceal dilation, and abscess cavity (Figure 14–5). An area of central calcification can often be seen surrounded by a contracted renal pelvis (Solomon et al, 1983; Goodman et al, 1984; Eastham, Ahlering, and Skinner, 1994). With administration of intravenous contrast, the parenchyma surrounding the cystic hypodense areas will enhance, but typically little excretion will be observed. CT also characterizes the ex-

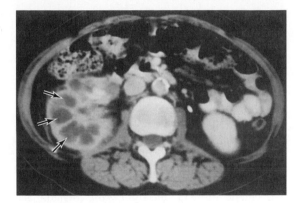

Figure 14–5. Xanthogranulomatous pyelonephritis. A contrast-enhanced computed tomography scan shows multiple centrally located hypodense areas in the right kidney (arrows) that correspond to areas of deposition of lipid-laden macrophages (xanthoma cells).

tent of invasion of the inflammatory mass into surrounding tissues. The psoas or quadratus lumborum might show involvement, as might the spleen, colon, and great vessels.

Other imaging studies are less sensitive than CT. Intravenous urography may show an enlarged renal shadow, renal calculi, poor contrast excretion, a renal mass, or calyceal deformity (Malek and Elder, 1978). Ultrasound usually shows renal enlargement and a stone in the renal pelvis. The hydronephrotic spaces are often filled with fluid of increased echogenicity, suggesting pyonephrosis (Van Kirk, Go, and Wedel, 1980; Eastham, Ahlering, and Skinner, 1994).

Management: Nephrectomy with excision of all involved tissue is usually required, but partial nephrectomy has been successfully performed in some patients with focal lesions, without relapse of disease (Tolia et al, 1980; Osca et al, 1997). Reports of association between xanthogranulomatous pyelonephritis and renal cell carcinoma, papillary transitional cell carcinoma, and infiltrating squamous cell carcinoma of the pelvis all support the approach of nephrectomy in the treatment of these patients (Schoborg et al, 1980; Pitts, Petersen, and Conley, 1981; Tolia et al, 1981). Incision and drainage alone do not eradicate the inflammatory and often infected mass. Furthermore, they can lead to the development of renocutaneous fistulae and make subsequent nephrectomy more difficult.

GENITOURINARY MALACOPLAKIA

Malacoplakia is a rare granulomatous disorder characterized by inflammatory, benign tumors composed primarily of macrophages and plasma cells.

Within the macrophages lie the lamellar inclusion bodies known as Michaelis-Guttman bodies, which are pathognomonic. These inclusion bodies are probably phagolysosomes, which harbor incompletely digested bacteria surrounded by a matrix of calcium apatite and iron salts. It appears that the granulomatous process responsible for malacoplakia results from defective bacterial digestion of phagocytosed bacteria by macrophages, which may be related to low intracellular levels of cyclic guanosine monophosphate (Abdou et al, 1977). The association between malacoplakia and chronic UTI is strong, with 90% of cases having positive cultures for gram-negative enteric bacteria, mostly *E coli* (Stanton and Maxted, 1981; Long and Althausen, 1989).

Malacoplakia is a disease that predominantly affects women, a fact largely reflected by its association with UTIs. Most patients are over 50 years old. Although these tumors can form throughout the body, 75% occur in the urinary tract, and within the urinary tract 70% of cases are found in the bladder, 15% in the upper tracts, and 15% in both (Stanton and Maxted, 1981). The clinical presentation of malacoplakia varies with the site of involvement. Concurrent systemic illness or an otherwise debilitating condition are not infrequent. Bladder involvement is suggested by hematuria and irritative voiding symptoms. Renal lesions may present with colicky flank pain, fever, and a flank mass. When renal involvement is bilateral, as in about 50% of cases (Stanton and Maxted, 1981), presentation with azotemia or uremia is not uncommon. In general, the symptoms of malacoplakia can mimic those of several other, more common UTIs, as well as genitourinary malignancy.

In patients with lower tract symptoms, cystoscopy usually reveals mucosal plaques or nodules. As the disease progresses, these lesions can become large, fungating masses. At this point, IVU may reveal filling defects in the affected portion of the collecting system. The inflammatory mass may also cause ureteral obstruction and hydronephrosis. On ultrasonography, multifocal renal involvement may display as renal enlargement and a general increase in parenchymal echotexture (Hartman et al, 1980). On CT, hypodense parenchymal masses may be seen focally or diffusely; CT can also demonstrate any extension outside the urinary tract (Hartman, 1985). Angiography generally shows a hypovascular mass with peripheral neovascularity (Cavins and Goldstein, 1977).

Successful medical therapy depends on treatment with antibiotics able to achieve adequate intracellular levels. TMP-SMX and the fluoroquinolones have been demonstrated to penetrate into cells (Maderazo, Berlin, and Marhardt, 1979; Easmon and Crane, 1985). The uptake of ciprofloxacin by macrophages is 2–3 times the extracellular values, making it the first choice in treatment of malacoplakia (Easmon

and Crane, 1985; Dohle, Zwartendijk, and van Krieken, 1993). Although somewhat controversial, bethanecol and ascorbic acid have been recommended to enhance phagolysosomal activity (Stanton and Maxted, 1981; Abdou et al, 1977). When malacoplakia is isolated to the lower urinary tract, medical therapy often suffices. The treatment of ureteral and renal disease, however, usually involves nephroureterectomy and antibiotic therapy (Long and Althausen, 1989). When renal disease is bilateral, the prognosis is poor and patients rarely survive beyond 6 months.

BLADDER INFECTIONS

Acute Cystitis

Etiology & Pathogenesis: Acute uncomplicated bacterial cystitis predominantly affects women. By definition, these are infections occurring in the absence of any anatomic or functional abnormality of the urinary tract. The ascending fecal-perineal-urethral route is the primary mode of infection. Men are somewhat protected from ascending infection by the antibacterial properties of prostatic secretions.

Reports consistently indicate that nearly 80% of bladder infections in women are caused by *E coli* (Jordan et al, 1980; Latham, Running, and Stamm, 1983; Stamm and Hooton, 1993). *Staphylococcus saprophyticus* and enterococci, representing the only significant participation of aerobic gram-positive organisms, are less frequent pathogens. Other coliform bacteria, including *Klebsiella* and *Proteus* spp., are sometimes found.

Clinical Features: Irritative voiding symptoms (frequency, urgency, and dysuria) are the hallmarks of acute cystitis. Low back and suprapubic pain are also frequent complaints. Occasionally the patient may note hematuria or cloudy, foul-smelling urine. In adults, fever and other constitutional symptoms are unusual. Physical examination reveals few characteristic signs, except occasional suprapubic tenderness.

Diagnosis: Urinalysis typically shows pyuria, bacteriuria, and occasionally hematuria. Urinary dipstick tests for the detection of bacterial nitrites or host leukocyte esterase are useful for making the presumptive diagnosis of bacteriuria, but urine culture is required for definitive confirmation of infection and identification of the pathogen. If the adult patient's symptoms and urinalysis are strongly suggestive of an uncomplicated infection, a urine culture may be avoided. Carlson and Mulley (1995) found that it may be more cost-effective to forego urine culture in routine cases, given the highly predictable nature of bacterial profiles in acute cystitis. When the diagnosis is not straightforward, or when the patient is a child, has recently received antibiotics, or has had other urinary infections, then the response to antibiotic therapy is less predictable and a pretherapy urine culture is required to diagnose and guide therapy.

Other laboratory tests or radiographic studies are rarely indicated in uncomplicated infections in adult women.

Management: For the treatment of routine acute UTI, almost any antibiotic that achieves adequate urinary levels is useful. TMP-SMX maintains excellent activity against the commonly infecting organisms. For patients with allergy to products containing sulfa, trimethoprim alone is probably just as efficacious as TMP-SMX (Harbord and Grueneberg, 1981). Nitrofurantoin is also effective and well tolerated, though it is more expensive than TMP-SMX. Resistance to nitrofurantoin is rare, and this makes it a good option for those patients who, through exposure to other antibiotics, have selected pathogens with resistant profiles; however, this agent may need to be reserved for those patients requiring long-term prophylaxis. Ampicillin and amoxicillin are more frequently associated with antibiotic resistance than TMP-SMX. Fluoroquinolones are expensive agents, but they have excellent activity against uropathogens.

Norrby (1990) analyzed 28 clinical trials conducted on women with uncomplicated cystitis to derive the optimal treatment duration. He found that, irrespective of which antibiotic agent is used, single-dose treatment is not as effective as 3-day treatment or treatment for 5 days or more, although the difference is less pronounced for TMP-SMX than for beta-lactams. Beta-lactams actually have unacceptably low cure rates when used as single-dose therapy. Beyond 3 days, all agents have higher incidences of adverse effects. A 3-day treatment course seems optimal.

Recurrent Urinary Tract Infection

Etiology & Pathogenesis: Either bacterial persistence or bacterial reinfection leads to recurrent UTIs. The recognition of this natural history of infections in any given patient is important in deciding on therapy. Bacterial persistence is usually curable by surgical removal of the infectious source, whereas reinfection is managed principally through medical prevention. Although reinfections are most often associated with ascending urethral infection, underlying urinary tract abnormalities can also cause them. Fistulas between the bladder and the bowel or vagina should be considered in any patient with reinfections who also complains of pneumaturia or fecaluria, or who has a history of diverticulitis, pelvic surgery, or pelvic irradiation. In these cases, surgical therapy may be curative.

Diagnosis: If bacterial persistence is suspected, a thorough investigation of the urinary tract should be undertaken. Typically, genitourinary imaging with ultrasonography can provide a primary survey of the lower and upper tracts; cystoscopy and IVU can provide more detailed assessments, if necessary. Occa-

sionally, retrograde studies of the upper tracts may be needed to visualize certain abnormalities, such as diverticulae and nonrefluxing ureteral stumps. Bacterial localization studies involving ureteral catheterization will confirm that the site of a detected abnormality corresponds to the source of bacteriuria. Additionally, localization studies for prostatitis should be undertaken in the appropriate clinical setting.

The evaluation of the patient with reinfection varies. If a vesicovaginal or vesicoenteric fistula is suspected, then CT imaging, cystoscopy, or radiocontrast GI studies may be employed. If ascending infection is suspected, and the patient does not exhibit signs of upper tract infection, then cystoscopy alone may be sufficient.

Management: The goal in cases of bacterial persistence should be the extirpation of any infectious source. Since the most common cause of persistence is infected calculi, SWL or endoscopic stone removal may be curative. Other congenital or acquired abnormalities usually require surgical correction.

In some patients, such as men with chronic bacterial prostatitis, the source of bacterial persistence may not be easily correctable. In these cases, long-term, low-dose suppressive antibiotic therapy with agents such as TMP-SMX, nitrofurantoin, or the fluoroquinolones may be necessary to prevent recurrent bacteriuria and recurrent symptoms.

Unless a fistula is present, the management of reinfections consists mainly of low-dose continuous prophylaxis. This regimen is employed once the urine is sterilized with a standard course of therapeutic antibiotics. The difference between prophylactic therapy and suppressive therapy is that prophylactic therapy aims to maintain a sterile urinary tract, whereas suppressive therapy keeps bacteria already present in the urinary tract from infecting the urine. Common prophylactic regimens are given in Table 14–6. Usually, the prophylactic regimen is continued for 6 months, during which the patient is monitored for reinfection. Remissions following the treatment course are not uncommon and require the reinstitution of prophylaxis.

Another variation of prophylaxis is the use of postintercourse dosing. Intercourse is a significant risk factor for reinfections (Nicolle et al, 1982). A

Table 14–6. Common low-dose prophylactic regimens for recurrent UTIs

---

Nitrofurantoin, 50 or 100 mg daily
Nitrofurantoin macrocrystals, 100 mg daily
TMP-SMX, 40/200 mg daily
Cephalexin, 250 mg daily
Ciprofloxacin, 250 mg daily
Trimethoprim, 100 mg daily

TMP-SMX = trimethoprim-sulfamethoxazole.

single dose of full-strength antibiotics taken after intercourse can reduce the incidence of reinfections in patients with a history of this problem (Pfau, Sacks, and Engelstein, 1983).

While antibiotic prophylactic regimens work, they are often associated with the emergence of bacterial resistance. As alternatives, intravaginal estriol, oral cranberry juice, and lactobacillus vaginal suppositories have been suggested (Raz and Stamm, 1993; Avorn et al, 1994; Reid, Bruce, and Taylor, 1992). Urinary tract infection vaccines have also been under development. The prime rationale for their development is the observation that urinary anti–*E coli* antibody prevents bacterial adherence to voided epithelial cells in vitro (Eden et al, 1976). A study using an intravaginal suppository containing heat-killed bacteria from 10 human uropathogenic isolates showed that the mean interval to reinfection was delayed from 8.7 weeks in control subjects to 13 weeks in patients receiving the vaccine, suggesting that vaginal mucosal immunization can enhance resistance in susceptible women (Uehling et al, 1997).

Research has also been aimed at using pili as vaccines to prevent bacterial infection. The development of antibodies directed at these bacterial adhesins would prevent mucosal colonization and subsequent infection. Along these lines, an adhesin-based systemic vaccination (using FimH, the adhesin that confers mannose-specific binding activity to type 1 pili) has been shown effective in blocking colonization in vivo in laboratory animals (Langermann et al, 1997).

BACTERIURIA IN PREGNANCY

During pregnancy, the urinary tract undergoes a number of anatomic and physiologic changes that are caused both by the gravid uterus and by an altered, progestational hormonal milieu. Ureteral peristalsis is generally dampened during pregnancy, and to some degree most women exhibit ureteral dilation, especially of the right side, by late in the gestation (Waltzer, 1981). Both progesterone's effect on smooth-muscle tone and ureteral compression from the gravid uterus have been cited as reasons for this hydroureter. Renal function is also affected. The renal plasma flow and the glomerular filtration rate increase significantly during pregnancy, the latter by 30–50% (Davison and Lindheimer, 1978; Waltzer, 1981). As a result, average values for serum creatinine and urea nitrogen are lower in pregnant women than in their nonpregnant counterparts (Davison and Lindheimer, 1978). The renal excretion of protein is also increased in pregnant women.

The anatomic and physiologic changes of pregnancy alter the natural history of bacteriuria in pregnant women. Pregnant women are more susceptible to pyelonephritis than their nonpregnant counterparts, even though the incidence of bacteriuria in both these groups is similar, ranging from 3% to 9% (Stamey, 1980; Sweet, 1977). Whereas acute bacterial pyelonephritis rarely develops from uncomplicated cases of bacteriuria found on screening in nonpregnant women, studies have shown that pregnant women found to have bacteriuria during screening have a 13.5–65% incidence of pyelonephritis (Sweet, 1977). Furthermore, treatment of bacteriuria found on screening during pregnancy reduces the incidence of acute pyelonephritis from 13.5–65% down to 0–5.3% (Sweet, 1977).

Untreated pyelonephritis during pregnancy is associated with a high rate of premature delivery and infant mortality. When pyelonephritis is recognized and treated, however, its effect on the fetus is controversial. Some studies indicate that renal infections treated antepartum, whether symptomatic or not, do not adversely affect the outcome of pregnancy (Gilstrap et al, 1981). Other studies have shown that the infant mortality rate more than doubles when the pregnancy is associated with UTI (McGrady, Daling, and Petersen, 1985). Although the effect on the fetus remains unclear, pyelonephritis does have potential complications for the mother. Bacteriuria in a pregnant woman should be treated regardless of symptoms.

Pregnant women should be systematically screened for bacteriuria to help prevent the development of pyelonephritis. Urine culture obtained at the first prenatal visit and again at week 16 reveals most women at risk for symptomatic UTI during pregnancy (Stenqvist et al, 1989). When bacteriuria is detected on screening, it should be treated. The choice of antibiotic is greatly limited by known antibiotic toxicities during pregnancy. In general, only the penicillins and cephalosporins can be regarded as safe throughout the gestation. A 3-day course of an oral agent in either class should be employed for screening bacteriuria. Bacterial eradication should then be documented with follow-up cultures. If reinfection or bacterial persistence is an issue, the woman should be placed on low-dose prophylaxis or suppression throughout the remainder of her pregnancy.

Acute bacterial pyelonephritis in a pregnant woman requires the administration of parenteral antibiotics. After therapy, periodic urine cultures should be obtained for the remainder of the pregnancy, as these women are at increased risk for repeated pyelonephritis (Gilstrap et al, 1981).

PROSTATITIS

Prostatitis is a prevalent and debilitating disease. A 1990 National Institutes of Health report tabulated more clinician visits for prostatitis than either benign prostatic hypertrophy or prostate cancer. A more recent national survey of physician visits showed that prostatitis is the most common urologic diagnosis in men under 50 years of age, and the third most common in older men, with 2 million outpatient visits yearly between the two groups (Collins et al, 1998). From 10% to 30% of men will have had a diagnosis of prostatitis by 79 years of age (Roberts et al, 1998; de la Rosette et al, 1992).

Despite its prevalence and its drain on health care resources, our understanding of the etiology, diagnosis, and treatment of prostatitis has not advanced with that of other prostate diseases. Only recently has a consensus been reached on the definition and classification of prostatitis syndromes. In 1995, the National Institute of Diabetes and Digestive and Kidney Diseases Workshop on Chronic Prostatitis proposed a new scheme, outlined in Table 14–7 (National Institutes of Health, 1995). Categories I and II represent the traditional forms of acute and chronic bacterial prostatitis, defined by the presence of both prostatic inflammation and uropathogenic bacteria in prostatic culture. Category III, chronic pelvic pain syndrome (CPPS), is characterized by prostatitislike symptoms in the absence of bacterial localization to the prostate. The 2 subcategories of CPPS are distinguished by the presence or absence of leukocytes in prostatic fluid or the urine voided after prostatic massage. Category IV, or asymptomatic prostatitis, is defined as pathologic evidence of prostatic inflammation in patients without symptoms and would include patients who have prostatic inflammation found incidentally on biopsies done for other prostate diseases.

Diagnostic Techniques

Meares and Stamey (1968) described the 4-glass test in 1968, and since then it has become the standard in prostatitis diagnosis. This technique allows localization of bacteria by examining specimens from the urethra, midstream urine, and prostatic secretions. The examiner obtains the first voided 10 mL of urine (urethral specimen), a late midstream sample (bladder specimen), a specimen of prostatic secretions following prostatic massage, and the first voided 10 mL of urine following massage. The specimens are labeled VB1, VB2, EPS, and VB3, respectively, and sent for bacterial identification and quantification using standard microbiologic methods. If

the VB2 is sterile or has very low colony counts, urethral colonization or infection would be suggested by a higher colony count in VB1 than in both EPS and VB3. Conversely, the EPS and VB3 specimens in patients with bacterial prostatitis demonstrate at least a 10-fold increase in bacterial growth over VB1.

Localization specimens can also be centrifuged and their sediments examined microscopically for assessment of prostatic inflammation. Most studies indicate that prostatic fluid normally contains ≤ 10 leukocytes per high-power field (HPF) (Anderson and Weller, 1979; Schaeffer, Jones, and Dunn, 1981). An increased density of leukocytes, particularly if accompanied by lipid-laden macrophages, implies prostatic inflammation. Despite these general findings, normal or near-normal EPS leukocyte densities may be seen in specimens from patients with chronic bacterial prostatitis undergoing antimicrobial therapy. Additionally, some 5–10% of normal men will have EPS specimens with leukocyte densities > 10 per HPF (Anderson and Weller, 1979; Schaeffer, Jones, and Dunn, 1981). For these reasons, examination of the sediment must be viewed as complementary to bacteriologic studies, and not as a replacement for them.

A simple alternative to the 4-glass test, designed to facilitate screening for prostatitis, is the pre- and postmassage test (Nickel, 1997). In patients with no clinical evidence of urethritis, urine specimens are obtained before and after prostatic massage. Comparing the presence and amount of bacteria and leukocytes in the 2 specimens allows almost as accurate a classification as the 4-glass test. This test works best in patients before any antibiotic therapy has begun. Examination and culture of the EPS, however, still remains the gold standard.

Acute Bacterial Prostatitis

Etiology & Pathogenesis: Aerobic gram-negative organisms principally cause acute bacterial prostatitis. The incidence of infection by various species and their antibiotic susceptibilities follow those of organisms that regularly infect the urine. *E coli* is implicated in 80% of infections (Stamey, 1980; Lopez-Plaza and Bostwick, 1990). *Pseudomonas aeruginosa, Serratia, Klebsiella,* and *Proteus* species account for 10–15% of cases and enterococci for

Table 14–7. NIDDK categorization and criteria for the prostatitis syndromes.

NIDDK Classification	Criteria
Category I: Acute bacterial prostatitis	Acute, symptomatic bacterial infection
Category II: Chronic bacterial prostatitis	Recurrent prostate infection
Category III: Chronic pelvic pain syndorme	No clearly identifiable infection
IIIA: Inflammatory type	Leukocytes present in prostatic fluid (> 10/HPF)
IIIB: Noninflammatory type	No leukocytes in prostatic fluid (< 10/HPF)
Category IV: Asymptomatic inflammatory prostatitis	No subjective symptoms; detected incidentally on biopsy or examination of prostate fluid

NIDDK = National Institute of Diabetes and Digestive and Kidney Diseases.

5–10% (Lopez-Plaza and Bostwick, 1990; Meares, 1987). Other than enterococci, the gram-positive bacteria become pathogenic only under special circumstances (eg, *S aureus* infection associated with catheterization) (Bergman, 1994). Anaerobes rarely cause prostate infections. Although most infections are caused by a single organism, they can be polymicrobial.

Bacterial prostatitis probably results from ascending urethral infection (Blacklock, 1974; Stamey, 1980) and from reflux of infected urine into prostatic ducts (Kirby et al, 1982; Meares, 1991). Intraprostatic reflux of urine may indeed play the most important role. Prostate anatomy has something to do with this (Blacklock, 1991). Most infections occur in the peripheral zone, where the ducts drain horizontally into the urethra, facilitating reflux of urine as well as intraductal stasis. Glands of the central zone empty obliquely and completely into the prostatic urethra, preventing easy reflux and stagnation. Invasion by rectal bacteria, either directly or via lymphogenous spread, has also been suggested to cause prostatitis.

Clinical Features: Acute bacterial prostatitis is marked by fever and chills; rectal, low back, and perineal pain; and urinary urgency, frequency, and dysuria. Prostatic swelling may produce acute urinary retention. Malaise, arthralgia, and myalgia are also common.

Digital rectal examination reveals an exquisitely tender, enlarged gland that is irregularly firm and warm. The urine may be cloudy and malodorous owing to concomitant urinary infection. Gross hematuria is observed occasionally.

Diagnosis: Acute bacterial prostatitis is often diagnosed on the basis of symptoms and physical examination alone. A complete blood count typically shows leukocytosis with a shift toward immature forms. The voided urine shows pyuria, microscopic hematuria, and bacteria. Culture of a voided urine sample usually identifies the infecting organism. The 4-glass test, or any prostate massage, is not recommended owing both to the extreme discomfort of the procedure and to the possibility of inducing bacteremia. For much the same reasons, transurethral catheterization should be avoided. Acute urinary retention requiring bladder drainage should be managed with a suprapubic tube.

Management: The intense inflammation and diffuse edema of acute prostatitis make it particularly susceptible to antibiotic therapy. Patients will often respond dramatically to agents that would otherwise diffuse poorly into prostatic tissue. The choice of antibiotic is ultimately guided by in vitro susceptibility testing. Empiric treatment should not be delayed, however, and should be directed primarily against gram-negative rods and enterococci. The fluoroquinolones work very well as initial therapy (Naber, 1989; Andriole, 1991), as does TMP-SMX. Supportive measures include antipyretics, analgesics, stool softeners, hydration, and bed rest. The recommended duration of antibiotic treatment is 4–6 weeks to prevent the development of such complications as prostatic abscess and chronic prostatitis (Childs, 1992). Most otherwise healthy men can be treated as outpatients. Several factors warrant hospital admission, however, including sepsis, immunodeficiency, and acute urinary retention. Patients with significant comorbidities also require close observation. In cases requiring admission, parenteral antibiotics, usually consisting of ampicillin and an aminoglycoside, should be used. A suitable oral agent can be substituted once antibiotic sensitivities are obtained.

Eradication of bacterial infection needs to be documented as part of routine patient management. A VB2 sample sent for quantitative culture 1 and 3 months after antibiotic therapy helps to identify those patients with persistent bacteriuria at risk for prostatic abscess and chronic prostatitis. If found, further treatment action, described below, would need to be implemented.

As mentioned previously, any transurethral catheterization or instrumentation is contraindicated during acute infection. Acute urinary retention should be managed with suprapubic drainage until the patient is able to void spontaneously.

Complications: Prostatic abscess can develop in the setting of acute prostatitis. Immunocompromised patients, diabetics, those with indwelling urethral catheters, or those on chronic dialysis are all at higher risk for this complication. Some patients may progress to chronic bacterial prostatitis if attention is not focused on bacterial eradication.

Chronic Bacterial Prostatitis

Etiology & Pathogenesis: The causative organisms in chronic bacterial prostatitis are the same as those in acute prostatitis, namely, the gram-negative enterics and enterococci. Most authorities agree that other gram-positive organisms probably do not play a significant role in this disease. When they are causative, they rarely lead to recurrent UTI. A lot of debate concerns the role of mycoplasmal, ureaplasmal, and chlamydial species in the etiology of prostatitis, and most of it is centered on the chronic pelvic pain syndromes. These organisms are not appreciable pathogens in chronic bacterial prostatitis.

Intraprostatic reflux and the ductal anatomy cited for acute prostatitis contribute to chronic bacterial infection. Some investigators feel that a secretory dysfunction may also play a role. Although argument exists over the pH of normal prostatic secretions, the secretions in men with chronic bacterial prostatitis are uniformly alkaline (Anderson and Fair, 1976; Fair et al, 1979). This alkalinity may hinder antibiotic activity in prostatic fluid by affecting passage of antimicrobial agents from plasma into prostatic fluid (Meares, 1997). Zinc has shown bactericidal activity against gram-negative organisms, as well as inhibition of viral, yeast, and chlamydial growth (Fair, Couch, and Wehner, 1976; Fridlender, Chejanovsky, and Becker, 1978; Mardh, Colleen, and Sylwan, 1980). Free zinc, otherwise known as prostatic antibacterial factor, is at low levels in men with chronic bacterial prostatitis (Fair, Couch, and Wehner, 1976).

Intraprostatic bacterial sequestration can hinder treatment of this disease. Bacterial microcolonies encased in a calyx of polysaccharides adhere to ductal and acinar walls and are impervious to antibiotics. Prostatic calculi also provide sanctuary for pathogens. A large proportion of men with chronic bacterial prostatitis have multiple large prostatic calculi demonstrable on transrectal ultrasonography that can serve as a source for bacterial persistence and recurrent UTIs (Meares, 1986). Bacterial reinfection of the prostate may occur in these men just as reinfection occurs in women susceptible to UTI (Shortliffe and Wehner, 1986).

Clinical Features: Most patients report dysuria as well as urgency, frequency, and nocturia. Low back and perineal pain or discomfort are also common. The natural history is marked by disease relapse with occasional acute exacerbations, at which time fever, chills, and malaise might manifest. Sometimes, however, the diagnosis is made in an asymptomatic patient in whom bacteriuria is found incidentally.

There are no characteristic findings on digital rectal examination. The prostate frequently feels normal, although tenderness, swelling, and firmness can be present. Large prostatic calculi may cause crepitation in part of the gland. Secondary epididymitis is sometimes associated. Hematuria, hematospermia, and urethral discharge are rare.

Diagnosis: Laboratory diagnosis of chronic bacterial prostatitis is based on the 4-glass test described above. If VB2 indicates a bladder infection, the patient should be treated for 4–5 days with an antibiotic that has poor penetration into the prostate, and then the segmental specimens should be recollected. To confirm the diagnosis, the colony counts in EPS and VB3 should exceed those of VB1 and VB2 by at least 10-fold (Meares and Stamey, 1968). Since prostatic infection is a focal process and sampling errors are inevitable, falsely negative results do occur. Two or more bacterial localization tests may then be required to identify the pathogenic bacteria. If no organisms can be cultured, and the prostatic fluid has an increased leukocyte count (> 10 per HPF), a diagnosis of chronic pelvic pain syndrome (inflammatory type) can be made.

These patients are prone to bacteriuria and recurrent episodes of cystitis caused by the same organism. Despite sterilization in the urine, the pathogen often remains sheltered in the prostate because most standard antibiotics diffuse poorly into prostatic fluid. After therapy, infection of the urine can arise again from prostatic sources. The recurrent UTI is indeed a hallmark of chronic bacterial prostatitis.

Serum analysis is rarely helpful. The complete blood count does not show leukocytosis unless the patient is experiencing a flare. The prostate-specific antigen may be elevated, probably because of disruption or increased permeability of prostatic glandular epithelium. However, there is no evidence that response to treatment corresponds with the level of prostate-specific antigen.

Management: Chronic bacterial prostatitis is a difficult and frustrating entity to treat. The course of therapy is long, and definitive cure is often not achieved. The greatest therapeutic difficulties stem from the poor penetration of most antibiotic agents into prostatic fluid and the stubborn foci of bacterial growth within the prostate.

Factors that promote antibiotic diffusion into prostatic fluid include lipid solubility, weak binding to plasma proteins, and an uncharged state. It appears from most recent testing that the newer fluoroquinolones have the most favorable diffusion characteristics. Other useful agents include TMP-SMX, carbenicillin, doxycycline, minocycline, amikacin, and carbenecillin. At least 3–4 months of treatment is generally recommended, although some studies have reported success with a 4-week course of a fluoroquinolone. Barbalias, Nikiforidis, and Liatsikos (1998) found that addition of an alpha blocker to antibiotic therapy significantly reduced the number of symptom recurrences over antibiotics alone.

Even with such therapy, relapses occur. At this point, suppressive therapy aimed at eliminating bacterial growth in the urine is often instituted. Most antibiotics are concentrated in the urine, allowing for drastically reduced dosing while maintaining bactericidal efficacy. The most common daily suppressive regimens are nitrofurantoin (100 mg daily), TMP-SMX (1 single-strength tablet daily), and ciprofloxacin (250 mg daily). Suppressive therapy can provide relief from symptoms for most men.

Surgical therapy often provides the only chance at cure in relapsing cases. Complete prostatectomy would likely be curative, but its morbidity limits its usefulness. TURP has been described as an alternative treatment. Since prostate infection primarily affects the peripheral zone, and since this area is most difficult to excise at TURP, this treatment appears disadvantaged. However, infected prostatic calculi and bacterial microcolonies (enclosed in biofilms and adherent to duct walls) may be removed transurethrally, thereby eliminating a nidus for reinfection of the peripheral zones. Studies of patients undergoing TURP for chronic bacterial prostatitis followed by 6–8 weeks of antibiotic therapy have had varying success rates, anywhere from 30% to 100%. Meares reported a 100% success rate using a "radical" TURP in 12 patients, yet he still could not recommend the procedure for most patients with the disease.

Complications: Recurrent UTIs (reinfections) are a major complication of chronic bacterial prostatitis. It may also lead to infertility. Reports of successful treatment of prostatitis leading to improvement in semen parameters and to pregnancy have been made. Although more difficult to quantify, the negative impact of chronic bacterial prostatitis on quality of life probably cannot be overstated.

Chronic Pelvic Pain Syndrome

Etiology & Pathogenesis: Chronic pelvic pain syndrome, category III in the NIDDK scheme (Table 14–7), is both the most common form of prostatitis and the most poorly understood. The category is divided into inflammatory (category IIIA) and noninflammatory (category IIIB) forms, based on the presence of leukocytes in prostatic fluid. The inflammatory type has previously been called nonbacterial prostatitis and is associated with elevated prostatic immunoglobulin levels; the noninflammatory type has been called prostatodynia and is not associated with increased immunoglobulins (Shortliffe and Wehner, 1986). Clinical symptoms between the two subgroups are essentially the same.

A lot of investigational activity has been focused on the role of fastidious organisms in the etiology of these diseases. *C trachomatis,* a common cause of urethritis in men, has been studied extensively. Several studies have demonstrated chlamydial antigen in prostatic fluid and antichlamydial antibodies in sera of men with CPPS (Abdelatif, Chandler, and McGuire, 1991; Weidner, Scheifer, and Krauss, 1988; Ostaszewska et al, 1998). Other studies, however, have not shown any link (Berger et al, 1989; Shortliffe, Seller, and Schachter, 1992; Doble et al, 1989). Shortliffe, Seller, and Schachter (1992) found no difference in the level of antibodies to chlamydiae in the prostatic fluid of normal men and those with CPPS. Doble et al (1989) performed transperineal prostate biopsy of men with CPPS and failed to detect chlamydiae by either immunofluorescence or culture. Other studies have examined the role of ureaplasmas and mycoplasmas and found varying results.

Berger and associates (1997) recently did urethral and urine cultures as well as transperineal biopsies to look for commensal, anaerobic, and fastidious organisms. They isolated bacteria from the biopsies of 32% of their 85 subjects. Nearly half of the isolates were anaerobes; of the aerobes, most were coagulase-negative staphylococcal and coryneform organisms. They found no difference in the number of positive cultures between men with prostate inflammation and men without. They did not biopsy a control group for comparison, however, so the positive biopsy rate in asymptomatic men is unknown. The role of any infectious organism is still controversial.

A mechanistic association has been claimed between backflow of urine into prostatic ducts and a subsequent chemically induced inflammatory reaction of the prostate. Kirby et al (1982) demonstrated evidence of more urinary backflow in patients with CPPS than in normal subjects. Persson and Ronquist (1996) found that backflow of urine could lead to high concentrations of urinary urate and creatinine in prostate fluid, inducing a chemical prostatitis. They saw a positive correlation between prostate pain, leukocyte count in prostate fluid, and urate concentration in prostate fluid. In both of these studies, however, patients with positive bacterial cultures were included in the analysis along with patients having no culture growth, greatly complicating the interpretation of their findings.

Urodynamic evaluations have prompted some to propose urethral hypertonia as a cause of CPPS, noninflammatory type. Barbalias, Nikiforidis, and Liatsikos (1998) found an increased maximal urethral closure pressure and a decreased urinary flow rate in patients with CPPS compared with control subjects. They attributed the high maximal urethral closure pressure to increased adrenergic stimulation in the proximal urethra and bladder neck and proposed that this might cause intraprostatic reflux of urine. Based on these observations they suggested "painful male urethral syndrome" as a more appropriate term for the disorder. In other patients, spasm of pelvic floor muscles may operate alone or in combination with bladder neck dysfunction to bring about chronic pelvic pain.

Could either form of CPPS be an autoimmune process? A subpopulation of men with this disorder had evidence of significant T-cell response to normal prostatic proteins found in seminal plasma, a response not seen in normal control subjects (Alexander, Brady, and Ponniah, 1997). Whether this autoimmune response was initiated by infection with microorganisms or came about by other means is unknown.

Clinical Features: Clinical features of CPPS are similar to those of chronic bacterial prostatitis. Pain symptoms predominate, especially in the perineum, penis, and testicles. Voiding dysfunction consisting of dysuria, slow stream, urgency, and frequency also occurs commonly. Sexual dysfunction has been described. Krieger et al (1996) found no difference in any symptom parameter between men with inflamed or uninflamed prostatic secretions.

These patients should have no history of bladder infection. On examination, their prostates can be normal or tender. They may have tenderness of pelvic floor musculature on palpation and a tight anal sphincter.

Diagnosis: Examination of the EPS in patients with inflammatory CPPS shows numerous leukocytes and lipid-laden macrophages. Anderson and Weller (1979) observed a 5-fold increase in leukocytes and an 8-fold increase in lipid-laden macrophages in prostate fluids of men with this type of prostatitis compared with control subjects. In noninflammatory CPPS there is a paucity of positive laboratory findings. Urodynamic evaluation may disclose urethral hypertonia and diminished flow in the absence of striated sphincter dyssynergia.

Management: Definitive treatment for CPPS is not available. Some patients do enjoy symptomatic improvement on antibiotics. This has prompted the recommendation of a trial of antibiotic therapy (Meares, 1987; de la Rosette and Debruyne, 1991). Generally, a fluoroquinolone is used. If chlamydia is suspected, then tetracycline, minocycline, doxycycline, or erythromycin should be chosen. Antibiotic therapy should probably continue for several weeks.

Alpha-adrenergic blocking agents have shown some usefulness. By decreasing adrenergic tone in the proximal urethra, alpha blockers would act to alleviate urethral hypertonia and might by extension help prevent intraprostatic reflux of urine. Barbalias et al actually found that patients with CPPS had a lower symptom recurrence rate when treated with alpha blockers alone compared with those treated with alpha blockers and antibiotics in combination (Barbalias, Nikiforidis, and Liatsikos, 1998).

High concentrations of urate in urine can be reduced with the use of allopurinol, a xanthine oxidase inhibitor. This may alleviate chemical irritation in the prostate caused by refluxed urine and reduce the symptoms of CPPS. Persson, Ronquist, and Ekblom (1996) observed a significant effect of allopurinol on urate concentration in prostatic fluid and a significant decrease in discomfort in treated patients compared with untreated controls. They did not, however, find any difference in the leukocyte counts in prostate fluid between the two groups.

Pelvic floor relaxation techniques, biofeedback, prostate physical therapy (massage), and muscle relaxants may all reduce pelvic floor spasticity and, in turn, chronic pain symptoms. Anti-inflammatory agents, sitz baths, and normal sexual activity may provide symptomatic relief. Surgical therapy using transurethral microwave thermotherapy and neodynium:YAG laser therapy has been described.

Complications: CPPS may have a significant effect on fertility. Lower sperm counts and abnormal morphologic and motility characteristics have been observed in affected patients (Leib et al, 1994; Christiansen, Tollefsrud, and Purvis, 1991). These parameters may worsen with time. As with chronic bacterial prostatitis, quality of life is adversely affected.

Granulomatous Prostatitis

Granulomatous prostatitis can result from bacterial, viral, or fungal infection; from iatrogenic causes such as the use of bacille Calmette-Guérin therapy for bladder cancer; from systemic granulomatous disease; from malacoplakia; or from some nonspecific cause. Two-thirds of cases are nonspecific (Lopez-Plaza and Bostwick, 1990). Of these, some have an eosinophilic infiltrate and others do not. The eosinophilic type usually occurs in men who are asthmatic or prone to allergy. The noneosinophilic type may result from a granulomatous reaction to extravasation of prostatic fluid into the stroma (O'Dea, Hunting, and Greene, 1977; Epstein and Hutchins, 1984).

A variety of symptoms are common. Granulomatous prostatitis may present as an acute illness, with fever, chills, and irritative and obstructive voiding symptoms, much like acute bacterial prostatitis. On digital rectal examination, the prostate is often hard, fixed, and variably indurated. These findings are often mistaken for carcinoma. Prostatic biopsy is required to confirm the diagnosis. Urine culture may help in patients with a history suggestive of tuberculosis or systemic mycotic disease.

The nonspecific cases may respond to corticosteroids, especially those that are eosinophilic (Meares, 1997). If a treatable pathogen can be identified, therapy should be appropriately targeted.

Prostatic Abscess

Most cases of prostatic abscess are probably complications of acute bacterial prostatitis, with *E coli* the predominant organism. An initial favorable response to the treatment of acute bacterial prostatitis followed by a recrudescence of symptoms suggests abscess formation. The clinical picture often mimics that of acute bacterial prostatitis but can be highly variable. On digital rectal examination, the gland is tender and swollen, and there may be fluctuance over the affected area.

Prostate imaging with either transrectal ultrasound or pelvic CT is essential in the diagnosis and for guiding therapy (Figure 14–6). These imaging techniques can guide transrectal or percutaneous aspiration and drainage of abscess cavities. Transurethral incision and resection may be required if needle drainage does not suffice. Pathogen-specific antibiotics are also required.

Most cases resolve without serious complications. The mortality rate before the advent of antibiotics was 30%; it is now about 5% (Weinberger et al, 1988).

EPIDIDYMITIS

Etiology & Pathogenesis: Inflammation of the epididymis most often results from ascent of pathogens from the lower urinary tract. An increased pressure in the prostatic urethra experienced during voiding may alter the urethrovasal closure mechanism enough to allow ingress of microorganisms into the vas deferens. Thind, Gerstenberg, and Bilde (1990) documented a higher intravesical voiding pressure in patients with a history of epididymitis compared with control subjects and postulated that this pressure might promote urethrovasal reflux. On occasion, urethral instrumentation or prostatic

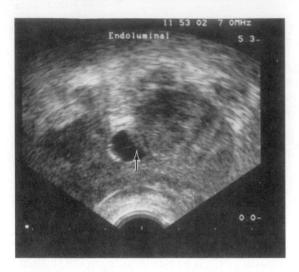

Figure 14–6. Prostatic abscess. Transrectal ultrasound in the transverse plane of a patient in left lateral decubitus position. Note layering of debris along the right side (patient's left side) of the hypoechoic cystic cavity.

surgery may result in bacterial ascent. The microorganisms that find their way into the vas deferens and epididymis vary with the age of the patient. Several extended microbiologic studies have shown that *C trachomatis* is the pathogen most frequently found in men less than 40 years old and that coliform bacteria are more common in older men (Berger et al, 1979; Melekos and Asbach, 1987). These data suggest that epididymitis in younger men is primarily a sexually transmitted disease, whereas in older men it is more often a result of bacteriuria and prostatitis. Epididymitis in an infant or young boy happens much less commonly than it does in adults and is often associated with genitourinary anomalies, such as ureteral drainage into a vas deferens or seminal vesicle.

After the onset of infection, the epididymis becomes swollen and indurated. As a result of venous congestion, the testis often becomes swollen as well. In cases of severe epididymitis, the testis may even become involved in the inflammatory process (epididymo-orchitis). A reactive hydrocele may also develop.

Clinical Features: The scrotal pain associated with epididymitis can be quite severe and can radiate along the inguinal canal and even to the flank. The patient often notes that scrotal size has increased rapidly, often doubling over a short time. Fever may be present. Additionally, symptoms of urethritis, cystitis, or prostatitis may precede or be intercurrent with the scrotal complaints.

On examination, the scrotum is usually enlarged and reddened. The epididymis is often indistinguishable from the testis, as the two become obscured by one large inflammatory mass. The spermatic cord is thickened. Tenderness may be elicited on lower abdominal palpation on the affected side. If urethritis is also present, urethral discharge may be noted.

Diagnosis: A complete blood count typically reveals leukocytosis. Gram's stain of a urethral smear and of a midstream urine often allows for presumptive diagnosis of the offending organism. *N gonorrhoeae* would show up as intracellular gram-negative diplococci on the urethral smear. The absence of these diplococci, in conjunction with leukocytes on the smear, would suggest nongonococcal urethritis, most often caused by *C trachomatis*. Gram-negative rods in the urine would indicate epididymitis caused by enteric organisms.

The most important aspect of diagnosing acute epididymitis is differentiating it from testicular torsion. Two scrotal imaging modalities typically employed for this end are Doppler ultrasonography and radionuclide scanning. Doppler ultrasonography is the more commonly used. In men with epididymitis, the objective with Doppler ultrasound is to demonstrate an arterial pulse within the affected testicle, which should be louder than the pulse on the contralateral side. Absence or attenuation of the pulse would warrant surgical exploration for torsion. Radionuclide scanning is probably more accurate than Doppler ultrasound, but it is less readily available in an emergency setting. In this study, distribution of radiotracer into the affected testicle relies on a patent testicular artery. Patients with torsion have a cold area on the symptomatic side, whereas patients with epididymitis have a hot area.

Management: Epididymitis associated with urethritis or the identification of *N gonorrhoeae* on urethral swab should be treated with single-dose coverage of *N gonorrhoeae* (usually ceftriaxone, 1 g intramuscularly) followed by a 10-day course of tetracycline or erythromycin to cover *C trachomatis*. Additionally, the patient's sexual partner should be screened and treated appropriately. If enteric bacteriuria is found, a 2-week course of broad-spectrum oral antibiotics should be initiated. Occasionally, patients with systemic illness or severe infection require admission and parenteral antibiotic therapy. Supportive measures include bed rest, scrotal elevation, and pain medications.

Complications: Severe epididymitis may lead to abscess formation requiring open drainage. Testicular infarction has also been reported. Patients may sometimes develop chronic epididymitis after an acute attack and repeated mild infections. Chronic epididymitis leads to induration and fibrosis of part or all of the organ, often with resulting tubular occlusion. As a consequence, these patients can become secondarily infertile. In addition, they may also have symptoms of chronic scrotal pain. Once they have reached this stage, epididymectomy may be the only therapeutic option.

REFERENCES

Abdelatif OM, Chandler FW, McGuire BS: *Chlamydia trachomatis* in chronic abacterial prostatitis: Demonstration by colorimetric in situ hybridization. Hum Pathol 1991;22:41.

Abdou NI et al: Malakoplakia: Evidence of monocyte abnormality correctable by cholinergic agonists in vitro and in vivo. N Engl J Med 1977;297:1413.

Ahlering TE et al: Emphysematous pyelonephritis: A 5-year experience with 13 patients. J Urol 1985;134:1086.

Alexander RB, Brady F, Ponniah S: Autoimmune prostatitis: Evidence of T cell reactivity with normal prostatic proteins. Urology 1997;50:893.

Anderson KA, McAninch JW: Renal abscesses: Classification and review of 40 cases. Urology 1980;16:333.

Anderson RU, Fair WR: Physical and chemical determinations of prostatic secretion in benign hyperplasia, prostatitis, and adenocarcinoma. Invest Urol 1976;3:137.

Anderson RU, Weller C: Prostatic secretion leukocyte studies in non-bacterial prostatitis (prostatosis). J Urol 1979;121:292.

Andriole VT: Use of quinolones in treatment of prostatitis and lower urinary tract infections. Eur J Clin Microbiol Infect Dis 1991;10:342.

Avorn J et al: Reduction of bacteriuria and pyuria after ingestion of cranberry juice. JAMA 1994;271:751.

Bailey RR et al: DMSA renal scans in adults with acute pyelonephritis. Clin Nephrol 1996;46:99.

Barbalias GA, Nikiforidis G, Liatsikos EN: α-Blockers for the treatment of chronic prostatitis in combination with antibiotics. J Urol 1998;159:883.

Behr MA et al: Fever duration in hospitalized acute pyelonephritis patients. Am J Med 1996;101:277.

Berger RE et al: Bacteria in the prostate tissue of men with idiopathic prostatic inflammation. J Urol 1997;157:863.

Berger RE et al: Case-control study of men with suspected chronic idiopathic prostatitis. J Urol 1989;141:328.

Berger RE et al: Etiology, manifestations and therapy of acute epididymitis: prospective study of 50 cases. J Urol 1979;121:750.

Bergman B: On the relevance of gram-positive bacteria in prostatitis. Infection 1994;22:S22.

Bhatia NN et al: Antibiotic prophylaxis following lower urinary tract instrumentation. Urology 1992;39:583.

Blacklock NJ: Anatomical factors in prostatitis. Br J Urol 1974;46:47.

Blacklock NJ: The anatomy of the prostate: Relationship with prostatic infection. Infection 1991;19:S111.

Breidahl WH et al: Power Doppler sonography in the assessment of musculoskeletal fluid collections. AJR 1996;166:1443.

Cardiff-Oxford Bacteriuria Study Group: The sequelae of urinary tract infections in schoolgirls: A 4-year follow-up study. Lancet 1978;1:889.

Carlson KJ, Mulley AG: Management of acute dysuria: A decision-analysis model of alternative strategies. Ann Intern Med 1985;102:244.

Cavins JA, Goldstein AMB: Renal malacoplakia. Urology 1977;10:155.

Chen M-T et al: Percutaneous drainage in the treatment of emphysematous pyelonephritis: 10-year experience. J Urol 1997;157:1569.

Childs SJ: Prostatitis: Current diagnosis and treatment. Contemp Urol 1992;4:31.

Christ W, Lehnert T, Ulbrich B: Specific toxologic aspects to the quinolones. Rev Infect Dis 1988;10:41.

Christiansen E, Tollefsrud A, Purvis K: Sperm quality in men with chronic abacterial prostatovesiculitis verified by rectal ultrasonography. Urology 1991;38:545.

Chuang C-K et al: Xanthogranulomatous pyelonephritis: Experience in 36 cases. J Urol 1992;147:333.

Claes H et al: Xanthogranulomatous pyelonephritis with emphasis on computerized tomography scan. Urology 1987;29:389.

Collins MM et al: How common is prostatitis? A national survey of physician visits. J Urol 1998;159:1224.

Davidson AJ, Talner LB: Urographic and angiographic abnormalities in adult-onset acute bacterial nephritis. Radiology 1973;106:249.

Davison JM, Lindheimer MD: Renal diseases in pregnant women. Clin Obstet Gynecol 1978;21:411.

de la Rosette JJMCH, Debruyne FMJ: Nonbacterial prostatitis: A comprehensive review. Urol Int 1991;46:121.

de la Rosette JJMCH et al: Results of a questionnaire among Dutch urologists and general practitioners concerning diagnostics and treatment of patients with prostatitis syndromes. Eur Urol 1992;22:14.

Doble A et al: The role of *Chlamydia trachomatis* in chronic abacterial prostatitis: A study using ultrasound guided biopsy. J Urol 1989;141:332.

Dohle GR, Zwartendijk J, van Krieken JHJM: Urogenital malacoplakia treated with fluoroquinolones. J Urol 1993;150:1518.

Duclos JM, Larrouturou P, Sarkis P: Timing of antibiotic prophylaxis with cefotaxime for prostatic resection: Better in the operative period or at urethral catheter removal? Am J Surg 1992;164:21S.

Easmon CSF, Crane JP: Uptake of ciprofloxacin by macrophages. J Clin Pathol 1985;38:442.

Eastham J, Ahlering T, Skinner E: Xanthogranulomatous pyelonephritis: Clinical findings and surgical considerations. Urology 1994;43:295.

Eden CS et al: Variable adherence to normal human urinary-tract epithelial cells of *Escherichia coli* strains associated with various forms of urinary tract infection. Lancet 1976;1:490.

Epstein JI, Hutchins GM: Granulomatous prostatitis: Distinction among allergic, nonspecific, and post-transurethral resection lesions. Hum Pathol 1984;15:818.

Fair WR, Couch J, Wehner N: Prostatic antibacterial factor: Identity and significance. Urology 1976;7:169.

Fair WR et al: A re-appraisal of treatment in chronic bacterial prostatitis. J Urol 1979;121:437.

Fernandez JA, Miles BJ, Buck AS: Renal carbuncle: Comparison between surgical open drainage and closed percutaneous drainage. Urology 1985;25:142.

Finn DJ, Palestrant AM, DeWolf WC: Successful percutaneous management of renal abscess. J Urol 1982;127:425.

Fowler JE, Stamey TA: Studies of introital colonization

in women with recurrent urinary infections. VII: The role of bacterial adherence. J Urol 1977;117:472.

Freiha FS, Messing EM, Gross DM: Emphysematous pyelonephritis. Urology 1979;18:9.

Fridlender B, Chejanovsky N, Becker Y: Selective inhibition of herpes simplex virus type I DNA polymerase by zinc ions. Virology 1978;84:551.

Gilstrap LC et al: Renal infection and pregnancy outcome. Am J Obstet Gynecol 1981;141:709.

Goodman SM et al: CT of xanthogranulomatous pyelonephritis: Radiologic-pathologic correlation. AJR 1984;141:963.

Haaga JR, Weinstein AJ: CT guided percutaneous aspiration and drainage of abscesses. AJR 1980;135:1187.

Hall JR, Choa RG, Wells IP: Percutaneous drainage in emphysematous pyelonephritis—an alternative to major surgery. Clin Radiol 1988;39:622.

Harbord RG, Grueneberg RN: Treatment of urinary tract infections with a single dose of amoxycillin, co-trimoxazole, or trimethoprim. Br Med J 1981;238:1301.

Hartman DS: Radiologic pathologic correlation of the infectious granulomatous diseases of the kidney: Parts I and II. Monogr Urol 1985;6:3.

Hartman DS et al: Renal parenchymal malakoplakia. Radiology 1980;136:33.

Hooton TM, Stamm WE: Management of acute uncomplicated urinary tract infections in adults. Med Clin North Am 1991;75:339.

Hoverman IV et al: Intrarenal abscesses: Report of 14 cases. Arch Intern Med 1980;140:914.

Huland H, Busch R: Chronic pyelonephritis as a cause of end stage renal disease. J Urol 1982;127:642.

Jacobson SH et al: P fimbriated *Escherichia coli* in adults with acute pyelonephritis. J Infect Dis 1985; 152:426.

Janknegt RA: Prophylaxis in urologic surgery. Infection 1992;20:S213.

Jenkins RD, Fenn JP, Matsen J: Review of urine microscopy for bacteriuria. JAMA 1986;255:3397.

Johnson JR: Virulence factors in *Escherichia coli* urinary tract infection. Clin Microbiol Rev 1991;4:80.

Johnson JR et al: Renal ultrasonographic correlates of acute pyelonephritis. Clin Infect Dis 1992;14:15.

Johnson JR et al: Therapy for women hospitalized with acute pyelonephritis: A randomized trial of ampicillin versus trimethoprim-sulfamethoxazole for 14 days. J Infect Dis 1991;163:325.

Jordan PA et al: Urinary tract infections caused by *Staphylococcus saprophyticus*. J Infect Dis 1980;142: 510.

Kallenius G et al: Occurrence of P fimbriated *Escherichia coli* in urinary tract infections. Lancet 1981;2:1369.

Kass EH: The role of asymptomatic bacteriuria in the pathogenesis of pyelonephritis. In: Quinn EL, Kass EH (editors): *Biology of Pyelonephritis*. Little, Brown, 1960.

Kass EH et al: The urographic findings in acute pyelonephritis: Non-obstructive hydronephrosis. J Urol 1976;116:544.

Kirby RS et al: Intra-prostatic urinary reflux: An aetiological factor in abacterial prostatitis. Br J Urol 1982; 54:729.

Klein FA et al: Emphysematous pyelonephritis: Diagnosis and treatment. South Med J 1986;79:41.

Krieger JN et al: Chronic pelvic pains represent the most prominent urogenital symptoms of "chronic prostatitis." J Urol 1996;48:715.

Lachs MS et al: Spectrum bias in the evaluation of diagnostic tests: Lessons from the rapid dipstick test for urinary tract infection. Ann Intern Med 1992;117: 135.

Langermann S et al: Prevention of mucosal *Escherichia coli* infection by FimH-Adhesin-based systemic vaccination. Science 1997;276:607.

Latham RH, Running K, Stamm WE: Urinary tract infections in young adult women caused by *Staphylococcus saprophyticus*. JAMA 1983;250:3036.

Leib Z et al: Reduced semen quality caused by chronic abacterial prostatitis: An enigma or reality? Fertil Steril 1994;61:1109.

Levin R et al: The diagnosis and management of renal inflammatory processes in children. J Urol 1984;132: 718.

Levy AH, Schwinger HN: Gas containing perinephric abscess. Radiology 1953;60:720.

Little PJ, McPherson DR, Wardener HE: The appearance of the intravenous pyelogram during and after acute pyelonephritis. Lancet 1965;1:1186.

Lomberg H et al: Correlation of P blood group, vesicoureteral reflux, and bacterial attachment in patients with recurrent pyelonephritis. N Engl J Med 1983; 308:1189.

Long JP, Althausen AF: Malacoplakia: A 25-year experience with a review of the literature. J Urol 1989;141:1328.

Lopez-Plaza I, Bostwick DG: Prostatitis. In: Bostwick DG (editor): *Pathology of the Prostate*. Churchill Livingstone, 1990.

Maderazo EG, Berlin BB, Marhardt C: Treatment of malacoplakia with trimethoprim-sulfamethoxazole. Urology 1979;13:70.

Malek RS, Elder JS: Xanthogranulomatous pyelonephritis: A critical analysis of 26 cases and the literature. J Urol 1978;119:589.

Manson AL: Is antibiotic administration indicated after outpatient cystoscopy? J Urol 1988;140:316.

Mardh PA, Colleen S, Sylwan J: Inhibitory effect on the formation of chlamydial inclusions in McCoy cells by seminal fluid and some of its components. Invest Urol 1980;17:510.

McGrady GA, Daling JR, Peterson DR: Maternal urinary tract infection and adverse fetal outcomes. Am J Epidemiol 1985;121:377.

Meares EM: Acute and chronic prostatitis: Diagnosis and treatment. Infect Dis Clin North Am 1987;1:855.

Meares EM: Chronic bacterial prostatitis: Role of transurethral prostatectomy (TURP) in therapy. In: Weidner W et al (editors): *Therapy of Prostatitis*. W. Zuckschwerdt Verlag, 1986.

Meares EM: Prostatitis. Med Clin North Am 1991;75: 405.

Meares EM: Prostatitis and related disorders. In: Walsh PC et al (editors): *Campbell's Urology*. Saunders, 1997.

Meares EM, Stamey TA: Bacteriologic localization patterns in bacterial prostatitis and urethritis. Invest Urol 1968;5:492.

Melekos MD, Asbach HW: Epididymitis: Aspects concerning etiology and treatment. J Urol 1987;138:86.

Michaeli J: Emphysematous pyelonephritis. J Urol 1984; 131:203.

Mitsumori K et al: Virulence characteristics and DNA fingerprints of *Escherichia coli* isolated from women with acute uncomplicated pyelonephritis. J Urol 1997;158:2329.

Murray T, Goldberg M: Chronic interstitial nephritis: Etiologic factors. Ann Intern Med 1975;82:453.

Naber KG: Use of quinolones in urinary tract infections and prostatitis. Rev Infect Dis 1989;11:S1321.

National Institutes of Health—National Institute of Diabetes and Digestive and Kidney Diseases Workshop on Chronic Prostatitis: *Summary Statement.* US Department of Health and Human Services, December 1995.

Navas EL et al: Blood group antigen expression on vaginal and buccal epithelial cells and mucus in secretor and nonsecretor women. J Urol 1993;149:1492.

Nickel JC: The pre and post massage test (PPMT): A simple screen for prostatitis. Tech Urol 1997;3:38.

Nicolle LE et al: The association of urinary tract infection with sexual intercourse. J Infect Dis 1982;146:579.

Norrby SR: Short-term treatment of uncomplicated lower urinary tract infections in women. Rev Infect Dis 1990;12:458.

O'Dea MJ, Hunting DB, Greene LF: Non-specific granulomatous prostatitis. J Urol 1977;118:58.

Osca JM et al: Focal xanthogranulomatous pyelonephritis: Partial nephrectomy as definitive treatment. Eur Urol 1997;32:375.

Ostaszewska I et al: Chlamydia trachomatis: Probable cause of prostatitis. Int J STD AIDS 1998;9:350.

Parsons MA et al: Fistula and sinus formation in xanthogranulomatous pyelonephritis. A clinicopathological review and report of four cases. Br J Urol 1986; 58:488.

Parsons MA et al: Xanthogranulomatous pyelonephritis: A pathological, clinical and aetiological analysis of 87 cases. Diagn Histopathol 1983;6:203.

Pearle MS, Roehrborn CG: Antimicrobial prophylaxis prior to shock wave lithotripsy in patients with sterile urine before treatment: A meta-analysis and cost-effectiveness analysis. Urology 1997;49:679.

Persson B-E, Ronquist G: Evidence for a mechanistic association between nonbacterial prostatitis and levels of urate and creatinine in expressed prostatic secretion. J Urol 1996;155:958.

Persson B-E, Ronquist G, Ekblom M: Ameliorative effect of allopurinol on nonbacterial prostatitis: A parallel double-blind controlled study. J Urol 1996;155:961.

Pezzlo M: Detection of urinary tract infection by rapid methods. Clin Microbiol Rev 1988;1:268.

Pfau A, Sacks T, Engelstein D: Recurrent urinary tract infections in premenopausal women: Prophylaxis based on an understanding of the pathogenesis. J Urol 1983;129:1153.

Pitts JC, Petersen NE, Conley MC: Calcified functionless kidney in a 51-year-old man. J Urol 1981;125:398.

Ransley PG, Ridson RA: The pathogenesis of reflux nephropathy. Contrib Nephrol 1979;16:90.

Raz R, Stamm WE: A controlled trial of intravaginal estriol in postmenopausal women with recurrent urinary tract infections. N Engl J Med 1993;329:753.

Reid G, Bruce AW, Taylor M: Influence of three-day antimicrobial therapy and lactobacillus vaginal suppositories on recurrence of urinary tract infections. Clin Ther 1992;14:11.

Roberts RO et al: Prevalence of a physician-assigned diagnosis of prostatitis: The Olmsted County study of urinary symptoms and health status among men. Urology 1998;51:578.

Rubin JM et al: Power Doppler: A potentially useful alternative to mean-frequency based color Doppler sonography. Radiology 1994;190:853.

Saiki J, Vaziri ND, Barton C: Perinephric and intranephric abscesses: A review of the literature. West J Med 1982;136:95.

Sakarya ME et al: The role of power Doppler ultrasonography in the diagnosis of acute pyelonephritis. Br J Urol 1998;81:360.

Schaeffer A: Infections of the urinary tract. In: Walsh PC et al (editors): *Campbell's Urology.* Saunders, 1997.

Schaeffer AJ, Jones JM, Dunn JK: Association of in vitro *Escherichia coli* adherence to vaginal and buccal epithelial cells with susceptibility of women to recurrent urinary tract infections. N Engl J Med 1981; 304:1062.

Schaeffer AJ et al: Prevalence and significance of prostatic inflammation. J Urol 1981;125:215.

Schainuck LI, Fouty R, Cutler RE: Emphysematous pyelonephritis. A new case and review of previous observations. Am J Med 1968;44:134.

Schoborg TW et al: Xanthogranulomatous pyelonephritis associated with renal carcinoma. J Urol 1980;124: 125.

Scholz M et al: Single-dose antibiotic prophylaxis in transurethral resection of the prostate: A prospective randomized trial. Br J Urol 1998;81:827.

Schultz HJ et al: Acute cystitis: A prospective study of laboratory tests and duration of therapy. Mayo Clin Proc 1984;59:391.

Sheinfeld J et al: Association of the Lewis blood-group phenotype with recurrent urinary tract infections in women. N Engl J Med 1989;320:804.

Shokeir AA et al: Emphysematous pyelonephritis: A 15 year experience with 20 cases. Urology 1997;49:343.

Shortliffe LD, Wehner N: The characterization of bacterial and non-bacterial prostatitis by prostatic fluid immunoglobulins. Medicine 1986;65:399.

Shortliffe LM, Seller RG, Schachter J: The characterization of nonbacterial prostatitis: Search for an etiology. J Urol 1992;148:1461.

Silver TM et al: The radiologic spectrum of acute pyelonephritis in adults and adolescence. Radiology 1976;118:65.

Solomon A et al: Computerized tomography in xanthogranulomatous pyelonephritis. J Urol 1983;130: 323.

Soulen MC et al: Bacterial renal infection: Role of CT. Radiology 1989;171:703.

Stamey TA: *Pathogenesis and Treatment of Urinary Tract Infections.* Williams & Wilkins, 1980.

Stamey TA, Govan DE, Palmer JM: The localization and treatment of urinary tract infections: The role of bactericidal urine levels as opposed to serum levels. Medicine 1965;44:1.

Stamey TA, Pfau A: Some functional, pathologic, bacteriologic, and chemotherapeutic characteristics of unilateral pyelonephritis in man. Invest Urol 1963;1:134.

Stamm WE, Hooton TM: Management of urinary tract infections in adults. N Engl J Med 1993;329:1328.

Stamm WE et al: Diagnosis of coliform infection in acutely dysuric women. N Engl J Med 1982;307:463.

Stamm WE et al: Treatment of acute urethral syndrome. N Engl J Med 1981;304:956.

Stanton MJ, Maxted W: Malacoplakia: A study of the literature and current concepts of pathogenesis, diagnosis and treatment. J Urol 1981;125:139.

Stenqvist K et al: Bacteriuria in pregnancy: Frequency and risk of acquisition. Am J Epidemiol 1989;129:372.

Sweet RL: Bacteriuria and pyelonephritis during pregnancy. Semin Perinatol 1977;1:25.

Talner LB, Davidson AJ, Lebowitz RL: Acute pyelonephritis: Can we agree on terminology? Radiology 1994;192:297.

Teplick JG et al: Urographic and angiographic changes in acute unilateral pyelonephritis. Clin Radiol 1978;30:59.

Thind P, Gerstenberg TC, Bilde T: Is micturition disorder a pathogenic factor in acute epididymitis? An evaluation of simultaneous bladder pressure and urine flow in men with previous acute epididymitis. J Urol 1990;143:323.

Thorley JD, Jones SR, Sanford JP: Perinephric abscess. Medicine 1974;53:441.

Timmons JW, Perlmutter AD: Renal abscess: A changing concept. J Urol 1976;115:299.

Tolia BM et al: Xanthogranulomatous pyelonephritis: Detailed analysis of 29 cases and a brief discussion of atypical presentations. J Urol 1981;126:437.

Tolia BM et al: Xanthogranulomatous pyelonephritis: Segmental or generalized disease? J Urol 1980;124:122.

Uehling DT et al: Vaginal mucosal immunization for recurrent urinary tract infection: Phase II clinical trial. J Urol 1997;157:2049.

Van Kirk OC, Go RT, Wedel VJ: Sonographic features of xanthogranulomatous pyelonephritis. AJR 1980;134:1035.

Waltzer WC: The urinary tract in pregnancy. J Urol 1981;125:271.

Wan Y-L et al: Predictors of outcome in emphysematous pyelonephritis. J Urol 1998;159:369.

Weidner W, Scheifer HG, Krauss H: Role of *Chlamydia trachomatis* and mycoplasmas in chronic prostatitis. A review. Urol Int 1988;43:167.

Weinberger M et al: Prostatic abscess in the antibiotic era. Rev Infect Dis 1988;10:239.

Wigton RS et al: Use of clinical findings in the diagnosis of urinary tract infection in women. Arch Intern Med 1985;145:2222.

Specific Infections of the Genitourinary Tract

15

Emil A. Tanagho, MD

Specific infections are those caused by specific organisms, each of which causes a clinically unique disease that leads to specific pathologic tissue reactions. See also Chapter 16.

TUBERCULOSIS

Tubercle bacilli may invade one or more (or even all) of the organs of the genitourinary tract and cause a chronic granulomatous infection that shows the same characteristics as tuberculosis in other organs. Urinary tuberculosis is a disease of young adults (60% of patients are between the ages of 20 and 40) and is a little more common in males than in females.

Etiology
The infecting organism is *Mycobacterium tuberculosis,* which reaches the genitourinary organs by the hematogenous route from the lungs. The primary site is often not symptomatic or apparent.

The kidney and possibly the prostate are the primary sites of tuberculous infection in the genitourinary tract. All other genitourinary organs become involved by either ascent (prostate to bladder) or descent (kidney to bladder, prostate to epididymis). The testis may become involved by direct extension from epididymal infection.

Pathogenesis
(Figure 15–1)
A. Kidney and Ureter: When a shower of tubercle bacilli hits the renal cortex, the organisms may be destroyed by normal tissue resistance. Evidence of this is commonly seen in autopsies of persons who have died of tuberculosis; only scars are found in the kidneys. However, if enough bacteria of sufficient virulence become lodged in the kidney and are not overcome, a clinical infection is established.

Tuberculosis of the kidney progresses slowly; it may take 15–20 years to destroy a kidney in a patient who has good resistance to the infection. As a rule,

therefore, there is no renal pain and little or no clinical disturbance of any type until the lesion has involved the calyces or the pelvis, at which time pus and organisms may be discharged into the urine. It is only at this stage that symptoms (of cystitis) are manifested. The infection then proceeds to the pelvic mucosa and the ureter, particularly its upper and vesical ends. This may lead to stricture and back pressure (hydronephrosis).

As the disease progresses, a caseous breakdown of tissue occurs until the entire kidney is replaced by cheesy material. Calcium may be laid down in the reparative process. The ureter undergoes fibrosis and tends to be shortened and therefore straightened. This change leads to a "golf-hole" (gaping) ureteral orifice, typical of an incompetent valve.

B. Bladder: Vesical irritability develops as an early clinical manifestation of the disease as the bladder is bathed by infected material. Tubercles form later, usually in the region of the involved ureteral orifice, and finally coalesce and ulcerate. These ulcers may bleed. With severe involvement, the bladder becomes fibrosed and contracted; this leads to marked frequency. Ureteral reflux or stenosis and, therefore, hydronephrosis may develop. If contralateral renal involvement occurs later, it is probably a separate hematogenous infection.

C. Prostate and Seminal Vesicles: The passage of infected urine through the prostatic urethra ultimately leads to invasion of the prostate and one or both seminal vesicles. There is no local pain.

On occasion, the primary hematogenous lesion in the genitourinary tract is in the prostate. Prostatic infection can ascend to the bladder and descend to the epididymis.

D. Epididymis and Testis: Tuberculosis of the prostate can extend along the vas or through the perivasal lymphatics and affect the epididymis. Because this is a slow process, there is usually no pain. If the epididymal infection is extensive and an abscess forms, it may rupture through the scrotal skin, thus establishing a permanent sinus, or it may extend into the testicle.

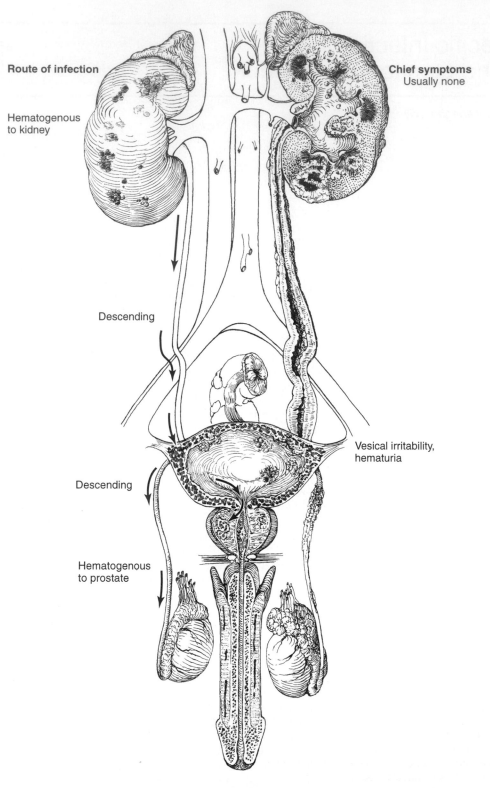

Figure 15–1. Pathogenesis of tuberculosis of the urinary tract.

Pathology

A. Kidney and Ureter: The gross appearance of the kidney with moderately advanced tuberculosis is often normal on its outer surface, although the kidney is usually surrounded by marked perinephritis. Usually, however, there is a soft, yellowish localized bulge. On section, the involved area is seen to be filled with cheesy material (caseation). Widespread destruction of parenchyma is evident. In otherwise normal tissue, small abscesses may be seen. The walls of the pelvis, calyces, and ureter may be thickened, and ulceration appears frequently in the region of the calyces at the point at which the abscess drains. Ureteral stenosis may be complete, causing "autonephrectomy." Such a kidney is fibrosed and functionless. Under these circumstances, the bladder urine may be normal and symptoms absent.

Tubercle foci appear close to the glomeruli. These are an aggregation of histiocytic cells possessing a vesicular nucleus and a clear cell body that can fuse with neighboring cells to form a small mass called an epithelioid reticulum. At the periphery of this reticulum are large cells with multiple nuclei (giant cells). This pathologic reaction, which can be seen macroscopically, is the basic lesion in tuberculosis. It can heal by fibrosis or coalesce and reach the surface and ulcerate, forming an ulcerocavernous lesion. Tubercles might undergo a central degeneration and caseate, creating a tuberculous abscess cavity that can reach the collecting system and break through. In the process, progressive parenchymal destruction occurs. Depending on the virulence of the organism and the resistance of the patient, tuberculosis is a combination of caseation and cavitation and healing by fibrosis and scarring.

Microscopically, the caseous material is seen as an amorphous mass. The surrounding parenchyma shows fibrosis with tissue destruction, small round cell and plasma cell infiltration, and epithelial and giant cells typical of tuberculosis. Acid-fast stains will usually demonstrate the organisms in the tissue. Similar changes can be demonstrated in the wall of the pelvis and ureter.

In both the kidney and ureter, calcification is common. It may be macroscopic or microscopic. Such a finding is strongly suggestive of tuberculosis but, of course, is also observed in bilharzial infection. Secondary renal stones occur in 10% of patients.

In the most advanced stage of renal tuberculosis, the parenchyma may be completely replaced by caseous substance or fibrous tissue. Perinephric abscess may develop, but this is rare.

B. Bladder: In the early stages, the mucosa may be inflamed, but this is not a specific change. The bladder is quite resistant to actual invasion. Later, tubercles form and can be seen easily, especially through the cystoscope, as white or yellow raised nodules surrounded by a halo of hyperemia. With mural fibrosis and severe vesical contracture, reflux may occur.

Microscopically, the nodules are typical tubercles. These break down to form deep, ragged ulcers. At this stage the bladder is quite irritable. With healing, fibrosis develops that involves the muscle wall.

C. Prostate and Seminal Vesicles: Grossly, the exterior surface of these organs may show nodules and areas of induration from fibrosis. Areas of necrosis are common. In rare cases, healing may end in calcification. Large calcifications in the prostate should suggest tuberculous involvement.

D. Spermatic Cord, Epididymis, and Testis: The vas deferens is often grossly involved; fusiform swellings represent tubercles that in chronic cases are characteristically described as beaded. The epididymis is enlarged and quite firm. It is usually separate from the testis, although occasionally it may adhere to it. Microscopically, the changes typical of tuberculosis are seen. Tubular degeneration may be marked. The testis is usually not involved except by direct extension of an abscess in the epididymis.

E. Female Genital Tract: Infections are usually carried by the bloodstream; rarely, they are the result of sexual contact with an infected male. The incidence of associated urinary and genital infection in females ranges from 1 to 10%. The uterine tubes may be affected. Other presentations include endarteritis, localized adnexal masses (usually bilateral), and tuberculous cervicitis, but granulomatous lesions of the vaginal canal and vulva are rare.

Clinical Findings

Tuberculosis of the genitourinary tract should be considered in the presence of any of the following situations: (1) chronic cystitis that refuses to respond to adequate therapy, (2) the finding of pus without bacteria in a methylene blue stain or culture of the urinary sediment, (3) gross or microscopic hematuria, (4) a nontender, enlarged epididymis with a beaded or thickened vas, (5) a chronic draining scrotal sinus, or (6) induration or nodulation of the prostate and thickening of one or both seminal vesicles (especially in a young man). A history of present or past tuberculosis elsewhere in the body should cause the physician to suspect tuberculosis in the genitourinary tract when signs or symptoms are present.

The diagnosis rests on the demonstration of tubercle bacilli in the urine by culture. The extent of the infection is determined by (1) the palpable findings in the epididymides, vasa deferentia, prostate, and seminal vesicles; (2) the renal and ureteral lesions as revealed by excretory urograms; (3) involvement of the bladder as seen through the cystoscope; (4) the degree of renal damage as measured by loss of function; and (5) the presence of tubercle bacilli in one or both kidneys.

A. Symptoms: There is no classic clinical picture of renal tuberculosis. Most symptoms of this disease, even in the most advanced stage, are vesical in origin (cystitis). Vague generalized malaise, fatigability, low-grade but persistent fever, and night sweats are some of the nonspecific complaints. Even vesical irritability may be absent, in which case only proper collection and examination of the urine will afford the clue. Active tuberculosis elsewhere in the body is found in less than half of patients with genitourinary tuberculosis.

1. Kidney and ureter–Because of the slow progression of the disease, the affected kidney is usually completely asymptomatic. On occasion, however, there may be a dull ache in the flank. The passage of a blood clot, secondary calculi, or a mass of debris may cause renal and ureteral colic. Rarely, the presenting symptom may be a painless mass in the abdomen.

2. Bladder–The earliest symptoms of renal tuberculosis may arise from secondary vesical involvement. These include burning, frequency, and nocturia. Hematuria is occasionally found and is of either renal or vesical origin. At times, particularly in a late stage of the disease, the vesical irritability may become extreme. If ulceration occurs, suprapubic pain may be noted when the bladder becomes full.

3. Genital tract–Tuberculosis of the prostate and seminal vesicles usually causes no symptoms. The first clue to the presence of tuberculous infection of these organs is the onset of a tuberculous epididymitis.

Tuberculosis of the epididymis usually presents as a painless or only mildly painful swelling. An abscess may drain spontaneously through the scrotal wall. A chronic draining sinus should be regarded as tuberculous until proved otherwise. In rare cases, the onset is quite acute and may simulate an acute nonspecific epididymitis.

B. Signs: Evidence of extragenital tuberculosis may be found (lungs, bone, lymph nodes, tonsils, intestines).

1. Kidney–There is usually no enlargement or tenderness of the involved kidney.

2. External genitalia–A thickened, nontender, or only slightly tender epididymis may be discovered. The vas deferens often is thickened and beaded. A chronic draining sinus through the scrotal skin is almost pathognomonic of tuberculous epididymitis. In the more advanced stages, the epididymis cannot be differentiated from the testis on palpation. This may mean that the testis has been directly invaded by the epididymal abscess.

Hydrocele occasionally accompanies tuberculous epididymitis. The idiopathic hydrocele should be tapped so that underlying pathologic changes, if present, can be evaluated (epididymitis, testicular tumor). Involvement of the penis and urethra is rare.

3. Prostate and seminal vesicles–These organs may be normal to palpation. Ordinarily, however, the tuberculous prostate shows areas of induration, even nodulation. The involved seminal vesicle is usually indurated, enlarged, and fixed. If epi-

didymitis is present, the ipsilateral seminal vesicle usually shows changes as well.

C. Laboratory Findings: Proper urinalysis affords the most important clue to the diagnosis of genitourinary tuberculosis.

1. Persistent pyuria without organisms on culture or on the smear stained with methylene blue means tuberculosis until proved otherwise. Acid-fast stains done on the concentrated sediment from a 24-h specimen are positive in at least 60% of cases. However, this must be corroborated by a positive culture.

About 15–20% of patients with tuberculosis have secondary pyogenic infection; the clue ("sterile" pyuria) is thereby obscured. If clinical response to adequate treatment fails and pyuria persists, tuberculosis must be ruled out by bacteriologic and roentgenologic means.

2. Cultures for tubercle bacilli from the first morning urine are positive in a very high percentage of cases of tuberculous infection. If positive, sensitivity tests should be ordered. In the face of strong presumptive evidence of tuberculosis, negative cultures should be repeated.

The blood count may be normal or may show anemia in advanced disease. The sedimentation rate is usually accelerated.

Tubercle bacilli often may be demonstrated in the secretions from an infected prostate. Renal function is normal unless there is bilateral damage; as one kidney is slowly injured, compensatory hypertrophy of the normal kidney develops. It can also be infected with tubercle bacilli, or it may become hydronephrotic from fibrosis of the bladder wall (ureterovesical stenosis) or vesicoureteral reflux.

If tuberculosis is suspected, the tuberculin test should be performed. A positive test, particularly in an adult, is hardly diagnostic, but a negative test in an otherwise healthy patient speaks against a diagnosis of tuberculosis.

D. X-Ray Findings (Figure 15–2): A chest film that shows evidence of tuberculosis should cause the physician to suspect tuberculosis of the urogenital tract in the presence of urinary signs and symptoms. A plain film of the abdomen may show enlargement of one kidney or obliteration of the renal and psoas shadows due to perinephric abscess. Punctate calcification in the renal parenchyma may be due to tuberculosis. Renal stones are found in 10% of cases. Calcification of the ureter may be noted, but this is rare (Figure 6–1). Small prostatic stones the size of grape seeds in the region of the pubic symphysis ordinarily are not due to tuberculosis, but large calcific bodies may be.

Excretory urograms can be diagnostic if the lesion is moderately advanced. The typical changes include (1) a "moth-eaten" appearance of the involved ulcerated calyces, (2) obliteration of one or more calyces, (3) dilatation of the calyces due to ureteral stenosis from fibrosis, (4) abscess cavities that connect with

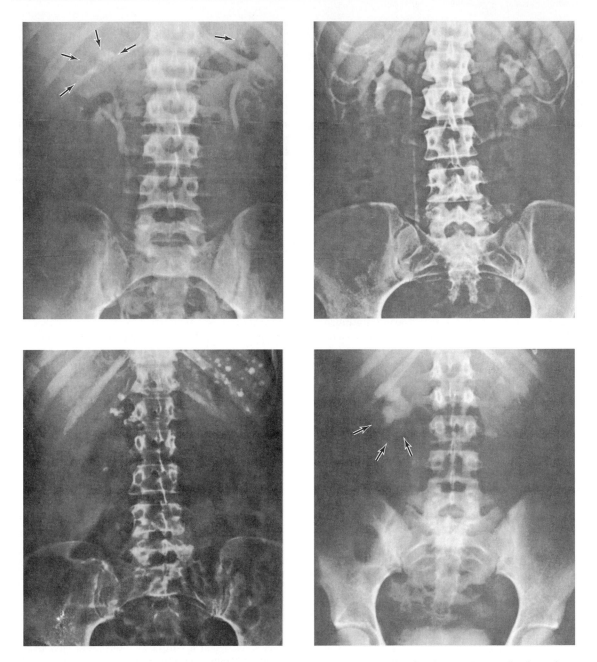

Figure 15–2. Radiologic evidence of tuberculosis. **Upper left:** Excretory urogram showing "moth-eaten" calyces in upper renal poles. Calcifications in upper calyces; right upper ureter is straight and dilated. **Upper right:** Excretory urogram showing ulcerated and dilated calyces on the left. **Lower left:** Plain film showing calcifications in right kidney, adrenals, and spleen (tuberculosis of right kidney and Addison disease). **Lower right:** Excretory urogram. Dilatation of calyces; upper right ureter dilated and straight. Arrows point to poorly defined parenchymal abscesses.

calyces, (5) single or multiple ureteral strictures, with secondary dilatation, with shortening and therefore straightening of the ureter, and (6) absence of function of the kidney due to complete ureteral occlusion and renal destruction (autonephrectomy).

If the excretory urograms demonstrate gross tuberculosis in one kidney, there is no need to do a retrograde urogram on that side. In fact, there is at least a theoretic danger of hematogenous or lymphogenous dissemination resulting from the increased intrapelvic pressure. Retrograde urography may be carried out on the unsuspected side, however, as a verification of its normality. This is further substantiated if the urine from that side is free of both pus cells and tubercle bacilli.

E. Instrumental Examination: Thorough cystoscopic study is indicated even when the offending organism has been found in the urine and excretory urograms show the typical renal lesion. This study clearly demonstrates the extent of the disease. Cystoscopy may reveal the typical tubercles or ulcers of tuberculosis. Biopsy can be done if necessary. Severe contracture of the bladder may be noted. A cystogram may reveal ureteral reflux. A clean specimen of urine should also be obtained for further study.

Differential Diagnosis

Chronic nonspecific cystitis or pyelonephritis may mimic tuberculosis perfectly, especially since 15–20% of cases of tuberculosis are secondarily invaded by pyogenic organisms. If nonspecific infections do not respond to adequate therapy, a search for tubercle bacilli should be made. Painless epididymitis points to tuberculosis. Cystoscopic demonstration of tubercles and ulceration of the bladder wall means tuberculosis. Urograms are usually definitive.

Acute or chronic nonspecific epididymitis may be confused with tuberculosis, since the onset of tuberculosis is occasionally quite painful. It is rare to have palpatory changes in the seminal vesicles with nonspecific epididymitis, but these are almost routine findings in tuberculosis of the epididymis. The presence of tubercle bacilli on a culture of the urine is diagnostic. On occasion, only the pathologist can make the diagnosis by microscopic study of the surgically removed epididymis.

Amicrobic cystitis usually has an acute onset and is often preceded by a urethral discharge. "Sterile" pyuria is found, but tubercle bacilli are absent. Cystoscopy may reveal ulcerations, but these are acute and superficial. Although urograms show mild hydroureter and even hydronephrosis, there is no ulceration of the calyces as seen in renal tuberculosis. Interstitial cystitis is typically characterized by frequency, nocturia, and suprapubic pain with vesical filling. The urine is usually free of pus. Tubercle bacilli are absent.

Multiple small renal stones or nephrocalcinosis seen by x-ray may suggest the type of calcification seen in the tuberculous kidney. In renal tuberculosis, the calcium is in the parenchyma, although secondary stones are occasionally seen.

Necrotizing papillitis, which may involve all of the calyces of one or both kidneys or, rarely, a solitary calyx, shows caliceal lesions (including calcifications) that simulate those of tuberculosis. Careful bacteriologic studies fail to demonstrate tubercle bacilli.

Medullary sponge kidneys may show small calcifications just distal to the calyces. The calyces are sharp, however, and no other stigmas of tuberculosis can be demonstrated.

In disseminated coccidioidomycosis, renal involvement may occur. The renal lesion resembles that of tuberculosis. Coccidioidal epididymitis may be confused with tuberculous involvement.

Urinary bilharziasis is a great mimic of tuberculosis. Both present with symptoms of cystitis and often hematuria. Vesical contraction, seen in both diseases, may lead to extreme frequency. Schistosomiasis must be suspected in endemic areas; the typical ova are found in the urine. Cystoscopic and urographic findings are definitive for making the differential diagnosis.

Complications

A. Renal Tuberculosis: Perinephric abscess may cause an enlarging mass in the flank. A plain film of the abdomen shows obliteration of the renal and psoas shadows. Sonograms and CT scans may be more helpful. Renal stones may develop if secondary nonspecific infection is present. Uremia is the end stage if both kidneys are involved.

B. Ureteral Tuberculosis: Scarring with stricture formation is one of the typical lesions of tuberculosis and most commonly affects the juxtavesical portion of the ureter. This may cause progressive hydronephrosis. Complete ureteral obstruction may cause complete nonfunction of the kidney (autonephrectomy).

C. Vesical Tuberculosis: When severely damaged, the bladder wall becomes fibrosed and contracted. Stenosis of the ureters or reflux occurs, causing hydronephrotic atrophy.

D. Genital Tuberculosis: The ducts of the involved epididymis become occluded. If this is bilateral, sterility results. Abscess of the epididymis may rupture into the testis, through the scrotal wall, or both, in which case the spermatogenic tubules may slough out.

Treatment

Tuberculosis must be treated as a generalized disease. Even when it can be demonstrated only in the urogenital tract, one must assume activity elsewhere. (It is theoretically possible, however, for the primary focus to have healed spontaneously.) This means that the basic treatment is medical. Surgical excision of an infected organ, when indicated, is merely an adjunct to overall therapy.

A. Renal Tuberculosis: A strict medical regimen should be instituted. A combination of drugs is usually desirable. The following drugs are effective in combination: (1) isoniazid, 200–300 mg orally once daily; (2) rifampin, 600 mg orally once daily; (3) ethambutol, 25 mg/kg daily for 2 months, then 15 mg/kg orally once daily; (4) streptomycin, 1 g intramuscularly once daily; and (5) pyrazinamide, 1.5–2 g orally once daily. It is preferable to begin treatment with a combination of isoniazid, rifampin, and ethambutol. If resistance to one of these drugs develops, one of the others listed should be chosen as a replacement. The following drugs are usually considered only in cases of resistance to first-line drugs and when expert medical personnel are available to treat toxic side effects, should they occur: aminosalicylic acid (PAS), capreomycin, cycloserine, ethionamide, pyrazinamide, viomycin. See note following on pyrazinamide.

While most authorities advise appropriate medication for 2 years (or longer if cultures remain positive), Gow (1979) finds that a 6-month course of drugs is adequate. He recommends 600 mg of rifampin, 300 mg of isoniazid, 1 g of pyrazinamide, and 1 g of vitamin C daily for 2 months, followed by 900 mg of rifampin, 600 mg of isoniazid, and 1 g of vitamin C 3 times/week for 4 months. *Pyrazinamide may cause serious liver damage.*

If, after 3 months, cultures are still positive and gross involvement of the affected kidney is radiologically evident, nephrectomy should be considered. Gow (1979) recommends that nonfunctioning kidneys be removed after 1–2 months of medical therapy.

If bacteriologic and radiographic studies demonstrate bilateral disease, only medical treatment can be considered. The only exceptions are (1) severe sepsis, pain, or bleeding from one kidney (may require nephrectomy as a palliative or lifesaving measure) and (2) marked advance of the disease on one side and minimal damage on the other (one may consider removal of the badly damaged organ).

B. Vesical Tuberculosis: Tuberculosis of the bladder is always secondary to renal or prostatic tuberculosis; it tends to heal promptly when definitive treatment for the "primary" genitourinary infection is given. Vesical ulcers that fail to respond to this regimen may require transurethral electrocoagulation. Vesical instillations of 0.2% monoxychlorosene (Clorpactin) may also stimulate healing.

Should extreme contracture of the bladder develop, it may be necessary to divert the urine from the bladder or perform augmentation cystoplasty after subtotal cystectomy (ileocystoplasty, ileocecocystoplasty, sigmoidocystoplasty) to increase bladder capacity (Abel and Gow, 1978).

C. Tuberculosis of the Epididymis: This condition never produces an isolated lesion; the prostate is always involved and usually the kidney as well. Only rarely does the epididymal infection break through into the testis. Treatment is medical. If after months of treatment an abscess or a draining sinus exists, epididymectomy is indicated.

D. Tuberculosis of the Prostate and Seminal Vesicles: Although a few urologists advocate removal of the entire prostate and the vesicles when they become involved by tuberculosis, the majority opinion is that only medical therapy is indicated.

Control can be checked by culture of the semen for tubercle bacilli.

E. General Measures for All Types: Optimal nutrition is no less important in treating tuberculosis of the genitourinary tract than in the treatment of tuberculosis elsewhere. Bladder sedatives may be given for the irritable bladder.

F. Treatment of Other Complications: Perinephric abscess usually occurs when the kidney is destroyed, but this is rare. The abscess must be drained, and nephrectomy should be done either then or later to prevent development of a chronic draining sinus. Prolonged antimicrobial therapy is indicated. If ureteral stricture develops on the involved side, ureteral dilatations offer a better than 50% chance of cure (Cos and Cockett, 1982). The severely involved bladder may cause incompetence of the ureterovesical junction on the uninvolved side. Ureteroneocystostomy cannot be done in such a bladder; some form of urinary diversion may be required. For this reason, serial excretory urograms are necessary even when the treatment is medical.

Prognosis

The prognosis varies with the extent of the disease and the organs involved, but the overall control rate is 98% at 5 years. The urine must be studied bacteriologically every 6 months during treatment and then every year for 10 years. Relapse indicates the need for reinstitution of treatment. Nephrectomy is rarely necessary. In the healing process, ureteral stenosis or vesical contraction may develop. Appropriate surgical intervention may be necessary.

AMICROBIC (ABACTERIAL) CYSTITIS

Amicrobic cystitis is a rare disease of abrupt onset with a marked local vesical reaction. Although it acts like an infectious disease, search for the usual urinary bacterial pathogens is negative. It affects adult men and occasionally children, usually boys.

Etiology

The patient usually gives a history of recent sexual exposure. Mycoplasmas and chlamydiae have been isolated or suspected as etiologic agents. An adenovirus has been isolated from the urine in children suffering from acute hemorrhagic cystitis.

Pathogenesis & Pathology

Whatever the source and identity of the invader, the disease is primarily manifested as an acute inflammation of the bladder. Vesical irritability is severe and often associated with terminal hematuria. The mucosa is red and edematous, and superficial ulceration is occasionally seen. A thin membrane of fibrin often lies on the wall. Similar changes may be noted in the posterior urethra. The renal parenchyma is not involved, although the pelvic and ureteral mucosa may show mild inflammatory changes. Some dilatation of the lower ureters is apt to develop. This may be due to an inflammatory reaction about the ureteral orifices, for these changes regress after successful treatment.

Microscopically, there is nothing specific about the reaction. The mucosa and submucosa are infiltrated with neutrophils, plasma cells, and eosinophils. Submucosal hemorrhages are common; superficial ulceration of the mucosa may be noted.

Clinical Findings

A. Symptoms: All symptoms are local. Urethral discharge, which is usually clear and mucoid but may be purulent, may be the initial symptom in men. Symptoms of acute cystitis come on abruptly. Urgency, frequency, and burning may be severe. Terminal hematuria is not uncommon. Suprapubic discomfort or even pain may be noted; it is most apt to be present as the bladder fills and is relieved somewhat by voiding. There is no fever or malaise.

B. Signs: Some suprapubic tenderness may be found. Urethral discharge may be profuse or scanty and may be purulent or thin and mucoid. The prostate is usually normal to palpation. Massage is contraindicated during the acute stage of urinary tract infection. When massage is done later, infection is usually not present.

C. Laboratory Findings: Some leukocytosis may develop. The urine is grossly purulent and may contain blood as well. Stained smears reveal an absence of bacteria. Routine cultures are uniformly negative. In a few cases, mycoplasmas and TRIC agent (*Chlamydia trachomatis*) have been identified, but the significance of this is not yet clear. Search for tubercle bacilli is not successful.

Urethral discharge reveals no bacteria. Renal function is not impaired.

D. X-Ray Findings: Excretory urograms may demonstrate some dilatation of the lower ureters, but these changes regress completely when the disease is cured. The bladder shadow is small because of its markedly diminished capacity. Cystograms may reveal reflux.

E. Instrumental Examination: Cystoscopy is not indicated in acute inflammation of the bladder. It has been done, however, when the diagnosis was obscure and tuberculosis suspected. In such cases it reveals redness and edema of the mucosa. Superficial ulceration may be noted. Bladder capacity is markedly diminished. Biopsy of the wall shows nonspecific changes.

Differential Diagnosis

Tuberculosis causes symptoms of cystitis, which usually come on gradually and become severe only in the stage of ulceration. A painless, nontender enlargement of an epididymis suggests tuberculosis.

Although both tuberculosis and amicrobic cystitis produce pus without bacteria, thorough laboratory study demonstrates tubercle bacilli only in the former. On cystoscopy, the tuberculous bladder may be studded with tubercles. The ulcers in this disease are deep and of a chronic type. The changes in amicrobic cystitis are more acute; ulceration, if present, is superficial. Excretory urograms in tuberculosis may show "moth-eaten" calyces typical of infection with acid-fast organisms.

Nonspecific (pyogenic) cystitis may mimic amicrobic cystitis perfectly, but pathogenic organisms are easily found on a smear stained with methylene blue or on culture.

Cystitis secondary to chronic nonspecific prostatitis occasionally produces pus without bacteria. The findings on rectal examination, the pus in the prostatic secretion, and the response to antibiotics point to the proper diagnosis.

Vesical neoplasm may ulcerate, become infected, and bleed; hence it may mimic amicrobic cystitis. Bacteriuria, however, is found. In case of doubt, cystoscopy is indicated.

Interstitial cystitis may be accompanied by severe symptoms of vesical irritability. However, it usually affects women past the menopause, and urinalysis is entirely negative except for a few red cells. Cystoscopy should be diagnostic.

Complications

Amicrobic cystitis is usually self-limited. Rarely, secondary contracture of the bladder develops. Under these circumstances, vesicoureteral reflux may be noted.

Treatment

A. Specific Measures: One of the tetracyclines or chloramphenicol, 1 g/d orally in divided doses for 3–4 days, is said to be curative in 75% of cases. Streptomycin, 1–2 g/d intramuscularly for 3–4 days, may be tried. Neoarsphenamine is also effective and appears to be the drug of choice, but arsenicals are hard to find. The first dose is 0.3 g intravenously; subsequent dosage is 0.45 g intravenously every 3–5 days for a total of 3–4 injections.

Penicillin and the sulfonamides are without effect.

In the cases reported in children, cure occurred spontaneously.

B. General Measures: Bladder sedatives are usually of little help if symptoms are severe. Analgesics or narcotics may prove necessary to combat pain. Hot sitz baths may relieve spasm.

The instillation of a 0.1% solution of sodium oxychlorosene (Clorpactin WCS-90) has been recommended.

Prognosis

The prognosis is excellent.

CANDIDIASIS

Candida albicans is a yeastlike fungus that is a normal inhabitant of the respiratory and gastrointestinal tracts and the vagina. The intensive use of potent modern antibiotics is apt to disturb the normal balance between normal and abnormal organisms, thus allowing fungi such as *Candida* to overwhelm an otherwise healthy organ. The bladder and, to a lesser extent, the kidneys have proved vulnerable; candidemia has been observed. Anogenital candidiasis is discussed in Chapter 43.

The patient may present with vesical irritability or symptoms and signs of pyelonephritis. Fungus balls may be passed spontaneously. The diagnosis is made by observing mycelial or yeast forms of the fungus microscopically in a properly collected urine specimen. The diagnosis may be confirmed by culture. Excretory urograms may show caliceal defects and ureteral obstruction (fungus masses).

Vesical candidiasis usually responds to alkalinization of the urine with sodium bicarbonate. A urinary pH of 7.5 is desired; the dose is regulated by the patient, who checks the urine with indicator paper. Should this fail, amphotericin B should be instilled via catheter 3 times a day. One dissolves 50 mg of the drug in 1 L of sterile water.

If there is renal involvement, irrigations of the renal pelvis with a similar concentration of amphotericin B are efficacious. In the presence of systemic manifestations or candidemia, flucytosine (Ancobon) is the drug of choice. The dose is 100 mg/kg/d orally in divided doses given for 1 week. In the face of serious involvement, 600 mg is given intravenously on the first day followed by a shift to the oral form of the drug. Nifuratel, a nitrofuran antibiotic, is superior to flucytosine. The recommended dose is 400 mg 3 times daily for 1 week. The dose must be modified in the face of renal impairment. The drug is more active in acid urine. Graybill et al (1983) reported good results with ketoconazole. The dose is 200–400 mg/d for 2–3 weeks or more depending on the effect as reflected by serial cultures. Its toxicity is relatively low. Amphotericin B (Fungizone) has the disadvantages of requiring parenteral administration and being highly nephrotoxic. It is given intravenously in a dosage of 1–5 mg/d in divided doses dissolved in 5% dextrose. The concentration of the solution should be 0.1 mg/mL.

ACTINOMYCOSIS

Actinomycosis is a chronic granulomatous disease in which fibrosis tends to become marked and spontaneous fistulas are the rule. On rare occasions, the disease involves the kidney, bladder, or testis by hematogenous invasion from a primary site of infection. The skin of the penis or scrotum may become involved through a local abrasion. The bladder may also become diseased by direct extension from the appendix, bowel, or oviduct.

Etiology

Actinomyces israelii (*A bovis*) is the causative organism.

Clinical Findings

There is nothing specifically pathognomonic about the symptoms or signs in actinomycosis. The microscopic demonstration of the organisms, which are visible as yellow bodies called "sulfur granules," makes the diagnosis. If persistently sought, these may be found in the discharge from sinuses or in the urine. Pollock et al (1978) recommend aspiration biopsy performed by a thin needle. They found that in addition to the discovery of sulfur granules, both Gram stain and a modified Ziehl-Neelsen stain were useful in diagnosis. Definitive diagnosis is established by culture.

Urographically, the lesion in the kidney may resemble tuberculosis (eroded calyces) or tumor (space-occupying lesion).

Treatment

Penicillin G is the drug of choice. The dosage is 10–20 million units/d parenterally for 4–6 weeks, followed by penicillin V orally for a prolonged period. If secondary infection is suspected, a sulfonamide is added; streptomycin is also efficacious. Broad-spectrum antibiotics are indicated only if the organism is resistant to penicillin. Surgical drainage of the abscess or, better, removal of the involved organ is usually indicated.

Prognosis

Removal of the involved organ (eg, kidney or testis) may be promptly curative. Drainage of a granulomatous abscess may cause the development of a chronic draining sinus. Chemotherapy is helpful.

SCHISTOSOMIASIS
(Bilharziasis)

Schistosomiasis, caused by a blood fluke, is a disease of warm climates. In its 3 forms, it affects about 350 million people. *Schistosoma mansoni* is widely distributed in Africa, South and Central America, Pakistan, and India; *Schistosoma japonicum* is found in the Far East; and *Schistosoma haematobium* (*Bilharzia haematobia*) is limited to Africa (especially along its northern coast), Saudi Arabia, Israel, Jordan, Lebanon, and Syria.

Schistosomiasis is on the increase in endemic areas because of the construction of modern irrigation systems that provide favorable conditions for the intermediate host, a freshwater snail. This disease principally affects the urogenital system, especially the bladder, ureters, seminal vesicles, and, to a lesser extent, the male urethra and prostate gland. Because of emigration of people from endemic areas, the disease is being seen with increasing frequency in both Europe and the United States. Infection with *S mansoni* and *S japonicum* mainly involves the colon.

Etiology

Humans are infected when they come in contact with larva-infested water in canals, ditches, or irrigation fields during swimming, bathing, or farming procedures. Fork-tailed larvae, the cercariae, lose their tails as they penetrate deep under the skin. They are then termed **schistosomules.** They cause allergic skin reactions that are more intense in people infected for the first time. These schistosomules enter the general circulation through the lymphatics and the peripheral veins and reach the lungs. If the infection is massive, they may cause pneumonitis. They pass through the pulmonary circulation, to the left side of the heart, and to the general circulation. The worms that reach the vesicoprostatic plexus of veins survive and mature, whereas those that go to other areas die.

Pathogenesis

The adult *S haematobium* worm, a digenetic trematode, lives in the prostatovesical plexus of veins. The male is about 10×1 mm in size, is folded upon itself, and carries the long, slim 20×0.25 mm female in its "schist," or gynecophoric canal. In the smallest peripheral venules, the female leaves the male and partially penetrates the venule to lay her eggs in the subepithelial layer of the affected viscus, usually in the form of clusters that form tubercles. The ova are seen only rarely within the venules; they are almost always in the subepithelial or interstitial tissues. The female returns to the male, which carries her to other areas to repeat the process.

The living ova, by a process of histolysis and helped by contraction of the detrusor muscle, penetrate the overlying urothelium, pass into the cavity of the bladder, and are extruded with the urine. If these ova reach fresh water, they hatch, and the contained larvae—ciliated miracidia—find a specific freshwater snail that they penetrate. There they form sporocysts that ultimately form the cercariae, which leave the snail hosts and pass into fresh water to repeat their life cycle in the human host.

Pathology

The fresh ova excite little tissue reaction when they leave the human host promptly through the urothelium. The contents of the ova trapped in the tissues and the death of the organisms cause a severe local reaction, with infiltration of round cells, monocytes, eosinophils, and giant cells that form tubercles, nodules, and polyps. These are later replaced by fibrous tissue that causes contraction of different parts of the bladder and strictures of the ureter. Fibrosis and massive deposits of eggs in subepithelial tissues interfere with the blood supply of the area and cause chronic bilharzial ulcerations. Epithelial metaplasia is common, and squamous cell carcinoma is a frequent sequela. Secondary infection of the urinary tract is a common complication and is difficult to overcome. The trapped dead ova become impregnated with calcium salts and form sheets of subepithelial calcified layers in the ureter, bladder, and seminal vesicles.

Clinical Findings

A. Symptoms: Penetration of the skin by the cercariae causes allergic reactions, with cutaneous hyperemia and itching that are more intense in people infected for the first time. During the stage of generalization or invasion, the patient complains of symptoms such as malaise, fatigue and lassitude, low-grade fever, excessive sweating, headache, and backache. When the ova are laid in the bladder wall and begin to be extruded, the patient complains of terminal, slightly painful hematuria that is occasionally profuse. This may remain the only complaint for a long time until complications set in, when vesical symptoms become exaggerated and progressive. Increasing frequency, suprapubic and back pain, urethralgia, profuse hematuria, pyuria, and necroturia are likely to occur, with secondary infection, ulceration, or malignancy. Renal pain may be due to ureteral stricture, vesicoureteral reflux, or secondary stones obstructing the ureter. Fever, rigor, toxemia, and uremia are manifestations of renal involvement.

B. Signs: In early uncomplicated cases, there are essentially no clinical findings. Later, a fibrosed, pitted, bilharzial glans penis, a urethral stricture or fistula, or a perineal fibrous mass may be found. A suprapubic bladder mass or a renal swelling may be felt abdominally. Rectal examination may reveal a fibrosed prostate, an enlarged seminal vesicle, or a thickened bladder base.

C. Laboratory Findings: Urinalysis usually reveals the terminal-spined dead or living ova, blood and pus cells, and bacteria. Malignant squamous cells may be seen. The hemogram usually shows leukocytosis with eosinophilia and hypochromic normocytic anemia. Serum creatinine and blood urea nitrogen measurements may demonstrate some degree of renal impairment.

A variety of immunologic methods have been used to confirm the diagnosis of schistosomiasis. Positive immunologic tests indicate previous exposure but not whether schistosomiasis is currently present. The cercariae, schistosomules, adult worms, and eggs are all potentially antigenic. Adult worms, however, acquire host antigen on their integument that circumvents the immunologic forces of the host. Antibody production may be manifested as hypergammaglobulinema.

D. X-Ray Findings: A plain film of the abdomen may show areas of grayness in the flank (enlarged hydronephrotic kidney) or in the bladder area (large tumor). Opacifications (stones) may be noted in the kidney, ureter, or bladder. Linear calcification may be seen in the ureteral and bladder walls (Figure 15–3). Punctate calcification of the ureter (ureteritis calcinosa) and a honeycombed calcification of the seminal vessels may be obvious (Figure 15–3).

Excretory urograms may show either normal or diminished renal function and varying degrees of dilatation of the upper urinary tracts (Figure 15–4). These changes include hydronephrosis, dilated and tortuous ureters, ureteral strictures, or a small contracted bladder having a capacity of only a few milliliters. Gross irregular defects of the bladder wall represent cancer (Figure 15–4).

Retrograde urethrography may reveal a bilharzial urethral stricture. Cystograms often reveal vesicoureteral reflux, particularly if the bladder is contracted.

E. Instrumental Examination: Urethral calibration with a sound may reveal stricture formation.

Cystoscopy may show fresh conglomerate, grayish tubercles surrounded by a halo of hyperemia, old calcified yellowish tubercles, sandy patches of mucous

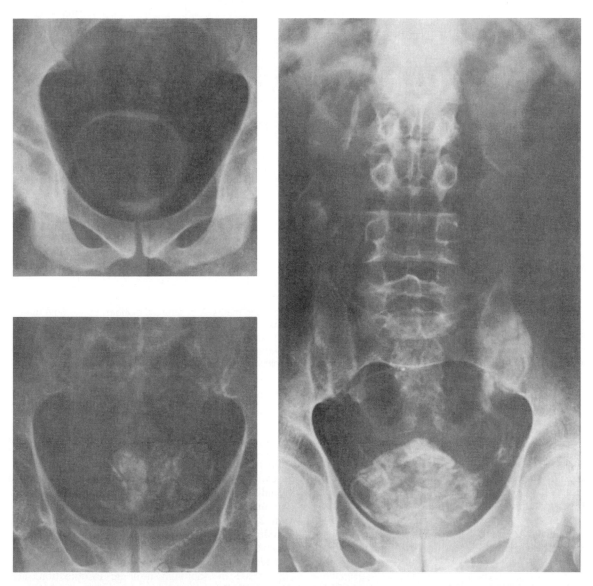

Figure 15–3. Schistosomiasis. Plain films. **Upper left:** Extensive calcification in the wall of a contracted bladder. **Right:** Extensive calcification of the bladder and both ureters up to the renal pelves. The ureters are dilated and tortuous. **Lower left:** Extensive calcification of seminal vesicles and ampullae of vasa.

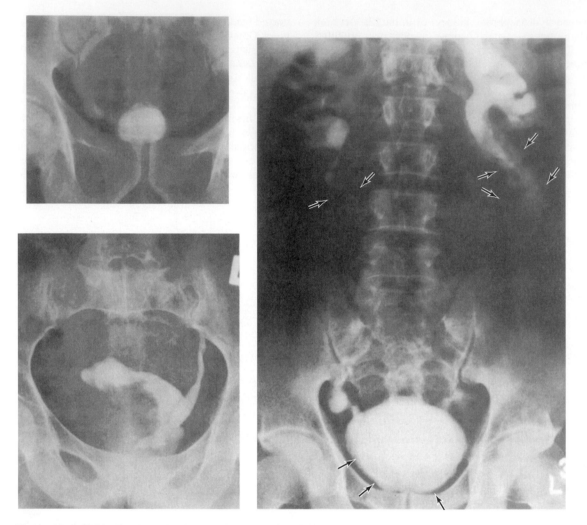

Figure 15–4. Schistosomiasis. **Upper left:** Excretory urogram showing markedly contracted bladder. Lower right ureter dilated probably secondary to vesicoureteral reflux. **Right:** Excretory urogram at 2 h showing a fairly normal right kidney. The upper ureter is distorted. Arrows point to calcified wall. The lower ureter is quite abnormal. The calyces and pelvis of the left kidney are dilated, but the kidney shows atrophy secondary to nonspecific infection. The upper ureter is dilated and displaced by elongation due to obstruction. Arrows show calcification. Linear calcification can be seen in the periphery of the lower half of the bladder wall (arrows). **Lower left:** Nodular squamous cell carcinoma of the bladder. Dilated left lower ureter probably secondary to obstruction by tumor. Nonvisualization of the right ureter caused by complete occlusion.

membrane, and a lusterless ground-glass mucosa that lacks the normal vascular pattern. Other obvious lesions include bilharzial polyps, chronic ulcers on the dome that bleed when the bladder is deflated (weeping ulcers), vesical stones, malignant lesions, stenosed or patulous ureteric orifices, and a distorted, asymmetric trigone. All are signs of schistosomal infestation.

Differential Diagnosis

Bilharzial cystitis is unmistakable in endemic areas. The presence of schistosomal ova in the urine,

together with radiographic and cystoscopic findings, usually confirms the diagnosis. Nonspecific cystitis usually responds to medical treatment unless there is a complicating factor. Tuberculous cystitis may mimic bilharzial cystitis; the detection of tubercle bacilli, together with the radiographic picture, is confirmatory, but tuberculosis may occur in a bilharzial bladder. Vesical calculi and malignancy should be diagnosed by thorough urologic examination, although both conditions are common in association with bilharzial bladder. Complications of schistosomiasis are the result of fibrosis, which may be extreme and causes contraction of the bladder neck as well as of the bladder itself. It also causes strictures of the urethra and ureter that are usually bilateral. Vesicoureteral reflux is a frequent sequela. Secondary persistent infection and stone formation usually complicate the picture still further. Squamous cell tumors of the bladder are common. They are seen as early as the second or third decade of life and are much more common in men than in women.

Treatment

A. Medical Measures: Praziquantel, metrifonate, and oxamniquine are the drugs of choice in treating schistosomiasis. These drugs do not have the serious side effects associated with the older drugs (eg, antimonials).

1. Praziquantel is unique in that it is effective against all human schistosome species. It is given orally and is effective in adults and children. Patients in the hepatosplenic stage of advanced schistosomiasis tolerate the drug well. The recommended dosage for all forms of schistosomiasis is 20 mg/kg 3 times in 1 day only.

2. Metrifonate is also a highly effective oral drug. It is the drug of choice for treatment of *S haematobium* infections but is not effective against *S mansoni* or *S japonicum*. For treatment of *S haematobium* infections, the dosage is 7.5–10 mg/kg (maximum 600 mg) once and then repeated twice at 2-week intervals.

3. Oxamniquine is a highly effective oral drug and is the drug of choice for treatment of *S mansoni* infections. It is safe and effective in advanced disease. It is not effective in *S haematobium* or *S japonicum* infections. The dosage is 12–15 mg/kg given once; for children under 30 kg, 20 mg/kg is given in 2 divided doses in 1 day, with an interval of 2–8 h between doses. Cure rates are 70–95%.

4. Niridazole, a nitrothiazole derivative, is effective in treating *S mansoni* and *S haematobium* infections. It may be tried against *S japonicum* infections. It is given orally and should be administered only under close medical supervision. The dosage is 25 mg/kg (maximum, 1.5 g) daily in 2 divided doses for 7 days. Side effects may include nausea, vomiting, anorexia, headache, T-wave depression, and temporary suppression of spermatogenesis.

5. Antimonial drugs are no longer used in the treatment of schistosomiasis if praziquantel, oxamniquine, or metrifonate is available. The antimonials (eg, sodium antimony dimercaptosuccinate [stibocaptate], stibophen, tartar emetic) are much more toxic, and a longer course of therapy is needed. Tartar emetic is nonetheless occasionally needed as a third alternative drug in the treatment of *S japonicum* infection.

B. General Measures: Antibiotics or urinary antiseptics are needed to overcome or control secondary infection. Supportive treatment in the form of iron, vitamins, and a high-calorie diet is indicated in selected cases.

C. Complications: Treatment of the complications of schistosomiasis of the genitourinary tract makes demands on the skill of the physician. Juxtavesical ureteral strictures require resection of the stenotic segment with ureteroneocystostomy. If the ureter is not long enough to reimplant, a tube of bladder may be fashioned, turned cephalad, and anastomosed to the ureter. Should the ureter be widely dilated, it must be tailored to approach normal size. Vesicoureteral reflux requires a suitable surgical repair. A contracted bladder neck may need transurethral anterior commissurotomy or a suprapubic Y-V plasty.

A chronic "weeping" bilharzial bladder ulcer necessitates partial cystectomy. The contracted bladder is treated by enteroplasty (placing a segment of bowel as a patch on the bladder), preferably with an isolated portion of sigmoid colon. This procedure, which significantly increases vesical capacity, is remarkably effective in lessening the severity of symptoms associated with contracted bladder. Preoperative vesicoureteral reflux may disappear.

The most dreaded complication, squamous cell carcinoma, requires total cystectomy with supravesical urinary diversion if the lesion is deemed operable. Unfortunately, late diagnosis is the rule.

Prognosis

With energetic treatment, mild and early cases of schistosomiasis are not likely to result in severe damage to the urinary tract. On the other hand, massive repeated infections undermine the function of the urinary tract to such an extent that patients are disabled and become chronic invalids whose life spans are shortened by 1 or 2 decades.

In many endemic areas, attempts have been made to control the disease by mass treatment of patients, proper education, mechanization of agriculture, and various methods of eradication or control of the snail population. All these efforts have failed to be fully effective.

FILARIASIS

Filariasis is endemic in the countries bordering the Mediterranean, in south China and Japan, the West Indies, and the South Pacific islands, particularly Samoa. Limited infection, as seen in American soldiers during World War II, gives an entirely different clinical picture from that seen in the frequent reinfections usually encountered among the native population.

Etiology

Wuchereria bancrofti is a threadlike nematode about 0.5 cm or more in length that lives in the human lymphatics. In the lymphatics, the female gives off microfilariae, which are found in the peripheral blood, particularly at night. The intermediate host (usually a mosquito) bites an infected person and becomes infested with microfilariae, which develop into larvae. These are in turn transferred to another human, in whom they reach maturity. Mating occurs, and microfilariae are again produced. *Brugia malayi,* a nematode that causes filariasis in Southeast Asia and adjacent Pacific islands, acts in a similar fashion.

Pathogenesis & Pathology

The adult nematode in the human host invades and obstructs the lymphatics; this leads to lymphangitis and lymphadenitis. In long-standing cases, the lymphatic vessels become thickened and fibrous; there is a marked reticuloendothelial reaction.

Clinical Findings

A. Symptoms: In mild cases (few exposures), the patient suffers recurrent lymphadenitis and lymphangitis with fever and malaise. Not infrequently, inflammation of the epididymis, testis, scrotum, and spermatic cord occurs. These structures then become edematous, boggy, and at times tender. Hydrocele is common. In advanced cases (many exposures), obstruction of major lymph channels may cause chyluria and elephantiasis.

B. Signs: Varying degrees of painless elephantiasis of the scrotum and extremities develop as obstruction to lymphatics progresses. Lymphadenopathy is common.

C. Laboratory Findings: Chylous urine may look normal if minimal amounts of fat are present, but in an advanced case or following a fatty meal, it is milky. On standing, the urine forms layers: the top layer is fatty, the middle layer is pinkish, and the lower layer is clear. In the presence of chyluria, large amounts of protein are to be expected. Hypoproteinemia is found, and the albumin-globulin ratio is reversed. Both white blood cells (leukocytes) and red blood cells (erythrocytes) are found.

Marked eosinophilia is the rule in the early stages. Microfilariae may be demonstrated in the blood, which should be drawn at night. The adult worm may be found by biopsy. When filariae cannot be found, an indirect hemagglutination titer of 1/128 and a bentonite flocculation titer of 1/5 in combination are considered diagnostic.

D. Cystoscopy: Following a fatty meal, endoscopy to observe the efflux of milky urine from the ureteral orifices may differentiate between unilateral and bilateral cases.

E. X-Ray Findings: Retrograde urography and lymphangiography may reveal the renolymphatic connections in patients with chyluria.

Prevention

In endemic areas, mosquito abatement programs must be intensively pursued.

Treatment

A. Specific Measures: Diethylcarbamazine (Hetrazan) is the drug of choice, but it is toxic (Nelson, 1979). The dose is 2 mg/kg orally 3 times daily for 12 days. This drug kills the microfilariae but not the adult worms. Several courses of the drug may be necessary. Antibiotics may be necessary to control secondary infection.

B. General Measures: Prompt removal of recently infected patients from the endemic area almost always results in regression of the symptoms and signs in early cases.

C. Surgical Measures: Elephantiasis of the external genitalia may require surgical excision.

D. Treatment of Chyluria: Mild cases require no therapy. Spontaneous cure occurs in 50% of cases. If nutrition is impaired, the lymphatic channels may be sealed off by irrigating the renal pelvis with 2% silver nitrate solution. Should this fail, renal decapsulation and resection of the renal lymphatics should be performed (Okamoto and Ohi, 1983).

Prognosis

If exposure has been limited, resolution of the disease is spontaneous and the prognosis is excellent. Frequent reinfection may lead to elephantiasis of the scrotum or chyluria.

ECHINOCOCCOSIS (Hydatid Disease)

Involvement of the urogenital organs by hydatid disease is relatively rare in the United States. It is common in Australia, New Zealand, South America, Africa, Asia, the Middle East, and Europe. Livestock are the intermediate hosts. Canines, especially dogs, are the final hosts.

Etiology

The adult tapeworm (*Echinococcus*) inhabits the intestinal tracts of carnivorous animals. Its eggs pass out with the feces and may be ingested by such animals as sheep, cattle, pigs, and occasionally humans. Larvae from these eggs pass through the intestinal wall of the various intermediate hosts and are disseminated throughout the body. In humans, the liver is principally involved, but about 3% of infected humans develop echinococcosis of the kidney.

If a cyst of the liver should rupture into the peritoneal cavity, the scoleces (tapeworm heads) may directly invade the retrovesical tissues, thus leading to the development of cysts in this area.

Clinical Findings

If renal hydatid disease is closed (not communicating with the pelvis), there may be no symptoms until a mass is found. With communicating disease, there

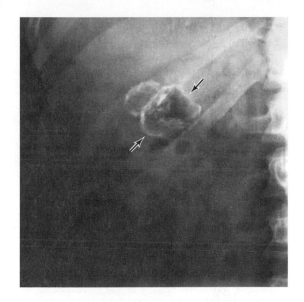

Figure 15–5. Hydatid disease, right kidney. Plain film showing 2 calcified hydatid cysts.

may be symptoms of cystitis, and renal colic may occur as cysts are passed from the kidney. X-ray films may show calcification in the wall of the cyst (Figure 15–5), and urograms often reveal changes typical of a space-occupying lesion. The cystic nature of the lesion may be demonstrated on sonograms and computed tomography scans. Calcification in the cyst wall may be noted. Scintillation scanning or angiography can also suggest the presence of a cyst. Serologic tests that should be done include immunoelectrophoresis and indirect hemagglutination. The Casoni intracutaneous procedure is unreliable.

Retroperitoneal (perivesical) cysts may cause symptoms of cystitis, or acute urinary retention may develop secondary to pressure. The presence of a suprapubic mass may be the only finding. It may rupture into the bladder and cause hydatiduria, which establishes the diagnosis.

Treatment

Nephrectomy is generally the treatment of choice for renal hydatid disease. Aspiration of the cyst is unwise; leakage or rupture may occur. Retroperitoneal cysts are best treated by marsupialization and curettage.

Prognosis

Echinococcosis of the kidney usually has a good prognosis. The problem presented by perivesical cysts is more troublesome. After surgical intervention, drainage may be prolonged. It must be remembered, too, that involvement of other organs, especially the liver, is usually present.

REFERENCES

TUBERCULOSIS

Abel BJ, Gow JG: Results of caecocystoplasty for tuberculous bladder contracture. Br J Urol 1978;50:511.

Carl P, Stark L: Indications for surgical management of genitourinary tuberculosis. World J Surg 1997;21:505.

Cos CR, Cockett ATK: Genitourinary tuberculosis revisited. Urology 1982;20:111.

Das KM, Indudhara R, Vaidyanathan S: Sonographic features of genitourinary tuberculosis. AJR 1992;158:327.

Ehrlich RM, Lattimer JK: Urogenital tuberculosis in children. J Urol 1971;105:461.

Gokalp A, Gultekin EY, Ozdamar S: Genito-urinary tuberculosis: A review of 83 cases. Br J Clin Pract 1990;44:599.

Gow JG: Genitourinary tuberculosis: A 7-year review. Br J Urol 1979;51:239.

Gow JG: The management of genitourinary tuberculosis. In: Hendry WF (editor): *Recent Advances in Urology/Andrology,* 3rd ed., p. 91. Churchill Livingstone, 1981.

Hamrick-Turner J, Abbitt PL, Ros PR: Tuberculosis of the lower genitourinary tract: Findings on sonography and MR. (Letter.) AJR 1992;158:919.

Jensen H, Nielsen K, Frimodt-Moller C: Abacterial cystitis in urinary incontinent females. Urol Int 1990;45:20.

Kollins SA et al: Roentgenographic findings in urinary tract tuberculosis: A 10-year review. AJR 1974;121:487.

Management of extra-pulmonary tuberculosis. Drug Ther Bull 1991;29:26.

Mehta JB et al: Epidemiology of extrapulmonary tuberculosis: A comparative analysis with pre-AIDS era. Chest 1991;99:1134.

Poulios C, Malovrouvas D: Progress in the approach of tuberculosis of the genitourinary tract: Remarks on a decade's experience over cases. Acta Urol Belg 1990;58:101.

Premkumar A, Lattimer J, Newhouse JH: CT and sonography of advanced urinary tract tuberculosis. AJR 1987;148:65.

Tikkakoski T et al: Tuberculosis of the lower genitourinary tract: Ultrasonography as an aid to diagnosis and treatment. J Clin Ultrasound 1993;21:269.

Valentini AL, Summaria V, Marano P: Diagnostic imaging of genitourinary tuberculosis. Rays 1998;23:126.

AMICROBIC (ABACTERIAL) CYSTITIS

Holm-Bentzen M et al: A prospective double-blind clinically controlled multicenter trial of sodium pentosanpolysulfate in the treatment of interstitial cystitis and related painful bladder disease. J Urol 1987;138:503.

Moore T, Parker C, Edwards EC: Sterile non-tuberculous pyuria. Br J Urol 1971;43:47.

Morgan MG et al: Controversies in the laboratory diagnosis of community-acquired urinary tract infection. Eur J Clin Microbiol Infect Dis 1993;12:491.

Parsons CL, Schmidt JD, Pollen JJ: Successful treatment of interstitial cystitis with sodium pentosanpolysulfate. J Urol 1983;130:51.

GENITOURINARY CANDIDIASIS

Fox GN: Single-dose therapy for genitourinary infections. Am Fam Physician 1987;36:111.

Freeman SB: Common genitourinary infections. J Obstet Gynecol Neonatal Nurs 1995;24:735.

Graybill JR et al: Ketoconazole therapy for fungal urinary tract infections. J Urol 1983;129:68.

Odds FC et al: *Candida* species and *C. albicans* biotypes in women attending clinics in genitourinary medicine. J Med Microbiol 1989;29:51.

Priestley CJ et al: What is normal vaginal flora? Genitourin Med 1997;73:23.

Rashid S, Collins M, Kennedy RJ: A study of candidosis: The role of fomites. Genitourin Med 1991;67:137.

Rivera L, Bellotti MG, Malighetti V: Morphotypes of *Candida albicans* and their associations with underlying diseases and source of samples. New Microbiol 1996;19:335.

Sandin KJ et al: Candida pyelonephritis complicating traumatic C5 quadriplegia: Diagnosis and management. Arch Phys Med Rehab 1991;72:243.

Wise GJ et al: Miconazole: A cost-effective antifungal genitourinary irrigant. J Urol 1987;138:1413.

Woolley PD, Higgins SP: Comparison of clotrimazole, fluconazole and itraconazole in vaginal candidiasis. Br J Clin Pract 1995;49:65.

ACTINOMYCOSIS

Jani AN, Casibang V, Mufarrij WA: Disseminated actinomycosis presenting as a testicular mass: A case report. J Urol 1990;143:1012.

Pollock PG et al: Rapid diagnosis of actinomycosis by thin-needle aspiration biopsy. Am J Clin Pathol 1978;70:27.

Rashid AM et al: Actinomycosis associated with pilonidal sinus of the penis. J Urol 1992;148:405.

Smego RA Jr et al: Actinomycosis. Clin Infect Dis 1998;26:1255.

SCHISTOSOMIASIS (BILHARZIASIS)

Abdel-Halim RE: Ileal loop replacement and restoration of kidney function in extensive bilharziasis of the ureter. Br J Urol 1980;52:280.

Al Ghorab MM: Radiological manifestations of genitourinary bilharziasis. Clin Radiol 1968;19:100.

Al Ghorab MM, El-Badawi AA, Effat H: Vesicoureteric reflux in urinary bilharziasis: A clinico-radiological study. Clin Radiol 1966;17:41.

Badawi AF et al: Role of schistosomiasis in human bladder cancer: Evidence of association, aetiological factors, and basic mechanisms of carcinogenesis. Eur J Cancer Prev 1995;4:45.

Barrou B et al: Resuls of renal transplantation in patients with Schistosoma infection. J Urol 1997;157:1232.

Bazeed MA, Nabeeh A, Atwan N: Xanthogranulomatous pyelonephritis in bilharzial patients: A report of 25 cases. J Urol 1989;141:261.

Bazeed MA et al: Partial flap ureteroneocystostomy for bilharzial strictures of the lower ureter. Urology 1982;20:237.

El-Feky HM et al: Histopathological study of the bilharzial affection on the bladder and ureter. J Egypt Soc Parasitol 1992;22:71.

El-Mahrouky A et al: The predictive value of 2, 4-dinitrochlorobenzene skin testing in patients with bilharzial bladder cancer. J Urol 1983;129:497.

Eltoum IA et al: Significance of eosinophiluria in urinary schistosomiasis: A study using Hansel's stain and electron microscopy. Am J Clin Pathol 1989;92:329.

Ghoneim MA et al: Staging of the carcinoma of bilharzial bladder. Urology 1974;3:40.

Hanafy MH, Youssef TK, Saad MS: Radiographic aspects of (bilharzial) schistosomal ureter. Urology 1975;6:118.

Helling-Giese G et al: Schistosomiasis in women: Manifestations in the upper reproductive tract. Acta Trop 1996;62:225.

Ibrahim A et al: Bilharzial vesicoureteric reflux and bladder neck stenosis: Fact or fiction? Br J Urol 1991;68:582.

Johansson SL, Cohen SM: Epidemiology and etiology of bladder cancer. Semin Surg Oncol 1997;13:291.

King CH et al: Urinary tract morbidity in schistosomiasis haematobia: Associations with age and intensity of infection in an endemic area of Coast Province, Kenya. Am J Trop Med Hyg 1988;39:361.

Lukacs T et al: Multiple urolithiasis in bilharziasis patients. Int Urol Nephrol 1989;21:269.

Patil KP et al: Specific investigations in chronic urinary bilharziasis. Urology 1992;40:117.

Sato K et al: Efficacy of metrifonate in a highly endemic area of urinary schistosomiasis in Kenya. Am J Trop Med Hyg 1988;38:81.

Sharfi AR, Rayis AB: The continuing challenge of bilharzial ureteric stricture. Scand J Urol Nephrol 1989;23:123.

Stock JA, Scherz HC, Kaplan GW: Urinary schistosomiasis in childhood. Urology 1994;44:305.

Tungekar MF, Gatter KC, Al-Adnani MS: Immunohistochemistry of cytokeratin proteins in squamous and transitional cell lesions of the urinary tract. J Clin Pathol 1988;41:1288.

FILARIASIS

Brunkwall J et al: Chyluria treated with renal autotransplantation: A case report. J Urol 1990;143:793.

Kohli V, Gulati S, Kumar L: Filarial chyluria. Indian Pediatr 1994;31:451.

Nelson GS: Current concepts in parasitology: Filariasis. N Engl J Med 1979;300:1136.

Okamoto K, Ohi Y: Recent distribution and treatment of filarial chyluria in Japan. J Urol 1983;129:64.

Pool MO et al: Bilateral excision of perinephric fat and fascia (Gerota's fasciectomy) in the treatment of intractable chyluria. J Urol 1991;146:1374.

Punekar SV et al: Surgical disconnection of lymphorenal communication for chyluria: A 15-year experience. Br J Urol 1997;80:858.

Thrasher JB, Snyder JA: Post-nephrolithotomy chyluria. J Urol 1990;143:578.

Xu YM et al: Microsurgical treatment of chyluria: A preliminary report. J Urol 1991;145:1184.

Yagi S et al: Endoscopic treatment of refractory filarial chyluria: A preliminary report. J Urol 1998;159:1615.

ONCHOCERCIASIS

Kumate J: Infectious diseases in the 21st century. Arch Med Res 1997;28:155.

Ottesen EA: Immune responsiveness and the pathogenesis of human onchocerciasis. J Infect Dis 1995;171:659.

Van Laethem Y, Lopes C: Treatment of onchocerciasis. Drugs 1996;52:861.

ECHINOCOCCOSIS (HYDATID DISEASE)

Birkhoff JD, McClennan BL: Echinococcal disease of the pelvis: Urologic complication, diagnosis and treatment. J Urol 1973;109:473.

Cirenei A: Histopathology, clinical findings and treatment of renal hydatidosis. Ann Ital Chir 1997;68:275.

Diamond HM et al: Echinococcal disease of the kidney. J Urol 1976;115:742.

Kumar PV, Jahanshahi S: Hydatid cyst of testis: A case report. J Urol 1987;137:511.

Martorana G, Giberi C, Pescatore D: Giant echinococcal cyst of the kidney associated with hypertension evaluated by computerized tomography. J Urol 1981;126:99.

Migaleddu V et al: Imaging of renal hydatid cysts. AJR 1997;169:1339.

Pasaoglu E et al: Hydatid cysts of the kidney, seminal vesicle and gluteus muscle. Australas Radiol 1997;41:297.

Ptasznik R, Hennessy OF: Pelvic hydatid disease presenting as acute urinary retention. Br J Radiol 1988;61:164.

16

Sexually Transmitted Diseases

John N. Krieger, MD

The didactic approach to discussing sexually transmitted diseases (STDs) is to consider the causative agents, emphasizing different classes, genera, and species of organisms. This fits with most medical school curricula, since the causative agents span the full spectrum of medical microbiology (viruses, bacteria, protozoa, ectoparasites, etc). Unfortunately, this classical approach may be of limited help in clinical practice, where many different types of agents must be considered in the differential diagnosis of an individual patient.

This chapter takes a selective and practical approach. Patients present with particular syndromes that may be caused by a variety of microorganisms, often from very different microbiologic classes. Therefore, I emphasize diagnosis and treatment of clinical syndromes in contrast to traditional teaching (Table 16–1). This is a large subject with much active research and a huge literature. I consider the most important conditions encountered in urology: urethritis, epididymitis, genital ulcers, genital warts, and a brief consideration of human immunodeficiency virus (HIV) infection.

The interested reader is referred to the reference list for discussion of other STD syndromes, including prevention messages and methods; STDs in special populations (children, adolescents, and pregnant women); vaginitis syndromes; pelvic inflammatory disease; cervical cancer screening; vaccine-preventable STDs; ectoparasitic infections; sexually transmitted proctitis, proctocolitis, and enteritis; and sexual assault and STDs.

URETHRITIS & CERVICITIS

Urethritis in Men

Urethritis, or urethral inflammation, is often caused by infection. Characteristically, patients complain of urethral discharge and dysuria. On examination the discharge may be purulent or mucopurulent. Asymptomatic infections are common. The common bacterial causes are *Neisseria gonorrhoeae* and *Chlamydia trachomatis.*

Testing is recommended to document a specific disease, because both of these infections are reportable to health departments. Specific diagnosis may also improve compliance and partner notification. The traditional diagnostic algorithm includes microscopic examination of the Gram's-stained urethral smear for gram-negative intracellular diplococci (*N gonorrhoeae*) and culture for *N gonorrhoeae*. New nucleic acid amplification tests have proved accurate for detection of *N gonorrhoeae* and *C trachomatis* in first-void urine in high-risk populations. If diagnostic testing is unavailable, patients should be treated empirically for both infections.

Complications of urethritis in men include epididymitis (see below), disseminated gonococcal infection, and Reiter's syndrome. Complications of urethritis in female sex partners include pelvic inflammatory disease, ectopic pregnancy, and infertility. Complications in children include neonatal pneumonia and ophthalmia neonatorum.

Etiology: Gonorrhea is diagnosed when *N gonorrhoeae* is detected by Gram's stain, culture, or nucleic acid amplification testing. Nongonococcal urethritis (NGU) is diagnosed when gram-negative intracellular organisms cannot be diagnosed on microscopic examination. *C trachomatis,* the most common infectious cause of NGU, is responsible for 23–55% of cases in reported studies, but the proportion of cases is substantially lower in urologic practice. The prevalence of chlamydial infection differs by age group, with a lower prevalence among older men. In addition, the proportion of cases of NGU caused by *C trachomatis* has been declining. Documentation of chlamydial NGU is important, because this diagnosis supports partner referral, evaluation, and treatment.

The causes of most cases of nonchlamydial NGU are unknown. The genital mycoplasmas, *Ureaplasma urealyticum* and perhaps *Mycoplasma genitalium* or *Mycoplasma hominis,* are implicated in 20–30% of cases in some studies. Specific diagnostic tests for these organisms are not indicated routinely. *Trichomonas vaginalis,* a protozoan parasite, and herpes simplex virus (HSV) may also cause NGU. Testing

Table 16–1. Sexually transmitted disease (STD) syndromes.[1]

Urethritis and cervicitis[2]	Nongonococcal urethritis
	Gonococcal infection
	Chlamydial infection
	Mucopurulent cervicitis
Epididymitis[2]	
Genital ulcers[2]	Genital herpes simplex virus (HSV)
	Syphilis
	Chancroid
	Lymphogranuloma venereum (LGV)
	Granuloma inguinale (donovanosis)
Human papillomavirus (HPV) infections[2]	Genital warts
	Subclinical genital HPV
HIV infection[2]	
Vaginal discharge	Trichomoniasis
	Vulvovaginal candidiasis
	Bacterial vaginosis
Pelvic inflammatory disease	
Ectoparasitic infections	Pediculosis pubis
	Scabies
Vaccine-preventable STDs	Hepatitis A
	Hepatitis B
Proctitis, proctocolitis, and enteritis	
Sexual assault and STDs	

[1] According to Centers for Disease Control and Prevention: 1998 guidelines for treatment of sexually transmitted diseases. MMWR Morb Mortal Wkly Rep 1998;47(RR–1):1.
[2] Considered in this chapter.

and treatment for these organisms should be considered when NGU is unresponsive to treatment.

Document Urethritis: It is important to document urethritis, because some patients have symptoms in the absence of inflammation. Urethritis may be documented by the presence of any of the following clinical signs: mucopurulent urethral discharge on physical examination, > 5 leukocytes per oil immersion microscopic field of the Gram's-stained urethral secretions, a positive leukocyte esterase test on first-void urine, or > 10 leukocytes per high-power microscopic field of the first-void urine. Gram's stain is the preferred diagnostic test for documenting urethritis and for evaluating the presence or absence of gonococcal infection, because it is highly sensitive and specific.

If none of the criteria for urethritis are met, then treatment should be deferred. The patient should be tested for both *N gonorrhoeae* and *C trachomatis* and followed up closely in the event of a positive test result.

Empiric treatment of symptoms without documenting urethritis is recommended only if the patient is at high risk for infection and is unlikely to return for follow-up. Empiric treatment should be appropriate for both gonococcal and chlamydial infection. Sex partners should be referred for appropriate evaluation and treatment.

Treatment of Gonococcal Infections: There are an estimated 600,000 new gonococcal infections per year in the United States. In men, most infections cause symptoms that motivate the patient to seek treatment soon enough to prevent serious sequelae. However, this may not be soon enough to prevent transmission of infection to sex partners. In contrast, many gonococcal (and also chlamydial) infections in women do not cause recognizable symptoms until the patient presents with complications, such as pelvic inflammatory disease. Both symptomatic and asymptomatic pelvic inflammatory disease result in tubal scarring, increased rates of ectopic pregnancy, and infertility.

Dual therapy is recommended for both gonococcal and chlamydial infection, because patients are often coinfected with both pathogens. Some authorities feel that routine use of dual therapy has led to substantial decreases in the prevalence of gonorrhea. Since most gonococci in the United States are susceptible to doxycycline and azithromycin, cotreatment may also limit development of antimicrobial resistant *N gonorrhoeae*. Quinolone-resistant *N gonorrhoeae* has been reported in many geographic areas, and such infections are becoming widespread in parts of Asia. To date, however, the prevalence of quinolone resistance has been exceedingly low in the United States. Although resistant strains will continue to be imported into this country, quinolones can still be recommended for treatment. Table 16–2 summarizes recommended treatment regimens that reliably cure > 97% of uncomplicated gonococcal infections. Pharyngeal infections are more difficult to treat, and few regimens reliably cure > 90% of infections. Patients who cannot tolerate cephalosporins or quinolones should be treated with spectinomycin (2 g as a single dose intramuscularly [IM]). However, this regimen is only 52% effective for pharyngeal infections.

Routine test-of-cure cultures are no longer recommended for patients treated with the recommended regimens. Such patients should refer their sex partners for evaluation and treatment. However, patients should be reevaluated if their symptoms persist after therapy. Any gonococci that persist should be evaluated for antimicrobial susceptibility, but infections identified after treatment are usually reinfections rather than treatment failures. Persistent inflammation may be caused by *C trachomatis* or other organisms.

A few patients develop complications such as disseminated gonococcal infection, perihepatitis, meningitis, or endocarditis. These infections result from gonococcal bacteremia. Disseminated gonococcal infection often causes petechial or pustular skin lesions, asymmetric arthralgias, tenosynovitis, or septic arthritis. Some patients develop perihepatitis or, rarely, endocarditis or meningitis. *N gonorrhoeae* strains that cause disseminated infection tend to

Table 16–2. Urethritis, cervicitis, and related infections: Recommended treatment regimens[1]

Gonococcal infections
  Uncomplicated urethral, cervical, and rectal infections
    Cefixime, 400 mg as a single dose; or ceftriaxone, 125 mg as a single IM dose; or ciprofloxacin, 500 mg as a single oral dose; or ofloxacin, 400 mg as a single oral dose, plus azithromycin, 1 g as a single oral dose; or doxycycline, 100 mg orally twice a day for 7 days
  Uncomplicated pharyngeal infections
    Ceftriaxone, 125 mg as a single IM dose; or ciprofloxacin, 500 mg as a single oral dose; or ofloxacin, 400 mg as a single oral dose, plus azithromycin, 1 g as a single oral dose; or doxycycline, 100 mg orally twice a day for 7 days
Nongonococcal urethritis (chlamydial infections)
  Azithromycin, 1 g as a single oral dose; or doxycycline, 100 mg orally twice a day for 7 days
Recurrent and persistent urethritis
  Metronidazole, 2 g as a single oral dose, plus erythromycin base, 500 mg orally 4 times a day for 7 days; or erythromycin ethylsuccinate, 800 mg orally 4 times a day for 7 days

[1] According to Centers for Disease Control and Prevention: 1998 guidelines for treatment of sexually transmitted diseases. MMWR Morb Mortal Wkly Rep 1998;47(RR–1):1.

cause minimal genital tract inflammation. The recommended treatment is ceftriaxone (1 g IM or intravenously [IV] every 24 h for disseminated infection or 1 g IV every 12 h for meningitis or endocarditis).

Treatment of Nongonococcal Urethritis (NGU): Treatment of NGU should be initiated as soon after diagnosis as possible (Table 16–2). Single-dose regimens of azithromycin or doxycycline are preferred because they offer the advantages of improved compliance and directly observed therapy. Alternative choices for patients who are allergic to or cannot tolerate these drugs include a 7-day course of either erythromycin or ofloxacin. Routine follow-up and repeat testing are no longer recommended for patients taking the recommended regimens. However, patients should return for reevaluation if symptoms persist or recur after completion of treatment. The presence of symptoms alone without documentation of signs or laboratory findings of inflammation is not sufficient for retreatment. Patients should refer their sex partners for appropriate evaluation and treatment.

Treatment of Recurrent and Persistent Urethritis: Objective signs of urethritis should be documented before a repeated course of empiric therapy is prescribed. Men with persistent or recurrent urethritis should be retreated with the initial regimen if they did not comply with treatment or if they were reexposed to an untreated sex partner. Other patients should have a wet-mount and urethral culture for *T vaginalis*. For patients who were compliant with the initial regimen and who were not reexposed, the regimen in Table 16–2 should be used. This regimen provides treatment for both *T vaginalis* and the genital mycoplasmas.

Mucopurulent Cervicitis in Women

Mucopurulent cervicitis has many parallels to urethritis in men. Characteristically, patients have a purulent or mucopurulent endocervical exudate visible in the endocervical canal or on an endocervical swab sample. Easily induced endocervical bleeding is also common, as is an increased number of polymorphonuclear cells on the Gram's-stained endocervical secretions. Patients may present with abnormal vaginal discharge or abnormal vaginal bleeding, such as after intercourse, but many are asymptomatic.

As with urethritis in men, *N gonorrhoeae* and *C trachomatis* are the most important infectious causes of mucopurulent cervicitis, but in many women neither pathogen is identified. Treatment should be guided by the results of testing for gonococcal and chlamydial infection, unless the patient is considered unlikely to return for follow-up. In such cases, empiric therapy should be given for both *C trachomatis* and *N gonorrhoeae*.

EPIDIDYMITIS

Epididymitis is caused by sexually transmitted pathogens or by organisms causing urinary tract infection. Among sexually active men < 35 years old, most cases of epididymitis are caused by sexually transmitted pathogens, particularly *C trachomatis* and *N gonorrhoeae*. Epididymitis may also be caused by *Escherichia coli* among men who are the insertive partners during anal intercourse. Sexually transmitted epididymitis is usually associated with urethritis, which is often asymptomatic. Patients with uncomplicated sexually transmitted epididymitis do not require thorough evaluation for anatomic abnormalities.

In men > 35 years old, most cases of epididymitis are associated with urinary tract infection. The most common pathogens are gram-negative enteric bacteria. Epididymitis associated with urinary infection is more common among men who have anatomic abnormalities or those who have recently had urinary tract instrumentation. Therefore, evaluation of genitourinary tract anatomy is indicated for men with epididymitis associated with urinary tract infection.

Epididymitis is typically associated with unilateral hemiscrotal pain and tenderness. An inflammatory hydrocele and palpable swelling of the epididymis are characteristic. Diagnostic recommendations include a Gram's-stained smear for evaluation of urethritis and for presumptive identification of gonococcal infection, diagnostic testing for *N gonorrhoeae* and *C trachomatis,* urine Gram's stain and culture, and syphilis serologic and HIV tests (if sexually transmitted epididymitis is likely).

Treatment: Outpatient management is appropriate for most patients with epididymitis. Hospitalization should be considered when severe pain suggests other possible diagnoses, such as testicular torsion, testicular infarction, or testicular abscess, when patients are febrile, or when noncompliance with medication is likely. Empiric antimicrobial regimens are summarized in Table 16–3. Adjunctive measures include bed rest, scrotal elevation, and analgesics until fever and local inflammation subside.

Routine follow-up is recommended. Failure to respond within 3 days requires reevaluation of both the diagnosis and treatment. Swelling and tenderness that persist after completion of antimicrobial therapy should be reevaluated to consider possible testicular tumor, abscess, infarction, tuberculosis, or fungal epididymitis. HIV-infected patients with epididymitis should receive the same initial therapy as HIV-negative men. However, fungi, atypical mycobacteria, and other opportunistic infections are more likely in immunosuppressed patients.

GENITAL ULCER DISEASES

In the United States, genital herpes (HSV) is the most common cause of genital ulcers. Other important considerations are syphilis and chancroid. In contrast, lymphogranuloma venereum (LGV) and granuloma inguinale (donovanosis) are uncommon causes of genital ulcers in this country. Each of these ulcerative STDs is associated with a 2- to 5-fold increased risk of HIV transmission.

Diagnostic Testing

Diagnosis based solely on the history and physical findings is often inaccurate. Patients may be infected with more than one agent simultaneously. Ideally,

Table 16–3. Epididymitis: Recommended treatment regimens[1]

Gonococcal or chlamydial infection likely
Ceftriaxone, 250 mg in a single IM dose, plus doxycyline, 100 mg orally twice a day for 10 days
Enteric infection likely
Ofloxacin, 300 mg orally twice a day for 10 days

[1] According to Centers for Disease Control and Prevention: 1998 guidelines for treatment of sexually transmitted diseases. MMWR Morb Mortal Wkly Rep 1998; 47(RR–1):1.

evaluation of patients with genital ulcers should include testing for the most common causes: HSV, syphilis, and chancroid. These tests include a culture or antigen test for HSV, a darkfield examination or direct immunofluorescence test for *Treponema pallidum* (syphilis), and a culture for *Haemophilus ducreyi* (chancroid). In the future, improved molecular detection tests for these organisms may become commercially available. After thorough diagnostic evaluation, 25% of patients with genital ulcers do not have a laboratory-confirmed diagnosis. HIV testing is also recommended for patients who have genital ulcers (see below).

Often, patients must be treated before test results become available. In this situation, treatment is recommended for both syphilis and chancroid.

Genital Herpes Virus Infection

Genital HSV is an incurable and recurrent viral infection. Characteristically, patients present with painful genital lesions that start as papules or vesicles. Often, the genital lesions have evolved into pustules or ulcers. With primary genital herpes, the ulcerative lesions persist for 4–15 days until crusting, reepithelization, or both. Pain, itching, vaginal or urethral discharge, and tender inguinal adenopathy are the predominant local symptoms. Primary HSV infection is associated with a high frequency and prolonged duration of systemic and local symptoms. Fever, headache, malaise, and myalgias are common. The clinical symptoms of pain and irritation from genital lesions gradually increase over the first 6–7 days, reach maximum intensity between days 7 and 11, then recede gradually during the second or third week.

In contrast to first episodes of genital infection, recurrent HSV infection is characterized by symptoms, signs, and anatomic sites localized to the genital region. Local symptoms, such as pain and itching, are mild compared with the symptoms of initial infection, and the duration of the usual episode ranges from 8–12 days or less.

Two HSV serotypes cause genital ulcers: HSV-1 and HSV-2. Both viruses infect the genital tract, but HSV-2 is substantially more likely to cause recurrent infections. Studies suggest that 5–30% of first episodes of genital HSV infection are caused by HSV-1. However, recurrences of HSV-1 infection are substantially less likely than recurrences of HSV-2. Therefore, HSV-2 cases predominate in the population of patients with recurrent genital lesions. Typing the infecting strain has prognostic importance and is useful for patient counseling. However, most commercially available antibody tests are not accurate enough to distinguish HSV-1 from HSV-2 infection. Better assays should become available in the future.

Serologic studies suggest that 45 million people in the United States are infected with genital HSV-2.

Most infections are mild or unrecognized. Therefore, most HSV-infected people do not receive this diagnosis. Asymptomatic or mildly symptomatic persons shed virus intermittently in their genital tracts and can infect their sex partners. First-episode genital HSV infections are more likely to cause symptoms than are recurrent infections. Occasional cases are severe enough to require hospitalization for complications such as disseminated infection, pneumonitis, hepatitis, meningitis, or encephalitis.

Treatment: Systemic antiviral therapy results in partial control of symptoms and signs of genital HSV infection. Treatment does not cure the infection or change the frequency or severity of recurrences after discontinuation of treatment. Three antiviral drugs have proved beneficial in randomized clinical trials: acyclovir, valacyclovir, and famciclovir (Table 16–4). Topical treatment with acyclovir has proved substantially less effective than systemic treatment.

Patients with first clinical episodes of genital HSV should receive antiviral treatment to speed healing of genital lesions and to shorten the duration of viral shedding. Patients should also be counseled about the natural history of genital herpes, the risks for sexual and perinatal transmission, and methods to reduce transmission. Patients with severe disease should receive IV treatment with acyclovir.

Most persons with first clinical episodes of genital HSV-2 experience recurrent episodes. Treatment can shorten the duration of lesions and decrease recurrences. Thus, many patients can benefit from antiviral therapy, and this option should be discussed. There are two approaches to antiviral therapy for recurrent HSV infection: episodic treatment and daily suppressive treatment. Episodic therapy is beneficial for many patients with occasional recurrences. Such therapy is started during the prodrome or first day of lesions. Thus, patients on episodic therapy should receive the medication or a prescription so that they can initiate treatment at the first symptom or sign of lesions.

Daily suppressive therapy is useful for patients who experience frequent recurrences (6 or more per year). Therapy reduces the frequency of recurrences by > 75%. Such treatment has been shown to be safe and effective for as long as 6 years with acyclovir

Table 16–4. Genital ulcers: Recommended treatment regimens.[1]

Genital herpes
  First episode
    Acyclovir, 400 mg orally 3 times a day for 7–10 days; or acyclovir, 200 mg orally 5 times a day for 7–10 days; or famciclovir, 250 mg orally 3 times a day for 7–10 days; or valacyclovir, 1 g orally twice a day for 7–10 days
  Severe disease
    Acyclovir, 5–10 mg/kg body weight IV every 8 h for 5–7 days or until clinical resolution
Recurrent episodes
  Episodic recurrences
    Acyclovir, 400 mg orally 3 times a day for 5 days; or acyclovir, 200 mg orally 5 times a day for 5 days; or acyclovir, 800 mg orally twice a day for 5 days; or famciclovir, 125 mg orally twice a day for 5 days; or valacyclovir, 500 mg orally twice a day for 5 days
  Daily suppressive therapy
    Acyclovir, 400 mg orally twice a day; or famciclovir, 250 mg orally twice a day; or valacyclovir, 250 mg orally twice a day; or valacyclovir, 500 mg orally twice a day; or valacyclovir, 1 g orally twice a day
Syphilis
  Primary and secondary
    Benzathine penicillin G, 2.4 million units IM as a single dose
  Tertiary (except neurosyphilis)
    Benzathine penicillin G, 2.4 million units IM weekly for 3 weeks
  Neurosyphilis
    Aqueous crystalline penicillin G, 3–4 million units IV every 4 hours for 10–14 days; or procaine penicillin, 2.4 million units IM daily for 10–14 days, plus probenecid, 500 mg orally 4 times a day for 10–14 days
  Latent syphilis
    Early
        Benzathine penicillin G, 2.4 million units IM as a single dose
    Late or of unknown duration
        Benzathine penicillin G, 2.4 million units IM weekly for 3 weeks
Chancroid
    Azithromycin, 1 g as a single oral dose; or ceftriaxone, 250 mg as a single IM dose; or ciprofloxacin, 500 mg orally twice a day for 3 days; or erythromycin base, 500 mg orally 4 times a day for 7 days
Granuloma inguinale
    Trimethoprim-sulfamethoxazole, 1 double-strength tablet orally twice a day for a minimum of 3 weeks; or doxycycline, 100 mg orally twice a day for a minimum of 3 weeks
Lymphogranuloma venereum
    Doxycycline, 100 mg orally twice a day for 21 days

[1] According to the Centers for Disease Control and Prevention: 1998 guidelines for treatment of sexually transmitted diseases. MMWR Morb Mortal Wkly Rep 1998;47(RR–1):1.

and for as long as 1 year with both valacyclovir and famciclovir. Daily therapy does not appear to be associated with clinically significant HSV drug resistance. After 1 year, discontinuation of treatment should be considered, since the frequency of recurrences often decreases with time.

Syphilis

Syphilis may be the deepest and darkest of all the infectious diseases. This complex illness is caused by *T pallidum,* a spirochete, and holds a special place in the history of medicine as "the great imposter" and "the great imitator." Sir William Osler in 1897 said, "Know syphilis in all its manifestations and relations, and all other things clinical will be added unto you."

Syphilis is a systemic disease. Patients may seek treatment for symptoms or signs of primary, secondary, or tertiary infection. Primary infection is characterized by an ulcer, or chancre, at the site of infection. Secondary manifestations include rash, mucocutaneous lesions, and adenopathy. Tertiary infection may present with cardiac, neurologic, ophthalmic, auditory, or gummatous lesions. In addition, syphilis may be diagnosed by serologic testing of asymptomatic patients; this is termed latent syphilis. Latent syphilis acquired within the preceding year is classified as early latent syphilis. All other cases of latent syphilis are classified as late latent syphilis or syphilis of unknown duration.

Sexual transmission of syphilis occurs only when mucocutaneous lesions are present. These manifestations are uncommon after the first year of infection in untreated patients. However, all persons exposed to a person with syphilis should be evaluated clinically and by serologic testing.

Definitive diagnosis of early syphilis is done by darkfield examination or direct immunofluorescent antibody tests of lesion exudate. Presumptive diagnosis depends on serologic testing. Serologic tests are either nontreponemal, such as the VDRL and rapid plasma reagin (RPR) tests, or treponemal, such as the fluorescent treponemal antibody absorption (FTA-ABS) test and microagglutination assay for antibody to *T pallidum* (MHA-TP). Use of only one type of serologic test is considered insufficient for diagnosis. False-positive nontreponemal test results occur with a variety of medical conditions. Nontreponemal tests correlate with disease activity, and results are reported quantitatively. In general, a 4-fold change in titer is considered significant. Most patients with reactive treponemal tests remain reactive for life. Treponemal test titers correlate poorly with disease activity. Thus, a combination of treponemal and nontreponemal tests is necessary for patient management.

Treatment: For more than 40 years, penicillin has been the treatment of choice for syphilis (Table 16–4). Patients who are allergic to penicillin should receive a 2-week course of doxycycline (100 mg orally twice a day) or tetracycline (500 mg orally 4 times a day). Treatment heals local lesions, prevents sexual transmission, and prevents late sequelae. Patients with syphilis should be tested for HIV infection. In geographic areas with a high prevalence of HIV, this test should be repeated after 3 months if the initial HIV test is negative. Patients with syphilis and symptoms or signs of ophthalmic disease should have a slit-lamp examination, and those with symptoms or signs of neurologic disease should have cerebrospinal fluid evaluation. Because treatment failures occur with any regimen, serologic testing should be repeated 6 and 12 months after initial treatment.

Chancroid

Chancroid is an acute ulcerative disease often associated with inguinal adenopathy ("bubo"). *H ducreyi,* a gram-negative facultative bacillus, is the causative agent. The infection is endemic in parts of the United States, and the disease also occurs in outbreaks. An estimated 10% of patients with chancroid are coinfected with either *T pallidum* or HSV. Each of these infections is associated with an increased rate of HIV transmission.

Definitive diagnosis of chancroid requires identification of the causative bacterium, *H ducreyi,* on specialized culture media that are not widely available. In addition, these media have an estimated sensitivity of < 80%. In practice, a probable diagnosis of chancroid can be based on the following: The patient has a painful genital ulcer; there is no evidence of *T pallidum* by darkfield examination or by syphilis serologic testing at least 7 days before the onset of ulcers; an HSV test is negative; and the clinical appearance is typical. The combination of a painful genital ulcer and tender inguinal adenopathy also suggests the diagnosis of chancroid. Unfortunately, this characteristic clinical appearance occurs in only one-third of cases. However, the combination of a painful genital ulcer and suppurative inguinal adenopathy is considered almost pathognomonic.

Treatment: Recommended antimicrobial regimens for chancroid are summarized in Table 16–4. Successful treatment cures the infection, resolves symptoms, and prevents transmission. However, scarring can continue despite successful treatment. Uncircumcised or HIV-infected patients may respond less well to treatment. Testing for HIV and syphilis is recommended at the time of diagnosis and again 3 months later, if the initial tests are negative.

Follow-up is recommended after 3–7 days. If there is minimal or no clinical improvement, another diagnosis or the possibility of coinfection with another STD should be considered. A few *H ducreyi* strains are resistant to antimicrobial agents. Large ulcers or fluctuant lymphadenopathy may take > 2 weeks for resolution. Occasionally, patients require incision and drainage or needle aspiration of fluctuant inguinal nodes.

Lymphogranuloma Venereum

LGV is caused by the invasive serovars of *C trachomatis* (L1, L2, and L3). The disease is a rare cause of genital ulcers in the United States. Tender inguinal or femoral lymphadenopathy, often unilateral, is the characteristic clinical presentation in heterosexual men. Women and homosexual men may present with inflammatory involvement of perirectal and perianal lymphatics, strictures, fistulas, or proctocolitis. Usually, the self-limited genital ulcers have healed when most patients seek medical care. In most clinical settings, diagnosis is made by serologic testing and exclusion of other causes of inguinal adenopathy or genital ulcers.

Treatment: Therapy causes microbiologic cure and prevents ongoing tissue destruction (Table 16–4). Doxycycline is preferred, but erythromycin and azithromycin are alternatives. Prolonged therapy, for a minimum of 3 weeks, is necessary with each of these drugs. However, tissue reaction and scarring can progress after effective treatment. Inguinal adenopathy may require needle aspiration through intact skin or incision and drainage to prevent inguinal or femoral ulcerations. Patients should be followed up until clinical symptoms and signs are resolved.

Granuloma Inguinale (Donovanosis)

Granuloma inguinale is caused by *Calymmatobacterium granulomatis,* a gram-negative intracellular bacillus. This infection is rare in the United States. Granuloma inguinale is an important cause of genital ulcers in tropical and developing countries, particularly India, Papua New Guinea, central Australia, and southern Africa.

Clinically, granuloma inguinale presents with painless, progressive genital ulcers. The genital lesions are highly vascular, with a beefy red appearance. These patients seldom have inguinal adenopathy. The causative organism cannot be cultured on standard microbiologic media. Diagnosis requires visualization of dark-staining Donovan bodies on tissue crush preparations or biopsy specimens. Secondary bacterial infections may develop in the lesions. In addition, coinfection with other STD agents may occur.

Treatment: Effective treatment halts progressive tissue destruction (Table 16–4). Trimethoprim-sulfamethoxazole or doxycycline is recommended. Alternative drugs are ciprofloxacin or erythromycin. Prolonged treatment is often necessary to facilitate granulation and reepithelization of the ulcers. Patients should be reevaluated after the first few days of treatment. Addition of an aminoglycoside, such as gentamicin, should be considered if lesions have not responded, and treatment should be continued until all lesions have healed. Relapse can occur 6–18 months after effective initial therapy.

Genital Warts

Genital warts are caused by human papillomavirus (HPV) infection. Of the more than 80 HPV genotypes, more than 20 infect the genital tract. Most of these genital HPV infections are asymptomatic, subclinical, or unrecognized. Depending on their size and anatomic location, visible external warts can be painful, friable, pruritic, or all three. Most visible genital warts are caused by HPV types 6 or 11. These HPV types can also cause exophytic warts on the cervix and within the vagina, urethra, and anus. HPV types 6 and 11 are only rarely associated with development of invasive squamous cell carcinoma of the external genitalia.

HPV types 16, 18, 31, 33, and 35 are uncommon in visible external genital warts. These HPV types are associated with cervical dysplasia, as well as vaginal, anal, and cervical squamous cell carcinoma. They have also been associated with external genital intraepithelial neoplastic lesions, including squamous cell carcinoma, carcinoma in situ, bowenoid papulosis, erythroplasia of Queyrat, and Bowen disease. Patients with external genital warts can be infected simultaneously with more than one HPV type.

Most often, the diagnosis of genital warts can be made by inspection. Diagnosis can be confirmed by biopsy, if necessary, but biopsy is rarely necessary. Biopsy is indicated only if the diagnosis is uncertain, if lesions do not respond to standard therapy, if the disease worsens during treatment, if the patient is immunocompromised, or if warts are pigmented, indurated, fixed, or ulcerated. Routine use of type-specific HPV nucleic acid tests is not indicated for diagnosis or management of visible genital warts.

Treatment: For visible genital warts, the primary goal of treatment is removal of symptomatic lesions. Treatment can induce wart-free periods in most patients. Genital warts are often asymptomatic, and lesions may resolve spontaneously. Currently, there are no data indicating that available therapy can eradicate HPV infection or change the natural history of infection. In theory, removal of exophytic warts may decrease infectivity, but there is no evidence that treatment changes the risk for development of dysplastic or cancerous lesions in the patient or in sex partners.

Treatment decisions should be guided by the health provider's experience and patient preferences. None of the recommended therapies is superior or ideal for every case. Treatments can be patient-applied or provider-administered (Table 16–5). Most patients with visible warts have lesions that respond to most treatment modalities. Many patients require a course of therapy. In general, lesions on moist surfaces or in intertriginous areas respond better to topical treatments, such as trichloroacetic acid, podophyllin, or imiquimod, than do warts on drier surfaces.

Podofilox is an antimitotic drug that destroys warts. Most patients experience pain or local irritation after treatment. Imiquimod is a topically active immune en-

Table 16–5. External genital warts: Recommended treatment regimens.[1]

Patient-applied
  Podofilox, 0.5% solution of gel to lesions twice a day for 3 days, followed by 4 days off therapy; repeat as needed for up to 4 cycles; or imiquimod, 5% cream to lesions at bedtime 3 times a week for up to 16 weeks; wash off after 6–10 h
Provider-administered
  Cryotherapy with liquid nitrogen or cryoprobe; repeat as necessary every 1–2 weeks; or podophyllin resin, 10–25% in tincture of benzoin; repeat weekly as necessary; or trichlor/bichloracetic acid, 80–90%; apply until white "frosting"; repeat weekly as necessary; or surgical removal

[1] According to Centers for Disease Control and Prevention: Guidelines for treatment of sexually transmitted diseases. MMWR Morb Mortal Wkly Rep 1998;47(RR–1):1.

hancer that stimulates production of cytokines, followed by local inflammation and resolution of warts. Effective use of cryotherapy requires training to avoid either overtreatment or undertreatment and poor results. Pain is common after application of liquid nitrogen, followed by necrosis of the warts. Podophyllin resin contains a number of antimitotic compounds. Resin preparations vary in the concentrations of active components and contaminants. Although both trichloroacetic acid and bichloroacetic acid are recommended and are used widely, these treatments are associated with a number of potential problems. The acid can spread rapidly if applied excessively, with damage to normal adjacent tissues. These solutions should be applied sparingly and allowed to dry before the patient stands. If the patient experiences excessive discomfort, the acid can be neutralized by using soap or sodium bicarbonate (baking soda). Treatment should be changed if the patient has not improved substantially after 3 provider-administered treatments or if warts do not resolve completely after 6 treatments.

Surgical removal offers the advantage of rendering the patient wart-free in a single visit. A number of approaches are possible, including tangential scissor or shave excision, curettage, electrosurgery, or laser surgery. All of these methods require local anesthesia and are more time-consuming and expensive than the methods discussed above. Surgical approaches are most useful if patients have a large number or large volume of genital warts, if the diagnosis is uncertain, or if patients have been unresponsive to other treatments. Patients should be warned that scarring, hypopigmentation, and hyperpigmentation are common after ablative therapies. Occasionally, patients develop chronic pain after such treatment.

Recurrence of warts is common after all therapies, most often within the first 3 months. Women should be counseled about the need for regular cervical cytologic screening. Examination of sex partners is unnecessary for management of external genital warts, because the role of reinfection is probably minimal. However, sex partners of patients with genital warts may benefit from evaluation for genital warts and other STDs.

Subclinical Genital HPV Infection

Subclinical HPV infection (without visible genital warts) is more common than visible genital lesions. Most cases are diagnosed indirectly by cervical cytologic testing, colposcopy, or biopsy of genital skin, or by routine use of acetic acid soaks and examination with magnification for "acetowhite" areas. The consensus of expert opinion is to discourage routine examination for acetowhiting. This test has poor specificity for HPV infection and has many false-positive results in low-risk populations. Definitive diagnosis of subclinical HPV infection requires detection of HPV nucleic acid or capsid protein, but this test is not recommended outside of research settings.

Treatment of subclinical HPV infection is not recommended in the absence of dysplasia. Diagnosis is often questionable because many of the diagnostic tests (e.g., cytologic, acetowhiting, colposcopy) correlate poorly with detection of HPV DNA or RNA. Furthermore, no therapy has been proved to eradicate infection. HPV has been demonstrated in normal-appearing tissue adjacent to treated areas after aggressive surgical treatment.

HIV INFECTION: OVERVIEW OF DETECTION, INITIAL EVALUATION, & REFERRAL

Infection with HIV produces a wide clinical spectrum, ranging from asymptomatic infection to AIDS. The rate of clinical progression is highly variable. Some persons progress from HIV infection to AIDS within a few months; others remain asymptomatic for decades. Overall, the median time from infection to AIDS is around 10 years. Adults with HIV infection can remain asymptomatic for prolonged periods. However, HIV viral replication continues during all stages of infection, with substantial increases in the viral burden during later stages of infection, accompanied by marked deterioration in immune function.

Increasing awareness of risk factors for HIV infection has led to increased testing and earlier diagnosis for many patients. The primary risk factors for HIV infection are sexual contact with an HIV-infected person and the sharing of injecting-drug equipment.

Early diagnosis is important, because treatment can slow the decline in immune function. HIV-infected persons with evidence of immune dysfunction are at risk for preventable infections. Prophylactic treatment can substantially reduce the risk of pneumonia (*Pneumocystis carinii* and bacterial), toxoplasma encephalitis, and mycobacterial disease (tuberculosis and *Mycobacterium avium* complex). Early diagnosis also facilitates patient counseling, which may reduce transmission. In addition, early diagnosis facilitates planning for referral to a health care provider or facility experienced in the care of HIV-infected persons.

Testing for HIV

Diagnostic testing for HIV should be offered to anyone at risk for infection, especially those seeking evaluation for STDs. Appropriate pre- and posttest counseling and informed consent should be included in the test procedure. Some states require documentation of informed consent.

Usually, HIV infection is documented by using HIV-1 antibody tests. HIV antibodies are detected in > 95% of infected persons within 6 months of infection. In most laboratories, this is a 2-stage procedure beginning with a sensitive screening test, such as an enzyme immunoassay. Reactive screening test results are then confirmed by a supplemental test, such as a Western blot or an immunofluorescence assay. Patients with positive results on both the screening and confirmatory tests are infected with HIV and can transmit the virus.

In the United States, almost all HIV infections are caused by HIV-1. Extremely rare cases are caused by a second virus, HIV-2. Thus, routine clinical testing for HIV-2 is not recommended. The only indications for this test are in blood centers and for persons who have specific demographic or behavioral risk factors for HIV-2. These persons include those from countries where HIV-2 is endemic (West Africa, Angola, Mozambique, France, and Portugal) and their sex partners. The possibility of HIV-2 infection should also be considered when there is clinical suspicion of HIV disease in the absence of a positive HIV-1 antibody test.

Acute Retroviral Syndrome

Acute retroviral syndrome occurs in many persons shortly after HIV infection, before antibody tests are positive. The syndrome is characterized by acute symptoms and signs, including fever, malaise, lymphadenopathy, and skin rash. Suspicion of acute retroviral syndrome should prompt nucleic acid testing to detect HIV. New data suggest that early initiation of treatment during this period can result in a lower HIV viral burden, delay HIV-related complications, and perhaps cause immune reconstitution.

Initial Management of HIV Infection

It is advisable to refer HIV-infected persons to a single clinical resource for comprehensive care. Because of the limited availability of these facilities, it is often advisable to initiate evaluation and provide access to psychosocial services while planning for referral and continuation of medical care. Thus, a brief consideration of initial management is in order.

Recently diagnosed HIV infection may not have been acquired recently. Persons with newly diagnosed HIV infection can be at any of the clinical stages of infection. Thus, it is important to be alert for signs and symptoms that suggest advanced infection, such as fever, weight loss, diarrhea, oral candidiasis, cough, or shortness of breath. These findings suggest the need for urgent referral.

In nonemergent situations the recommended evaluation of a person with newly diagnosed HIV infection includes a detailed medical history that emphasizes sexual and substance abuse history, previous STDs, and specific HIV-related symptoms or diagnoses. The physical examination should include a pelvic examination in women, with Pap smear, and testing for gonorrhea and chlamydial infection. Recommended blood work includes complete blood cell with platelet count; chemistry profile; testing for toxoplasma antibody and hepatitis viral markers; syphilis serologic test; and a CD4+ T-lymphocyte count. Other evaluations should include a tuberculin skin test and chest x-ray. Finally, provision should be made for evaluation and management of sex and injecting-drug partners.

REFERENCES

Centers for Disease Control and Prevention: 1998 guidelines for treatment of sexually transmitted diseases. MMWR Morb Mortal Wkly Rep 1998;47(RR-1). (Copies available from the US Government Printing Office, Washington, D.C.; 202-512-1800.)

Holmes K et al: *Sexually Transmitted Diseases,* 2nd ed. McGraw-Hill, 1990.

Krieger J: Acquired immunodeficiency syndrome and related conditions. In: Walsh PC et al (editors): *Campbell's Urology,* 7th ed., vol. 1, p. 685. Saunders, 1998.

Krieger JN: Urethritis: Etiology, diagnosis, treatment, and complications. In: Gillenwater JY et al (editors): *Adult and Pediatric Urology,* vol. 2, p. 1879. Mosby, 1996.

Mandell GE, Bennett DR, Dolin R: *Mandell, Douglas and Bennett's Principles and Practice of Infectious Diseases,* 4th ed., vols. 1–2, especially Chapters 87–91. Churchill Livingstone, 1990.

Rein MF (editor): *Sexually Transmitted Diseases.* Churchill Livingstone, 1996. Mandell JF (editor): *Atlas of Infectious Diseases,* vol. 5.

Urinary Stone Disease

17

Marshall L. Stoller, MD, & Damien M. Bolton, MD

Urinary calculi are the third most common affliction of the urinary tract, exceeded only by urinary tract infections and pathologic conditions of the prostate. They are common in both animals and humans. The nomenclature associated with urinary stone disease arises from a variety of disciplines. Struvite stones, for example, composed of magnesium ammonium phosphate hexahydrate, are named in honor of H.C.G. von Struve (1772–1851), a Russian naturalist. Before the time of von Struve, the stones were referred to as guanite, because magnesium ammonium phosphate is prominent in bat droppings. Calcium oxalate dihydrate is frequently referred to as weddellite, because it was commonly found in floor samples collected from the Weddell Sea in Antarctica. The history of the nomenclature associated with urinary stone disease is as intriguing as that of the development of the interventional techniques used in their treatment.

Urinary stones have plagued humans since the earliest records of civilization. The etiology of stones remains speculative. If urinary constituents are similar from each kidney and if there is no evidence of obstruction, why do most stones present in a unilateral fashion? Why don't small stones pass uneventfully down the ureter early in their development? Why do some people form one large stone and others form multiple small calculi? Recent preliminary evidence has suggested a potential association of nanobacteria with urinary stones. There is much speculation concerning these and other questions.

Advances in the surgical treatment of urinary stones have outpaced our understanding of their etiology. As clinicians we are concerned with an expedient diagnosis and efficient treatment. Equally important is a thorough metabolic evaluation directing appropriate medical therapy and lifestyle changes to help reduce recurrent stone disease. Without such follow-up and medical intervention, stone recurrence rates can be as high as 50% within 5 years. Uric acid calculi can recur even more frequently. Physicians look forward to gaining a better understanding of this multifactorial disease process in hopes of developing more effective prophylaxis.

RENAL & URETERAL STONES

Etiology

Mineralization in all biologic systems has a common theme in that the crystals and matrix are intertwined. Urinary stones are no exception; they are polycrystalline aggregates composed of varying amounts of crystalloid and organic matrix. Theories to explain urinary stone disease are incomplete.

Stone formation requires supersaturated urine. Supersaturation depends on urinary pH, ionic strength, solute concentration, and complexation. Urinary constituents may change dramatically during different physiologic states from a relatively acid urine in a first morning void to an alkaline tide noted after meals. Ionic strength is determined primarily by the relative concentration of monovalent ions. As ionic strength increases, the activity coefficient decreases. The activity coefficient reflects the availability of a particular ion.

The role of solute concentrations is clear: The greater the concentration of 2 ions, the more likely they are to precipitate. Low ion concentrations result in undersaturation and increased solubility. As ion concentrations increase, their activity product reaches a specific point termed the **solubility product (K_{sp})**. Concentrations above this point are metastable and are capable of initiating crystal growth and heterogeneous nucleation. As solutions become more concentrated, the activity product eventually reaches the formation product (K_{fp}). Supersaturation levels beyond this point are unstable, and spontaneous homogeneous nucleation may occur.

Multiplying 2 ion concentrations reveals the concentration product. The concentration products of most ions are greater than established solubility products. Other factors must play major roles in the development of urinary calculi, including complexation. Complexation influences the availability of specific ions. For instance, sodium complexes with oxalate and decreases its free ionic form, while sulfates can complex with calcium. Crystal formation is modified by a variety of other substances found in the urinary tract, including magnesium, citrate, pyrophosphate, and a variety of trace metals. These inhibitors may act at the active crystal growth sites or as inhibitors in solution (as with citrate).

The nucleation theory suggests that urinary stones originate from crystals or foreign bodies immersed in supersaturated urine. This theory is challenged by the same arguments that support it. Stones do not always form in patients who are hyperexcretors or who are at risk for dehydration. Additionally, many stone formers' 24-h urine collections are completely normal with respect to stone forming ion concentrations.

The crystal inhibitor theory claims that calculi form owing to the absence or low concentration of natural stone inhibitors, including magnesium, citrate, pyrophosphate, acid glycoprotein, and a variety of trace metals. This theory does not have absolute validity since many people lacking such inhibitors may never form stones, and others with an abundance of inhibitors may, paradoxically, form them.

A. Crystal Component: Stones are composed primarily of a crystalline component. Crystals of adequate size and transparency are easily identified under a polarizing microscope. X-ray diffraction is preferred to assess the geometry and architecture of calculi. A group of stones from the same geographic location or the same historical time period typically have crystalline constituents that are common.

Multiple steps are involved in crystal formation, including nucleation, growth, and aggregation. Nucleation initiates the stone process and may be induced by a variety of substances, including proteinaceous matrix, crystals, foreign bodies, and other particulate tissues. Heterogeneous nucleation (epitaxy), which requires less energy and may occur in less saturated urine, is a common theme in stone formation. It should be suspected whenever an oriented conglomerate is found. A crystal of one type thereby serves as a nidus for the nucleation of another type with a similar crystal lattice. This is frequently seen with uric acid crystals initiating calcium oxalate formation. It takes time for these early nidi to grow or aggregate to form a stone incapable of passing with ease through the urinary tract.

How these early crystalline structures are retained in the upper urinary tract without uneventful passage down the ureter is unknown. The theory of mass precipitation or intranephronic calculosis suggests that the distal tubules or collecting ducts, or both, become plugged with crystals, thereby establishing an environment of stasis, ripe for further stone growth. This explanation is unsatisfactory; tubules are conical in shape and enlarge as they enter the papilla, thereby reducing the possibility of ductal obstruction. Additionally, urine transit time from the glomerulus into the renal pelvis is only a few minutes, making crystal aggregation and growth within the uriniferous tubules unlikely.

The fixed particle theory postulates that formed crystals are somehow retained within cells or beneath tubular epithelium. Randall noted whitish-yellow precipitations of crystalline substances occurring on the tips of renal papillae as submucosal plaques. These can be appreciated during endoscopy of the upper urinary tract. Carr hypothesized that calculi form in obstructed lymphatics and then rupture into adjacent fornices of a calyx. Arguing against Carr's theory are the grossly visible early stone elements in areas remote from fornices.

B. Matrix Component: The amount of the noncrystalline, matrix component of urinary stones varies with stone type, commonly ranging from 2 to 10% by weight. It is composed predominantly of protein, with small amounts of hexose and hexosamine. An unusual type of stone called a matrix calculus can be associated with previous kidney surgery or chronic urinary tract infections and has a gelatinous texture (Figure 17–1). Histologic inspection reveals laminations with scant calcifications. On plain abdominal radiographs, matrix calculi are usually radiolucent and can be confused with other filling defects, including blood clots, upper-tract tumors, and fungal bezoars. Computed tomography (CT) reveals calcifications and can help to confirm the diagnosis. The role of matrix in the initiation of ordinary urinary stones as well as matrix stones is unknown. It may serve as a nidus for crystal aggregation or as a naturally occurring glue to adhere small crystal components and thereby hinder uneventful passage down the urinary tract. Alternatively, matrix may have an inhibitory role in stone formation or may be an innocent bystander, playing no active role in stone formation.

Urinary Ions

A. Calcium: Calcium is a major ion present in urinary crystals. Only 50% of plasma calcium is ionized and available for filtration at the glomerulus.

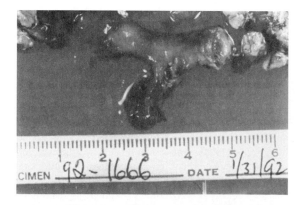

Figure 17–1. Gross picture of matrix calculus percutaneously extracted after extracorporeal shock wave lithotripsy failure.

Well over 95% of the calcium filtered at the glomerulus is reabsorbed at both the proximal and distal tubules and limited amounts in the collecting tube. Less than 2% is excreted in the urine. Diuretic medications may exert a hypocalciuric effect by further decreasing calcium excretion. Many factors influence the availability of calcium in solution, including complexation with citrate, phosphate, and sulfate. An increase in monosodium urates and a decrease in urinary pH further interfere with this complexation and therefore promote crystal aggregation.

B. Oxalate: Oxalate is a normal waste product of metabolism and is relatively insoluble. Normally, approximately 10–15% of oxalate found in the urine originates from the diet; the vast majority is a metabolic by-product. Most of the oxalate that enters the large bowel is consumed by bacterial decomposition. Diet, however, can have an impact on the amount of oxalate found in the urine. Once absorbed from the small bowel, oxalate is not metabolized and is excreted almost exclusively by proximal tubule. The presence of calcium within the bowel lumen is an important factor influencing the amount of oxalate that is absorbed. The control of oxalate in the urine plays a pivotal role in the formation of calcium oxalate calculi. Urinary magnesium and sodium may complex with oxalate. Normal excretion ranges from 20 to 45 mg/d and does not change significantly with age. Excretion is higher during the day when one eats. Small changes in oxalate levels in the urine can have a dramatic impact on the supersaturation of calcium oxalate. The principal precursors of oxalate are glycine and ascorbic acid; however, the impact of ingested vitamin C on urinary oxalate levels is unknown at present.

Hyperoxaluria may develop in patients with bowel disorders, particularly inflammatory bowel disease, small-bowel resection, and jejunoileal bypass (previously used for morbid obesity). Renal calculi develop in 5–10% of patients with these conditions. Chronic diarrhea with fatty stools results in a saponification process. Intraluminal calcium binds to the fat, thereby becoming unavailable to bind to oxalate. The unbound oxalate is readily absorbed.

Excessive oxalate may occur secondary to the accidental or deliberate ingestion of ethylene glycol (partial oxidation to oxalate). This may result in diffuse and massive deposition of calcium oxalate crystals and may occasionally lead to renal failure.

C. Phosphate: Phosphate is an important buffer and complexes with calcium in urine. It is a key component in calcium phosphate and magnesium ammonium phosphate stones. The excretion of urinary phosphate in normal adults is related to the amount of dietary phosphate (especially in meats, dairy products, and vegetables). The small amount of phosphate filtered by the glomerulus is predominantly reabsorbed in the proximal tubule. Parathyroid hormone inhibits this reabsorption. The predominant crystal found in those with hyperparathyroidism is phosphate, in the form of hydroxyapatite, amorphous calcium phosphate, and carbonate apatite.

D. Uric Acid: Uric acid is the by-product of purine metabolism. The pKa of uric acid is 5.75. Undissociated uric acid predominates with pH values less than this. Elevated pH values increase urate, which is soluble. Approximately 10% of the filtered uric acid finds its way into the urine. Other defects in purine metabolism may result in urinary stone disease. Rarely, a defect in xanthine oxidase results in increased levels of xanthine; the xanthine may precipitate in urine, resulting in stone formation. Unusual alterations in adenine metabolism may result in the production of 2,8-dihydroxyadeninuria, which is poorly soluble in urine and may develop into a urinary stone. This results from a deficiency of adenine phosphoribosyltransferase (APRT). Pure uric acid crystals and calculi are typically radiolucent in nature and may not be identified on plain abdominal films (Figure 17–2). They are visible on noncontrast CT images. Some uric acid calculi may be partially radiopaque, however, because of associated calcium deposits.

E. Sodium: Although not identified as one of the major constituents of most urinary calculi, sodium plays an important role in regulating the crystallization of calcium salts in urine. Sodium is found in higher than expected concentrations in the core of renal calculi and may play a role in initiating crystal development and aggregation. High dietary sodium intake increases urinary calcium excretion, decreases urinary pH, and decreases urinary excretion of citrate. These factors reduce the ability of urine to inhibit calcium oxalate crystal agglomeration. These effects are thought to be due to a sodium-induced increase in bicarbonaturia and decrease in serum bicarbonate. Con-

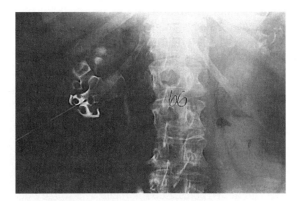

Figure 17–2. Radiolucent right staghorn renal calculus appreciated after percutaneous injection of radiocontrast material. This uric acid stone was effectively removed in a single percutaneous procedure. Postoperative urinary alkalinization has been effective prophylaxis.

versely, a reduction in dietary sodium helps to reduce recurrent calcium nephrolithiasis.

F. Citrate: Citrate is a key factor affecting the development of calcium urinary stones. A deficiency commonly is associated with stone formation in those with chronic diarrhea or renal tubular acidosis type I (distal tubular defect) and in patients undergoing chronic thiazide therapy. Citrate plays a pivotal role in the citric acid cycle in renal cells. Metabolic stimuli that consume this product (as with intracellular metabolic acidosis due to fasting, hypokalemia, or hypomagnesemia) reduce the urinary excretion of citrate. Estrogen increases citrate excretion and may be a factor that decreases the incidence of stones in women, especially during pregnancy. Alkalosis also increases citrate excretion.

G. Magnesium: Dietary magnesium deficiency is associated with an increased incidence of urinary stone disease. Magnesium is a component of struvite calculi. Experimentally, lack of dietary magnesium is associated with increased calcium oxalate stone formation and calcium oxalate crystalluria. The exact mechanism whereby magnesium exerts its effect is undefined. Dietary magnesium supplements do not protect against stone formation in normal people.

H. Sulfate: Urinary sulfates may help prevent urinary calculi. They can complex with calcium. These sulfates occur primarily as components of longer urinary proteins, such as chondroitin sulfate and heparin sulfate.

I. Other Urinary Stone Inhibitors: Inhibitors of urinary stone formation other than citrate, magnesium, and sulfates have been identified. These consist predominantly of urinary proteins and other macromolecules such as glycosaminoglycans, pyrophosphates, and uropontin. Although citrate appears to be the most active inhibitory component in urine, these substances demonstrate a substantial role in preventing urine crystal formation. The N-terminal amino acid sequence and the acidic amino acid content of these protein inhibitors, especially their high aspartic acid content, appear to play pivotal inhibitory roles. Fluoride may be an inhibitor of urinary stone formation.

Stone Varieties

A. Calcium Calculi: Calcifications can occur and accumulate in the collecting system, resulting in nephrolithiasis. Eighty to eighty-five percent of all urinary stones are calcareous.

Calcium nephrolithiasis is most commonly due to elevated urinary calcium, elevated urinary uric acid, elevated urinary oxalate, or a decreased level of urinary citrate. Hypercalciuira is found as a solitary defect in 12% of patients and in combination with other defects in an additional 18%. Hyperuricosuria is identified as a solitary defect in 8% of patients and associated with additional defects in 16%. Elevated urinary oxalate is found as a solitary finding in 5% of

patients and as a combined defect in 16%. Finally, decreased urinary citrate is found as an isolated defect in 17% of patients and as a combined defect in an additional 10%. Approximately one-third of patients undergoing a full metabolic evaluation will find no identiable metabolic defect.

Symptoms are secondary to obstruction, with resultant pain, infection, nausea, and vomiting, and rarely culminate in renal failure. Asymptomatic hematuria or repetitive urinary tract infections recalcitrant to apparently appropriate antibiotics should lead one to suspect a urinary stone. Calcifications within the parenchyma of the kidney, known as nephrocalcinosis, rarely cause symptoms, however, and usually are not amenable to traditional therapies appropriate for urinary stone disease (Figure 17–3). Nephrocalcinosis is frequently encountered with renal tubular acidosis and hyperparathyroidism. Nephrolithiasis and nephrocalcinosis frequently coexist. Most patients with nephrolithiasis, however, do not have obvious nephrocalcinosis.

Nephrocalcinosis may result from a variety of pathologic states. Ectatic collecting tubules as seen with medullary sponge kidney, are common. This is frequently a bilateral process. Increased calcium absorption from the small bowel is common with sarcoidosis, milk-alkali syndrome, hyperparathyroidism, and excessive vitamin D intake. Disease processes resulting in bony destruction, including hyperparathyroidism, osteolytic lesions, and multiple myeloma, are a third mechanism. Finally, dystrophic calcifications forming on necrotic tissue may develop after a renal insult.

1. Absorptive hypercalciuric nephrolithiasis—Normal calcium intake averages approximately 900–1000 mg/d. Approximately one-third is absorbed by the small bowel, and of that portion approximately 150–200 mg is obligatorily excreted in

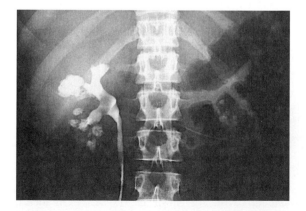

Figure 17–3. Retrograde pyelogram demonstrating multiple punctate calcifications within the renal parenchyma establishing the diagnosis of nephrocalcinosis. Renal pelvis and infundibula are free of calculi.

the urine. A large reservoir of calcium remains in the bone. Most dietary calcium is excreted in the stool. Absorptive hypercalciuria is secondary to increased calcium absorption from the small bowel, predominantly from the jejunum. This results in an increased load of calcium filtered from the glomerulus. The result is suppression of parathyroid hormone, leading to decreased tubular reabsorption of calcium, culminating in hypercalciuria. This physiologic cascade is in response to the primary defect, an increased absorption of calcium from the small bowel.

Absorptive hypercalciuria can be subdivided into 3 types. Type I absorptive hypercalciuria is independent of diet and represents 15% of all calcareous calculi. There is an elevated urinary calcium (> 150–200 mg/24 h; 4 mg/kg) even during a calcium-restricted diet. Cellulose phosphate is an effective nonabsorbable exchange resin. This effectively binds the calcium in the gut, preventing bowel absorption. Cellulose phosphate has no impact on the calcium transport defect. Urinary calcium excretion returns to normal values with therapy.

Cellulose phosphate must be taken with meals to be available when calcium is ingested. A typical dose is 10–15 g orally in 3 divided doses and is well tolerated. This therapy is relatively contraindicated in postmenopausal women and in children during their active growth cycles. Inappropriate use may lead to a negative calcium balance and a secondary hyperparathyroid state. As with all stone formers, long-term follow-up is required. Cellulose phosphate may bind other cations besides calcium, including magnesium. Secondary hyperoxaluria may develop owing to decreased calcium in the gut. See the section on hyperoxaluria for a more detailed discussion.

Hydrochlorothiazides are an alternative treatment for type I absorptive hypercalciuria. Initially there is a reduction in renal excretion of calcium. The increased absorbed calcium is likely deposited in bone. Eventually the bone reservoir reaches its capacity and the drug becomes ineffective. Hydrochlorothiazides have limited long-term efficacy (approximately 3–5 years). These drugs have no effect on the defective bowel transport system. Hydrochlorothiazides may be alternated with cellulose phosphate as an effective treatment regimen.

Type II absorptive hypercalciuria is dietary dependent and is a common cause of urinary stone disease. There is no specific medical therapy. Calcium excretion returns to normal on a calcium restricted diet. Patients should limit their calcium intake to 400–600 mg/d. Type II absorptive hypercalciuria is not as severe as type I.

Type III absorptive hypercalciuria is secondary to a phosphate renal leak and accounts for 5% of all urinary calculi. Decreased serum phosphate leads to an increase in 1,25-dihydroxyvitamin D synthesis. The physiologic cascade culminates in an increased absorption of phosphate and calcium from the small bowel (predominantly the jejunum) and an increased renal excretion of calcium—hence its classification as absorptive hypercalciuria. Successful treatment replaces bioavailable phosphate. Orthophosphate (Neutra-Phos) inhibits vitamin D synthesis and is administered as 250–2000 mg 3–4 times daily. It is best taken after meals and before bedtime. Orthophosphates do not alter intestinal calcium absorption.

2. Resorptive hypercalciuric nephrolithiasis–About half the patients with clinically obvious primary hyperparathyroidism present with nephrolithiasis. This group represents less than 5–10% of all patients with urinary stones. Patients with calcium phosphate stones, women with recurrent calcium stones, and those with both nephrocalcinosis and nephrolithiasis should be suspected of having hyperparathyroidism. Hypercalcemia is the most consistent sign of hyperparathyroidism.

Parathyroid hormone results in a cascade of events starting with an increase in urinary phosphorus and a decrease in plasma phosphorus, followed by an increase in plasma calcium and a decrease in urinary calcium. Its action on the kidney and on the bone are independent of each other. Ultimately renal damage is secondary to the hypercalcemia. It limits the concentrating ability of the kidney and impairs the kidney's ability to acidify urine. Surgical removal of the offending parathyroid adenoma is the only effective way of treating this disease. Attempts at medical management are futile.

3. Renal induced hypercalciuric nephrolithiasis–Hypercalciuria of renal origin is due to an intrinsic renal tubular defect in calcium excretion. This creates a physiologically vicious cycle. Excessive urinary calcium excretion results in a relative decrease in serum calcium, which leads to a secondarily increased parathyroid hormone level that mobilizes calcium from the bone and increases calcium absorption from the gut. This step completes the pathologic cycle by delivering increased levels of calcium back to the kidney, whereby the renal tubules excrete large amounts of calcium. These patients have an elevated fasting urinary calcium level, normal serum calcium level, and an elevated parathyroid hormone level.

Renal hypercalciuria is effectively treated with hydrochlorothiazides. Unlike their role in type I absorptive hypercalciuria, in this setting hydrochlorothiazides have a durable long-term effect. Hydrochlorothiazides affect both the proximal and distal renal tubules. As a diuretic, they decrease the circulating blood volume and subsequently stimulate proximal tubular absorption of calcium as well as other constituents. They also increase reabsorption at the distal tubule. Both mechanisms correct the secondary hyperparathyroid state.

Hypercalciuric states may result in elevated parathyroid levels. To differentiate primary from secondary hyperparathyroidism in patients with urinary stone disease, one can prescribe a hydrochlorothiazide challenge of 50 mg twice a day for approximately 10 days. Patients with secondary hyperparathyroidism will have normal serum parathyroid levels, while those with primary hyperparathyroism will continue to have elevated serum values.

4. Hyperuricosuric calcium nephrolithiasis—Hyperuricosuric calcium nephrolithiasis is due to either an excessive dietary intake of purines or an increase in endogenous uric acid production. In both situations there is an increase in urinary monosodium urates. Monosodium urates absorb and adsorb urinary stone inhibitors and facilitate heterogeneous nucleation.

Patients have elevated urinary uric acid levels (> 600 mg/24 h in women and > 750 mg/24 h in men) and consistently have a urinary pH > 5.5. The urinary pH helps to differentiate hyperuricosuric calcium from hyperuricosuric uric acid stone formation.

Patients with excessive purine intake can be effectively treated by changing their diet to one with low purines. Those with excessive endogenous uric acid production can be successfully treated with allopurinol. Allopurinol is a xanthine oxidase inhibitor. It inhibits the production of uric acid without interfering with purine anabolism. Allopurinol reduces uric acid synthesis and renal excretion of uric acid. It also inhibits uric acid–calcium oxalate crystallization. Allopurinol has many potential side effects, including a variety of skin rashes and liver toxicity, and should be administered with careful monitoring. Dosing can start at 100 mg and can be advanced to 300 mg daily. Potassium citrate is an alternative treatment, especially when associated with hypocitraturia.

5. Hyperoxaluric calcium nephrolithiasis—Hyperoxaluric calcium nephrolithiasis is secondary to increased urinary oxalate levels (> 40 mg/24 h). It is frequently found in patients with inflammatory bowel disease or other chronic diarrheal states that result in severe dehydration. It is rarely associated with excessive oxalate intake as seen in poisoning with ethylene glycol, methoxyflurane, or oxalic acid or in pyridoxine deficiency, phenylketonuria, or endogenous overproduction. The role of ascorbic acid is unknown.

Chronic diarrheal states alter oxalate metabolism. Malabsorption leads to increased luminal fat and bile. Intraluminal calcium readily binds to fat, resulting in a saponification process. Urinary calcium levels are usually low (< 100 mg/24 h). The intraluminal gut calcium that normally would have bound to oxalate is decreased. The unbound oxalate is readily absorbed by a diffusion mechanism that is unaffected by the usual metabolic inhibitors of energy dependent pumps. Bile salts may increase the passive bowel absorption of oxalate. A small increase in oxalate absorption and subsequent urinary excretion dramatically increases the formation product of calcium-oxalate. This increases the potential for heterogeneous nucleation and crystal growth in this metastable environment. All patients with increased urinary excretion of oxalate do not form calcium oxalate calculi. Other factors must be contributory, therefore, including dehydration, hypocitraturia (associated with an acidosis), decreased excretion of urinary inhibitors including magnesium, and protein malabsorption.

Enteric hyperoxaluric calcium nephrolithiasis is successfully treated with oral calcium supplementation. The calcium binds to the intraluminal oxalate and limits its absorption. It must be given with meals when the oxalate is present. Other oral cations are effective, including magnesium supplements. An alternative therapy includes a diet limited to medium-chain fatty acids and triglycerides; however, it is poorly tolerated by patients. Equally difficult is an attempt to alter oxalate intake. Unless large amounts of specific oxalate-rich foods can be excluded, an alternative diet may result in *increased* oxalate levels.

Primary hyperoxaluria is a rare hereditary disease. It is associated with calcium oxalate renal calculi, nephrocalcinosis, and other distant deposits of oxalate, culminating in progressive renal failure and eventual death. Type I is associated with an enzyme deficiency of 2-oxoglutarate:glyoxylate carboligase, resulting in elevated urinary levels of glycolic acid and oxalic acid. Type II has increased excretory levels of L-glyceric acid rather than elevated levels of glycolic acid. It is associated with a D-glycerate dehydrogenase enzyme deficiency. This ultimately results in the accumulation of hydroxypyruvate, which is eventually converted to oxalate. Oxalate crystal deposits develop rapidly in transplanted kidneys. Combined liver and renal transplantation has cured this previously fatal rare disease.

6. Hypocitraturic calcium nephrolithiasis—Citrate is an important inhibitor of urinary stone disease. Increased metabolic demands on the mitochondria of renal cells decrease the excretion of citrate. Such conditions include intracellular metabolic acidosis, hypokalemia (as with thiazide therapy), fasting, hypomagnesemia, androgens, gluconeogenesis, and an acid-ash diet. Citrate may be consumed in the urine by bacteria during a urinary tract infection. The cause of hypocitraturia may be unknown in some cases. In contrast, alkalosis, alkaline-ash diet, estrogen, growth hormone, parathyroid hormone, and vitamin D increase urinary citrate levels.

Citrate has its action in solution. It complexes with calcium, thereby decreasing the ionic calcium concentration and thus the activity product and thereby decreasing the energy for crystallization. Citrate decreases agglomeration, spontaneous nucleation, and crystal growth of calcium oxalate. Citrate also decreases calcium oxalate calculi by decreasing monosodium urates that can absorb inhibitors and facilitate heterogeneous nucleation.

Hypocitraturic (< 320 mg/24 h) calcium nephrolithiasis is associated commonly with renal tubular acidosis type I (distal tubule) (Figure 17–4), thiazide

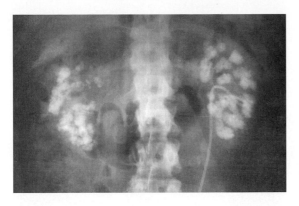

Figure 17–4. Scout abdominal radiograph demonstrating bilateral, multiple renal calculi in a patient with renal tubular acidosis, type I.

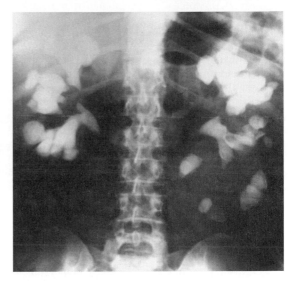

Figure 17–5. Scout abdominal radiograph demonstrating large bilateral struvite staghorn calculi. Patient was treated for many years with numerous antibiotics for recurrent urinary tract infections. Only after this radiograph were calculi identified and removed and the infections resolved.

therapy (accompanied by potassium wastage), and chronic diarrhea; it also is found in the rare idiopathic calcium stone former. Treatment is successful with potassium citrate supplementation. Routine dosage is 20–30 mEq 2–3 times daily and is usually well tolerated. Six to 8 glasses of lemonade can increase urinary citrate excretion by approximately 150 mg/24 h and thus either limit or eliminate the need for pharmacologic citrate supplementation.

B. Noncalcium Calculi:

1. Struvite–Struvite stones are composed of magnesium, ammonium, and phosphate (MAP). They are found most commonly in women and may recur rapidly. They frequently present as renal staghorn calculi and rarely present as ureteral stones except after surgical intervention (Figure 17–5). Struvite stones are infection stones associated with urea-splitting organisms, including *Proteus, Pseudomonas, Providencia, Klebsiella, Staphylococci,* and *Mycoplasma.* The high ammonium concentration derived from the urea-splitting organisms results in an alkaline urinary pH. The urinary pH of a patient with a MAP stone ranges from 6.8 to 8.3 and rarely is below 7.0 (normal urinary pH is 5.85). It is only at this elevated urinary pH (> 7.19) that MAP crystals precipitate. MAP crystals are soluble in the normal urinary pH range of 5–7. Preoperative bladder cultures do not necessarily reflect the bacteriologic composition found in calculi. Foreign bodies and neurogenic bladders may predispose patients to urinary infections and subsequent struvite stone formation. Massive diuresis does not prevent struvite calculi. Women with recurrent infections despite apparently appropriate antibiotic therapy should be evaluated for struvite calculi with a conventional kidney-ureter-bladder (KUB) film or renal ultrasound, or both. It is impossible to sterilize such calculi with antibiotics. Culture-specific antibiotics can reduce urease levels by 99% and help reduce stone recurrence. Stone removal is therapeutic.

Long-term management is optimized with the removal of all foreign bodies, including catheters of all varieties. A short ileal loop helps decrease the risk of stones in those with supravesical urinary diversion. All stone fragments should be removed with or without the aid of follow-up irrigations. Hemiacidrin (Renacidin) irrigations should be used with caution if at all. Rapid magnesium toxicity can result in death even with a low pressure irrigation setup (< 20 cm water pressure), negative daily urine cultures, and no evidence of upper-tract extravasation. Acetohydroxamic acid inhibits the action of bacterial urease, thereby reducing the urinary pH and decreasing the likelihood of precipitation. Most patients have a difficult time tolerating this medication.

2. Uric acid–Uric acid stones compose less than 5% of all urinary calculi and are usually found in men. Patients with gout, myeloproliferative diseases, or rapid weight loss, and those treated for malignant conditions with cytotoxic drugs have a high incidence of uric acid lithiasis. Most patients with uric acid calculi, however, do not have hyperuricemia. Elevated uric acid levels are frequently due to dehydration and excessive purine intake. Patients present with a urinary pH consistently < 5.5, in contrast to patients with hyperuricosuric calcium nephrolithiasis, who have a urinary pH > 5.5. As the urinary pH increases above the dissociation constant pKa of 5.75, it dissociates into a relatively soluble urate ion. Treatment is centered on maintaining a urine volume

> 2 L/d and a urinary pH > 6.0. Reducing dietary purines or the administration of allopurinol also helps reduce uric acid excretion. Alkalinization (with oral sodium bicarbonate, potassium bicarbonate, potassium citrate, or intravenous 1/6 normal sodium lactate) may dissolve calculi and is dependent on the stone surface area. Stone fragments after lithotripsy have a dramatically increased surface area and will dissolve more rapidly. Dissolution proceeds at approximately 1 cm of stone (as seen on KUB) per month, with compliance regarding alkalinization.

3. Cystine—Cystine lithiasis is secondary to an inborn error of metabolism resulting in abnormal intestinal (small bowel) mucosal absorption and renal tubular absorption of dibasic amino acids, including cystine, ornithine, lysine, and arginine. The genetic defects associated with cystinuria have now been mapped to chromosome 2p.16 and more recently to 19q13.1. Cystine lithiasis is the only clinical manifestation of this defect. Classic cystinuria is inherited in an autosomal recessive fashion. Homozygous expression has a prevalence of 1:20,000, while the heterozygous expression is 1:2000. It represents 1–2% of all urinary stones, with a peak incidence in the second or third decade. Homozygous cystinurics excrete more than 250 mg/d, resulting in constant supersaturation. Heterozygous patients usually excrete 100–150 mg/d. Unaffected patients typically excrete less than 40 mg/d. Approximately 400 mg/L of cystine can remain in solution at a urinary pH of 7.0. As the urinary pH increases above 7.0, the amount of soluble cystine increases exponentially.

The solubility of cystine is pH-dependent, with a pK of approximately 8.1. There is no difference in the solubility curves in normal versus cystinuric patients. There is no known inhibitor for cystine calculi, and cystine stone formation is completely dependent on excessive cystine excretion. Cystine stones are frequently associated with calcium calculi and their related metabolic abnormalities. They may present as single, multiple, or staghorn stones. The diagnosis is suspected in patients with a family history of urinary stones and the radiographic appearance of a faintly opaque, ground glass, smooth-edged stone (Figure 17–6). Urinalysis frequently reveals hexagonal crystals. Stone analysis confirms the diagnosis.

A qualitative sodium cyanide nitroprusside urine test produces a purple color when positive. If positive, a quantitative urinary cystine evaluation helps confirm the diagnosis and differentiate heterozygous from homozygous states. It is also important to titrate medical therapy.

Medical therapy includes high fluid intake (> 3 L/d) and urinary alkalinization. Patients should monitor their pH with nitrazine indicator paper and keep their pH values above 7.5. It is difficult or impossible to maintain levels higher than 8.0. A low-methionine (precursor to cystine) diet has limited impact, as most of the cystine is endogenous and most of the ingested

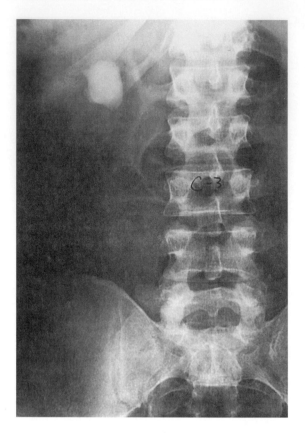

Figure 17–6. Scout radiograph demonstrating a right cystine calculus. Note ground-glass appearance with smooth edges.

methionine is incorporated into protein. A low-sodium diet may reduce recurrence rates, as seen with other stones. Glutamine, ascorbic acid, and captopril are effective in some patients. Penicillamine can reduce urinary cystine levels. It complexes with the amino acid, and this complex is dramatically more soluble. Treatment should be titrated with quantitative urinary cystine values. Many patients poorly tolerate penicillamine, reporting skin rashes (discrete or confluent macules with occasional itching), loss of taste, nausea, vomiting, and anorexia. It may inhibit pyridoxine, which should be supplemented during treatment (50 mg/d). Mercaptopropionylglycine (Thiola), 300–1200 mg in divided doses, forms a soluble complex with cystine and can reduce stone formation. Side effects and frequent dosing decrease patient compliance rates. It is better tolerated than penicillamine and is now the first drug of choice in these difficult cases.

Surgical treatment is similar to that for other stones except that most stones are recalcitrant to extracorporeal shock wave lithotripsy (ESWL). One should have a low threshhold to proceed with percutaneous stone extraction in symptomatic patients. Two populations of cystine stones have been described, including the rough and smooth varieties, and may reflect subpopulations: those that are effectively treated with ESWL and those that require more invasive therapy. Despite optimum medical therapy, a high stone recurrence rate frequently frustrates both patient and physician. Minimally invasive techniques and optimum medical therapy are paramount.

4. Xanthine–Xanthine stones are secondary to a congenital deficiency of xanthine oxidase. This enzyme normally catalyzes the oxidation of hypoxanthine to xanthine and of xanthine to uric acid. It is of interest that allopurinol, used to treat hyperuricosuric calcium nephrolithiasis and uric acid lithiasis, produces iatrogenic xanthinuria. Blood and urine levels of uric acid are lowered, and hypoxanthine and xanthine levels are increased; however, there are no case reports of xanthine stone formation resulting from allopurinol treatment. It is unlikely that allopurinol completely inhibits xanthine oxidase. Approximately 25% of patients with a xanthine oxidase deficiency develop urinary stones. The stones are radiolucent and are tannish-yellow in color. Treatment should be directed by symptoms and evidence of renal obstruction. High fluid intake and urinary alkalinization are required for prophylaxis. If stones recur, a trial of allopurinol and a purine-restricted diet is appropriate.

5. Indinavir–Protease inhibitors are now a popular and effective treatment in patients with acquired immunodeficiency syndrome. Indinavir is the most common protease inhibitor that results in radiolucent stones in up to 6% of patients who are prescribed this medication. Indinavir calculi are the only urinary stones to be radiolucent on noncontrast CT scans. They may be associated with calcium components and in these situations will be visible on noncontrast CT images. Temporary cessation of the medication with intravenous hydration frequently allows these stones to pass. The stones are tannish red and usually fall apart during basket extraction.

6. Rare–Silicate stones are very rare and are usually associated with long-term use of antacids containing silica, such as products containing magnesium silicate and magnesium aluminometasilicate. Surgical treatment is similar to that of other calculi.

Triamterene stones are radiolucent and have been identified with an increased frequency. They are associated with antihypertensive medications containing triamterene, such as Dyazide. Discontinuing the medication eliminates stone recurrences. Other medications that may become stone constituents include glafenine and antrafenine.

Rarely, patients arrive at an emergency room at an odd hour feigning signs and symptoms of passing a urinary stone in hopes of obtaining pain medications. They may add blood to their urine and give a believable story of a severe allergy to intravenous contrast medium. Occasionally, patients present a fake urinary stone, with specks of paint or other obvious curiosities. Such patients suffer from Munchausen syndrome, and the diagnosis is difficult and made by exclusion.

Symptoms & Signs at Presentation

Upper-tract urinary stones usually eventually cause pain. The character of the pain depends on the location. Calculi small enough to venture down the ureter usually have difficulty passing through the ureteropelvic junction, over the iliac vessels, or entering the bladder at the ureterovesical junction (Figure 17–7).

A. Pain: Renal colic and noncolicky renal pain are the 2 types of pain originating from the kidney. Renal colic usually is caused by stretching of the collecting system or ureter, while noncolicky renal pain is caused by distention of the renal capsule. These symptoms may overlap, making a clinical differentiation difficult or impossible. Urinary obstruction is the main mechanism responsible for renal colic. This may be mimicked by the pain a patient experiences when a retrograde ureteropyelogram is performed under local anesthesia, with excessive pressure resulting in overdistention of the collecting system. This pain is due to a direct increase in intraluminal pressure, stretching nerve endings.

Renal colic does not always wax and wane or come in waves like intestinal or biliary colic but may be relatively constant. Renal colic implies an intraluminal origin. Extrinsic compression of the ureter in an acute manner can produce similar symptoms. Patients with renal calculi suffer pain primarily due to urinary obstruction.

Local mechanisms such as inflammation, edema, hyperperistalsis, and mucosal irritation may contribute to the perception of pain in patients with renal calculi. Edema can lead to stretching of free nerve endings with resultant perception of renal colic. In the collecting system, local pain is difficult to differentiate from renal colic caused by urinary obstruction; they may be perceived as one and the same by the central nervous system due to common ascending pathways. Further down the ureter, however, local pain is referred to the distribution of the ilioinguinal nerve and the genital branch of the genitofemoral nerve, whereas pain from obstruction is referred to the same areas as for collecting system calculi (flank and costovertebral angle), thereby allowing discrimination.

The vast majority of urinary stones present with the acute onset of pain due to acute obstruction and distention of the upper urinary tract. The severity and location of the pain can vary from patient to patient due to stone size, stone location, degree of obstruction, acuity of obstruction, and variation in individual anatomy (intrarenal versus extrarenal pelvis, for example). The stone burden does not correlate with the severity of the

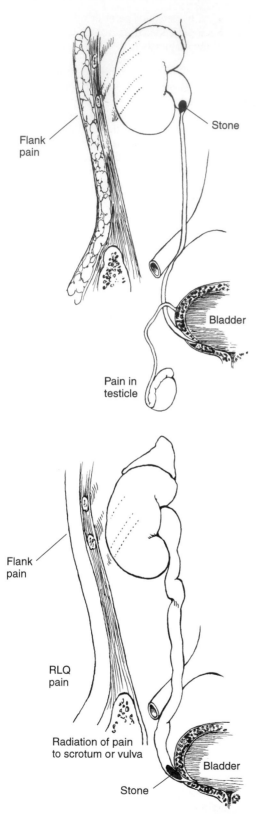

Figure 17–7. Radiation of pain with various types of ureteral stone. **Upper left:** Ureteropelvic stone. Severe costovertebral angle pain from capsular and pelvic distention; acute renal and urethral pain from hyperperistalsis of smooth muscle of calyces, pelvis, and ureter, with pain radiating along the course of the ureter (and into the testicle, since the nerve supply to the kidney and testis is the same.) The testis is hypersensitive. **Upper right:** Midureteral stone. Same as above but with more pain in the lower abdominal quadrant. **Left:** Low ureteral stone. Same as above, with pain radiating into bladder, vulva, or scrotum. The scrotal wall is hyperesthetic. Testicular sensitivity is absent. When the stone approaches the bladder, urgency and frequency with burning on urination develop as a result of inflammation of the bladder wall around the ureteral orifice.

symptoms. Small ureteral stones frequently present with severe pain, while large staghorn calculi may present with a dull ache or flank discomfort.

The pain frequently is abrupt in onset and severe and may awaken a patient from sleep. The severity of the pain is worsened by the unexpected nature of its onset. Patients frequently move constantly into unusual positions in an attempt to relieve the pain. This movement is in contrast to the lack of movement of someone with peritoneal signs; such a patient lies in a stationary position.

The symptoms of acute renal colic depend on the location of the calculus; several regions may be involved: renal calyx, renal pelvis, upper and mid ureter, and distal ureter. An orderly progression of symptoms as a stone moves down the urinary tract is the exception.

1. Renal calyx—Stones or other objects in calyces or caliceal diverticula may cause obstruction and renal colic. In general, nonobstructing stones cause pain only periodically, owing to intermittent obstruction. The pain is a deep, dull ache in the flank or back that can vary in intensity from severe to mild. The pain may be exacerbated after consumption of large amounts of fluid. An intravenous pyelogram may not reveal evidence of obstruction despite the patient's complaints of intermittent symptoms. It remains unclear how much of this pain is related to local mucosal irritation with activation of chemoreceptors due to edema or exudation. The presence of infection or inflammation in the calyx or diverticulum (milk of calcium, for example) in addition to obstruction may contribute to pain perception. Caliceal calculi occasionally result in spontaneous perforation with urinoma, fistula, or abscess formation.

Caliceal calculi are frequently small and numerous and appear to be able to pass spontaneously. Long-term retention against the flow of urine and against the forces of gravity and antegrade peristalsis suggests a significant element of obstruction. Effective long-term treatment requires stone extraction and elimination of the obstructive component.

Pain relief has been reported in most patients following ESWL for small symptomatic caliceal calculi. Thus, if a patient continues to complain of pain in the face of a small caliceal calculus, ESWL treatment may be justified for both diagnosis and treatment. Percutaneous, retrograde, and laparoscopic techniques have been successful in the management of calculi in calyces or caliceal diverticula.

2. Renal pelvis—Stones in the renal pelvis > 1 cm in diameter commonly obstruct the ureteropelvic junction, generally causing severe pain in the costovertebral angle, just lateral to the sacrospinalis muscle and just below the 12th rib. This pain may vary from dull to excruciatingly sharp and is usually constant, boring, and difficult to ignore. It often radiates to the flank and also anteriorly to the upper ipsilateral abdominal quadrant. It may be confused with biliary colic or cholecystitis if on the right side and with gastritis, acute pancreatitis, or peptic ulcer disease if on the left, especially if the patient has associated anorexia, nausea, or emesis. Acquired or congenital ureteropelvic junction obstruction may cause a similar constellation of symptoms. Symptoms frequently occur on an intermittent basis following a drinking binge or consumption of large quantities of fluid.

Partial or complete staghorn calculi that are present in the renal pelvis are not necessarily obstructive. In the absence of obstruction, these patients often have surprisingly few symptoms such as flank or back pain. Recurrent urinary tract infections frequently culminate in radiographic evaluation with the discovery of a staghorn calculus. If untreated, these "silent" staghorn calculi can often lead to significant morbidity, including renal deterioration, infectious complications, or both.

3. Upper and mid ureter—Stones or other objects in the upper or mid ureter often cause severe, sharp back (costovertebral angle) or flank pain. The pain may be more severe and intermittent if the stone is progressing down the ureter and causing intermittent obstruction. A stone that becomes lodged at a particular site may cause less pain, especially if it is only partially obstructive. Stationary calculi that result in high-grade but constant obstruction may allow autoregulatory reflexes and pyelovenous and pyelolymphatic backflow to decompress the upper tract, with diminution in intraluminal pressure gradually easing the pain. Pain associated with ureteral calculi often projects to corresponding dermatomal and spinal nerve root innervation regions. The pain of upper ureteral stones thus radiates to the lumbar region and flank. Midureteral calculi tend to cause pain that radiates caudally and anteriorly toward the mid and lower abdomen in a curved, bandlike fashion. This band initially parallels the lower costal margin but deviates caudad toward the bony pelvis and inguinal ligament. The pain may mimic acute appendicitis if on the right or acute diverticulitis if on the left side, especially if concurrent gastrointestinal symptoms are present.

4. Distal ureter—Calculi in the lower ureter often cause pain that radiates to the groin or testicle in males and the labia majora in females. This referred pain is often generated from the ilioinguinal or genital branch of the genitofemoral nerves. Diagnosis may be confused with testicular torsion or epididymitis. Stones in the intramural ureter may mimic cystitis, urethritis, or prostatitis by causing suprapubic pain, pain at the tip of the penis, urinary frequency and urgency, dysuria, stranguria, or gross hematuria. Bowel symptoms are not uncommon. In women the diagnosis may be confused with menstrual pain, pelvic inflammatory disease, and ruptured or twisted ovarian cysts. Strictures of the distal ureter from radiation, operative injury, or previous endoscopic procedures can present with similar symptoms. This pain pattern is likely due to the similar innervation of the intramural ureter and bladder.

B. Hematuria: A complete urinalysis helps to confirm the diagnosis of a urinary stone by assessing for hematuria and crystalluria and documenting urinary pH. Patients frequently admit to intermittent gross hematuria or occasional tea-colored urine (old blood). Most patients will have at least microhematuria. Rarely (in 10–15% of cases), complete ureteral obstruction presents without microhematuria.

C. Infection: Magnesium ammonium phosphate (struvite) stones are synonymous with infection stones. They are commonly associated with *Proteus, Pseudomonas, Providencia, Klebsiella,* and *Staphylococcus* infections. They are rarely if ever associated with *Escherichia coli* infections. Calcium phosphate stones are the second variety of stones associated with infections. Calcium phosphate stones with a urine pH < 6.6 are frequently referred to as brushite stones, whereas infectious apatite stones have a urinary pH > 6.6. Rarely, matrix stones with minimal crystalline components are associated with urinary tract infections. All stones, however, may be associated with infections secondary to obstruction and stasis proximal to the offending calculus. Culture-directed antibiotics should be administered before elective intervention.

Infection may be a contributing factor to pain perception. Uropathogenic bacteria may alter ureteral peristalsis by the production of exotoxins and endotoxins. Local inflammation from infection can lead to chemoreceptor activation and perception of local pain with its corresponding referral pattern.

1. Pyonephrosis–Obstructive calculi may culminate in the development of pyonephrosis. Unlike pyelonephritis, pyonephrosis implies gross pus in an obstructed collecting system. It is an extreme form of infected hydronephrosis. Presentation is variable and may range from asymptomatic bacteriuria to florid urosepsis. Bladder urine cultures may be negative. Radiographic investigations are frequently nondiagnostic. Renal ultrasonography may be misguiding because of the nonspecific and variable appearance of pyonephrosis. Renal urine aspiration is the only way to make the definitive diagnosis. If the condition is noted at the time of a percutaneous nephrolithotomy, the procedure should be postponed to allow for adequate percutaneous drainage and treatment with appropriate intravenous antibiotics (Figure 17–8). If unrecognized and untreated, pyonephrosis may develop into a renocutaneous fistula.

2. Xanthogranulomatous pyelonephritis– Xanthogranulomatous pyelonephritis is associated with upper-tract obstruction and infection. One-third of patients present with calculi; two-thirds present with flank pain, fever, and chills. Fifty percent present with persistent bacteriuria. Urinalysis usually shows numerous red and white cells. This condition

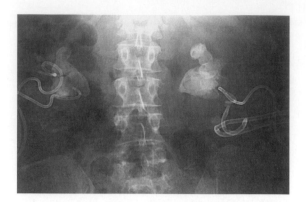

Figure 17–8. Bilateral renal calculi seen on scout radiograph with numerous bilateral percutaneous nephrostomy tubes to drain severe bilateral pyonephrosis.

is a common imitator of other pathologic states of the kidney. It usually presents in a unilateral fashion. Open surgical procedures, such as a simple nephrectomy for minimal or nonrenal function, can be challenging owing to marked and extensive reactive tissues.

D. Associated Fever: The association of urinary stones with fever is a relative medical emergency. Signs of clinical sepsis are variable and include fever, tachycardia, hypotension, and cutaneous vasodilation. Costovertebral angle tenderness may be marked with acute upper-tract obstruction; however, it cannot be relied on to be present in instances of long-term obstruction. In such instances a mass may be palpable resulting from a grossly hydronephrotic kidney. Fever associated with urinary tract obstruction requires prompt decompression. This may be accomplished with a retrograde catheter (double-J, or an externalized variety to serve as a port for selective urine collections, injection of contrast material, or both). If retrograde manipulations are unsuccessful, insertion of a percutaneous nephrostomy tube is required.

E. Nausea and Vomiting: Upper-tract obstruction is frequently associated with nausea and vomiting. Intravenous fluids are required to restore a euvolemic state. Intravenous fluids should not be used to force a diuresis in an attempt to push a ureteral stone down the ureter. Effective ureteral peristalsis requires coaptation of the ureteral walls and is most effective in a euvolemic state.

Special Situations

A. Renal Transplantation: Urinary stones associated with renal transplantation are rare. Perirenal nerves are severed at the time of renal harvesting. Classic renal colic is not found in these patients. The patients usually are admitted with the presumptive diagnosis of graft rejection. Only after appropriate radiographic and ultrasonic evaluation is the correct diagnosis made (Figure 17–9).

B. Pregnancy: Renal colic is the most common nonobstetric cause of acute abdominal pain during pregnancy (Figure 17–10). Despite marked hypercalciuria associated with pregnancy, calculi are relatively rare, with an incidence approximating 1:1500 pregnancies. Women with known urinary stone disease do not have an increased risk of stones during pregnancy. The increased filtered load of calcium, uric acid, and sodium from the 25–50% increase in glomerular filtration rate associated with pregnancy has been thought to be a responsible factor in stone development.

The fetus demands special considerations regarding the potential dangers of radiation exposure (especially during the first trimester), medications, anesthesia, and surgical intervention. About 90% of symptomatic calculi present during the second and third trimesters. Initial investigations can be undertaken with renal ultrasonography and limited abdominal x-rays with appropriate shielding. Treatment requires balancing the safety of the fetus with the health of the mother. Temporizing measures to relieve upper-tract obstruction with a double-J ureteral stent or a percutaneous nephrostomy tube can be performed under local anesthesia. Treatment usually can be delayed until after delivery.

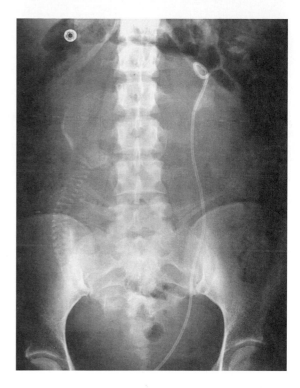

Figure 17–10. Scout radiograph demonstrating left renal calculus with double-J ureteral stent in place. Skeletal fetal structures can be appreciated in this pregnant patient.

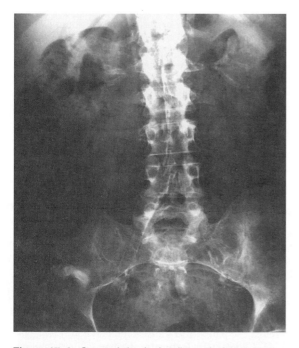

Figure 17–9. Scout abdominal radiograph demonstrating renal calculus in a renal transplant in the right iliac fossa. Note native renal vasculature with marked calcifications secondary to malignant diabetes mellitus.

C. Dysmorphia: Patients with severe skeletal dysmorphia that is either congenital (spina bifida, myelomeningocele, cerebral palsy) or acquired (arthritis, traumatic spinal cord injuries) and concurrent urinary calculi represent a unique clinical situation requiring special considerations (Figure 17–11). These skeletal abnormalities may preclude appropriate positioning for ESWL or percutaneous approaches. Calculi on the concave side in a patient with severe scoliosis may eliminate percutaneous puncture access between the rib and the posterosuperior iliac spine. Retrograde manipulations may need to be performed with flexible endoscopes due to marked contractures, making conventional dorsal lithotomy positioning impossible. Many such patients have undergone supravesical urinary diversion, so that retrograde access may be limited. Risks that need to be addressed include hypercalciuria associated with immobilization, relative dehydration due to patients' or attendants' attempts to reduce urinary output into external collecting devices, and the potential inability to drink without assistance. A full metabolic evaluation is even more important because these social and physical restrictions may be difficult or impossible to remedy.

D. Obesity: Obesity is a risk factor for the de-

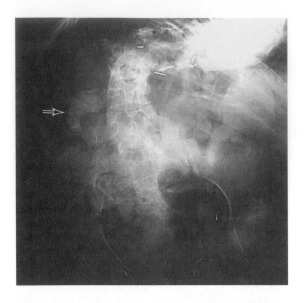

Figure 17–11. Scout abdominal radiograph demonstrating a right renal calculus (arrow) in a patient with severe kyphoscoliosis. Respiratory compromise limited patient positioning for surgery.

velopment of urinary calculi. Surgical bypass procedures can cause hyperoxaluria. Massive weight gain or loss also may precipitate stone development. Obesity limits diagnostic and treatment options. A large pannus may limit the physical examination and misguide incisions. Ultrasound examination is hindered by the attenuation of ultrasound beams. Computed tomography, magnetic resonance imaging, fluoroscopy tables, and lithotripters all have weight limitations, and patients weighing more than 300 pounds may be unsuited for diagnosis and treatment with these resources. Standard lithotripters have focal lengths less than 13 cm between the energy source and the F2 target, frequently making treatment of obese patients impossible. A large anterior pannus limits prone positioning on lithotripters. Standard Amplatz nephrostomy sheaths may not be long enough to enter the collecting system. Such sheaths may need to be advanced well below the skin. A preplaced heavy suture eases removal of such sheaths.

Risks of anesthesia are increased and special high pressure respirators may be required if patients are placed in a prone position for a percutaneous procedure. Careful positioning for open procedures helps to reduce the likelihood of crush injuries and associated rhabdomyolysis. These patients are at increased risk of anesthetic complications. Postoperative prophylaxis for thromboembolic complications should be considered.

E. Medullary Sponge Kidney: Medullary sponge kidney is a common condition characterized by tubular ectasia associated with parenchymal cysts and clefts that predispose to nephrolithiasis in 50% of affected patients. It is most often an asymptomatic condition; however it may present with renal colic, hematuria, or urinary tract infection. Diagnosis is easily made during excretory urography with the classic caliceal blush representing contrast collections within the ectatic tubules. The condition can involve select papillae or, more frequently, can be global. A full metabolic evaluation helps direct appropriate medical therapy.

F. Renal Tubular Acidosis: There are 3 main types of renal tubular acidosis: types I, II, and IV. Type I, associated with renal calculi, results from either a distal tubular hydrogen ion excretion defect or a hydrogen ion gradient defect. Both types of defect result in decreased hydrogen excretion and increased potassium and sodium excretion. Type II is secondary to a proximal tubular defect, resulting in bicarbonate wastage. Type IV occurs with chronic renal insufficiency and is associated with a metabolic acidosis, hyperkalemia, and hypoaldosteronemia.

Patients with type I renal tubular acidosis present with persistent acidemia with a low serum bicarbonate value unexplained by hyperventilation or known renal failure. The diagnosis should be suspected in those with a known family history, severe hypocitraturia, nephrocalcinosis, medullary sponge kidney, or a fasting urine pH > 6.0 in the absence of infection. Patients usually present with nephrolithiasis (calcium phosphate), nephrocalcinosis, or osteomalacia (or a combination). This disease can be acquired as an adult or inherited with an autosomal dominant pattern. The diagnosis is confirmed by assessing the patient's response to an acid load. This is frequently produced by a rapid oral ammonium chloride load (0.1 g/kg over 1 h). The dose can be given before bedtime in the evening; the patient is instructed to fast until a second morning voided urine sample and a serum bicarbonate level are obtained. A normal person responds by eliminating the acid load in the urine, resulting in a urinary pH below 5.3. Those who do not respond in this fashion can be said to have type I renal tubular acidosis. Additionally, the diagnosis should be challenged in those with normal citrate values. Treatment is centered on base replacement with potassium citrate or potassium bicarbonate solutions. Urinary citrate levels can be used to monitor effective treatment.

G. Associated Tumors: Squamous cell carcinoma of the upper urinary tract is uncommon but has been associated with calculi in more than 50% of cases. Chronic irritation from calculi or infection may be contributory factors. Upper-tract calculi may predispose patients to transitional cell carcinoma.

H. Pediatric Patients: Urinary calculi are unusual in children. A full and thorough metabolic evaluation should be undertaken. Stone analysis is particularly helpful in directing these investigations.

Children born prematurely and given furosemide while in the neonatal intensive care unit are at increased risk of developing urinary stone disease. Treatment may be limited by endoscope size. Preliminary data show no change in renal growth after ESWL.

I.   Caliceal Diverticula: Pyelocaliceal diverticula are cystic urine containing eventrations of the upper tract lying within the renal parenchyma; they communicate through a narrow channel into the main collecting system (Figure 17–12). These diverticula occur in approximately 0.2–0.5% of the population and are congenital in origin; up to 40% are associated with calculi. Type I diverticula are the most common and are closely related to minor calyces. Type II have a direct communication with the renal pelvis and tend to be larger and symptomatic. Caliceal diverticuli are usually asymptomatic, but patients may complain of flank pain or recurrent urinary tract infections. Diagnosis is usually made with intravenous pyelography (IVP). Frequently many small calculi, rather than a solitary stone, are found in these obstructed cavities. When intervention was required in the past, treatment was with nephrectomy, heminephrectomy, or open surgical unroofing. Less invasive means are used today. Communications with the collecting system are commonly pinpoint and may be difficult to locate through a retrograde approach. Retrograde access into superior pole diverticula has been successful. Surprisingly, treatment may be successful with ESWL if stone fragments are small enough to pass uneventfully. More commonly, percutaneous access and, more recently, laparoscopic means are used with success. Dilation of the caliceal neck or direct cauterization and/or sclerosis of the caliceal epithelium can help reduce stone recurrence rates.

J.   Renal Malformations: Anatomic renal variants such as ectopic kidneys, including the horseshoe kidney, predispose to renal calculi due to impaired urinary drainage. Pain symptoms appear to be no different from those reported in patients with normally positioned kidneys. Radiographic diagnosis may be difficult due to the unexpected location of the ureters and kidneys (Figure 17–13). If calculi can be targeted with ESWL, most stone fragments pass surprisingly uneventfully. Large stone burdens should be approached percutaneously as in normally positioned kidneys. Severe outlet obstruction should be corrected with open surgery, and concurrent calculi can be removed at the same setting. Aberrant vasculature should be appreciated before percutaneous and open procedures are undertaken.

Evaluation

A.   Differential Diagnosis: Urinary stones can mimic other retroperitoneal and peritoneal pathologic states. A full differential diagnosis of the acute abdomen should be made, including acute appendicitis, ectopic and unrecognized pregnancies, ovarian pathologic conditions including twisted ovarian cysts, diverticular disease, bowel obstruction, biliary stones with and without obstruction, peptic ulcer disease, acute renal artery embolism, and abdominal aortic aneurysm—to mention a few. Peritoneal signs should be sought during physical examination.

B.   History: A proper evaluation requires a thorough medical history. The nature of the pain should be evaluated, including its onset; character; potential

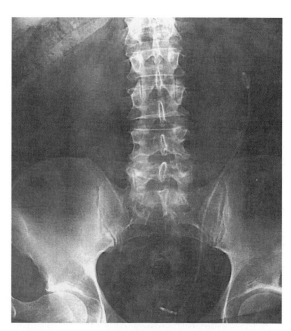

Figure 17–13. Scout abdominal radiograph demonstrating horseshoe kidney with lateral ureteral deviation and double-J ureteral stent. Extraosseous calcifications are left lower calyceal stones.

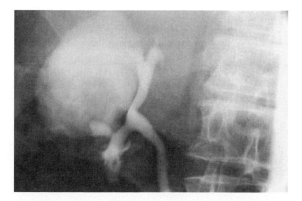

Figure 17–12. Intravenous pyelogram demonstrating symptomatic right calyceal diverticula with numerous small calculi.

radiation; activities that exacerbate or ease the pain; associated nausea, vomiting, or gross hematuria; and a history of similar pain. Patients with previous stones frequently have had similar types of pain in the past, but not always.

C. Risk Factors:

1. Crystalluria–Crystalluria is a risk factor for stones. Stone formers, especially those with calcium oxalate stones, frequently excrete more calcium oxalate crystals, and those crystals are larger than normal (> 12 μm). The rate of stone formation is proportional to the percentage of large crystals and crystal aggregates. Crystal production is determined by the saturation of each salt and the urinary concentration of inhibitors and promoters. Urine samples should be fresh; they should be centrifuged and examined immediately for optimum results. Cystine crystals are hexagonal; struvite stones appear as coffin lids; brushite ($CaHPO_4$) stones are splinterlike and may aggregate with a spokelike center; calcium apatite—$(Ca)_5(PO_4)_3(OH)$—and uric acid crystals appear as amorphous powder because the crystals are so small; calcium oxalate dihydrate stones are bipyramids; and calcium oxalate monohydrate stones are small biconcave ovals that may appear as a dumbbell. Cystine and struvite crystals are always abnormal and require further investigations. Other crystals are frequently found in normal urinalyses.

2. Socioeconomic factors–Renal stones are more common in affluent, industrialized countries. Immigrants from less industrialized nations gradually increase their stone incidence and eventually match that of the indigenous population. Use of soft water does not decrease the incidence of urinary stones.

3. Diet–Diet may have a significant impact on the incidence of urinary stones. As per capita income increases the average diet changes, with an increase in saturated and unsaturated fatty acids, an increase in animal protein and sugar, and a decrease in dietary fiber, vegetable protein, and unrefined carbohydrates. A less energy-dense diet may decrease the incidence of stones. This fact has been documented during war years when diets containing minimal fat and protein resulted in a decreased incidence of stones. Vegetarians may have a decreased incidence of urinary stones. High sodium intake is associated with increased urinary sodium, calcium, and pH, and a decreased excretion of citrate; this increases the likelihood of calcium salt crystallization because the urinary saturation of monosodium urate and calcium phosphate (brushite) is increased. Fluid intake and urine output may have an effect on urinary stone disease. The average daily urinary output in stone formers is 1.6 L/d.

4. Occupation–Occupation can have an impact on the incidence of urinary stones. Physicians and other white-collar workers have an increased incidence of stones compared with manual laborers. This finding may be related to differences in diet but also

may be related to physical activity; physical activity may agitate urine and dislodge crystal aggregates. Individuals exposed to high temperatures may develop higher concentrations of solutes owing to dehydration, which may have an impact on the incidence of stones.

5. Climate–Individuals living in hot climates are prone to dehydration, which results in an increased incidence of urinary stones, especially uric acid calculi. Although heat may cause a higher fluid intake, sweat loss results in lowered voided volumes. Hot climates usually expose people to more ultraviolet light, increasing vitamin D_3 production. Increased calcium and oxalate excretion has been correlated with increased exposure time to sunlight. This factor has more impact on light-skinned people and may help explain why African Americans in the United States have a decreased stone incidence.

6. Family history–A family history of urinary stones is associated with an increased incidence of renal calculi. A patient with stones is twice as likely as a stone-free cohort to have at least one first-degree relative with renal stones (30% versus 15%). Those with a family history of stones have an increased incidence of multiple and early recurrences. Spouses of patients with calcium oxalate stones have an increased incidence of stones; this may be related to environmental or dietary factors.

7. Medications–A thorough history of medications taken may provide valuable insight into the cause of urinary calculi. The antihypertensive medication triamterene is found as a component of several medications, including Dyazide, and has been associated with urinary calculi with increasing frequency. Long-term use of antacids containing silica has been associated with the development of silicate stones. Carbonic anhydrase inhibitors may be associated with urinary stone disease (10–20% incidence). The long-term effect of sodium- and calcium-containing medications on the development of renal calculi is not known. Protease inhibitors in immunocompromised patients are associated with radiolucent calculi.

D. Physical Examination: A detailed physical examination is an essential component of the evaluation of any patient suspected of having a urinary calculus. The patient presenting with acute renal colic typically is in severe pain, often attempting to find relief in multiple, frequently bizarre, positions. This fact helps differentiate patients with this condition from those with peritonitis, who are afraid to move. Systemic components of renal colic may be obvious, with tachycardia, sweating, and nausea often prominent. Costovertebral angle tenderness may be apparent. An abdominal mass may be palpable in patients with long-standing obstructive urinary calculi and severe hydronephrosis.

Fever, hypotension, and cutaneous vasodilation may be apparent in patients with urosepsis. In such instances there is an urgent need for decompression of the obstructed urinary tract, massive intravenous fluid resuscitation, and intravenous antibiotics. Occasionally, intensive care support is needed.

A thorough abdominal examination should exclude other causes of abdominal pain. Abdominal tumors, abdominal aortic aneurysms, herniated lumbar disks, and pregnancy may mimic renal colic. Referred pain may be similar owing to common afferent neural pathways. Intestinal ileus may be associated with renal colic or other intraperitoneal or retroperitoneal processes. Bladder palpation should be performed because urinary retention may present with pain similar to renal colic. Incarcerated inguinal hernias, epididymitis, orchitis, and female pelvic pathologic states may mimic urinary stone disease. A rectal examination helps exclude other pathologic conditions.

E. Radiologic Investigations:

1. Computed tomography–Noncontrast spiral CT scans are now the imaging modality of choice in patients presenting with acute renal colic. It is rapid and is now less expensive than an IVP. It images other peritoneal and retroperitoneal structures and helps when the diagnosis is uncertain. It does not depend on an experienced radiologic technician to obtain appropriate oblique views when there is confusion with overlying bowel gas in a nonprepped abdomen. There is no need for intravenous contrast. Distal ureteral calculi can be confused with phleboliths. These images do not give anatomic details as seen on an IVP (for example, a bifid collecting system) that may be important in planning intervention. If intravenous contrast material is used during the study, a KUB film can give additional helpful information. Uric acid stones are visualized no differently from calcium oxalate stones. Matrix calculi have adequate amounts of calcium to be visualized easily by CT.

2. Intravenous pyelography–An intravenous pyelogram can document simultaneously nephrolithiasis and upper-tract anatomy. Extraosseous calcifications on radiographs may be erroneously assumed to be urinary tract calculi (Figure 17–14). Oblique views easily differentiate gallstones from right renal calculi. Static hard-copy films can be interpreted by most clinicians. Anecdotally, small ureteral stones have passed spontaneously during such studies. An inadequate bowel preparation, associated ileus and swallowed air, and lack of available technicians may result in a less than ideal study when obtained during acute renal colic. A delayed, planned IVP may result in a superior study.

Acute forniceal rupture is not uncommonly associated with a highly obstructive ureteral calculus. It may result in dramatic radiographs but is of no clinical significance, and no intervention is required. The rupture may be precipitated by the osmotic diuresis of the intravenous contrast agent.

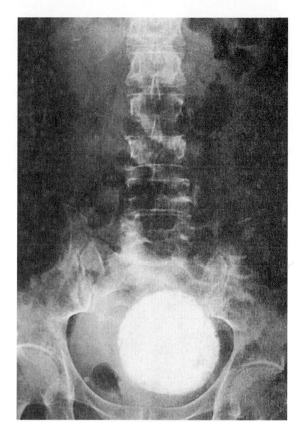

Figure 17–14. Scout abdominal radiograph demonstrating large extraosseous calcification that represents a uterine fibroid. This easily could be confused with a large bladder calculus.

3. Tomography–Renal tomography is useful to identify calculi in the kidney when oblique views are not helpful. It visualizes the kidney in a coronal plane at a set distance from the top of the x-ray table. This study may help identify poorly opacified calculi, especially when interfering abdominal gas or morbid obesity make KUB films suboptimal.

4. KUB films and directed ultrasonography–A KUB film and renal ultrasound may be as effective as an IVP in establishing a diagnosis. The ultrasound examination should be directed by notation of suspicious areas seen on a KUB film; it is, however, operator-dependent. The distal ureter is easily visualized through the acoustic window of a full bladder. Edema and small calculi missed on an IVP can be appreciated with such studies.

5. Retrograde pyelography–Retrograde pyelography occasionally is required to delineate upper-tract anatomy and localize small or radiolucent offending calculi. Bulb ureterograms frequently leak contrast back into the bladder, resulting in a suboptimal study. Advancing an angiographic exchange catheter with or without the aid of a guide wire 3–4 cm into the ureter is an alternative technique. Intermittent fluoroscopic images direct appropriate injection volumes and help reduce the likelihood of pyelolymphatic, pyelosinus, and pyelovenous reflux.

6. Magnetic resonance imaging–Magnetic resonance imaging is a poor study to document urinary stone disease.

7. Nuclear scintigraphy–Nuclear scintigraphic imaging of stones has recently been appreciated. Bisphosphonate markers can identify even small calculi that are difficult to appreciate on a conventional KUB film (Figure 17–15). Differential radioactive uptake dependent on stone composition appreciated during in vitro studies cannot be appreciated on in vivo studies. Nuclear scintigraphy cannot delineate upper-tract anatomy in sufficient detail to help direct a therapeutic plan.

Intervention

A. Conservative Observation: Most ureteral calculi pass and do not require intervention. Spontaneous passage depends on stone size, shape, location, and associated ureteral edema (which is likely to depend on the length of time that a stone has not progressed). Ureteral calculi 4–5 mm in size have a 40–50% chance of spontaneous passage. In contrast, calculi > 6 mm have a less than 5% chance of spontaneous passage. This does not mean that a 1-cm stone will not pass or that a 1- to 2-mm stone will always pass uneventfully.

The vast majority of stones that pass do so within a 6-week period after the onset of symptoms. Ureteral calculi discovered in the distal ureter at the time of presentation have a 50% chance of spontaneous passage, in contrast to a 25% and 10% chance in the mid and proximal ureter, respectively.

B. Dissolution Agents: The effectiveness of dissolution agents depends on stone surface area, stone type, volume of irrigant, and mode of delivery. Oral alkalinizing agents include sodium or potassium bicarbonate and potassium citrate. Extra care should be employed in patients susceptible to congestive heart failure or renal failure. Citrate is metabolized to bicarbonate and comes in a variety of preparations. Polycitra contains potassium and sodium citrate and citric acid. Bictra contains only sodium citrate and citric acid. Food does not alter the effectiveness of these agents. Alternatively, orange juice alkalinizes urine. Intravenous alkalinization is effective with 1/6 molar sodium lactate.

Intrarenal alkalinization may be performed successfully under a low-pressure system (< 25 cm water pressure). This may be achieved through a percutaneous nephrostomy tube or an externalized retrograde catheter. A manometer, similar to those used for central venous pressure monitoring, is cheap, available, and practical. Agents include sodium bicarbonate, 2–4 ampules in 1 L of normal saline, producing a urinary

pH between 7.5 and 9.0. Tromethamine-E and tromethamine can produce urinary pHs of 8.0–10.5 and are especially effective with pH-sensitive calculi as in uric acid and cystine lithiasis.

Cystine calculi can be dissolved with a variety of thiols, including D-penicillamine (0.5% solution), N-acetylcysteine (2–5% solution), and alpha-mercapto-propionylglycine (Thiola) (5% solution).

Struvite stone dissolution requires acidification and may be achieved successfully with Suby's G solution and hemiacidrin (Renacidin). Urinary pH may get down to 4.0. Hemiacidrin must be used with sterile urine and careful monitoring of serum magnesium levels is required. The Food and Drug Administration has not approved hemiacidrin for upper-tract irrigations, and thus appropriate informed consent is required.

C. Relief of Obstruction: Urinary stone disease may result in significant morbidity and possible mortality in the presence of obstruction, especially with concurrent infection. A patient with obstructive urinary calculi with fever and infected urine requires emergent drainage. Retrograde pyelography to define upper-tract anatomy is logically followed by retrograde placement of a double-J ureteral stent. On occasion such catheters are unable to bypass the offending calculus or may perforate the ureter. In such situations one must be prepared to place a percutaneous nephrostomy tube.

D. Extracorporeal Shock Wave Lithotripsy: Ureteral calculi that fail to progress with conservative measures require intervention. Proximal ureteral stones and distal calculi in women past the childbearing age can be treated with in situ ESWL (no stone manipulations). Stones poorly visible overlying the sacroiliac joint may not be amenable to ESWL. Renal calculi less than 2.0–2.5 cm in aggregate length are best treated with ESWL. Inferior caliceal calculi have suboptimal stone-free rates. Double-J stents do not facilitate stone passage but ensure kidney drainage. Most stone fragments that pass do so within a 2-week period. A 3-month follow-up KUB film helps direct the need for additional therapy. A full discussion is found in Chapter 18.

E. Ureteroscopic Stone Extraction: Ureteroscopic stone extraction is highly efficacious for lower ureteral calculi. The use of small-caliber ureteroscopes and the advent of balloon dilation have increased stone-free rates dramatically. Even relatively large-caliber endoscopes without balloon dilation are effective in lower ureteral stone retrieval. Stone-free rates range from 66 to 100% and are dependent on stone burden and location, length of time the stone has been impacted, history of retroperitoneal surgery, and the experience of the operator. Complication rates range from 5 to 30%; the rates increase when manipulations venture into the proximal ureter. Ureteral stricture rates are less than 5%. Postopera-

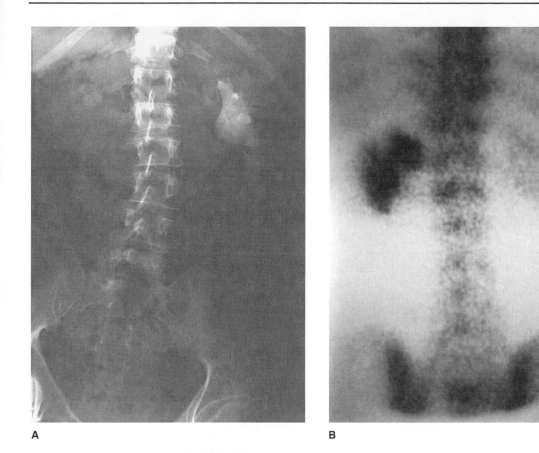

A

B

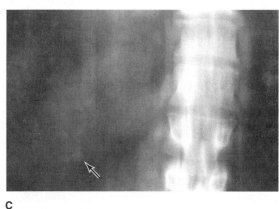

C

Figure 17–15. A: Scout abdominal radiograph demonstrating large left staghorn renal calculus. **B:** Nuclear scintigraphic evaluation of renal calculi. Posterior view demonstrating uptake on large left staghorn calculus after furosemide (lasix) diuresis. Note right kidney with uptake in lower pole. **C:** Follow-up tomogram confirms calculus (arrow) in right lower pole missed on initial radiograph.

tive vesicoureteral reflux is extremely rare. Calculi that measure less than 8 mm are frequently removed intact. Round wire stone baskets can be torqued to help entrap stone or stone fragments. Flat wire baskets should be used with caution; if twisted, they can develop sharp, knifelike edges resulting in ureteral injury. Excessive force with any instrument in the ureter may result in ureteral injury.

A variety of lithotrites can be placed through an ureteroscope, including electrohydraulic; solid, and hollow-core ultrasonic probes; a variety of laser systems; electromechanical impactors; and pneumatic systems such as the Swiss lithoclast. Electrohydraulic lithotrites have power settings as high as 120 V that result in a cavitation bubble, followed by collapse of this bubble causing subsequent shock waves. Care should be taken to keep the tip of the electrode away from surrounding tissue and the tip of the endoscope. Ultrasonic lithotrites have a piezoceramic energy source that converts electrical energy into ultrasonic waves in the range of 25,000 Hz. This vibratory action is effective in fragmenting calculi. Hollow probes can suction stone fragments and debris simultaneously. Laser systems are discussed elsewhere in this book. The electromechanical impactors are similar to jackhammers with a movable pistonlike tip that fragments calculi.

F. Percutaneous Nephrolithotomy: Percutaneous removal of renal and proximal ureteral calculi is the treatment of choice for large (> 2.5 cm) calculi, those resistant to ESWL, select lower pole calyceal stones with a narrow, long infundibulum and an acute infundibulo-pelvic angle, and instances with evidence of obstruction; the method can rapidly establish a stone-free status. Needle puncture is directed by fluoroscopy, ultrasound or both, and is routinely placed from the posterior axillary line into a posterior inferior calyx. Superior caliceal puncture may be required, and in such situations care should be taken to avoid injury to the pleura, lungs, spleen, and liver. Tract dilation is performed by sequential plastic dilators (Amplatz system), telescoping metal dilators (Alken), or balloon dilation with a back-loaded Amplatz system. Tracts placed during open renal procedures are frequently tortuous and suboptimal for subsequent endourologic procedures.

Percutaneous extraction of calculi requires patience and perseverance. Hard-copy radiographs help to confirm a stone-free status. Remaining calculi can be retrieved with the aid of flexible endoscopes, additional percutaneous puncture access, follow-up irrigations, ESWL, or additional percutaneous sessions. Realistic goals should be established. Patients should be informed that complex calculi frequently require numerous procedures.

Maintenance of body temperature with appropriate blankets during preoperative patient positioning and with warmed irrigation fluids helps to prevent bleeding diatheses associated with hypothermia. Autologous blood donation is reasonable in such elective procedures. The average blood loss during a percutaneous nephrolithotomy is 2.0–2.8 g/dL of hemoglobin. Multiple percutaneous punctures and renal pelvic perforations are associated with a greater blood loss. Overall, such procedures are safe and effective and have a transfusion rate well below 10%.

G. Open Stone Surgery: Open stone surgery is the classic way to remove calculi. The morbidity of the incision, the possibility of retained stone fragments, and the ease and success of less invasive techniques have made these procedures relatively uncommon when instruments and surgical experience are available. It is mandatory to obtain a radiograph before the incision is made; calculi frequently move. A variety of incisions to access the kidney are available, including a thoracoabdominal approach for superior pole access; flank incisions to remain retroperitoneal, especially in the setting of concurrent infection; lumbodorsal incision; and a Gibson incision.

H. Pyelolithotomy: Pyelolithotomy is effective, especially with an extrarenal pelvis. A transverse pyelotomy is effective and does not require interruption of the renal arterial blood supply. Inspection with flexible endoscopes helps ensure a stone-free status. Multiple, small renal pelvic calculi and difficult-to-access caliceal calculi can be retrieved with the aid of a coagulum. Coagulum was initially produced from pooled human fibrinogen. The risks of hepatitis and other viral infections have made this method unacceptable. Cryoprecipitate can be obtained from rapid freezing of plasma. Autologous plasma may be used to decrease the incidence of bloodborne infections. The tensile strength of cryoprecipitate is approximately 10 times that of a blood clot. Injected into the renal pelvis, endogenous clotting factors result in a jellolike coagulum of the collecting system. Small stones are entrapped and removed with the coagulum. A variety of Randall stone forceps help gain access into most of the collecting system.

I. Anatrophic Nephrolithotomy: Anatrophic nephrolithotomy is used with complex staghorn calculi. A complete staghorn calculi is a cast of the renal pelvis and calyces (Figure 17–16). A partial staghorn calculus involves the renal pelvis and extends into at least 2 infundibula. To gain access to the entire collecting system, a longitudinal incision is made on the convex surface of the kidney just posterior to the line of Brödel, taking advantage of the converging anterior and posterior renal blood supplies. Occlusion of the renal artery followed by renal cooling with slushed ice gives a relatively bloodless surgical field. A nerve hook is helpful to tease out calculi. Careful inspection of the entire collecting system helps remove all stones. Repair of narrowed infundibula helps reduce stone recurrence rates. The collecting system is closed followed by the renal capsule. Intraoperative placement of a nephrostomy tube for possible follow-up irrigations or endoscopic inspection or stone retrieval makes hemostasis difficult. Open stone surgery becomes progressively more difficult after the first procedure owing to reactive scar tissue.

J. Radial Nephrotomy: Radial nephrotomy gives access to limited calyces of the collecting system. An appropriate approach to localized calculi, it is frequently used in blown-out calyces with thin overlying parenchyma. Intraoperative ultrasound helps to localize the calyx and the calculi. Once the kidney has been opened, the introduction of air can make interpre-

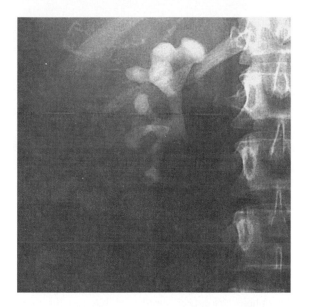

Figure 17–16. Plain abdominal radiograph demonstrating complete staghorn calculus with renal pelvic extension into all infundibula and calyces.

tation of subsequent ultrasound scans confusing. A shallow incision of the renal capsule can be followed by puncture into the collecting system. Brain retractors provide excellent exposure. Care should be taken not to force stones through narrow infundibula. Stones may be cut with heavy Mayo scissors, and remaining fragments can be retrieved. Inspection with flexible endoscopes is helpful. Intraoperative radiographs help document a stone-free status.

K. Other Renal Procedures: Partial nephrectomy is appropriate with a large stone burden in a renal pole with marked parenchymal thinning. Caution should be taken with a simple nephrectomy even with a normal contralateral kidney, as stones are frequently associated with a systemic metabolic defect that may recur in the contralateral kidney. What may seem prudent and simple today may be regretted tomorrow.

Other unusual procedures include ileal ureter substitution performed with the hope of decreasing pain with frequent stone passage. Autotransplantation with pyelocystostomy is another option for patients with rare malignant stone disease.

L. Ureterolithotomy: Long-standing ureteral calculi—those inaccessible with endoscopy and those resistant to ESWL—can be extracted with a ureterolithotomy. Again, a preoperative radiograph documents stone location and directs an appropriate incision. The proximal ureter may be approached with a dorsal lumbotomy. An incision lateral to the sacrospinalis muscles allows medial retraction of the quadratus lumborum. The anterior fascicle of the dorsal lumbar fascia must be incised to gain proper exposure despite the appearance of potentially opening the peritoneum. Once the ureter is identified, a vessel loop or a Babcock clamp should be placed proximal to the stone to prevent frustrating stone migration. Extension of this incision is limited superiorly by the 12th rib and inferiorly by the iliac crest. A longitudinal incision over the stone with a hooked blade exposes the calculus. The nerve hook is excellent to help tease out the stone. A flank or anterior abdominal muscle splitting incision gives excellent exposure to mid and distal ureteral stones.

Prevention

In general, 50% of patients experience recurrent urinary stones within 5 years without prophylactic intervention. Appropriate education and preventive measures are best instituted with a motivated patient after spontaneous stone passage or surgical stone removal. Risk factors as described previously should be identified and modified, if possible. Irrespective of the final metabolic evaluation and stone analysis, the patient's fluid intake should be about 1.6 L/24 h. Fluids should be encouraged during mealtime. Additionally, liquids should be increased approximately 2 h after meals. Water produced as a metabolic by-product reaches its nadir at this time, and thus the body is relatively dehydrated. Fluid ingestion also should be encouraged to force a nighttime diuresis adequate to awaken the patient to void. Awakening and ambulating to void limit urinary stasis and offer an opportunity to ingest additional fluids. These lifestyle changes are difficult to maintain and should be encouraged during subsequent office visits. Motivated patients who regularly return to a urinary stone clinic have a reduced stone recurrence rate that is probably due to increased compliance.

A. Metabolic Evaluation: A systematic metabolic evaluation should be instituted after a patient has recovered from urinary stone intervention or spontaneous stone passage. Stone analysis should be obtained to help direct the workup. An outpatient urine collection during typical activities and fluid intake helps unmask significant abnormalities. An initial 24-h urine collection for calcium stone formers should include tests for calcium, uric acid, oxalate, citrate, sodium, volume, and pH. An open dialog with local laboratories helps to standardize collection routines and determine whether an outside laboratory is preferred. Baseline serum levels for blood urea nitrogen, creatinine, calcium, phosphorous, and uric acid are appropriate.

Hypercalciuria is the most common abnormality. To differentiate among hypercalciuria types I, II, and III, a patient should be placed on a sodium- and calcium-restricted diet for a few days to a week. This is easily achieved (100 mEq/d) by eliminating table salt and reducing obviously salty foods. Calcium is restricted (400–500 mg) by excluding dairy products.

A repeat 24-h urine collection is evaluated for calcium. A urinary calcium level < 250 mg/d confirms a diagnosis of dietary-dependent hypercalciuria, type II. Type I and type III hypercalciuria must be differentiated in patients with urinary calcium levels > 250 mg/d. A calcium binder such as cellulose phosphate is prescribed (5 g 3 times daily with meals) for a few days. This is followed by a repeat 24-h urine calcium level and parathyroid hormone blood value. Patients who have type I absorptive hypercalciuria have at least a 50% drop in urinary calcium levels and normal parathyroid hormone levels.

Hyperuricosuria, hyperoxaluria, and hypocitraturia calcium stone formers can be treated appropriately and followed with repeat 24-h urine collections. Many calcium stone formers have multiple defects; although one treatment may reverse one defect, it may exacerbate others. Subsequent 24-h urine collections are critical for effective long-term follow-up and stone prevention. Treatment of cystinuria should be titrated with repeat 24-h cystine levels. Repeat urine cultures should be obtained in patients with infectious calculi.

B. Oral Medications:

1. Alkalinizing pH agents–Potassium citrate is an oral agent that elevates urinary pH effectively by 0.7–0.8 pH units. Typical dosing is 60 mEq in 3 or 4 divided doses daily. It is available in wax-matrix 5- and 10-mEq tablets, liquid preparations, and crystals that must be mixed with fluids. The effect is maintained over many years. Care should be taken in patients susceptible to hyperkalemia, those with renal failure, and those taking potassium-sparing diuretics. Although the medication is usually well tolerated, some patients may complain of abdominal discomfort, especially with tablet preparations. Potassium citrate also raises urinary citrate excretion by 400 mg/d. This reduces the urinary saturation of calcium oxalate. It is indicated, therefore, in those with calcium oxalate calculi secondary to hypocitraturia (< 320 mg/d), including those with renal tubular acidosis. Potassium citrate also may be used effectively to treat uric acid lithiasis and nonsevere forms of hyperuricosuric calcium nephrolithiasis.

Sodium and potassium bicarbonate and orange juice are alternative alkalinizing agents. There are no effective long term urinary acidifying agents.

2. Gastrointestinal absorption inhibitor–Cellulose phosphate binds calcium in the gut and thereby inhibits calcium absorption and urinary excretion. It is a popular drug in the treatment of absorptive hypercalciuria type I with recurrent calcium nephrolithiasis, although it only prevents new stone formation. Patients should have normal parathyroid hormone values, normal serum calcium and phosphate values, no evidence of bone disease, and evidence of increased intestinal calcium absorption. The drug decreases the urinary saturation of calcium phosphate and calcium oxalate. It may increase urinary oxalate and urinary phosphate levels. A typical starting dosage is 5 g 3 times daily with meals; the dosage may be titrated by following 24-h urinary calcium levels. Urinary magnesium, calcium, oxalate, and sodium levels and serum parathyroid hormone should be monitored 1–2 times yearly. Magnesium supplements are frequently required and should be taken at least 1 h before or after cellulose phosphate is taken. Cellulose phosphate is associated with a sodium load and should be used with caution in those with congestive heart failure. Gastrointestinal side effects are infrequent; they include dyspepsia and loose bowel movements.

Cellulose phosphate may be suboptimal treatment for postmenopausal women who are at risk for bone disease. An alternative treatment for such patients would be hydrochlorothiazides supplemented with potassium citrate to offset the potential hypokalemia and hypocitraturia.

3. Phosphate supplementation–Renal phosphate leak is best treated by replacing phosphate. Phosphate absorption may be inhibited in the presence of aluminum-, magnesium-, or calcium-containing antacids. This treatment should be used with caution in digitalized patients and in those with severe renal failure, Addison disease, or severe hepatic dysfunction. It is generally well tolerated. Dosing can begin with 250 mg 3–4 times daily and may be doubled depending on follow-up serum electrolyte, calcium, and phosphorus levels.

4. Diuretics–Thiazides can correct the renal calcium leak associated with renal hypercalciuria. This prevents a secondary hyperparathyroid state and its associated elevated vitamin D synthesis and intestinal calcium absorption. A rapid decrease in urinary calcium excretion is appreciated and is sustained long-term (> 10 years). A starting dose of 25 mg may be titrated based on urinary calcium levels. Side effects are usually well tolerated. Potassium levels should be monitored. Hypokalemia induces a hypocitraturic state; potassium replacement corrects the hypokalemia and its associated hypocitraturia.

Thiazides result in a transient decrease in urinary calcium excretion in absorptive hypercalciurics. Urinary calcium excretion rebounds to pretreatment values in 50% of such patients after 4–5 years of therapy. Dietary changes are not believed to be responsible for this phenomenon. Thiazides do not restore normal intestinal absorption of calcium.

Diuretics containing triamterene, such as Dyazide, are associated with triamterene urinary stones. Individuals taking such diuretics who are found on analysis to have triamterene stones should be given an alternative antihypertensive medication.

5. Calcium supplementation–Enteric hyperoxaluric calcium nephrolithiasis is effectively treated with calcium supplements. Calcium gluconate and calcium citrate are better absorbed and are more effective in increasing serum calcium availability than are other forms of calcium. Calcium carbonate, calcium phosphate, and oyster shell are forms of calcium that are less efficiently absorbed; they remain in the intestinal lumen, available to bind oxalate, thus reducing its absorption. These less efficiently absorbed forms of calcium are optimal to treat enteric hyperoxaluric calcium nephrolithiasis and must be given with meals to be effective.

6. Uric acid-lowering medications–Allopurinol is used to treat hyperuricosuric calcium nephrolithiasis with or without hyperuricemia. Unlike uricosuric agents that reduce serum uric acid levels by increasing urinary uric acid excretion, allopurinol is a xanthine-oxidase inhibitor and reduces both serum and urinary levels of uric acid. It has no impact on the biosynthesis of purines; rather, it acts exclusively on purine catabolism. Elevated levels of xanthine and hypoxanthine in the urine secondary to allopurinol have not been associated with nephrolithiasis. Allopurinol is a potentially dangerous drug and should be discontinued at the first appearance of a skin rash, which infrequently may be fatal. Therapy can be started at 100 mg daily and titrated up to 300 mg daily in divided doses or as a single dose by monitoring 24-h urinary uric acid levels. It is tolerated best when taken after meals.

7. Urease inhibitor–Acetohydroxamic acid is an effective adjunctive treatment in those with chronic urea-splitting urinary tract infections associated with struvite stones. Acetohydroxamic acid reversibly inhibits bacterial urease, decreasing urinary ammonia levels, and will subsequently acidify urine. It is best used as prophylaxis after removal of struvite stones. It also may be used after unsuccessful attempts at curative surgical removal of calculi or culture-specific antibiotic therapy. Patients with serum creatinine > 2.5 mg/dL are unable to achieve therapeutic urinary levels. Acetohydroxamic acid is not effective with non-urease-producing bacteria. Long-term data (> 7 years) are unavailable. A significant number of patients complain of side effects, including headaches that are usually short-lived and responsive to aspirin compounds. Other frequent complaints include nausea, vomiting, anorexia, nervousness, and depression. A typical dosing regimen is one 250 mg tablet 3 or 4 times daily (total dosage: 10–15 mg/kg/d).

8. Prevention of cystine calculi–Conservative measures, including massive fluid intake and urinary alkalinization, are frequently inadequate to control cystine stone formation. Penicillamine, the same drug that is used to chelate excess copper in the treatment of Wilson disease, undergoes a thiol-disulfide exchange with cystine. This reduces the amount of urinary cystine that is relatively insoluble. Cystine solubility is pH-dependent (pH 5.0: 150–300 mg/L; pH 7.0: 200–400 mg/L; pH 7.5: 220–500 mg/L). D-Penicillamine is associated with numerous and frequent side effects, including rashes and hematologic, renal, and hepatic abnormalities. An initial dosage of 250 mg daily in 3–4 divided doses may help reduce

severe side effects. It may be increased gradually to 2 g/d. Dosage should be titrated with quantitative urinary cystine values. Penicillamine increases the requirement of pyridoxine (vitamin B_6), which should be supplemented with 25–50 mg/d.

Mercaptopropionylglycine (Thiola) is better tolerated by patients than is penicillamine. Mercaptopropionylglycine, a reducing agent, binds to the sulfide portion of cystine, forming a mixed disulfide (Thiola-cysteine) water-soluble compound. It may retard the rate of new stone formation. The dosage should be titrated with repeat 24-h urinary cystine values. An initial dosage may be 200–300 mg 3 times daily, either 1 h before or 2 h after each meal. Side effects are not infrequent and may include drug fever; nausea, vomiting, and gastrointestinal upset; rash, wrinkling, or friable skin; lupuslike symptoms, decreased taste perception; and a variety of hematologic disorders.

BLADDER STONES

Bladder calculi usually are a manifestation of an underlying pathologic condition, including voiding dysfunction or a foreign body. Voiding dysfunction may be due to a urethral stricture, benign prostatic hyperplasia, bladder neck contracture, or flaccid or spastic neurogenic bladder, all of which result in static urine. Foreign bodies such as Foley catheters and forgotten double-J ureteral catheters can serve as nidi for stones (Figure 17–17). Most bladder calculi are seen in men. In developing countries, they are frequently found in prepubescent boys. Stone analysis frequently reveals ammonium urate, uric acid, or calcium oxalate stones. A solitary bladder stone is the rule, but there are numerous stones in 25% of patients (Figure 17–18). Patients present with irritative voiding symptoms, intermittent urinary stream, urinary tract infections, hematuria, or pelvic pain. Physical examination is unrevealing. A large percentage of bladder stones are radiolucent (uric acid). Ultrasound of the bladder identifies the stone with its characteristic shadowing. The stone moves with changing body position.

Stones within a ureterocoele do not move with body position (Figure 17–19) as seen on ultrasound examination. They frequently are nonobstructive. Endoscopic incision and stone removal rarely result in vesicoureteral reflux. The mode of stone removal for other bladder stones should be directed by the underlying cause.

Early instruments used to remove bladder calculi were both clever and bizarre. Simple mechanical crushing devices are still used today. Mechanical lithotrites should be used with caution to prevent bladder injury when the jaws are closed. Ensuring partially full bladder and endoscopic visualization of unrestricted lateral movement before forceful crushing of the stones helps reduce this troublesome complication.

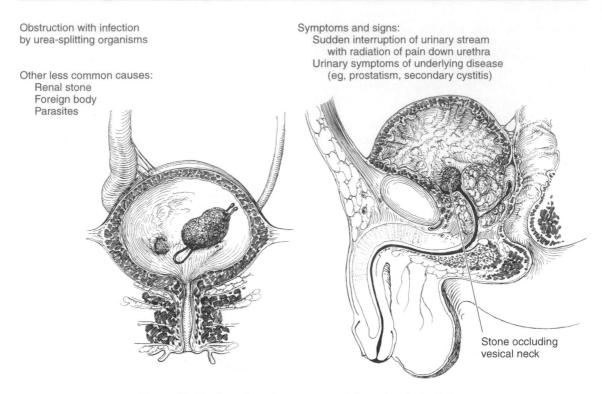

Obstruction with infection
by urea-splitting organisms

Other less common causes:
    Renal stone
    Foreign body
    Parasites

Symptoms and signs:
    Sudden interruption of urinary stream
        with radiation of pain down urethra
    Urinary symptoms of underlying disease
        (eg, prostatism, secondary cystitis)

Stone occluding
vesical neck

Figure 17–17. Genesis and symptoms and signs of vesical calculus.

Cystitholapaxy allows most stones to be broken and subsequently removed through a cystoscope. Electrohydraulic, ultrasonic, and pneumatic lithotrites similar to those used through a nephroscope are effective. Cystolithotomy can be performed through a small abdominal incision. A Turner-Warwick urethral sound may be used to tent up the bladder to help reduce the size of the incision.

PROSTATIC AND SEMINAL VESICLE STONES

Prostatic calculi are found within the prostate gland per se and are found uncommonly within the prostatic urethra. They are thought to represent calcified corpora amylacea and are rarely found in boys. Usually small and numerous, they are noted to be

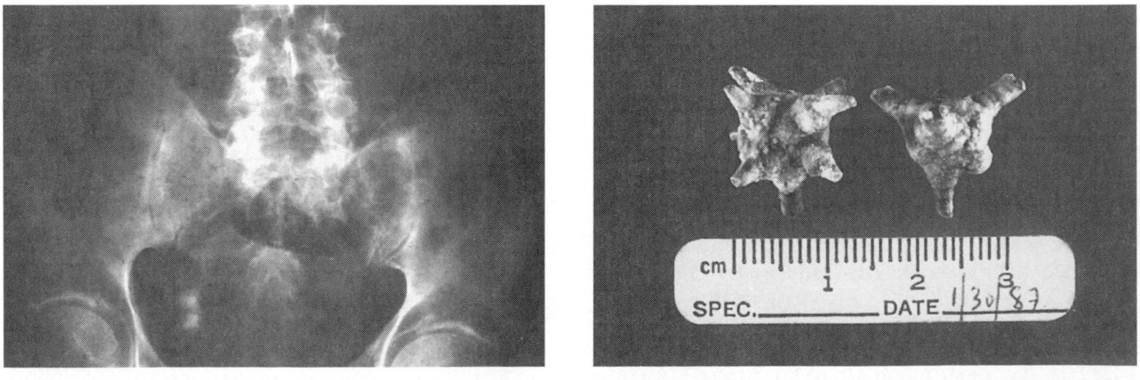

A

B

Figure 17–18. A: Plain abdominal radiograph demonstrating 2 bladder calculi. **B:** Gross picture of removed bladder calculi. Note the characteristic shape of jack-stones typically composed of uric acid.

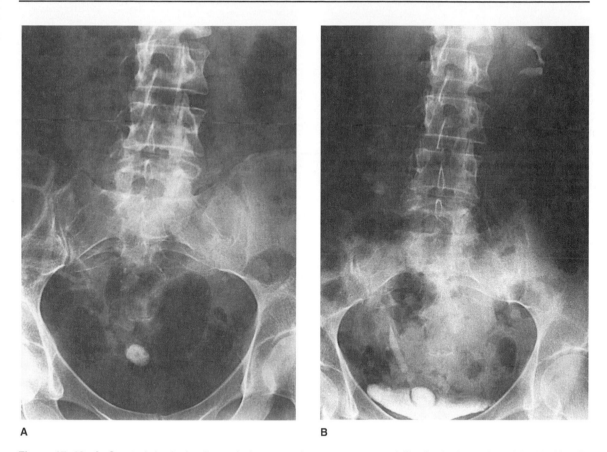

A   B

Figure 17–19. A: Scout abdominal radiograph demonstrating extraosseous calcification in the region of the bladder. **B:** Intravenous pyelogram demonstrates stone to be within a ureterocele.

tannish-gray in color during transurethral resection of the prostate. They are commonly located at the margin of the surgically resected adenoma and are composed of calcium phosphate. Although usually of no clinical significance, rarely they are associated with chronic prostatitis. Large prostatic calculi may be misinterpreted as a carcinoma. The prostate is usually mobile, however, and a radiograph or transrectal ultrasound help to confirm the diagnosis.

Seminal vesicle stones are smooth and hard and are extremely rare. They may be associated with hematospermia. Physical examination reveals a stony hard gland, and when multiple stones are present, a crunching sensation may be noted. These stones occasionally are confused with tuberculosis of the seminal vesicle.

URETHRAL AND PREPUCIAL STONES

Urethral calculi usually originate from the bladder and rarely from the upper tracts. Most ureteral stones

that pass spontaneously into the bladder can pass through the urethra unimpeded. Urethral stones may develop secondary to urinary stasis, secondary to a urethral diverticulum, near urethral strictures, or at sites of previous surgery. Most urethral stones in men present in the prostatic or bulbar regions and are solitary. Patients with recurrent pendulous urethral calculi without evidence of other pathologic conditions should be suspected of self-introduction of such stones in an attempt to obtain pain medications or for attention, as seen in Munchausen syndrome.

Females rarely develop urethral calculi owing to their short urethra and a lower incidence of bladder calculi. Most urethral stones found in women are associated with urethral diverticula.

Symptoms are similar to bladder calculi—intermittent urinary stream, terminal hematuria, and infection. The stones may present with dribbling or during acute urinary retention. Pain may be severe and, in men, may radiate to the tip of the penis. The diagnosis may be confirmed by palpation, endoscopic visualization, or radiographic study.

Treatment should be directed by the underlying

cause. Stones associated with a dense urethral stricture or complex diverticula can be removed during definitive open surgical repair. Small stones may be grasped successfully and removed intact. More frequently they need to be fragmented and removed. Long-standing, large impacted stones are best removed through a urethrotomy.

Preputial calculi are rare and usually occur in adults. They develop secondary to a severe obstructive phimosis. They may occur secondary to poor hygiene with inspissated smegma. Diagnosis is confirmed by palpation. Treating the underlying cause with a dorsal preputial slit or a formal circumcision prevents recurrent calculi.

REFERENCES

IONS IN URINARY STONE FORMATION

Calcium

Ackermann D et al: Influence of calcium content in mineral water on chemistry and crystallization conditions in urine of calcium stone formers. Eur Urol 1988;14: 305.

Breslau NA et al: Relationship of animal protein-rich diet to kidney stone formation and calcium metabolism. J Clin Endocrinol Metab 1988;66:140.

Fellstrom B et al: Dietary habits in renal stone patients compared with healthy subjects. Br J Urol 1989;63: 575.

Fuss M et al: Calcitonin secretion in idiopathic renal stone formers. J Bone Miner Res 1991;6:35.

Fuss M et al: Low calcium diet in idiopathic urolithiasis: A risk factor for osteopenia as great as in primary hyperparathyroidism. Br J Urol 1990;65:560.

Gentle DL et al: Geriatric nephrolithiasis. J Urol 1997; 158:2221.

Harvey JA, Pak CY: Gouty diathesis and sarcoidosis in patient with recurrent calcium nephrolithiasis. J Urol 1988;139:1287.

Iguchi M et al: Glucose metabolism in renal stone patients. Urol Int 1993;51:185.

Jabbour N et al: The natural history of renal stone disease after parathyroidectomy for primary hyperparathyroidism. Surg Gynecol Obstet 1991;172:25.

Jahnen A et al: Dietary fibre: The effectiveness of a high bran intake in reducing renal calcium excretion. Urol Res 1992;20:3.

Jarrar K et al: Relationship between 1,25-dihydroxyvitamin-D, calcium and uric acid in urinary stone formers. Urol Int 1996;56:16.

Khanam A, Rahman B, Rahman MA: Role of vitamins in urolithiasis. Biomed Pharmacother 1988;42:609.

Langley SE, Fry CH: The influence of pH on urinary ionized [Ca2+]: Differences between urinary tract stone formers and normal subjects. Br J Urol 1997; 79:8.

Litin RB, Diessner GR, Keating FR: Urinary excretion of calcium in patients with renal lithiasis. J Urol 1961;86:17.

Menon M: Value of repeated analyses of 24-hour urine in recurrent calcium urolithiasis. J Urol 1995;153: 555.

Milosevic D et al: Determination of urine saturation with computer program EQUIL 2 as a method for estimation of the risk of urolithiasis. J Chem Inf Comput Sci 1998;38:646.

Parivar F, Low RK, Stoller ML: The influence of diet on urinary stone disease. J Urol 1996;155:432.

Preminger GM, Sakhaee K, Pak CY: Alkali action on the urinary crystallization of calcium salts: Contrasting responses to sodium citrate and potassium citrate. J Urol 1988;139:240.

Tiselius HG: Metabolic evaluation of patients with stone disease. Urol Int 1997;59:131.

Trinchieri A et al: The influence of diet on urinary risk factors for stones in healthy subjects and idiopathic renal calcium stone formers. Br J Urol 1991;67: 230.

Urivetzky M et al: Biochemical evaluation of calcium stone patients: How soon can it be done after stone surgery/passage? Urology 1990;36:410.

Urivetzky M et al: Urinary excretion of oxalate by patients with renal hypercalciuric stone disease: Effect of chronic treatment with hydrochlorothiazide. Urology 1991;37:327.

Oxalate

Bataille P et al: Diet, vitamin D and vertebral mineral density in hypercalciuric calcium stone formers. Kidney Int 1991;39:1193.

Brown JM et al: The variability and dietary dependence of urinary oxalate excretion in recurrent calcium stone formers. Ann Clin Biochem 1987;24:385.

Grases F, Millan A, Sohnel O: Role of agglomeration in calcium oxalate monohydrate urolith development. Nephron 1992;61:145.

Grases F, Sohnel O: Mechanism of oxalocalcic renal calculi generation. Int Urol Nephrol 1993;25:209.

Hatch M: Oxalate status in stone-formers: Two distinct hyperoxaluric entities. Urol Res 1993:21:55.

Kohri K, Garside J, Blacklock NJ: The role of magnesium in calcium oxalate urolithiasis. Br J Urol 1988; 61:107.

Koide T et al: Promotive effect of urine from patients with primary hyperparathyroidism on calcium oxalate crystal aggregation in an in vitro whole urine system. J Urol 1988;140:1571.

Kok DJ, Papapoulos SE, Bijvoet OL: Crystal agglomeration is a major element in calcium oxalate urinary stone formation. Kidney Int 1990;37:51.

Kok DJ et al: The effects of dietary excesses in animal protein and in sodium on the composition and the crystallization kinetics of calcium oxalate monohydrate in urines of healthy men. J Clin Endocrinol Metab 1990;71:861.

Laminski NA et al: Hyperoxaluria in patients with recurrent calcium oxalate calculi: Dietary and other risk factors. Br J Urol 1991;68:454.

Lanzalaco AC et al: The influence of urinary macromolecules on calcium oxalate monohydrate crystal growth. J Urol 1988;139:190.

Morse RM, Resnick MI: A new approach to the study of urinary macromolecules as a participant in calcium oxalate crystallization. J Urol 1988;139:869.

Nakada T et al: Effect of high-calcium diet on urinary oxalate excretion in urinary stone formers. Eur Urol 1988;15:264.

Ryall RL: The scientific basis of calcium oxalate urolithiasis: Predilection and precipitation, promotion and proscription. World J Urol 1993;11:59.

Ryall RL et al: Urinary risk factors in calcium oxalate stone disease: Comparison of men and women. Br J Urol 1987;60:480.

Tiselius HG: Standardized estimate of the ion activity product of calcium oxalate in urine from renal stone formers. Eur Urol 1989;16:48.

Williams HE, Wandzilak TR: Oxalate synthesis, transport and the hyperoxaluric syndromes. J Urol 1989; 141:742.

Phosphate

Gault MH et al: Bacteriology of urinary tract stones. J Urol 1995;153:1164.

Harmelin DL, Martin FI, Wark JD: Antacid-induced phosphate depletion syndrome presenting as nephrolithiasis. Aust N Z J Med 1990;20:803.

Kohri K et al: Relationship between metabolic acidosis and calcium phosphate urinary stone formation in women. Int Urol Nephrol 1991;23:307.

Lingeman JE, Siegel YI, Steele B: Metabolic evaluation of infected renal lithiasis: Clinical relevance. J Endourol 1995;9:51.

Ohman S, Larsson L, Tiselius HG: Clinical significance of phosphate in calcium oxalate renal stones. Ann Clin Biochem 1992;29:59.

Schwille PO et al: Urinary phosphate excretion in the pathophysiology of idiopathic recurrent calcium urolithiasis: Hormonal interactions and lipid metabolism. Urol Res 1997;25:417.

Tiselius HG, Larsson L: Calcium phosphate: An important crystal phase in patients with recurrent calcium stone formation? Urol Res 1993;21:175.

Tozuka K et al: Study of calcium phosphate crystalluria. J Urol 1987;138:326.

Uric Acid

Asplin JR: Uric acid stones. Semin Nephrol 1996;16: 412.

Fukushima T et al: Prophylaxis of uric acid stone in patients with inflammatory bowel disease following extensive colonic resection. Gastroenterol Jpn 1991;26: 430.

Gutman AB, Yu TF: Uric acid nephrolithiasis. Am J Med 1968;45:756.

Jarrar K et al: Relationship between 1,25-dihydroxyvitamin-D, calcium and uric acid in urinary stone formers. Urol Int 1996;56:16.

Stoller ML: Gout and stones or stones and gout? J Urol 1995;154:1670.

Teichman JM et al: Holmium:YAG lithotripsy: Pho-
tothermal mechanism converts uric acid calculi to cyanide. J Urol 1998;160:320.

Yu TF: Urolithiasis in hyperuricemia and gout. J Urol 1981;126:424.

Cystine

Chow GK, Streem SB: Contemporary urological intervention for cystinuric patients: Immediate and long-term impact and implications. J Urol 1998;160:341, 344.

Gupta M, Bolton DM, Stoller ML: Etiology and management of cystine lithiasis. Urology 1995;45:344.

Kachel TA, Vijan SR, Dretler SP: Endourological experience with cystine calculi and a treatment algorithm. J Urol 1991;145:25.

Katz G et al: Place of extracorporeal shock-wave lithotripsy (ESWL) in management of cystine calculi. Urology 1990;36:124.

Rutchik SD, Resnick MI: Cystine calculi. Diagnosis and management. Urol Clin North Am 1997;24:163.

Sakhaee K, Poindexter JR, Pak CY: The spectrum of metabolic abnormalities in patients with cystine nephrolithiasis. J Urol 1989;141:819.

Stoller ML et al: Acalculous cystinuria. J Endourol 1997; 11:235.

Xanthine

Badertscher E et al: Xanthine calculi presenting at 1 month of age. Eur J Pediatr 1993;152:252.

Kario K, Matsuo T, Tankawa H: Xanthine urolithiasis: Ultrastructure analysis of renal and bladder calculi. Int Urol Nephrol 1991;23:317.

Maynard J, Benson P: Hereditary xanthinuria in 2 Pakistani sisters: Asymptomatic in one with beta-thalassemia but causing xanthine stone, obstructive uropathy and hypertension in the other. J Urol 1988; 139:338.

Triamterene

Dooley DP, Callsen ME, Geiling JA: Triamterene nephrolithiasis. Milit Med 1989;154:126.

Silicate

Lee MH et al: Silica stone—Development due to long time oral trisilicate intake. Scand J Urol Nephrol 1993; 27:267.

Matrix Urinary Calculi

Binette JP, Binette MB: The matrix of urinary tract stones: Protein composition, antigenicity, and ultrastructure. Scanning Microsc 1991;5:1029.

Iwata H et al: The organic matrix of urinary uric acid crystals. J Urol 1988;139:607.

Morse RM, Resnick MI: Urinary stone matrix. J Urol 1988;139:602.

URINARY STONE INHIBITORS

Citrate

Alvarez Arroyo MV, Traba ML, Rapado A: Hypocitraturia as a pathogenic risk factor in the mixed (calcium oxalate/uric acid) renal stones. Urol Int 1992;48:342.

Alvarez-Arroyo MV et al: Role of citric acid in primary

hyperparathyroidism with renal lithiasis. Urol Res 1992;20:88.

Berg C: Alkaline citrate in prevention of recurrent calcium oxalate stones. Scand J Urol Nephrol [Suppl] 1990;130:1.

Coe FL, Nakagawa Y, Parks JH: Inhibitors within the nephron. Am J Kidney Dis 1991;17:407.

Goldberg H et al: Urine citrate and renal stone disease. Can Med Assoc J 1989;141:217.

Grases F et al: Evolution of lithogenic urinary parameters with a low dose potassium citrate treatment. Int Urol Nephrol 1998;30:1.

Hojgaard I, Tiselius HG: The effects of citrate and urinary macromolecules on the aggregation of hydroxyapatite crystals in solutions with a composition similar to that in the distal tubule. Urol Res 1998;26:89.

Mandel NS, Mandel GS, Hasegawa AT: The effect of some urinary stone inhibitors on membrane interaction potentials of stone crystals. J Urol 1987;138:557.

Pak CY: Citrate and renal calculi: New insights and future directions. Am J Kidney Dis 1991;17:420.

Pak CY: Southwestern Internal Medicine Conference: Medical management of nephrolithiasis—a new, simplified approach for general practice. Am J Med Sci 1997;313:215.

Sakhaee K et al: Alkali absorption and citrate excretion in calcium nephrolithiasis. J Bone Miner Res 1993;8:789.

Seltzer MA et al: Dietary manipulation with lemonade to treat hypocitraturic calcium nephrolithiasis. J Urol 1996;156:907.

Singh RK et al: Circadian periodicity of urinary inhibitor of calcium oxalate crystallization in healthy Indians and renal stone formers. Eur Urol 1993;24:387.

Orthophosphates & Pyrophosphates

Conte A et al: The relation between orthophosphate and pyrophosphate in normal subjects and in patients with urolithiasis. Urol Res 1989;17:173.

Schwille PO et al: Urinary pyrophosphate in patients with recurrent calcium urolithiasis and in healthy controls: A re-evaluation. J Urol 1988;140:239.

Wolf JS, Stoller ML: Inhibition of calculi fragment growth by metal bisphosphonate complexes demonstrated with a new assay measuring the surface activity of urolithiasis inhibitors. J Urol 1994;152:1609.

Urinary Proteins

Baggio B et al: Correction of erythrocyte abnormalities in idiopathic calcium-oxalate nephrolithiasis and reduction of urinary oxalate by oral glycosaminoglycans. Lancet 1991;338:403.

Buck AC, Davies RL, Harrison T: The protective role of eicosapentaenoic acid (EPA) in the pathogenesis of nephrolithiasis. J Urol 1991;146:188.

Edyvane KA et al: Macromolecules inhibit calcium oxalate crystal growth and aggregation in whole human urine. Clin Chim Acta 1987;167:329.

Hesse A, Wuzel H, Vahlensieck W: Significance of glycosaminoglycans for the formation of calcium oxalate stones. Am J Kidney Dis 1991;17:414.

Hwang TI et al: Urinary glycosaminoglycans in normal subjects and patients with stones. J Urol 1988;139:995.

Khan SR: Interactions between stone-forming calcific crystals and macromolecules. Urol Int 1997;59:59.

Siddiqui AA et al: Low molecular weight proteoglycans from renal stones. Biochem Soc Trans 1992;20: 209S.

Singhal GD et al: Urinary mucoprotein in pediatric urolithiasis. J Pediatr Surg 1987;22:218.

Winter P et al: Extracorporeal shock wave lithotripsy and glycosaminoglycans in urine. Int Urol Nephrol 1998;30:113.

Trace Elements

Gentle DL et al: Protease inhibitor-induced urolithiasis. Urology 1997;50:508.

Komleh K et al: Zinc, copper and manganese in serum, urine and stones. Int Urol Nephrol 1990;22:113.

Li LC et al: Inhibitory effect of fluoride on renal stone formation in rats. Urol Int 1992;48:336.

Puche RC et al: Increased fractional excretion of sulphate in stone formers. Br J Urol 1993;71:523.

Rangnekar GV, Gaur MS: Serum and urinary zinc levels in urolithiasis. Br J Urol 1993;71:527.

Su CJ et al: Effect of magnesium on calcium oxalate urolithiasis. J Urol 1991;145:1092.

Wandt MA, Underhill LG: Covariance biplot analysis of trace element concentrations in urinary stones. Br J Urol 1988;61:474.

2,8-DIHYDROXYADENINE UROLITHIASIS

Fye KH et al: Adenine phosphoribosyltransferase deficiency with renal deposition of 2,8-dihydroxyadenine leading to nephrolithiasis and chronic renal failure. Arch Int Med 1993;153:767.

Hesse A et al: 2,8-Dihydroxyadeninuria: Laboratory diagnosis and therapy control. Urol Int 1988;43:174.

Kamatani N et al: Identification of a compound heterozygote for adenine phosphoribosyltransferase deficiency (APRT*J/APART*Q0) leading to 2,8-dihydroxyadenine urolithiasis. Hum Gen 1990;85:500.

Sevcik J, Adam T, Mazacova H: A fast and simple screening method for detection of 2,8-dihydroxyadenine urolithiasis by capillary zone electrophoresis. Clin Chim Acta 1996;245:85.

RENAL TUBULAR ACIDOSIS

Buckalew VM Jr: Nephrolithiasis in renal tubular acidosis. J Urol 1989;141:731.

Caruana RJ, Buckalew VM Jr: The syndrome of distal (type 1) renal tubular acidosis: Clinical and laboratory findings in 58 cases. Medicine 1988;67:84.

Homayoon K: Spontaneous steinstrasse due to renal tubular acidosis. Br J Urol 1996;77:610.

Ito H, Kotake T, Suzuki F: Incidence and clinical features of renal tubular acidosis-1 in urolithiasis. Urol Int 1993;50:82.

Osther PJ et al: Pathophysiology of incomplete renal tubular acidosis in recurrent renal stone formers: Evidence of disturbed calcium, bone and citrate metabolism. Urol Res 1993;21:169.

Schneeberger W, Hesse A, Vahlensieck W: Recurrent nephrolithiasis in renal tubular acidosis: Metabolic profiles, therapy and course. Urol Res 1992;20:98.

Singh PP et al: A study of recurrent stone formers with

special reference to renal tubular acidosis. Urol Res 1995;23:201.

Van Savage JG, Fried FA: Bilateral spontaneous steinstrasse and nephrocalcinosis associated with distal renal tubular acidosis. J Urol 1993;150:467.

URINARY STONE DISEASE IN UNCOMMON SITUATIONS

Spinal Cord Dysfunction

Burr RG, Nuseibeh I: Citrate excretion in spinal cord patients. Paraplegia 1990;28:496.

Hall MK et al: Renal calculi in spinal cord–injured patient: Association with reflux, bladder stones, and Foley catheter drainage. Urology 1989;34:126.

Nath M, Wheeler JS Jr, Walter JS: Urologic aspects of traumatic central cord syndrome. J Am Paraplegia Soc 1993;16(3):160.

Vaidyanathan S et al: Recurrent bilateral renal calculi in a tetraplegic patient. Spinal Cord 1998;36:454.

Wan J et al: Urinary tract status of patients with neurogenic dysfunction presenting with upper tract stone disease. J Urol 1992;148:1126.

Pregnancy

Denstedt JD, Razvi H: Management of urinary calculi during pregnancy. J Urol 1992;148:1072, 1074.

Erturk E, Ptak AM, Monaghan J: Fertility measures in women after extracorporeal shockwave lithotripsy of distal ureteral stones. J Endourol 1997;11:315.

Gorton E, Whitfield HN: Renal calculi in pregnancy. Br J Urol 1997;80:(Suppl 1):4.

Peer A et al: Use of percutaneous nephrostomy in hydronephrosis of pregnancy. Eur J Radiol 1992;15:220.

Shokeir AA, Mutabagani H: Rigid ureteroscopy in pregnant women. Br J Urol 1998;81:678.

Strothers L, Lee LM: Renal colic in pregnancy. J Urol 1992;148:1383.

Wolf MC et al: A new technique for ureteral stent placement during pregnancy using endoluminal ultrasound. Surgery Gynecol Obstet 1992;175:575.

Renal Transplantation

Benoit G et al: Treatment of kidney graft lithiasis. Transplantation Proc 1995;27:1743.

Caldwell TC, Burns JR: Current operative management of urinary calculi after renal transplantation. J Urol 1988;140:1360.

Cho DK et al: Urinary calculi in renal transplant recipients. Transplantation 1988;45:899.

Dumoulin G et al: Lack of increased urinary calcium-oxalate supersaturation in long-term kidney transplant recipients. Kidney Int 1997;51:804.

Hayes JM et al: Renal transplant calculi: A reevaluation of risks and management. Transplantation 1989;47:949.

Makisalo H et al: Urological complications after 2084 consecutive kidney transplantations. Transplantation Proc 1997;29:152.

Obesity

Hofmann R, Stoller ML: Endoscopic and open stone surgery in morbidly obese patients. J Urol 1992;148:1108.

Anatomic Renal Anomalies

Baskin LS, Floth A, Stoller ML: The horseshoe kidney: Therapeutic considerations with urolithiasis. J Endourol 1989;(3):51.

Cussenot O et al: Anatomical bases of percutaneous surgery for calculi in horseshoe kidney. Surg Radiol Anat 1992;14:209.

Locke DR et al: Extracorporeal shock-wave lithotripsy in horseshoe kidneys. Urology 1990;35:407.

Torres VE et al: Renal stone disease in autosomal dominant polycystic kidney disease. Am J Kidney Dis 1993;22:513.

Renal Failure

Daudon M et al: Urolithiasis in patients with end stage renal failure. J Urol 1992;147:977.

Pediatrics

MacDonald I, Azmy AF: Recurrent and residual renal calculi in children. Br J Urol 1988;61:395.

Perrone HC et al: Urolithiasis in childhood: Metabolic evaluation. Pediatr Nephrol 1992;6:54.

Voskaki I et al: The diagnosis of hypercalciuria in children. Br J Urol 1988;61:385.

Caliceal Diverticulae

Ellis JH et al: Stones and infection in renal caliceal diverticula: Treatment with percutaneous procedures. AJR 1991;156:995.

Hedelin H et al: Percutaneous surgery for stones in pyelocaliceal diverticula. Br J Urol 1988;62:206.

Lang EK: Percutaneous infundibuloplasty: Management of calyceal diverticula and infundibular stenosis. Radiology 1991;181:871.

Tumors

Mhiri MN et al: Association between squamous cell carcinoma of the renal pelvis and calculi. Br J Urol 1989;64:201.

MEDICAL THERAPY

Burns JR, Cargill JG III: Kinetics of dissolution of calcium oxalate calculi with calcium-chelating irrigating solutions. J Urol 1987;137:530.

Griffith DP et al: A randomized trial of acetohydroxamic acid for the treatment and prevention of infection-induced urinary stones in spinal cord injury patients. J Urol 1988;140:318.

Hallson PC, Rose GA: Reduction of the urinary risk factors of urolithiasis with magnesium and tartrate mixture: A new treatment. Br J Urol 1988;61:382.

Hymes LC, Warshaw BL: Thiazide diuretics for the treatment of children with idiopathic hypercalciuria and hematuria. J Urol 1987;138:1217.

Insogna KL et al: Trichlormethiazide and oral phosphate therapy in patients with absorptive hypercalciuria. J Urol 1989;141:269.

Mitwalli A et al: Control of hyperoxaluria with large doses of pyridoxine in patients with kidney stones. Int Urol Nephrol 1988;20:353.

Pak CY: Prevention and treatment of kidney stones: Role of medical prevention. J Urol 1989;141:798.

Palmqvist E, Tiselius HG: Phosphate treatment of patients with renal calcium stone disease. Urol Int 1988; 43:24.

Preminger GM: The metabolic evaluation of patients with recurrent nephrolithiasis: A review of comprehensive and simplified approaches. J Urol 1989;141:760.

Stegmayr B et al: Urinary tract calculi dissolved by means of Renacidin: An experimental study. Scand J Urol Nephrol 1990;24:215.

SURGICAL THERAPY

Assimos DG et al: A comparison of anatrophic nephrolithotomy and percutaneous nephrolithotomy with and without extracorporeal shock wave lithotripsy for management of patients with staghorn calculi. J Urol 1991;145:710.

EXTRACORPOREAL SHOCK WAVE LITHOTRIPSY

Cass AS: Do upper ureteral stones need to be manipulated (push back) into the kidneys before extracorporeal shock wave lithotripsy? J Urol 1992;147:349.

Delacretaz G et al: Importance of the implosion of ESWL-induced cavitation bubbles. Ultrasound Med Biol 1995;21:97.

Jenkins AD, Gillenwater JY: Extracorporeal shock wave lithotripsy in the prone position: Treatment of stones in the distal ureter or anomalous kidney. J Urol 1988;139:911.

Michaels EK, Fowler JE Jr: Extracorporeal shock wave lithotripsy for struvite renal calculi: Prospective study with extended followup. J Urol 1991;146:728.

Montgomery BS et al: Does extracorporeal shockwave lithotripsy cause hypertension? Br J Urol 1989;64:567.

Pettersson B, Tiselius HG: Extracorporeal shock wave lithotripsy of proximal and distal ureteral stones. Eur Urol 1988;14:184.

Selli C, Carini M: Treatment of lower ureteral calculi with extracorporeal shock wave lithotripsy. J Urol 1988;140:280.

Shigeta M, Hayashi M, Igawa M: Fever after extracorporeal shock wave lithotripsy for patients with upper urinary tract calculi associated with bacteriuria before treatment. Eur Urol 1995;27:121.

PERCUTANEOUS NEPHROSTOLITHOTOMY

Candela J et al: "Tubeless" percutaneous surgery: A new advance in the technique of percutaneous renal surgery. Tech Urol 1997;3:6.

Knoll LD et al: Long-term followup in patients with cystine urinary calculi treated by percutaneous ultrasonic lithotripsy. J Urol 1988;140:246.

Lam HS et al: Staghorn calculi: Analysis of treatment results between initial percutaneous nephrostolithotomy and extracorporeal shock wave lithotripsy monotherapy with reference to surface area. J Urol 1992;147:1219.

Lingeman JE et al: Comparison of results and morbidity of percutaneous nephrostolithotomy and extracorporeal shock wave lithotripsy. J Urol 1987;138:485.

Meretyk S et al: Complete staghorn calculi: Random prospective comparison between extracorporeal shock wave lithotripsy monotherapy and combined with percutaneous nephrostolithotomy. J Urol 1997;157:780.

Mokulis JA, Peretsman SJ: Retrograde percutaneous nephrolithotomy using the Lawson technique for management of complex nephrolithiasis. J Endourol 1997;11:125.

Streem SB: Long-term incidence and risk factors for recurrent stones following percutaneous nephrostolithotomy or percutaneous nephrostolithotomy/extracorporeal shock wave lithotripsy for infection related calculi. J Urol 1995;153:584.

URETEROSCOPY

Bagley DH: Removal of upper urinary tract calculi with flexible ureteropyeloscopy. Urology 1990;35:412.

Seeger AR, Rittenberg MH, Bagley DH: Ureteropyeloscopic removal of ureteral calculi. J Urol 1988;139:1180.

Stoller ML et al: Ureteroscopy without routine balloon dilatation: An outcome assessment. J Urol 1992;147:1238.

Watson G et al: The pulsed dye laser for fragmenting urinary calculi. J Urol 1987;138:195.

PROSTATIC URETHRAL CALCULI

Kato H, Ogawa A: Large brushite stone in a dilated prostatic urethra. J Urol 1987;138:154.

Extracorporeal Shock Wave Lithotripsy

18

Marshall L. Stoller, MD

Extracorporeal shock wave lithotripsy has revolutionized the treatment of urinary stones. The concept of using shock waves to fragment stones was noted in the 1950s in Russia. However, it was during the investigation of pitting on supersonic aircraft that Dornier, a German aircraft corporation, rediscovered that shock waves originating from passing debris in the atmosphere can crack something that is hard. It was the ingenious application of a model developed in hopes of understanding such shock waves that extracorporeal (outside the body) shock wave lithotripsy (ESWL) emerged. The first clinical application with successful fragmentation of renal calculi was in 1980. The HM-1 (Human Model-1) underwent modifications in 1982 leading to the HM-2 and, finally, to the widespread application of the HM-3 in 1983 (Figure 18–1). It is the acceptance of the HM-3 in Europe, Japan, and the United States (with formal Food and Drug Administration approval in December 1984) that transformed the approach to urinary calculi. Since then, thousands of lithotriptors have been put into use around the world, with millions of patients successfully treated.

Since the development of HM-3, Dornier has made modifications of the reflective semiellipsoid disc and computerized the gantry movements to facilitate stone localization. Many other manufacturers have continued to introduce various machines. All require an energy source to create the shock wave, a coupling mechanism to transfer the energy from outside to inside the body, and either fluoroscopic or ultrasonic modes, or both, to identify and position the calculi at a focus of converging shock waves. They differ in generated pain and anesthetic or anesthesiologist requirements, consumable components, size, mobility, cost, and durability. Focal peak pressures (400–1500 bar), focal dimensions (6 × 28 mm to 50 × 15 mm), modular design, possible biliary applications, utilization to help increase mobility of frozen joints, varied distances (12–17.0 cm) between focus 1 (the shock wave source) and focus 2 (the target), and purchase price differentiate the various machines available today.

Shock Wave Physics

In contrast to the familiar ultrasonic wave with sinusoidal characteristics and longitudinal mechanical properties, acoustic shock waves are unharmonic and have nonlinear pressure characteristics. There is a steep rise in pressure amplitude that results in compressive forces (Figure 18–2). There are two basic types of shock wave sources, supersonic and finite amplitude emitters.

Supersonic emitters release energy in a confined space, thereby producing an expanding plasma and an acoustic shock wave. Such shock waves occur in nature—the familiar thunderstorm with lightning (an electrical discharge) followed by thunder (an acoustic sonic boom) is an analogous situation. Under controlled conditions, such an acoustic shock wave can successfully fragment calculi. The initial compression wave travels faster than the speed of sound in water and rapidly slows down to that speed. The traveling pressure wave is reduced in a nonlinear fashion. The physics of such shock waves has been extensively studied during underwater explosions. Medical applications have focused such waves to concentrate energy on a calculus (Figure 18–3). Optimal focusing uses a slight deviation from the geometric ellipsoid.

Finite amplitude emitters, in contrast to point source energy systems, create pulsed acoustic shock waves by displacing a surface activated by electrical discharge. There are 2 major types of finite amplitude emitters, piezoceramic and electromagnetic. The piezoceramic variety results in a shock wave after an electrical discharge causes the ceramic component to elongate in such a manner that the surface is displaced and an acoustic pulse is generated. Thousands of such components placed on the concave side of a spheric surface directed toward a focus result in high stress, strain, and cavitation pressures (Figure 18–4). Electromagnetic systems are similar in concept to a stereo speaker system. An electrical discharge to a slab, adjacent to an insulating foil, creates an electric current that repulses a metal membrane, displacing it and generating an acoustic pulse into an adjacent

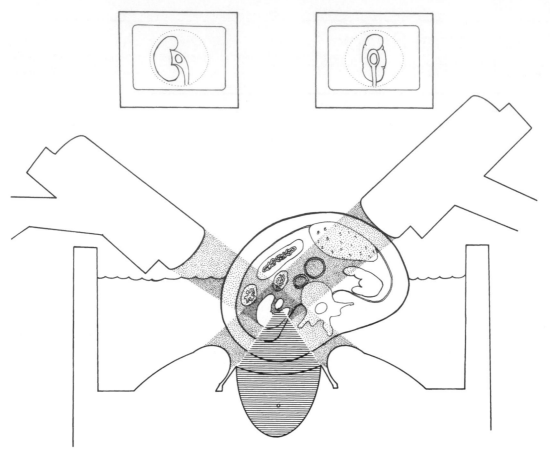

Figure 18–1. Diagrammatic representation of a Dornier HM-3 lithotriptor.

medium. These waves need to be focused toward the offending stone.

All shock waves, despite their source, are capable of fragmenting stones when focused. Fragmentation is achieved by erosion and shattering (Figure 18–5). Cavitational forces result in erosion at the entry and exit sites of the shock wave. Shattering results from energy absorption with stress, strain, and shear forces. Surrounding biologic tissues are resilient because they are not brittle nor are the shock waves focused on them.

PREOPERATIVE EVALUATION

A careful history and physical examination should be followed by an evaluation of stone size, number, and location. Renal anatomy must be known to formulate realistic therapeutic goals. An intravenous urogram, a plain abdominal radiograph (KUB) combined with reliable renal ultrasonography, or spiral computed tomography (CT) imaging with or without con-

trast helps to identify calculi, delineate upper tract anatomy including degree of dilation, and rule out distal obstruction. Without previous stone analysis, preoperative stone composition cannot be definitively known. Such knowledge is invaluable as stones have great variability in the ease with which they fragment. Stones with a ground-glass appearance with smooth edges, combined with an acidic urinary pH, are suggestive of cystine composition. Cystine and calcium oxalate monohydrate stones are hard and recalcitrant to fragmentation. In contrast, calcium oxalate dihydrate usually has a spiculated appearance on radiographs and frequently fragments well.

Therapeutic options should be addressed with all patients. Percutaneous access and extraction with or without subsequent ESWL is the most efficient way to render a patient with a stone burden greater than 2.5–3.0 cm stone-free. Alternatively, such large stones may be treated with repeated shock wave sessions, or monotherapy. Dilated collecting systems are less efficient at discharging such large amounts of gravel. Additionally, monosurgery may not render the patient

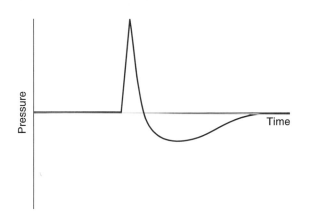

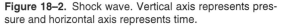

Figure 18–2. Shock wave. Vertical axis represents pressure and horizontal axis represents time.

stone-free. A very lucent central core surrounded by calcification with poor fragmentation after previous lithotripsy suggests a matrix composition (Figure 18–6). Matrix stones are soft, like a gelatinous plug, and usually do not crack with ESWL (Figure 18–7). Percutaneous extraction, rather than repeated shock wave sessions, is the treatment of choice in such a situation. Painful calculi in a caliceal diverticulum with a narrow-necked infundibulum may not pass after adequate fragmentation. To render the patient stone-free, percutaneous extraction or retrograde dilation of the infundibulum with stone extraction may be required.

Imaging studies should be performed close to the anticipated treatment time because calculi do not remain stationary. Not all patients with urinary calculi require immediate therapy. Asymptomatic patients may be followed. Chemolysis of uric acid stones in an asymptomatic, motivated patient is a reasonable option.

Physical examination should be as thorough as in preparation for any other surgical procedure. Vital signs including blood pressure should be noted. Body habitus including any gross skeletal abnormalities, contractures, or excessive weight (> 300 lb) may severely limit or preclude ESWL. Borderline individuals require simulation before treatment. Pregnant women and patients with large abdominal aortic aneurysms or uncorrectable bleeding disorders should not be treated with ESWL. Individuals with cardiac pacemakers should be thoroughly evaluated by a cardiologist. If ESWL is contemplated, a cardiologist with thorough knowledge and with the ability to override the pacemaker should be present in the lithotripsy suite.

Laboratory evaluation should include blood urea nitrogen, creatinine, a complete blood count, and uri-

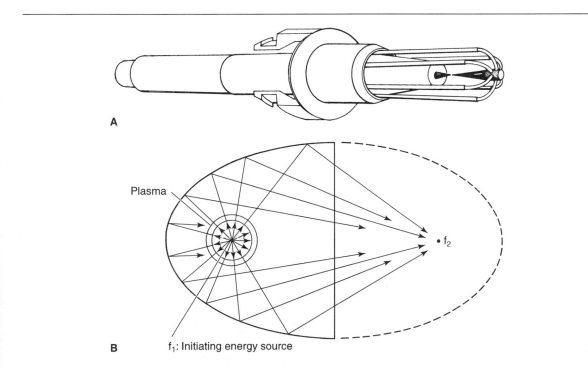

Figure 18–3. A: Supersonic shock wave emission from a spark gap electrode. **B:** Reflecting the shock wave from focus 1 to focus 2 allows for stone fragmentation.

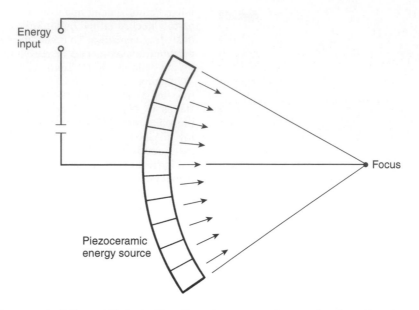

Figure 18–4. Piezoceramic finite amplitude emitter. Ceramic components are placed on the concave surface of a sphere and each component is directed to an identified focus.

nalysis with culture and sensitivities. Elderly patients should have a baseline electrocardiogram. Complete informed consent should be obtained.

INTRAOPERATIVE CONSIDERATIONS

After a thorough review of recent radiographs, offending calculi should be identified. Distal calculi need to be addressed first to eliminate potential obstructive problems. Ureteral calculi can be treated in situ or after pushback procedures to place the stone in a more capacious chamber to potentially increase the efficiency of fragmentation. Pushback procedures may be unsuccessful owing to long-standing impaction with associated tortuosity, kinking, or both, and should be performed under fluoroscopic imaging. Most ureteral stones are now treated with in situ

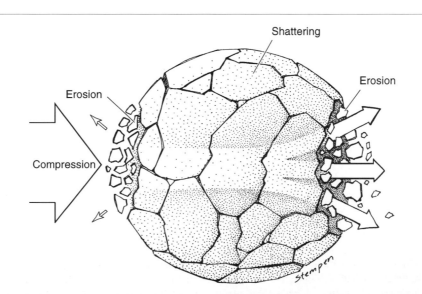

Figure 18–5. Incoming shock waves result in fragmentation from erosion and shattering.

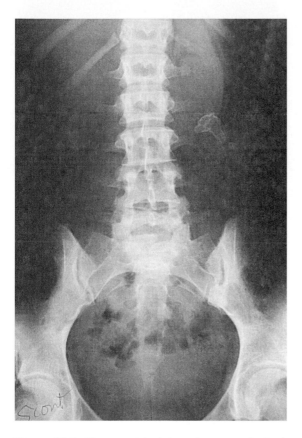

Figure 18–6. Stone resistant to extracorporeal shock wave lithotripsy. Note left renal calculus with a lucent center and an opaque rim.

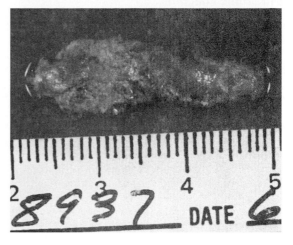

Figure 18–7. Matrix stone resistant to extracorporeal shock wave lithotripsy and subsequently percutaneously extracted.

Small or poorly calcified calculi can be difficult to image with fluoroscopy, irrespective of their location. Placing a ureteral catheter identifies known anatomy and supplies an injection port for radiocontrast agents. A poorly calcified caliceal calculus can be identified by injection of dilute contrast agents into the collecting system and then focusing on the appropriate calyx or filling defect. Retrograde catheters can be difficult to place in patients with tubularized urinary diversions. In patients who cannot have retrograde stents placed, intravenous contrast agents may be used to help localize and thus focus on such stones.

Fluoroscopic Imaging

The conditions for fluoroscopic imaging include appropriate collimation, dimmed room lighting, and adequate bowel preparation to decrease bothersome bowel gas and thus decrease radiation exposure and improve the quality of the fluoroscopic image. Intermittent fluoroscopy reveals movement of calculi with respiration and is helpful in locating and focusing on offending calculi. After the stone is roughly in focus, image intensifiers should be brought as close to the x-ray source as possible. In water bath units, balloons should be adjusted to decrease the amount of water through which x-ray beams must travel. Such balloons should not push the patient because when the balloons are deflated during treatment, the patient will "fall out of focus." "Quick-pics" improve resolution and are helpful in determining stone geometry before treatment and adequate fragmentation after treatment. However, every "quick-pic" is equivalent to approximately 30 s of fluoroscopy time.

ESWL or ureteroscopic stone extraction; pushback procedures are much less popular.

Stone Localization

Proper patient positioning is a prerequisite for successful lithotripsy. Palpating the patient's ribs and pelvic bony girdle can approximate appropriate positioning. When fluoroscopic imaging with the standard Dornier HM-3 is used, patients with medially located stones or ureteral calculi need to be rotated with the stone side down to help visualize them away from overlying midline bony structures. Lower ureteral stones require a prone or a sitting position to direct the shock waves accurately. Females of childbearing potential should not be treated in this fashion because short- and long-term consequences to ovarian function remain unknown. Anterior located kidneys, medial oriented portions of a horseshoe kidney, or transplant kidneys are best treated in the prone position. Understanding positioning options with the various lithotriptors available today is required to optimize therapy.

Ultrasonic Imaging

Ultrasound localization has the advantage of eliminating radiation exposure to the patient or lithotripsy team. There are 2 basic types: the coaxial unit, aligned with the shock wave generator, and the articulating arm unit with a mobile transducer. Ultrasound can easily identify radiolucent or small calculi that are difficult to visualize with fluoroscopy. However, ureteral or other medially located calculi may be difficult or impossible to identify, especially in nonobstructive collecting systems. Visualization may be difficult or impossible with obese patients. Proficiency in ultrasound localization and assessment of fragmentation has a longer learning curve than that of fluoroscopy. Ultrasound images may be confusing when multiple stones or stone fragments are present.

Coupling

Successful fragmentation requires effective coupling. Coupling devices should have properties similar to those of human skin. Optimal systems should prevent pain, ecchymoses, hematomas, or skin breakdown. Interfaces between gas and tissue can result in tissue damage. Air bubbles entrapped by hair, by bandages from prior percutaneous procedures, or by inadequately degassed fluid, or air in coupling cushions can significantly impede directed shock waves and result in skin ecchymoses or breakdown. If shock waves traverse through lung tissue, catastrophic consequences can occur. Despite adequate coupling, fragmentation may be inadequate owing to refraction and reflection of shock waves at tissue interfaces, especially with obese patients.

The water bath provides good coupling. Submersion of patients can result in profound hemodynamic changes including peripheral venous compression resulting in increased right atrial pressure, increased pulmonary capillary wedge pressure, and increased cardiac index. These hemodynamic changes should be appreciated and appropriate monitoring should be used in individuals with marginal cardiovascular reserve. Electrical hazards must be considered. Safe practice with respect to possible transfer of body fluids requires that water be evacuated and the tub cleansed between treatments. This can be time consuming. In areas where water conservation is necessary owing to drought conditions, this may be a drain on a precious resource.

In contrast, water cushion coupling systems have decreased water demands. A coupling gel like those used with ultrasonography provides an excellent interface with skin. The volume of such water cushions can frequently be adjusted to help focus calculi when patients are either extremely thin (eg, children) or obese. Very small patients may require an interposed bag (1–3 L) of normal saline to help with coupling. Both water coupling systems require degassed water to decrease water bubbles.

Shock Wave Triggering

Triggering shock waves with the electrocardiogram was originally performed to decrease cardiac dysrhythmias. The lithotriptor would sense the large swing of the QRS complex and initiate the shock wave 20 ms later; this would decrease shock waves during the repolarization phase of the cardiac cycle (myocardium is most sensitive during this time). If cardiac dysrhythmias occur, interruption of the procedure frequently stops them. However, if they continue, standard medical therapy is effective. Conceptually, it makes more sense to trigger the shock waves in response to the respiratory cycle to optimize accurate focusing on the offending calculi that move with respiratory motion. Such systems are available. Many lithotriptors are now triggered without electrocardiogram gating and with unusual associated cardiac dysrhythmias. This can speed up therapy, especially in those with slow heart rates that are not amenable to pharmacologic manipulation.

Pain

Anesthetic requirements were initially unknown. Early procedures were performed under general endotracheal or epidural anesthesia. High-frequency jet ventilation was tried to decrease stone movement by limiting diaphragm motion. It is now recognized that even the unmodified HM-3 can be successfully used with intravenous analgesia and sedation, even during periprocedure endoscopic manipulations. Newer machines have reduced or eliminated requirements for medications. Pain is subjective, and initial shock waves should be delivered after patients are informed as to what to expect. This eliminates the surprise factor, increases patient cooperation, and decreases the likelihood of patient movement. Without a formal anesthetic, initial shock waves should be delivered at a low kilovoltage and gradually increased.

Fragmentation

Safe shock wave dosage is unknown. In practice, manufacturer recommendations are frequently exceeded. Shock waves induce trauma, including intrarenal and perirenal hemorrhage and edema, and thus the minimal shocks needed to achieve fragmentation should be given. Long sessions of shock wave therapy may not be efficient because surrounding fragments may impede incoming shock waves from effectively fragmenting remaining large particles. Casual overtreatment should be avoided since long-term complications are not yet known.

Solitary stones are approached by focusing on the segment of the stone closest to the ureteropelvic junction. Low kilovolt settings decrease the likelihood of the stone caroming into a different part of the collecting system and requiring refocusing. When multiple stones in a kidney are treated, a strategy must be formulated. Renal pelvic stones or centrally located stones must be fragmented first to eliminate potentially obstructing fragments. Those in a more peripheral location can be treated next. Adequate fragmentation must be achieved prior to moving to the next stone.

Large stone burdens or infected stones are best treated after placement of double-J ureteral catheters. Such catheters may not ease the passage of fragments; rather they increase the likelihood of adequate drainage. This is especially advantageous when treated patients live great distances away from the treatment center. Additionally, double-J catheters keep large fragments from entering into the ureter.

Determination of adequate fragmentation during treatment may be difficult. Initial sharp edges become fuzzy or blurred and have a shotgun-blast-like appearance. Stones that were initially visualized may disappear after successful fragmentation. Intermittent visualization ensures accurate focusing and assessment of progress and eventual termination of the procedure. Numerous caliceal stones should be approached from the bottom up. Inferior caliceal stones should be fragmented before treatment of middle and superior caliceal stones because fragments from middle and superior caliceal stones may migrate to the inferior calyx. Such fragments may surround and impede incoming shock waves from effectively fragmenting the inferior caliceal stone.

Bilateral nephrolithiasis may be treated in the same setting. One must first approach the side that is symptomatic or potentially more troublesome. If there is uncertainty concerning a large stone burden, one or more double-J catheters should be placed to decrease the likelihood of bilateral obstruction.

POSTOPERATIVE CARE

The ultimate goal of ESWL is stone fragmentation and eventual elimination, resulting in a stone-free patient. Preoperative education of the patient and possibly the referring physician with respect to realistic expectations helps facilitate a smooth postoperative course. During outpatient treatment, the patient should be monitored postoperatively until the treating physician is convinced that the patient is hemodynamically stable and ready for discharge. Examination should reveal a benign abdomen and an occasional ecchymosis at the entry site of the shock waves. Gross hematuria is the rule. Ureteral catheters placed to help localize calculi or as a contrast injection port and Foley catheters should be removed, and the patient should void before discharge.

Upon discharge, patients should be instructed to contact a specified physician who is part of the lithotripsy team for persistent nausea or vomiting, fever, or pain uncontrolled by routine oral pain medications. Such symptoms are suggestive of urinary obstruction. Infected urine with an obstructing fragment may lead to sepsis. ESWL has no impact on the microbiologic flora of infected calculi. Patients should strain their urine for stone fragments for future stone analysis. Patients who form stones recurrently should consider metabolic evaluation after calculi have passed.

Patients should be encouraged to maintain an active ambulatory status to facilitate stone passage. Gross hematuria should resolve during the first postoperative week. Fluid intake should be encouraged. Follow-up in approximately 2 weeks for discussion and evaluation of a KUB and renal ultrasonography will help assess success of fragmentation and passage of gravel. Patients may return to work as soon as they feel comfortable in doing so.

Abdominal pain may be related to the shock waves. Severe pain unresponsive to routine intravenous or oral medications should alert the physician for possible rare (0.66%) perirenal hematomas. In such a situation a KUB may disclose evidence of hemorrhage including loss of psoas shadow or renal outline. As in the management of other blunt renal trauma, CT should then be undertaken to stage the injury. Uncontrolled hemorrhage noted by tachycardia and hypotension may on rare occasions necessitate open surgical exploration. Pancreatitis is a rare complication but should be considered, especially in left-side stones.

Nerve palsies have been reported and are usually related to improper, poorly padded positioning. Positioning and transfer of patients onto and off gantries can result in falls and fractures.

The potential association of ESWL with the development of hypertension has not been substantiated. Long-term data are still being collected.

Patients with double-J ureteral catheters should be informed that such foreign bodies were placed and eventually need to be removed, usually after the 2-week evaluation. If the majority of gravel has passed, the double-J catheter may be removed at this time. If significant gravel persists, the double-J catheter should be left in place to help ensure drainage; serial KUBs should be obtained every 2–4 weeks.

Stone burden correlates with postoperative complications. Steinstrasse (stone street) or columnation of stone gravel in a ureter can be frustrating. It should be specifically ruled out when postoperative radiographs are evaluated. Asymptomatic individuals can be followed up with serial KUBs and ultrasonography. Severe pain or fever requires intervention. Percutaneous nephrostomy drainage is usually uncomplicated owing to the associated hydronephrosis. Decompressing the collecting system allows for effective coaptation of the ureteral walls and encourages resolution of the problem. It is only in the rare patient that steinstrasse does not resolve with the procedures outlined; such cases require retrograde endoscopic manipulations to relieve the obstructed stone fragments. Usually one finds one or two relatively large fragments that are obstructing. With their removal the columnation of fragments resolves.

One of the most frustrating complications is inadequate fragmentation or passage of the offending calculi. Success is related to stone burden, location, and composition. Stone-free rates are usually evaluated 3 months postoperatively and require the use of imaging techniques. Routine assessment involves an abdominal KUB and renal ultrasonography. Careful inspection along the course of the ureter, including over the sacroiliac joint, and at the ureterovesical junction should be undertaken. Questionable distal ureteral fragments can be differentiated from phleboliths via suprapubic ultrasonography (using a full bladder as an acoustic window). A final KUB and renal ultrasound or an intravenous urogram to rule out silent hydronephrosis may be scheduled a few months hence.

Large renal pelvic calculi (> 1.5 cm) have a stone-free rate at 3 months approximating 75%, in comparison with that of a similar stone in a lower calyx, which approximates only 50%. Patients with small renal pelvic stones (< 1.5 cm) have approximately a 90% stone-free rate in comparison to similar stones in a middle calyx (approximately 75%) or lower calyx (approximately 70%). Lower calyceal stone-free rates are increased with small stone burdens, short and wide infundibulum, and a nonacute infundibulo-pelvic angle. Overall, approximately 75% of patients with renal calculi treated with ESWL become stone-free in 3 months. As stones increase in size, stone-free rates decrease, more so in the lower and middle calyces than in superior calyceal and renal pelvic locations.

REFERENCES

Barcena M et al: EMLA cream for renal extracorporeal shock wave lithotripsy in ambulatory patients. Eur J Anaesthesiol 1996;13:373.

Baskin LS, Floth A, Stoller ML: Monitored anesthesia care with the standard Dornier HM3 lithotriptor. J Endourol 1990;4:49.

Bush WH, Brannen GE: Extracorporeal shock wave lithotripsy (ESWL) of pelvic kidney calculus. Urology 1987;29:357.

Chaussy CG (editor): *Extracorporeal Shock Wave Lithotripsy: Technical Concept, Experimental Research, and Clinical Application.* Karger, 1986.

Chaussy CG et al: Extracorporeal shock wave lithotripsy (ESWL) for treatment of urolithiasis. Urology 1984; 23:59.

Chaussy CG et al: First clinical experience with extracorporeally induced destruction of kidney stones by shock waves. J Urol 1982;127:417.

Coleman AJ, Choi MJ, Saunders JE: Detection of acoustic emission from cavitation in tissue during clinical extracorporeal lithotripsy. Ultrasound Med Biol 1996;22:1079.

Drach GW et al: Report of the United States cooperative study of extracorporeal shock wave lithotripsy. J Urol 1986;135:1127.

Dretler SP: Stone fragility: A new therapeutic distinction. In: Lingeman JE, Newman DM (editors): *Shock Wave Lithotripsy: State of the Art.* Plenum Press, 1988.

Elbahnasy AM et al: Lower caliceal stone clearance after shock wave lithotripsy or ureteroscopy: The impact of lower pole radiographic anatomy. J Urol 1998;159:676.

Gleeson MJ, Shabsigh R, Griffith DP: Outcome of extracorporeal shock wave lithotripsy in patients with multiple renal calculi based on stone burden and location. J Endourol 1988;2:145.

Grenabo L et al: Stone fragmentation pattern of piezo-electric shockwave lithotripsy in vitro. J Endourol 1998;12:247.

Heine G: Physical aspects of shock-wave treatment. In:

Gravenstein JS, Peter K (editors): *Extracorporeal Shock Wave Lithotripsy for Renal Stone Disease.* Butterworths, 1986.

Hepp W: *Survey of the Development of Shock Wave Lithotripsy.* Dornier Medizintechnik GmbH, 1984.

Hunter PT et al: Geometry of and pressures with ESWL. In: Gravenstein JS, Peter K (editors): *Extracorporeal Shock Wave Lithotripsy for Renal Stone Disease.* Butterworths, 1986.

Jewett MA et al: A randomized controlled trial to assess the incidence of new onset hypertension in patients after shock wave lithotripsy for asymptomatic renal calculi. J Urol 1998;160:1241.

Kahnoski RJ et al: Combined percutaneous and extracorporeal shock wave lithotripsy for staghorn calculi: An alternative to anatrophic nephrolithotomy. J Urol 1986;135:679.

Kamihira O et al: Long-term stone recurrence rate after extracorporeal shock wave lithotripsy. J Urol 1996; 156:1267.

Kaude JV et al: Renal morphology and function immediately after extracorporeal shock wave lithotripsy. AJR 1985;145:305.

Knapp PM et al: Extracorporeal shock wave lithotripsy induced perirenal hematomas. J Urol 1988;139:700.

Kramolowsky EV, Willoughby BL, Loening SA: Extracorporeal shock wave lithotripsy in children. J Urol 1987;137:939.

Lingeman JE, Woods JR, Toth PD: Blood pressure changes following extracorporeal shock wave lithotripsy and other forms of treatment for nephrolithiasis. JAMA 1990;263:1789.

Lingeman JE et al: Comparison of results and morbidity of percutaneous nephrolithotomy and extracorporeal shock wave lithotripsy. J Urol 1987;138:485.

Lingeman JE et al: Management of upper ureteral calculi with extracorporeal shock wave lithotripsy. J Urol 1987;138:720.

Lingeman JE et al: Shock wave lithotripsy with the Dornier MFL 5000 lithotriptor using an external fixed rate signal. J Urol 1995;154:951.

Low RL et al: Outcome assessment of double-J stents during extracorporeal shock wave lithotripsy of small, solitary renal calculi. J Endourol 1996;10:341.

Meretyk S et al: Complete staghorn calculi: Random prospective comparison between extracorporeal shock wave lithotripsy monotherapy and combined with percutaneous nephrostolithotomy. J Urol 1997;157:780.

Nakada SY et al: Extracorporeal shock-wave lithotripsy of middle ureteral stones: Are ureteral stents necessary? Urology 1995;46:649.

Newman DM et al: Extracorporeal shock wave lithotripsy experience in children. J Urol 1986;136:238.

Politis G, Griffith DP: ESWL: Stone-free efficacy based on stone size and location. World J Urol 1987;5:255.

Psihramis KE, Dretler SP: Extracorporeal shock wave lithotripsy of calyceal diverticula calculi. J Urol 1987;138:707.

Reichenberger H: Lithotriptor systems. IEEE Proc 1988; 76(9):1236.

Remer EM et al: Spiral noncontrast CT versus combined plain radiography and renal US after extracorporeal shock wave lithotripsy: Cost-identification analysis. Radiology 1997;204:33.

Rubin JI et al: Kidney changes after extracorporeal shock wave lithotripsy: CT evaluation. Radiology 1987;162: 21.

Sen S et al: Effect of extracorporeal shock wave lithotripsy on glomerular and tubular functions. Int Urol Nephrol 1996;28:309.

Smith LH et al: National High Blood Pressure Education Program (NHBPEP) review paper on complications of shock wave lithotripsy for urinary calculi. Am J Med 1991;91:635.

Stoller ML, Litt L, Salazar RG: Severe hemorrhage after extracorporeal shock-wave lithotripsy. Ann Intern Med 1989;111:612.

Stoller ML et al: Extracorporeal shock wave lithotripsy performed on woman with a cardiac pacemaker. J Urol 1988;140:1510.

Streem SB, Yost A, Mascha E: Clinical implications of clinically insignificant stone fragments after extracorporeal shock wave lithotripsy. J Urol 1996;155:1186.

Winfield HN, Clayman RV, Chaussy CG: Monotherapy of staghorn renal calculi: Comparative study between percutaneous nephrolithotomy and extracorporeal shock wave lithotripsy. J Urol 1988;139:895.

19 Injuries to the Genitourinary Tract

Jack W. McAninch, MD

EMERGENCY DIAGNOSIS & MANAGEMENT

About 10% of all injuries seen in the emergency room involve the genitourinary system to some extent. Many of them are subtle and difficult to define and require great diagnostic expertise. Early diagnosis is essential to prevent serious complications.

Initial assessment should include control of hemorrhage and shock along with resuscitation as required. Resuscitation may require intravenous lines and a urethral catheter in seriously injured patients. In men, before the catheter is inserted, the urethral meatus should be examined carefully for the presence of blood. Once the intravenous lines are established, if any suspicion of renal or ureteral injury is entertained, contrast material should be injected intravenously for later x-ray study.

The history should include a detailed description of the accident. In cases involving gunshot wounds, the type and caliber of the weapon should be determined, since high-velocity projectiles cause much more extensive damage.

The abdomen and genitalia should be examined for evidence of contusions or subcutaneous hematomas, which might indicate deeper injuries to the retroperitoneum and pelvic structures. Fractures of the lower ribs are often associated with renal injuries, and pelvic fractures often accompany bladder and urethral injuries. Diffuse abdominal tenderness is consistent with perforated bowel, free intraperitoneal blood or urine, or retroperitoneal hematoma. As an aid to diagnosis of intraperitoneal injuries, a small catheter inserted percutaneously into the abdomen followed by irrigation will help detect free intraperitoneal blood.

Initial radiographic studies should be done in the trauma unit, if possible, before the patient is moved. Plain films of the abdomen disclose early excretion of contrast material injected at the time intravenous lines were inserted. Lower rib fractures, vertebral body and transverse process fractures, and pelvic fractures may be associated with severe urinary tract injuries. Early extravasation of contrast material may be noted with renal, ureteral, or bladder injuries.

Patients who do not have life-threatening injuries and whose blood pressure is stable can undergo more deliberate radiographic studies. This provides more definitive staging of the injury.

Special Examinations (Figures 19–1 through 19–3)

When genitourinary tract injury is suspected on the basis of the history and physical examination, additional studies are required to establish its extent.

A. Catheterization and Assessment of Injury: Assessment of the injury should be done in an orderly fashion so that accurate and complete information is obtained. This process of defining the extent of injury is termed **staging.** The algorithms (Figures 19–1 through 19–3) outline the staging process for urogenital trauma.

1. Catheterization–Blood at the urethral meatus in men indicates urethral injury; catheterization should not be attempted if blood is present, but retrograde urethrography should be done immediately. If no blood is present at the meatus, a urethral catheter can be carefully passed to the bladder to recover urine; microscopic or gross hematuria indicates urinary system injury. If catheterization is traumatic despite the greatest care, the significance of hematuria cannot be determined, and other studies must be done to investigate the possibility of urinary system injury.

2. Excretory urography–Immediately after intravenous lines have been established and the resuscitation process has begun, 150 mL (2 mL/kg) of contrast material can be injected intravenously by the push technique. As hypotension is overcome and renal perfusion improves, plain abdominal films permit adequate visualization of the kidneys. This technique allows evaluation of renal injuries without undue delay before emergency operations, if indicated. If renal injury seems likely from the urogram, nephrotomography should be done immediately. In most cases, it is not necessary to inject more contrast medium, since adequate contrast medium remains, and tomography gives additional information regarding parenchymal injuries.

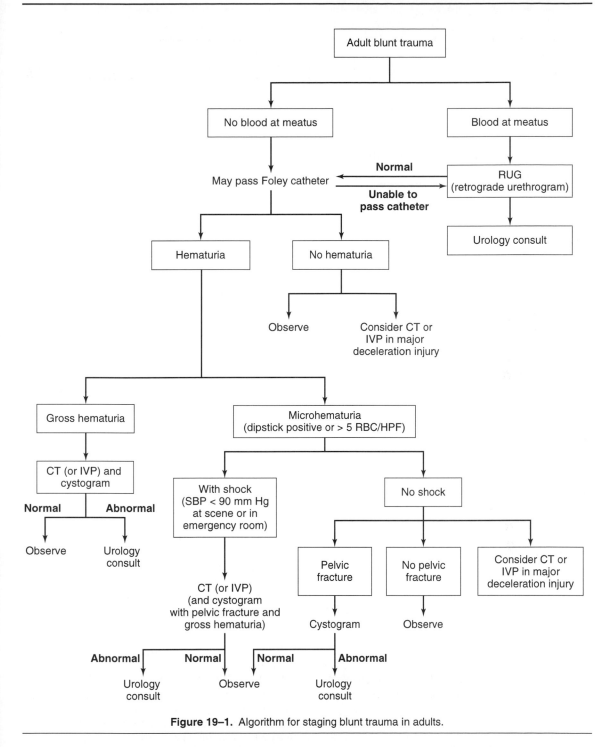

Figure 19–1. Algorithm for staging blunt trauma in adults.

3. Retrograde cystography–Filling of the bladder with contrast material is essential to establish whether bladder perforations exist. At least 300 mL of contrast medium should be instilled for full vesical distention. A film should be obtained with the bladder filled and a second one after the bladder has emptied itself by gravity drainage. These 2 films establish the degree of bladder injury as well as the size of the surrounding pelvic hematomas.

4. Urethrography–A small (12F) catheter can be inserted into the urethral meatus and 3 mL of water placed in the balloon to hold the catheter in posi-

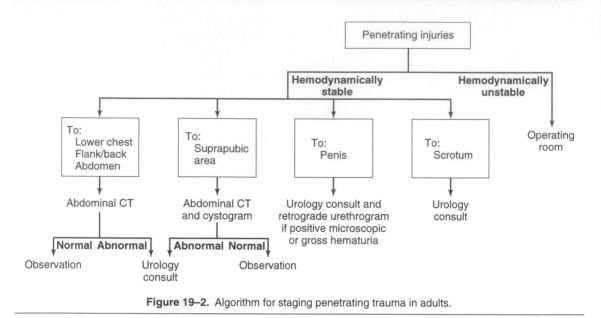

Figure 19–2. Algorithm for staging penetrating trauma in adults.

tion. After retrograde injection of 20 mL of water-soluble contrast material, the urethra will be clearly outlined on film, and extravasation in the deep bulbar area in case of straddle injury—or free extravasation into the retropubic space in case of prostatomembranous disruption—will be visualized.

5. Arteriography–Arteriography may help define renal parenchymal and renal vascular injuries. It is also useful in the detection of persistent bleeding from pelvic fractures for purposes of embolization with Gelfoam or autologous clot.

6. Computed tomography (CT)–CT scans can help in assessing the size and extent of retroperitoneal hematomas and renal parenchymal trauma. CT is a noninvasive test that gives accurate and fast information. Currently, CT is the definitive study for staging renal injuries.

B. Cystoscopy and Retrograde Urography: Cystoscopy and retrograde urography are seldom necessary, since information can be obtained by less invasive techniques.

C. Abdominal Sonography: Abdominal sonography has not been shown to add substantial information during initial evaluation of severe abdominal trauma.

INJURIES TO THE KIDNEY

Renal injuries are the most common injuries of the urinary system. The kidney is well protected by heavy lumbar muscles, vertebral bodies, ribs, and the viscera anteriorly. Fractured ribs and transverse vertebral processes may penetrate the renal parenchyma or vasculature. Most injuries occur from automobile accidents or sporting mishaps, chiefly in men and boys. Kidneys with existing pathologic conditions such as hydronephrosis or malignant tumors are more readily ruptured from mild trauma.

Etiology
(Figure 19–4)

Blunt trauma directly to the abdomen, flank, or back is the most common mechanism, accounting for 80–85% of all renal injuries. Trauma may result from motor vehicle accidents, fights, falls, and contact sports. Vehicle collisions at high speed may result in major renal trauma from rapid deceleration and cause major vascular injury. Gunshot and knife wounds cause most penetrating injuries to the kidney; any such wound in the flank area should be regarded as a cause of renal injury until proved otherwise. Associated abdominal visceral injuries are present in 80% of renal penetrating wounds.

Pathology & Classification
(Figure 19–5)

A. Early Pathologic Findings: Lacerations from blunt trauma usually occur in the transverse plane of the kidney. The mechanism of injury is thought to be force transmitted from the center of the impact to the renal parenchyma. In injuries from rapid deceleration, the kidney moves upward or downward, causing sudden stretch on the renal pedicle and sometimes complete or partial avulsion. Acute thrombosis of the renal artery may be caused by an intimal tear from rapid deceleration injuries owing to the sudden stretch.

Pathologic classification of renal injuries is as follows (Moore et al, 1989):

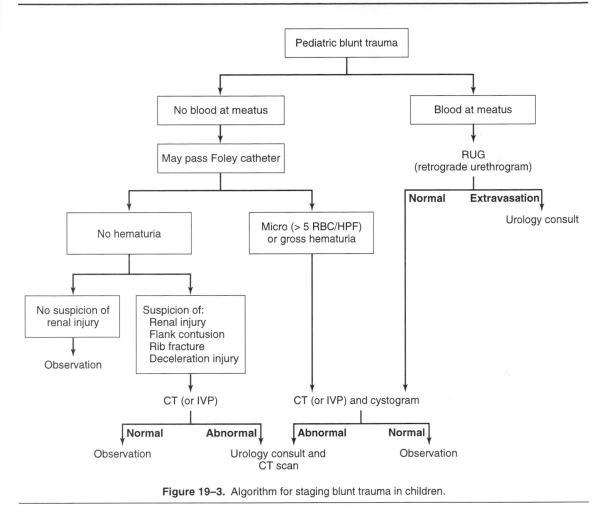

Figure 19–3. Algorithm for staging blunt trauma in children.

1. Minor renal trauma (85% of cases)–Renal contusion or bruising of the parenchyma is the most common lesion. Subcapsular hematoma in association with contusion is also noted. Superficial cortical lacerations are also considered minor trauma. These injuries rarely require surgical exploration.

2. Major renal trauma (15% of cases)–Deep corticomedullary lacerations may extend into the collecting system, resulting in extravasation of urine into the perirenal space. Large retroperitoneal and perinephric hematomas often accompany these deep lacerations. Multiple lacerations may cause complete destruction of the kidney. Laceration of the renal pelvis without parenchymal laceration from blunt trauma is rare.

3. Vascular injury (about 1% of all blunt trauma cases)–Vascular injury of the renal pedicle is rare but may occur, usually from blunt trauma. There may be total avulsion of the artery and vein or partial avulsion of the segmental branches of these vessels. Stretch on the main renal artery without avulsion may result in renal artery thrombosis. Vas-

cular injuries are difficult to diagnose and result in total destruction of the kidney unless the diagnosis is made promptly.

B. Late Pathologic Findings (Figure 19–6):

1. Urinoma–Deep lacerations that are not repaired may result in persistent urinary extravasation and late complications of a large perinephric renal mass and, eventually, hydronephrosis and abscess formation.

2. Hydronephrosis–Large hematomas in the retroperitoneum and associated urinary extravasation may result in perinephric fibrosis engulfing the ureteropelvic junction, causing hydronephrosis. Follow-up excretory urography is indicated in all cases of major renal trauma.

3. Arteriovenous fistula–Arteriovenous fistulas may occur after penetrating injuries but are not common.

4. Renal vascular hypertension–The blood flow in tissue rendered nonviable by injury is compromised; this results in renal vascular hypertension in about 1% of cases. Fibrosis from surrounding

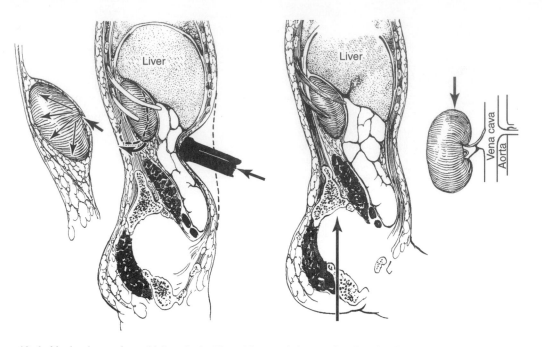

Figure 19–4. Mechanisms of renal injury. **Left:** Direct blow to abdomen. Smaller drawing shows force of blow radiating from the renal hilum. **Right:** Falling on buttocks from a height (contrecoup of kidney). Smaller drawing shows direction of force exerted on the kidney from above. Tear of renal pedicle.

trauma has also been reported to constrict the renal artery and cause renal hypertension.

Clinical Findings & Indications for Studies

Microscopic or gross hematuria following trauma to the abdomen indicates injury to the urinary tract. It bears repeating that stab or gunshot wounds to the flank area should alert the physician to possible renal injury whether or not hematuria is present. Some cases of renal vascular injury are not associated with hematuria. These cases are almost always due to rapid deceleration accidents and are an indication for intravenous urography.

The degree of renal injury does not correspond to the degree of hematuria, since gross hematuria may occur in minor renal trauma and only mild hematuria in major trauma. However, not all adult patients sustaining blunt trauma require full imaging evaluation of the kidney (Figure 19–1). Miller and McAninch (1995) made the following recommendations based on findings in over 1800 blunt renal trauma injuries: Patients with gross hematuria or microscopic hematuria with shock (systolic blood pressure < 90 mm Hg) should undergo radiographic assessment; patients with microscopic hematuria without shock need not. However, should physical examination or associated injuries prompt reasonable suspicion of a

renal injury, renal imaging should be undertaken. This is especially true of patients with rapid deceleration trauma, who may have renal injury without the presence of hematuria.

A. Symptoms: There is usually visible evidence of abdominal trauma. Pain may be localized to one flank area or over the abdomen. Associated injuries such as ruptured abdominal viscera or multiple pelvic fractures also cause acute abdominal pain and may obscure the presence of renal injury. Catheterization usually reveals hematuria. Retroperitoneal bleeding may cause abdominal distention, ileus, and nausea and vomiting.

B. Signs: Initially, shock or signs of a large loss of blood from heavy retroperitoneal bleeding may be noted. Ecchymosis in the flank or upper quadrants of the abdomen is often noted. Lower rib fractures are frequently found. Diffuse abdominal tenderness may be found on palpation; an "acute abdomen" indicates free blood in the peritoneal cavity. A palpable mass may represent a large retroperitoneal hematoma or perhaps urinary extravasation. If the retroperitoneum has been torn, free blood may be noted in the peritoneal cavity but no palpable mass will be evident. The abdomen may be distended and bowel sounds absent.

C. Laboratory Findings: Microscopic or gross hematuria is usually present. The hematocrit may be normal initially, but a drop may be found when serial studies are done. This finding represents persistent

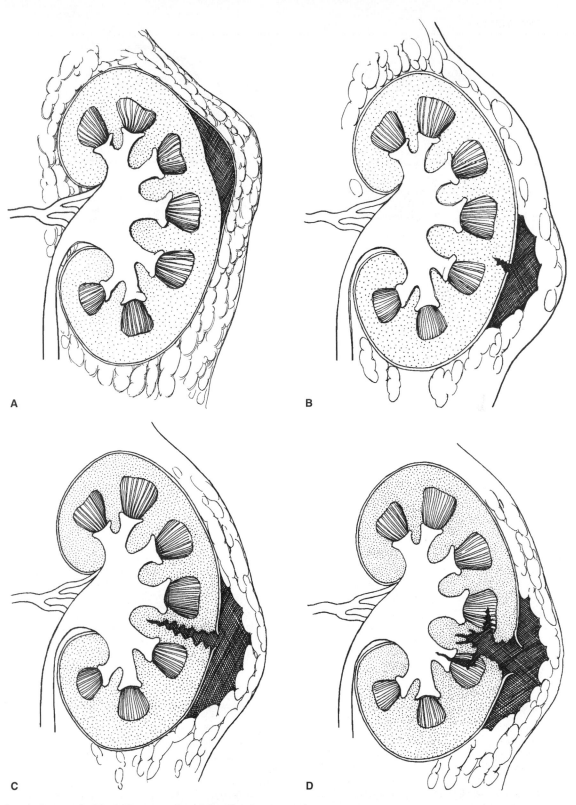

Figure 19–5. Classification of renal injuries. Grades I and II are minor. Grades III, IV, and V are major. **A:** Grade I—microscopic or gross hematuria; normal findings on radiographic studies; contusion or contained subcapsular hematoma without parenchymal laceration. **B:** Grade II—nonexpanding, confined perirenal hematoma or cortical laceration less than 1 cm deep without urinary extravasation. **C:** Grade III—parenchymal laceration extending less than 1 cm into the cortex without urinary extravasation. **D:** Grade IV—parenchymal laceration extending through the corticomedullary junction and into the collecting system. A laceration at a segmental vessel may also be present. (continued)

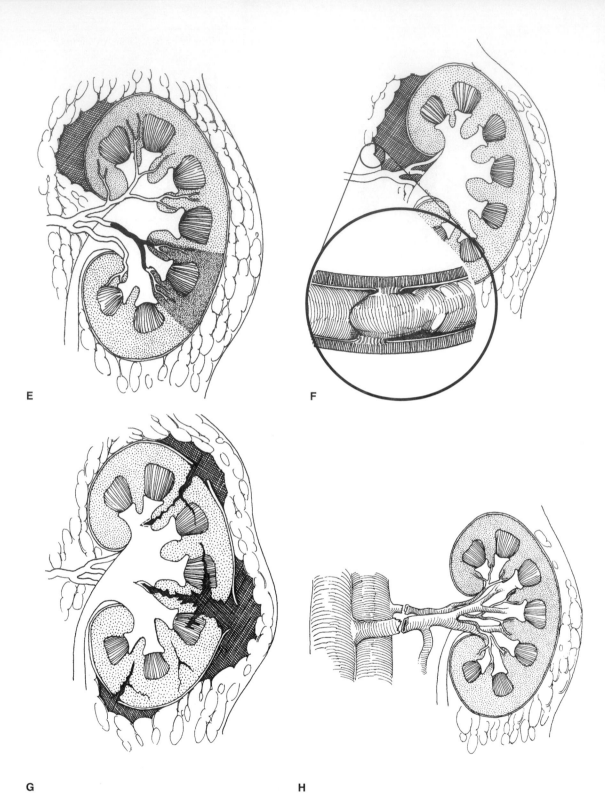

Figure 19–5 (cont'd). E: Grade IV—thrombosis of a segmental renal artery without a parenchymal laceration. Note the corresponding parenchymal ischemia. **F:** Grade V—thrombosis of the main renal artery. The inset shows the intimal tear and distal thrombosis. **G:** Grade V—multiple major lacerations, resulting in a "shattered" kidney. **H:** Grade V—avulsion of the main renal artery and/or vein.

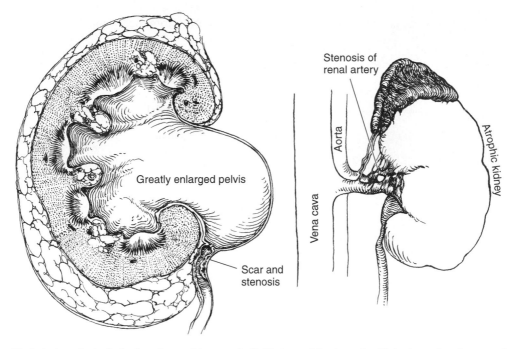

Figure 19–6. Late pathologic findings in renal trauma. **Left:** Ureteropelvic stenosis with hydronephrosis secondary to fibrosis from extravasation of blood and urine. **Right:** Atrophy of kidney caused by injury (stenosis) of arterial blood supply.

retroperitoneal bleeding and development of a large retroperitoneal hematoma. Persistent bleeding may necessitate operation.

    D. Staging and X-Ray Findings: Staging of renal injuries allows a systematic approach to these problems (Figures 19–1 through 19–3). Adequate studies help define the extent of injury and dictate appropriate management. For example, blunt trauma to the abdomen associated with gross hematuria and a normal urogram requires no additional renal studies; however, nonvisualization of the kidney requires immediate arteriography or CT scan to determine whether renal vascular injury exists. Ultrasonography and retrograde urography are of little use initially in the evaluation of renal injuries.

    Staging begins with an abdominal CT scan, the most direct and effective means of staging renal injuries. This noninvasive technique clearly defines parenchymal lacerations and urinary extravasation, shows the extent of the retroperitoneal hematoma, identifies nonviable tissue, and outlines injuries to surrounding organs such as the pancreas, spleen, liver, and bowel (Figure 19–7). (If CT is not available, an intravenous pyelogram can be obtained [Figure 19–8].)

    Arteriography defines major arterial and parenchymal injuries when previous studies have not fully done so. Arterial thrombosis and avulsion of the renal pedicle are best diagnosed by arteriography and

are likely when the kidney is not visualized on imaging studies (Figure 19–9). The major causes of nonvisualization on an excretory urogram are total pedicle avulsion, arterial thrombosis, severe contusion causing vascular spasm, and absence of the kidney (either congenital or from operation).

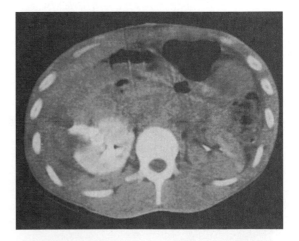

Figure 19–7. Computed tomography scan of right kidney following knife stab wound. Laceration with urine extravasation is seen. Large right retroperitoneal hematoma is present.

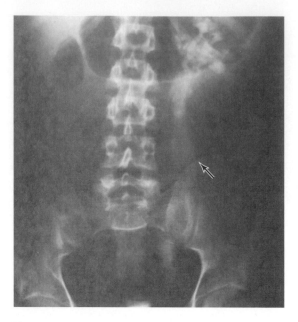

Figure 19–8. Blunt renal trauma to left kidney demonstrating extravasation (at arrow) on intravenous urogram.

Radionuclide renal scans have been used in staging renal trauma. However, in emergency management, this technique is less sensitive than arteriography or CT.

Differential Diagnosis

Trauma to the abdomen and flank areas is not always associated with renal injury. In such cases, there is no hematuria, and the results of imaging studies are normal.

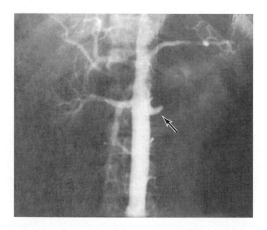

Figure 19–9. Arteriogram following blunt abdominal trauma shows typical findings of acute renal artery thrombosis (arrow) of left kidney.

Complications

A. Early Complications: Hemorrhage is perhaps the most important immediate complication of renal injury. Heavy retroperitoneal bleeding may result in rapid exsanguination. Patients must be observed closely, with careful monitoring of blood pressure and hematocrit. Complete staging must be done early (Figures 19–1 through 19–3). The size and expansion of palpable masses must be carefully monitored. Bleeding ceases spontaneously in 80–85% of cases. Persistent retroperitoneal bleeding or heavy gross hematuria may require early operation.

Urinary extravasation from renal fracture may show as an expanding mass (urinoma) in the retroperitoneum. These collections are prone to abscess formation and sepsis. A resolving retroperitoneal hematoma may cause slight fever (38.3 °C [101 °F]), but higher temperatures suggest infection. A perinephric abscess may form, resulting in abdominal tenderness and flank pain. Prompt operation is indicated.

B. Late Complications: Hypertension, hydronephrosis, arteriovenous fistula, calculus formation, and pyelonephritis are important late complications. Careful monitoring of blood pressure for several months is necessary to watch for hypertension. At 3–6 months, a follow-up excretory urogram or CT scan should be obtained to be certain that perinephric scarring has not caused hydronephrosis or vascular compromise; renal atrophy may occur from vascular compromise and is detected by follow-up urography. Heavy late bleeding may occur 1–4 weeks after injury.

Treatment

A. Emergency Measures: The objectives of early management are prompt treatment of shock and hemorrhage, complete resuscitation, and evaluation of associated injuries.

B. Surgical Measures:

1. Blunt injuries–Minor renal injuries from blunt trauma account for 85% of cases and do not usually require operation. Bleeding stops spontaneously with bed rest and hydration. Cases in which operation is indicated include those associated with persistent retroperitoneal bleeding, urinary extravasation, evidence of nonviable renal parenchyma, and renal pedicle injuries (less than 5% of all renal injuries). Aggressive preoperative staging allows complete definition of injury before operation.

2. Penetrating injuries–Penetrating injuries should be surgically explored. A rare exception to this rule is when staging has been complete and only minor parenchymal injury, with no urinary extravasation, is noted. In 80% of cases of penetrating injury, associated organ injury requires operation; thus, renal exploration is only an extension of this procedure.

C. Treatment of Complications: Retroperitoneal urinoma or perinephric abscess demands prompt surgical drainage. Malignant hypertension requires vascular repair or nephrectomy. Hydronephrosis may require surgical correction or nephrectomy.

Prognosis

With careful follow-up, most renal injuries have an excellent prognosis, with spontaneous healing and return of renal function. Follow-up excretory urography and monitoring of blood pressure ensure detection and appropriate management of late hydronephrosis and hypertension.

INJURIES TO THE URETER

Ureteral injury is rare but may occur, usually during the course of a difficult pelvic surgical procedure or as a result of gunshot wounds. Rapid deceleration accidents may avulse the ureter from the renal pelvis. Endoscopic basket manipulation of ureteral calculi may result in injury. Injury to the intramural ureter during transurethral resections also may occur.

Etiology

Large pelvic masses (benign or malignant) may displace the ureter laterally and engulf it in reactive fibrosis. This may lead to ureteral injury during dissection, since the organ is anatomically malpositioned. Inflammatory pelvic disorders may involve the ureter in a similar way. Extensive carcinoma of the colon may invade areas outside the colon wall and directly involve the ureter; thus, resection of the ureter may be required along with resection of the tumor mass. Devascularization may occur with extensive pelvic lymph node dissections or after radiation therapy to the pelvis for pelvic cancer. In these situations, ureteral fibrosis and subsequent stricture formation may develop along with ureteral fistulas.

Endoscopic manipulation of a ureteral calculus with a stone basket or ureteroscope may result in ureteral perforation or avulsion. Passage of a ureteral catheter beyond an area of obstruction may perforate the ureter. This is usually secondary to the acute inflammatory process in the ureteral wall and surrounding the calculus.

Pathogenesis & Pathology

The ureter may be inadvertently ligated and cut during difficult pelvic surgery. In such cases, sepsis and severe renal damage usually occur postoperatively. If a partially divided ureter is unrecognized at operation, urinary extravasation and subsequent buildup of a large urinoma will ensue, which usually leads to ureterovaginal or ureterocutaneous fistula formation. Intraperitoneal extravasation of urine can also occur, causing ileus and peritonitis. After partial transection of the ureter, some degree of stenosis and reactive fibrosis develops, with concomitant mild to moderate hydronephrosis.

Clinical Findings

A. Symptoms: If the ureter has been completely or partially ligated during operation, the postoperative course is usually marked by fever of 38.3–38.8 °C (101–102 °F) as well as flank and lower quadrant pain. Such patients often experience paralytic ileus with nausea and vomiting. If ureterovaginal or cutaneous fistula develops, it usually does so within the first 10 postoperative days. Bilateral ureteral injury is manifested by postoperative anuria.

Ureteral injuries from external violence should be suspected in patients who have sustained stab or gunshot wounds to the retroperitoneum. The mid portion of the ureter seems to be the most common site of penetrating injury. There are usually associated vascular and other abdominal visceral injuries.

B. Signs: The acute hydronephrosis of a totally ligated ureter results in severe flank pain and abdominal pain with nausea and vomiting early in the postoperative course and with associated ileus. Signs and symptoms of acute peritonitis may be present if there is urinary extravasation into the peritoneal cavity. Watery discharge from the wound or vagina may be identified as urine by determining the creatinine concentration of a small sample—urine has many times the creatinine concentration found in serum—and by intravenous injection of 10 mL of indigo carmine, which will appear in the urine as dark blue.

C. Laboratory Findings: Ureteral injury from external violence is manifested by microscopic hematuria in 90% of cases. Urinalysis and other laboratory studies are of little use in diagnosis when injury has occurred from other causes. The serum creatinine level usually remains normal except in bilateral ureteral obstruction.

D. X-Ray Findings: Diagnosis is by excretory urography. A plain film of the abdomen may demonstrate a large area of increased density in the pelvis or in an area of retroperitoneum where injury is suspected. After injection of contrast material, delayed excretion is noted with hydronephrosis. Partial transection of the ureter results in more rapid excretion, but persistent hydronephrosis is usually present, and contrast extravasation at the site of injury is noted on delayed films (Figure 19–10).

In acute injury from external violence, the excretory urogram usually appears normal, with very mild fullness down to the point of extravasation at the ureteral transection.

Retrograde ureterography demonstrates the exact site of obstruction or extravasation.

E. Ultrasonography: Ultrasonography outlines hydroureter or urinary extravasation as it develops into a urinoma and is perhaps the best means of ruling out ureteral injury in the early postoperative period.

It has the advantages of being noninvasive and rapid.

F. Radionuclide Scanning: Radionuclide scanning demonstrates delayed excretion on the injured

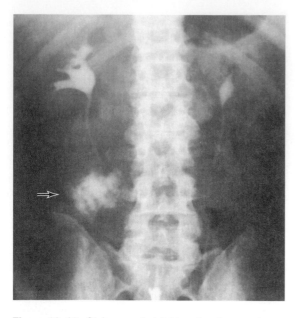

Figure 19–10. Stab wound of right ureter shows extravasation (at arrow) on intravenous urogram.

side, with evidence of increasing counts owing to accumulation of urine in the renal pelvis. Its great benefit, however, is in the assessment of renal function after surgical correction.

Differential Diagnosis

Postoperative bowel obstruction and peritonitis may cause symptoms similar to those of acute ureteral obstruction from injury. Fever, "acute abdomen," and associated nausea and vomiting following difficult pelvic surgery are definite indications for screening sonography or excretory urography to establish whether ureteral injury has occurred.

Deep wound infection must be considered postoperatively in patients with fever, ileus, and localized tenderness. The same findings are consistent with urinary extravasation and urinoma formation.

Acute pyelonephritis in the early postoperative period may also result in findings similar to those of ureteral injury. Sonography is normal, and urography shows no evidence of obstruction.

Drainage of peritoneal fluid through the wound from impending evisceration may be confused with ureteral injury and urinary extravasation. The creatinine concentration of the transudate is similar to that of serum, whereas urine contains very high creatinine levels.

Complications

Ureteral injury may be complicated by stricture formation with resulting hydronephrosis in the area of injury. Chronic urinary extravasation from unrecog-

nized injury may lead to formation of a large retroperitoneal urinoma. Pyelonephritis from hydronephrosis and urinary infection may require prompt proximal drainage.

Treatment

Prompt treatment of ureteral injuries is required. The best opportunity for successful repair is in the operating room when the injury occurs. If the injury is not recognized until 7–10 days after the event and no infection, abscess, or other complications exist, immediate reexploration and repair are indicated. Proximal urinary drainage by percutaneous nephrostomy or formal nephrostomy should be considered if the injury is recognized late or if the patient has significant complications that make immediate reconstruction unsatisfactory. The goals of ureteral repair are to achieve complete debridement, a tension-free spatulated anastomosis, watertight closure, ureteral stenting (in selected cases), and retroperitoneal drainage.

A. Lower Ureteral Injuries: Injuries to the lower third of the ureter allow several options in management. The procedure of choice is reimplantation into the bladder combined with a psoas-hitch procedure to minimize tension on the ureteral anastomosis. An antireflux procedure should be done when possible. Primary ureteroureterostomy can be used in lower-third injuries when the ureter has been ligated without transection. The ureter is usually long enough for this type of anastomosis. A bladder tube flap can be used when the ureter is shorter.

Transureteroureterostomy may be used in lower-third injuries if extensive urinoma and pelvic infection have developed. This procedure allows anastomosis and reconstruction in an area away from the pathologic processes.

B. Midureteral Injuries: Midureteral injuries usually result from external violence and are best repaired by primary ureteroureterostomy or transureteroureterostomy.

C. Upper Ureteral Injuries: Injuries to the upper third of the ureter are best managed by primary ureteroureterostomy. If there is extensive loss of the ureter, autotransplantation of the kidney can be done as well as bowel replacement of the ureter.

D. Stenting: Most anastomoses after repair of ureteral injury should be stented. The preferred technique is to insert a silicone internal stent through the anastomosis before closure. These stents have a J memory curve on each end to prevent their migration in the postoperative period. After 3–4 weeks of healing, stents can be endoscopically removed from the bladder. The advantages of internal stenting are maintenance of a straight ureter with a constant caliber during early healing, the presence of a conduit for urine during healing, prevention of urinary extravasation, maintenance of urinary diversion, and easy removal.

Prognosis

The prognosis for ureteral injury is excellent if the diagnosis is made early and prompt corrective surgery is done. Delay in diagnosis worsens the prognosis because of infection, hydronephrosis, abscess, and fistula formation.

INJURIES TO THE BLADDER

Bladder injuries occur most often from external force and are often associated with pelvic fractures. (About 15% of all pelvic fractures are associated with concomitant bladder or urethral injuries.) Iatrogenic injury may result from gynecologic and other extensive pelvic procedures as well as from hernia repairs and transurethral operations.

Pathogenesis & Pathology (Figure 19–11)

The bony pelvis protects the urinary bladder very well. When the pelvis is fractured by blunt trauma, fragments from the fracture site may perforate the bladder. These perforations usually result in extraperitoneal rupture. If the urine is infected, ex-

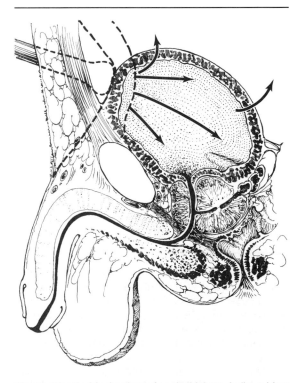

Figure 19–11. Mechanism of vesical injury. A direct blow over the full bladder causes increased intravesical pressure. If the bladder ruptures, it will usually rupture into the peritoneal cavity.

traperitoneal bladder perforations may result in deep pelvic abscess and severe pelvic inflammation.

When the bladder is filled to near capacity, a direct blow to the lower abdomen may result in bladder disruption. This type of disruption ordinarily is intraperitoneal. Since the reflection of the pelvic peritoneum covers the dome of the bladder, a linear laceration will allow urine to flow into the abdominal cavity. If the diagnosis is not established immediately and if the urine is sterile, no symptoms may be noted for several days. If the urine is infected, immediate peritonitis and acute abdomen will develop.

Clinical Findings

Pelvic fracture accompanies bladder rupture in 90% of cases. The diagnosis of pelvic fracture can be made initially in the emergency room by lateral compression on the bony pelvis, since the fracture site will show crepitus and be painful to the touch. Lower abdominal and suprapubic tenderness is usually present. Pelvic fracture and suprapubic tenderness with acute abdomen suggest intraperitoneal bladder disruption.

A. Symptoms: There is usually a history of lower abdominal trauma. Blunt injury is the usual cause. Patients ordinarily are unable to urinate, but when spontaneous voiding occurs, gross hematuria is usually present. Most patients complain of pelvic or lower abdominal pain.

B. Signs: Heavy bleeding associated with pelvic fracture may result in hemorrhagic shock, usually from venous disruption of pelvic vessels. Evidence of external injury from a gunshot or stab wound in the lower abdomen should make one suspect bladder injury, manifested by marked tenderness of the suprapubic area and lower abdomen. An acute abdomen indicates intraperitoneal bladder rupture. A palpable mass in the lower abdomen usually represents a large pelvic hematoma. On rectal examination, landmarks may be indistinct because of a large pelvic hematoma.

C. Laboratory Findings: Catheterization usually is required in patients with pelvic trauma but not if bloody urethral discharge is noted. Bloody urethral discharge indicates urethral injury, and a urethrogram is necessary before catheterization (Figures 19–1 through 19–3). When catheterization is done, gross or, less commonly, microscopic hematuria is usually present. Urine taken from the bladder at the initial catheterization should be cultured to determine whether infection is present.

D. X-Ray Findings: A plain abdominal film generally demonstrates pelvic fractures. There may be haziness over the lower abdomen from blood and urine extravasation. An intravenous urogram should be obtained to establish whether kidney and ureteral injuries are present.

Bladder disruption is shown on cystography. The bladder should be filled with 300 mL of contrast material and a plain film of the lower abdomen obtained. Contrast medium should be allowed to drain out completely, and a second film of the abdomen should be obtained. The drainage film is extremely important, because it demonstrates areas of extraperitoneal extravasation of blood and urine that may not appear on the filling film (Figure 19–12). With intraperitoneal extravasation, free contrast medium is visualized in the abdomen, highlighting bowel loops (Figure 19–13).

CT cystography is an excellent method for detecting bladder rupture; however, retrograde filling of the bladder with 300 mL of contrast medium is necessary to distend the bladder completely. Incomplete distention with consequent missed diagnosis of bladder rupture often occurs when the urethral catheter is clamped during standard abdominal CT scan with intravenous contrast injection.

E. Instrumental Examination: If urethral injury is suspected (bloody discharge), a urethrogram should be obtained before any attempt is made to catheterize the patient. If there is no evidence of urethral injury, catheterization can be safely accomplished.

Cystoscopy is not indicated, since bleeding and clots obscure visualization and prevent accurate diagnosis.

Differential Diagnosis

Abdominal trauma with hematuria may cause injury to the kidney and ureter as well as the bladder. A urogram is indicated for all patients with trauma-related hematuria. Associated injuries to the pelvic vessels and bowel also should be considered.

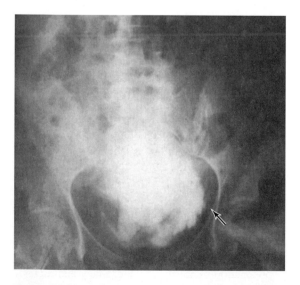

Figure 19–12. Extraperitoneal bladder rupture. Extravasation (at arrow) seen outside the bladder in the pelvis on cystogram.

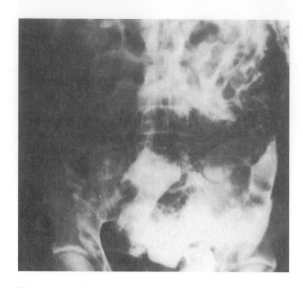

Figure 19–13. Intraperitoneal bladder rupture. Cystogram shows contrast surrounding loops of bowel.

The urethra may be injured as well as the bladder; this possibility should be considered in any patient with blunt trauma and pelvic fractures. Urethrography demonstrates disruption of the urethra.

Complications

A pelvic abscess may develop from extraperitoneal bladder rupture; if the urine becomes infected, the pelvic hematoma becomes infected too.

Intraperitoneal bladder rupture with extravasation of urine into the abdominal cavity causes delayed peritonitis.

Partial incontinence may result from bladder injury when the laceration extends into the bladder neck. Meticulous repair may ensure normal urinary control.

Treatment

A. Emergency Measures: Shock and hemorrhage should be treated.

B. Surgical Measures: A lower midline abdominal incision should be made. As the bladder is approached in the midline, a pelvic hematoma, which is usually lateral, should be avoided. Entering the pelvic hematoma can result in increased bleeding from release of tamponade and in infection of the hematoma, with subsequent pelvic abscess. The bladder should be opened in the midline and carefully inspected. After repair, a suprapubic cystostomy tube is usually left in place to ensure complete urinary drainage and control of bleeding.

1. Extraperitoneal rupture–Extraperitoneal rupture should be repaired intravesically. As the bladder is opened in the midline, it should be carefully inspected and lacerations closed from within. Polyglycolic acid or chromic absorbable sutures should be used.

Extraperitoneal bladder lacerations occasionally extend into the bladder neck and should be repaired meticulously. Fine absorbable sutures should be used to ensure complete reconstruction so that the patient will have urinary control after injury. Such injuries are best managed with indwelling urethral catheterization and suprapubic diversion.

Peritoneotomy should be done and the intra-abdominal fluid inspected before the procedure is completed. If abdominal fluid is bloody, complete abdominal exploration should be done to rule out associated injuries.

2. Intraperitoneal rupture–Intraperitoneal bladder ruptures should be repaired via a transperitoneal approach after careful transvesical inspection and closure of any other perforations. The peritoneum must be closed carefully over the area of injury. The bladder is then closed in separate layers by absorbable suture. All extravasated fluid from the peritoneal cavity should be removed before closure. At the time of closure, care should be taken that the suprapubic cystostomy is in the extraperitoneal position.

3. Pelvic fracture–Stable fracture of the pubic rami is usually present. In such cases, the patient can be ambulatory within 4–5 days without damage or difficulty. Unstable pelvic fractures requiring external fixation have a more protracted course.

4. Pelvic hematoma–There may be heavy uncontrolled bleeding from rupture of pelvic vessels even if the hematoma has not been entered at operation. At exploration and bladder repair, packing the pelvis with laparotomy tapes often controls the problem. If bleeding persists, it may be necessary to leave the tapes in place for 24 h and operate again to remove them. Embolization of pelvic vessels with Gelfoam or skeletal muscle under angiographic control is useful in controlling persistent pelvic bleeding.

C. Medical Measures: The patient whose cystogram shows only a small degree of extravasation can be managed by placing a urethral catheter into the bladder, without operation or suprapubic cystostomy. The urine must be free of infection. Corriere and Sandler (1988) have reported success with such management. Careful observation is necessary because of the potential for pelvic hematoma infection, continued bleeding from the bladder, and clot retention.

Prognosis

With appropriate treatment, the prognosis is excellent. The suprapubic cystostomy tube can be removed within 10 days, and the patient can usually void normally. Patients with lacerations extending into the bladder neck area may be temporarily incontinent, but full control is usually regained. At the time of discharge, urine culture should be performed to determine whether catheter-associated infection requires further treatment.

INJURIES TO THE URETHRA

Urethral injuries are uncommon and occur most often in men, usually associated with pelvic fractures or straddle-type falls. They are rare in women.

Various parts of the urethra may be lacerated, transected, or contused. Management varies according to the level of injury. The urethra can be separated into 2 broad anatomic divisions: the posterior urethra, consisting of the prostatic and membranous portions, and the anterior urethra, consisting of the bulbous and pendulous portions.

INJURIES TO THE POSTERIOR URETHRA

Etiology
(Figure 19–14)

The membranous urethra passes through the urogenital diaphragm and is the portion of the posterior urethra most likely to be injured. The urogenital diaphragm contains most of the voluntary urinary sphincter. It is attached to the pubic rami inferiorly, and when pelvic fractures occur from blunt trauma, the membranous urethra is sheared from the prostatic apex at the prostatomembranous junction. The urethra can be transected by the same mechanism at the interior surface of the membranous urethra.

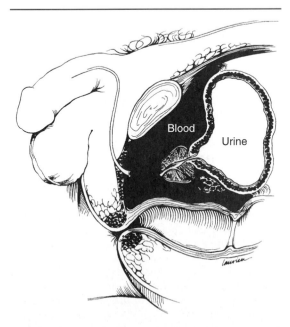

Figure 19–14. Injury to the posterior (membranous) urethra. The prostate has been avulsed from the membranous urethra secondary to fracture of the pelvis. Extravasation occurs above the triangular ligament and is periprostatic and perivesical.

Pathogenesis & Pathology

Injuries to the posterior urethra commonly occur from blunt trauma and pelvic fractures. The urethra usually is sheared off just proximal to the urogenital diaphragm, and the prostate is displaced superiorly by the developing hematoma in the periprostatic and perivesical spaces.

Clinical Findings

A. Symptoms: Patients usually complain of lower abdominal pain and inability to urinate. A history of crushing injury to the pelvis is usually obtained.

B. Signs: Blood at the urethral meatus is the single most important sign of urethral injury. The importance of this finding cannot be overemphasized, because an attempt to pass a urethral catheter may result in infection of the periprostatic and perivesical hematoma and conversion of an incomplete laceration to a complete one. The presence of blood at the external urethral meatus indicates that immediate urethrography is necessary to establish the diagnosis.

Suprapubic tenderness and the presence of pelvic fracture are noted on physical examination. A large developing pelvic hematoma may be palpated. Perineal or suprapubic contusions are often noted. Rectal examination may reveal a large pelvic hematoma with the prostate displaced superiorly. Rectal examination can be misleading, however, because a tense pelvic hematoma may resemble the prostate on palpation. Superior displacement of the prostate does not occur if the puboprostatic ligaments remain intact. Partial disruption of the membranous urethra (currently 10% of cases) is not accompanied by prostatic displacement.

C. Laboratory Findings: Anemia due to hemorrhage may be noted. Urine usually cannot be obtained initially, since the patient should not void and catheterization should not be attempted.

D. X-Ray Findings: Fractures of the bony pelvis are usually present. A urethrogram (using 20–30 mL of water-soluble contrast material) shows the site of extravasation at the prostatomembranous junction. Ordinarily, there is free extravasation of contrast material into the perivesical space (Figure 19–15). Incomplete prostatomembranous disruption is seen as minor extravasation, with a portion of contrast material passing into the prostatic urethra and bladder.

E. Instrumental Examination: The only instrumentation involved should be for urethrography. Catheterization or urethroscopy should not be done, because these procedures pose an increased risk of hematoma, infection, and further damage to partial urethral disruptions.

Differential Diagnosis

Bladder rupture may be associated with posterior urethral injuries. An intravenous urogram should be considered part of the assessment. Delayed films

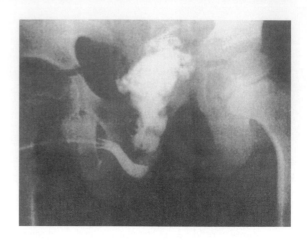

Figure 19–15. Ruptured prostatomembranous urethra shows free extravasation on urethrogram. No contrast medium is seen entering the prostatic urethra.

should be obtained to demonstrate the bladder and note extravasation. Cystography cannot be done preoperatively, since a urethral catheter should not be passed. Careful evaluation of the bladder at operation is necessary. The anterior portion of the urethra may be injured as well as the prostatomembranous urethra.

Complications

Stricture, impotence, and incontinence as complications of prostatomembranous disruption are among the most severe and debilitating mishaps that result from trauma to the urinary system. Stricture following primary repair and anastomosis occurs in about one-half of cases. If the preferred suprapubic cystostomy approach with delayed repair is used, the incidence of stricture can be reduced to about 5%.

The incidence of impotence after primary repair is 30–80% (mean, about 50%). This figure can be reduced to 10–15% by suprapubic drainage with delayed urethral reconstruction.

Incontinence in primary reanastomosis is noted in one-third of patients. Delayed reconstruction reduces the incidence to less than 5%.

Treatment

A. Emergency Measures: Shock and hemorrhage should be treated.

B. Surgical Measures: Urethral catheterization should be avoided.

1. Immediate management–Initial management should consist of suprapubic cystostomy to provide urinary drainage. A midline lower abdominal incision should be made, care being taken to avoid the large pelvic hematoma. The bladder and prostate are usually elevated superiorly by large periprostatic and perivesical hematomas. The bladder often is distended by a large volume of urine accumulated during the period of resuscitation and operative preparation. The urine is often clear and free of blood, but gross hematuria may be present. The bladder should be opened in the midline and carefully inspected for lacerations. If a laceration is present, the bladder should be closed with absorbable suture material and a cystostomy tube inserted for urinary drainage. This approach involves no urethral instrumentation or manipulation. The suprapubic cystostomy is maintained in place for about 3 months. This allows resolution of the pelvic hematoma, and the prostate and bladder will slowly return to their anatomic positions.

Incomplete laceration of the posterior urethra heals spontaneously, and the suprapubic cystostomy can be removed within 2–3 weeks. The cystostomy tube should not be removed before voiding cystourethrography shows that no extravasation persists.

2. Urethral reconstruction–Reconstruction of the urethra after prostatic disruption can be undertaken within 3 months, assuming there is no pelvic abscess or other evidence of persistent pelvic infection. Before reconstruction, a combined cystogram and urethrogram should be done to determine the exact length of the resulting urethral stricture. This stricture usually is 1–2 cm long and situated immediately posterior to the pubic bone. The preferred approach is a single-stage reconstruction of the urethral rupture defect with direct excision of the strictured area and anastomosis of the bulbous urethra directly to the apex of the prostate. A 16F silicone urethral catheter should be left in place along with a suprapubic cystostomy. Catheters are removed within a month, and the patient is then able to void (Figure 19–16).

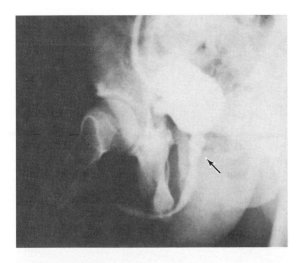

Figure 19–16. Delayed repair of urethral injury. Normal voiding urethrogram after transpubic repair of stricture following prostatomembranous urethral disruption. Arrow indicates area of repair.

3. Immediate urethral realignment–Some surgeons prefer to realign the urethra immediately. Direct suture reconstruction of the prostatomembranous disruption in the acute injury is extremely difficult. Persistent bleeding and surrounding hematoma create technical problems. The incidence of stricture, impotence, and incontinence appears to be higher than with immediate cystostomy and delayed reconstruction. However, several authors have reported success with immediate urethral realignment.

C. General Measures: After delayed reconstruction by a perineal approach, patients are allowed ambulation on the first postoperative day and usually can be discharged within 3 days.

D. Treatment of Complications: Approximately 1 month after the delayed reconstruction, the urethral catheter can be removed and a voiding cystogram obtained through the suprapubic cystostomy tube. If the cystogram shows a patent area of reconstruction free of extravasation, the suprapubic catheter can be removed; if there is extravasation or stricture, suprapubic cystostomy should be maintained. A follow-up urethrogram should be obtained within 2 months to watch for stricture development.

Stricture, if present (< 5%), is usually very short, and urethrotomy under direct vision offers easy and rapid cure.

The patient may be impotent for several months after delayed repair. Impotence is permanent in about 10% of patients. Implantation of a penile prosthesis is indicated if impotence is still present 2 years after reconstruction (see Chapter 47).

Incontinence seldom follows transpubic or perineal reconstruction. If present, it usually resolves slowly.

Prognosis

If complications can be avoided, the prognosis is excellent. Urinary infections ultimately resolve with appropriate management.

INJURIES TO THE ANTERIOR URETHRA

Etiology
(Figure 19–17)

The anterior urethra is the portion distal to the urogenital diaphragm. Straddle injury may cause laceration or contusion of the urethra. Self-instrumentation or iatrogenic instrumentation may cause partial disruption.

Pathogenesis & Pathology

A. Contusion: Contusion of the urethra is a sign of crush injury without urethral disruption. Perineal hematoma usually resolves without complications.

B. Laceration: A severe straddle injury may result in laceration of part of the urethral wall, allowing extravasation of urine. If the extravasation is unrecognized, it may extend into the scrotum, along the

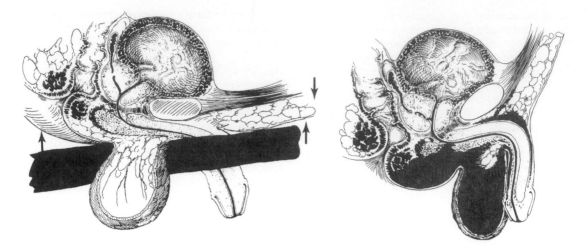

Figure 19–17. Injury to the bulbous urethra. **Left:** Mechanism: Usually a perineal blow or fall astride an object; crushing of urethra against inferior edge of pubic symphysis. **Right:** Extravasation of blood and urine enclosed within Colles' fascia (see Figure 1–9).

penile shaft, and up to the abdominal wall. It is limited only by Colles' fascia and often results in sepsis, infection, and serious morbidity.

Clinical Findings

A. Symptoms: There is usually a history of a fall, and in some cases a history of instrumentation. Bleeding from the urethra is usually present. There is local pain into the perineum and sometimes massive perineal hematoma. If voiding has occurred and extravasation is noted, sudden swelling in the area will be present. If diagnosis has been delayed, sepsis and severe infection may be present.

B. Signs: The perineum is very tender, and a mass may be found. Rectal examination reveals a normal prostate. The patient usually has a desire to void, but voiding should not be allowed until assessment of the urethra is complete. No attempt should be made to pass a urethral catheter, but if the patient's bladder is overdistended, percutaneous suprapubic cystostomy can be done as a temporary procedure.

When presentation of such injuries is delayed, there is massive urinary extravasation and infection in the perineum and the scrotum. The lower abdominal wall may also be involved. The skin is usually swollen and discolored.

C. Laboratory Findings: Blood loss is not usually excessive, particularly if secondary injury has occurred. The white count may be elevated with infection.

D. X-Ray Findings: A urethrogram, with instillation of 15–20 mL of water-soluble contrast material, demonstrates extravasation and the location of injury (Figure 19–18). A contused urethra shows no evidence of extravasation.

E. Instrumental Examination: If there is no evidence of extravasation on the urethrogram, a urethral catheter may be passed into the bladder. Extravasation is a contraindication to further instrumentation at this time.

Differential Diagnosis

Partial or complete disruption of the prostatomembranous urethra may occur if pelvic fracture is present. Urethrography usually demonstrates the location and extent of extravasation and its relationship to the urogenital diaphragm.

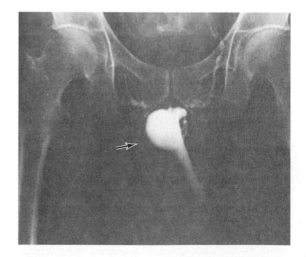

Figure 19–18. Ruptured bulbar (anterior) urethra following straddle injury. Extravasation (at arrow) on urethrogram.

Complications

Heavy bleeding from the corpus spongiosum injury may occur in the perineum as well as through the urethral meatus. Pressure applied to the perineum over the site of the injury usually controls bleeding. If hemorrhage cannot be controlled, immediate operation is required.

The complications of urinary extravasation are chiefly sepsis and infection. Aggressive debridement and drainage are required if there is infection.

Stricture at the site of injury is a common complication, but surgical reconstruction may not be required unless the stricture significantly reduces urinary flow rates.

Treatment

A. General Measures: Major blood loss usually does not occur from straddle injury. If heavy bleeding does occur, local pressure for control, followed by resuscitation, is required.

B. Specific Measures:

1. Urethral contusion–The patient with urethral contusion shows no evidence of extravasation, and the urethra remains intact. After urethrography, the patient is allowed to void; and if the voiding occurs normally, without pain or bleeding, no additional treatment is necessary. If bleeding persists, urethral catheter drainage can be done.

2. Urethral lacerations–Instrumentation of the urethra following urethrography should be avoided. A small midline incision in the suprapubic area readily exposes the dome of the bladder so that a suprapubic cystostomy tube can be inserted, allowing complete urinary diversion while the urethral laceration heals. Percutaneous cystostomy may also be used in such injuries. If only minor extravasation is noted on the urethrogram, a voiding study can be performed within 7 days after suprapubic catheter drainage to search for extravasation. In more extensive injuries, one should wait 2–3 weeks before doing a voiding study through the suprapubic catheter. Healing at the site of injury may result in stricture formation. Most of these strictures are not severe and do not require surgical reconstruction. The suprapubic cystostomy catheter may be removed if no extravasation is documented. Follow-up with documentation of urinary flow rates will show whether there is urethral obstruction from stricture.

3. Urethral laceration with extensive urinary extravasation–After major laceration, urinary extravasation may involve the perineum, scrotum, and lower abdomen. Drainage of these areas is indicated. Suprapubic cystostomy for urinary diversion is required. Infection and abscess formation are common and require antibiotic therapy.

4. Immediate repair–Immediate repair of urethral lacerations can be performed, but the procedure is difficult and the incidence of associated stricture is high.

C. Treatment of Complications: Strictures at the site of injury may be extensive and require delayed reconstruction.

Prognosis

Urethral stricture is a major complication but in most cases does not require surgical reconstruction. If, when stricture resolves, urinary flow rates are poor and urinary infection and urethral fistula are present, reconstruction is required.

INJURIES TO THE PENIS

Disruption of the tunica albuginea of the penis (penile fracture) can occur during sexual intercourse. At presentation, the patient has penile pain and hematoma. This injury should be surgically corrected.

Gangrene and urethral injury may be caused by obstructing rings placed around the base of the penis. These objects must be removed without causing further damage. Penile amputation is seen occasionally, and in a few patients, the penis can be surgically replaced successfully by microsurgical techniques.

Total avulsion of the penile skin occurs from machinery injuries. Immediate debridement and skin grafting are usually successful in salvage.

Injuries to the penis should suggest possible urethral damage, which should be investigated by urethrography.

INJURIES TO THE SCROTUM

Superficial lacerations of the scrotum may be debrided and closed primarily. Blunt trauma may cause local hematoma and ecchymosis, but these injuries resolve without difficulty. One must be certain that testicular rupture has not occurred.

Total avulsion of the scrotal skin may be caused by machinery accidents or other major trauma. The testes and spermatic cords are usually intact. It is important to provide coverage for these structures: this is best done by immediate surgical debridement and by placing the testes and spermatic cords in the subcutaneous tissues of the upper thighs. Later reconstruction of the scrotum can be done with a skin graft or thigh flap.

INJURIES TO THE TESTIS

Blunt trauma to the testis causes severe pain and, often, nausea and vomiting. Lower abdominal tenderness may be present. A hematoma may surround the testis and make delineation of its margin difficult. Ultrasonography can be used as an aid to better define the organ. If rupture has occurred, the sonogram will delineate the injury, which should be surgically repaired.

REFERENCES

EMERGENCY DIAGNOSIS & MANAGEMENT

Breaux CW et al: The first two years' experience with major trauma at a pediatric trauma center. J Trauma 1990;30:37.

Carroll PR, McAninch JW: Staging of renal trauma. Urol Clin North Am 1989;16:193.

Franko ER, Ivatury RR, Schwalb DM: Combined penetrating rectal and genitourinary injuries: A challenge in management. J Trauma 1993;34:347.

Grüssner R et al: Sonography versus peritoneal lavage in blunt abdominal trauma. J Trauma 1989;29:242.

Jacobs DG et al: Peritoneal lavage white count: A reassessment. J Trauma 1990;30:607.

Knudson MM et al: Hematuria as a predictor of abdominal injury after blunt trauma. Am J Surg 1992;164: 482, 485.

Sims DW et al: Urban trauma: A chronic recurrent disease. J Trauma 1989;29:940.

INJURIES TO THE KIDNEY

Baumann L et al: Nonoperative management of major blunt renal trauma in children: In-hospital morbidity and long-term followup. J Urol 1992;148:691.

Bretan PN Jr et al: Computerized tomographic staging of renal trauma: 85 consecutive cases. J Urol 1986; 136:561.

Carroll PR et al: Renovascular trauma: Risk assessment, surgical management, and outcome. J Trauma 1990; 30:547.

Cass AS: Renovascular injuries from external trauma: Diagnosis, treatment, and outcome. Urol Clin North Am 1989;16:213.

Husmann DA et al: Major renal lacerations with a devitalized fragment following blunt abdominal trauma: A comparison between nonoperative (expectant) versus surgical management. J Urol 1993;150:1774. [See comments.]

McAninch JW, Carroll PR: Renal exploration after trauma: Indications and reconstructive techniques. Urol Clin North Am 1989;16:203.

McAninch JW et al: Renal gunshot wounds: Methods of salvage and reconstruction. J Trauma 1993;35:279, 283.

McAninch JW et al: Renal reconstruction after injury. J Urol 1991;145:932.

Miller KS, McAninch JW: Radiographic assessment of renal trauma: Our 15-year experience. J Urol 1995; 154:352.

Moore EE et al: Organ injury scaling: Spleen, liver, and kidney. J Trauma 1989;29:1664.

Morey AF, Bruce JE, McAninch JW: Efficacy of radiographic imaging in pediatric blunt renal trauma. J Urol 1996;156:2014.

Peterson NE: Complications of renal trauma. Urol Clin North Am 1989;16:221.

Wessells H et al: Criteria for nonoperative treatment of significant penetrating renal lacerations. J Urol 1996; 157:24.

INJURIES TO THE URETER

Guerriero WG: Ureteral injury. Urol Clin North Am 1989;16:237.

Presti JC Jr, Carroll PR, McAninch JW: Ureteral and renal pelvic injuries from external trauma: Diagnosis and management. J Trauma 1989;29:370.

Rober PE, Smith JB, Pierce JM Jr: Gunshot injuries of the ureter. J Trauma 1990;30:83.

Toporoff B et al: Percutaneous antegrade ureteral stenting as an adjunct for treatment of complicated ureteral injuries. J Trauma 1992;32:534.

INJURIES TO THE BLADDER

Cass AS: Diagnostic studies in bladder rupture: Indications and techniques. Urol Clin North Am 1989;16: 267.

Corriere JN Jr, Sandler CM: Mechanisms of injury, patterns of extravasation and management of extraperitoneal bladder rupture due to blunt trauma. J Urol 1988;139:43.

Mee SL, McAninch JW, Federle MP: Computerized tomography in bladder rupture: Diagnostic limitations. J Urol 1987;137:207.

Peters PC: Intraperitoneal rupture of the bladder. Urol Clin North Am 1989;16:279.

Rehm CG et al: Blunt traumatic bladder rupture: The role of retrograde cystogram. Ann Emerg Med 1991; 20:845.

INJURIES TO THE URETHRA

al-Rifaei MA, Gaafar S, Abdel-Rahman M: Management of posterior urethral strictures secondary to pelvic fractures in children. J Urol 1991;145:353.

Armenakas NA, McAninch JW: Acute anterior urethral injuries: Diagnosis and initial management. In: McAninch JW (editor): Traumatic and Reconstructive Urology. Saunders, 1996.

Armenakas NA et al: Posttraumatic impotence: Magnetic resonance imaging and duplex ultrasound in diagnosis and management. J Urol 1993;149:1272.

de la Rosette JJ et al: Urethroplasty using the pedicled island flap technique in complicated urethral strictures. J Urol 1991;146:40.

Devine CJ Jr, Jordan GH, Devine PC: Primary realignment of the disrupted prostatomembranous urethra. Urol Clin North Am 1989;16:291.

Dixon CM, McAninch JW: Preoperative staging of posterior urethral disruptions. In: McAninch JW (editor): Traumatic and Reconstructive Urology. Saunders, 1996.

Husmann DA, Boone TB, Wilson WT: Management of low velocity gunshot wounds to the anterior urethra: The role of primary repair versus urinary diversion alone. J Urol 1993;150:70.

Jenkins BJ et al: Long-term results of treatment of urethral injuries in males caused by external trauma. Br J Urol 1992;70:73.

McAninch JW: Pubectomy in repair of membranous urethral stricture. Urol Clin N Am 1989;16:297.

McAninch JW, Morey AF: Penile circular fasciocutaneous skin flap in one-stage reconstruction of complex anterior urethral strictures. J Urol 1998;159:1209.

Morey AF, McAninch JW: Reconstruction of posterior urethral disruption injuries: Outcome analysis in 82 patients. J Urol 1997;157:506.

Scherz HC, Kaplan GW: Etiology, diagnosis, and management of urethral strictures in children. Urol Clin North Am 1990;17:389.

Webster GD, Ramon J: Repair of pelvic fracture posterior urethral defects using an elaborated perineal approach: Experience with 74 cases. J Urol 1991;145:744.

INJURIES TO THE PENIS

Gomez RG, Castanheira AC, McAninch JW: Gunshot wounds to the male external genitalia. J Urol 1993;150:1147.

Jordon GH, Gilbert DA: Management of amputation injuries of the male genitalia. Urol Clin North Am 1989;16:359.

McAninch JW, Armenakas NA: Genital reconstruction after major skin loss. In: McAninch JW (editor): *Traumatic and Reconstructive Urology.* Saunders, 1996.

Nicolaisen GS et al: Rupture of corpus cavernosum: Surgical management. J Urol 1983;130:917.

Orvis BR, McAninch JW: Penile rupture. Urol Clin North Am 1989;16:369.

Tsang T, Demby AM: Penile fracture with urethral injury. J Urol 1992;147:466.

INJURIES TO THE SCROTUM

Aboseif S, Gomez R, McAninch JW: Genital self-mutilation. J Urol 1993;150:1143.

McAninch JW: Management of genital skin loss. Urol Clin North Am 1989;16:387.

McAninch JW et al: Major traumatic and septic genital injuries. J Trauma 1984;24:291.

INJURIES TO THE TESTIS

Baskin LS, McAninch JW: Reconstruction of testicular rupture. In: McAninch JW (editor): *Traumatic and Reconstructive Urology.* Saunders, 1996.

Fournier GR Jr, Laing FC, McAninch JW: Scrotal ultrasonography in the management of testicular trauma. Urol Clin North Am 1989;16:377.

Gerscovich EO: High-resolution ultrasonography in the diagnosis of scrotal pathology: 1. Normal scrotum and benign disease. J Clin Ultrasound 1993;21:355.

Martinez-Pineiro L Jr et al: Value of testicular ultrasound in the evaluation of blunt scrotal trauma without haematocele. Br J Urol 1992;69:286.

20

Immunology & Immunotherapy of Urologic Cancers

Eric J. Small, MD

Both experimental and naturally occurring tumors are capable of stimulating a specific antitumor immune response. This observation suggests that there are foreign proteins (antigens) on tumor cells that classically have been described as resulting in humoral and cellular immune responses. However, experimental models suggest that a T-cell (cell-mediated) response may be more important in the killing of tumor cells than a B-cell (humoral) response.

A detailed description of the components of the immune system is beyond the scope of this chapter, but certain features of the immune system as they pertain to diagnostic and therapeutic issues will be reviewed.

Tumor Antigens

Tumor antigens can be divided into tumor-specific antigens and tumor-associated antigens. Tumor-specific antigens are not found on normal tissue, and they permit the host to recognize a tumor as foreign. Tumor-specific antigens have been shown to exist in oncogenesis models utilizing chemical, physical, and viral carcinogens but appear to be less common in models of spontaneous tumor development.

The identification of tumor-specific antigens led to the theory of immune surveillance, which suggests that the immune system is continuously trolling for foreign (tumor-specific) antigens. This theory is supported by the observation that at least some cancers are more common in immune-suppressed patients such as transplant patients or human immunodeficiency virus-infected individuals. However, many cancers are not overrepresented in these patient populations. Furthermore, spontaneous tumor models, which more closely resemble human carcinogenesis, appear to have a less extensive repertoire of tumor-specific antigens but instead have been found to express many tumor-associated antigens.

Tumor-associated antigens are found on normal cells but either become less prevalent in normal tissue after embryogenesis (eg, alpha-fetoprotein [AFP]) or remain present on normal tissue but are overexpressed on cancer cells (eg, prostate-specific

antigen [PSA]). In either case, the more ubiquitous nature of these antigens appears to cause reduced immune reactivity (also known as tolerance) to the specific antigen. The mechanisms of tolerance are complex and may be due in part to the absence of other required costimulatory molecules (such as B7, a molecule required for T-cell stimulation).

The development of monoclonal (hybridoma) technology has allowed the development of many antibodies against many tumor-associated antigens and has provided insight into the regulation and expression of these antigens. The re-expression or upregulation of these tumor-associated antigens during carcinogenesis may lead to immune response (or loss of tolerance). Many novel therapeutic approaches have sought to break this tolerance, and approaches to enhance a patient's immune response will be discussed.

Humoral Immunity

A large number of monoclonal antibodies have been developed against a variety of tumor-associated antigens. Oncofetal antigens such as AFP and beta-human chorionic gonadotropin (β-hCG) are important markers in germ cell tumors. β-hCG is also expressed in a small percentage of patients with bladder carcinoma. Growth factor receptors constitute another group of tumor-associated antigens that show promise as therapeutic targets as well as prognostic factors. For example, the receptor for fibroblastic growth factor appears to be expressed on prostate cancer cells, and therapies against growth factors such as fibroblastic growth factor, platelet-derived growth factor, and vascular endothelial growth factor are under investigation. The growth factor receptor HER2-neu has proved to be a strong predictive and prognostic marker, as well as a therapeutic target in breast cancer, and its utility in several urologic cancers is currently being evaluated.

Antibodies in Cancer Diagnosis & Detection

A. Prostate Cancer: Immunoassays are used to test both body fluids and tissues for the presence of tumor-associated antigens. In the urologic cancers, the most obvious example is the development of monoclonal antibodies against PSA. The utility and limitations of PSA are described elsewhere in this volume. Other antigens that have been tested in prostate cancer include prostatic acid phosphatase, which has largely been replaced by PSA in screening programs and in patients with low tumor burden. Prostatic acid phosphatase may be of some use in detecting or following up bone metastases and as a predictive marker of response to therapy for metastatic disease, both hormone-sensitive and -insensitive. More recently, antibodies to prostate-specific membrane antigen (PSMA) have been used, primarily for immunohistochemistry.

B. Renal Cell Carcinoma: Unfortunately, there are as yet no well-established antigens (or antibodies) that can be used to reliably evaluate and monitor renal cell carcinoma, although a variety of target antigens are being evaluated.

C. Bladder Cancer: Two oncofetal antigens, β-hCG and carcinoembryonic antigen, are expressed by a minority (20% or less) of transitional cell carcinomas. These markers are not routinely used, but in diagnostic dilemmas, measurement of serum levels of β-hCG or staining of tissue for this antigen may be useful. Trophoblastic differentiation in transitional cell carcinoma is associated with a poor prognosis.

D. Germ Cell Tumors: As described in Chapter 24, antibodies to hCG and AFP are routinely used to detect shed antigen from germ cell tumors in the bloodstream. These antigens can also be detected on tissue samples in the setting of some diagnostic dilemmas. While the use of serum markers in germ cell tumors is reviewed elsewhere, it is worth noting that the presence of the oncofetoprotein AFP, either in serum or on tissue specimens, is pathognomic for a nonseminomatous germ cell tumor, regardless of results of routine pathologic evaluation. In addition to their diagnostic utility, AFP and hCG can be used as markers of response to therapy and as predictive factors of outcome. For example, the international germ cell tumor risk classification schema for patients with metastatic disease relies heavily on AFP and hCG levels as well as levels of a nonspecific marker, lactate dehydrogenase, to assign patients with nonseminomatous germ cell tumors to one of 3 risk levels. Thus, patients can be classified as low-risk (92% 5-year survival) only if AFP is < 1000 ng/mL and hCG is < 5000 IU/L (with other criteria evaluating extent and location of tumor). By contrast, AFP > 1000 and < 10,000 or hCG > 5000 and < 50,000 immediately places a patient in an intravesicle risk category (80% 5-year survival), and AFP > 10,000 and hCG > 50,000 has an ominous prognosis (48% 5-year survival).

E. Radioimmunodetection: A growing field is the use of monoclonal antibodies for radioimmunodetection. Monoclonal antibodies to a specific antigen are radiolabeled, and the preferential binding of the monoclonal antibody to tumor cells can be exploited. Theoretically, such an approach could be used for the presurgical evaluation of disease, postsurgical evaluation for minimal residual disease, confirmation of cancer identified by other imaging modalities, and detection of recurrent disease. Unfortunately, these potential uses have not been successfully developed in the urologic cancers, with one possible exception. There are several potential impediments to successful tumor radioimmunodetection. These include dilution of antibody in the bloodstream; metabolism of the antibody; nonspecific binding in liver, reticuloendothelial system, bone marrow, and elsewhere; binding of antibody by circulating or shed antigen; and the development of neutralizing human antimouse antibodies.

The only radioimmunodetection system for urologic cancers at this time is ^{111}In-capromab pendetide, a murine monoclonal antibody to PSMA. Its use has been hampered by a fairly laborious administration process, tremendous operator dependence in interpretation of scans, and a less than satisfactory positive predictive value. The use of ^{111}In-capromab pendetide is described in Chapter 10.

Immunotherapy With Monoclonal Antibodies

Immunotherapy with monoclonal antibodies alone ("naked antibodies") has been fairly extensively evaluated. The use of monoclonal antibodies against tumor-associated antigens has met with only limited success in patients with solid tumors. In lymphoproliferative disorders such as leukemia and lymphoma, some antibodies to tumor-associated surface antigens appear to result in cell death. The mechanism for these effects is certainly multifactorial but may in part be mediated by resultant complement fixation.

Direct antiproliferative effects of antibodies on cancer cells can be achieved by antibodies against functionally important antigens. Thus, the inhibition of growth factors and growth factor receptors and the activation or inhibition of signal transducing molecules are attractive therapeutic targets. As noted above, an anti-HER2-neu antibody has been shown to have activity in breast cancer and has recently obtained US Food and Drug Administration (FDA) approval for use. In the urologic cancers, while no approved monoclonal antibody therapy exists, trials of antibodies against growth factors, vascular endothelial growth factor (an angiogenic molecule), and signal transduction molecules are being undertaken. In addition to the problems cited above in the discussion on radioimmunodetection, with the administration of any monoclonal antibody, one additional reason that naked antibody therapy could prove unsuccessful is that antigenic heterogeneity may result in only a small percentage of cancer cells being recognized, resulting in incomplete cell killing.

An alternative approach to naked antibodies is to conjugate any of a variety of cytotoxic agents to an antibody. The advantage of this approach is a "bystander effect," making it unnecessary to use an antibody that binds each and every cell. This can be achieved in a variety of ways. The most straightforward is to use the monoclonal antibody as a means of providing some targeting specificity for the cytotoxic agent used. Cytotoxic agents used include radioisotopes, chemotherapy, and toxins such as ricin. Other means of providing some specificity is to bind a prodrug (with an antibody) to the tumor site and then to activate the bound prodrug. (Conversely, a nontoxic prodrug administered systemically could be activated in situ by the addition of an activating enzyme bound to a localizing antibody.) Finally, targeting with bispecific antibodies (eg, to antigen and to an effector T cell, or to antigen and toxin) has been undertaken. These approaches have all been tested in prostate cancer, but all remain investigational at this point. Considerable difficulties remain with nonspecific binding and the development of human antimouse antibodies. Humanization of antibodies largely prevents the development of human antimouse antibodies and allows repetitive dosing.

Cell-Mediated Immunity

There is considerable evidence, both clinical and preclinical, that tumor-associated antigens can elicit a cell-mediated immune response. In some models, when carcinogen-induced tumors in mice are resected and the mouse is reinoculated with tumor cells, the tumor fails to regrow, suggesting the development of immunity to specific antigens. Specific antigens that are rejected in immunized hosts are termed transplantation antigens. The specificity of tumor rejection has since been demonstrated to reside in T lymphocytes (at a minimum). Lymphocytes of cancer patients can sometimes be stimulated in vitro to recognize specific tumor-associated antigens and consequently demonstrate properties of cytolytic T lymphocytes. Unfortunately, the phenomenon of tumor rejection is by no means universal, either in the laboratory or clinically, and it is unusual to detect cytolytic-T-lymphocyte activity against many tumor-associated antigens.

Nevertheless, there are several clinical scenarios that suggest that cell-mediated antitumor responses exist. These observations have promoted a broad search for the means of enhancing patients' immune responses to tumor-associated antigens. Renal cell carcinoma (RCC) is in many ways the prototypical immune-mediated tumor and, along with melanoma, has until recently been the primary target of immune manipulations. A dramatic example of such an immune-mediated response is the phenomenon of spontaneous regression of metastatic RCC deposits after nephrectomy. While classically this has been described in less than 1% of patients, recent data suggest that the spontaneous regression rate may approach 6–8%. The impact of tumor debulking may also explain why a subset of RCC patients with lymph node or renal vein involvement that undergo resection are seemingly cured. The exact mechanism of this phenomenon is not well understood but may involve elimination of inhibitors of cell-mediated immunity. Indeed, tumor-infiltrating lymphocytes in RCC have been shown to exhibit mutant or faulty T-cell-receptor components, and it is not unreasonable to speculate that involvement in the tumor milieu in some fashion results in "deactivation" of such lymphocytes.

Immunotherapy Involving Cell-Mediated Immunity

Additional evidence of cell-mediated immunity playing a role in tumor rejection lies in the results of a variety of immunotherapeutic interventions. Immunotherapy can be broadly classified as active or passive. This classification refers to the role the host's immune system plays. Thus, the passive transfer of preformed antibodies is contrasted to a vaccination program in which the host's immune system must be capable of mounting an immune response. Adoptive therapy refers to a middle ground in which efforts are made to reconstitute, modify, or bolster one of the effector cells involved ex vivo, followed by reinfusion into the patient, where the rest of the immune cascade must then be recruited.

Active Immunotherapy: Vaccination

Vaccine therapy is a type of active specific immunotherapy. This approach remains experimental, and, while occasional dramatic responses are seen, consistent efficacy is elusive. Autologous vaccination programs (the vaccination of patients with their own tumor cells) have been extensively explored. The advantage of autologous vaccination is that the vaccine bears the antigens of the patient's tumor, although the distinct disadvantage is that not every patient has tumor available for vaccine preparation, and the preparation of each vaccine is tremendously labor-intensive. By contrast, allogeneic vaccines (the use of a generic vaccine or antigen) have the benefit of mass production and ease of use, and the identification of specific tumor rejection antigens allows specific antigenic targeting. However, this approach runs the risk of a more narrow shared antigenic spectrum with the patient's tumor.

Several means exist to undertake vaccination. The simplest is to use intact but inactivated tumor cells. Inactivation can be achieved with UV radiation, external beam (photon) radiation, or freeze-thawing. Crude extracts of cells can also be used. The advantage of using cell extracts is that inactivation is not necessary and small particles and proteins that might be more easily phagocytosed are available. One can also enhance the immunogenicity of inoculated cells by growing the cells in cytokines, coinjecting with cytokines (nonspecific active immunotherapy, described below), or transfecting these cells with the genes for immune stimulatory cytokines or the costimulatory molecule B7. An example of an active immunotherapy trial in a urologic cancer is a current clinical trial under way that uses prostate cancer cell lines transfected with the GM-CSF gene for vaccination in patients with prostate cancer. Purified protein or peptides represent a second potential vaccination schema. In prostate cancer, trials of vaccination with PSMA and PSA are under way. A third way of undertaking specific vaccination is to attempt to bypass the antigen-presenting function of the immune system and to directly stimulate professional antigen-presenting cells, such as dendritic cells, ex vivo. These cells can be stimulated by pulsing them with protein or peptides of interest or by transfecting them with a gene encoding the antigenic peptide of interest before reinfusion. The utility of antigen-pulsed dendritic cells in prostate cancer (the antigens used have included PSMA and PAP) is currently being evaluated but appears promising.

Nonspecific Active Immunotherapy: Cytokines & Biologic Response Modifiers

BCG (bacillus Calmette-Guérin) is a live attenuated form of tubercle bacillus that appears to have local activity against some tumors but has been largely disappointing as systemic therapy. The utility of BCG in the treatment of superficial bladder cancer is well described and is beyond the scope of this chapter. The mechanism by which BCG can elicit a local immune response in the uroepithelium and thereby exhibit impressive anticancer activity is not well delineated. However, possible mechanisms of action include macrophage activation, lymphocyte activation, recruitment of dendritic cells, and natural killer cells. It is intriguing that this is strictly a local phenomenon and that BCG has no role in the treatment of muscle-invasive or metastatic disease.

Interleukin-2 (IL-2) is a naturally occurring cytokine that has multiple immunoregulatory properties. The observation that exogenously administered IL-2 could result in tumor regression in patients with RCC and melanoma was the first unequivocal indication that cancer regression could be mediated by immune manipulations. IL-2 stimulates lymphocyte proliferation, enhances cytolytic-T-cell activity, induces natural killer cell activity, and induces gamma interferon and tumor necrosis factor production. IL-2 has no direct cytotoxicity, but when administered endogenously will activate effector cells of the host immune system, including lymphocytes, natural killer cells, lymphokine-activated killer cells, and tumor-infiltrating lymphocytes. As noted above, in many ways RCC is the prototypical immunologically reactive cancer. The details of immunotherapy for RCC

are beyond the scope of this chapter. Nevertheless, in brief, IL-2 has been administered in RCC in several different schemas, including high-dose intravenous bolus (IL-2 is FDA-approved with this schedule), continuous intravenous infusion, and at lower doses subcutaneously. The high-dose regimens must be administered on an inpatient basis and are characterized by significant, albeit manageable, toxicities, including fever, malaise, vascular leak syndrome, hypotension, and cardiac, renal, and hepatic dysfunction. Subcutaneous IL-2 is self-administered by patients in the outpatient setting, and while clearly less toxic, still has associated malaise and constitutional symptoms. The optimal dosing regimen is not well established, and overall response proportions rarely exceed 20%. Durable complete responses of 5–8% have been reported with some of the high-dose regimens. IL-2 has also been combined with other active agents such as alpha interferon and chemotherapy, although it is not clear if these combinations provide additional benefit.

Alpha interferon is a naturally occurring cytokine that has direct cytotoxic and possibly antiproliferative properties, but also has immunoregulatory properties. It enhances major histocompatibility complex expression, thereby potentially increasing the efficiency of antigen processing and recognition. Alpha interferon has anticancer activity in both RCC and superficial bladder cancer. Its primary toxicity is fever, malaise, and constitutional symptoms, although at higher doses it can result in bone marrow toxicity, central nervous system toxicity, and hepatic toxicity. In RCC, as a single agent, alpha interferon can result in clinical responses in up to 20% of patients. In contradistinction to IL-2 as a single agent, durable complete responses are quite rare. Alpha interferon is also used as an intravesicle treatment in superficial bladder cancer, where it has established activity, and is not infrequently used as second-line therapy after BCG (see Chapter 27).

Adoptive Immunotherapy

Adoptive immunotherapy is the transfer of cellular products (effector cells) to the host or patient in an effort to develop an immune response. The use of adoptive immunotherapy was prompted by the observation that T cells derived from patients with melanoma or RCC had the ability to recognize antigens on the primary tumor. Thus, it was hoped that these cells could be harvested, activated ex vivo, and then reinfused into patients. Lymphokine-activated killer cells and tumor-infiltrating lymphocytes have been used to treat patients with metastatic RCC in the investigational setting, frequently along with IL-2. However, randomized trials comparing IL-2 alone with IL-2 plus cellular products have failed to demonstrate an improvement in response proportions or survival. Chapter 22 gives specific details of immunotherapy in RCC.

REFERENCES

Agarwala SS, Kirkwood JM: Interferons in the treatment of solid tumors. Oncology 1994;51:129.

Anichini A, Fossati G, Parmiani G: Clonal analysis of the cytolytic T-cell response to human tumors. Immunol Today 1987;8:385.

Berd D: Cancer vaccines: Reborn or just recycled? Semin Oncol 1998;25:605.

Berd D, Maguire HC Jr, Mastrangelo MJ: Induction of cell-mediated immunity to autologous melanoma cells and regression of metastases after treatment with a melanoma cell vaccine preceded by cyclophosphamide. Cancer Res 1986;46:2572.

Berd D et al: Treatment of metastatic melanoma with an autologous tumor-cell vaccine: Clinical and immunologic results in 64 patients. J Clin Oncol 1990;11:1858.

Bukowski RM: Natural history and therapy of metastatic renal cell carcinoma: The role of interleukin-2. Cancer 1997;80:1198.

Fyfe G et al: Results of treatment of 255 patients with metastatic RCC who received high-dose recombinant interleukin-2 therapy. J Clin Oncol 1995;13:688.

Gitlitz BJ, Belldegrun A. Figlin R: Immunotherapy and gene therapy. Semin Urol Oncol 1996;14:237.

Goedegebuure PS, Eberlen TJ: Vaccine trials for the clinician: Prospects for viral and non-viral vectors. Oncologist 1997;2:300.

Hewitt H, Blake E, Walder A: A critique of the evidence for active host defense against cancer based on personal studies of 27 murine tumors of spontaneous origin. Br J Cancer 1976;33:241.

Hoover HC Jr et al: Adjuvant active specific immunotherapy for human colorectal cancer: 6.5-year median follow-up of a phase III prospectively randomized trial. J Clin Oncol 1993;11:390.

Hsu FJ, Engleman EG, Levy R: Dendritic cells and their application in immunotherapeutic approaches to cancer therapy. PPO Updates 1997;11:1.

International Germ Cell Cancer Collaborative Group: International germ cell consensus classification: A prognostic factor-based staging system for metastatic germ cell cancers. J Clin Oncol 1997;15:594.

Lamm DL: Long-term results of intravesical therapy for superficial bladder cancer. Urol Clin North Am 1992; 19:573.

Morales A, Nickel JC: Immunotherapy for superficial bladder cancer. Urol Clin North Am 1992;19:549.

Morton DL et al: Prolongation of survival in metastatic after active specific immunotherapy with a new polyvalent melanoma vaccine. Ann Surg 1992;216:463.

Osanto S: Vaccine trials for the clinician: Prospects for tumor antigens. Oncologist 1997;2:284.

Rosenberg SA: New opportunities for the development of cancer immunotherapies. Cancer J 1998;4(Suppl 1):S1.

Rosenberg SA et al: Observations on the systemic administration of autologous lymphokine-activated killer cells and recombinant interleukin-2 to patients with metastatic cancer. N Engl J Med 1985;313:1485.

Rosenberg SA et al: Treatment of 283 consecutive patients with metastatic melanoma or renal cell cancer using high-dose bolus interleukin-2. JAMA 1994; 271:907.

Rosenberg SA et al: Use of tumor-infiltrating lymphocytes and interleukin-2 in the immunotherapy of patients with metastatic melanoma. N Engl J Med 1988; 319:1676.

Schlag P et al: Active specific immunotherapy with Newcastle-disease-virus-modified autologous tumor cells following resection of liver metastases in colorectal cancer. Cancer Immunol Immunother 1992;35:325.

Shepard HM et al: Monoclonal antibody therapy of human cancer: Taking the HER2 protooncogene to the clinic. J Clin Immunol 1991;11:117.

Simons JW, Mikhak B: Ex vivo gene therapy using cytokine-transduced tumor vaccines: Molecular and clinical pharmacology. Semin Oncol 1998;25:661.

Texter JH Jr, Neal CE: The role of monoclonal antibody in the management of prostate adenocarcinoma. J Urol 1998;160:2393.

Vanky F, Klein E: Specificity of auto-tumor cytotoxicity exerted by fresh, activated and propagated human T lymphocytes. Int J Cancer 1982;29:547.

Velders MP, Schreiber H, Kast WM: Active immunization against cancer cells: Impediments and advances. Semin Oncol 1998;25:697.

Urothelial Carcinoma: Cancers of the Bladder, Ureter, & Renal Pelvis

21

Peter R. Carroll, MD

BLADDER CARCINOMAS

Incidence

The male-female ratio for bladder carcinoma is 2.7:1 (7% of new cancer cases occur in men, and 3% in women), and the disease is more common in whites than in blacks. Bladder cancer is the second most common cancer of the genitourinary tract. The average age at diagnosis is 65 years. At that time, approximately 85% are localized to the bladder and 15% have spread to regional lymph nodes or distant sites.

Pathogenesis

A neoplastic change in the urothelium is a multistep phenomenon (Shirai, 1993). An initiator or its metabolite induces an alteration in a single normal cell's DNA, which allows its transformation into a malignant cell. An alteration in the normal transfer of genetic information from DNA to RNA and ultimately to protein formation occurs. Promoters, which are not carcinogenic, bind to receptors on the cell surface to cause already transformed cells to proliferate.

Human bladder cancer initiators or promoters have been identified. Cigarette smoking accounts for 50% and 31% of cases in men and women, respectively (Wynder and Goldsmith, 1977). The association is independent of country, appears to be dose-related, and increases with occupational exposure to certain chemicals (Thompson and Fair, 1990; Mommsen and Aagaard, 1983). The causative agents are thought to be alpha- and beta-naphthylamine, which are secreted into the urine of smokers.

Occupational exposure accounts for 15–35% of cases in men and 1–6% in women (Matanoski and Elliott, 1981). Workers in the chemical, dye, rubber, petroleum, leather, and printing industries are at increased risk. Specific occupational carcinogens include benzidine, beta-naphthylamine, and 4-aminobiphenyl, and the latency period between exposure and tumor development may be prolonged. Patients who have received cyclophosphamide (Cytoxan) for the management of various malignant diseases are

also at increased risk (Fairchild et al, 1979). Ingestion of artificial sweeteners has been proposed to be a risk factor, but several studies have failed to confirm any association (Howe et al, 1977; Najem et al, 1982; Elcock and Morgan, 1993). Physical trauma to the urothelium induced by infection, instrumentation, and calculi increases the risk of malignancy (Hicks, 1982).

The exact genetic events leading to this multistep transformation are unknown, but they are likely to be multiple and may involve the activation of oncogenes and inactivation or loss of cancer suppressor genes (Olumi et al, 1990b). Increased expression of the c-Ha-ras oncogene product, p21, has been noted in high-grade bladder cancers (Viola et al, 1985). Tumor suppressor genes regulate cell proliferation, and the loss or inactivation of both alleles results in unrestrained activity (Knudson, 1985). Because the loss of genetic material on the long arm of chromosome 9 occurs in all grades of bladder carcinoma, this is probably an early event in its development (Olumi et al, 1990a; Dalbagni et al, 1993; Miyao et al, 1993). In contrast, deletion of material from the short arms of chromosomes 11 and 17 is more common in high-grade neoplasms, suggesting that loss of suppressor genes in these locations is associated with tumor progression. The nuclear phosphoprotein p53 is encoded by the gene often deleted along chromosome 17, and a mutation of p53 commonly occurs in colon and bladder cancers (Sidransky et al, 1991; Miyao et al, 1993). (See Molecular Markers.)

Although little is known regarding the histologic changes in the urothelium that accompany neoplastic transformation, considerable information has been gained with animal models (Soloway and Hardeman, 1990). Exposure of rodents to the compound N-[(4-(5-nitro-2-furyl)-2-thiazoy]-formamide (FANFT) induces bladder cancers in a large number. The earliest change identified is urothelial hyperplasia, an increase in the number of cell layers. Polarity and differentiation are maintained. Similar proliferative changes in human urothelium include cystitis cystica and Von Brunn's nests, an outpocketing of epithelium into the lamina propria. Examination of the rodent bladder at a later time may show metaplastic changes, transformation of transitional cell epithelium into mature glandular, tubular, or squamous epithelium. In the animal model, dysplasia and neoplasia may follow. Although such a process occurs in at least some human tumors, it must be remembered that cancers may be derived from normal, hyperplastic, or metaplastic epithelium.

Once neoplastic change has occurred, the cancer may remain superficial or progress to invasive or metastatic disease. The exact nature of events responsible for tumor progression is unknown, but a 3-step theory of invasion has been proposed (Liotta, 1986). Initially, the tumor cell must bind the basement membrane. The laminin receptor is a cell-surface protein that binds to laminin, a glycoprotein component of the basement membrane. The number of laminin receptors is greater along the surface of invasive tumor cells than noninvasive cells (Wewer et al, 1986). Once tumor cells have bound to the basement membrane, degradation of the membrane is facilitated by the production of proteases such as type IV collagenase. Tumor progression is completed in those cells that secrete cytokines, the autocrine motility factors that induce cell motility and allow for invasion and eventual metastasis. Indeed, the concentration of autocrine motility factor is higher in the urine of patients with invasive tumors than of those with superficial tumors (Guirguis et al, 1988).

Staging

Two staging systems for bladder cancer are currently in widespread use. One proposed initially by Jewett and Strong (1946) was based on the relationship of the depth of tumor penetration into the bladder wall with the incidence of lymph node or distant metastases. Whereas submucosal (stage A) or muscular invasion (stage B) had a low incidence of metastases (0 and 13%), perivesical tumor infiltration had a high incidence (87%). Marshall modified this system in 1952 to allow segregation of superficial tumors invading the lamina propria (stage A) from those confined to the mucosa (stage 0) and to include lymph node metastases (stage D1) and distant metastases (stage D2) as separate stages (Marshall, 1952). The Union Internationale Centre le Cancer (UICC) recommended a staging system that allows a precise and simultaneous description of the primary tumor (T stage), the status of lymph nodes (N stage), and metastatic sites (M stage). The 2 staging systems are compared in Figure 21–1. Although either provides a reasonable estimate of a given tumor's biologic potential and the need for and type of treatment, significant staging errors exist when one compares the clinical stage (that based on physical examination and imaging) with the pathologic stage (that based on removal of the bladder and regional lymph nodes). Overstaging is relatively uncommon, but clinical understaging occurs in up to 53% of patients (Skinner, 1977; Skinner et al, 1982).

Histopathology

Ninety-eight percent of all bladder cancers are epithelial malignancies, with the majority being transitional cell carcinomas.

A. Normal Urothelium: The normal urothelium is composed of 3–7 layers of transitional cell epithelium resting on a basement membrane composed of extracellular matrix (collagen, adhesive glycoproteins, glycosaminoglycans) (Figure 21–2A). The epithelial cells vary in appearance: the basal cells are actively proliferating cells resting on the basement membrane; the luminal cells, perhaps the most important feature of a normal bladder epithelium, are larger umbrellalike cells that are bound together by tight junctions. Beyond the basement membrane is loose connective tissue, the lamina propria, in which occasionally smooth-muscle fibers can be identified. These fibers should be distinguished from deeper, more extensive muscle elements defining the true muscularis propria. The muscle wall of the bladder is composed of muscle bundles coursing in multiple directions. As these converge near the bladder neck, 3 layers can be recognized: inner and outer longitudinally oriented layers and a middle, circularly oriented layer.

B. Papilloma: The World Health Organization recognizes a papilloma as a papillary tumor with a fine fibrovascular stalk supporting an epithelial layer of normal transitional cells maintaining polarity. Papillomas are uncommon, accounting for approximately 2% of all transitional cell tumors (Friedell et al, 1976). The prognosis is very favorable: only a small number, approximately 16%, progress to higher grade cancers (Lerman, Hutter, and Whitmore, 1970).

C. Transitional Cell Carcinoma: Approximately 90% of all bladder cancers are transitional cell carcinomas. These tumors most commonly appear as papillary, exophytic lesions (Figure 21–2B); less commonly, they may be sessile or ulcerated. Whereas the former group are usually superficial in nature, sessile growths are often invasive. The World Health Organization has proposed that transitional cell carcinomas be divided into 3 grades on the basis of urothelial architecture; cell size, pleomorphism, nuclear polarization, and hyperchromatism; and the number of mitoses present (Mostofi, Sorbin, and Torloni, 1973).

Carcinoma in situ (CIS) is recognizable as flat, nonpapillary anaplastic epithelium. The urothelium lacks the normal cellular polarity, and cells are large and have prominent nucleoli (Figure 21–2C). Carcinoma in situ may occur either close to or remote from an exophytic lesion or, rarely, it may occur as focal or diffuse lesions in a patient without macroscopic tumors. It has a variable natural history, but many cases progress to invasive disease. In addition, exophytic lesions occurring with CIS are more likely to recur and invade.

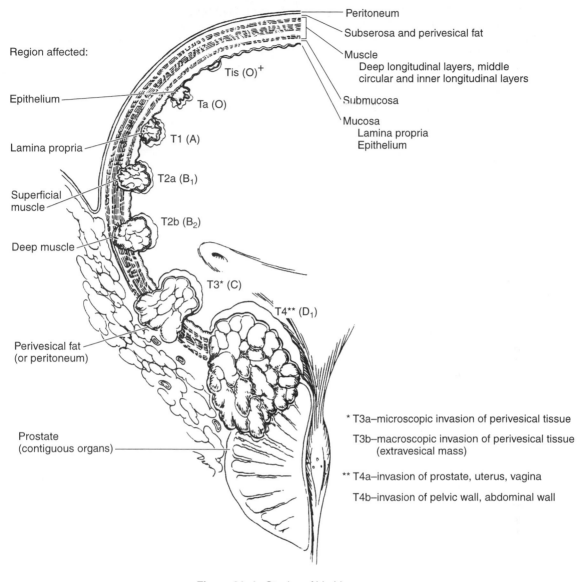

Figure 21–1. Staging of bladder cancer.

The frequency of tumor invasion, recurrence, and progression is strongly correlated with tumor grade: progression is noted in 10–20% of grade 1 tumors, 19–37% of grade 2, and 33–67% of grade 3 (Lutzeyer, Rubben, and Dahm, 1982; Torti et al, 1987). Survival rates are similarly affected. Whereas patients with low-grade tumors have an excellent 10-year survival (98%), those with high-grade tumors have a reduced survival (35%) (Jordan, Weingarten, and Murphy, 1987).

D. Nontransitional Cell Carcinomas:

1. Adenocarcinoma–Adenocarcinomas account for less than 2% of all bladder cancers. Primary adenocarcinomas of the bladder may be preceded by

cystitis and metaplasia. Histologically, adenocarcinomas are mucus-secreting and may have glandular, colloid, or signet-ring patterns. Whereas primary adenocarcinomas often arise along the floor of the bladder, adenocarcinomas arising from the urachus occur at the dome. Both tumor types are often localized at the time of diagnosis, but muscle invasion is usually present. Five-year survival is usually less than 40%, despite aggressive surgical management (Kramer et al, 1979; Malek, Rosen, and O'Dea, 1983; Abenoza, Manivel, and Fraley, 1987; Bernstein et al, 1988).

2. Squamous cell carcinoma–Squamous cell carcinoma accounts for between 5 and 10% of all

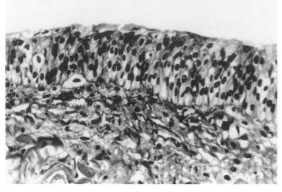

A

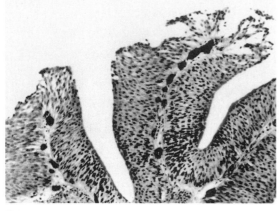

B

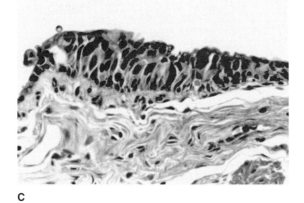

C

Figure 21–2. A: Normal urothelium (125×). **B:** Moderately well-differentiated, papillary bladder cancer (60×).

bladder cancers in the United States and is often associated here with a history of chronic infection, vesical calculi, or chronic catheter use. It may also be associated with bilharzial infection owing to *Schistosoma haematobium,* because squamous cell carcinoma accounts for approximately 60% of all bladder cancers in Egypt, parts of Africa, and the Middle East, where this infection is prevalent (El-Bolkainy et al, 1981). These tumors are often nodular and invasive at the time of diagnosis. Histologically they appear as poorly differentiated neoplasms composed of polygonal cells with characteristic intercellular bridges. Keratinizing epithelium is present, although often in small amounts.

3. Undifferentiated carcinomas–Undifferentiated bladder carcinomas, which are rare (accounting for less than 2%), have no mature epithelial elements. A small-cell type has been described, which histologically resembles similar lesions of the lung (Mills et al, 1987).

4. Mixed carcinoma–Mixed carcinomas constitute 4–6% of all bladder cancers and are composed of a combination of transitional, glandular, squamous, or undifferentiated patterns. The most common type comprises transitional and squamous cell elements (Murphy, 1989). Most mixed carcinomas are large and infiltrating at the time of diagnosis.

E. Rare Epithelial and Nonepithelial Cancers: Rare epithelial carcinomas identified in the bladder include villous adenomas, carcinoid tumors, carcinosarcomas, and melanomas. Rare nonepithelial cancers of the urinary bladder include pheochromocytomas, lymphomas, choriocarcinomas, and various mesenchymal tumors (hemangioma, osteogenic sarcoma, and myosarcoma) (Murphy, 1989). Cancers of the prostate, cervix, and rectum may involve the bladder by direct extension. The most common tumors metastatic to the bladder include (in order of incidence) melanoma, lymphoma, stomach, breast, kidney, and lung (Murphy, 1989; Goldstein, 1967).

Clinical Findings

A. Symptoms:

Hematuria is the presenting symptom in 85–90% of patients with bladder cancer. It may be gross or microscopic, intermittent rather than constant. In a smaller percentage of patients, it is accompanied by symptoms of vesical irritability: frequency, urgency, and dysuria. Irritative voiding symptoms seem to be more common in patients with diffuse CIS (Farrow et al, 1977). Symptoms of advanced disease include bone pain from bone metastases or flank pain from retroperitoneal metastases or ureteral obstruction.

B. Signs: The majority of patients with bladder cancer have no pertinent physical signs, owing to the superficial nature of their disease. However, patients with large-volume or invasive tumors may be found to have bladder wall thickening or a palpable mass—

findings that may be detected on a careful bimanual examination under anesthesia. Masses palpable before transurethral resection but not identifiable thereafter are most often either very large superficial lesions or tumors that have penetrated the more superficial layers of the bladder wall (ie, T2–3a). Those that remain palpable are often locally extensive (> T3a). Tumors that are movable anteroposteriorly are classified as a lower stage than T3b, whereas those that are fixed or are invading contiguous organs (rectum, prostate, vagina) are considered to be stage T4.

Hepatomegaly and supraclavicular lymphadenopathy are signs of metastatic disease. Lymphedema from occlusive pelvic lymphadenopathy may be seen occasionally.

C. Laboratory Findings:

1. Routine testing–The most common laboratory abnormality is hematuria. It may be accompanied by pyuria, which on occasion may result from concomitant urinary tract infection. Azotemia may be noted in patients with ureteral occlusion owing to the primary bladder tumor or lymphadenopathy. Anemia may be a presenting symptom owing to chronic blood loss, or replacement of the bone marrow with metastatic disease.

2. Urinary cytology and flow cytometry–Exfoliated cells from both normal and neoplastic urothelium can be readily identified in voided urine. Larger quantities of cells can be obtained by gently irrigating the bladder with isotonic saline solution through a catheter or cystoscope. Examination of cytologic specimens obtained in either fashion allows for tumor detection either at the time of initial presentation or during follow-up. Cytologic examination of exfoliated cells may be especially useful in screening high-risk populations and assessing response to treatment. Detection rates vary depending on the adequacy of the specimen and the grade and volume of the tumor.

Cytologic preparations are made by fixing exfoliated cells, placing them on glass slides, and staining them. High-grade and infiltrating carcinomas are commonly detected, but low-grade or superficial carcinomas may be missed. Because the majority of bladder cancers will possess at least one cell population with an increased DNA content, many institutions have examined exfoliated urothelial cells with flow cytometry (Traganos, 1984; Wheeless et al, 1993). Exfoliated cells are collected, centrifuged, passed through a sieve to remove tissue fragments, and stained with DNA-binding dyes. The cells are processed by a flow cytometer, which measures emission at specific wavelengths for each cell. Cell populations may be negative, suspicious, or positive for cancer, depending on the presence of aneuploidy and degree of hyperdiploidy. Flow cytometry detects approximately 80% of all bladder cancers (Badalament et al, 1988). As in cytologic study, the detection

rates are better for lesions of higher grade and stage: Papillomas are detected in only 50% of patients; Ta, Tis, and invasive lesions are detected in approximately 82%, 89%, and 90% of patients, respectively. The specificity of flow cytometry may be improved by enriching the proportion of urothelial cells in the sample by using monoclonal antibodies that recognize urothelial cells (Wheeless et al, 1991). Contaminating inflammatory cells are excluded from analysis. Both flow cytometry and cytology can be used to detect recurrence in patients with a previous history of bladder cancer and to monitor response to intravesical chemotherapy or irradiation (Badalament et al, 1986; Klein et al, 1982; Klein, Whitmore, and Wolf, 1983).

3. Other markers–The sensitivity of voided urine cytologic tests depends on a variety of factors, including the number of urine specimens examined, the stage and grade of the bladder tumor, and the expertise of the cytopathologist. Consequently, newer tests that are also performed on voided urine specimens are currently being developed and validated to determine their ability to reliably predict the presence of bladder cancer. These tests include the BTA test (Bard Urological, Covington, GA), the BTA stat test (Bard Diagnostic Sciences, Inc, Redmond, WA), the BTA TRAK assay (Bard Diagnostic Sciences, Inc), determination of urinary nuclear matrix protein (NMP22; Matritech Inc, Newton, MA), quantification of urinary fibrinogen/fibrin degradation products (AuraTek FDP; PerImmune Inc, Rockville, MD), identification of the Lewis X antigen on exfoliated urothelial cells, and the determination of telomerase activity in exfoliated cells. Several studies have examined the performance of these voided urinary markers for the detection and follow-up of patients with bladder cancer (Ellis et al, 1997; Johnston et al, 1997; Van der Poel et al, 1998; Soloway et al, 1996; Ianari et al, 1997; Yoshida et al, 1997; Landman et al, 1998; Planz et al, 1998; Stampfer et al, 1998; Wiener et al, 1998; Pode et al, 1999; Zippe et al, 1999) (Table 21–1).

Most of the studies performed to date have evaluated these voided markers in patients with known bladder cancer, either primary or recurrent, and have compared the results with those obtained in a control group without bladder cancer. Although these tests may, in many clinical situations, complement traditional evaluation and surveillance techniques, more information on their performance is needed before they are performed routinely. Such exfoliated markers, if they prove to be both specific and sensitive, may play an important role in the initial evaluation and follow-up of patients with bladder cancer. In addition to enhancing the detection of bladder cancer, such tests may give important information on the natural history of the bladder cancer detected.

The loss of blood group antigens may correlate with bladder cancer stage and risk of progression.

Table 21–1. Exfoliated markers for the detection of bladder cancer.

Marker	Number of Studies	Sensitivity (%)	Specifity (%)	PPV (%)	NPV (%)
BTA	8	28–65	73–96	33–80	52–94
NMP22	6	48–100	61–85	29–58	66–100
BTA stat	2	57–67	33–95	20–56	70–95
BTA TRAK	1	72	73		
Lewis X antigen	3	80–97	73–86	72–81	83–98
Telomerase	2	62–80	80–96	84	89

PPV, positive predictive value; NPV, negative predictive value.

Fradet and colleagues (1990) identified a set of bladder carcinoma cell antigens detected by monoclonal antibodies whose expression correlates not only with tumor stage, but also with progression rates.

D. Imaging: Although bladder cancers may be detected by various imaging techniques, their presence is confirmed by cystoscopy and biopsy. Imaging is therefore used to evaluate the upper urinary tract and, when infiltrating bladder tumors are detected, to assess the depth of muscle wall infiltration and the presence of regional or distant metastases (See and Fuller, 1992). Intravenous urography remains the most common imaging test for the evaluation of hematuria. Bladder tumors may be recognized as pedunculated, radiolucent filling defects projecting into the lumen (Figure 21–3); nonpapillary, infiltrating tumors may result in fixation or flattening of the bladder wall. Hydronephrosis from ureteral obstruction is usually associated with deeply infiltrating lesions (Hatch and Barry, 1986).

Abdominal or endovesical ultrasound may also detect bladder tumors and upper urinary tract abnormalities (Singer, Itzchak, and Fiselovitch, 1981; Schuller et al, 1982). The bladder is examined when full, and tumors appear as echogenic foci projecting into the lumen. Bladder wall invasion is recognized when the normal bladder wall, which is intensely echogenic, is interrupted by less echogenic tumor tissue. Although transurethral ultrasound may be more accurate than abdominal ultrasound, it is invasive and may give little more information than that gained by cystoscopy and transurethral resection.

Superficial (Ta, Tis) bladder cancers staged with a properly performed transurethral resection and examination under anesthesia do not require additional imaging of the bladder or pelvic organs. However, higher stage lesions are often understaged, and the addition of imaging may be useful. Both computed tomography (CT) and magnetic resonance imaging (MRI) (Figure 21–4) have been used to characterize the extent of bladder wall invasion and detect enlarged pelvic lymph nodes, with overall staging accuracy ranging from 40% to 85% for CT and from 50% to 90% for MRI (Amendola et al, 1986; Koss et al, 1981; Fisher, Hricak, and Tanagho,

1985; Husband et al, 1989; Wood et al, 1988). Magnetic resonance imaging offers several potential advantages over CT: Neoplastic tissue may be better differentiated from normal bladder wall; scanning in multiple planes is possible; lymph nodes may be better differentiated from blood vessels; and intravenous contrast is not necessary. However, motion artifacts may make scans uninterpretable; patients may become claustrophobic; and patients with pacemakers, intracranial vascular clips, and other metallic implants may be ineligible for MRI. Neither technique can reliably distinguish Ta from T1 or T2 from T3a tumors.

The main advantage of both CT and MRI is in distinguishing organ-confined disease from extravesical extension. Both techniques rely on size criteria for the detection of lymphadenopathy: Lymph nodes larger than 1 cm are thought to be suggestive of metastases; unfortunately, small-volume pelvic lymph node metastases are often missed. Because invasive bladder cancers may metastasize to the lung or bones, staging of advanced lesions is completed with chest x-ray and radionuclide bone scan.

E. Cystourethroscopy and Tumor Resection: The diagnosis and initial staging of bladder cancers is made by cystoscopy and transurethral resection. Cystoscopy can be done with either flexible or rigid instruments, although the former may be associated with less discomfort. For either, topical anesthetic solutions are injected directly into the urethra. Superficial, low-grade tumors usually appear as single or multiple papillary lesions; most measure less than 3 cm in diameter. Higher grade lesions are larger and sessile. Carcinoma in situ may appear as flat areas of erythema and mucosal irregularity.

Once a tumor is visualized or suspected, the patient is scheduled for examination under anesthesia and transurethral resection or biopsy of the suspicious lesion. The objectives are tumor diagnosis, assessment of the degree of bladder wall invasion (staging), and complete excision of the low-stage lesions amenable to such treatment.

Patients are placed in the lithotomy position. Before instrumentation is begun, a bladder wash com-

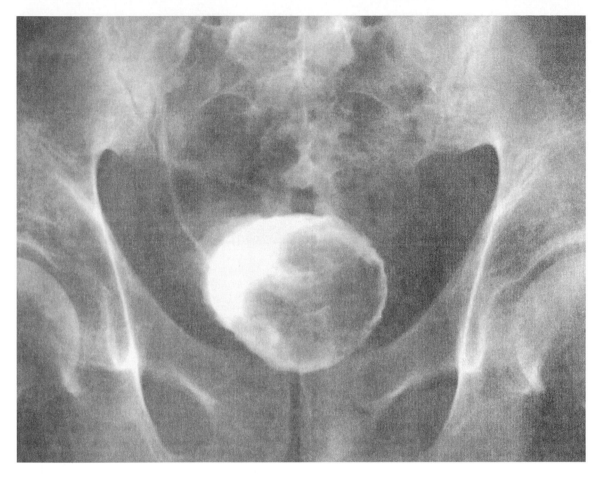

Figure 21–3. Image of the urinary bladder obtained on an intravenous urogram. The filling defect represents a papillary bladder cancer.

monly is obtained to allow for cytologic examination of exfoliated cells. A careful bimanual examination is then performed. The presence, position, and size of any mass are noted, along with any degree of fixation to contiguous structures. Cystoscopy is repeated with a lens that permits complete visualization of the entire bladder surface. A resectoscope is then placed into the bladder, and visible tumors are removed by electrocautery. Suspicious areas may be biopsied with cup biopsy forceps and the areas cauterized with an electrode. Some clinicians routinely perform random bladder biopsies of normal-appearing urothelium both close to and remote from the tumor. Others believe that disruption of the urothelium may promote implantation of tumor cells floating in the bladder at the time of tumor resection (Hicks, 1982). Although detection of dysplasia or CIS occurs in up to 65% of selected patients, probably less than 15% of all patients with initial bladder tumors have such lesions (Althausen, Prout, and Dal, 1976; Wallace et al, 1979; Wolf and Hojgaard, 1983). Those who do

are at a greater risk of both recurrence and progression to a higher stage.

Natural History & Selection of Treatment

A. Standard Histopathological Assessment: The natural history of bladder cancers is defined by 2 separate but related processes: tumor recurrence and progression. Progression, including metastasis, represents the greater biologic risk. However, recurrence, even without progression, represents substantial patient morbidity in that it requires periodic reevaluation (cytology, cystoscopy, etc), repeat endoscopic ablation, and often intravesical chemotherapy (which may be costly, uncomfortable, and associated with complications). Treatment decisions are made after tumor staging has been completed. Such decisions are based variously on tumor stage (TNM), grade, size, multiplicity, and recurrence pattern (Table 21–2).

At initial presentation, approximately 50–70% of

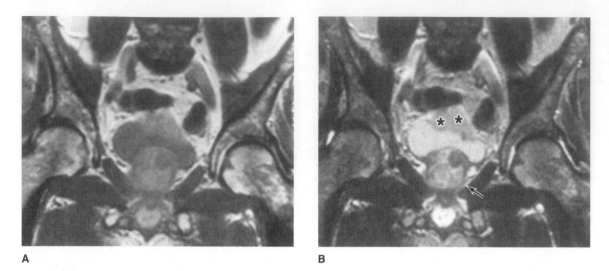

A   **B**

Figure 21–4. MRI scan of invasive bladder carcinoma: **Left:** T1-weighted image; **Right:** T2-weighted image. Bladder wall invasion is best assessed on T2-weighted images because of heightened contrast between tumor (asterisks) and detrusor muscle along with ability to detect interruption of the thin high-intensity line representing normal bladder wall. The heterogeneous appearance of the prostate (arrow) on the T2-weighted image owes to benign prostatic hypertrophy, confirmed at cystectomy.

bladder tumors are superficial—stage Tis or Ta (Cutler, Heney, and Friedell, 1982). Invasion into the lamina propria or muscle wall is identified in a smaller number of patients, approximately 28% and 24%, respectively; regional or distant metastases are found in approximately 15%. Unfortunately, 80% of

Table 21–2. Initial treatment options for bladder cancers.

Cancer Stage	Initial Treatment Options
Tis	Complete TUR followed by intravesical BCG
Ta (single, low-to-moderate grade, not recurrent)	Complete TUR
Ta (large, multiple, high-grade, or recurrent)	Complete TUR followed by intravesical chemo- or immunotherapy
T1	Complete TUR followed by intravesical chemo- or immunotherapy
T2–T4	Radical cystectomy Neoadjuvant chemotherapy followed by radical cystectomy Radical cystectomy followed by adjuvant chemotherapy Neoadjuvant chemotherapy followed by concomitant chemotherapy and irradiation
Any T, N+, M+	Systemic chemotherapy followed by selective surgery or irradiation

TUR, transurethral resection.

patients with invasive or metastatic disease have no previous history of bladder cancer (Brawn, 1982; Kaye and Lange, 1982). Bladder carcinomas also may be stratified at the time of initial presentation on the basis of grade: Approximately 43% of tumors are classified as grade I; 25% grade II; and 32% grade III (Gilbert et al, 1978). There are strong correlations between tumor grade and stage and tumor recurrence, progression, and survival (Frazier et al, 1993). Whereas survival is excellent for patients with superficial disease (PO, PI, PIS, 81%), it falls substantially for patients with P2 (53%), P3 (39%), and P4 (25%) tumors (Skinner et al, 1982; Frazier et al, 1993; Thrasher et al, 1994)—owing to the greater likelihood of metastasis in tumors of higher stage. Whereas lymph node metastases are uncommon (5%) in tumors of low stage, they are increasingly more common in P3A, P3B, and P4 tumors: 10–30%, 31–35%, and 35–64%, respectively (Skinner et al, 1982; Frazier et al, 1993). In patients with organ-confined disease, the presence of pelvic lymph node metastases appears to be the most important prognostic factor (Vieweg et al, 1999).

Although metastasis is less common with superficial bladder cancers, such tumors may progress; the majority recur and require additional treatment. Stratification of superficial disease into different grades and stages (Ta and T1) is of clinical benefit, because progression and recurrence are related to both. Tumor progression occurs in less than 6% of patients with Ta disease, but in up to 46% of those with T1 disease (Heney et al, 1983; Pauwels et al, 1988; Abel et al, 1988). It occurs in 10–20% of patients with grade I tumors, 19–37% with grade II tumors, and 33–64% with grade III tumors (Torti et al, 1987; Lutzeyer, Rubben, and Dahm, 1982).

Tumor recurrence is related to grade, number, size, and history of disease. It is more common in the first 12 months after diagnosis (but can become manifest many years later), and patients with one recurrence are more likely to have another. Patients with T1, multiple (> 4), large (> 5 cm), or high-grade tumors are at greater risk, as are those with either CIS or severe dysplasia in normal-appearing urothelium remote from the tumor site (Heney et al, 1983; Wolf, Olsen, and Hojgaard, 1985).

B. Molecular Markers: Conventional histopathologic analysis of bladder tumors, including determination of tumor grade and stage, may not reliably predict the behavior of many bladder cancers. Assessment of molecular markers of disease, most often with immunohistochemical methods, may complement traditional assessment of cancer stage and grade and better predict outcome. Some markers may be assessed in biopsy specimens, whereas others may be prognostic only when evaluating cystectomy specimens.

Blood group–related antigens are a group of carbohydrate determinants that are present on membrane lipids and proteins (Newman et al, 1980). These antigens, including the ABH and Lewis antigens ($Le^{a,b,x,y}$) on the cell surface of erythrocytes, have been identified on various epithelial tissues, including transitional urothelium. Loss of ABH antigens has been associated with increased recurrence rates and progression to muscle invasive disease for patients with superficial bladder cancer (Weinstein et al, 1979). However, the secretory status of the individual must be considered when interpreting blood group antigen status. Although the majority of normal urothelium is rich in A, B, H, Le^b, and Le^y blood group antigens (secretors), 20% of individuals with normal urothelium lack expression of these antigens (nonsecretors). Thus, loss of ABH antigen expression can be reliably determined only in secretory individuals. Similarly, the related Lewis antigens ($Le^{a,b,x,y}$) are absent in 20% of patients with normal urothelium, limiting their prognostic application. Immunohistochemical evaluation of Le^x on fresh frozen and formalin-fixed bladder tissues have demonstrated that most tumors (90%) express this blood group antigen, whereas only an occasional umbrella cell of normal urothelium will express this antigen. Not only may evaluation of Le^x antigen expression on exfoliated bladder cells enhance the detection of bladder cancer, but Le^x may also be a useful clinical marker in predicting tumor recurrence or progression in patients with superficial bladder cancer.

Tumor growth and metastasis require the growth of new blood vessels, a process called angiogenesis. New vessel growth is tightly regulated by both an-

giogenic stimulators, such as the fibroblastic growth factors and vascular endothelial growth factor, and angiogenic inhibitors, such as thrombospondin-1 and angiostatin. Immunohistochemical methods have been developed for quantification of angiogenesis in a given tumor by measuring microvessel density. Microvessel density is a useful prognostic indicator for a variety of human malignancies, including bladder cancer. In bladder cancer, microvessel density has been associated with lymph node metastases, disease progression, and overall survival in patients with invasive bladder cancer treated with radical cystectomy (Dickinson et al, 1994; Jaeger et al, 1995; Bochner et al, 1997). Furthermore, immunohistochemical expression of thrombospondin-1 has been reported to be significantly associated with both tumor recurrence and overall survival (Grossfeld et al, 1997).

Normal cellular proliferation is the result of an orderly progression through the cell cycle, whereas malignancy is characterized by uncontrolled cell growth. Cell cycle–associated protein complexes composed of cyclins and cyclin-dependent kinases tightly regulate this progression. These protein complexes phosphorylate key proteins involved in cell cycle transition points, including the protein encoded by the retinoblastoma (pRB) and p53 genes. Loss of cell cycle control may be an early step in the development of carcinogenesis. The most extensively characterized molecular marker in patients with invasive bladder cancer is p53 expression. The p53 gene is a tumor suppressor gene that plays a key role in the regulation of the cell cycle. When DNA damage occurs, the level of p53 protein increases, causing cell cycle arrest and repair of DNA. Mutations in the p53 gene result in the production of an abnormal protein product, allowing cells with damaged DNA to continue through the cell cycle. The altered p53 protein has a prolonged half-life compared with the wild-type protein, allowing for its detection by immunohistochemical techniques. Increased p53 immunoreactivity has been found in high-grade and high-stage bladder cancers, and it is associated with disease progression and decreased overall and disease-specific survival. Patients with altered p53 expression (indicating possible mutation of the p53 gene) appear to have an increased risk for disease recurrence and a decreased overall survival when compared with patients with normal p53 expression (Esrig et al, 1995). pT1, pT2, and P3a cancers that are p53 positive are associated with recurrence rates of 62%, 56%, and 80%, respectively, compared with 7%, 12%, and 11% for cancers without p53 reactivity. This information has recently led to a clinical trial in which patients are assigned to adjuvant treatment after radical cystectomy based on the p53 status of their tumor. Assessment of p21, another cell cycle protein, may complement knowledge gained from assessment of p53 expression (Stein et al, 1998).

The retinoblastoma (Rb) gene, a tumor suppressor gene, is expressed in a number of human tumors, including transitional cell carcinoma of the bladder. Rb alteration, as determined by immunohistochemical methods, is associated with high-grade, high-stage bladder cancers. In addition, Rb alteration appears to be significantly associated with decreased overall survival in such patients (Cordon-Cardo et al, 1992; Logothetis et al, 1992). Studies in which both p53 and Rb have been examined in patients with invasive bladder cancer suggest that bladder tumors with alterations in both genes have a poorer prognosis and decreased overall survival when compared with tumors with wild-type p53 and Rb. Tumors with an alteration of only one of these genes behave in an intermediate fashion.

Other markers that may correlate with outcome in patients with bladder cancer include assessment of tumor growth fraction (proliferative index) and cellular adhesion molecule expression (E-cadherin) (Okamura et al, 1990; Lipponen and Eskelinen, 1995).

C. Treatment Selection: Patients with superficial bladder cancers can be treated with transurethral resection followed by selective intravesical chemotherapy. Patients with initial low-grade, small tumors are at low risk of progression and may be treated by transurethral resection alone followed by surveillance. Patients with T1, multiple, large, recurrent tumors or those associated with CIS in remote bladder biopsies are at a higher risk of progression and recurrence and should be considered candidates for intravesical chemotherapy after complete and careful transurethral resection. Management of T1 tumors is somewhat controversial; some clinicians advise radical cystectomy, especially for grade III lesions, which are associated with a high rate of progression. However, progression rates can be reduced by intravesical chemotherapy (Herr et al, 1989; Cookson and Sarosdy, 1992). Recurrence of T1 disease after a trial of intravesical therapy warrants more aggressive therapy (Herr, 1991).

Patients with more invasive, but still localized, tumors (T2, T3) are candidates for more aggressive local treatment, including partial or radical cystectomy, irradiation, or a combination of either irradiation or surgery and systemic chemotherapy. (It has been suggested that selected patients with stage T2 disease may be treated adequately with transurethral resection alone. However, this mode of treatment leaves residual disease in most patients [Henry et al, 1988; Herr, 1988; Solsona et al, 1998].) Superficial ductal or acinar in situ carcinoma of the prostatic urethra, not invading the basement membrane or prostatic stroma, may be treated with transurethral resection and intravesical chemotherapy rather than cystectomy (Bretton et al, 1989). However, patients with more extensive involvement of the prostatic urethra by transitional cell carcinomas require more aggressive therapy (Schellhammer, Bean, and Whitmore,

1977). Patients with unresectable local tumors (T4B) are candidates for either systemic or, more rarely, intra-arterial chemotherapy, followed by irradiation or surgery. Patients with either local or distant metastases should receive systemic chemotherapy followed by the selective use of either irradiation or surgery, depending on the response.

Treatment

A. Intravesical Chemotherapy: In the majority of patients with superficial bladder cancer, tumors recur. Because a certain percentage of these are of higher stage or grade, attempts to reduce recurrence should be undertaken.

Immuno- or chemotherapeutic agents can be instilled into the bladder directly via catheter, thereby avoiding the morbidity of systemic administration in most cases. Intravesical therapy can have a prophylactic or therapeutic objective, either to reduce recurrence in patients whose tumors have been completely resected or to eradicate existing disease in patients whose superficial tumors are so extensive that complete transurethral resection is not possible. Therefore, intravesical chemotherapy or immunotherapy may be delivered in 3 different fashions to achieve individual goals (Table 21–3). Considerable experience has been gained, but comparison of different agents is difficult owing to the paucity of randomized trials and variations in dose, contact time, patient population, and intervals between treatments. Most agents are administered weekly for 6 weeks. Maintenance therapy (ie, monthly or bimonthly intravesical therapy) may decrease recurrence rates further. Although local toxicity is relatively common—primarily irritative voiding symptoms—systemic toxicity is rare because of the limited absorption of drugs across the lumen of the bladder. Severe systemic complications can be avoided by not administering intravesical chemotherapy in patients with gross hematuria. Efficacy may be improved by increasing contact time and drug concentration, ie, by restricting fluid intake before administration, asking the patient to lie in different positions during treatment, avoiding instillation of air during drug administration, and requiring the patient to avoid urinating for 1–2 h thereafter. The most common agents in the United States are mitomycin C, thiotepa, doxorubicin, and bacillus Calmette-Guérin. Patients in whom treatment with one agent fails may respond to another.

1. Mitomycin C–Mitomycin C (MMC) is an antitumor, antibiotic, alkylating agent that inhibits DNA synthesis. With a molecular weight of 329, systemic absorption is minimal. Between 39 and 78% of patients with residual tumor experience a complete response to intravesical MMC (Kowalkowski and Lamm, 1988), and recurrence is reduced in 2–33% after complete transurethral resection (Herr, Laudone, and Whitmore, 1987). Side effects are

Table 21–3. Delivery of intravesical chemotherapy or immunotherapy.

Use	Timing	Goal
Adjunctive	At TUR	Prevent implantation
Prophylactic	After complete TUR	Prevent or delay recurrence or progression
Therapeutic	After incomplete TUR	Cure residual disease

TUR, transurethral resection.

noted in 10–43% and consist largely of irritative voiding symptoms including urinary frequency, urgency, and dysuria (Soloway, 1989). Unique to this drug is the appearance of a rash on the palms and genitalia in approximately 6%, but this effect can be alleviated if patients wash their hands and genitalia at the time of voiding after intravesical administration.

2. Thiotepa–Thiotepa is an alkylating agent with a molecular weight of 189. Although various doses have been used, 30 mg weekly seems to be sufficient. Up to 55% of patients respond completely. Most series show significantly lower recurrence rates in patients taking thiotepa than in those taking a placebo (Herr, Laudone, and Whitmore, 1987; Kowalkowski and Lamm, 1988; Prout et al, 1983). Cystitis is not uncommon after instillation but is usually mild and self-limited. Myelosuppression manifested as leukopenia and thrombocytopenia occurs in up to 9% of patients owing to systemic absorption. A complete blood count should be obtained in all patients before successive instillations.

3. Doxorubicin–Doxorubicin is an intercalating agent of high molecular weight (580). Complete response rates vary among series, with a mean of 38% (Kowalkowski and Lamm, 1988). As a prophylactic agent, the benefit of intravesical administration ranges from 10 to 23% (Herr, Laudone, and Whitmore, 1987). Cystitis is not uncommon, but systemic toxicity is rare.

4. Bacillus Calmette-Guérin (BCG)–Bacillus Calmette-Guérin (BCG) is an attenuated strain of *Mycobacterium bovis*. Many different strains of BCG exist, and the marketed preparations vary in the number, pathogenicity, viability, and immunogenicity of organisms (Catalona and Ratliff, 1990). The exact mechanism by which BCG exerts its antitumor effect is unknown, but it seems to be immunologically mediated. Mucosal ulceration and granuloma formation are commonly seen after intravesical instillation. Activated helper T lymphocytes can be identified in the granulomas, and interleukin-2 reportedly can be detected in the urine of treated patients (Haaf, Catalona, and Ratliff, 1986). BCG has been shown to be very effective both therapeutically and prophylactically. BCG appears to be the most efficacious intravesical agent for the management of CIS. Complete responses are recorded in 36–71% of patients with residual carcinoma (Herr, Laudone, and Whitmore, 1987; Catalona and Ratliff, 1990); recurrence rates

are reduced substantially in patients treated after endoscopic resection (11–27% versus a 70% recurrence after endoscopic resection alone) (Catalona and Ratliff, 1990; Herr, Laudone, Whitmore, 1987; Camacho et al, 1980; Herr et al, 1985; Lamm, 1985). Although the optimal schedule of intravesical BCG is not known with certainty, the most commonly recommended induction regimen is BCG weekly for 6 weeks followed by a period of 6 weeks where no BCG is given. At 12 weeks, if no cancer is identified, BCG is given weekly for 3 weeks. Continuous administration of BCG for more than 6 weeks may be immunosuppressive. Maintenance therapy at 3- to 6-month intervals should be considered in high-risk patients. Combining dermal scarification with intravesical instillation appears to result in no enhanced benefit (Badalament et al, 1987; Hudson et al, 1987). Side effects of intravesical BCG administration are relatively common, although severe complications are uncommon. Most patients experience some degree of urinary frequency and urgency. Hemorrhagic cystitis occurs in approximately 7% of patients, and evidence of distant infection is found in less than 2%. Patients with mild systemic or moderate local symptoms should be treated with isoniazid (300 mg daily), and the dosage of BCG should be reduced. Isoniazid is continued while symptoms persist and restarted 1 day before the next instillation.

Patients with severe systemic symptoms should have instillations stopped. Patients with prolonged high fever (> 103 °F), symptomatic granulomatous prostatitis, or evidence of systemic infection require treatment with isoniazid and rifampin (600 mg daily). Patients with signs and symptoms of BCG sepsis (eg, high fever, chills, confusion, hypotension, respiratory failure, jaundice) should be treated with isoniazid, rifampin, and ethambutol (1200 mg). The addition of cycloserine (500 mg twice daily) or prednisolone (40 mg daily) increases survival rates (Lamm, 1992).

5. New intravesical agents and approaches–The rate of metachronous tumor recurrence is high compared with that of low-grade cancers occurring in other organs (eg, nasopharynx, colon). Recurrence of superficial bladder cancer is related to cancer stage, grade, number, associated dysplasia, and DNA content. Recurrent tumors may be due to regrowth of previously resected cancers, growth of new cancers at remote sites, or implantation and subsequent proliferation of cells released into the bladder at the time of endoscopic treatment of the original tumor. Several investigators have studied the efficacy of single-dose therapy delivered at the time of complete transurethral resection (Tolley et al, 1988; Oosterlinck et al, 1993). Such therapy has been shown to decrease recurrence rates, probably by decreasing the risk of tumor cell implantation at the time of initial cancer resection. Clinical trials are currently under way to test the hypothesis that instillation of a single dose of intravesical chemotherapy at the time of initial transurethral resection will decrease recurrence and, it is hoped, cancer progression rates in patients with superficial bladder cancer.

Trials of alpha interferon, bropiramine (an oral immunomodulator), and AD-32 (an antracycline derivative) suggest that these agents, either alone or perhaps in combination with other agents, may be effective in either high-risk patients or those who fail to respond to first-line therapy (Belldegrun et al, 1998; Sarosdy et al, 1998). Given the relatively easy accessibility of bladder cancer cells to direct application of therapeutic agents, such cancers may be ideal targets for genetic manipulation (Miyake et al, 1998).

B. Surgery:

1. Transurethral resection or laser vaporization–Transurethral resection is the initial form of treatment for all bladder cancers. It allows a reasonably accurate estimate of tumor stage and grade and the need for additional treatment. Patients with single, low-grade, noninvasive tumors may be treated with transurethral resection alone. Laser energy for tumor vaporization has been used to treat a limited number of patients (see Chapter 26). Its advantages are that it may be less likely to promote tumor dissemination within the bladder, it often can be performed under sedation alone, and local (but not remote) recurrence rates may be lower than those with standard transurethral resection. It has the disadvantage that no tumor tissue is retrieved for histologic examination unless a separate biopsy specimen is obtained beforehand. Laser energy has been combined with systemic use of hematoporphyrin derivative (photodynamic therapy) in selected cases (Prout et al, 1987).

Careful follow-up of patients with superficial bladder cancers is mandatory, as disease will recur in 30–80% of patients, depending on cancer grade, tumor stage, and number. Disease status at 3 months after initial resection is an important predictor of the risk of subsequent recurrence (Fitzpatrick et al, 1986). All patients who undergo transurethral resection should undergo cystoscopy at 3 months. For patients who presented initially with solitary, low-grade lesions and who are free of recurrence at 3 months, repeat cystoscopy at 1 year is suggested. Patients who presented initially with multiple and/or higher grade lesions and those who develop recurrences at 3 months require

more careful surveillance. In such patients, cystoscopy at 3-month intervals is necessary. Although periodic cystoscopy is suggested for all patients with a history of bladder cancer, the risk of recurrence decreases as the tumor-free interval increases. After 5 and 10 years without recurrence, the risk of recurrence has been estimated to be 22% and 2%, respectively (Morris et al, 1995).

2. Partial cystectomy–Patients with solitary, infiltrating tumors (T1–T3) localized along the posterior lateral wall or dome of the bladder are candidates for partial cystectomy, as are patients with cancers in a diverticulum. Associated in situ disease remote from the primary tumor must be excluded by random bladder biopsies preoperatively. Few patients with invasive transitional cell carcinomas are candidates (Utz et al, 1973). Tumor implantation as a result of contamination of the wound with cancer cells at the time of surgery can be minimized by using short-course, limited-dose (1000 to 1600 cGy) irradiation and instilling an intravesical chemotherapeutic agent preoperatively (Ojeda and Johnson, 1983; Van der Werf–Messing, 1969). Although survival rates approach those for patients with similar stage tumors treated by radical cystectomy, local recurrences are common (Whitmore, 1983; Cummings et al, 1978; Merrell, Brown, and Rose, 1979; Schoborg, Sapolsky, and Lewis, 1979; Sweeney et al, 1992). Given current techniques of bladder replacement surgery, partial cystectomy is performed less commonly than in the past.

3. Radical cystectomy–Radical cystectomy implies removal of the anterior pelvic organs: in men, the bladder with its surrounding fat and peritoneal attachments, the prostate, and the seminal vesicles; in women, the bladder and surrounding fat and peritoneal attachments, cervix, uterus, anterior vaginal vault, urethra, and ovaries. The risk of urethral occurrence or recurrence in men who undergo radical cystectomy is 6.1–10.6%. Patients with cancers in the prostate or at the bladder neck are more likely to have urethral disease, either initially or in a delayed fashion. Such patients are candidates for urethrectomy at the time of radical cystectomy (Zabbo and Montie, 1984; Schellhammer and Whitmore, 1976).

Although prostatic urethral disease is a risk factor for urethral recurrence, recent evidence suggests that urethrectomy may be omitted and orthotopic urinary diversion performed safely in men with only proximal prostatic urethral involvement (Iselin et al, 1997). Urethrectomy was once routinely performed in all women undergoing radical cystectomy. However, recent clinical experience suggests that bladder replacement may be an acceptable procedure in women as well as men. Women with bladder cancer whose cancers are not located at the bladder neck and have a clear urethral margin at the time of cystectomy are candidates for this procedure. Approximately 66% of women undergoing radical cystectomy for the management of bladder cancer fall into this group (Stein et al, 1995; Stenzl et al, 1995; Stein et al, 1998).

External beam radiation therapy in various doses, usually 2000–4000 cGy, has been used before radical cystectomy to decrease local recurrence rates. The advantage of preoperative irradiation has been most apparent in patients with deeply infiltrating tumors (T3B) and tumors that are downstaged by irradiation (Whitmore and Batata, 1984; Whitmore et al, 1977; Van der Werf–Messing, 1979; Slack, Bross, and Prout, 1977). More recently, however, its value has been questioned (Radwin, 1980; Droller, 1983). Contemporary series of patients treated with radical cystectomy alone suggest that preoperative irradiation may not be beneficial in the majority of patients judged to be candidates for the procedure (Skinner and Lieskovsky, 1984; Montie, Straffon, and Stewart, 1984).

A bilateral pelvic lymph node dissection is usually performed simultaneously with radical cystectomy. Lymph node metastases are identified in approximately 20–35% (Lieskovsky, Aherling, and Skinner, 1988)—an incidence that reflects the inability of any imaging mode to identify consistently small-volume lymph node metastases preoperatively. Patients with lymph node metastases have a poor prognosis, and all but a few develop distant metastases despite lymphadenectomy. However, a small percentage of patients (10–33%) with limited disease in regional lymph nodes may be cured by radical cystectomy and lymphadenectomy (Dretler, Ragsdale, and Leadbetter, 1973; Whitmore and Marshall, 1962; Skinner, 1982). Other patients may benefit from adjuvant chemotherapy (see section following).

Urinary diversion may be accomplished using a variety of techniques. Methods have been developed that allow construction of reservoirs that are continent and do not require the patient to wear an external appliance for collection of urine (see Chapter 25).

C. Radiotherapy: External beam irradiation (5000–7000 cGy), delivered in fractions over a 5- to 8-week period, is an alternative to radical cystectomy in patients with deeply infiltrating bladder cancers. Treatment is generally well tolerated, but approximately 15% of patients may suffer significant bowel, bladder, or rectal complications. Five-year survival rates for stages T2 and T3 disease range from 18% to 41% (Timmer, Hartliff, and Hooijkaas, 1985; Goffinet et al, 1975; Corcoran et al, 1985; Miller, 1977; Woon et al, 1985; Quilty and Duncan, 1986; Rider and Evans, 1976; Cummings et al, 1976). Unfortunately, local recurrence is common, occurring in approximately 33–68% of patients. Irradiation alone seems to be associated with a lower survival rate than planned, preoperative irradiation followed by radical cystectomy (Miller, 1977; Wallace and Bloom, 1976; Bloom et al, 1982). Some investigators recommend radiother-

apy as initial treatment in all patients and radical cystectomy only in those who fail to respond (Blandy et al, 1980). However, one must bear in mind that radical cystectomy performed after definitive irradiation is associated with higher complication rates, and many patients who fail to improve after irradiation never come to surgery.

D. Chemotherapy: Approximately 15% of patients who present with bladder cancer are found to have regional or distant metastases; approximately 30–40% of patients with invasive disease develop distant metastases despite radical cystectomy or definitive radiotherapy. Without treatment, survival is limited. Early results with single chemotherapeutic agents and, more recently, combinations of drugs have shown that a significant number of patients with metastatic bladder cancer respond partially or completely (Scher and Sternberg, 1985). The single most active agent is cisplatin, which, when used alone, produces responses in approximately 30% (Yagoda, 1983). Other effective agents include methotrexate, doxorubicin, vinblastine, cyclophosphamide, and 5-fluorouracil. Response rates improve when active agents are combined: eg, methotrexate, vinblastine, doxorubicin, and cisplatin (MVAC); cisplatin, methotrexate, and vinblastine (CMV); and cisplatin, doxorubicin, and cyclophosphamide (CISCA) (Sternberg et al, 1988; Harker et al, 1985; Logothetis et al, 1985; Tannock et al, 1989). Approximately 13–35% of patients receiving such regimens attain a complete response. However, the median survival time is approximately 1 year, and the sustained survival rate is 20–25%.

Other agents demonstrating activity in this disease include ifosfamide, gemcitabine, paclitaxel, and gallium nitrate (Fagbemi and Stadler, 1998). Phase II trials are under way to examine the efficacy of new agents either alone or in combination.

E. Combination Therapy: Once it became apparent that patients with metastatic bladder cancer could benefit from combination chemotherapy, investigators began treating patients with locally invasive (T2–T4), but not metastatic, cancer similarly. Chemotherapy can be given before planned radical cystectomy (neoadjuvant) in an attempt to decrease recurrence rates and, in selected cases, allow for bladder preservation. Approximately 22–43% of patients achieve a complete response to chemotherapy alone (Scher, 1990; Scher et al, 1988). However, additional treatment is still indicated because a substantial number of patients believed to be free of tumors after chemotherapy alone are found to have infiltrating disease at the time of surgery (Scher et al, 1989). Alternatively, adjuvant chemotherapy may be offered to selected patients after radical cystectomy because of an increased risk of recurrence due to the presence of locally advanced disease, ie, P3, P4, or N+ (Skinner et al, 1991; Logothetis et al,1988; Scher, 1990; Stockle et al, 1992; Stockle et al, 1995; Freiha et al, 1996). These studies suggest that patients initially managed with radical cystectomy who are found to be at an increased risk of systemic relapse due to the presence of lymph node metastases or regionally advanced disease are candidates for adjuvant chemotherapy.

Owing to high local and systemic failure rates after definitive irradiation, several investigators have explored the possibility of combining irradiation with systemic chemotherapy to decrease recurrence rates, improve patient survival, and allow bladder preservation. Trials of single-agent chemotherapy and irradiation have shown better local response rates than are found in historical series of irradiation alone (Shipley et al, 1984; Jakse, Fritsch, and Frommhold, 1985; Pearson and Raghaven, 1985).

More recently, investigators have treated patients with invasive bladder cancer with complete transurethral resection and intravenously administered combination chemotherapy followed by concomitant chemotherapy and radiation (Given et al, 1995; Chauvet et al, 1996; Shipley et al, 1997; Zietman et al, 1997; Cervek et al, 1998). Early cystectomy is offered to those who do not tolerate chemotherapy and/or radiation owing to toxicity and those whose cancers fail to respond to such therapy. Complete response rates to chemoradiation may be as high as 50–70% initially with 5-year overall survival rates approaching 50–60%. However, local recurrence is common, exceeding 50% in many of these studies. Owing to invasive local recurrences, only 18–44% of patients may be alive with an intact bladder 5 years after chemoradiation. Predictors of poor outcome after combined chemoradiation for invasive bladder cancer include hydronephrosis at presentation, advanced clinical tumor stage, inability to complete the entire treatment protocol, and poor performance status. A recent study has suggested that chemoradiation may also be inappropriate for patients with bladder tumors that are p53-positive (Herr et al, 1999).

Systemic chemotherapy for locally invasive, but not metastatic, bladder cancer should not yet be considered standard therapy. The durability of the response, ultimate survival rates, and optimal candidates for the treatment regimens described will be determined only after completion of randomized studies.

URETERAL & RENAL PELVIC CANCERS

Incidence

Carcinomas of the renal pelvis and ureter are rare, accounting for only 4% of all urothelial cancers. The ratio of bladder–renal pelvic–ureteral carcinomas is approximately 51:3:1 (Williams and Mitchell, 1973). Mean age at diagnosis is 65 years, and the male-female ratio is 2–4:1 (Babaian and Johnson, 1980; Hawtrey, 1971). Urothelial cancer often presents as a widespread urothelial abnormality: Patients with a single upper-tract carcinoma are at risk of developing bladder carcinomas (30–50%) and contralateral upper-tract carcinoma (2–4%). Conversely, patients with primary bladder cancer are at low risk (< 2%) of developing upper urinary tract cancers (Oldbring et al, 1989). However, patients with multiple, recurrent superficial and in situ bladder cancers that are successfully treated by transurethral resection and BCG are at a substantial, lifelong risk of developing upper-tract cancers (Herr, 1998). The cumulative risks of such cancers have been estimated to be 10%, 26%, and 34% at 5, 5–10, and > 10 years of follow-up.

Etiology

As with bladder carcinoma, smoking and exposure to certain industrial dyes or solvents are associated with an increased risk of upper urinary tract transitional cell carcinomas (Shinka et al, 1988). However, these tumors also occur with increased frequency in patients with a long history of excessive analgesic intake, those with Balkan nephropathy, and those exposed to Thorotrast, a contrast agent previously used for retrograde pyelography. Patients with carcinomas associated with analgesic abuse are more likely to be women, have higher stage disease, and be younger than others (Taylor, 1972; Mahoney et al, 1977). All the major constituents of the analgesic compounds consumed (acetaminophen, aspirin, caffeine, and phenacetin) may be associated with an increased risk of upper urinary tract cancer (Ross et al, 1989; Jensen et al, 1989). Balkan nephropathy is an interstitial inflammatory disease of the kidneys that affects Yugoslavians, Rumanians, Bulgarians, and Greeks (Markovic, 1972); associated upper-tract carcinomas are generally superficial and more likely to be bilateral. The exact mechanism of tumor induction in these patients remains unknown.

Pathology

The mucosal lining of the renal pelvis and ureter is similar to that of the urinary bladder, being composed of transitional cell epithelium. Thus, the majority of renal pelvic and ureteral cancers (90% and 97%, respectively) are transitional cell carcinomas. Grading is similar to that for bladder carcinomas. Papillomas account for approximately 15–20% of cases (Grabstald, Whitmore, and Melamed, 1971; Bennington and Beckwith, 1975). They are isolated in just over 50% of patients and multiple in others, and approximately 25% and 50% of these patients, respectively, eventually develop carcinomas. Among patients with carcinomas of the ureter, multicentricity approaches 50% (Bennington and Beckwith, 1975). There is a relationship between tumor grade and the likelihood of urothelial abnormalities elsewhere: Low-grade cancers are associated with a low incidence of urothelial atypia or CIS in remote sites; however, these abnormalities are common with high-grade neoplasms (McCarron, Chasko, and Bray, 1982). The majority of upper urinary tract transitional cell carcinomas are localized at the time of diagnosis; the most common metastatic sites include regional lymph nodes, bone, and lung (Abeshouse, 1956).

Squamous carcinomas account for approximately 10% of renal pelvic cancers and are much rarer in the ureter. The majority of carcinomas are usually sessile and infiltrating at the time of diagnosis. Such tumors are commonly identified in patients with a history of chronic inflammation from infection or calculous disease. Adenocarcinomas are very rare tumors of the upper urinary tract and, like squamous carcinomas, tend to be far advanced at the time of diagnosis.

Mesodermal tumors of the renal pelvis and ureter are quite rare. Benign tumors include fibroepithelial polyps (the most common), leiomyomas, and angiomas. Fibroepithelial polyps occur most commonly in young adults and are characterized radiographically by a long, slender, and polyploid filling defect within the collecting system. The most common malignant mesodermal tumors are leiomyosarcomas. The ureter and renal pelvis may be invaded by cancers of contiguous structures, such as primary renal, ovarian, or cervical carcinomas. True metastases to the ureter are rare. The most common metastatic tumors include those of stomach, prostate, kidney, and breast and lymphomas (Bennington and Beckwith, 1975).

Staging & Natural History

Staging of both renal pelvic and ureteral carcinomas (Table 21–4) is based on an accurate assessment of the degree of tumor infiltration and parallels the staging system developed for bladder cancer (Batata et al, 1975; Grabstald, Whitmore, and Melamed, 1971; American Joint Committee on Cancer, 1988). Tumor stage and grade correlate with survival (Cummings et al, 1975; Batata et al, 1975; Batata and Grabstald, 1976; Bloom, Vidone, and Lytton, 1970; Reitelman et al, 1987): low-grade and low-stage cancers of the renal pelvis and ureter are associated with survival rates between 60% and 90%, compared with 0% and 33% for tumors of higher grade or those that

Table 21–4. Staging of ureteral and renal pelvic carcinoma.

	System	
	Batata[1]	TNM[2]
Confined to mucosa	O	Ta, Tis
Invasion of lamina propria	A	T1
Invasion of muscularis	B	T2
Extension through muscularis into fat or renal parenchyma	C	T3
Spread to adjacent organs	D	T4
Lymph node metastases	D	N+
Metastases	D	M+

[1] Drawn from Batata et al, 1975.
[2] Drawn from American Joint Committee on Cancer, 1988.

have penetrated deep into or through the renal pelvic or ureteral wall (Hall et al, 1998). The latter figures reflect a high likelihood of regional or distant metastases—40% and 75% in patients with stages B and C (T2–T4) cancers, respectively.

Clinical Findings

A. Symptoms and Signs: Gross hematuria is noted in 70–90% of patients. Flank pain, present in 8–50%, is the result of ureteral obstruction from blood clots or tumor fragments, renal pelvic or ureteral obstruction by the tumor itself, or regional invasion by the tumor. Irritative voiding symptoms are present in approximately 5–10% of patients. Constitutional symptoms of anorexia, weight loss, and lethargy are uncommon and are usually associated with metastatic disease. A flank mass owing to hydronephrosis or a large tumor is detected in approximately 10–20% (Geerdsen, 1979), and flank tenderness may be elicited as well. Supraclavicular or inguinal adenopathy or hepatomegaly may be identified in a small percentage of patients with metastatic disease.

B. Laboratory Findings: Hematuria is identified in the majority of patients but may be intermittent. Elevated liver function levels due to liver metastases are noted in a small number of patients. Pyuria and bacteriuria may be identified in patients with concomitant urinary tract infection from obstruction and urinary stasis.

As with bladder cancers, upper urinary tract cancers may be identified by examining exfoliated cells in the urinary sediment. In addition, specimens may be obtained directly with a ureteral catheter or by passing a small brush through the lumen of an open-ended catheter (Gill, Lu, and Thomsen, 1973; Blute, Gittes, and Gittes, 1981; Dodd et al, 1997). Detection depends on the grade of the tumor and the adequacy of the specimen obtained: 20–30% of low-grade cancers may be detected by cytologic testing compared with more than 60% of higher grade lesions (McCarron, Mullis, and Vaughn, 1983); using barbotage or a ureteral brush increases diagnostic accuracy (Zincke et al, 1976). The utility of the newer voided markers, such as the BTA stat test (Bard Diagnostic Sciences, Inc, Redmond, WA) in detecting upper-tract urothelial cancers has not yet been determined (Zimmerman et al, 1998).

C. Imaging: Findings on intravenous urography (IVU) in patients with upper urinary tract cancers are usually abnormal. The most common abnormalities identified include an intraluminal filling defect, unilateral nonvisualization of the collecting system, and hydronephrosis (Williams and Mitchell, 1973; Batata et al, 1975; Almgard, Freedman, and Ljungqvist, 1973). Ureteral and renal pelvic tumors must be differentiated from nonopaque calculi, blood clots, papillary necrosis, and inflammatory lesions such as ureteritis cystica, fungus infections, or tuberculosis.

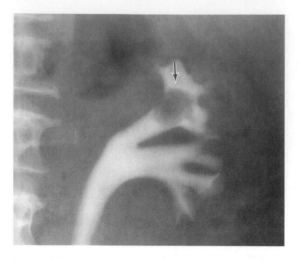

Figure 21–5. Filling defect representing a transitional cell carcinoma (arrow) on retrograde pyelography

The IVU is often indeterminate, requiring retrograde pyelography for more accurate visualization of collecting system abnormalities and simultaneous collection of cytologic specimens. Contrast material is injected into the ureteral orifice with a bulb or acorn tip catheter. Intraluminal filling defects may then be identified in the ureter or renal pelvis (Figure 21–5). Ureteral tumors are often characterized by dilation of the ureter distal to the lesion, creating the appearance of a "goblet." Nonopaque ureteral calculi appear as a narrowing of the ureter distal to the calculus. A ureteral catheter passed up the ureter may coil distal to a ureteral tumor (Bergman's sign) (Bergman, Friedenberg, and Sayegh, 1961). Ultrasonography, CT, and MRI frequently identify soft tissue abnormalities of the renal pelvis but may fail to identify ureteral filling defects directly, although they may show hydronephrosis (Figure 21–6). All 3 imaging techniques differentiate blood clot and tumor from nonopaque calculi. In addition, CT and MRI allow simultaneous examination of abdominal and retroperitoneal structures for signs of regional (lymph node) or more distant metastases.

D. Ureteropyeloscopy: The use of rigid and flexible ureteropyeloscopes has allowed direct visualization of upper urinary tract abnormalities. These instruments are passed transurethrally through the ureteral orifice; in addition, they (and the similarly constructed but larger nephroscopes), can be passed percutaneously into renal calyces and the pelvis directly. The latter instrument carries with it the theoretic possibility of tumor spillage along the percutaneous tract. Indications for ureteroscopy include evaluation of filling defects within the upper urinary tract and after positive results on cytologic study or after noting unilateral gross hematuria in the absence of a filling defect. In addition, it is also performed as a surveillance procedure in patients who have undergone conservative surgery for removal of a ureteral or renal pelvic tumor. Visualization, biopsy, and, on occasion, complete tumor resection, fulguration, or laser vaporization of the tumor are possible endoscopically. Detection of renal pelvic and ureteral tumors with these methods seems to be superior to that from conventional methods (Blute et al, 1989).

Treatment

Treatment of renal pelvic and ureteral tumors

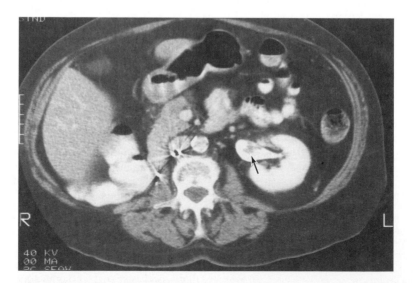

Figure 21–6. Computed tomography scan showing the presence of a renal pelvic tumor (arrow).

should be based primarily on grade, stage, position, and multiplicity. Renal function and anatomy should be assessed. The standard therapy for both tumor types has been nephroureterectomy owing to the possibility of multifocal disease within the ipsilateral collecting system. When the operation is performed for proximal ureteral or renal pelvic cancers, the entire distal ureter with a small cuff of bladder needs to be removed to avoid recurrence within this segment (Strong et al, 1976; Reitelman et al, 1987). Tumors of the distal ureter may be treated with distal ureterectomy and ureteral reimplantation into the bladder if no proximal defects suggestive of cancer have been noted (Babaian and Johnson, 1980).

Indications for more conservative surgery, including open or endoscopic excision, are not well defined. Absolute indications for renal-sparing procedures include tumor within the collecting system of a single kidney and bilateral urothelial tumors of the upper urinary tract or in patients with 2 kidneys but marginal renal function. In patients with 2 functioning kidneys, endoscopic excision alone should be considered only for low-grade and noninvasive tumors. One must realize that endoscopic examination may fail to detect the degree of infiltration adequately and therefore may understage some tumors. Limited experience with endoscopic resection, fulguration, or vaporization suggests that the procedure is safe in properly selected patients (Blute et al, 1989). However, recurrences have been noted in 15–80% of patients treated with open or endoscopic excision (Maier et al, 1990; Blute et al, 1989; Wallace et al, 1981; Orihuela and Smith, 1988; Keeley et al, 1997; Stoller et al, 1997). The rate of recurrence may be avoided by treating with instillation of immuno- or chemotherapeutic agents such as BCG or mitomycin C (Orihuela and Smith, 1988). Recurrence may be avoided by treating with instillation of immuno- or chemotherapeutic agents (Orihuela and Smith, 1988; Studer et al, 1989). These agents can be delivered to the upper urinary tract through single or double-J ureteral catheters (Patel and Fuchs, 1998).

Radiotherapy plays a limited role in upper urinary tract cancers. Although controversial, postoperative irradiation is believed by some investigators to decrease recurrence rates and improve survival in patients with deeply infiltrating cancers (Brookland and Richter, 1985; Batata et al, 1975). Patients with metastatic, transitional cell cancers of the upper urinary tract should receive cisplatin-based chemotherapeutic regimens as described for patients with metastatic bladder cancers.

Future Directions

Urothelial cancers represent a spectrum of disease defined by various recurrence and progression rates. A greater understanding of tumor induction and progression may allow the clinician to select treatments more wisely. Further development of biologic markers such as tumor proliferation or antigen expression may permit a better estimate of the biologic potential of individual tumors. More refined imaging techniques, perhaps with monoclonal antibodies, would allow clinicians to identify more advanced disease earlier and thereby select treatment strategies better. An assessment of the true benefit, if any, of either neoadjuvant or adjuvant chemotherapy awaits completion of large clinical trials. New agents for the management of the majority of patients with metastatic disease who do not respond to conventional chemotherapy need to be developed. Mechanisms of drug resistance and the means to circumvent them need to be investigated.

REFERENCES

BLADDER CARCINOMAS

Abel PD, Hall RR, Williams G: Should pT1 transitional cell cancers of the bladder still be classified as superficial? Br J Urol 1988;62:235.

Abenoza P, Manivel C, Fraley EE: Primary adenocarcinoma of urinary bladder. Urology 1987;29:2.

Althausen AF, Prout GR, Dal JJ: Non-invasive papillary carcinoma of the bladder associated with carcinoma-in-situ. J Urol 1976;116:575.

Amendola MA et al: Staging of bladder carcinoma: MRI-CT surgical correlation. AJR 1986;146:1179.

Badalament RA et al: Monitoring intravesical BCG treatment of superficial bladder carcinoma by serial flow cytometry. Cancer 1986;58:2751.

Badalament RA et al: A prospective randomized trial of maintenance versus non-maintenance intravesical bacillus Calmette-Guérin therapy of superficial bladder cancer. J Clin Oncol 1987;55:441.

Badalament RA et al: The relative value of cytometry and cytology in the management of bladder cancer: The Memorial Sloan-Kettering Cancer Center experience. Semin Urol 1988;6:22.

Belldegrun A et al: Superficial bladder cancer: The role of interferon-alpha. J Urol 1998;159:1793.

Bernstein SA et al: Primary signet-ring cell carcinoma of urinary bladder. Urology 1988;31:432.

Blandy JP et al: T3 bladder cancer—the case for salvage cystectomy. Br J Urol 1980;52:506.

Bloom HJG et al: Treatment of T3 bladder cancer: Controlled trial of preoperative radiotherapy and radical cystectomy versus radical radiotherapy (second report and review). Br J Urol 1982;54:136.

Bochner BH et al: Relationship of tumor angiogenesis and nuclear p53 accumulation in invasive bladder cancer. Clin Cancer Res 1997;3:1615.

Brawn PN: The origin of invasive carcinoma of the bladder. Cancer 1982;50:515.

Bretton PR et al: Intravesical bacillus Calmette-Guérin therapy for in situ transitional cell carcinoma involving the prostatic urethra. J Urol 1989;141:853.

Camacho F et al: Treatment of superficial bladder cancer with intravesical BCG. Proc Am Soc Clin Oncol 1980; 21:359.

Catalona WJ, Ratliff TL: Bacillus Calmette-Guérin and superficial bladder cancer. Surg Annu 1990;22:363.

Cervek J et al: Invasive bladder cancer: Our experience with bladder sparing approach. Int J Radiat Oncol Biol Phys 1998;41:273.

Chauvet B et al: Concurrent cisplatin and radiotherapy for patients with muscle invasive bladder cancer who are not candidates for radical cystectomy. J Urol 1996; 156:1258.

Cookson MS, Sarosdy M: Management of stage T1 bladder cancer with intravesical bacillus Calmette-Guérin therapy. J Urol 1992;148:797.

Corcoran MO et al: Invasive bladder cancer treated by radical external radiotherapy. Br J Urol 1985;57:40.

Cordon-Cardo C et al: Altered expression of the retinoblastoma gene product: Prognostic indicator in bladder cancer [see comments]. J Natl Cancer Inst 1992; 84:1251.

Cummings KB et al: Observations on definitive cobalt radiation for cure in bladder carcinoma: 15 year followup. J Urol 1976;115:152.

Cummings KB et al: Segmental resection in the management of bladder carcinoma. J Urol 1978;118:56.

Cutler SJ, Heney NM, Friedell GH: Longitudinal study of patients with bladder cancer: Factors associated with disease recurrence and progression. In: Bonney WW, Prout GR (editors): Bladder Cancer, AUA Monographs. Williams & Wilkins, 1982.

Dalbagni G et al: Genetic alterations in bladder cancer. Lancet 1993;342:469.

Dickinson AJ et al: Quantification of angiogenesis as an independent predictor of prognosis in invasive bladder carcinomas. Br J Urol 1994;74:762.

Dretler SP, Ragsdale BD, Leadbetter WR: The value of pelvic lymphadenectomy in the surgical treatment of bladder cancer. J Urol 1973;109:414.

Droller MJ: The controversial role of radiation as an adjunctive treatment of bladder cancer. J Urol 1983;129: 897.

El-Bolkainy MN et al: The impact of schistosomiasis on the pathology of bladder carcinoma. Cancer 1981;48: 2643.

Elcock M, Morgan RW: Update on artificial sweeteners and bladder cancer. Regul Toxicol Pharmacol 1993;17: 35.

Ellis WJ et al: Clinical evaluation of the BTA TRAK assay and comparison to voided urine cytology and the Bard BTA test in patients with recurrent bladder tumors. The Multi Center Study Group. Urology 1997; 50:882.

Esrig D et al: Prognostic importance of p53 and Rb alterations in transitional cell carcinoma of the bladder. J Urol 1995;153(Pt 2):362A.

Fagbemi S, Stadler W: New chemotherapy regimens for advanced bladder cancer. Semin Urol Oncol 1998;16: 23.

Fairchild WV et al: The incidence of bladder cancer after cyclophosphamide therapy. J Urol 1979;122: 163.

Farrow GM et al: Clinical observations in 69 cases of in situ carcinoma of the urinary bladder. Cancer Res 1977;37:2794.

Fisher MR, Hricak H, Tanagho EA: Urinary bladder MR imaging. 2. Neoplasm. Radiology 1985;157:471.

Fitzpatrick J et al: Superficial bladder tumors (stage pTa grades 1 and 2): The importance of recurrence pattern following initial resection. J Urol 1986;135:920.

Fradet Y et al: Clinical cancer progression in urinary bladder tumors evaluated by multiparameter flow cytometry with monoclonal antibodies. Laval University Urology Group. Cancer Res 1990;50:432.

Frazier HA et al: The value of pathologic factors in predicting cancer-specific survival among patients treated with radical cystectomy for transitional cell carcinoma of the bladder and prostate. Cancer 1993;71:3993.

Freiha F et al: A randomized trial of radical cystectomy versus radical cystectomy plus cisplatin, vinblastine and methotrexate chemotherapy for muscle invasive bladder cancer [see comments]. J Urol 1996;155: 495.

Friedell GH et al: Histopathology and classification of urinary bladder carcinomas. Urol Clin North Am 1976; 3:53.

Gilbert HA et al: The natural history of papillary transitional cell carcinoma of the bladder and its treatment in an unselected population on the basis of histologic grading. J Urol 1978;119:488.

Given RW et al: Bladder-sparing multimodality treatment of muscle-invasive bladder cancer: A five-year follow-up. Urology 1995;46:499.

Goffinet DR et al: Bladder cancer: Results of radiation therapy in 384 patients. Radiology 1975;117:149.

Goldstein AG: Metastatic carcinoma to the bladder. J Urol 1967;98:209.

Grossfeld GD et al: Thrombospondin-1 expression in bladder cancer: Association with p53 alterations, tumor angiogenesis, and tumor progression. J Natl Cancer Inst 1997;89:219.

Guirguis R et al: Detection of autocrine motility factor(s) in urine as markers of bladder cancer. JCMNI 1988;80:1203.

Haaf EO, Catalona WJ, Ratliff TL: Detection of interleukin 2 in urine of patients with superficial bladder tumors after treatment with intravesical BCG. J Urol 1986;136:970.

Harker WG et al: Cisplatin methotrexate and vinblastine (CMV): An effective chemotherapy regimen for metastatic transitional cell carcinoma of the urinary tract. A Northern California Oncology Group study. J Urol 1985;134:118.

Hatch TR, Barry JM: Value of excretory urography in staging bladder cancer. J Urol 1986;135:49.

Heney NM et al: Superficial bladder cancer: Progression and recurrence. J Urol 1983;130:1083.

Henry K et al: Comparison of transurethral resection to radical therapies for stage B bladder tumors. J Urol 1988;140:964.

Herr HW: Conservative management of muscle infiltrating bladder cancer: Prospective experience. J Urol 1988;138:1162.

Herr HW: Progression of stage T1 bladder tumors after intravesical bacillus Calmette-Guérin. J Urol 1991; 145:40.

Herr HW, Laudone VP, Whitmore WF: An overview of

intravesical therapy for superficial bladder tumors. J Urol 1987;138:1363.

Herr HW et al: Can p53 help select patients with invasive bladder cancer for bladder preservation? J Urol 1999;161:20.

Herr HW et al: Experience with intravesical bacillus Calmette-Guérin therapy of superficial bladder tumors. Urology 1985;25:119.

Herr HW et al: Superficial bladder cancer treated with bacillus Calmette-Guérin: A multivariate analysis of factors affecting tumor progression. J Urol 1989;141:22.

Hicks RM: Promotion in bladder cancer. Carcinogenesis 1982;7:139.

Howe GR et al: Artificial sweeteners and bladder cancer. Lancet 1977;2:578.

Hudson MA et al: Single course versus maintenance bacillus Calmette-Guérin therapy for superficial bladder tumours: A prospective randomized trial. J Urol 1987;138:295.

Husband JES et al: Bladder cancer: Staging with CT and MR imaging. Radiology 1989;173:435.

Ianari A et al: Results of Bard BTA test in monitoring patients with a history of transitional cell cancer of the bladder. Urology 1997;49:786.

Iselin C et al: Does prostate transitional cell carcinoma preclude orthotopic bladder reconstruction after radical cystoprostatectomy for bladder cancer? J Urol 1997;158:2123.

Jaeger TM et al: Tumor angiogenesis correlates with lymph node metastasis in invasive bladder cancer. J Urol 1995;154:69.

Jakse G, Fritsch E, Frommhold H: Combination of chemotherapy and irradiation for non-resectable bladder carcinoma. World J Urol 1985;3:121.

Jewett HJ, Strong GH: Infiltrating carcinoma of the bladder: Relation of the depth of penetration of the bladder wall to incidence of local extension and metastasis. J Urol 1946;55:366.

Johnston B et al: Rapid detection of bladder cancer: A comparative study of point of care tests [see comments]. J Urol 1997;158:2098.

Jordan AM, Weingarten J, Murphy WM: Transitional cell neoplasms of the urinary bladder: Can biologic potential be predicted from tumor grade? Cancer 1987;60:2766.

Kaye KW, Lange PH: Mode of presentation of invasive bladder cancer: Reassessment of the problem. J Urol 1982;128:31.

Klein FA, Whitmore WF, Wolf RM: Presumptive downstaging from preoperative irradiation for bladder cancer as determined by flow cytometry: Preliminary report. Int J Radiat Oncol Biol Physiol 1983;9:487.

Klein FA et al: Flow cytometry follow-up in patients with low stage bladder tumors. J Urol 1982;128:88.

Knudson AG: Hereditary cancer oncogenes and antioncogenes. Cancer Res 1985;45:1437.

Koss JC et al: CT staging of bladder carcinoma. AJR 1981;137:359.

Kowalkowski TS, Lamm DL: Intravesical chemotherapy of superficial bladder cancer. In: Resnick M (editor): *Current Trends in Urology.* Williams & Wilkins, 1988.

Kramer SA et al: Primary non-urachal adenocarcinoma of the bladder. J Urol 1979;121:278.

Lamm DL: Bacillus Calmette-Guérin immunotherapy for bladder cancer. J Urol 1985;134:40.

Lamm DL: Complications of bacillus Calmette-Guérin immunotherapy. Urol Clin North Am 1992;19:565.

Landman J et al: Sensitivity and specificity of NMP-22, telomerase, and BTA in the detection of human bladder cancer. Urology 1998;52:398.

Lerman RI, Hutter RVP, Whitmore WF Jr: Papilloma of the urinary bladder. Cancer 1970;25:333.

Lieskovsky G, Aherling T, Skinner DG: Diagnosis and staging of bladder cancer. In: Skinner DR, Lieskovsky G (editors): *Diagnosis and Management of Genitourinary Cancer.* Saunders, 1988.

Liotta LA: Tumor invasion and metastases. Cancer Res 1986;46:1.

Lipponen PK, Eskelinen MJ: Reduced expression of E-cadherin is related to invasive disease and frequent recurrence in bladder cancer. J Cancer Res Clin Oncol 1995;121:303.

Logothetis CJ et al: Adjuvant cyclophosphamide, doxorubicin, and cisplatin chemotherapy for bladder cancer: An update. J Clin Oncol 1988;6:1590.

Logothetis CJ et al: Altered expression of retinoblastoma protein and known prognostic variables in locally advanced bladder cancer [see comments]. J Natl Cancer Inst 1992;84:1256.

Logothetis CJ et al: Cyclophosphamide, doxorubicin and cisplatin chemotherapy for patients with locally advanced urothelial tumors with or without nodal metastases. J Urol 1985;134:460.

Lutzeyer W, Rubben H, Dahm H: Prognostic parameters in superficial bladder cancer: An analysis of 315 cases. J Urol 1982;127:250.

Malek RS, Rosen JS, O'Dea MJ: Adenocarcinoma of bladder. Urology 1983;21:357.

Marshall VF: The relation of the preoperative estimate to the pathologic demonstration of the extent of vesical neoplasms. J Urol 1952;68:714.

Matanoski GM, Elliott EA: Bladder cancer epidemiology. Epidemiol Rev 1981;3:203.

Merrell RW, Brown HE, Rose JF: Bladder carcinoma treated by partial cystectomy: A review of 54 cases. J Urol 1979;122:471.

Miller LS: Bladder cancer: Superiority of preoperative irradiation and cystectomy in clinical stages B2 and C. Cancer 1977;39(Suppl):973.

Mills SE et al: Small cell undifferentiated carcinoma of the urinary bladder. Am J Surg Pathol 1987;79:728.

Miyake H et al: Enhancement of chemosensitivity in human bladder cancer cells by adenoviral-mediated p53 gene transfer. Anticancer Res 1998;18:3087.

Miyao N et al: Role of chromosome 9 in human bladder cancer. Cancer Res 1993;53:4066.

Mommsen S, Aagaard J: Tobacco as a risk factor in bladder cancer. Carcinogenesis 1983;4:335.

Montie JE, Straffon RA, Stewart BH: Radical cystectomy without radiation therapy for carcinoma of the bladder. J Urol 1984;131:477.

Morris S et al: Superficial bladder cancer: How long should a tumor-free patient have check cystoscopies? Br J Urol 1995;75:193.

Mostofi FK, Sorbin LH, Torloni H: *Histological Typing of Urinary Bladder Tumours: International Classification of Tumours.* World Health Organization, 1973.

Murphy WM: Diseases of the urinary bladder, urethra,

ureters, and renal pelvis. In: Murphy WM (editor): *Urological Pathology.* Saunders, 1989.

Najem GR et al: Life time occupation, smoking, caffeine, saccharine, hair dyes, and bladder carcinogenesis. Int J Epidemiol 1982;11:212.

Newman AJ et al: Cell surface A, B, or O(H) blood group antigens as an indicator of malignant potential in stage A bladder carcinoma. J Urol 1980;124:27.

Ojeda L, Johnson DE: Partial cystectomy: Can it be incorporated into an integrated therapy program? Urology 1983;22:115.

Okamura K et al: Growth fractions of transitional cell carcinomas of the bladder defined by the monoclonal antibody Ki-67. J Urol 1990;144:875.

Olumi AF et al: Allelic loss of chromosome 17p distinguishes high grade from low grade transitional cell carcinoma of the bladder. Cancer Res 1990a;50:7081.

Olumi AF et al: Molecular analysis of human bladder cancer. Semin Urol 1990b;4:270.

Oosterlinck W et al: A prospective European Organization for Research and Treatment of Cancer Genitourinary Group Randomized trial comparing transurethral resection followed by a single intravesical instillation of epirubicin or water in single stage Ta, T1 papillary carcinoma of the bladder. J Urol 1993;149:749.

Pauwels RPE et al: Grading in superficial bladder cancer. 1. Morphological criteria. Br J Urol 1988;61:129.

Pearson BS, Raghaven D: First line intravenous cisplatin for deeply invasive bladder cancer: Update on 70 cases. Br J Urol 1985;57:690.

Planz B et al: Use of Lewis X antigen and deoxyribonucleic acid image cytometry to increase sensitivity of urinary cytology in transitional cell carcinoma of the bladder. J Urol 1998;159:384.

Pode D et al: Noninvasive detection of bladder cancer with the BTA stat test. J Urol 1999;161:443.

Prout GR et al: Long-term fate of 90 patients with superficial bladder cancer randomly assigned to receive or not to receive thiotepa. J Urol 1983;130:677.

Prout GR et al: Photodynamic therapy with hematoporphyrin derivative in the treatment of superficial transitional cell carcinoma of the bladder. N Engl J Med 1987;317:1251.

Quilty PM, Duncan W: Primary radical radiotherapy for T3 transitional cell cancer of the bladder: Analysis of survival and control. Int J Radiat Oncol Biol Phys 1986;12:853.

Radwin HM: Radiotherapy and bladder cancer: A critical review. J Urol 1980;124:43.

Rider WD, Evans DH: Radiotherapy in the treatment of recurrent bladder cancer. Br J Urol 1976;48:595.

Ruppert JM, Tokino K, Sidransky D: Evidence for two bladder cancer suppressor loci on human chromosome 9. Cancer Res 1993;53:5093.

Sarosdy M et al: Oral bropiramine immunotherapy of bladder carcinoma in situ after prior intravesical bacille Calmette-Guérin. Urology 1998;51:226.

Schellhammer PF, Bean MA, Whitmore WF: Prostatic involvement by transitional cell carcinoma: Pathogenesis patterns and prognosis. J Urol 1977;118:399.

Schellhammer PF, Whitmore WF: Transitional cell carcinoma of the urethra in men having cystectomy for bladder cancer. J Urol 1976;115:56.

Scher HI: Neoadjuvant therapy of invasive bladder tumors. In: Williams R, Carroll PR (editors): *Treatment Perspectives in Urologic Oncology.* Pergamon Press, 1990.

Scher HI, Sternberg CN: Chemotherapy of urologic malignancies. Semin Urol 1985;3:239.

Scher HI et al: Neoadjuvant chemotherapy for invasive bladder cancer: Experience with the M-VAC regimen. Br J Urol 1989;64:250.

Scher HI et al: Neoadjuvant M-VAC (methotrexate, vinblastine, doxorubicin and cisplatin) effect on the primary bladder lesion. J Urol 1988;139:470.

Schoborg TW, Sapolsky JL, Lewis CW: Carcinoma of the bladder treated by segmental resection. J Urol 1979;122:473.

Schuller J et al: Intravesical ultrasound tomography in staging bladder carcinoma. J Urol 1982;128:264.

See WA, Fuller JR: Staging of advanced bladder cancer. Current concepts and pitfalls. Urol Clin North Am 1992;19:663.

Shipley WU et al: Cisplatin and full dose irradiation for patients with invasive bladder carcinoma: A preliminary report of tolerance and local response. J Urol 1984;132:899.

Shipley WU et al: Invasive bladder cancer: Treatment strategies using transurethral surgery, chemotherapy and radiation therapy with selection for bladder conservation. Int J Radiat Oncol Biol Phys 1997;39:937.

Shirai T: Etiology of bladder cancer. Semin Urol 1993;3:113.

Sidransky D et al: Identification of p53 gene mutations in bladder cancers and urine samples. Science 1991;252:706.

Singer D, Itzchak Y, Fiselovitch Y: Ultrasonographic assessment of bladder tumors. II Clinical staging. J Urol 1981;126:34.

Skinner DG: Current state of classification and staging of bladder cancer. Cancer Res 1977;37:2838.

Skinner DG: Management of invasive bladder cancer: A meticulous lymph node dissection can make a difference. J Urol 1982;128:34.

Skinner DG, Lieskovsky G: Contemporary cystectomy with pelvic node dissection compared with preoperative radiation therapy plus cystectomy in the management of invasive bladder cancer. J Urol 1984;131:1069.

Skinner DG et al: High dose short course preoperative radiation therapy and immediate single stage radical cystectomy with pelvic node dissection in the management of bladder cancer. J Urol 1982;127:671.

Skinner DG et al: The role of adjuvant chemotherapy following cystectomy for invasive bladder cancer: A prospective comparative trial. J Urol 1991;145:459.

Slack NH, Bross IDJ, Prout GR: Five-year followup results of a collaborative study of therapies for carcinoma of the bladder. J Surg Oncol 1977;9:393.

Soloway MS: Diagnosis and management of superficial bladder cancer. Semin Surg Oncol 1989;5:247.

Soloway MS, Hardeman SW: Animal models in bladder cancer research. In: Chisolm GD, Fair WR (editors): *Scientific Foundations of Urology,* 2nd ed. Heinemann Medical Books, 1990.

Soloway MS et al: Use of a new tumor marker, urinary NMP22, in the detection of occult or rapidly recurring transitional cell carcinoma of the urinary tract following surgical treatment. J Urol 1996;156(2 Pt 1):363.

Solsona E et al: Feasibility of transurethral resection for muscle infiltrating carcinoma of the bladder: Long-term followup of a prospective study. J Urol 1998; 159:95.

Stampfer DS et al: Evaluation of NMP22 in the detection of transitional cell carcinoma of the bladder [see comments] [published erratum appears in J Urol 1998 May;159(5):1650]. J Urol 1998;159:394.

Stein JP et al: Effect of p21WAF1/CIP1 expression on tumor progression in bladder cancer [see comments]. J Natl Cancer Inst 1998;90:1072.

Stein JP et al: Indications for lower urinary tract reconstruction in women after cystectomy for bladder cancer: A pathological review of female cystectomy specimens [see comments]. J Urol 1995;154:1329.

Stein JP et al: Prospective pathologic analysis of female cystectomy specimens: Risk factors for orthotopic diversion in women. Urology 1998;51:951.

Stenzl A et al: The risk of urethral tumors in female bladder cancer: Can the urethra be used for orthotopic reconstruction of the lower urinary tract? J Urol 1995;153(3 Pt 2):950.

Sternberg CN et al: M-VAV (methotrexate vinblastine doxorubicin and cisplatin) for advanced transitional cell carcinoma of the urothelium. J Urol 1988;139: 461.

Stockle M et al: Adjuvant polychemotherapy of nonorgan-confined bladder cancer after radical cystectomy revisited: Long-term results of a controlled prospective study and further clinical experience. J Urol 1995;153:47.

Stockle M et al: Advanced bladder cancer (stages pT3b, pT4a, pN1 and pN2): Improved survival after radical cystectomy and 3 adjuvant cycles of chemotherapy. Results of a controlled prospective trial. J Urol 1992; 148:302.

Sweeney P et al: Partial cystectomy. Urol Clin North Am 1992;19:701.

Tannock I et al: M-VAC (methotroxate vinblastine doxorubicin and cisplatin) chemotherapy for transitional cell carcinoma: The Princess Margaret Hospital experience. J Urol 1989;142:289.

Thompson I, Fair W: Occupational and environmental factors in bladder cancer. In: Chisolm GD, Fair WR (editors): *Scientific Foundations of Urology,* 2nd ed. Heinemann Medical Books, 1990.

Thrasher JB et al: Clinical variables which serve as predictors of cancer-specific survival among patients treated with radical cystectomy for transitional cell carcinoma of the bladder and prostate. Cancer 1994;73:1708.

Timmer PR, Hartliff HA, Hooijkaas JAP: Bladder cancer: Pattern of recurrence in 142 patients. Int J Radiat Oncol Biol Phys 1985;11:899.

Tolley D et al: Effect of mitomycin C on recurrence of newly diagnosed superficial bladder cancer: Interim report from the Medical Research Council Subgroup on Superficial Bladder Cancer. Br Med J 1988;296: 1759.

Torti FM et al: Superficial bladder cancer: The primacy of grade in the development of invasive disease. J Clin Oncol 1987;5:125.

Traganos F: Flow cytometry: Principles and applications. Cancer Invest 1984;2:149.

UICC Staff et al (editors): *TNM Classification of Malignant Tumors,* 4th ed. (UICC International Union Against Cancer Series.) Springer-Verlag, 1989.

Utz DC et al: A clinicopathologic evaluation of partial cystectomy for carcinoma of the urinary bladder. Cancer 1973;32:1075.

Van der Poel HG et al: Bladder wash cytology, quantitative cytology, and the qualitative BTA test in patients with superficial bladder cancer. Urology 1998;51:44.

Van der Werf–Messing B: Carcinoma of the bladder treated by suprapubic radium implants. Eur J Cancer 1969;5:27.

Van der Werf–Messing B: Preoperative irradiation followed by cystectomy to treat carcinoma of the urinary bladder category T3NX0-4M0. Int J Radiat Oncol Biol Phys 1979;5:3975.

Vieweg J et al: Impact of primary stage on survival in patients with lymph node positive bladder cancer. J Urol 1999;161:72.

Viola MV et al: Ras oncogene p21 expression is increased in premalignant lesions and high grade bladder carcinoma. J Exp Med 1985;161:1213.

Wallace DM, Bloom HJG: The management of deeply infiltrating (T3) bladder carcinoma: Controlled trial of radical radiotherapy versus preoperative radiotherapy and radical cystectomy. Br J Urol 1976;48:587.

Wallace DM et al: The role of multiple mucosal biopsies in the management of patients with bladder cancer. Br J Urol 1979;51:535.

Weinstein RS et al: Blood group isoantigen deletion in carcinoma in situ of the urinary bladder. Cancer 1979;43:661.

Wewer UM et al: Altered levels of laminin receptor RNA in various human carcinoma cells that have different abilities to bind laminin. Proc Natl Acad Sci USA 1986;83:7137.

Wheeless LL et al: Consensus review of the clinical utility of DNA cytometery in bladder caner. Cytometry 1993;14:478.

Wheeless LL et al: DNA slit-scan flow cytometry of bladder irrigation specimens and the importance of recognizing urothelial cells. Cytometry 1991;12: 140.

Whitmore WF: Management of invasive bladder neoplasms. Semin Urol 1983;1:34.

Whitmore WF, Batata MA: Status of integrated irradiation and cystectomy for bladder cancer. Urol Clin North Am 1984;11:681.

Whitmore WF, Marshall VF: Radical total cystectomy for cancer of the bladder: 230 consecutive cases 5 years later. J Urol 1962;87:853.

Whitmore WF et al: Radical cystectomy with or without irradiation in the treatment of bladder cancer. J Urol 1977;118:184.

Wiener HG et al: Can urine bound diagnostic tests replace cystoscopy in the management of bladder cancer? J Urol 1998;159:1876.

Wolf H, Hojgaard K: Prognostic factors in local surgical treatment of invasive bladder cancer with special reference to the presence of urothelial dysplasia. Cancer 1983;51:1710.

Wolf H, Olsen PR, Hojgaard K: Urothelial dysplasia concomitant with bladder tumours: A determinant for future new occurrences in patients treated by full course radiotherapy. Lancet 1985;I:1005.

Wood DP et al: The role of magnetic resonance imaging

in the staging of bladder carcinoma. J Urol 1988; 140:741.

Woon SY et al: Bladder carcinoma: Experience with radical and preoperative radiotherapy in 421 patients. Cancer 1985;56:1293.

Wynder EL, Goldsmith K: The epidemiology of bladder cancer: A second look. Cancer 1977;40:1246.

Yagoda A: Chemotherapy for advanced urothelial cancer. Semin Urol 1983;1:60.

Yoshida K et al: Telomerase activity in bladder carcinoma and its implication for noninvasive diagnosis by detection of exfoliated cancer cells in urine. Cancer 1997;79:362.

Zabbo A, Montie JE: Management of the urethra in men undergoing radical cystectomy for bladder cancer. J Urol 1984;131:267.

Zietman A et al: The case for radiotherapy with or without chemotherapy in high-risk superficial and muscle-invading bladder cancer. Semin Urol Oncol 1997;15:161.

Zippe C et al: NMP22 is a sensitive, cost-effective test in patients at risk for bladder cancer. J Urol 1999; 161:62.

URETERAL & RENAL PELVIC CANCER

Abeshouse BS: Primary benign and malignant tumors of the ureter: A review of the literature and report of one benign and 12 malignant tumors. Am J Surg 1956;91: 237.

Almgard LE, Freedman D, Ljungqvist A: Carcinoma of the ureter with special reference to malignancy grading and prognosis. Scand J Urol Nephrol 1973;7:165.

American Joint Committee on Cancer: *Manual for Staging of Cancer.* Lippincott, 1988.

Babaian RJ, Johnson DE: Primary carcinoma of the ureter. J Urol 1980;123:357.

Batata M, Grabstald H: Upper urinary tract urothelial tumors. Urol Clin North Am 1976;3:79.

Batata MA et al: Primary carcinoma of the ureter: A prognostic study. Cancer 1975;35:1626.

Bennington J, Beckwith JB: Tumors of the renal pelvis and ureter. In: *Atlas of Tumor Pathology.* Armed Forces Institute of Pathology, Fasc 12, 1975.

Bergman H, Friedenberg RM, Sayegh V: New roentgenologic signs of carcinoma of the ureter. Am J Roentgenol 1961;86:707.

Bloom NA, Vidone RA, Lytton B: Primary carcinoma of the ureter: A report of 102 new cases. J Urol 1970; 103:590.

Blute ML et al: Impact of endourology on diagnosis and management of upper urinary tract urothelial cancer. J Urol 1989;141:1298.

Blute RD, Gittes RR, Gittes RF: Renal brush biopsy: Survey of indications, techniques, and results. J Urol 1981;126:146.

Brookland RK, Richter MP: The postoperative irradiation of transitional cell carcinoma of the renal pelvis and ureter. J Urol 1985;133:952.

Cummings KB et al: Renal pelvic tumors. J Urol 1975; 113:158.

Dodd L et al: Endoscopic brush cytology of the upper urinary tract. Evaluation of its efficacy and potential limitations in diagnosis. Acta Cytol 1997;41:377.

Geerdsen J: Tumours of the renal pelvis and ureter. Symptomatology, diagnosis, treatment, and prognosis. Scand J Urol Nephrol 1979;13:287.

Gill WB, Lu CT, Thomsen S: Retrograde brushing: A new technique for obtaining histologic and cytologic material from ureteral renal pelvic and renal caliceal lesions. J Urol 1973;109:573.

Grabstald H, Whitmore WF, Melamed MR: Renal pelvic tumors. JAMA 1971;218:845.

Hall M et al: Prognostic factors, recurrence, and survival in transitional cell carcinoma of the upper urinary tract: A 30-year experience in 252 patients. Urology 1998; 52:594.

Hawtrey CE: Fifty-two cases of primary ureteral carcinoma: A clinical-pathologic study. J Urol 1971;105: 188.

Herr H: Long-term results of BCG therapy: Concern about upper tract tumors. Semin Urol Oncol 1998; 16:13.

Jensen OM et al: The Copenhagen case-control study of renal pelvis and ureter cancer: Role of analgesics. Int J Cancer 1989;44:965.

Keeley F et al: Ureteroscopic treatment and surveillance of upper urinary tract transitional cell carcinoma. J Urol 1997;157:1560.

Mahoney JF et al: Analgesic abuse renal parenchymal disease and carcinoma of the kidney or ureter. Aust NZ J Med 1977;7:463.

Maier U et al: Organ-preserving surgery in patients with urothelial tumors of the upper urinary tract. Eur Urol 1990;18:197.

Markovic B: Endemic nephritis and urinary tract cancer in Yugoslavia Bulgaria and Rumania. J Urol 1972; 107:212.

McCarron JP, Chasko SB, Bray GF: Systematic mapping of nephroureterectomy specimens removed for urothelial cancer: Pathological findings and clinical correlations. J Urol 1982;128:243.

McCarron JP, Mullis C, Vaughn ED: Tumors of the renal pelvis and ureter: Current concepts and management. Semin Urol 1983;1:75.

Oldbring J et al: Carcinoma of the renal pelvis and ureter following bladder carcinoma: Frequency risk factors and clinicopathological findings. J Urol 1989;141: 1311.

Orihuela E, Smith AD: Percutaneous treatment of transitional cell carcinoma of the upper urinary tract. Urol Clin North Am 1988;15:425.

Patel A, Fuchs G: New techniques for the administration of topical adjuvant therapy after endoscopic ablation of upper urinary tract transitional cell carcinoma. J Urol 1998;159:71.

Reitelman C et al: Prognostic variables in patients with transitional cell carcinoma of the renal pelvis and proximal ureter. J Urol 1987;138:1144.

Ross RK et al: Analgesics, cigarette smoking, and other risk factors for cancer of the renal pelvis and ureter. Cancer Res 1989;49:1045.

Shinka T et al: Occurrence of uroepithelial tumors of the upper urinary tract after the initial diagnosis of bladder cancer. J Urol 1988;140:745.

Stoller M et al: Endoscopic management of upper tract urothelial tumors. Tech Urol 1997;3:152.

Strong DW et al: The ureteral stump after nephroureterectomy. J Urol 1976;115:654.

Studer UE et al: Percutaneous bacillus Calmette-Guérin

perfusion of the upper urinary tract for carcinoma in situ. J Urol 1989;142:975.

Taylor JS: Carcinoma of the urinary tract and analgesic abuse. Med J Aust 1972;1:407.

Wallace DMA et al: The late results of conservative surgery for upper tract urothelial carcinomas. Br J Urol 1981;53:537.

Williams CB, Mitchell JP: Carcinoma of the ureter: A review of 54 cases. Br J Urol 1973;45:377.

Zimmerman R et al: Utility of the Bard BTA test in detecting upper urinary tract transitional cell carcinoma. Urology 1998;51:956.

Zincke H et al: Significance of urinary cytology in the early detection of transitional cell cancer of the upper urinary tract. J Urol 1976;116:781.

22

Renal Parenchymal Neoplasms

Robert Dreicer, MD, MS, FACP, & Richard D. Williams, MD

BENIGN TUMORS

Prior to routine use of abdominal computed tomography (CT) scans, benign tumors of the kidney were infrequently detected because they rarely cause significant symptoms or morbidity. The liberal use of CT and magnetic resonance imaging (MRI) and the recognition of new syndromes, such as neoplasia associated with acquired renal cystic disease, will increasingly require the clinician to differentiate benign from malignant renal tumors.

Benign renal tumors include adenoma, oncocytoma, angiomyolipoma, leiomyoma, lipoma, hemangioma, and juxtaglomerular tumors.

Renal Adenomas

The adenoma is the most common benign renal parenchymal lesion (Williams, 1992). These are small, well-differentiated glandular tumors of the renal cortex. They are typically asymptomatic and usually identified incidentally at autopsy after a nephrectomy is performed for an unrelated disease. The true incidence of renal adenomas is unknown; however, 7–22% of patients exhibit them at autopsy (Bonsib, 1985). Despite the classification of adenoma as a benign tumor, no clinical, histologic, or immunohistochemical criteria differentiate renal adenoma from renal carcinoma. Therefore, the incidental finding of a renal adenoma has significant clinical implications for the patient and clinician. Adenomas of any size should be treated as a fortuitous finding representative of an early renal cancer, and the patient should be evaluated and treated appropriately.

Renal Oncocytoma

Renal oncocytoma has a spectrum of behavior ranging from benign to malignant. Composed of large epithelial cells with finely granular eosinophilic cytoplasm (oncocytes), oncocytomas occur in various organs and organ systems including adrenal, salivary, thyroid, and parathyroid glands as well as the kidney (Hamperl, 1962). An estimated 3–5% of renal tumors are oncocytomas, accounting for approxi-

mately 500 cases per year (Lieber and Tsukamoto, 1986). Men are affected twice as often as women.

Renal oncocytomas have a gross appearance significantly different from that of most renal adenocarcinomas. Oncocytomas generally occur within a well-defined fibrous capsule, with tumor tissue rarely penetrating the renal capsule, pelvis, collecting system, or perinephric fat. On cut section, the surface of the tumor is usually tan or light brown. A central stellate scar is often present, especially in larger tumors, but necrosis typical of renal adenocarcinoma is absent. The tumors are usually solitary and unilateral, although several bilateral cases and even multiple sites within one kidney have been reported.

Histologically, well-differentiated oncocytomas are made up of large, uniform cells containing an intensely eosinophilic cytoplasm, which on ultrastructural studies is found to be packed with mitochondria. Mitotic activity is absent, and nuclear pleomorphism is uncommon. The cellular origin of renal oncocytes has not been fully elucidated, although some early evidence suggested that oncocytes resemble proximal convoluted tubular cells (Merino and Librelsi, 1982). Recent findings suggest their origin may be a precursor stem cell (Cohen, McCue, and Derose, 1988) or the intercalated cells of the collecting ducts (Storkel et al, 1989).

Histological grading of oncocytomas, although a subjective process, has clinical relevance. Grade I neoplasms are composed of similar, regular cells possessing rounded smooth nuclei and abundant eosinophilic granular cytoplasm (Figure 22–1). Grade II neoplasms have larger, irregular nuclei and more variation in cell size and configuration. Grade III neoplasms have significant nuclear atypia and may have abundant mitotic figures (Lieber, Tomera, and Farrow, 1981).

The diagnosis of oncocytoma is predominantly pathologic because there are no reliable distinguishing clinical characteristics. Gross hematuria and flank pain occur in less than 20% of patients (Lieber and Tsukamoto, 1986). No characteristic features of the tumors appear on CT, ultrasound (US), intravenous urography (IVU), or MRI. Ambos et al (1978) and

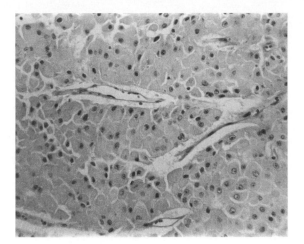

Figure 22–1. Histologic section of a grade I (benign) renal oncocytoma (original magnification, × 100).

Weiner and Bernstein (1977) have described angiographic features of oncocytomas, including the "spoke-wheel" appearance of tumor arterioles, the "lucent rim sign" of the capsule, and a homogeneous capillary nephrogram phase. Unfortunately, these findings are not invariable (Older et al, 1978), and similar findings have been reported in patients with renal cell carcinoma (Maatman et al, 1984).

High-grade oncocytomas may be intermixed with elements of renal cell carcinoma (Davis et al, 1991) and can be found as coexisting lesions within the same or opposite kidney (Licht et al, 1993). Additionally, renal oncocytoma is associated with various premalignant or malignant conditions including angiomyolipoma, tuberous sclerosis, multiple myeloma, lung cancer, and carcinoid (Morra and Das, 1993). Grade I oncocytomas were generally believed to have a benign natural history; however, several well-described case reports documenting malignant transformation in patients with grade I tumors suggest that a small subset of these tumors may have malignant potential (Morra and Das, 1993).

The current inability to definitively diagnose oncocytomas preoperatively complicates consideration of renal-sparing surgery (subtotal nephrectomy) in patients with grade I tumors. The role of fine-needle aspiration in the preoperative diagnosis of oncocytomas remains controversial. Cytologic features characteristic of oncocytomas have been described (Alanen, Tyrkkö, and Nurmi, 1985), and some investigators have proposed the use of preoperative diagnosis to allow nephron-sparing surgery (Morra and Das, 1993).

Angiomyolipoma
(Renal Hamartoma)

Angiomyolipoma is a rare benign tumor of the kidney seen in 2 distinct clinical populations. An-

giomyolipomas are found in approximately 45–80% of patients with tuberous sclerosis and are typically bilateral and asymptomatic. In patients without tuberous sclerosis, renal angiomyolipomas can be unilateral and tend to be larger than those associated with tuberous sclerosis (Anderson and Hatcher, 1990). There is no known histologic difference between the lesions seen in these 2 populations. As many as 25% of cases can present with spontaneous rupture and subsequent hemorrhage into the retroperitoneum (Wong, McGeorge, and Clark, 1981).

Angiomyolipomas are unencapsulated yellow-to-gray lesions, typically round to oval, that elevate the renal capsule, producing a bulging smooth or irregular mass (Bennington and Beckwith, 1975). They are characterized by 3 major histologic components: mature fat cells, smooth muscle, and blood vessels. Renal hamartomas may extend to perirenal or renal sinus fat and involve regional lymphatics (Bush, Bark, and Clyde, 1976) and other visceral organs (Ditonno et al, 1992). The presence of renal hamartomas in extrarenal sites is a manifestation of multicentricity rather than metastatic potential, because only one well-documented case of malignant transformation of angiomyolipoma has been reported (Lowe et al, 1992).

The diagnosis of renal hamartoma has evolved with the widespread use of US and CT. Arteriography can reveal neovascularity similar to that of renal cancer and therefore is not helpful in differential diagnosis. Ultrasonography and CT are frequently diagnostic in lesions with high fat content. Fat visualized on US appears as very high intensity echoes. Fat imaged by CT has a negative density (–20 to – 80 Hounsfield units), which is pathognomonic for angiomyolipomas when observed in the kidney (Figure 22–2) (Pitts et al, 1980). The role of MRI as a diagnostic tool has been investigated; as in CT, the high fat content makes this lesion suitable for MRI diagnosis (Uhlenbrock, Fischer, and Beyer, 1988); however, because the presence

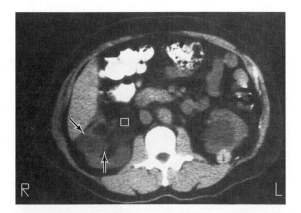

Figure 22–2. Computed tomogram of an angiomyolipoma (arrows).

of bleeding in any renal tumor can mimic the typical pattern of angiomyolipoma, MRI should not be considered the diagnostic method of choice until additional clinical experience is gained.

The management of angiomyolipomas historically has been correlated with symptoms. Steiner and colleagues (1993) reported a long-term follow-up study of 35 patients with angiomyolipomas. They proposed that patients with isolated lesions less than 4 cm be followed with yearly CT or US. Patients with asymptomatic or mildly symptomatic lesions greater than 4 cm should be followed with semiannual US. Patients with lesions greater than 4 cm with moderate or severe symptoms (bleeding or pain) should undergo renal-sparing surgery or renal arterial embolization. Given the difference in the natural history of angiomyolipomas in patients with tuberous sclerosis, Steiner et al advocate prophylactic intervention in patients with lesions greater than 4 cm irrespective of symptoms, with close follow-up of smaller lesions.

Other Rare Benign Renal Tumors

Several other benign renal tumors are quite rare, including leiomyomas, hemangiomas, lipomas, and juxtaglomerular cell tumors. Most benign tumors are not a diagnostic or therapeutic dilemma since they are rarely encountered during the patient's lifetime. With the exception of juxtaglomerular tumors, there are no features that unequivocally establish the diagnosis prior to surgery; therefore, the pathologist most often provides the diagnosis following total nephrectomy.

Leiomyomas are rare small tumors typically found in smooth-muscle-containing areas of the kidney including the renal capsule and renal pelvis. Two groups of renal leiomyomas have been described (Steiner et al, 1990). The more common group comprises cortical tumors that are less than 2 cm and may be multiple. These tumors are typically found at autopsy and are not clinically significant. A larger, commonly solitary leiomyoma has been described, which may cause symptoms and is confirmed pathologically following nephrectomy.

Hemangiomas are small vascular tumors occurring in the kidney with a frequency second only to that in the liver among visceral organs (White and Braunstein, 1946). Multiple lesions in one kidney occur in approximately 12% of cases; however, they are rarely bilateral. They can occasionally be the elusive source of hematuria in an otherwise well-evaluated patient. The diagnosis may be determined by angiography or by direct visualization by endoscopy (Ekelund and Gothlin, 1975).

Renal lipomas are very uncommon deposits of mature adipose cells without evident mitosis that arise from the renal capsule or perirenal tissue. They are seen primarily in middle-aged females and, owing to the characteristic CT differentiation of fat, are best detected radiographically on CT scanning.

The juxtaglomerular cell tumor is the most clinically significant member of this subgroup of rare benign tumors because it causes significant hypertension that can be cured by surgical treatment. It is a very rare lesion, with less than 20 reported cases. The tumors originate from the pericytes of afferent arterioles in the juxtaglomerular apparatus and can be shown to contain renin secretory granules. They are typically encapsulated and located in the cortical area. The diagnosis is suspected when there is secondary hyperaldosteronism and is confirmed by selected renal vein sampling for renin (Bonnin et al, 1977). While a subtotal nephrectomy might be possible with adequate radiographic localization, in most reported cases complete nephrectomy has been curative (Bonsib, 1985).

ADENOCARCINOMA OF THE KIDNEY (RENAL CELL CARCINOMA)

In the United States in 1999, an estimated 30,000 new cases of adenocarcinoma of the kidney will be diagnosed, and 11,900 deaths will occur from this disease (Landis et al, 1999). Renal cell carcinoma (RCC) accounts for roughly 3% of adult cancers and constitutes approximately 85% of all primary malignant renal tumors. Renal cell carcinoma occurs most commonly in the fifth to sixth decade and has a male-female ratio of 2:1. The incidence of renal cancer is equivalent between whites and blacks; however, Hispanic men and women have kidney cancer rates more than one-third higher than those of white Americans.

Multiple terms have been used to describe renal adenocarcinoma, including hypernephroma, clear cell carcinoma, and alveolar carcinoma. This diversity reflects the historical controversy over the histogenesis of RCC. It was not until 1960 that Oberling and associates, using electron microscopy, demonstrated the similarities between cells from the proximal renal tubule epithelium and RCC.

Etiology

The cause of renal adenocarcinoma is unknown. There are various etiologic hypotheses encompassing a range of environmental and occupational exposures in addition to the role of both chromosomal aberrations and tumor suppressor genes. Cigarette smoking is the only risk factor consistently linked to RCC by both epidemiologic case-control and cohort studies (La Vecchia, 1990), with most investigations demonstrating at least a 2-fold increase in risk for the development of RCC in smokers (Yu et al, 1986). Exposure to asbestos and tanning products has also been associated with an increased incidence of RCC (Maclure, 1987; Malker et al, 1984).

RCC occurs in two forms, inherited and sporadic. In 1979, Cohen and colleagues described a pedigree with hereditary RCC in which the pattern of inheritance was consistent with an autosomal dominant gene with a balanced reciprocal translocation between the short arm of chromosome 3 and the long arm of chromosome 8 (Cohen et al, 1979). Subsequent work has documented that both the hereditary and sporadic form of RCC are associated with structural changes in chromosome 3 (Kovacs et al, 1988; Erlandsson, 1998).

Two other hereditary forms of RCC have been described. Von Hippel-Lindau disease is a familial cancer syndrome in which affected individuals have a predisposition to develop tumors in multiple organs, including cerebellar hemangioblastoma, retinal angiomata, and bilateral clear cell RCC. In 1993, Latif and colleagues identified the von Hippel-Lindau gene, leading to the detection of a germ line mutation in approximately 75% of von Hippel-Lindau families (Chen et al, 1995).

Hereditary papillary renal carcinoma was described in 1994 and is characterized by a predisposition to develop multiple bilateral renal tumors with a papillary histologic appearance (Zbar et al, 1994). In contrast to von Hippel-Lindau patients, the major neoplastic manifestations appear to be confined to the kidney.

Acquired cystic disease of the kidneys is a well-recognized entity of multiple bilateral cysts in the native kidneys of uremic patients (Dunnill, Millard, and Oliver, 1977; Hughson, Hennigar, and McManus, 1980; Reichard, Roubidoux, and Dunnick, 1998). The risk of developing RCC has been estimated to be greater than 30 times higher in dialysis patients with cystic changes in their kidney than in the general population (Brennan et al, 1991). Several series reported in the literature suggest that RCC occurs in 3–9% of patients with acquired cystic disease of the kidneys (Gardner and Evan, 1984; Gulanikar et al, 1998). Most RCC cases have been described in patients undergoing hemodialysis, but it has been reported in association with peritoneal dialysis (Smith et al, 1987) and successful renal transplants (Vaziri et al, 1984) and in patients with long-term renal insufficiency not requiring dialysis (Bretan et al, 1986; Fallon and Williams, 1989).

Pathology

As previously noted, RCC originates from the proximal renal tubular epithelium as evidenced by electron microscopy (Makay, Ordonez, and Khoursland, 1987) and immunohistochemical analysis (Holthöfer, 1990). These tumors occur with equal frequency in either kidney and are randomly distributed in the upper and lower poles. RCCs originate in the cortex and tend to grow out into perinephric tissue, causing the characteristic bulge or mass effect that aids in their detection by diagnostic imaging studies. These tumors average 7–8 cm in diameter but can grow to fill the entire retroperitoneum. Grossly, the tumor is characteristically yellow to orange because of the abundance of lipids, particularly

in the clear cell type (25%). The granular cell type (25%) contains cells that have large nuclei that stain darker than the clear cell variety and tend to be more gray to white. The rest of the tumors are mixed cell types, with approximately 2% being a sarcomatoid variety that is typically less pigmented and appears gray or tan. Small tumors are homogeneous on a cut surface, but larger tumors can exhibit hemorrhage, necrosis with secondary cystic areas, and, occasionally, calcification. RCCs do not have true capsules but may have a pseudocapsule of compressed renal parenchyma, fibrous tissue, and inflammatory cells.

Histologically, RCC is most often a mixed adenocarcinoma containing clear cells, granular cells, and, occasionally, sarcomatoid-appearing cells. Clear cells are rounded or polygonal with abundant cytoplasm which contains cholesterol, triglycerides, glycogen, and lipids (Figure 22–3). Granular cells contain less glycogen and lipids, and electron microscopy reveals that the granular cytoplasm contains large numbers of mitochondria and cytosomes. Sarcomatoid cells are spindle-shaped and form sheets or bundles. This cell type rarely occurs as a pure form and is most commonly a small component of either the clear cell or granular cell type (or both).

Pathogenesis

RCCs are vascular tumors that tend to spread either by direct invasion through the renal capsule into perinephric fat and adjacent visceral structures or by direct extension into the renal vein. Approximately one-third of patients have evidence of metastatic disease at presentation (Middleton, 1967). The most common site of distant metastases is the lung. However, liver, bone, ipsilateral adjacent lymph nodes, adrenal gland, and the opposite kidney are frequent sites of disease spread.

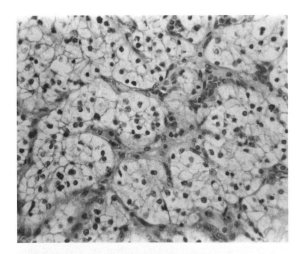

Figure 22–3. Photomicrograph of clear cell renal adenocarcinoma (original magnification, × 125).

Tumor Staging & Grading

A. Tumor Staging: The ultimate goal of staging is to select appropriate therapy and obtain prognostic information. Appropriate studies for a complete clinical staging evaluation include history and physical examination, complete blood count, serum chemistries (renal and hepatic function), urinalysis, chest x-ray (chest CT scan for an equivocal exam), CT scan of abdomen and pelvis, and a radionuclide bone scan (with x-rays of abnormal areas).

Owing to the lack of useful diagnostic studies and effective therapy for metastatic disease, early staging systems were primarily geared toward evaluation of operative findings for prognostic information. Flocks and Kadesky (1958) proposed a staging system based on gross physical characteristics of the tumor. Robson (1969) proposed modifications to the Flocks and Kadesky staging scheme, taking into account the degree of vascular involvement (Figure 22–4).

Stage I: Tumor is confined within the kidney parenchyma (no involvement of perinephric fat, renal vein, or regional lymph nodes).

Stage II: Tumor involves the perinephric fat but is confined within Gerota's fascia (including the adrenal).

Stage IIIA: Tumor involves the main renal vein or inferior vena cava.

Stage IIIB: Tumor involves regional lymph nodes.

Stage IIIC: Tumor involves both local vessels and regional lymph nodes.

Stage IVA: Tumor involves adjacent organs other than the adrenal (colon, pancreas, etc).

Stage IVB: Distant metastases.

Although the Robson system is easy to use, long-term evaluation of patients, especially those with stage III disease, has determined that it does not relate di-

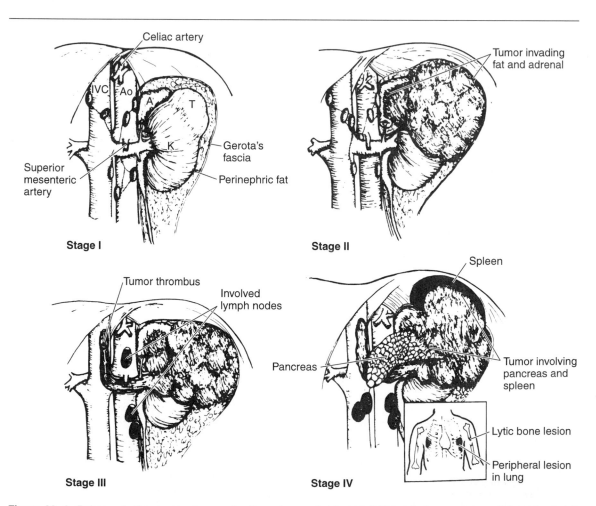

Figure 22–4. Robson staging system for renal cell carcinoma. In stage I, IVC is inferior vena cava; Ao, aorta; A, left suprarenal gland; T, tumor; K, left kidney. (Adapted with permission from Williams RD: Renal, perirenal, and ureteral neoplasms. In: *Adult and Pediatric Urology,* 2nd ed. Yearbook Medical Publishers, 1991.)

rectly to prognosis. Patients with renal vein (or proximal vena cava) involvement (stage IIIA), but without disease extension into perinephric fat and lymph nodes, have survival rates comparable to those of patients with disease confined to the kidney (stages I and II) (Siminovitch, Montie, and Straffon, 1983).

The Tumor-Node-Metastasis (TNM) system more accurately classifies the extent of tumor involvement. The TNM classification system for RCC was redefined and simplified in 1997 (Sobin and Wittekind) (Table 22–1).

While the Robson system is still the most widely used system in the United States, the recent modification of the TNM system has simplified its use. The 1987 modification of the TNM renal carcinoma staging system has generated considerable controversy regarding its clinical usefulness (Shröder et al, 1988). A recent retrospective comparison of the available staging systems suggests that none of them are totally satisfactory and that additional modifications will likely be required (Hermanek and Schrott, 1990).

B. Tumor Grading: The existence of multiple grading schemes emphasizes the considerable controversy regarding tumor grading as a prognostic factor. Recently, Fuhrman grading has become commonly used by pathologists in North America (Fuhrman, Lasky, and Limas, 1982; Goldstein, 1997). The system uses four grades based on nuclear size and irregularity and nucleolar prominence. The system is most effective in predicting metastasis (50% of high-grade tumors within 5 years). When high-grade, predominantly granular tumors are corrected for grade and stage, there is no apparent difference between clear cell and granular cell tumor prognosis (McNichols, Segura, and DeWeerd, 1981). However, patients presenting with advanced disease do poorly irrespective of tumor grade. Until effective adjuvant therapy is available, grading early-stage tumors will continue to have minimal clinical utility.

Clinical Findings

A. Symptoms and Signs: RCCs along with malignant melanomas are the great masqueraders among the more common neoplasms. Dubbed the "internists' tumor," RCC is associated with a wide variety of presenting signs and symptoms. The classically described triad of gross hematuria, flank pain, and a palpable mass occurs in only 10–15% of patients and is frequently a manifestation of advanced disease. Sixty percent of patients present with gross or microscopic hematuria. Pain, an abdominal mass, or both, are seen in approximately 40% of patients (Skinner et al, 1971). Symptoms secondary to metastatic disease such as dyspnea and cough, seizure and headache, or bone pain from lung, brain, and bone metastases, respectively, lead to a diagnosis in up to 30% of patients. With the routine use of CT scanning, renal tumors are increasingly detected incidentally; therefore, older literature describing RCC presentation may no longer be accurate.

B. Paraneoplastic Syndromes: RCC is associated with a wide spectrum of paraneoplastic syndromes including erythrocytosis, hypercalcemia, hypertension, and nonmetastatic hepatic dysfunction.

RCC is the most common cause of paraneoplastic erythrocytosis, which is reported to occur in 3–10% of patients with this tumor (Sufrin et al, 1989). In patients with RCC, the elevated erythrocyte mass is physiologically inappropriate and may result either from enhanced production of erythropoietin from the

Table 22–1. TNM classification system for renal cell carcinoma.[a]

Classification	Definition
T—Primary tumor	
TX	Primary tumor cannot be assessed.
T0	No evidence of primary tumor.
T1	Tumor 7.0 cm or less limited to the kidney.
T2	Tumor more than 7.0 cm limited to the kidney.
T3	Tumor extends into major veins or invades adrenal gland or perinephric tissues but not beyond Gerota's fascia.
T3a	Tumor invades adrenal gland or perinephric tissues but not beyond Gerota's fascia.
T3b	Tumor grossly extends into renal vein(s) or vena cava.
T3c	Tumor grossly extends into vena cava above diaphragm.
T4	Tumor invades beyond Gerota's fascia.
N—Regional lymph nodes	
NX	Regional lymph nodes cannot be assessed.
N0	No regional lymph node metastasis.
N1	Metastasis in a single regional lymph node 2 cm or less.
N2	Metastasis in more than a single regional lymph node.
M—Distant metastases	
MX	Distant metastasis cannot be assessed.
M0	No distant metastasis.
M1	Distant metastasis.

[a] All sizes measured in greatest dimension.

tumor or as a consequence of regional renal hypoxia promoting erythropoietin production from nonneoplastic renal tissue (Hocking, 1987).

Hypercalcemia has been reported to occur in up to 20% of patients with RCC (Muggia, 1990). Two subsets of hypercalcemia are seen in patients with localized RCC. Humoral hypercalcemia of malignancy has been the subject of considerable research efforts over the past two decades. Various investigators have identified and subsequently cloned a molecule called parathyroid hormone-related peptide that mimics the function of parathyroid hormone (Strewler et al, 1987). Tumor-produced parathyroid hormone-related peptide mimics many of the effects of parathyroid hormone, leading to alterations in normal calcium homeostasis. Other humoral factors such as osteoclast-activating factor, tumor necrosis factor, and transforming growth factor-alpha are known to contribute to humoral hypercalcemia (Muggia, 1990).

Hypertension associated with RCC has been reported in up to 40% of patients (Sufrin et al, 1989), and renin production by the neoplasm has been documented in 37%. The excess renin and hypertension associated with RCC are typically refractory to antihypertensive therapy but may respond following nephrectomy (Gold et al, 1996).

In 1961, Stauffer described a reversible syndrome of hepatic dysfunction in the absence of hepatic metastases associated with RCC (Stauffer, 1961). Hepatic function abnormalities include elevation of alkaline phosphatase and bilirubin, hypoalbuminemia, prolonged prothrombin time, and hypergammaglobulinemia. Stauffer syndrome tends to occur in association with fever, fatigue, and weight loss and typically resolves after nephrectomy. The reported incidence of Stauffer syndrome varies from 3 to 20% (Gold et al, 1996). The cause is unknown but is suspected to be a hepatotoxic product of the tumor.

RCC is known to produce a multitude of other biologically active products that result in clinically significant syndromes, including adrenocorticotropic hormone (Cushing syndrome), enteroglucagon (protein enteropathy), prolactin (galactorrhea), insulin (hypoglycemia), and gonadotropins (gynecomastia and decreased libido; or hirsutism, amenorrhea, and male pattern balding) (Sufrin, Golio, and Murphy, 1986).

A paraneoplastic syndrome present at the time of disease diagnosis does not in and of itself confer a poor prognosis. However, patients whose paraneoplastic metabolic disturbances fail to normalize following nephrectomy (suggesting the presence of clinically undetectable metastatic disease) have very poor prognoses (Hanash, 1982; Robson, 1982).

C. Laboratory Findings: In addition to the laboratory abnormalities associated with the various RCC paraneoplastic syndromes, anemia, hematuria, and an elevated sedimentation rate are frequently observed.

Anemia occurs in about 30% of RCC patients. The anemia typically is not secondary to blood loss or hemolysis and is commonly normochromic. The serum iron and total iron-binding capacity are usually low, as in the anemia of chronic disease. Iron therapy is usually ineffective; however, surgical removal of early-stage tumors usually leads to physiologic correction of the anemia. The potential role of recombinant erythropoietin for patients with unresectable disease represents a potential, but untested, option.

Gross or microscopic hematuria can be seen in up to 60% of patients presenting with RCC. An elevated erythrocyte sedimentation rate is also commonly seen with reported incidence as high as 75%. These findings are nonspecific, and normal findings do not rule out a diagnosis of RCC.

D. X-Ray Findings: While a large number of radiologic techniques are available to aid in the detection and diagnosis of renal masses, CT scanning remains the primary technique with which others must be compared. Other radiologic techniques used include US, MRI, and arteriography. In this era of cost containment, selecting the appropriate studies for an efficient, cost-effective evaluation is mandatory.

The most appropriate diagnostic method is to some extent dictated by the clinical presentation. Patients presenting with hematuria should have intravenous urography as their initial radiologic evaluation; however, patients with a suspicious renal mass found during either a US evaluation or IVU for other indications would best be evaluated with CT scanning.

E. Intravenous Urography: When used alone, IVU is only 75% accurate, and additional studies are needed for confirmation. Calcification overlying the renal shadow is an important diagnostic finding because its presence significantly increases the probability of cancer. Daniel and colleagues (1972) found that 87% of renal masses with central calcification and 20% of those with peripheral calcification were malignant. Less than 1% of simple benign renal cysts contain calcium; therefore, calcium-containing masses require additional diagnostic studies and probably surgical definition as well.

F. Ultrasonography: Ultrasound examination is a noninvasive, relatively inexpensive technique able to further delineate a renal mass seen on IVU. Approximately 98% accurate in defining simple cysts, US spares the majority of patients the need for needle biopsy. Strict ultrasonographic criteria for a simple cyst include through transmission, a well-circumscribed mass without internal echoes, and adequate visualization of a strong posterior wall (Figure 22–5).

G. CT Scanning: CT scanning has been shown to be more sensitive than US or IVU for renal cancer detection (Warshauer et al, 1988). A typical finding of RCC on CT is a mass that becomes enhanced with the use of intravenous contrast media. In general,

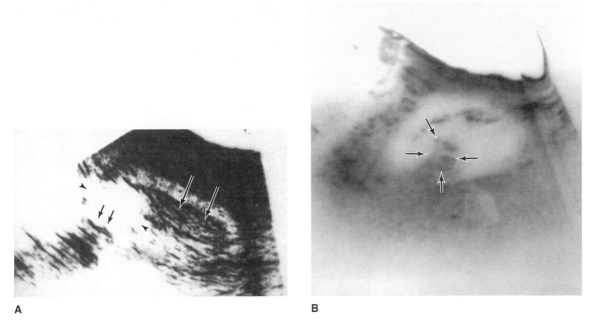

A

B

Figure 22–5. A: Ultrasound of a simple renal cyst showing renal parenchyma (long arrows), cyst wall (arrow heads), and a strong posterior wall (short arrows). **B:** Ultrasound of a solid renal mass (arrows).

RCC exhibits an overall decreased density in Hounsfield units compared with normal renal parenchyma but shows a heterogeneous pattern of enhancement or increased attenuation (slightly decreased from the surrounding parenchyma) when contrast is used (Figure 22–6) (Kosko, Lipuma, and Resnick, 1984). In addition to defining the primary lesion, CT scanning is also the method of choice in staging the patient by visualizing the renal hilum, perinephric space, renal

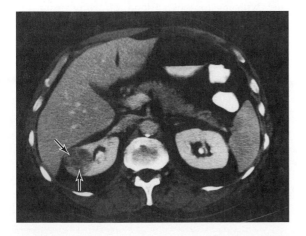

Figure 22–6. Computed tomogram (contrast enhancement) of a renal cell carcinoma (arrows).

vein and vena cava, adrenals, regional lymphatics, and adjacent organs. In patients with equivocal chest x-ray findings, a CT scan of the chest is indicated. Patients who present with symptoms consistent with brain metastases should be evaluated with either CT or MRI. Spiral CT has become useful for evaluating tumors prior to nephron-sparing surgery to delineate the 3-dimensional extent of the tumor and thus to aid the surgeon in preventing positive surgical margins (Holmes et al, 1997).

H. Renal Angiography: With the widespread availability of CT scanners, the role of renal angiography in the diagnostic evaluation of RCC has markedly diminished. Angiography is capable of demonstrating neovascularity and arteriovenous fistulas as well as renal vein and vena caval tumor involvement, but it is of limited usefulness in the approximately 10% of patients whose tumors are not hypervascular (Figure 22–7). In addition, angiography is invasive and carries a small but real risk of complications, including hemorrhage, pseudoaneurysm formation at the puncture site, arterial emboli, and contrast-related nephrotoxicity. Furthermore, renal angiography is relatively expensive and may require hospitalization. There remain specific clinical situations in which angiography may be useful, for example, guiding the operative approach in a patient with an RCC in a solitary kidney when attempts to perform a partial nephrectomy may be indicated.

I. Radionuclide Imaging: Radionuclide renal

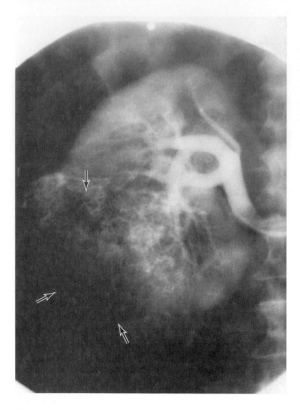

Figure 22–7. Right renal angiogram showing typical neo-vascularity (arrows) in a large lower pole renal cell cancer.

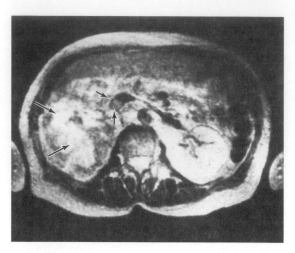

Figure 22–8. Transaxial magnetic resonance image (T2) of a renal cell carcinoma (long arrows) with vena caval tumor thrombus (short arrows).

scans may occasionally be useful in the evaluation of patients unable to receive contrast material for IVU. Determination of metastases to bones is most accurate by radionuclide bone scan, although the study is nonspecific and requires confirmation with bone x-rays of identified abnormalities to verify the presence of the typical osteolytic lesions. There is evidence that patients without bone pain and with a normal alkaline phosphatase level have a very low incidence of bone metastases (Henriksson et al, 1992), and thus a routine bone scan is not necessary in such patients.

J. Magnetic Resonance Imaging: MRI is equivalent to CT for staging of RCC (Hricak et al, 1988). Its primary advantage is in the evaluation of patients with suspected vascular extension (Figure 22–8). Prospective trials have demonstrated that MRI is superior to CT in assessing inferior vena caval involvement (Kabala et al, 1991) and is at least as accurate as venacavography (Horan et al, 1989). In contrast to both CT and cavography, MRI evaluation does not require either iodinated contrast material or ionizing radiation. Recent studies using MRI angiography with gadolinium or CT angiography have improved vascular evaluation of renal neoplasms (Bluemke and Chambers, 1995).

K. Fine-Needle Aspiration: Fine-needle aspiration has a limited role in the evaluation of RCC. Patients with radiologic findings consistent with RCC require definitive surgical management. Fine-needle aspiration of renal lesions is the diagnostic approach of choice in those patients with clinically apparent metastatic disease who may be candidates for nonsurgical therapy. Other settings in which fine-needle aspiration may be appropriate include establishing a diagnosis in patients who are not surgical candidates, differentiating a primary RCC from a renal metastasis in patients with known primary cancers of nonrenal origin, and evaluating some radiographically indeterminate lesions (Renshaw, Granter, and Cibas, 1997).

L. Instrumental and Cytologic Examination: Patients presenting with hematuria should be evaluated with cystoscopy. Blood effluxing from the ureteral orifice identifies the origin of bleeding from the upper tract. Most renal pelvis tumors can be distinguished radiographically from RCC; however, endoscopic evaluation of the bladder, ureters, and renal pelvis is occasionally helpful in making a diagnosis. Additionally, while urine cytologic study is rarely helpful in the diagnosis of RCC, cytologic study of urine with renal pelvis washing is frequently diagnostic in renal pelvis tumors.

M. Tumor Markers: As noted previously, RCC is associated with numerous biologically active substances. However, at present there are no clinically relevant tumor markers to aid in screening, diagnosis, or evaluating response to therapy.

Differential Diagnosis

When a patient presents with clinical findings consistent with metastatic disease and is found to have a renal mass, a diagnosis of RCC can be straightforward. The majority of patients present with a renal mass discovered after an evaluation of hematuria or pain or as an incidental finding during an imaging workup of an unrelated problem. The differential diagnosis of RCC includes other solid renal lesions. The great majority of renal masses are simple cysts. Once the diagnosis of a cyst is confirmed by US, no additional evaluation is required if the patient is asymptomatic. Equivocal findings or the presence of calcification within the mass warrant further evaluation by CT. There are a wide variety of pathologic entities that appear as solid masses on CT scans, and differentiation of benign from malignant lesions is frequently difficult. Findings on CT scan that suggest malignancy include amputation of a portion of the collecting system, presence of calcification, a poorly defined interface between the renal parenchyma and the lesion, invasion into perinephric fat or adjacent structures, and the presence of abnormal periaortic adenopathy or distant metastatic disease (Kosko, Lipuma, and Resnick, 1984).

Some characteristic lesions can be defined using CT criteria in combination with clinical findings. Angiomyolipomas (with large fat components) can easily be identified by the low attenuation areas classically produced by substantial fat content. A renal abscess may be strongly suspected in a patient presenting with fever, flank pain, pyuria, and leukocytosis, and an early needle aspiration and culture should be performed. Other benign renal masses (in addition to those previously described) include granulomas and arteriovenous malformations. Renal lymphoma (both Hodgkin disease and non-Hodgkin disease), transitional cell carcinoma of the renal pelvis, adrenal cancer, and metastatic disease are additional diagnostic possibilities that may be suspected based on CT and clinical findings.

Treatment

A. Specific Measures:

1. Localized disease–Surgical removal of the early-stage lesion remains the only potentially curative therapy available for RCC patients. Appropriate therapy depends almost entirely on the stage of tumor at presentation and therefore requires a thorough staging evaluation. The prognoses of patients with stages I, II, and IIIA (renal vein only) are very similar after surgical removal of the kidney and enveloping fascia are accomplished (Skinner, Vermillion, and Colvin, 1972).

Radical nephrectomy is the primary treatment for localized RCC. Its goal is to achieve the removal of tumor and to take a wide margin of normal tissue. Radical nephrectomy (Robson, 1963) entails en bloc removal of the kidney and its enveloping fascia (Gerota's) including the ipsilateral adrenal, proximal

one-half of the ureter, and lymph nodes up to the area of transection of the renal vessels (Figure 22–9).

Various incisions provide optimal access for the radical nephrectomy, including an anterior subcostal (unilateral chevron) or thoracoabdominal incision, and, occasionally, a midline incision or the classic flank incision (Droller, 1992).

The role of regional lymphadenectomy in RCC remains controversial. Between 18 and 33% of patients undergoing radical nephrectomy with lymph node dissection for RCC have metastatic disease identified (Skinner, Lieskovsky, and Pritchett, 1988). While there are several retrospective studies (Thrasher and Paulson, 1993) and a prospective, nonrandomized study (Herrlinger et al, 1991) suggesting that regional lymphadenectomy can improve survival in patients with Robson stages I and II RCCs, this subject remains highly controversial, and the definitive answer will require a prospective, randomized clinical trial. Removal of the adrenal is unnecessary if the tumor is not in the upper pole, as adrenal involvement is uncommon in this instance.

Preoperative renal artery embolization (angioinfarction) has been used as a surgical adjunct to facilitate radical nephrectomy, purportedly by decreasing operative blood loss and by causing edema in tissue planes (McLean and Meranze, 1985). Various substances have been used for embolization, including

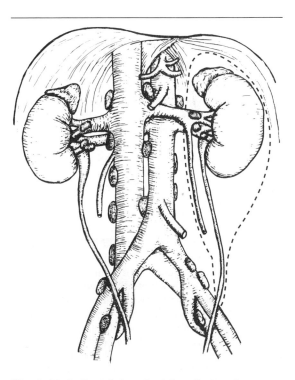

Figure 22–9. Boundaries of a left radical nephrectomy. Dotted line represents both the surgical margin and Gerota's fascia.

barium, polyvinyl alcohol sponge, particulate Gel-foam, subcutaneous fat, detachable balloons, and steel coils. Absolute ethanol has been recommended because it causes superior occlusion in less time and minimizes the resultant postinfarction syndrome. Reported complications of embolization include migration of coils or balloons to the opposite kidney or distant sites, damage to the contralateral kidney by excessive use of contrast material during the procedure, and ischemic injury to the lower limbs or bowel from an overflow of the embolization agent. The postinfarction syndrome is characterized by flank pain, fever, and leukocytosis typically lasting an average of 3 days.

As there is no conclusive evidence that preoperative embolization actually decreases blood loss or facilitates surgery, its use should be limited to patients with very large tumors in which the renal artery may be difficult to reach early in the procedure. Additionally, this technique may be useful to palliate patients with nonresectable tumors and significant symptoms such as hemorrhage, flank pain, or paraneoplastic symptoms.

Radiation therapy has been advocated as a neoadjuvant (preoperative) or adjuvant method to radical nephrectomy, but there has been controversy over its effectiveness (Rafla, 1970; van der Werf-Messing, 1973; Juusela, 1977). There is no evidence that post-surgical radiation therapy to the renal bed, whether or not residual tumor is present, contributes to prolonged survival.

RCC may invade renal vascular spaces and produce tumor thrombi extending into renal veins, inferior vena cava, hepatic veins, and, occasionally, the right atrium. Between 5 and 10% of patients presenting with RCC have some degree of vena caval involvement (Figure 22–10) (Skinner, Lieskovsky, and Pritchett, 1988). As previously described, patients presenting with involvement of the renal vein and vena cava below the hepatic veins (stage IIIA or T3aN0M0) but without evidence of regional or distant metastases have a prognosis similar to patients with stage II (T2) disease when treated by radical excision. The surgical approach to the removal of caval thrombi depends entirely on the level of cephalad extension. In general, these thrombi do not invade the cava and therefore can be removed without resection of the caval wall. For tumor thrombi that have reached the level of the right atrium, the use of cardiopulmonary bypass is typically required.

Laparoscopic radical nephrectomy and even partial nephrectomy has been accomplished successfully and safely in several hundred patients. Early reports indicate a highly satisfactory long-term outcome similar to that of open surgery (Caddedu et al, 1998; Janetschek et al, 1998).

The approach to the patient with either bilateral RCC or disease in a solitary kidney differs from the standard approach of radical nephrectomy. Bilateral

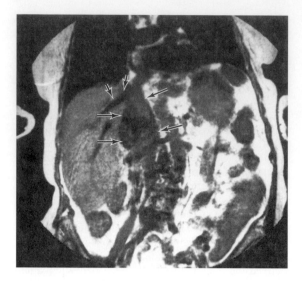

Figure 22–10. Coronal magnetic resonance image (T1) of a large vena caval tumor thrombus (long arrows) in a patient with renal cell carcinoma. Thrombus extends just to entrance of hepatic veins (short arrows).

RCC occurs with a frequency as high as 3% (Smith, 1986). Radical nephrectomy in these patients or in those with solitary kidneys obviously commits patients to long-term dialysis or renal transplantation and the morbidities of these conditions. Staging these patients is essentially the same as previously outlined, with the notable exception that angiography is often used to assess the extent of tumor within the kidney and the renal artery anatomy. Surgical alternatives to radical nephrectomy include partial nephrectomy, ex vivo partial nephrectomy (bench surgery followed by autotransplantation) (Novick, Stewart, and Straffon, 1980), and enucleation of multiple lesions (Marshall et al, 1986). Given the lack of effective adjuvant therapy and the risk of inadequate excision and subsequent recurrence from various renal-sparing approaches, partial nephrectomy with an adequate parenchymal margin remains the preferred treatment.

Recent studies have shown that even for patients with a normal contralateral kidney and a single lesion of 4 cm or less, partial nephrectomy has a similar outcome as radical nephrectomy (Herr, 1999).

Observation as treatment should also be mentioned for small (< 3.0 cm) lesions particularly in elderly patients. One recent study noted a growth rate of 0–1.3 cm per year in 40 patients followed for a mean of 3.5 years (Bosniak, 1995), indicating that with careful follow-up, watchful waiting may be appropriate in selected patients.

2. Disseminated disease—Approximately 30% of patients with RCC will present with metastatic disease. Metastatic RCC is a disease whose natural history is typically aggressive and rapidly progressive but alternatively may have a more protracted course. The biological diversity of RCC is illustrated by the 6.6% response rate (including 3% complete responders) in the placebo arm of a recently completed phase III trial of interferon-gamma in advanced RCC (Gleave et al, 1998).

a. Surgery–The role of radical nephrectomy in the management of patients with advanced disease is limited. Historically, some asymptomatic patients with metastatic RCC have undergone radical nephrectomy for various presumptive indications, including an attempt to improve survival by inducing regression of metastatic disease and to prevent potential morbidity from the primary neoplasm. There is little evidence to support the role of nephrectomy in inducing spontaneous regression of metastases, with one large series demonstrating a 0.8% incidence of disease regression following nephrectomy (Montie et al, 1977). Radical nephrectomy as a palliative procedure can be helpful in managing patients with severe hemorrhage, unremitting pain despite appropriate use of opioids, and occasionally in the management of paraneoplastic syndromes.

Patients presenting with a solitary metastatic site (synchronous metastases) that is amenable to surgical resection may be candidates for combined nephrectomy and removal of the metastatic foci. In carefully selected patients, 5-year survival has approached 30% in some series (O'Dea et al, 1978; Toho and Whitmore, 1975). Several reports in the literature have suggested that patients who undergo resection of metastatic disease presenting after nephrectomy (metachronous) have better outcomes than those with synchronous resections (O'Dea et al, 1978; Tally et al, 1969); however, this is not a universally held opinion (Pontes et al, 1989).

The important role of surgical resection of solitary brain metastases has been highlighted by several randomized trials demonstrating an improvement in survival in patients with solitary brain metastases who undergo both surgical resection and whole-brain radiotherapy compared with patients who receive only radiation therapy (Patchell et al, 1990; Vecht et al, 1993).

The role of nephrectomy as a means of reducing tumor burden prior to the administration of biological response modifier therapy and the more recent use of adjuvant nephrectomy in patients with evidence of clinical response to biological response modifier therapy remains controversial and the subject of ongoing clinical trials.

b. Radiation therapy–Radiation therapy is an important method in the palliation of patients with metastatic RCC. Despite the belief that RCC is a relatively radioresistant tumor, effective palliation of metastatic disease to the brain, bone, and lungs is reported in up to two-thirds of patients (Fossa,

Kjolseth, and Lund, 1982; Onufrey and Mohiuddin, 1985). External-beam radiation therapy has been occasionally used in lieu of nephrectomy to palliate patients with gross hematuria or pain, but without significant efficacy.

c. Hormonal therapy–The use of various hormonal agents in the treatment of metastatic RCC is based on studies demonstrating an enhanced rate of renal cancer formation in hamsters exposed to estrogen and the prevention of similar tumors in animals receiving concomitant progesterone (Kirkman and Bacon, 1949). There are numerous uncontrolled trials of progestational, androgenic, and antiestrogenic agents in the literature with responses ranging from 0 to 33% (Bono, 1986). More recent studies in large numbers of patients have shown response rates of 1–2%, with responses typically being partial and of brief duration (Kjaer, 1988).

d. Chemotherapy–RCC is among the most chemotherapy-resistant epithelial cancers. The mechanism of drug resistance is complex and may in part be a consequence of the presence of the mulitdrug resistance-associated P-glycoprotein (Mickish et al, 1990). A review of over 4000 RCC patients treated in 83 phase II trials over a 10-year span demonstrated only a 6% overall response rate (Yagoda et al, 1995). Vinblastine, once believed to have single-agent activity in the 15–20% range, in more recent series has been reported to have response rates less than 10% (Fossa et al, 1992; Yagoda et al, 1995).

e. Radioimmunotherapy–A monoclonal antibody to G250, an RCC-associated antigen, has been attached to iodine-131 and used for treatment of metastatic RCC. Results in 33 patients thus far showed tumor volume decreased in 2 and stable disease in 17 (Divgi et al, 1998). These phase I/II studies are promising; however, much more research is required to determine the efficacy of this approach.

f. Biologic response modifiers–The use of metastatic RCC as a model for the investigation of various biologic response modifiers is a consequence of both the lack of effective therapy and the long-recognized biologic "eccentricities" of this tumor. Spontaneous regression of metastatic RCC is a well-recognized, albeit rare, event (Kavoussi et al, 1986; Vogelzang et al, 1992). While no specific evidence exists, many believe this phenomenon to be immunologically mediated.

A variety of clinical approaches to the immunotherapy of RCC have been tested, including the administration of bacillus Calmette-Guérin, infusion of autologous tumor cells, and use of immune RNA. The results from these and other early trials led to the more recent experience with interferons (alpha, beta, gamma); adoptive cellular therapy with lymphokine-activated cells and tumor-infiltrating lymphocytes; autolymphocyte therapy and the only approved agent for the treatment of metastatic renal carcinoma, interleukin-2 (IL-2).

Early studies with interferon-alpha provided evidence for reproducible response rates in 15–20% of patients (Krown, 1987; Quesada, Swanson, and Gutterman, 1985). The characteristics of patients responding to interferon include a minimal tumor burden (ie, primary kidney tumor removed), lung metastases only, and an excellent performance status. A recent report of 159 patients with advanced RCC treated with various doses of interferon-alpha demonstrated an overall response proportion of 10% with a median response duration of 12.2 months. The median survival time was 11.4 months, and only 3% of patients were alive after 5 or more years (Minasian et al, 1993). The observation that most responses are seen in patients with a small tumor burden led to a randomized multi-institutional adjuvant therapy trial comparing interferon-alpha with observation after nephrectomy in patients at high risk for recurrent disease. With a median follow-up of 4.4 years, there was a higher relapse rate in the interferon-treated patients, suggesting that adjuvant interferon in the dose and schedule administered was not effective adjuvant therapy for high-risk patients (Trump et al, 1996). The experience with beta and gamma interferons has been less extensive. In 1989, Aulitzky and colleagues reported a 30% response rate in a trial of low-dose interferon-gamma (Aulitzky et al, 1989). Unfortunately, subsequent trials, including a phase III trial, have demonstrated response rates of less than 10% (Gleave et al, 1998).

IL-2 is a cytokine produced by activated T cells that has considerable immunostimulatory and antineoplastic activity. In patients with metastatic RCC, response rates to high-dose bolus IL-2 have ranged from 0 to 27% (Linehan, Shipley, and Parkinson, 1993). A multi-institutional trial comparing high-dose bolus IL-2 alone with IL-2 and lymphokine-activated cells demonstrated comparable response rates (8 and 13%, respectively) between the two therapies (McCabe, Stabler, and Hawkins, 1992). Based primarily on the response rates from the high-dose bolus experience, IL-2 was approved by the US Food and Drug Administration for treatment of metastatic RCC, although the optimal dose and administration schedule of IL-2 has not been established.

The wide variability in response rates to IL-2 is likely a function of patient selection. Atkins and colleagues recently reported a phase II experience of 71 patients treated with high-dose IL-2 (17% response rate) in which almost all responses occurred in patients with excellent performance status and metastases limited to one lung, lymph nodes, or small-volume extrahepatic abdominal disease (Atkins et al, 1993).

A recently reported, large phase III trial compared IL-2 administered intravenously at a dose of 18×10^6 IU per square meter, with interferon alfa-2a administered subcutaneously at a dose of 18×10^6 with a combination of IL-2 and interferon alfa-2a in patients with advanced RCC. The overall response rates were 6.5, 7.5, and 18.6%, respectively. Although a higher response rate to the IL-2 and interferon combination was observed, there were no differences in overall survival and, not surprisingly, the toxicity of the IL-2 plus interferon-alfa combination was significant (Negrier et al, 1998).

B. Follow-up Care: There is no universal agreement on the frequency or studies required in the follow-up care of patients with RCC. Patients who have undergone radical nephrectomy should be seen at regular intervals (3-month periods in the first year is suggested) to evaluate progress and assess for new disease-related signs and symptoms. These follow-up examinations should include a history and physical examination and laboratory and radiographic studies as clinically indicated (ie, chest x-ray for progressive cough or dyspnea, liver chemistries, and US for palpably enlarged liver). Patients with metastatic disease who are not undergoing therapy need continued follow-up to provide appropriate supportive care.

Prognosis

The prognosis of patients is most clearly related to the stage of disease at presentation. Recent studies report 5-year survival rate for patients with T1 disease in the 88–100% range and approximately 60% for stages T2 and T3a. As previously noted, patients with stage T3b have a markedly worsened 5-year survival rate (15–20%). Patients presenting with metastatic disease have a dismal prognosis with 0–20% 5-year survival rates (Cherrie et al, 1982; Selli et al, 1983; Golimbu et al, 1986).

NEPHROBLASTOMA (WILMS TUMOR)

Nephroblastoma, also known as Wilms tumor, is the most common solid renal tumor of childhood, accounting for roughly 5% of childhood cancers. Between 450 and 500 new cases are reported annually. The peak age for presentation is during the third year of life, and there is no sex predilection. The disease is seen worldwide with a similar age of onset and sex distribution. Tumors are commonly unicentric, but they occur in either kidney with equal frequency. In 5% of cases the tumors are bilateral.

Wilms tumor occurs in familial and nonfamilial forms. The National Wilms' Tumor Study (NWTS) group documented the occurrence of a familial Wilms tumor in approximately 1% of cases (Breslow and Beckwith, 1982). Although a relatively rare neoplasm, Wilms tumor has become a very important model for the study of tumorigenesis and has become a prototypical neoplasm for collaborative clinical trials, with approximately 85% of all new cases diagnosed in North America enrolled in NWTS group protocols (Beckwith, 1997). Approximately 10% of patients with Wilms tumors have recognized congenital malformations. Among the more common disorders associated with Wilms tumor are the overgrowth syndromes, such as Beckwith-Wiedemann syndrome and isolated hemihypertrophy, and nonovergrowth disorders, such as isolated aniridia and trisomy 18 (Weiner, Coppes, and Ritchey, 1998). Genitourinary abnormalities such as hypospadias, cryptorchidism, and renal fusion are found in 4.5–7.5% of patients with unilateral Wilms tumor and in up to 13.4% of those with bilateral disease (Breslow et al, 1993).

Etiology

In 1972 Knudson and Strong proposed a two-hit hypothesis to explain the earlier age of onset and bilateral presentation in children with a familial history of Wilms tumor. In this hypothesis, the pathogenesis of the sporadic form of Wilms tumor results from two postzygotic mutations in a single cell. In contrast, the familial form of the disease arises after one prezygotic mutation and a subsequent postzygotic event. Karyotypic analyses of Wilms tumor patients with various congenital malformations and loss of heterozygosity studies helped identify a region on the short arm of chromosome 11 (11p13) (Riccardi et al, 1978; Huff, 1994). This work ultimately led to the identification of a gene associated with Wilms tumor development (WT1), which maps to chromosome 11p13 (Coppes, Haber, and Grundy, 1994). Although alterations in this gene have been associated with Wilms tumor and genitourinary abnormalities, only 5–10% of sporadic Wilms tumors have been demonstrated to have WT1 mutations (Varanasi et al, 1994). Genetic linkage studies of families with an inherited susceptibility to Wilms tumors suggest that other Wilms tumor genes exist (Weiner, Coppes, and Ritchey, 1998).

Pathogenesis & Pathology

In 1990 Beckwith and colleagues proposed a simplified nomenclature and classification of Wilms tumor precursor lesions known as nephrogenic rests (NR). Two distinct categories of NR were identified and designated as perilobar NR and intralobar NR. One concept of Wilms tumor development proposed that some NR remain dormant for many years, with some undergoing involution and sclerosis and others giving rise to Wilms tumors (Beckwith, Kiviat, and Bonadio, 1990; Beckwith, 1997). The typical Wilms tumor consists of blastemal, epithelial, and stromal elements in varying proportions (Figure 22–11). Tumors composed of blastema and stroma or blastema alone have been described.

The NWTS correlated pathologic specimens with clinical outcome and divided various histologic features into favorable and unfavorable prognostic groups. The unfavorable subgroup includes tumors that contain focal or diffuse elements of anaplastic cells or two other neoplastic entities considered not

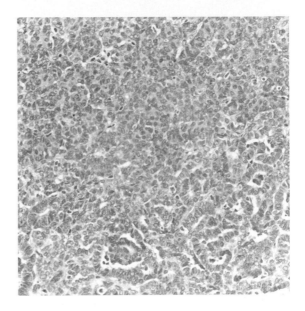

Figure 22–11. Wilms tumor with characteristic tubular/glomerulid structures and blastema (original magnification, × 40).

to be Wilms tumor variants, clear cell sarcoma of the kidney and rhabdoid tumor of the kidney (Beckwith and Palmer, 1978; Beckwith, 1997). Favorable histology tumors comprise all Wilms tumor patients without anaplasia. Anaplastic tumors are characterized by extreme nuclear atypia, hyperdiploidy, and numerous complex translocations.

Grossly, Wilms tumors are generally large, multilobulated, and gray or tan in color with focal areas of hemorrhage and necrosis. A fibrous pseudocapsule is occasionally seen.

Tumor dissemination can occur by direct extension through the renal capsule, hematogenously via the renal vein and vena cava, or via lymphatic spread. Metastatic disease is present at diagnosis in 10–15% of patients, with the lungs (85–95%) and liver (10–15%) the most common sites of involvement. Regional lymphatics are involved in as many as 25% of patients. Metastases to liver, bone, and brain are uncommon.

Tumor Staging

The NWTS staging system is most widely used and is based on surgical and pathologic findings. The original classification was used in the first and second NWTS trials and was modified for NWTS III (D'Angio et al, 1989).

Stage I: Tumor limited to kidney and completely excised. The surface of the renal capsule is intact. Tumor was not ruptured before or during removal.

There is no residual tumor apparent beyond the margins of resection.

Stage II: Tumor extends beyond the kidney but is completely removed. There is regional extension of the tumor, ie, penetration through the outer surface of the renal capsule into perirenal soft tissues. Vessels outside the kidney substance are infiltrated or contain tumor thrombus. The tumor may have been biopsied or there has been local spillage of tumor confined to the flank. There is no residual tumor apparent at or beyond the margins of excision.

Stage III: Residual nonhematogenous tumor confined to abdomen. Any one or more of the following occur: a. Lymph nodes on biopsy are found to be involved in the hilus, the periaortic chains, or beyond. b. There has been diffuse peritoneal contamination by tumor, such as spillage of tumor beyond the flank before or during surgery, or by tumor growth that has penetrated through the peritoneal surface. c. Implants are found on the peritoneal surfaces. d. The tumor extends beyond the surgical margins either microscopically or grossly. e. The tumor is not completely resectable because of local infiltration into vital structures. f. Tumor spill not confined to the flank occurred either before or during surgery.

Stage IV: Hematogenous metastases. Deposits beyond stage III, eg, lung, liver, bone, and brain.

Stage V: Bilateral renal involvement at diagnosis. An attempt should be made to stage each side according to the previously given criteria on the basis of extent of disease before biopsy.

Clinical Findings

A. Symptoms and Signs: The diagnosis of Wilms tumor is most commonly made after the discovery of an asymptomatic mass by a family member or a physician during a routine physical examination. Common symptoms at presentation include abdominal pain and distention, anorexia, nausea and vomiting, fever, and hematuria. The most common sign is an abdominal mass. Hypertension is seen in 25–60% of cases and is caused by elevated renin levels (D'Angio et al, 1982; Pizzo et al, 1989).

B. Laboratory Analysis: Urinalysis may show evidence of hematuria, and anemia may be present, particularly in patients with evidence of subcapsular hemorrhage. Patients with liver metastases may have abnormal serum chemistries.

C. X-Ray Imaging: Historically, IVU was the initial diagnostic study of choice to assess a suspected renal mass, but it has been replaced by newer modalities. Chest x-ray remains the initial examination of choice to evaluate for the presence of lung metastases.

Renal arteriography is typically indicated only in the patients with bilateral Wilms tumors or an involved horseshoe kidney. Chest x-ray remains the initial examination of choice for detection of metastatic disease. The role of a chest CT scan is controversial, and it is probably not indicated for routine use in low-risk patients; however, when done concomitantly with an abdominal CT, chest CT may provide clinically useful information in high-risk patients.

D. Ultrasonography, CT Scanning, and MRI: Ultrasonography is the current initial study of choice to evaluate palpable abdominal masses because it is accurate, does not require sedation, and is both widely available and cost-effective (Babyn et al, 1995).

CT of the abdomen is performed with suspected Wilms tumor and can be useful in providing information regarding tumor extension, the status of the contralateral kidney, and the presence of regional adenopathy. CT scanning remains an imperfect technique with a relatively high false-positive rate for hepatic invasion in right-sided tumors, and 7% of cases of surgically confirmed synchronous bilateral Wilms tumors were missed by preoperative CT imaging in the NWTS IV (Ritchey et al, 1995).

If pulmonary metastases are seen on chest x-ray, CT of the chest will not alter current therapy. However, the need for chest CT imaging in patients with negative chest x-rays remains controversial, as it is not clear whether those lesions detected by CT alone require more aggressive treatment (Weiner, Coppes, and Ritchey, 1998).

Magnetic resonance imaging can provide important information in defining the extent of tumor into the inferior vena cava, including those with intracardiac extension. It is limited in that there is no bowel contrast agent, and its use in children requires sedation (Babyn et al, 1995).

E. Radionuclide Imaging: Radionuclide bone scanning is rarely indicated. Abdominal CT scans essentially have taken the place of liver-spleen imaging.

F. Needle Biopsy: Preoperative biopsy is indicated routinely only in tumors deemed too large for safe primary surgical resection and for which preoperative chemotherapy or radiation therapy is planned.

Differential Diagnosis

The differential diagnosis of a flank mass in a child includes hydronephrosis, cystic kidneys, intrarenal neuroblastoma, mesoblastic nephroma, and various very rare sarcomas.

Ultrasonography can confirm the presence of hydronephrosis and evaluate for the presence of cystic kidneys. Neuroblastoma, while pathologically distinct from Wilms tumor, frequently presents in the abdomen as a mass arising from the adrenal glands or paraspinal ganglion. Neuroblastomas are radiographically indistinguishable from Wilms tumors, but there are several features that may aid in the differentiation. In contrast to Wilms tumors, which are typically confined to one side of the abdomen, neuroblastomas usually cross the midline. Wilms tumors are intrarenal masses and rarely cause a change in the axis of the kidney, while neuroblastomas may cause an outward and downward displacement of the kidney (drooping lily). Children with neuroblastomas are more likely to present with metastatic disease, and these tumors have a higher frequency of calcification observed radiographically. In addition, neuroblastomas may produce various tumor markers including vanillylmandelic acid and other catecholamines that are not seen in patients with Wilms tumor (Pizzo et al, 1989).

Mesoblastic nephromas are benign hamartomas and cannot be preoperatively distinguished from Wilms tumors. They are most commonly seen in the neonatal period and are typically identified by surgical pathology after nephrectomy. The tumor can occur in adults (Truong et al, 1998).

Treatment

The goal of therapy is to provide the highest possible cure rate with the lowest treatment-related morbidity. Significant improvements in survival rates for children with Wilms tumor have been achieved by an improved understanding of the disease and a multimodality approach to therapy, advocated by the NWTS, that incorporates surgery, radiation therapy, and chemotherapy.

A. Surgical Measures: For patients with unilateral kidney involvement deemed surgically resectable (tumors not crossing the midline or involving adjacent visceral organs), radical nephrectomy via a transabdominal incision is the procedure of choice.

Retroperitoneal lymph node dissection is not of proven value and is not recommended. However, biopsy of regional lymphatics (renal hilum and para-aortic nodes) and careful examination of the opposite kidney and the remainder of the abdomen provide crucial data for staging and prognosis. Tumor extending into the vena cava should be removed unless there is evidence of total obstruction. A major point of emphasis during surgical extirpation is to avoid spillage because there is evidence that this increases abdominal recurrence of disease (Shamberger et al, 1999; Ross and Kay, 1999).

A child with bilateral Wilms tumor, like an adult with bilateral RCC, requires an individualized approach. Patients with favorable histology tumors can frequently be managed with preoperative chemotherapy followed by renal-sparing surgery (Kumar, Fitzgerald, and Breatnach, 1998). In patients for whom preoperative chemotherapy is planned, a biopsy for diagnosis and staging is indicated (Blute et al, 1987). In some centers, needle aspiration biopsy has proved to be a reliable diagnostic tool when evaluated by experienced pathologists (Hanash, 1989). In patients with unfavorable histology, the therapeutic approach consists of aggressive surgery followed by chemotherapy and radiation therapy.

B. Radiation Therapy: Wilms tumor has long been recognized as a radiosensitive tumor. Despite the proven efficacy of radiation therapy in children, however, its use is complicated by its potential for growth disturbances and recognized cardiac, pulmonary, and hepatic toxicities. The development of effective chemotherapy combinations has practically replaced radiation therapy in the preoperative setting. The first and second NWTS trials demonstrated that postoperative radiotherapy was not required for patients with favorable histology stage I disease. NWTS III failed to show an advantage for postoperative radiotherapy in patients with favorable stage II disease and demonstrated that the relapse rate of patients with stage III disease was no different for patients receiving 1000 cGy compared with the traditional 2000 cGy (D'Angio et al, 1989). Postoperative radiation is recommended for patients with stage III or IV with favorable histology, stages II to IV with focal anaplasia and clear cell sarcoma, and all stages of rhabdoid tumor of the kidney (Weiner, Coppes, and Ritchey, 1998).

C. Chemotherapy: Wilms tumor is a chemosensitive neoplasm and is responsive to various single agents, including actinomycin D, vincristine, doxorubicin, cyclophosphamide, etoposide, and cisplatin. The first NWTS study demonstrated that the combination of actinomycin D plus vincristine was more effective in reducing the risk of relapse than either drug used alone (D'Angio et al, 1976). In an orderly fashion, the NWTS has used each successive study to evaluate new approaches to improving response and decreasing toxicity. Summarized below by stage and histologic findings are therapy recommendations used in NWTS V. (FH = favorable histology; UH = unfavorable histology.)

No chemotherapy or radiation.
- Stage I FH (<2 years and <550 g)

Pulse-intensive actinomycin D and vincristine for 18 weeks, no radiation.
- Stage I FH (>2 years or >550 g)
- Stage II FH
- Stage I anaplasia

Pulse-intensive actinomycin D, vincristine and doxorubicin for 24 weeks, plus radiation.
- Stage III-IV FH
- Stage II-IV focal anaplasia

Actinomycin D, vincristine, doxorubicin, cyclophosphamide, and etoposide, plus radiation in all clear cell sarcomas and selected anaplasia patients based on local tumor stage.
- Stage II–IV diffuse anaplasia and clear cell sarcoma kidney

Carboplatin, etoposide, and cyclophosphamide, plus radiation.
- Stage I–IV rhabdoid tumor of kidney

Prognosis

The multimodality approach to the treatment of children with Wilms tumors has significantly improved outcomes. The 4-year survival of patients with favorable histology Wilms tumor now approaches 90% (Weiner, Coppes, and Ritchey, 1998). The most important negative prognostic factors remain the unfavorable histologic subtypes (clear cell sarcoma, rhabdoid, and anaplastic tumors). While the addition of doxorubicin in NWTS III significantly improved the 2-year survival rate for patients with clear cell sarcomas (61.5–90.3%), it did not impact the survival of children with rhabdoid tumors. Analysis of patients with bilateral Wilms tumors registered with NWTS II and III revealed a 3-year survival rate of 82% (Blute et al, 1987).

Future challenges include improvements in therapy for patients with anaplastic tumors (stages II–IV), clear cell sarcoma, and rhabdoid tumors, and efforts to improve outcomes in favorable histology tumors while decreasing both short-term and late toxicities.

SARCOMA OF THE KIDNEY

Primary sarcomas of the kidney are rare, with a reported incidence ranging from 1 to 3% of all malignant renal neoplasms (Vogelzang et al, 1993; Srinivas et al, 1984). Renal sarcomas are most commonly present in patients in the fifth decade of life and there is a slight male predominance. Flank or abdominal pain and weight loss are the most frequent presenting symptoms. Primary renal sarcomas may be difficult to distinguish histologically from the sarcomatoid variant of renal carcinoma (Bonsib et al, 1987). Leiomyosarcomas compose approximately 50% of all renal sarcomas and occur with a female predominance of 2:1 (Loomis, 1972). The remaining 40–50% of renal sarcomas consist of fibrosarcomas, liposarcomas, and hemangiopericytomas. Extremely rare presentations of osteogenic sarcoma (Micolonghi et al, 1984) and malignant schwannomas (Farrow et al, 1968) have been reported. Renal sarcomas are typically of renal capsular origin. They present with symptoms analogous to those of other renal masses and tend to exhibit aggressive local spread with distant metastases to lung and liver as late findings.

Radical nephrectomy for localized disease is the only effective therapy. Adjuvant radiotherapy has been demonstrated to decrease the incidence of local recurrence in patients with resectable retroperitoneal sarcomas; however, there is no improvement in overall survival (Kinsella et al, 1988). Various chemotherapeutic agents, including doxorubicin, decarbazine, and ifosfamide, have activity in the treatment of metastatic disease, but responses are typically partial and of brief duration.

SECONDARY RENAL TUMORS

The kidney is a frequent site for metastatic spread of both solid and hematologic tumors. Wagle, Moore, and Murphy (1975) surveyed 4413 autopsies at a major cancer center and found 81 (18%) cases of secondary carcinoma of the kidney (hematologic tumors were excluded). The most frequent primary site of cancer was lung (20%), followed by breast (12%), stomach (11%), and renal (9%). The authors noted that metastases to the renal parenchyma typically demonstrated capsular and stromal invasion with sparing of the renal pelvis and that bilateral secondary renal involvement was found in approximately 50% of cases.

Albuminuria and hematuria are relatively common findings in patients with secondary renal metastases; however, pain and renal insufficiency are rare (Wagle, Moore, and Murphy, 1975; Olsson, Moyer, and Laferte, 1971). Secondary metastatic disease to the kidneys tends to be a late event, frequently in the setting of widely disseminated disease, which typically portends a poor prognosis. Therapy is dictated by the responsiveness of the primary neoplasm; ie, patients with breast and ovarian cancers for which there is effective therapy are more likely to respond than patients with primary lung or gastric cancers.

Autopsy series have reported clinically evident renal invasion by lymphoma to be in the range of 0.5–7%, with the rates of Hodgkin and non-Hodgkin lymphoma distributed equally (Goffinet et al, 1977; Weimar et al, 1981). In one series, renal involvement was usually in the form of bilateral, multiple, discrete tumor nodules (Martinez-Maldonado et al, 1966). Renal involvement by non-Hodgkin lymphoma is typically characterized by diffuse, aggressive histologic findings (ie, diffuse large cell) in the setting of extensive disease. Therapy typically consists of combination chemotherapy, with the prognosis of patients similar to that of patients without renal involvement but with widely disseminated, aggressive lymphomas (Geffen et al, 1985).

REFERENCES

Alanen KA, Tyrkkö JES, Nurmi MJ: Aspiration biopsy cytology of renal oncocytoma. Acta Cytol 1985;29: 859.

Ambos MA et al: Angiographic pattern in renal oncocytomas. Radiology 1978;129:615.

Anderson EE, Hatcher PA: Renal angiomyolipoma. Probl Urol 1990;4:230.

Atkins MB et al: Randomized phase II trial of high-dose interleukin-2 either alone or in combination with interferon alpha-2b in advanced renal cell carcinoma. J Clin Oncol 1993;11:661.

Aulitzky W et al: Successful treatment of metastatic renal cell carcinoma with a biologically active dose of recombinant interferon-gamma. J Clin Oncol 1989;7: 1875.

Babyn P et al: Imaging patients with Wilms' tumor. Hematol Oncol Clin North Am 1995;9:1217.

Beckwith JB: New developments in the pathology of Wilms' tumor. Cancer Invest. 1997;15:153.

Beckwith JB: Wilms' tumor and other renal tumors of childhood: A selective review from the National Wilms' Tumor Study Pathology Center. Human Pathol 1983;14:481.

Beckwith JB, Kiviat NB, Bonadio JF: Nephrogenic rests, nephroblastomatosis, and the pathogenesis of Wilms' tumor. Pediatr Pathol 1990;10:1.

Beckwith JB, Palmer NF: Histopathology and prognosis of Wilms' tumor: Results from the first National Wilms' Tumor Study. Cancer 1978;41:1937.

Bluemke DA, Chambers TP: Spiral CT angiography: An alternative to conventional angiography. Radiology 1995;195:317.

Blute ML et al: Bilateral Wilms' tumor. J Urol 1987; 138:968.

Bonnin JM et al: Hypertension due to a renin-secreting tumour localized by segmental renal vein sampling. Aust NZ J Med 1977;7:630.

Bono AV: Steroid hormones and hormonal treatment in renal cell carcinoma. In: deKernion JB, Pavone-Macaluso M (editors): *Tumors of the Kidney.* Williams & Wilkins, 1986.

Bonsib SM: Pathologic features of renal parenchymal tumors. In: Culp DA, Loening SA (editors): *Genitourinary Oncology.* Lea and Febiger, 1985.

Bonsib SM et al: Sarcomatoid renal tumors: Clinicopathologic correlation of three cases. Cancer 1987; 59:527.

Bosniak MA: Observation of small incidentally detected renal masses. Semin Urol Oncol 1995;13:267.

Brennan JF et al: Acquired renal cystic disease: Implications for the urologist. Br J Urol 1991;67:342.

Breslow N et al: Epidemiology of Wilms' tumor. Med Ped Oncol 1993;21:172.

Breslow NE, Beckwith JB: Epidemiological features of Wilms' tumor: Results of the National Wilms' Tumor Study. J Natl Cancer Inst 1982;68:429.

Bretan PN Jr et al: Chronic renal failure: A significant risk factor in the development of acquired renal cysts and renal cell carcinoma: Case reports and a review of the literature. Cancer 1986;57:1971.

Busch FM, Bark CC, Clyde HR: Benign renal angiomyolipoma with regional lymph node involvement. J Urol 1976;116:715.

Caddedu JA et al: Laparoscopic nephrectomy for renal cell cancer: Evaluation of efficacy and safety: A multicenter experience. Urology 1998;52:773.

Call KM et al: Isolation and characterization of a zinc finger polypeptide gene at the human chromosome 11 Wilms' tumor locus. Cell 1990;60:509.

Chen F et al: Germline mutations in the von Hippel-Lindau disease tumor suppressor gene: Correlation with phenotype. Hum Mutat 1995;5:66.

Cherri RJ et al: Prognostic implications of vena caval extension of renal cell carcinoma. J Urol 1982;128:910.

Cohen AJ et al: Hereditary renal-cell carcinoma associated with a chromosomal translocation. N Engl J Med 1979;301:592.

Cohen C, McCue PA, Derose PB: Histogenesis of renal cell carcinoma and renal oncocytoma: An immunohistochemical study. Cancer 1988;62:1946.

Coppes MJ, Haber DA, Grundy PE: Genetic events in the development of Wilms' tumor. N Engl J Med 1994;331:586.

D'Angio GJ et al: Treatment of Wilms' tumor: Results of the Third National Wilms' Tumor Study. Cancer 1989;64:349.

D'Angio GJ et al: Wilms' tumor: Genetic aspects and etiology: A report of the National Wilms' Tumor Study (NWTS) Committee of the NWTS Group. In: Kuss R et al (editors): *Renal Tumors: Proceedings of the First International Symposium on Kidney Tumors.* Alan R. Liss, 1982.

D'Angio GJ et al: The treatment of Wilms' tumor: Results of the National Wilms' Tumor Study. Cancer 1976;38:633.

Daniel WW et al: Calcified renal masses: A review of 10 years experience at Mayo Clinic. Radiology 1972; 103:503.

Davis CJ et al: Renal oncocytoma. Clinicopathological study of 166 patients. J Urogen Pathol 1991;1:42.

deKernion JB, Ramming KP, Smith RB: The natural history of metastatic renal cell carcinoma: A computer analysis. J Urol 1978;120:148.

Ditonno P et al: Extrarenal angiomyolipomas of the perinephric space. J Urol 1992;147:447.

Divgi CR et al: Phase I/II radioimmunotherapy trial with iodine-131-labeled monoclonal antibody G250 in metastatic renal cell carcinoma. Clin Cancer Res 1998;4:2729.

Droller MJ: *Surgical Management of Urologic Disease: An Anatomic Approach.* Mosby–Year Book, 1992.

Dunnill MS, Millard PR, Oliver D: Acquired cystic disease of the kidneys: A hazard of long-term intermittent hemodialysis. J Clin Pathol 1977;30:868.

Ekelund L, Gothlin J: Renal hemangiomas: An analysis of 13 cases diagnosed by angiography. Am J Roentgenol Radium Ther Nucl Med 1975;125:788.

Erlandsson R: Molecular genetics of renal cell carcinoma. Cancer Genet Cytogenet 1998;104:1.

Fallon B, Williams RD: Renal cancer associated with acquired cystic disease of the kidney and chronic renal failure. Semin Urol 1989;4:228.

Farrow GW et al: Sarcomas and sarcomatoid and mixed malignant tumors of the kidney in adults (parts 1–3). Cancer 1968;22:545.

Flocks RH, Kadesky MC: Malignant neoplasms of the

kidney: An analysis of 353 patients followed 5 years or more. J Urol 1958;79:196.

Fossa SD, Kjolseth I, Lund G: Radiotherapy of metastasis from renal cancer. Eur Urol 1982;8:340.

Fossa SD et al: Vinblastine in metastatic renal cell carcinoma: EORTC phase II trial 30882. Eur J Cancer 1992;28A:878.

Fuhrman SA, Lasky LC, Limas C: Prognostic significance of morphologic parameters in renal cell carcinoma. Am J Surg Pathol 1982;6:655.

Gardner KD, Evan AP: Cystic kidneys: An enigma evolves. Am J Kidney Dis 1984;3:403.

Geffen DB et al: Renal involvement in diffuse aggressive lymphomas: Results of treatment with combination chemotherapy. J Clin Oncol 1985;3:646.

Gleave ME et al: Interferon gamma-1b compared with placebo in metastatic renal cell carcinoma. N Engl J Med 1998;338:1265.

Goffinet DR et al: Clinical and surgical (laparotomy) evaluation of patients with non-Hodgkin's lymphomas. Cancer Treat Rep 1977;61:981.

Gold PJ et al: Paraneoplastic manifestations of renal cell carcinoma. Semin Urol Oncol 1996;14:216.

Goldstein NS: The current state of renal cell carcinoma grading. Cancer 1997;80:977.

Golimbu M et al: Renal cell carcinoma: Survival and prognostic factors. Urology 1986;27:291.

Gulanikar AC et al: Prospective pretransplant ultrasound screening in 206 patients for acquired renal cysts and renal cell carcinoma. Transplantation 1998;66:1669.

Hamperl H: Benign and malignant oncocytoma. Cancer 1962;15:1019.

Hanash KA: Recent advances in the surgical treatment of bilateral Wilms' tumor. In: Murphy GP, Khoury S (editors): *Therapeutic Progress in Urological Cancers.* Alan R. Liss, 1989.

Hanash KA: The nonmetastatic hepatic dysfunction syndrome associated with renal cell carcinoma (hypernephroma): Stauffer's syndrome. Prog Clin Biol Res 1982;100:301.

Henriksson C et al: Skeletal metastases in 102 pateints evaluated before surgery for renal cell carcinoma. Scand J Urol Nephrol 1992;26:363.

Hermanek P, Schrott KM: Evaluation of the new tumor, nodes and metastases classification of renal cell carcinoma. J Urol 1990;144:238.

Herr HW: Partial nephrectomy for unilateral renal carcinoma and a normal contralateral kidney: 10-year followup. J Urol 1999;161:33.

Herrlinger A et al: What are the benefits of extended dissecton of the regional lymph nodes in the therapy of renal cell carcinoma? J Urol 1991;146:1224.

Hocking WG: Hematologic abnormalities in patients with renal diseases. Hematol Oncol Clin North Am 1987;1:229.

Holmes NM et al: Renal imaging with spiral CT scan: Clinical applications. Tech Urol 1997;3:202.

Holthöfer H: Immunohistology of renal cell carcinoma. Eur Urol 1990;18(Suppl):15.

Horan JJ et al: The detection of renal cell carcinoma extension into the renal vein and inferior vena cava: A prospective comparison of venocavography and MRI. J Urol 1989;142:943.

Hricak H et al: Detection and staging of renal neo-

plasms: A reassessment of MR imaging. Radiology 1988;166:643.

Hricak H et al: MRI in the diagnosis and staging of renal and perirenal neoplasms. Radiology 1985;154:709.

Huff V: Inheritance and functionality of Wilms' tumor genes. Cancer Bull 1994;46:254.

Hughson MD, Hennigar GR, McManus JFA: Atypical cysts, acquired renal cystic disease, and renal cell tumors in end stage dialysis kidneys. Lab Invest 1980; 42:475.

Janetschek G et al: Laparoscopic nephron sparing surgery for small renal cell carcinoma. J Urol 1998; 159:1152.

Juusela H et al: Preoperative irradiation in the treatment of renal cell carcinoma. Scand J Urol Nephrol 1977;11:277.

Kabala JE et al: Magnetic resonance imaging in the staging of renal cell carcinoma. Br J Radiol 1991;64:683.

Kaneko Y, Eguel MC, Rowley JD: Interstitial deletion of short arm of chromosome-11 limited to Wilms' tumor patient cells in a patient without aniridia. Cancer Res 1981;41:4577.

Kavoussi LR et al: Regression of metastatic renal cell carcinoma: A case report and literature review. J Urol 1986;125:1005.

Kinsella TJ et al: Preliminary results of a randomized study of adjuvant radiation therapy in resectable adult retroperitoneal soft-tissue sarcomas. J Clin Oncol 1988;6:18.

Kirkman H, Bacon RL: Renal adenomas and carcinomas in diethylstilbestrol treated male golden hamsters. Anat Rec 1949;103:475.

Kjaer M: The role of medroxyprogesterone acetate (MPA) in the treatment of renal adenocarcinoma. Cancer Treat Rev 1988;15:195.

Knudson AG Jr, Strong LC: Mutation and cancer; A model for Wilms' tumor of the kidney. J Natl Cancer Inst 1972;48:313.

Kosko JW, Lipuma JP, Resnick MI: Radiological evaluation of renal mass. In: Javadpour N (editor): *Cancer of the Kidney.* Thieme-Stratton, 1984.

Kovacs G et al: Consistent chromosome 3p deletion and loss of heterozygosity in renal cell carcinoma. Proc Natl Acad Sci USA 1988;85:1571.

Krown SE: Interferon treatment of renal cell carcinoma. Cancer 1987;59:647.

Kumar R, Fitzgerald R, Breatnach F: Conservative surgical management of bilateral Wilms' tumor: Results of the United Kingdom Children's Cancer Study Group. J Urol 1998;160:1450.

Landis SH et al: Cancer Statistics 1999. CA Cancer J Clin 1999;49:8.

Latif F et al: Identification of the von Hippel-Lindau disease tumor suppressor gene. Science 1993;260:1317.

La Vecchia C et al: Smoking and renal cell carcinoma. Cancer Res 1990;50:5231.

Licht MR et al: Renal oncocytoma: Clinical and biological correlates. J Urol 1993;150:1380.

Lieber MM, Tomera KM, Farrow GM: Renal oncocytoma. J Urol 1981;124:481.

Lieber MM, Tsukamoto T: Renal oncocytoma. In: deKernion JB, Pavone-Macaluso M (editors): *Tumors of the Kidney.* Williams & Wilkins, 1986.

Linehan WM, Shipley WU, Parkinson DR: Cancer of the kidney and ureter. In: Devita VT Jr, Hellman S,

Rosenberg SA (editors): *Cancer Principles and Practice of Oncology.* Lippincott, 1993.

Loomis RC: Primary leiomyosarcoma of the kidney: Report of a case and a review of the literature. J Urol 1972;107:557.

Lowe BA et al: Malignant transformation of angiomyolipoma. J Urol 1992;147:1356.

Maatman TJ et al: Renal oncocytoma: A diagnostic and therapeutic dilemma. J Urol 1984;132:878.

Maclure M: Asbestos and renal adenocarcinoma: A case-control study. Environ Res 1987;42:353.

Makay B, Ordonez NG, Khousrsland J: The ultrastructure and immunocytochemistry of renal cell carcinoma. Ultrastruct Pathol 1987;11:483.

Malker HR et al: Kidney cancer among leather workers. Lancet 1984;1:56.

Marshall FF et al: The feasibility of surgical enucleation for renal cell carcinoma. J Urol 1986;135:231.

McCabe M, Stabler D, Hawkins M: The modified group C experience: Phase III randomized trials of IL-2 versus IL-2/LAK in advanced renal cell carcinoma and advanced melanoma. Proc Am Soc Clin Oncol 1991; 10:213.

Mclean GK, Meranze SG: Embolization techniques in the urinary tract. Urol Clin North Am 1985;12:743.

McNichols DW, Segura JW, DeWeerd JH: Renal cell carcinoma: Long term survival and late recurrence. J Urol 1981;126:17.

Merino MJ, Librelsi VA: Oncocytomas of the kidney. Cancer 1982;50:1952.

Mickish G et al: P-170 glycoprotein glutathione and associated enzymes in relation to chemoresistance of primary human renal cell carcinomas. Urol Int 1990; 45:170.

Micolonghi TS et al: Primary osteogenic sarcoma of the kidney. J Urol 1984;131:1164.

Middleton RG: Surgery for metastatic renal cell carcinoma. J Urol 1967;97:973.

Minasian LM et al: Interferon alpha-2a in advanced renal cell carcinoma: Treatment results and survival in 159 patients with long-term follow-up. J Clin Oncol 1993;11:1368.

Montie JE et al: The role of adjunctive nephrectomy in patients with metastatic renal cell carcinoma. J Urol 1977;117:272.

Morra MN, Das S: Renal oncocytoma: A review of histogenesis, histopathology, diagnosis and treatment. J Urol 1993;150:295.

Muggia FM: Overview of cancer-related hypercalcemia: Epidemiology and etiology. Semin Oncol 1990;17:3.

Negrier S et al: Recombinant human interleukin-2, recombinant human interferon alfa-2a, or both in metastatic renal cell carcinoma. N Engl J Med 1998; 338:1272.

Novick AC, Stewart BH, Straffon RA: Extracorporeal renal surgery and autotransplantation: Indications, techniques and results. J Urol 1980;123:806.

Oberling C, Riviere M, Haguenau F: Ultrastructure of the clear cells in renal carcinomas and its importance for the demonstration of their renal origin. Nature 1960;186:402.

O'Dea MJ et al: The therapy of renal cell carcinoma with solitary metastasis. J Urol 1978;120:540.

Older RA et al: Spoke-wheel angiographic pattern in renal masses: Nonspecificity. Radiology 1978;128:836.

Olsson CA, Moyer JD, Laferte RO: Pulmonary cancer metastatic to the kidneys: A common renal neoplasm. J Urol 1971;105:492.

Onufrey V, Mohiuddin M: Radiation therapy in the treatment of metastatic renal cell carcinoma. Int J Radiat Oncol Biol Phys 1985;11:2007.

Patchell RA et al: A randomized trial of surgery in the treatment of single metastases to the brain. N Engl J Med 1990;322:494.

Pitts WR et al: Ultrasonography, computed tomography and pathology of angiomyolipoma of the kidney: Solution to a diagnostic dilemma. J Urol 1980;124: 907.

Pizzo PA et al: Solid tumors of childhood. In: Devita VT Jr, Hellman S, Rosenberg SA (editors): *Cancer Principles and Practice of Oncology.* Lippincott, 1989.

Pontes JE et al: Salvage surgery for renal cell carcinoma. Semin Surg Oncol 1989;5:282.

Quesada JR, Swanson DA, Gutterman JU: Phase II study of alpha interferon in metastatic renal cell carcinoma: A progress report. J Clin Oncol 1985;3: 1086.

Quesada JR et al: Renal cell carcinoma: Antitumor effects of leukocyte interferon. Cancer Res 1983;43:940.

Rafla S: Renal cell carcinoma: Natural history and results of treatment. Cancer 1970;25:26.

Reichard EAP, Roubidoux MA, Dunnick NR: Renal neoplasms in patients with renal cystic disease. Abdom Imaging 1998;23:237.

Renshaw AA, Granter SR, Cibas ES: Fine-needle aspiration of the adult kidney. Cancer (Cancer Cytopathol) 1997;81:71.

Riccardi VM et al: Chromosomal imbalance in the Aniridia-Wilms' tumor association: 11p interstitial deletion. Pediatrics 1978;61:604.

Ritchey ML et al: Accuracy of current imaging modalities in the diagnosis of synchronous bilateral Wilms tumor. A report from the National Wilms' Tumor Study Group. Cancer 1995;75:600.

Robson CJ: The natural history of renal cell carcinoma. Prog Clin Biol Res 1982;100:447.

Robson CJ: Radical nephrectomy for renal cell carcinoma. J Urol 1963;89:37.

Robson CJ, Churchill BM, Anderson W: The results of radical nephrectomy for renal cell carcinoma. J Urol 1969;101:297.

Ross JH, Kay R: Surgical considerations for patients with Wilms' tumor. Semin Urol Oncol 1999;17:33.

Selli C et al: Stratification of risk factors in renal cell carcinoma. Cancer 1983;52:899.

Shamberger RC et al: Surgery-related factors and local recurrence of Wilms' tumor in National Wilms' Tumor Study 4. Ann Surg 1999;229:292.

Shröder FH: TNM classification of genitourinary tumors 1987—position of the EORTC Genitourinary Group. Br J Urol 1988;62:502.

Siminovitch JMP, Montie JE, Straffon RA: Prognostic indicators in renal adenocarcinoma. J Urol 1983;130:20.

Skinner DG, Lieskovsky G, Pritchett TR: Technique of radical nephrectomy. In: Skinner DG, Lieskovsky G (editors): *Genitourinary Cancer.* Saunders, 1988.

Skinner DG, Vermillion CD, Colvin RB: The surgical management of renal cell carcinoma. J Urol 1972a; 107:705.

Skinner DG et al: Diagnosis and management of renal

cell carcinoma: A clinical and pathologic study of 309 cases. Cancer 1971;28:1165.

Smith JW et al: Acquired renal cystic disease: Two cases of associated adenocarcinoma and a renal ultrasound survey of a peritoneal dialysis population. Am J Kidney Dis 1987;10:41.

Smith RB: The treatment of bilateral renal cell carcinoma or renal cell carcinoma in the solitary kidney. In: deKernion JB, Pavone-Macaluso M (editors): *Tumors of the Kidney.* Williams & Wilkins, 1986.

Sobin LH, Wittekind C for the International Union Against Cancer: *TNM Classification of Malignant Tumors,* 5th ed. John Wiley & Sons, 1997.

Srinivas V et al: Sarcomas of the kidney. J Urol 1984; 32:13.

Stauffer MH: Nephrogenic hepatosplenomegaly. (Abstract.) Gastroenterology 1961;40:694.

Steiner MS et al: The natural history of renal angiomyolipoma. J Urol 1993;150:1782.

Steiner MS et al: Leiomyoma of the kidney: Presentation of 4 new cases and the role of computerized tomography. J Urol 1990;143:994.

Storkel S et al: The human chromophobe cell renal carcinoma: Its probable relation to intercalated cells of the collecting duct. Virchows Arch [B] 1989;56:237.

Strewler GJ et al: Parathyroid hormone–like protein from human renal carcinoma cells: Structural and functional homology with parathyroid hormone. J Clin Invest 1987;80:1803.

Sufrin G, Golio A, Murphy GP: Serologic markers, paraneoplastic syndromes, and ectopic hormone production in renal adenocarcinoma. In: deKernion JB, Pavone-Macaluso M (editors): *Tumors of the Kidney.* Williams & Wilkins, 1986.

Sufrin G et al: Paraneoplastic and serologic syndromes of renal adenocarcinoma. Semin Urol 1989;7:158.

Tally RW et al: Treatment of metastatic hypernephroma. JAMA 1969;207:322.

Thrasher JB, Paulson DF: Prognostic factors in renal cancer. Urol Clin North Am 1993;20:247.

Toho BM, Whitmore WE Jr: Solitary metastases from renal cell carcinoma. J Urol 1975;114:836.

Trump DL et al: Randomized controlled trial of adjuvant therapy with lymphblastoid interferon in resected, high-risk renal cell carcinoma. (Abstract.) Proc Am Soc Clin Oncol 1996;15:648.

Truong LD et al: Adult mesoblastic nephroma: Expansion of the morphologic spectrum and review of literature. Am J Surg Pathol 1998;22:827.

Uhlenbrock D, Fischer C, Beyer HK: Angiomyolipoma of the kidney: Comparison between magnetic resonance imaging, computed tomography, and ultrasonography for diagnosis. Acta Radiol 1988;29:523.

van der Werf-Messing B: Carcinoma of the kidney. Cancer 1973;32:1056.

Varanasi R et al: Fine structure analysis of the WT1 gene in sporadic Wilms' tumors. Proc Natl Acad Sci USA 1994;91:3554.

Vaziri ND et al: Acquired renal cystic disease in renal transplant recipients. Nephron 1984;37:203.

Vecht CJ et al: Treatment of single brain metastases: Radiotherapy alone or combined with neurosurgery? Ann Neurol 1993;33:583.

Vogelzang NJ et al: Primary renal sarcoma in adults. Cancer 1993;71:804.

Vogelzang NJ et al: Spontaneous regression of histologically proved pulmonary metastases from renal cell carcinoma: A case with 5-year followup. J Urol 1992; 148:1247.

Wagle DG, Moore RH, Murphy GP: Secondary carcinomas of the kidney. J Urol 1975;114:30.

Warshauer DM et al: Detection of renal masses: Sensitivities and specificities of excretory urography/linear tomography, US and CT. Radiology 1988;169:363.

Weimar G et al: Urogenital involvement by malignant lymphomas. J Urol 1981;125:230.

Weiner JS, Coppes MJ, Ritchey ML: Current concepts in the biology and management of Wilms' tumor. J Urol 1998;159:1316.

Weiner SN, Bernstein RG: Renal oncocytoma: Angiographic features of two cases. Radiology 1977;125: 633.

White EW, Braunstein LE: Cavernous hemangioma: A renal vascular tumor requiring nephrectomy, an unusual entity. J Urol 1946;56:183.

Williams RD: Tumors of the kidney, ureter and bladder. In: Wyngaarden JB, Smith LH, Bennett JC (editors): *Cecil's Textbook of Medicine.* Saunders, 1992.

Wong AL, McGeorge A, Clark AH: Renal angiomyolipoma: A review of the literature and a report of 4 cases. Br J Urol 1981;53:406.

Yagoda A et al: Chemotherapy for advanced renal cell carcinoma: 1983–1993. Semin Oncol 1995;22:42.

Yu MC et al: Cigarette smoking, obesity, diuretic use and coffee consumption as risk factors for renal cell carcinoma. J Natl Cancer Inst 1986;77:351.

Yunis JJ, Ramsay NKC: Familial occurrence of the aniridia-Wilms' tumor syndrome with deletion 11p13-14.1. J Pediatr 1980;96:1027.

Zbar B et al: Hereditary papillary renal cell carcinoma. J Urol 1994;151:561.

Neoplasms of the Prostate Gland

23

Joseph C. Presti, Jr., MD

The prostate gland is the male organ most commonly afflicted with either benign or malignant neoplasms. It comprises the most proximal aspect of the urethra. Anatomically it resides in the true pelvis, separated from the pubic symphysis anteriorly by the retropubic space (space of Retzius). The posterior surface of the prostate is separated from the rectal ampulla by Denovillier's fascia. The base of the prostate is continuous with the bladder neck, and the apex of the prostate rests on the upper surface of the urogenital diaphragm. Laterally, the prostate is related to the levator ani musculature. Its arterial blood supply is derived from branches of the internal iliac artery (inferior vesical and middle rectal arteries). Venous drainage is via the dorsal venous complex, which receives the deep dorsal vein of the penis and vesical branches before draining into the internal iliac veins. Innervation is from the pelvic plexus. The normal prostate measures 3–4 cm at the base, 4–6 cm in cephalocaudad, and 2–3 cm in anteroposterior dimensions.

McNeal (1968) has popularized the concept of zonal anatomy of the prostate. Three distinct zones have been identified (Figure 23–1). The **peripheral zone** accounts for 70% of the volume of the young adult prostate, the **central zone** accounts for 25%, and the **transition zone** accounts for 5%. These anatomic zones have distinct ductal systems but, more important, are differentially afflicted with neoplastic processes. Sixty to 70 percent of carcinomas of the prostate (CaP) originate in the peripheral zone, 10–20% in the transition zone, and 5–10% in the central zone (McNeal et al, 1988). Benign prostatic hyperplasia uniformly originates in the transition zone (Figure 23–2).

BENIGN PROSTATIC HYPERPLASIA (BPH)

Incidence and Epidemiology

BPH is the most common benign tumor in men, and its incidence is age-related. The prevalence of histologic BPH in autopsy studies rises from approximately 20% in men aged 41–50, to 50% in men aged 51–60, and to over 90% in men older than 80 (Berry et al, 1984). Although clinical evidence of disease occurs less commonly, symptoms of prostatic obstruction are also age-related. At age 55, approximately 25% of men report obstructive voiding symptoms. At age 75, 50% of men complain of a decrease in the force and caliber of their urinary stream.

Risk factors for the development of BPH are poorly understood. Some studies have suggested a genetic predisposition, and some have noted racial differences. Approximately 50% of men under the age of 60 who undergo surgery for BPH may have a heritable form of the disease. This form is most likely an autosomal dominant trait, and first-degree male relatives of such patients carry an increased relative risk of approximately 4-fold (Sanda et al, 1994).

Etiology

The etiology of BPH is not completely understood, but it seems to be multifactorial and endocrine controlled. The prostate is composed of both stromal and epithelial elements, and each, either alone or in combination, can give rise to hyperplastic nodules and the symptoms associated with BPH. Each element may be targeted in medical management schemes.

Laboratory and clinical studies have identified two factors necessary for the development of BPH: dihydrotestosterone (DHT) and aging (McConnell, 1995). Animal studies in the dog have demonstrated that with aging, the prostate becomes more sensitive to androgens. Of interest is that prostatic growth in aging dogs appears to be more related to a decrease in cell death than to an increase in cell proliferation. Laboratory studies have suggested several theories in this area, including (1) stromal-epithelial interactions (stromal cells may regulate the growth of epithelial cells or other stromal cells via a paracrine or autocrine mechanism by secreting growth factors such as basic fibroblast growth factor or transforming growth factor-β); (2) aging may result in stem cells' undergoing a block in the maturation process that prevents them from entering into programmed cell

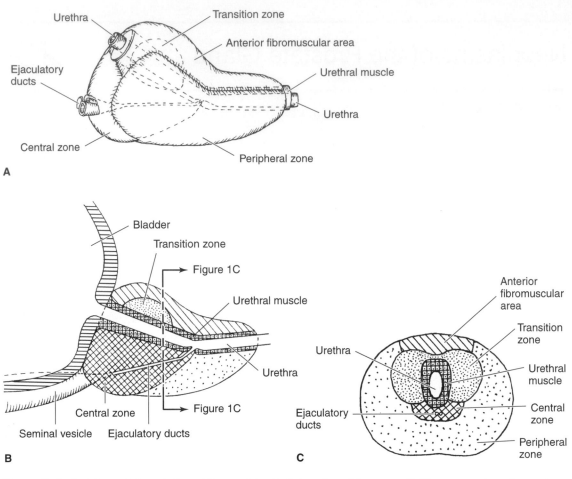

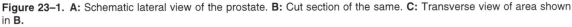

Figure 23–1. A: Schematic lateral view of the prostate. **B:** Cut section of the same. **C:** Transverse view of area shown in **B.**

death (apoptosis) (Cunha et al, 1983; Tenniswood, 1986). The impact of aging in animal studies appears to be mediated via estrogen synergism. In dogs, estrogens have been shown to induce the androgen receptor, alter steroid metabolism resulting in higher levels of intraprostatic DHT, inhibit cell death when given in the presence of androgens, and stimulate stromal collagen production (Berry and Isaacs, 1984; Berry et al, 1986; Barrack and Berry, 1987).

Observations and clinical studies in men have clearly demonstrated that BPH is under endocrine control. Castration results in the regression of established BPH and improvement in urinary symptoms. Administration of a luteinizing hormone-releasing hormone (LHRH) analog in men reversibly shrinks established BPH, resulting in objective improvement in flow rate and subjective improvement in symptoms (Peters and Walsh, 1987). Additional investigations have demonstrated a positive correlation between levels of free testosterone and estrogen and the

volume of BPH (Partin et al, 1991). The latter may suggest that the association between aging and BPH might result from the increased estrogen levels of aging causing induction of the androgen receptor, which thereby sensitizes the prostate to free testosterone. However, no studies to date have been able to demonstrate elevated estrogen receptor levels in human BPH.

Pathology

As discussed above, BPH develops in the transition zone (McNeal, 1978). It is truly a hyperplastic process resulting from an increase in cell number. Microscopic evaluation reveals a nodular growth pattern that is composed of varying amounts of stroma and epithelium. Stroma is composed of varying amounts of collagen and smooth muscle. The differential representation of the histologic components of BPH explains, in part, the potential responsiveness to medical therapy. Thus alpha-blocker therapy may re-

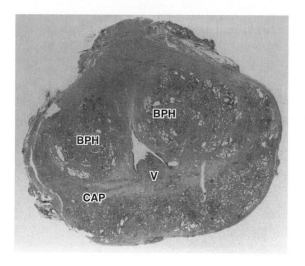

Figure 23–2. Whole mount of prostate at level of midprostatic urethra. Note verumontanum (V) and areas of prostate cancer (CAP) in peripheral zone and areas of benign prostatic hyperplasia (BPH) in transition zone.

sult in excellent responses in patients with BPH that has a significant component of smooth muscle, while those with BPH predominantly composed of epithelium might respond better to 5α-reductase inhibitors. Patients with significant components of collagen in the stroma may not respond to either form of medical therapy. Unfortunately, one cannot reliably predict responsiveness to a specific therapy (see below).

As BPH nodules in the transition zone enlarge, they compress the outer zones of the prostate, resulting in the formation of a so-called surgical capsule. This boundary separates the transition zone from the peripheral zone and serves as a cleavage plane for open enucleation of the prostate during open simple prostatectomies performed for BPH.

Pathophysiology

One can relate the symptoms of BPH to either the obstructive component of the prostate or the secondary response of the bladder to the outlet resistance. The obstructive component can be subdivided into the mechanical and the dynamic obstruction.

As prostatic enlargement occurs, mechanical obstruction may result from intrusion into the urethral lumen or bladder neck, leading to a higher bladder outlet resistance. Prior to the zonal classification of the prostate, urologists often referred to the "3 lobes" of the prostate, namely, the median and the two lateral lobes. A BPH autopsy study from the 1930s classified the gross changes of BPH into 5 categories: (1) isolated median lobe enlargement (30%); (2) isolated lateral lobe enlargement (15%); (3) lateral and median lobe (trilobar) enlargement (23%); (4) posterior com-

missure (posterior vesical lip or elevated bladder neck) hyperplasia (15%); (5) lateral and posterior commissure hyperplasia (17%) (Randall, 1931). Prostatic size on digital rectal examination (DRE) correlates poorly with symptoms, in part because the median lobe and posterior commissure are not readily palpable.

The dynamic component of prostatic obstruction explains the variable nature of the symptoms experienced by patients. The prostatic stroma, composed of smooth muscle and collagen, is rich in adrenergic nerve supply. The level of autonomic stimulation thus sets a tone to the prostatic urethra. Use of alphablocker therapy decreases this tone, resulting in a decrease in outlet resistance.

The irritative voiding complaints (see below) of BPH result from the secondary response of the bladder to the increased outlet resistance. Bladder outlet obstruction leads to detrusor muscle hypertrophy and hyperplasia as well as collagen deposition. Although the latter is most likely responsible for a decrease in bladder compliance, detrusor instability is also a factor. On gross inspection, thickened detrusor muscle bundles are seen as trabeculation on cystoscopic examination. If left unchecked, mucosal herniation between detrusor muscle bundles ensues, causing diverticula formation (so-called false diverticula composed of only mucosa and serosa).

Clinical Findings

A. Symptoms: As discussed above, the symptoms of BPH can be divided into obstructive and irritative complaints. Obstructive symptoms include hesitancy, decreased force and caliber of stream, sensation of incomplete bladder emptying, double voiding (urinating a second time within 2 h of the previous void), straining to urinate, and post-void dribbling. Irritative symptoms include urgency, frequency, and nocturia.

The self-administered questionnaire developed by the American Urological Association (AUA) is both valid and reliable in identifying the need to treat patients and in monitoring their response to therapy (Barry et al, 1992). The AUA Symptom Score questionnaire (Table 23–1) is perhaps the single most important tool used in the evaluation of patients with BPH and is recommended for all patients before the initiation of therapy. This assessment focuses on 7 items that ask patients to quantify the severity of their obstructive or irritative complaints on a scale of 0–5. Thus, the score can range from 0 to 35. A symptom score of 0–7 is considered mild, 8–19 is considered moderate, and 20–35 is considered severe. The relative distribution of scores for BPH patients and control subjects is, respectively, 20% and 83% in those with mild scores, 57% and 15% in those with moderate scores, and 23% and 2% in those with severe scores (McConnell et al, 1994).

A detailed history focusing on the urinary tract ex-

Table 23–1. Questionnaire for American Urological Association Score.

URINARY SYMPTOMS (SYMPTOM SCORE CRITERIA)	AUA Score					
	Not at all	Less than 1 time in 5	Less than half the time	About half the time	More than half the time	Almost always
1. Incomplete emptying Over the past month, how often have you had a sensation of not emptying your bladder completely after you finished urinating?	0	1	2	3	4	5
2. Frequency Over the past month, how often have you had to urinate again less than two hours after you finished urinating?	0	1	2	3	4	5
3. Intermittency Over the past month, how often have you found you stopped and started again several times when you urinate?	0	1	2	3	4	5
4. Urgency Over the past month, how often have you found it difficult to postpone urination?	0	1	2	3	4	5
5. Weak stream Over the past month, how often have you had a weak urinary stream?	0	1	2	3	4	5
6. Straining Over the past month, how often have you had to push or strain to begin urination?	0	1	2	3	4	5
	None	1 time	2 times	3 times	4 times	5 or more times
7. Nocturia Over the past month, how many times did you most typically get up to urinate from the time you went to bed at night until the time you got up in the morning?	0	1	2	3	4	5

AUA Symptom Score = sum of questions A1 to A7

QUALITY OF LIFE DUE TO URINARY PROBLEMS

	Delighted	Pleased	Mostly satisfied	Mixed— about equally satisfied and un-satisfied	Mostly dis-satisfied	Unhappy	Terrible
If you were to spend the rest of your life with your urinary condition just the way it is now, how would you feel about that?	0	1	2	3	4	5	6

Source: McConnell JD: *Benign Prostatic Hyperplasia; Diagnosis and Treatment.* Clinical Practice Guideline No. 8. AHCPR Publication No. 94-0582. Rockville, MD: Agency for Health Care Policy and Research, Public Health Serivce, US Department of Health and Human Services, 1994.

cludes other possible causes of symptoms that may not result from the prostate, such as urinary tract infection, neurogenic bladder, urethral stricture, or prostate cancer.

B. Signs: A physical examination, DRE, and focused neurologic examination are performed on all patients. The size and consistency of the prostate is noted, even though prostate size, as determined by DRE, does not correlate with severity of symptoms or degree of obstruction. BPH usually results in a smooth, firm, elastic enlargement of the prostate. Induration, if detected, must alert the physician to the possibility of cancer and the need for further evaluation (ie, prostate-specific antigen [PSA], transrectal ultrasound, and biopsy).

C. Laboratory Findings: A urinalysis to exclude infection or hematuria and serum creatinine measurement to assess renal function are required. Renal insufficiency may be observed in 10% of patients with prostatism and warrants upper-tract imaging. Patients with renal insufficiency are at an increased risk of developing postoperative complications following surgical intervention for BPH. Serum PSA is considered optional, but most physicians will include it in the initial evaluation. PSA, compared with DRE alone, certainly increases the ability to detect CaP, but because there is much overlap between levels seen in BPH and CaP, its use remains controversial (see Screening for CaP).

D. Imaging: Upper-tract imaging (intravenous pyelogram or renal ultrasound) is recommended only in the presence of concomitant urinary tract disease or complications from BPH (eg, hematuria, urinary tract infection, renal insufficiency, history of stone disease).

E. Cystoscopy: Cystoscopy is not recommended to determine the need for treatment but may assist in choosing the surgical approach in patients opting for invasive therapy.

F. Additional Tests: Cystometrograms and urodynamic profiles are reserved for patients with suspected neurologic disease or those who have failed prostate surgery. Measurement of flow rate, determination of post-void residual urine, and pressure-flow studies are considered optional.

Differential Diagnosis

Other obstructive conditions of the lower urinary tract, such as urethral stricture, bladder neck contracture, bladder stone, or CaP, must be entertained when evaluating men with presumptive BPH. A history of previous urethral instrumentation, urethritis, or trauma should be elucidated to exclude urethral stricture or bladder neck contracture. Hematuria and pain are commonly associated with bladder stones. CaP may be detected by abnormalities on the DRE or an elevated PSA (see below).

A urinary tract infection, which can mimic the irritative symptoms of BPH, can be readily identified by urinalysis and culture; however, a urinary tract infection can also be a complication of BPH. Although irritative voiding complaints are also associated with carcinoma of the bladder, especially carcinoma in situ, the urinalysis usually shows evidence of hematuria. Likewise, patients with neurogenic bladder disorders may have many of the signs and symptoms of BPH, but a history of neurologic disease, stroke, diabetes mellitus, or back injury may be present as well. In addition, examination may show diminished perineal or lower extremity sensation or alterations in rectal sphincter tone or the bulbocavernosus reflex.

Simultaneous alterations in bowel function (constipation) might also alert one to the possibility of a neurologic origin.

Treatment

After patients have been evaluated, they should be informed of the various therapeutic options for BPH. It is advisable for patients to consult with their physicians to make an educated decision on the basis of the relative efficacy and side effects of the treatment options.

Specific treatment recommendations can be offered for certain groups of patients. For those with mild symptoms (symptom score 0–7), watchful waiting only is advised. On the other end of the therapeutic spectrum, absolute surgical indications include refractory urinary retention (failing at least one attempt at catheter removal), recurrent urinary tract infection from BPH, recurrent gross hematuria from BPH, bladder stones from BPH, renal insufficiency from BPH, or large bladder diverticula (McConnell et al, 1994).

A. Watchful Waiting: Very few studies on the natural history of BPH have been reported. The risk of progression or complications is uncertain. However, in men with symptomatic BPH, it is clear that progression is not inevitable and that some men undergo spontaneous improvement or resolution of their symptoms.

Retrospective studies on the natural history of BPH are inherently subject to bias, related to patient selection and the type and extent of follow-up. Very few prospective studies addressing the natural history of BPH have been reported (Barry et al, 1997). One small series demonstrated that the progression to urinary retention occurred in approximately 10% of symptomatic men, while 50% of patients showed marked improvement or resolution of symptoms (Craigen et al, 1969). Recently, a large randomized study compared finasteride with placebo in men with moderately to severely symptomatic BPH and enlarged prostates on DRE (McConnell et al, 1998). Patients in the placebo arm of the study had a 7% risk of developing urinary retention over 4 years.

As mentioned above, watchful waiting is the appropriate management of men with mild symptom scores (0–7). Men with moderate or severe symptoms can also be managed in this fashion if they so choose. Neither the optimal interval for follow-up nor specific end points for intervention have been defined.

B. Medical Therapy

1. Alpha blockers–The human prostate and bladder base contains alpha-1-adrenoreceptors, and the prostate shows a contractile response to corresponding agonists (Hieble et al, 1985). The contractile properties of the prostate and bladder neck seem to be mediated primarily by the subtype α_1a receptors (Forray et al, 1994). Alpha blockade has been shown to result in both objective and subjective degrees of improvement in the symptoms and signs of

BPH in some patients. Alpha blockers can be classified according to their receptor selectivity as well as their half-life (Table 23–2).

Phenoxybenzamine and prazosin have comparable efficacy with respect to symptomatic relief, but the higher side-effect profile of phenoxybenzamine, associated with its lack of alpha-receptor specificity, precludes its use in BPH patients. Dose titration is necessary with prazosin, with typical therapy started at 1 mg at bedtime for 3 nights, then increased to 1 mg twice a day, which is titrated up to 2 mg twice a day if necessary. At higher doses, little additional symptomatic improvement is observed and side-effect profiles worsen. Typical side effects include orthostatic hypotension, dizziness, tiredness, retrograde ejaculation, rhinitis, and headache.

Long-acting alpha blockers make once-a-day dosing possible, but dose titration is still necessary. Terazosin is initiated at 1 mg daily for 3 days and increased to 2 mg daily for 11 days and then to 5 mg per day. Dosage can be escalated to 10 mg daily if necessary. Therapy with doxazosin is started at 1 mg daily for 7 days and increased to 2 mg daily for 7 days, and then to 4 mg daily. Dosage can be escalated to 8 mg daily if necessary. Side effects are similar to those described for prazosin.

The most recent advance in alpha-blocker therapy is related to the identification of subtypes of alpha-1-receptors. Selective blockade of the α_1a receptors, which are localized in the prostate and bladder neck, results in fewer systemic side effects (orthostatic hypotension, dizziness, tiredness, rhinitis, and headache), thus obviating the need for dose titration. Tamsulosin is initiated at 0.4 mg daily and can be increased to 0.8 mg daily if necessary.

Several randomized, double-blind, placebo-controlled trials, individually comparing terazosin, doxazosin, or tamsulosin with placebo (Roehrborn et al, 1996; Elhilali et al, 1996; Lepor et al, 1997; Lepor, 1998), have demonstrated the safety and efficacy of all of these agents. Comparative trials of various alpha blockers are ongoing.

Table 23–2. Classification of medical therapy and recommended dosage in BPH.

Classification	Oral Dosage
Alpha blockers	
Nonselective	
Phenoxybenzamine	10 mg twice a day
Alpha-1, short-acting	
Prazosin	2 mg twice a day
Alpha-1, long-acting	
Terazosin	5 or 10 mg daily
Doxazosin	4 or 8 mg daily
Alpha-1a selective	
Tamsulosin	0.4 or 0.8 mg daily
5α-reductase inhibitors	
Finasteride	5 mg daily

2. 5α-Reductase inhibitors–Finasteride is a 5α-reductase inhibitor that blocks the conversion of testosterone to dihydrotestosterone. This drug affects the epithelial component of the prostate, resulting in a reduction in the size of the gland and improvement in symptoms. Six months of therapy are required to see the maximum effects on prostate size (20% reduction) and symptomatic improvement.

Several randomized, double-blind, placebo-controlled trials have compared finasteride with placebo (Gormley et al, 1992; Nickel et al, 1996). Efficacy, safety, and durability are well established. However, symptomatic improvement is seen only in men with enlarged prostates (> 40 cm^3) (Boyle et al, 1996). Side effects include decreased libido, decreased ejaculate volume, and impotence. Serum PSA is reduced by approximately 50% in patients being treated with finasteride, but individual values may vary, thus complicating cancer detection.

A recent report suggests that finasteride therapy may decrease the incidence of urinary retention and the need for surgical intervention in men with enlarged prostates and moderate to severe symptoms (McConnell et al, 1998). However, optimal identification of appropriate patients for prophylactic therapy remains to be determined.

3. Combination therapy–The first randomized, double-blind, placebo-controlled study investigating combination alpha-blocker and 5α-reductase inhibitor therapy was recently reported (Lepor et al, 1996). This was a four-arm Veterans Administration Cooperative Trial comparing placebo, finasteride alone, terazosin alone, and combination finasteride and terazosin. Over 1200 patients participated, and significant decreases in symptom score and increases in urinary flow rates were seen only in the arms containing terazosin. However, one must note that enlarged prostates were not an entry criterion; in fact, prostate size in this study was much smaller than that in previous controlled trials using finasteride (32 versus 52 cm^3). Additional combination therapy trials are ongoing.

4. Phytotherapy–Phytotherapy refers to the use of plants or plant extracts for medicinal purposes. The use of phytotherapy in BPH has been popular in Europe for years, and its use in the United States is growing as a result of patient-driven enthusiasm. Several plant extracts have been popularized, including the saw palmetto berry, the bark of *Pygeum africanum,* the roots of *Echinicea purpurea* and *Hypoxis rooperi,* pollen extract, and the leaves of the trembling poplar. The mechanisms of action of these phytotherapies are unknown, and the efficacy and safety of these agents have not been tested in multicenter, randomized, double-blind, placebo-controlled studies (Lowe and Ku, 1996).

C. Conventional Surgical Therapy

1. Transurethral resection of the prostate (TURP)–Ninety-five percent of simple prostatectomies can be done endoscopically. Most of these procedures involve the use of a spinal anesthetic and require a 1- to 2-day hospital stay. Symptom score and flow rate improvement with TURP is superior to that of any minimally invasive therapy. The length of hospital stay of patients undergoing TURP, however, is greater. Much controversy revolves around possible higher rates of morbidity and mortality associated with TURP in comparison with those of open surgery, but the higher rates observed in one study were probably related to more significant comorbidities in the TURP patients than in the patients undergoing open surgery (Roos et al, 1989). Several other studies could not confirm the difference in mortality when results were controlled for age and comorbidities (Concato et al, 1992; Montorsi et al, 1993). Risks of TURP include retrograde ejaculation (75%), impotence (5–10%), and incontinence (< 1%). Complications include bleeding, urethral stricture or bladder neck contracture, perforation of the prostate capsule with extravasation, and if severe, TUR syndrome resulting from a hypervolemic, hyponatremic state due to absorption of the hypotonic irrigating solution. Clinical manifestations of the TUR syndrome include nausea, vomiting, confusion, hypertension, bradycardia, and visual disturbances. The risk of the TUR syndrome increases with resection times over 90 min. Treatment includes diuresis and, in severe cases, hypertonic saline administration (Mebust et al, 1989).

2. Transurethral incision of the prostate–Men with moderate to severe symptoms and a small prostate often have posterior commissure hyperplasia (elevated bladder neck). These patients will often benefit from an incision of the prostate. This procedure is more rapid and less morbid than TURP. Outcomes in well-selected patients are comparable, although a lower rate of retrograde ejaculation with transurethral incision has been reported (25%). The technique involves two incisions using the Collins knife at the 5 and 7 o'clock positions. The incisions are started just distal to the ureteral orifices and are extended outward to the verumontanum (Orandi, 1973).

3. Open simple prostatectomy–When the prostate is too large to be removed endoscopically, an open enucleation is necessary. What constitutes "too large" is subjective and will vary depending upon the surgeon's experience with TURP. Glands over 100 g are usually considered for open enucleation. Open prostatectomy may also be initiated when concomitant bladder diverticulum or a bladder stone is present or if dorsal lithotomy positioning is not possible.

Open prostatectomies can be done with either a suprapubic or retropubic approach. A **simple suprapubic prostatectomy** is performed transvesically and is the operation of choice in dealing with concomitant bladder pathology. After the bladder is opened, a semicircular incision is made in the bladder mucosa, distal to the trigone. The dissection plane is initiated sharply, and then blunt dissection with the finger is performed to remove the adenoma. The apical dissection should be done sharply to avoid injury to the distal sphincteric mechanism. After the adenoma is removed, hemostasis is attained with suture ligatures, and both a urethral and a suprapubic catheter are inserted before closure.

In a **simple retropubic prostatectomy,** the bladder is not entered. Rather, a transverse incision is made in the surgical capsule of the prostate, and the adenoma is enucleated as described above. Only a urethral catheter is needed at the end of the procedure.

D. Minimally Invasive Therapy

1. Laser therapy–Many different techniques of laser surgery for the prostate have been described. Two main energy sources of lasers have been utilized—Nd:YAG and holmium:YAG.

Several different **coagulation necrosis** techniques have been described. Transurethral laser-induced prostatectomy (TULIP) is done with transrectal ultrasound guidance. The TULIP device is placed in the urethra, and transrectal ultrasound is used to direct the device as it is slowly pulled from the bladder neck to the apex. The depth of treatment is monitored with ultrasound (McCullough, 1993).

Most urologists prefer to use visually directed laser techniques. **Visual coagulative necrosis** techniques have been popularized by Kabalin (Kabalin, Bite, and Doll, 1996). Under cystoscopic control, the laser fiber is pulled through the prostate at several designated areas, depending upon the size and configuration of the prostate. Four quadrant and sextant approaches have been described for lateral lobes, with additional treatments directed at enlarged median lobes. Coagulative techniques do not create an immediate visual defect in the prostatic urethra, but rather tissue is sloughed over the course of several weeks and up to 3 months following the procedure.

Visual contact ablative techniques are more time-consuming procedures because the fiber is placed in direct contact with the prostate tissue, which is vaporized. An immediate defect is obtained in the prostatic urethra, similar to that seen during TURP (Narayan et al, 1994).

Interstitial laser therapy places fibers directly into the prostate, usually under cystoscopic control. At each puncture, the laser is fired, resulting in submucosal coagulative necrosis. This technique may result in fewer irritative voiding symptoms, because the urethral mucosa is spared and prostate tissue is resorbed by the body rather than sloughed (Muschter et al, 1994).

Advantages of laser surgery include (1) minimal blood loss, (2) rare instances of TUR syndrome, (3) ability to treat patients receiving anticoagulation therapy, and (4) ability to be done as an outpatient procedure. Disadvantages include (1) lack of availability of tissue for pathologic examination, (2) longer postoperative catheterization time, (3) more irritative voiding complaints, and (4) high cost of laser fibers and generators.

Large-scale, multicenter, randomized studies with long-term follow-up are needed to compare laser prostate surgery with TURP and other forms of minimally invasive surgery.

2. Transurethral electrovaporization of the prostate–Transurethral electrovaporization uses the standard resectoscope but replaces a conventional loop with a variation of a grooved rollerball (Kaplan and Te, 1995). High current densities cause heat vaporization of tissue, resulting in a cavity in the prostatic urethra. Because the device requires slower sweeping speeds over the prostatic urethra, and the depth of vaporization is approximately one-third of a standard loop, the procedure usually takes longer than a standard TURP. Long-term comparative data are needed.

3. Hyperthermia–Microwave hyperthermia is most commonly delivered with a transurethral catheter. Some devices cool the urethral mucosa to decrease the risk of injury. However, if temperatures do not exceed 45 °C, cooling is unnecessary. Improvement in symptom score and flow rate is obtained, but as with laser surgery, large-scale, randomized studies with long-term follow-up are needed to assess durability and cost-effectiveness (Ogden et al, 1993).

4. Transurethral needle ablation of the prostate–Transurethral needle ablation uses a specially designed urethral catheter that is passed into the urethra. Interstitial radiofrequency needles are then deployed from the tip of the catheter, piercing the mucosa of the prostatic urethra. The use of radio frequencies to heat the tissue results in a coagulative necrosis. This technique is not adequate treatment for bladder neck and median lobe enlargement. Subjective and objective improvement in voiding occurs, but as mentioned above, comparative long term randomized studies are lacking (Schulman and Zlotta, 1995).

5. High-intensity focused ultrasound–High-intensity focused ultrasound is another means of performing thermal tissue ablation. A specially designed, dual-function ultrasound probe is placed in the rectum. This probe allows transrectal imaging of the prostate and also delivers short bursts of high-intensity focused ultrasound energy, which heats the prostate tissue and results in coagulative necrosis. Bladder neck and median lobe enlargement are not adequately treated with this technique. Although ongoing clinical trials demonstrate some improvement in symptom score and flow rate, the durability of response is unknown (Foster et al, 1993).

6. Intraurethral stents–Intraurethral stents are devices that are endoscopically placed in the prostatic fossa and are designed to keep the prostatic ure-

thra patent. They are usually covered by urothelium within 4–6 months after insertion. These devices are typically used for patients with limited life expectancy who are not deemed to be appropriate candidates for surgery or anesthesia. With the advent of other minimally invasive techniques requiring minimal anesthesia (conscious sedation or prostatic blocks), their application has become more limited.

7. Transurethral balloon dilation of the prostate–Balloon dilation of the prostate is performed with specially designed catheters that enable dilation of the prostatic fossa alone or the prostatic fossa and bladder neck (Castaneda et al, 1987). The technique is most effective in small prostates (< 40 cm^3). Although it may result in improvement in symptom score and flow rates, the effects are transient and the technique is rarely used today.

CARCINOMA OF THE PROSTATE (CaP)

Incidence and Epidemiology

Prostate cancer is the most common cancer diagnosed and is the second leading cause of cancer death in American men. Of all cancers, the prevalence of CaP increases the most rapidly with age. However, unlike most cancers, which have a peak age of incidence, the incidence of CaP continues to increase with advancing age. The lifetime risk of a 50-year-old man for latent CaP (detected as an incidental finding at autopsy, not related to the cause of death) is 40%; for clinically apparent CaP, 9.5%; and for death from CaP, 2.9%. Thus, many prostate cancers are indolent and inconsequential to the patient while others are virulent, and if detected too late or left untreated, they result in a patient's death. This broad spectrum of biological activity can make decision making for individual patients difficult.

Several risk factors for prostate cancer have been identified. As discussed above, increasing age heightens the risk for CaP. Which of the factors associated with the aging process are responsible for this observation are unknown. The probability of CaP developing in a man under the age of 40 is 1 in 10,000; for men 40–59 it is 1 in 103, and for men 60–79 it is 1 in 8 (Wingo et al, 1995). African Americans are at a higher risk for CaP than whites. In addition, African American men tend to present at a later stage of disease than whites. Controversial data have been reported suggesting that mortality from this disease may also be higher for African Americans (Morton, 1994; Moul et al, 1996; Fowler and Terrell, 1996). A positive family history of CaP also increases the relative risk for CaP. The age of disease onset in the family member with the diagnosis of CaP affects a patient's relative risk (Carter et al, 1993). If the age of onset is 70, the relative risk is increased 4-fold; if the age of onset is 60, the relative risk is increased 5-fold; and if the age of onset is 50, the relative risk is increased 7-fold. High dietary fat intake increases the relative risk for CaP by almost a factor of 2 (Whittemore et al, 1995). Another exposure that may increase the risk for CaP involves cadmium, which is found in cigarette smoke, alkaline batteries, and in the welding industry (Elghany et al, 1990). Previous vasectomy has been suggested as a factor that heightens the risk for CaP, but these data are controversial (Giovannucci et al, 1993; Rosenberg et al, 1994).

Etiology

The specific molecular mechanisms involved in the development and progression of CaP are an area of intense interest in the laboratory. The gene responsible for familial CaP resides on chromosome 1. Several regions of the human genome have been identified as possible areas that harbor tumor suppressor genes that may be involved in CaP. The regions most commonly identified are chromosomes 8p, 10q, 13q, 16q, 17p, and 18q (Carter et al, 1990; Kunimi et al, 1991). Epithelial-stromal interactions under the influence of growth factors such as transforming growth factor-β, platelet-derived growth factor, and neuroendocrine peptides modulate prostate cell development, differentiation, and metastasis.

Pathology

Over 95% of the cancers of the prostate are adenocarcinomas. Of the other 5%, 90% are transitional cell carcinomas, and the remaining cancers are neuroendocrine ("small cell") carcinomas or sarcomas. This discussion will address only adenocarcinomas.

The cytologic characteristics of CaP include hyperchromatic, enlarged nuclei with prominent nucleoli. Cytoplasm is often abundant; thus, nuclear-to-cytoplasmic ratios are not often helpful in making a diagnosis of CaP, unlike their usefulness in diagnosing many other neoplasms. Cytoplasm is often slightly blue-tinged or basophilic, which may assist in the diagnosis. The diagnosis of CaP is truly an architectural one. The basal cell layer is absent in CaP, although it is present in normal glands, BPH glands, and the precursor lesions of CaP. If the diagnosis of CaP is in question, high-molecular-weight keratin immunohistochemical staining is useful, as it preferentially stains basal cells. Absence of staining is thus consistent with CaP.

Prostatic intraepithelial neoplasia (PIN) is the precursor to invasive CaP. The critical distinguishing feature of invasive CaP is that the basal cell layer of the glandular architecture is absent. While PIN has the cytologic characteristics of CaP, the basal cell layer is present. PIN is usually classified into two categories, high grade (HGPIN) and low grade (LGPIN). The clinical importance of this distinction is that, when detected on prostate needle biopsy, HGPIN is usually associated with invasive CaP in approximately 80% of cases, whereas LGPIN is associated with invasive CaP only about 20% of the

time (Brawer et al, 1991; Aboseif et al, 1995). Thus, if a patient has needle biopsies showing only HGPIN, a repeat biopsy is critical to exclude the possibility of having missed an invasive cancer.

Sixty to 70 percent of cases of CaP originate in the peripheral zone, while 10–20% originate in the transition zone and 5–10% in the central zone. Radical prostatectomy series often demonstrate multifocal cancers within the prostate, with some variation in tumor grade.

Grading and Staging

The Gleason grading system is the most commonly employed grading system in the United States (Gleason et al, 1974). It is truly a system that relies upon the low-power appearance of the glandular architecture under the microscope. In assigning a grade to a given tumor, pathologists assign a primary grade to the pattern of cancer that is most commonly observed and a secondary grade to the second most commonly observed pattern in the specimen. Grades range from 1 to 5. If the entire specimen has only one pattern present, then both the primary and secondary grade are reported as the same grade. The **Gleason score** or **Gleason sum** is obtained by adding the primary and secondary grades together. As Gleason grades range from 1 to 5, Gleason scores or sums thus range from 2 to 10. Well-differentiated tumors have a Gleason sum of 2–4; moderately differentiated tumors have a Gleason sum of 5–6; and poorly differentiated tumors have a Gleason sum of 8–10. Historically, tumors having a Gleason sum of 7 have sometimes been grouped with the moderately differentiated tumors and at other times with the poorly differentiated tumors. One point that needs to be clarified is that the primary Gleason grade is perhaps the most important with respect to placing patients in prognostic groups (McNeal et al, 1990b; Epstein et al, 1996). This is most important in assessing patients with a Gleason sum of 7. Patients with a Gleason sum of 7 who have a primary Gleason grade of 4 (4 + 3) tend to have a worse prognosis than those who have a primary Gleason grade of 3 (3 + 4). Many clinical series have failed to distinguish between these two populations and, therefore, caution must be exercised in reviewing these series.

Gleason grades 1 and 2 are characterized by small, uniformly shaped glands, closely packed, with little intervening stroma. Gleason grade 3 is characterized by variable sized glands that percolate between normal stroma. A variant of Gleason grade 3 is referred to as a cribriform pattern. Here a small mass of cells is perforated by several gland lumens with no intervening stroma. This results in a cookie-cutterlike appearance of cell nests. The border of these cribriform glands is smooth. Gleason grade 4 has several histologic appearances. The characteristic observation common to all Gleason grade 4 patterns is **incomplete gland formation.** Sometimes glands appear fused, sharing a common cell border. At other times sheets of cell nests are seen or long cords of cells are observed. Cribriform glands can also occur in Gleason grade 4 but the cell masses are large and borders tend to appear ragged with infiltrating fingerlike projections. Gleason grade 5 usually has single infiltrating cells, with no gland formation or lumen appearance. Comedocarcinoma is an unusual variant of Gleason grade 5 carcinoma that has the appearance of cribriform glands with central areas of necrosis.

The TNM staging system for CaP is presented in Table 23–3 (American Joint Committee on Cancer, 1997). Note that with respect to the primary tumor categorization (T stage), the clinical staging system uses results of the DRE and transrectal ultrasound (TRUS), but not the results of the biopsy. Some examples to illustrate this staging system follow. If a patient has a palpable abnormality on one side of the prostate, even though biopsies demonstrate bilateral disease, his clinical stage remains T2a. If a patient has a normal DRE, with TRUS demonstrating a lesion on one side and a biopsy confirming cancer, his clinical stage is also T2a (using results of DRE and TRUS). A T1c cancer must have *both* a normal DRE and a normal TRUS.

Another popular staging system from a historical perspective is the Whitmore-Jewett staging system. One modification of this system is presented in Table 23–4 to assist the reader in the review of older published series. This system predates the use of TRUS and thus does not incorporate its findings.

Patterns of Progression

The pattern of CaP progression has been well de-fined. The likelihood of local extension outside the prostate (extracapsular extension) or seminal vesicle invasion and distant metastases increases with increasing tumor volume and more poorly differentiated cancers. Small and well-differentiated cancers (grades 1 and 2) are usually confined to the prostate, whereas large-volume (> 4 cm^3) or poorly differentiated (grades 4 and 5) cancers are more often locally extensive or metastatic to regional lymph nodes or bone (McNeal et al, 1990a). Penetration of the prostatic capsule by cancer is a common event and often occurs along perineural spaces. Seminal vesicle invasion is associated with a high likelihood of regional or distant disease. Locally advanced CaP may invade the bladder trigone, resulting in ureteral obstruction. Of note, rectal involvement is rare as Denovillier's fascia represents a strong barrier.

Lymphatic metastases are most often identified in the obturator lymph node chain. Other sites of nodal involvement include the common iliac, presacral, and periaortic lymph nodes. The axial skeleton is the most usual site of distant metastases, with the lumbar spine being most frequently implicated. The next most common sites in decreasing order are proximal femur, pelvis, thoracic spine, ribs, sternum, skull, and humerus (Saitoh et al, 1984). The bone lesions of metastatic CaP are typically osteoblastic. Involvement of long bones can lead to pathologic fractures. Vertebral body involvement with significant tumor masses extending into the epidural space can result in cord compression. Visceral metastases most commonly involve the lung, liver, and adrenal gland. Central nervous system involvement is usually a result of direct extension from skull metastasis.

Table 23–3. TNM staging system for prostate cancer.

T—Primary tumor	
Tx	Cannot be assessed
T0	No evidence of primary tumor
Tis	Carcinoma in situ (PIN)
T1a	≤ 5% of tissue in resection for benign disease has cancer, normal DRE
T1b	> 5% of tissue in resection for benign disease has cancer, normal DRE
T1c	Detected from elevated PSA alone, normal DRE and TRUS
T2a	Tumor palpable by DRE or visible by TRUS on one side only, confined to prostate
T2b	Tumor palpable by DRE or visible by TRUS on both sides, confined to prostate
T3a	Extracapsular extension on one or both sides
T3b	Seminal vesicle involvement
T4	Tumor directly extends into bladder neck, sphincter, rectum, levator muscles, or into pelvic sidewall
N—Regional lymph nodes (obturator, internal iliac, external iliac, presacral lymph nodes)	
Nx	Cannot be assessed
N0	No regional lymph node metastasis
N1	Metastasis in a regional lymph node or nodes
M—Distant metastasis	
Mx	Cannot be assessed
M0	No distant metastasis
M1a	Distant metastasis in nonregional lymph nodes
M1b	Distant metastasis to bone
M1c	Distant metastasis to other sites

DRE, digital rectal examination; PIN, prostatic intraepithelial neoplasia; PSA, prostate-specific antigen; TRUS, transrectal ultrasound.
Source: American Joint Committee on Cancer: *Cancer Staging Manual,* 5th ed. Lippincott-Raven, 1997.

Table 23–4. Whitmore-Jewett staging system for prostate cancer.

A1	≤ 3 foci of carcinoma and ≤ 5% of tissue in resection for benign disease has cancer, Gleason sum < 7
A2	> 3 foci of carcinoma and > 5% of tissue in resection for benign disease has cancer, Gleason sum ≥ 7
B1	Palpable nodule ≤ 1.5 cm, confined to prostate
B2	Palpable nodule > 1.5 cm, confined to prostate
C1	Palpable extracapsular extension
C2	Palpable seminal vesicle involvement
D0	Clinically localized disease, with negative bone scan but elevated serum acid phosphatase
D1	Pelvic lymph node metastases
D2	Bone metastases
D3	Hormone-refractory prostate cancer

Clinical Findings

A. Symptoms: Most patients with early-stage CaP are asymptomatic. The presence of symptoms often suggests locally advanced or metastatic disease. Obstructive or irritative voiding complaints can result from local growth of the tumor into the urethra or bladder neck or from its direct extension into the trigone of the bladder. Metastatic disease to the bones may cause bone pain. Metastatic disease to the vertebral column with impingement on the spinal cord may be associated with symptoms of cord compression, including paresthesias and weakness of the lower extremities and urinary or fecal incontinence.

B. Signs: A physical examination, including a DRE, is needed. Induration, if detected, must alert the physician to the possibility of cancer and the need for further evaluation (ie, PSA, TRUS, and biopsy). Locally advanced disease with bulky regional lymphadenopathy may lead to lymphedema of the lower extremities. Specific signs of cord compression relate to the level of the compression and may include weakness or spasticity of the lower extremities and a hyperreflexic bulbocavernosus reflex.

C. Laboratory Findings: Azotemia can result from bilateral ureteral obstruction either from direct extension into the trigone or from retroperitoneal adenopathy. Anemia may be present in metastatic disease. Alkaline phosphatase may be elevated in the presence of bone metastases. Serum acid phosphatase may be elevated with disease outside the confines of the prostate.

D. Tumor Markers—Prostate-Specific Antigen (PSA): Serum PSA has revolutionized our ability to detect CaP. Current detection strategies include the efficient use of the combination of DRE, serum PSA, and TRUS with systematic biopsy. Unfortunately, PSA is not specific for CaP, as other factors such as BPH, urethral instrumentation, and infection can cause elevations of serum PSA. Although the last two factors can usually be clinically ascertained, distinguishing between elevations of serum PSA resulting from BPH and those related to CaP remains the most problematic.

Numerous strategies to refine PSA for cancer detection have been explored. Their common goal is to decrease the number of false-positive test results. This would increase the specificity and positive predictive value of the test and lead to fewer unnecessary biopsies, lower costs, and reduced morbidity of cancer detection. Attempts at refining PSA have included PSA velocity (change of PSA over time), PSA density (standardizing levels in relation to the size of the prostate), age-adjusted PSA reference ranges (accounting for age-dependent prostate growth and occult prostatic disease), and PSA forms (free versus protein-bound molecular forms of PSA).

1. PSA velocity–PSA velocity refers to the rate of change of serum PSA. A retrospective study has shown that men with prostate cancer have a more rapidly rising serum PSA in the years before diagnosis than do men without prostate cancer. Patients whose serum PSA increases by 0.75 ng/mL/y appear to be at an increased risk of harboring cancer (Carter et al, 1992). In one study, the sensitivity and specificity of PSA velocity were 72% and 90%, respectively. Elevated PSA alone had a sensitivity of 78% and specificity of 60% (Mettlin et al, 1994). However, PSA velocity must be interpreted with caution. An elevated PSA velocity should be considered significant only when several serum PSA assays are carried out by the same laboratory over a period of at least 18 months.

2. PSA density–PSA levels are elevated approximately 0.12 ng/mL per gram of BPH tissue. Thus, patients with enlarged glands due to BPH may have elevated PSA levels. The ratio of PSA to gland volume is termed the PSA density. Some investigators advocate prostate biopsy only if the PSA density exceeds 0.1 or 0.15, while others have not found PSA density to be useful (Benson et al, 1992; Catalona et al, 1994; Cookson et al, 1995; Bazinet et al, 1994; Presti et al, 1996b). Problems with this approach include the facts that (1) epithelial-stromal ratios vary from gland to gland and only the epithelium produces PSA, and (2) errors in calculating prostatic volume may approach 25%. The relative performance of PSA and PSA density in the detection of nonpalpable prostate cancer in several series is summarized in Table 23–5.

3. Age-adjusted reference ranges for PSA–Age-adjusted PSA values for normal men are presented in Table 23–6 (Oesterling JE et al, 1993). It is

Table 23–5. Positive predictive values of PSA and PSA density for cancer detection in patients with a normal DRE and PSA level of 4–10 ng/mL.

Study (year)	n	TRUS	PSA > 4 (%)	PSAD > 0.1 (%)	PSAD > 0.15 (%)
Catalona et al (1994)	161	Negative	21	28	42
Cookson et al (1995)	44	NA	22	NA	7
Bazinet et al (1994)	142	Negative	16	20	32
Presti et al (1996b)	81	Negative	26	29	31

DRE, digital rectal examination; NA, not available; PSA, prostate-specific antigen; PSAD, PSA density; TRUS, transrectal ultrasound.

thought that the rise in PSA with increasing age results from prostate gland growth from BPH, the higher incidence of subclinical prostatitis, and the growing prevalence of microscopic, clinically insignificant prostate cancers. Concerns over the general applicability of these reference ranges have been raised because they were derived from US midwestern white men.

4. Racial variations in CaP detection–Although much evidence of racial variations in the incidence and mortality of CaP has been noted, little information is available on possible racial variations for cancer detection strategies. A recent retrospective study proposed different age-specific reference ranges for PSA for African Americans and whites (Morgan et al, 1996).

We prospectively evaluated racial variations in PSA and PSA density in 297 consecutive patients (97 African Americans and 200 whites) (Presti et al, 1997). In our population of patients with a normal DRE, use of a PSA density cutoff of 0.1 would have missed only one cancer (5%) in the African Americans while avoiding the need for biopsy in 20 (67%). Such favorable outcomes were not seen in whites, in whom 14% of cancers would have been missed while unnecessary biopsies would have been avoided in 76% by using a PSA density cutoff of 0.1. If these results are confirmed, application of PSA density may be appropriate in African Americans and may result in more efficient detection strategies in this high-risk population.

5. Molecular forms of PSA–The most recent refinement in PSA has been the recognition of the various molecular forms of PSA—free and protein-bound. Approximately 90% of the serum PSA

Table 23–6. Age-adjusted reference ranges for PSA.

Age (y)	PSA Normal Ranges (ng/mL)
40–49	0–2.5
50–59	0–3.5
60–69	0–4.5
70–79	0–6.5

Data from Oesterling JE et al: Serum prostate-specific antigen in a community-based population of healthy men. Establishment of age-specific reference ranges. JAMA 1993; 270:860.

is bound to alpha-1-antichymotrypsin, and lesser amounts are free or are bound to alpha-2-macroglobulins. In the latter form, no epitopes to the antibodies used in the current assays are available, while PSA bound to alpha-1-antichymotrypsin may have 3 of its 5 epitopes masked. Early studies suggest that prostate cancer patients demonstrate a lower percentage of free PSA than do patients with benign disease. Several investigators have reported early results using the free-to-total (F-T) PSA ratio in CaP detection, as shown in Table 23–7 (Oesterling et al, 1995; Demura et al, 1996). A large multicenter study has reported that in men with a normal DRE and a total PSA level between 4 and 10 ng/mL, a 25% free PSA cutoff would detect 95% of cancers while avoiding 20% of unnecessary biopsies. The cancers associated with greater than 25% free PSA were more prevalent in older patients and generally were less threatening in terms of tumor grade and volume (Catalona et al, 1998). Further validation studies with definition of optimal cutoff levels for different assays are needed, and issues such as possible racial variations in these levels must be addressed.

E. Prostate Biopsy: Systematic sextant prostate biopsy is the most commonly employed technique used in detecting CaP. Biopsies are usually obtained under TRUS guidance, from the apex, midsection, and base of each side of the prostate at the midsagittal line halfway between the lateral border and midline of the gland (Hodge et al, 1989). Information from sextant biopsies has mainly focused on cancer detection and has been underutilized for cancer staging. Along with other investigators, we have demonstrated some utility of systematic sextant biopsies in predicting extracapsular extension and risk of relapse following radical prostatectomy (Ravery et al, 1994; Peller et al, 1995; Huland et al, 1996; Borirakchanyavat et al, 1997; Presti et al, in press).

Refinement in systematic biopsy strategies to increase cancer detection rates is ongoing. We recently reported the utility of laterally directed biopsies of the peripheral zone in the base and mid sectors in addition to conventional sextant biopsies for the detection of CaP (Chang et al, in press). Two hundred thirty-five consecutive patients referred for an abnormal DRE or PSA > 4 ng/mL completed the protocol, and cancer was detected in 103 (44%). Lateral biop-

Table 23–7. Comparison between PSA and free to total (F-T) PSA ratios in cancer detection.

Study (year)	Biopsy result		PSA > 4 (%)		PSA (F-T < 0.2) (%)	
	Cancer	Benign	Sensitivity	Specificity	Sensitivity	Specificity
Demura et al (1996)	57	228	75	57	79	76
Oesterling et al (1995)	188	248	82	19	87	37

sies increased the sensitivity of cancer detection by 14% and obviated the need for lesion-directed biopsies.

We recently reported the role of systematic transition zone biopsies in prostates larger than 50 cm^3 (Chang et al, 1998). Two hundred thirteen consecutive patients referred for an abnormal DRE or PSA > 4.0 ng/mL had a calculated prostate size greater than 50 cm^3 by TRUS. These patients underwent TRUS-guided sextant biopsies of the peripheral zone and transition zone, for a total of 12 biopsies. The transition zone biopsies increased the sensitivity of cancer detection by 13%.

F. Imaging
1. TRUS–TRUS is useful in performing prostatic biopsies and in providing some useful local staging information if cancer is detected. Almost all prostate needle biopsies are performed under TRUS guidance. This allows uniform spatial separation and sampling of the regions of the prostate and also makes lesion-directed biopsies possible. If visible, CaP tends to appear as a hypoechoic lesion in the peripheral zone.

TRUS provides more accurate local staging than does DRE (Perrapato et al, 1989). The sonographic criteria for extracapsular extension are bulging of the prostate contour or angulated appearance of the lateral margin. The criteria for seminal vesicle invasion are a posterior bulge at the base of the seminal vesicle or asymmetry in echogenicity of the seminal vesicle associated with hypoechoic areas at the base of the prostate.

TRUS also enables measurement of the prostate volume, which is needed in the calculation of PSA density. Typically, a prolate ellipsoid formula is used: $(\pi/6) \times$ (anterior-posterior diameter) $\times$ (transverse diameter) $\times$ (sagittal diameter). TRUS is also used in the performance of cryosurgery and brachytherapy (see below).

2. Endorectal magnetic resonance imaging–The reported staging accuracy of endorectal coil magnetic resonance imaging (MRI) varies from 51% to 92% (Schnall et al, 1989; Hricak et al, 1994; Tempany et al, 1994). While rendering high image quality, the endorectal coil MRI appears to be operator dependent, requiring education and expertise. One prospective comparative trial assessing the relative merit of TRUS and endorectal MRI in evaluating the local stage of CaP failed to demonstrate any significant difference in the imaging modalities (Presti et al,

1996a). Costs associated with endorectal MRI are also high, and until this methodology demonstrates superiority in providing clinical information that alters patient management, its use should be limited. Attempts to identify patients who could potentially benefit from this imaging are ongoing.

3. Axial imaging (CT, MRI)–Cross-sectional imaging of the pelvis in patients with CaP is selectively performed to exclude lymph node metastases in high-risk patients who are thought to be candidates for definitive local therapy, whether it be surgery or irradiation. Both MRI and computed tomography (CT) are used for this purpose. Patients identified as having lymphadenopathy on imaging may undergo CT-guided fine-needle aspiration. If lymph node metastases are confirmed, such patients may be candidates for alternative treatment regimens. However, the incidence of lymph node metastases in contemporary radical prostatectomy series is low (< 10%). In addition, imaging is costly and its sensitivity is limited. A thorough review of the literature encompassing 15 series and 1354 patients with an incidence of lymph node metastases of 22% revealed a sensitivity of CT and MRI of 36% and a specificity of 97% (Wolf et al, 1995). Various criteria can be used to identify such patients, including negative bone scans and either T3 cancers or a PSA > 20 ng/mL and primary Gleason grade 4 or 5 cancers.

Analyses of several contemporary series of patients with clinically localized prostate cancer suggest that the risk of lymph node metastases is low and that its risk can be quantified on the basis of serum PSA, local tumor stage, and tumor grade. The serum concentration of PSA correlates well with cancer volume and stage. However, considerable overlap exists, making the use of serum PSA alone inaccurate for clinical staging in most patients. Use of serum PSA in conjunction with tumor grade and stage adds considerable sensitivity and specificity to the prediction of lymph node status compared with the use of PSA alone. Several investigators have published nomograms and probability curves that aid in predicting pathologic stage (Partin et al, 1993, 1997; Narayan et al, 1995; Bostwick et al, 1996).

4. Bone scan–When prostate cancer metastasizes, it most commonly does so to the bone. Soft tissue metastases (eg, lung and liver) are rare at the time of initial presentation. Although a bone scan has been considered a standard part of the initial evaluation of men with newly diagnosed prostate cancer, good evidence has been accumulated that it can be excluded in most of these men on the basis of serum PSA. Oesterling and colleagues have conducted studies to assess the ability of serum PSA to predict bone scan findings (Oesterling JE et al, 1993). On the basis of their results, bone scans can be omitted in patients with newly diagnosed, untreated prostate cancer who are asymptomatic and have serum PSA concentrations < 10 ng/mL. Sixty-six percent of the newly diagnosed patients in their study had PSA concentrations < 10 ng/mL, and the cancer stages were representative of the population of newly diagnosed patients in the United States currently. The serum PSA level was the best predictor of bone scan results. Use of tumor grade, local tumor stage, or a combination of these variables did not enhance the predictive power of PSA concentration.

G. Molecular Staging: Molecular staging refers to the detection of circulating prostate cells in the peripheral blood of men with CaP. The application of reverse transcription–polymerase chain reaction (RT-PCR) uses peripheral blood samples and attempts to identify the presence of the messenger RNA to PSA (Moreno et al, 1992; Katz et al, 1994). If detected, this is indirect evidence of prostate cells in the peripheral circulation. However, the clinical significance of positive RT-PCR test results at the present time is unknown. Numerous tumor systems have been identified that shed tumor cells into the circulation, but this finding is not always indicative of metastatic disease or treatment failure. Further studies are needed before the widespread application of this methodology.

Differential Diagnosis

Not all patients with an elevated PSA concentration have CaP. Other factors that elevate serum PSA include BPH, urethral instrumentation, infection, prostatic infarction, or vigorous prostate massage. Induration of the prostate is associated not only with CaP, but also with chronic granulomatous prostatitis, previous TURP or needle biopsy, or prostatic calculi. Sclerotic lesions on plain x-ray films and elevated levels of alkaline phosphatase can be seen in Paget disease and can often be difficult to distinguish from metastatic CaP. In Paget disease, PSA levels are usually normal and x-ray findings demonstrate subperiosteal cortical thickening.

Screening for CaP

The case for CaP screening is supported by the following: The disease is burdensome in this country; PSA improves detection of clinically important tumors without significantly increasing the detection of unimportant tumors; most PSA-detected tumors are curable; and curative treatments are available (Catalona et al, 1993; Littrup, Goodman, and Mettlin, 1993). Although the benefit of screening was recently shown in one randomized Canadian study,

several questions have been raised about the data analysis (Labrie et al, 1998). Currently, there are few data confirming that screening reduces morbidity and mortality (Krahn et al, 1994). Without these data, the net benefit of screening cannot be calculated or predicted. Several studies are currently in progress. In the Prostate, Lung, Colon and Ovarian (PLCO) trial supported by the National Cancer Institute, men are randomized to screening (with DRE and PSA) and no screening, with cancer-specific mortality as the end point. However, the fact that therapy is not standardized and that screening will be done over a limited period may make interpretation of results difficult. The efficacy of treatment is being examined in Scandinavia, where two randomized trials compare watchful waiting with radiation therapy or radical prostatectomy. A similar trial, Prostate Cancer Intervention Versus Observation Trial (PIVOT), is now under way in the United States. Such trials, although imperfect, may give us the information we need before prostate cancer screening and treatment can be recommended with confidence.

In summary, many factors must be considered by both clinicians and their patients who are contemplating screening for prostate cancer. Recently, editorials have called for standardized informed consent before ordering a screening test such as serum PSA (Hahn and Roberts, 1993). The information provided should attempt to answer such questions as the likelihood that an unscreened asymptomatic man will be adversely affected by prostate cancer in his lifetime, whether the screening test will lengthen or improve the quality of life, the chances of having a false-positive result and its consequences, the value of a normal result, and the recommendations of various experts. Based on available data, our bias has been that relatively young, healthy, asymptomatic men are encouraged to undergo screening. Screening is highly encouraged in certain populations with a higher disease prevalence or higher mortality rates, such as African American men or men with a significant family history of CaP. If CaP is detected, patients are carefully counseled regarding the benefits and risks of all treatment options, including watchful waiting. At the present time the data suggest that if screening is done, the combination of DRE and serum PSA is best.

Treatment

A. Localized Disease

1. General considerations–The optimal form of therapy for all stages of CaP remains a subject of great debate. Well-designed, randomized trials comparing various modalities for localized disease are lacking. Treatment dilemmas persist in the management of localized disease (T1 and T2) because of the uncertainty surrounding the relative efficacy of various modalities, including radical prostatectomy, radiation therapy, and surveillance. Currently, treatment decisions are based on the grade and stage of the tumor, the life expectancy of the patient, the ability of each therapy to ensure disease-free survival, its associated morbidity, and patient and physician preferences.

2. Watchful waiting–No randomized trial has demonstrated the therapeutic benefit of radical treatment for early-stage prostate cancer. Patients with prostate cancer are often older and may have concomitant illnesses. In addition, the small, well-differentiated prostate cancers commonly found in this population are often associated with very slow growth rates. Several studies have shown that surveillance alone may be an appropriate form of management for highly selected patients with prostate cancer (Table 23–8). However, most patients in such series are older and have very small, well-differentiated cancers. Even in such a selected population, cancer death rates approach 10%. In addition, end points for intervention in patients on surveillance regimens have not been defined.

3. Radical prostatectomy–The first radical perineal prostatectomy was performed by Hugh Hampton Young in 1904, and Millin first described the radical retropubic approach in 1945. However, the procedure remained unpopular because of frequent complications of incontinence and impotence. The rebirth of radical prostatectomy has resulted from a better understanding of the surgical anatomy of the pelvis. Description of the anatomy of the dorsal vein complex resulted in modifications in the surgical technique leading to reduced operative blood loss (Reiner and Walsh, 1979). In addition, improved visualization made possible a more precise apical dissection, allowing better reconstruction of the urinary tract and improved continence. Eversion of the bladder mucosa before anastomosis ensures a mucosa-to-mucosa apposition. Anatomic dissections have led to a better understanding of the prostate apex anatomy and its relationship to the distal urethral sphincteric mechanism (Meyers, Goellner, and Cahill, 1987). Description of the course of the cavernous nerves enabled modifications of the surgical technique, resulting in preservation of potency (Walsh and Donker, 1982).

The prognosis of patients treated by radical prostatectomy correlates with the pathologic stage of the specimen. Distant metastasis is inevitable in patients with positive lymph nodes. A high percentage of patients with seminal vesical involvement at radical prostatectomy are destined to distant failure. Fortunately, the number of patients with these adverse prognostic factors undergoing surgery is decreasing because of better candidate selection based on appropriate use of preoperative clinical parameters. Several investigators have established nomograms to predict final pathologic stage at radical prostatectomy based on the serum PSA level, clinical DRE stage, and Gleason sum derived from the biopsy.

Patients with organ-confined cancer have 10-year disease-free survival ranging from 70% to 85% in several series (Walsh, Partin, and Epstein, 1994; Paulson, 1994; Trapasso et al, 1994). Those with focal extracapsular extension demonstrate 85% and 75% disease-free survival at 5 and 10 years, respectively. Patients with more extensive extracapsular extension demonstrate 70% and 40% disease-free survival at 5 and 10 years, respectively (Epstein et al, 1993). High-grade tumors (Gleason sum > 7) have a higher risk of progression than do low-grade tumors. Disease-free survival at 10 years for patients with Gleason sum 2–6 tumors is in excess of 70%; for Gleason sum 7, 50%; and for Gleason sum > 8, 15%. Positive surgical margins significantly affect only tumors with extensive extracapsular extension.

The role of neoadjuvant hormonal therapy in men with localized CaP is currently being studied. Several investigators have reported a decrease in the number of positive surgical margins and the incidence of extracapsular extension. However, the largest randomized study to date demonstrated comparable serologic relapse rates at 4 years (Soloway et al, 1995; Witjes, Schulman, and Debruyne, 1997). Long-term data are still needed, and trials are ongoing.

The management of patients with positive surgical margins at radical prostatectomy remains controversial. Not all such patients relapse, but the identification of appropriate candidates for adjuvant radiation therapy remains problematic. A large multicenter randomized trial was recently closed to accrual to determine whether adjuvant radiation therapy in this setting is superior to radiation therapy at the time of relapse. Results of this study will not be available for several years.

Table 23–8. Results of watchful waiting studies.

Study (year)	n	Follow-up (y)	Overall Mortality (%)	Disease-Specific Mortality (%)	CaP Progression (%)
Johansson et al (1992)	223	10.2	56	8	34
Whitmore, Warner, and Thompson (1991)	75	9.5	39	15	69
Hanash et al (1972)	179	15	55	45	NA
George (1988)	120	7	44	4	83
Madsen et al (1988)	50	10	52	6	18

Morbidity associated with radical prostatectomy can be significant and is in part related to the experience of the surgeon. Immediate intraoperative complications include blood loss, rectal injury, and ureteral injury. Blood loss is more common with the retropubic approach than with the perineal approach because in the former, the dorsal venous complex must be divided. Rectal injury is rare with the retropubic approach and more common with the perineal approach but usually can be immediately repaired without long-term sequelae. Ureteral injury is exceedingly rare. Perioperative complications include deep venous thrombosis, pulmonary embolism, lymphocele formation, and wound infection. Late complications include urinary incontinence and impotence. Although total urinary incontinence tends to be rare (< 3%), stress urinary incontinence may be seen in up to 20% of patients. The return of continence after surgery is gradual, with 50% of patients continent at 3 months, 75% at 6 months, and the remainder at 9–12 months (Steiner et al, 1991). Age is the single most important factor in the restoration of continence. Preservation of one or both neurovascular bundles may allow maintenance of erectile function in men who are potent and sexually active before the procedure. However, the nerve-sparing procedure should be used selectively, for extracapsular extension is a common finding in patients with presumed localized CaP. If extracapsular extension is present, preservation of the neurovascular bundle may increase the likelihood that the tumor will recur. Preservation of potency varies as a function of age, preoperative sexual function, and preservation of one or both neurovascular bundles. Reported rates of potency preservation vary from 40% to 82% in men under the age of 60 when both nerves are preserved and drops to 20–60% when only one nerve is preserved. For men between the ages of 60 and 69, comparable rates are 25–75% with bilateral nerve-sparing and 10–50% with unilateral nerve-sparing (Walsh, Partin, and Epstein, 1994; Geary et al, 1995). Recovery of sexual function generally occurs within 6–12 months following surgery.

4. Radiation therapy—external beam therapy–Traditional external beam radiotherapy (XRT) techniques allow the safe delivery of 6500–7000 cGy to the prostate. Standard XRT techniques depend upon bony landmarks to define treatment borders or a single CT slice to define the target volume. These standard XRT techniques generally involve the use of open square or rectangular fields with minimal to no blocking and are characterized by the use of relatively small boost fields. Often, these XRT techniques fail to provide adequate coverage of the target volume in as many as 20–41% of patients with CaP irradiated.

Improved imaging and the use of 3-dimensional treatment planning software can now guarantee that the treatment field is accurately placed. This software can also allow higher doses of radiation to be given without exceeding the tolerances of surrounding normal tissues by causing the high-dose envelope of radiation to conform to the shape of the prostate. Conformal radiotherapy involves designing blocks from reconstructed CT images as viewed from the vantage point of the beam source. When viewed from the central axis, they are usually referred to as a "beam's-eye view." Computer-assisted beam's-eye views can be generated to design oblique and out-of-plane or noncoplanar beam arrangements. The approach is commonly referred to as 3-dimensional conformal radiotherapy. Additional benefits of this technique include the ability to calculate dose in 3 dimensions (to account more accurately for scattered radiation) and the ability to generate 3-dimensional dose displays and dose volume histograms. Three-dimensional dose displays allow so-called hot and cold spots (areas of overdosing and underdosing, respectively) to be recognized, while dose volume histograms allow different techniques to be compared and ranked for the relative sparing of surrounding normal tissues. Compared with standard XRT, considerably less normal tissue is irradiated because of the use of multiple complex fields.

Retrospective studies from several centers suggest that acute toxicity is reduced with the use of conformal radiotherapy compared with standard therapy (Soffen et al, 1992; Vijayakumar et al, 1993). Possible improvement in PSA response rates has also been reported in several retrospective studies using 3-dimensional conformal radiotherapy (Hanks et al, 1995; Roach et al, 1996). Although these results are encouraging, randomized trials and longer follow-up are required to determine if these improvements in PSA responses will translate into improved survival for these patients.

Readers are referred to Chapter 28 for a more detailed discussion of XRT in CaP.

5. Radiation therapy—brachytherapy–A resurgence in the interest in brachytherapy has occurred because of the technologic developments making it possible to place radioactive seeds under TRUS guidance. Previously, freehand seed placement techniques were used; however, very high failure rates were observed and the technique was virtually abandoned. Currently, with the use of computer software, one can preplan a precise dose of radiotherapy to be delivered by TRUS guidance.

Several investigators have reported their initial results using modern techniques. One study treated 197 patients with stages T1 and T2 prostatic cancer using TRUS-guided iodine-125 seed implantation (Blasko et al, 1995). The treatment group response was favorable, with 30% having a PSA < 4.0 ng/mL; 53%, a Gleason score of 2–4; and 88%, a cancer stage of < T2a. The actuarial rate of biochemical failure or local recurrence at 5 years following implantation was 7%. In another study 92 patients with stages T1 and

T2 cancer were treated with CT-based transperineal ^{125}I implantation (Wallner, Roy, and Harrison, 1996). Patients were monitored for a mean of 3 years (range 1–7). The overall actuarial freedom from biochemical failure at 4 years after implantation was 63%. The strongest predictors of failure were a PSA > 10 ng/mL, Gleason score 5–7, and T2 stage. A third study reported the results of TRUS-guided ^{125}I prostate implantation in 130 patients (Beyer and Priestley, 1997). Ninety-five percent had stage T2 cancers. Sixty-five percent had pretreatment PSA levels < 10 ng/mL, and only 9% had Gleason scores of 2–4. The median follow-up was only 9 months. Seventy-six percent of the 76 patients available for follow-up at 21 months had normal PSA levels.

Early data in men with low-volume, low-grade CaP are encouraging, but randomized studies comparing brachytherapy with other forms of radiotherapy are needed, as are studies assessing morbidity (impotence and urinary tract obstruction).

Readers are referred to Chapter 28 for a more detailed discussion of brachytherapy in CaP.

6. Cryosurgery–There has been a resurgence of interest in cryosurgery as a treatment for localized CaP in the past several years (Onik et al, 1993). This is due to an increased interest in less invasive forms of therapy for localized CaP as well as several recent technical innovations, including improved percutaneous techniques, expertise in TRUS, improved cryotechnology, and better understanding of cryobiology.

Freezing of the prostate is carried out by using a multiprobe cryosurgical device. Multiple hollow-core probes are placed percutaneously under TRUS guidance. Generally, 5 probes are placed: 2 anteromedially, 2 posterolaterally, and 1 posteriorly. Most surgeons routinely perform 2 freeze-thaw cycles in all patients, and if the iceball does not adequately extend to the apex of the prostate, the cryoprobes are pulled backwards into the apex and a third freeze-thaw cycle is undertaken. The temperature at the edge of the iceball is 0 to –2 °C, while actual cell destruction requires –25 to –50 °C. Therefore, actual tissue destruction occurs a few millimeters inside the iceball edge and cannot be monitored precisely by ultrasound imaging. Double freezing creates a larger tissue destruction area and theoretically brings the iceball edge and destruction zone edge closer together.

At the University of California at San Francisco (UCSF), we performed 107 cryosurgical procedures on patients with localized or locally advanced prostate cancer between July 1993 and February 1995 (Shinohara, 1996). Forty-four patients (41%) had tumors that appeared confined within the prostatic capsule (T1 and T2 lesions) on clinical examination and TRUS at the time of cryosurgery. The remaining patients had more extensive local disease: 31 patients (29%) had T3a tumors, 27 patients (25%) had T3b tumors, and 3 patients (3%) had involve-

ment of adjacent organs (T4). Two patients (2%) underwent cryosurgery for the management of local recurrence following radical prostatectomy.

PSA values were assessed at > 6 months after cryosurgery in 74 patients. PSA was undetectable (ie, < 0.1 ng/mL) in 35 patients (48%). In 22 patients (30%) the PSA was between 0.1 and 0.5 ng/mL, and in 17 patients (22%) it was > 0.5 ng/mL. Postoperative biopsies were carried out in 91 patients 3–6 months following cryosurgery. Twenty-one patients (23%) had residual cancer seen on one or more biopsies, and in the remaining 70 patients (77%) there was no evidence of tumor. The best results with cryosurgery were seen in patients with T1c disease and in those with a pretreatment PSA of < 10 ng/mL.

In total, 55 complications (excluding impotence) were seen in 107 patients giving a complication rate of 51%. Apart from impotence, the most frequently encountered complication following cryosurgery was urinary tract obstruction, which occurred in 25 patients and required transurethral resection of necrotic prostate tissue.

Studies to date indicate that, in the short term at least, cryosurgery can result in negative post-treatment prostatic biopsies and low or undetectable serum PSA levels. However, the morbidity of cryosurgery is significant and the long-term results are unknown. Currently, very few of these procedures are being performed, because other minimally invasive therapies are becoming more popular (brachytherapy).

B. Locally Advanced Disease

1. Radiation therapy–Most patients with T3 CaP are, at the present time, treated with neoadjuvant hormonal therapy followed by XRT. This approach has proved to be superior to XRT alone in several randomized trials. One study reported on 456 evaluable patients, with high-volume T2, T3, and T4 patients randomized to receive 4 months of neoadjuvant complete androgen blockade with XRT (2 months before and 2 months during XRT) compared with XRT alone. The study demonstrated an improvement in local control and disease-free survival in the patients treated with neoadjuvant therapy (Pilepich et al, 1995). Another study reported on 401 evaluable patients with locally advanced CaP (predominantly T3) randomized to receive 3 years of androgen ablation therapy and XRT compared with XRT alone. This study also demonstrated improved survival in patients receiving combination therapy (Bolla et al, 1997). The optimal duration of hormonal therapy, both before and after radiation therapy, still needs to be defined.

C. Recurrent Disease

1. Following radical prostatectomy–The likelihood of recurrence following radical prostatectomy is related to cancer grade, pathologic stage, and the extent of extracapsular extension. Cancer recurrence is more common in those with positive surgical margins, established extracapsular extension, seminal vesicle invasion, and high-grade disease. For those patients who develop a detectable PSA level after radical prostatectomy, the site of recurrence (local versus distant) can be established with reasonable certainty based on the interval from surgery to the detectable PSA concentration, PSA doubling time, selective use of imaging studies, and a local biopsy.

Patients with persistently detectable serum PSA levels immediately after surgery, those with PSA levels that become detectable in the early postoperative period, and those with serum PSA levels that double rapidly are more likely to have systemic relapse. Patients with initially undetectable serum PSA concentrations that become detectable a long time after radical prostatectomy, especially if PSA doubling times are prolonged, are more likely to have local recurrence. The average time to a detectable PSA level is longer in those with local versus distant relapse (33 and 20 months, respectively) (Partin et al, 1994). A PSA doubling time of 6 months or less is most consistent with metastatic disease after radical prostatectomy (Trapasso et al, 1994). We recently evaluated 114 patients with a detectable level of PSA after radical prostatectomy and no evidence of distant recurrence (Connolly et al, 1996). A local recurrence was documented in 53% of patients. Several biopsy sessions were often needed to document the local recurrence. The diagnosis was made on the first biopsy in 67% of patients, on the second biopsy in 18%, on the third biopsy in 10%, and on the fourth biopsy in 5%. Radiation therapy should be offered to patients with documented, isolated local recurrence.

2. Following radiation therapy–A rising PSA level following definitive radiotherapy is indicative of cancer recurrence. Biopsies of the prostate can identify local recurrences, while imaging with bone scans and possibly CT scans can identify distant recurrences. Irrespective of the site of recurrence, most patients receive androgen ablation therapy. While pa-

tients with clinical evidence of only local recurrence might be considered candidates for salvage radical prostatectomy or cryotherapy, morbidity remains high in this setting as well as subsequent clinical failure.

D. Metastatic Disease

1. Initial endocrine therapy–Since death due to CaP is almost invariably a result of failure to control metastatic disease, a great deal of research has concentrated on efforts to improve control of distant disease. It is well known that most prostatic carcinomas are hormone dependent and that approximately 70–80% of men with metastatic CaP respond to various forms of androgen deprivation. Testosterone, the major circulating androgen, is produced by the Leydig cells in the testes (95%), with a smaller amount being produced by peripheral conversion of other steroids. Although 98% of serum testosterone is protein bound, free testosterone enters prostate cells and is converted to DHT, the major intracellular androgen. DHT binds a cytoplasmic receptor protein and the complex moves to the cell nucleus, where it modulates transcription. Androgen deprivation may be induced at several levels along the pituitary-gonadal axis using a variety of methods or agents (Table 23–9). Use of a class of drugs (LHRH agonists) delivered as depot injections either monthly or, more recently, at 3-month intervals has allowed induction of androgen deprivation without orchiectomy or administration of diethylstilbestrol. Currently, administration of LHRH agonists and orchiectomy are the most common forms of primary androgen blockade used. Because of its rapid onset of action, ketoconazole should be considered in patients with advanced prostate cancer who present with spinal cord compression or disseminated intravascular coagulation. Although testosterone is the major circulating androgen, the adrenal gland secretes the androgens dehydroepiandrosterone, dehydroepiandrosterone sulfate, and androstenedione. Some investigators believe that

Table 23–9. Androgen ablation therapy for prostate cancer.

Level	Agent	Dose Route	Dose (mg)	Frequency
Pituitary				
	Diethylstilbestrol	Oral	1–3	Daily
	Goserelin	Subcutaneous	10.8	Every 3 months
	Goserelin	Subcutaneous	3.6	Every month
	Leuprolide	Intramuscular	22.5	Every 3 months
	Leuprolide	Intramuscular	7.5	Every month
Adrenal				
	Ketoconazole	Oral	400	Daily
	Aminoglutethimide	Oral	250	Four times a day
Testicle				
	Orchiectomy			
Prostate cell				
	Bicalutamide	Oral	50	Daily
	Flutamide	Oral	250	Three times a day
	Nilutamide	Oral	150	Daily

suppressing both testicular and adrenal androgens (**complete androgen blockade**) allows for a better initial and a longer response compared with those methods that inhibit production of only testicular androgens. Complete androgen blockade can be achieved by combining an antiandrogen with the use of an LHRH agonist or orchiectomy. Antiandrogens appear to act by competitively binding the receptor for DHT, the intracellular androgen responsible for prostatic cell growth and development. When patients with metastatic prostate cancer are stratified with regard to extent of disease and performance status, those patients with limited disease and a good performance status who are treated with combined androgen blockade (an LHRH agonist and antiandrogen agent) seem to survive longer than those treated with an LHRH agonist alone (Crawford et al, 1989). However, another study comparing the use of an antiandrogen with and without an orchiectomy failed to demonstrate a survival difference between the two arms (Crawford et al, 1997). Ongoing trials are studying the use of intermittent androgen deprivation to determine whether this might result in a delay in the appearance of the hormone-refractory state (Goldenberg et al, 1995).

The timing of initial endocrine therapy in CaP has been an area of great debate for many years. Data from the Veterans Administration Cooperative Studies from the 1960s did not demonstrate a clear survival advantage for early intervention with androgen ablation therapy in patients with advanced CaP (Byar, 1983). However, a randomized study from the Medical Research Council comparing early with delayed endocrine therapy in patients with advanced CaP demonstrated improved survival as well as lower complication rates (cord compression, ureteric obstruction, bladder outlet obstruction, and pathologic fractures) in patients treated with early endocrine therapy (Medical Research Council, 1997).

2. Early manipulations for endocrine therapy failure–Patients receiving complete androgen blockade therapy who demonstrate a rise in serum PSA levels are currently managed by discontinuing the antiandrogen. Approximately 20–30% of such patients have a secondary PSA response (Scher and Kelly 1993). Responses are not just serologic, as regression of soft tissue disease has been reported. The pathophysiology underlying this secondary response, referred to as the antiandrogen withdrawal syndrome, is not understood. Some investigators have postulated that emergence of the hormone-refractory state results from mutations in the androgen receptor (Veldscholte et al, 1992). Typically, antiandrogens competitively inhibit the androgen receptor, but it is possible that these agents actually stimulate a mutant androgen receptor. Removal of this stimulus (stopping the antiandrogen), thus leads to a secondary response.

Patients receiving monotherapy (LHRH agonist or orchiectomy) whose PSA level starts rising may respond to the addition of an antiandrogen. Response rates are approximately 20–30% in this setting.

3. Hormone-refractory disease–Readers are referred to Chapter 27 for a detailed discussion of the therapy for hormone-refractory disease.

REFERENCES

PROSTATE GLAND

McNeal JE: Normal histology of the prostate. Am J Surg Pathol 1988;12:619.

McNeal JE et al: Zonal distribution of prostatic adenocarcinoma. Am J Surg Pathol 1988;12:897.

BENIGN PROSTATIC HYPERPLASIA

Barrack ER, Berry SJ: DNA synthesis in the canine prostate. Effects of androgen and estrogen treatment. Prostate 1987;10:45.

Barry MJ et al: The American Urological Association Symptom Index for benign prostatic hyperplasia. J Urol 1992;148:1549.

Barry MJ et al: The natural history of patients with benign prostatic hyperplasia as diagnosed by North American urologists. J Urol 1997;157:10.

Berry SJ et al: The development of human benign prostatic hyperplasia with age. J Urol 1984;132:474.

Berry SJ, Isaacs JT: Prostatic growth and androgen metabolism with aging in the dog versus the rat. Endocrinology 1984;114:511.

Berry SJ et al: Effect of age, castration and testosterone replacement on the development and restoration of canine benign prostatic hyperplasia. Prostate 1986;9:295.

Boyle P, Gould AL, Roehrborn CG: Prostate volume predicts outcome of treatment of benign prostatic hyperplasia with finasteride: Meta-analysis of randomized clinical trials. Urology 1996;48:398.

Castaneda F et al: Benign prostatic hypertrophy, retrograde transurethral dilation of the prostate urethra in humans. Radiology 1987;163:645.

Concato J et al: Problems of comorbidity in mortality after prostatectomy. JAMA 1992;267:1077.

Craigen AA et al: The natural history of prostatic obstruction: A prospective survey. J R Coll Gen Pract 1969;18:226.

Cunha GR et al: Hormone-induced morphogenesis and growth: Role of mesenchymal–epithelial interactions. Recent Prog Horm Res 1983;39:559.

Elhilali MM et al: A multicenter, randomized, double-blind, placebo-controlled study to evaluate the safety and efficacy of terazosin in the treatment of benign prostatic hyperplasia. Urology 1996;47:335.

Forray C et al: The alpha-1 adrenergic receptor that mediates smooth muscle contraction in the human prostate has the pharmacologic properties of a cloned human alpha-1c subtype. Pharmacology 1994;45:703.

Foster RS et al: High-energy focused ultrasound in the treatment of prostatic disease. Eur Urol 1993;23:29.

Gormley GJ et al: The effect of finasteride in men with benign prostatic hyperplasia. N Engl J Med 1992; 327:1185.

Hieble JP et al: In vitro characterization of the alpha-adrenoreceptors in human prostate. Eur J Pharmacol 1985;107:111.

Kabalin JN, Bite G, Doll S: Neodymium:YAG laser coagulation prostatectomy: 3 years of experience with 227 patients. J Urol 1996;155:181.

Kaplan SA, Te AE: Transurethral electrovaporization of the prostate: A novel method for treating men with benign prostatic hyperplasia. Urology 1995;45:566.

Lepor H: Long-term evaluation of tamsulosin in benign prostatic hyperplasia: Placebo-controlled, double-blind extension of phase III trial. Tamsulosin Investigator Group. Urology 1998;51:901.

Lepor H et al: Doxazosin for benign prostatic hyperplasia: Long-term efficacy and safety in hypertensive and normotensive patients. The Multicenter Study Group. J Urol 1997;157:525.

Lepor H et al: The efficacy of terazosin, finasteride, or both in benign prostatic hyperplasia. Veterans Affairs Cooperative Studies Benign Prostatic Hyperplasia Study Group. N Engl J Med 1996;8:533.

Lowe FC, Ku JC: Phytotherapy in treatment of benign prostatic hyperplasia: A critical review. Urology 1996;48:12.

McConnell JD: Prostatic growth—new insights into hormonal regulation. Br J Urol 1995;76:5.

McConnell JD et al: *Benign Prostatic Hyperplasia; Diagnosis and Treatment.* Clinical Practice Guideline No. 8. AHCPR Publication No. 94-0582. Rockville, MD: Agency for Health Care Policy and Research, Public Health Service, US Department of Health and Human Services, 1994.

McConnell JD et al: The effect of finasteride on the risk of acute urinary retention and the need for surgical treatment among men with benign prostatic hyperplasia. N Engl J Med 1998;338:557.

McCullough DL: Transurethral ultrasound-guided laser-induced prostatectomy: National human cooperative study results. J Urol 1993;150:1607.

McNeal JE: Origin and evolution of benign prostatic enlargement. Invest Urol 1978;15:340.

Mebust WK et al: Transurethral prostatectomy: Immediate and postoperative complications. A cooperative study of thirteen participating institutions evaluating 3885 patients. J Urol 1989;141:243.

Montorsi F et al: Long-term clinical reliability of transurethral and open prostatectomy for benign prostatic obstruction: A term of comparison for nonsurgical procedures. Eur Urol 1993;23:262.

Muschter R et al: Interstitial laser coagulation of the prostate: Experiences in the treatment of benign prostatic hyperplasia. Prog Clin Biol Res 1994;386:521.

Narayan P et al: Transurethral evaporation of prostate (TUEP) with Nd:YAG laser using a contact free beam technique: Results in 61 patients with benign prostatic hyperplasia. Urology 1994;43:813.

Nickel JC et al: Efficacy and safety of finasteride therapy for benign prostatic hyperplasia: Results of a 2-year randomized controlled trial (the PROSPECT Study). Can Med Assoc J 1996;155:1251.

Ogden CW et al: Sham versus transurethral microwave thermotherapy in patients with symptoms of benign prostatic outflow obstruction. Lancet 1993;341:14.

Orandi A: Transurethral incision of the prostate. J Urol 1973;110:229.

Partin AW et al: The influence of age and endocrine factors on the volume of benign prostatic hyperplasia. J Urol 1991;145:405.

Peters CA, Walsh PC: The effect of nafarelinacetate, a luteinizing hormone-releasing hormone agonist on benign prostatic hyperplasia. N Engl J Med 1987; 317:599.

Randall A: *Surgical Pathology of Prostatic Obstruction.* Williams & Wilkins, 1931.

Roehrborn CG et al: The Hytrin Community Assessment Trial study: A one-year study of terazosin versus placebo in the treatment of men with symptomatic benign prostatic hyperplasia. HYCAT Investigator Group. Urology 1996;47:159.

Roos NP et al: Mortality and reoperation after open and transurethral resection of the prostate for benign prostatic hyperplasia. N Engl J Med 1989;320:1120.

Sanda MG et al: Genetic susceptibility of benign prostatic hyperplasia. J Urol 1994;152:115.

Schulman CC, Zlotta AR: Transurethral needle ablation of the prostate for treatment of benign prostatic hyperplasia: Early clinical experience. Urology 1995; 45:28.

Tenniswood M: Role of epithelial–stromal interactions in the control of gene expression in the prostate. An hypothesis. Prostate 1986;9:375.

CARCINOMA OF THE PROSTATE

Aboseif S et al: The significance of prostatic intra-epithelial neoplasia. Br J Urol 1995;76:355.

American Joint Committee on Cancer: *Cancer Staging Manual,* 5th ed. Lippincott-Raven, 1997.

Bazinet M et al: Prospective evaluation of prostate-specific antigen density and systematic biopsies for early detection of prostatic carcinoma. Urology 1994;43: 44.

Benson MC et al: Prostate-specific antigen density: A means of distinguishing benign prostatic hypertrophy and prostate cancer. J Urol 1992;147:815.

Beyer DC, Priestley JB Jr: Biochemical disease-free survival following ^{125}I prostate implantation. Int J Radiat Oncol Biol Phys 1997;37:559.

Blasko JC et al: Prostate specific antigen based disease control following ultrasound guided [125]iodine implantation for stage T1/T2 prostatic carcinoma. J Urol 1995;154:1096.

Bolla M et al: Improved survival in patients with locally advanced prostate cancer treated with radiotherapy and goserelin. N Engl J Med 1997;337:295.

Borirakchanyavat S et al: Systematic sextant biopsies in the prediction of extracapsular extension at radical prostatectomy. Urology 1997;50:373.

Bostwick DG et al: Prediction of capsular perforation and seminal vesicle invasion in prostate cancer. J Urol 1996;155:1361.

Brawer MK et al: Significance of prostatic intraepithelial neoplasia on prostate needle biopsy. Urology 1991;38:103.

Byar DP: The Veterans Administration Cooperative Research Group's studies of cancer of the prostate. Cancer 1983;32:1126.

Carter BS et al: Allelic loss of chromosomes 10q and 16q in human prostate cancer. Proc Natl Acad Sci USA 1990;87:8751.

Carter HB et al: Hereditary prostate cancer: Epidemiologic and clinical features. J Urol 1993;150:797.

Carter HB et al: Longitudinal evaluation of prostate specific antigen levels in men with and without prostate disease. JAMA 1992;267:2215.

Catalona WJ et al: Comparison of prostate specific antigen concentration versus prostate specific antigen density in the early detection of prostate cancer: Receiver operating characteristic curves. J Urol 1994; 152:2031.

Catalona WJ et al: Detection of organ-confined prostate cancer is increased through prostate-specific antigen-based screening. JAMA 1993;270:948.

Catalona WJ et al: Use of the percentage of free prostate-specific antigen to enhance differentiation of prostate cancer from benign prostatic disease: A prospective multicenter clinical trial. JAMA 1998;279:1542.

Chang JJ et al: Prospective evaluation of lateral biopsies of the peripheral zone for prostate cancer detection. J Urol, in press.

Chang JJ et al: Prospective evaluation of systematic sextant transition zone biopsies in large prostates for cancer detection. Urology 1998;52:89.

Connolly JA et al: Local recurrence after radical prostatectomy: Characteristics in size, location, and relationship to prostate specific antigen and surgical margins. Urology 1996;47:225.

Cookson MS et al: The lack of predictive value of prostate specific antigen density in the detection of prostate cancer in patients with normal rectal examinations and intermediate prostate specific antigen levels. J Urol 1995;154:1070.

Crawford ED et al: Comparison of bilateral orchiectomy with or without flutamide for the treatment of patients with stage D2 adenocarcinoma of the prostate: Results of NCI Intergroup Study 0105. Br J Urol 1997; 80:1092A.

Crawford ED et al: A controlled trial of leuprolide with and without flutamide in prostatic carcinoma. N Engl J Med 1989;321:419.

Demura T et al: The proportion of free to total prostate specific antigen: A method of detecting prostate carcinoma. Cancer 1996;77:1137.

Elghany NA et al: Occupation, cadmium exposure and prostate cancer. Epidemiology 1990;1:107.

Epstein JI et al: Influence of capsular penetration on progression following radical prostatectomy: A study of 196 cases with long term follow-up. J Urol 1993;150: 135.

Epstein JI et al: Prediction of progression following radical prostatectomy: A multivariate analysis of 721 men with long-term follow-up. Am J Surg Pathol 1996;20:286.

Fowler JE Jr, Terrell F: Survival in blacks and whites after treatment for localized prostate cancer. J Urol 1996;156:133.

Geary ES et al: Nerve sparing radical prostatectomy: A different view. J Urol 1995;154:145..

George NJR: Natural history of localized prostatic cancer managed by conservative therapy alone. Lancet 1988;(March 5):494.

Giovannucci E et al: A prospective cohort study of vasectomy and prostate cancer in US men. JAMA 1993; 269:873.

Gleason DF et al: Prediction of prognosis for prostatic adenocarcinoma by combined histologic grading and clinical staging. J Urol 1974;111:58.

Goldenberg SL et al: Intermittent androgen suppression in the treatment of prostate cancer: A preliminary report. Urology 1995;45:839.

Hahn DL, Roberts RG: PSA screening for asymptomatic prostate cancer: Truth in advertising. J Fam Pract 1993;37:432.

Hanash KA et al: Carcinoma of the prostate: A 15 year follow-up. J Urol 1972;107:450.

Hanks GE et al: External beam irradiation of prostate cancer: Conformal treatment techniques and outcomes for the 1990s. Cancer 1995;75:1972.

Hodge KK et al: Random systematic versus directed ultrasound guided transrectal core biopsies of the prostate. J Urol 1989;142:71.

Hricak H et al: Carcinoma of the prostate gland: MR imaging with pelvic phased-array coils versus integrated endorectal-pelvic phased-array coils. Radiology 1994;193:703.

Huland H et al: Preoperative prediction of tumor heterogeneity and recurrence after radical prostatectomy for localized prostatic carcinoma with digital rectal examination, prostate specific antigen and the results of 6 systematic biopsies. J Urol 1996;155:1344.

Johansson JE et al: High 10-year survival rate in patients with early, untreated prostatic cancer. JAMA 1992; 267:2191.

Katz AE et al: Molecular staging of prostate cancer with the use of an enhanced reverse-transcriptase PCR assay. Urology 1994;43:765.

Krahn MD et al: Screening for prostate cancer: A decision analytic view. JAMA 1994;272:773.

Kunimi K et al: Allelotyping of human prostatic adenocarcinoma. Genomics 1991;11:530.

Labrie F et al: Decrease of prostate cancer death by screening: First data from the Quebec prospective and randomized study. Proc ASCO 1998;17:2A.

Littrup PJ, Goodman AC, Mettlin CJ: The benefit and cost of prostate cancer early detection. The Investigators of the American Cancer Society–National Prostate Cancer Detection Project. CA Cancer J Clin 1993;43:134.

Madsen PO et al: Treatment of localized prostatic cancer: Radical prostatectomy versus placebo: A 15 year follow-up. Scand J Urol Nephrol Suppl 1988;110:95.

McNeal JE et al: Capsular penetration in prostate cancer: Significance for natural history and treatment. Am J Surg Pathol 1990a;14:240.

McNeal JE et al: Histologic differentiation, cancer volume, and pelvic lymph node metastases in adenocarcinoma of the prostate. Cancer 1990b;66:1225.

Medical Research Council Prostate Cancer Working Party Investigators Group: Immediate versus deferred treatment for advanced prostatic cancer: Initial results of the Medical Research Council trial. Br J Urol 1997;79:235.

Mettlin C et al: Relative sensitivity and specificity of serum prostate specific antigen (PSA) level compared with age-referenced PSA, PSA density and PSA change. Cancer 1994;74:1615.

Meyers RP, Goellner JR, Cahill DR: Prostate shape, external striated urethral sphincter and radical prostatectomy—the apical dissection. J Urol 1987;138:543.

Moreno JG et al: Detection of hematogenous micrometastases in patients with prostate cancer. Cancer Res 1992;52:6110.

Morgan TO et al: Age-specific reference ranges for serum prostate-specific antigen in Black men. N Engl J Med 1996;335:304.

Morton RA Jr: Racial differences in adenocarcinoma of the prostate in North American men. Urology 1994; 44:637.

Moul JW et al: Black race is an adverse prognostic factor for prostate cancer recurrence following radical prostatectomy in an equal access health care setting. J Urol 1996;155:1667.

Narayan P et al: The role of transrectal ultrasound-guided biopsy-based staging, preoperative serum prostate-specific antigen, and biopsy Gleason score in prediction of final pathologic diagnosis in prostate cancer. Urology 1995;46:205.

Oesterling J et al: The use of prostate-specific antigen in staging patients with newly diagnosed prostate cancer. JAMA 1993;269:57.

Oesterling JE et al: Free, complexed and total serum prostate specific antigen: The establishment of appropriate reference ranges for their concentrations and ratios. J Urol 1995;154:1090.

Oesterling JE et al: Serum prostate-specific antigen in a community-based population of healthy men. Establishment of age-specific reference ranges. JAMA 1993;270:860.

Onik GM et al: Transrectal ultrasound-guided percutaneous radical cryosurgical ablation of the prostate. Cancer 1993;72:1291.

Partin AW et al: Combination of prostate-specific antigen, clinical stage, and Gleason score to predict pathological stage of localized prostate cancer. JAMA 1997;277:1445.

Partin AW et al: Evaluation of serum prostate-specific antigen velocity after radical prostatectomy to distinguish local from distant metastases. Urology 1994; 43:649.

Partin AW et al: The use of prostate-specific antigen, clinical stage and Gleason score to predict pathological stage in men with localized prostate cancer. J Urol 1993;150:110.

Paulson DF: Impact of radical prostatectomy in the management of clinically localized disease. J Urol 1994; 152:1826.

Peller PA et al: Sextant prostate biopsies. A histopathologic correlation with radical prostatectomy specimens. Cancer 1995;75:530.

Perrapato SD et al: Comparing clinical staging plus transrectal ultrasound with surgical-pathological staging of prostate cancer. Urology 1989;33:103.

Pilepich MV et al: Androgen deprivation with radiation therapy compared with radiation therapy alone for locally advanced prostatic carcinoma: a randomized comparative trial of the Radiation Therapy Oncology Group. Urology 1995;45:616.

Presti JC Jr et al: Local staging of prostatic carcinoma: comparison of transrectal sonography and endorectal MR imaging. AJR 1996a;166:103.

Presti JC Jr et al: The positive fraction of systematic biopsies predicts risk of relapse following radical prostatectomy. Urology, in press.

Presti JC Jr et al: Prospective evaluation of prostate specific antigen and prostate specific antigen density in the detection of carcinoma of the prostate: Ethnic variations. J Urol 1997;157:907.

Presti JC Jr et al: Prospective evaluation of prostate specific antigen and prostate specific antigen density in the detection of nonpalpable and stage T1c carcinoma of the prostate. J Urol 1996b;156:1685.

Ravery V et al: Systematic biopsies accurately predict extracapsular extension of prostate cancer and persistent/recurrent detectable PSA after radical prostatectomy. Urology 1994;44:371.

Reiner WG, Walsh PC: An anatomical approach to the surgical management of the dorsal vein and Santorini's plexus during radical retropubic surgery. J Urol 1979;121:198.

Roach M III et al: Radiotherapy for high grade clinically localized adenocarcinoma of the prostate. J Urol 1996;156:1719.

Rosenberg L et al: The relation of vasectomy to the risk of cancer. Am J Epidemiol 1994;140:431.

Saitoh H et al: Metastatic patterns of prostate cancer: Correlation between sites and number of organs involved. Cancer 1984;54:3078.

Scher HI, Kelly WK: The flutamide withdrawal syndrome: Its impact on clinical trials in hormone-refractory prostatic carcinoma. J Clin Oncol 1993;11:1566.

Schnall MD et al: Prostate: MR imaging with an endorectal surface coil. Radiology 1989;172:570.

Shinohara K et al: Cryosurgical treatment of localized prostate cancer (stages T1–T4): Preliminary results. J Urol 1996;156:115.

Soffen EM et al: Conformal static field radiation therapy treatment of early prostate cancer versus non-conformal techniques: A reduction in acute morbidity. Int J Radiat Oncol Biol Phys 1992;24:485.

Soloway MS et al: Randomized prospective study comparing radical prostatectomy alone versus radical prostatectomy preceded by androgen blockade in clinical stage B2 (T2bNxM0) prostate cancer. The Lupron Depot Neoadjuvant Prostate Cancer Study Group. J Urol 1995;154:424.

Steiner MS, Morton RA, Walsh PC: Impact of anatomical radical prostatectomy on urinary incontinence. J Urol 1991;145:512.

Tempany CM et al: Staging of prostate cancer: Results of Radiology Diagnostic Oncology Group Project comparison of three MR imaging techniques. Radiology 1994;192:47.

Trapasso JG et al: The incidence and significance of detectable levels of serum prostate specific antigen after radical prostatectomy. J Urol 1994;152:1821.

Veldscholte J et al: Anti-androgens and the mutated androgen receptor of LNCaP cells: Differential effects on binding affinity, heat shock protein interaction, and transcription activation. Biochemistry 1992;31: 2393.

Vijayakumar S et al: Acute toxicity during external-beam radiotherapy for localized prostate cancer:

Comparison of different techniques. Int J Radiat Oncol Biol Phys 1993;25:359.

Wallner K, Roy J, Harrison L: Tumor control and morbidity following transperineal iodine 125 implantation for stage T1/T2 prostatic carcinoma. J Clin Oncol 1996;14:449.

Walsh PC, Donker PJ: Impotence following radical prostatectomy: Insight into etiology and prevention. J Urol 1982;128:492.

Walsh PC, Partin AW, Epstein JI: Cancer control and quality of life following anatomical radical retropubic prostatectomy: Results at 10 years. J Urol 1994;152:1831.

Whitmore WF, Warner JA, Thompson IM: Expectant management of localized prostatic cancer. Cancer 1991;67:1091.

Whittemore AS et al: Prostate cancer in relation to diet, physical activity and body size in blacks, whites and Asians in the United States and Canada. J Natl Cancer Inst 1995;87:652.

Wingo PA et al: Cancer statistics. Cancer J Clin 1995;45:8.

Witjes WP, Schulman CC, Debruyne FM: Preliminary results of a prospective randomized study comparing radical prostatectomy versus radical prostatectomy associated with neoadjuvant hormonal combination therapy in T2–3 N0 M0 prostatic carcinoma. The European Study Group on Neoadjuvant Treatment of Prostate Cancer. Urology 1997;49:65.

Wolf JS Jr et al: Use and accuracy of cross-sectional imaging and fine needle aspiration cytology for detection of pelvic lymph node metastases before radical prostatectomy. J Urol 1995;153:993.

Genital Tumors

Joseph C. Presti, Jr., MD

TUMORS OF THE TESTIS

GERM CELL TUMORS OF THE TESTIS

Epidemiology and Risk Factors

Malignant tumors of the testis are rare, with approximately 2–3 new cases per 100,000 males reported in the United States each year. Of all primary testicular tumors, 90–95% are germ cell tumors (seminoma and nonseminoma), while the remainder are nongerminal neoplasms (Leydig cell, Sertoli cell, gonadoblastoma). The lifetime probability of developing testicular cancer is 0.2% for a white male in the United States. Survival of patients with testicular cancer has improved dramatically in recent years, reflecting the development and refinement of effective combination chemotherapy. Overall 5-year survival rates have increased from 78% in 1974–1976 to 91% in 1980–1985 ($P < .05$).

The incidence of testicular cancer shows marked variation among different countries, races, and socioeconomic classes. Scandinavian countries report up to 6.7 new cases per 100,000 males annually with 0.8 per 100,000 males in Japan. In the United States, the incidence of testicular cancer in blacks is approximately one-fourth that in whites. Within a given race, individuals in the higher socioeconomic classes have approximately twice the incidence of those in the lower classes.

Testicular cancer is slightly more common on the right side than on the left, which parallels the increased incidence of cryptorchidism on the right side. Of primary testicular tumors, 1–2% are bilateral, and about 50% of these tumors occur in men with a history of unilateral or bilateral cryptorchidism. Primary bilateral tumors of the testis may happen synchronously or asynchronously but tend to be of the same histologic type. Seminoma is the most common germ cell tumor in bilateral *primary* testicular tumors, while malignant lymphoma is the most common bilateral tumor of the testis.

While the cause of testicular cancer is unknown, both congenital and acquired factors have been associated with tumor development. The strongest association has been with the cryptorchid testis. Approximately 7–10% of testicular tumors develop in patients who have a history of cryptorchidism; seminoma is the most common form of tumor these patients develop. However, 5–10% of testicular tumors occur in the contralateral, normally descended testis. The relative risk of malignancy is highest for the intra-abdominal testis (1 in 20) and is significantly lower for the inguinal testis (1 in 80). Placement of the cryptorchid testis into the scrotum (orchiopexy) does not alter the malignant potential of the cryptorchid testis; however, it does facilitate examination and tumor detection.

Exogenous estrogen administration to the mother during pregnancy has been associated with an increased relative risk for testicular tumors in the fetus, ranging from 2.8 to 5.3 over the expected incidence. Other acquired factors such as trauma and infection-related testicular atrophy have been associated with testicular tumors; however, a causal relationship has not been established.

Classification

Numerous classification systems have been proposed for germ cell tumors of the testis. Classification by histologic type proves to be the most useful with respect to treatment. The 2 major divisions are seminoma and nonseminomatous germ cell tumors (NSGCT), which include embryonal, teratoma, choriocarcinoma, and mixed tumors.

Tumorigenic Hypothesis for Germ Cell Tumor Development

The current model for germ cell tumor development resulted from the work of Dixon and Moore (1952), Teilum (1976), and Mostofi (1973). During embryonal development, the totipotential germ cells can travel down normal differentiation pathways and become spermatocytes. However, if these totipotential germ cells travel down abnormal developmental pathways, seminoma or embryonal carcinomas (totipotential tumor cells) develop. If the embryonal cells undergo further differentiation along intraembryonic pathways, teratoma will result. If the embryonal cells undergo further differentiation along extraembryonic pathways, either choriocarcinoma or yolk sac tumors are formed (Figure 24–1). This model helps to explain why specific histologic patterns of testicular tumors produce certain tumor markers. Note that yolk sac tumors produce alpha-fetoprotein (AFP) just as the yolk sac produces AFP in normal development. Likewise, choriocarcinoma produces human chorionic gonadotropin (hCG) just as the normal placenta produces hCG.

Pathology

A. Seminoma (35%): Three histologic subtypes of pure seminoma have been described. However, stage for stage, there is no prognostic significance to any of these subtypes. Classic seminoma accounts for 85% of all seminomas and is most common in the fourth decade of life. Grossly, coalescing gray nodules are observed. Microscopically, monotonous sheets of large cells with clear cytoplasm and densely staining nuclei are seen. It is noteworthy that syncytiotrophoblastic elements are seen in approximately 10–15% of cases, an incidence that corresponds approximately to the incidence of hCG production in seminomas.

Anaplastic seminoma accounts for 5–10% of all seminomas. Diagnosis requires the presence of 3 or more mitoses per high-power field, and the cells demonstrate a higher degree of nuclear pleomorphism

than the classic types. Anaplastic seminoma tends to present at a higher stage than the classic variety. When stage is taken into consideration, however, this subtype does not convey a worse prognosis.

Spermatocytic seminoma accounts for 5–10% of all seminomas. Microscopically, cells vary in size and are characterized by densely staining cytoplasm and round nuclei that contain condensed chromatin. More than half the patients with spermatocytic seminoma are over the age of 50.

B. Embryonal Cell Carcinoma (20%): Two variants of embryonal cell carcinoma are common: the adult type and the infantile type, or yolk sac tumor (also called endodermal sinus tumor). Histologic structure of the adult variant demonstrates marked pleomorphism and indistinct cellular borders. Mitotic figures and giant cells are common. Cells may be arranged in sheets, cords, glands, or papillary structures. Extensive hemorrhage and necrosis may be observed grossly.

The infantile variant, or yolk sac tumor, is the most common testicular tumor of infants and children. When seen in adults, it usually occurs in mixed histologic types and possibly is responsible for AFP production in these tumors. Microscopically, cells demonstrate vacuolated cytoplasm secondary to fat and glycogen deposition and are arranged in a loose network with large intervening cystic spaces. Embryoid bodies are commonly seen and resemble 1- to 2-week-old embryos consisting of a cavity surrounded by syncytio- and cytotrophoblasts.

C. Teratoma (5%): Teratomas may be seen in both children and adults. They contain more than one germ cell layer in various stages of maturation and differentiation. Grossly, the tumor appears lobulated

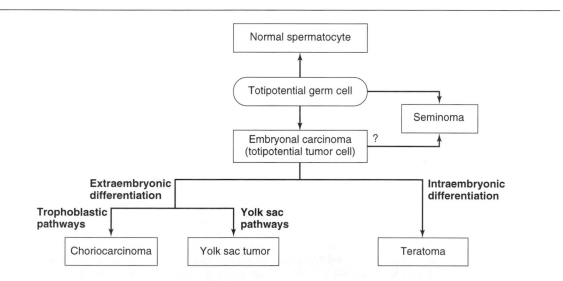

Figure 24–1. Tumorigenic model for germ cell tumors of the testis.

and contains variable-sized cysts filled with gelatinous or mucinous material. Mature teratoma may have elements resembling benign structures derived from ectoderm, mesoderm, and endoderm, while immature teratoma consists of undifferentiated primitive tissue. In contrast to its ovarian counterpart, the mature teratoma of the testis does not attain the same degree of differentiation as teratoma of the ovary. Microscopically, ectoderm may be represented by squamous epithelium or neural tissue; endoderm by intestinal, pancreatic, or respiratory tissue; and mesoderm by smooth or skeletal muscle, cartilage, or bone.

D. Choriocarcinoma (< 1%): Pure choriocarcinoma is rare. Lesions tend to be small within the testis and usually demonstrate central hemorrhage on gross inspection. Microscopically, syncytio- and cytotrophoblasts must be visualized. The syncytial elements are typically large, multinucleated cells with vacuolated, eosinophilic cytoplasm; the nuclei are large, hyperchromatic, and irregular. Cytotrophoblasts are uniform cells with distinct cell borders, clear cytoplasm, and a single nucleus.

Clinically, choriocarcinomas behave in an aggressive fashion characterized by early hematogenous spread. Paradoxically, small intratesticular lesions can be associated with widespread metastatic disease.

E. Mixed Cell Type (40%): Within the category of mixed cell types, the majority (up to 25% of all testicular tumors) are teratocarcinomas, which are a combination of teratoma and embryonal cell carcinoma. Up to 6% of all testicular tumors are of the mixed cell type, with seminoma being one of the components. Treatment for these mixtures of seminoma and NSGCT is similar to that of NSGCT alone.

F. Carcinoma in Situ (CIS): In a series of 250 patients with unilateral testicular cancer, Berthelsen et al (1982) demonstrated the presence of CIS in 13 (5.2%) of the contralateral testes. This is approximately twice the overall incidence of bilateral testicular cancer. While the natural history of this entity is incompletely defined, it should be noted that 5 of these 13 patients were followed for 3 years and that 2 of these 5 developed invasive disease. Presently, the ideal treatment of CIS of the testis remains unclear.

Patterns of Metastatic Spread

With the exception of choriocarcinoma, which demonstrates early hematogenous spread, germ cell tumors of the testis typically spread in a stepwise lymphatic fashion. Lymph nodes of the testis extend from T1 to L4 but are concentrated at the level of the renal hilum because of their common embryologic origin with the kidney. The primary landing site for the right testis is the interaortocaval area at the level of the right renal hilum. Stepwise spread, in order, is to the precaval, preaortic, paracaval, right common iliac, and right external iliac lymph nodes. The primary landing site for the left testis is the para-aortic area at the level of the left renal hilum. Stepwise spread, in order, is to the preaortic, left common iliac, and left external iliac lymph nodes. In the absence of disease on the left side, no crossover metastases to the right side have ever been identified. However, right-to-left crossover metastases are common. These observations by Donahue, Zachary, and Magnard (1982) and others have resulted in modified surgical dissections to preserve ejaculation in selected patients (see section on treatment, following).

Certain factors may alter the primary drainage of a testis neoplasm. Invasion of the epididymis or spermatic cord may allow spread to the distal external iliac and obturator lymph nodes. Scrotal violation or invasion of the tunica albuginea may result in inguinal metastases.

While the retroperitoneum is the most commonly involved site in metastatic disease, visceral metastases may be seen in advanced disease. The sites involved in decreasing frequency include lung, liver, brain, bone, kidney, adrenal, gastrointestinal tract, and spleen (Bredael, Vugrin, and Whitmore 1982).

As mentioned previously, choriocarcinoma is the exception to the rule and is characterized by early hematogenous spread, especially to the lung. Choriocarcinoma also has a predilection for unusual sites of metastasis such as the spleen.

Clinical Staging

Many clinical staging systems have been proposed for testicular cancer. Most, however, are variations of the original system proposed by Boden and Gibb (1951). In this system, a stage A lesion was confined to the testis, stage B demonstrated regional lymph node spread, and stage C was spread beyond retroperitoneal lymph nodes. In the Memorial Sloan-Kettering Cancer Center staging system for NSGCT, stage B has been subcategorized into B1 (retroperitoneal nodes less than 5 cm in maximum diameter), B2 (retroperitoneal nodes greater than 5 cm yet less than 10 cm in maximum diameter), and B3 (retroperitoneal nodes greater than 10 cm in maximum diameter or clinically palpable). Numerous clinical staging systems have also been suggested for seminoma. A stage I lesion is confined to the testis. Stage II has retroperitoneal nodal involvement (IIA is < 2 cm, IIB is > 2 cm). Stage III has supradiaphragmatic nodal involvement or visceral involvement.

The TNM classification of the American Joint Committee (1996) has attempted to standardize clinical stages as in Table 24–1.

Clinical Findings

A. Symptoms: The most common symptom of testicular cancer is a painless enlargement of the testis. Enlargement is usually gradual, and a sensation of testicular heaviness is not unusual. The typical delay in treatment from initial recognition of the lesion by the patient to definitive therapy (orchiec-

Table 24–1. TNM classification of tumors of the testis.

T—Primary tumor
TX: Cannot be assessed.
T0: No evidence of primary tumor.
Tis: Intratubular cancer (CIS).
T1: Limited to testis and epididymis, no vascular invasion.
T2: Invades beyond tunica albuginea or has vascular invasion.
T3: Invades spermatic cord.
T4: Invades scrotum.
N—Regional lymph nodes
NX: Cannot be assessed.
N0: No regional lymph node metastasis.
N1: Lymph node metastasis ≤ 2 cm and ≤ 5 lymph nodes.
N2: Metastasis in > 5 nodes, nodal mass > 2 cm and < 5 cm.
N3: Nodal mass > 5 cm.
M—Distant metastasis
MX: Cannot be assessed.
M0: No distant metastasis.
M1: Distant metastasis present.
S—Serum tumor markers
SX: Markers not available.
S0: Marker levels within normal limits.
S1: Lactic acid dehydrogenase (LDH) < 1.5 × normal and hCG < 5000 mIU/mL and AFP < 1000 ng/mL.
S2: LDH 1.5–10 × normal or hCG 5000–50,000 mIU/mL or AFP 1000–10,000 ng/mL.
S3: LDH > 10 × normal or hCG > 50,000 mIU/mL or AFP > 10,000 ng/mL.

Source: American Joint Committee on Cancer: *TNM Classification—Genitourinary Sites,* 1996.

tomy) ranges from 3 to 6 months. The length of delay correlates with the incidence of metastases (Oliver, 1985). The importance of patient awareness and self-examination is apparent. Acute testicular pain is seen in approximately 10% of cases and may be the result of intratesticular hemorrhage or infarction.

Approximately 10% of patients present with symptoms related to metastatic disease. Back pain (retroperitoneal metastases involving nerve roots) is the most common symptom. Other symptoms include cough or dyspnea (pulmonary metastases); anorexia, nausea, or vomiting (retroduodenal metastases); bone pain (skeletal metastases); and lower extremity swelling (venacaval obstruction).

Approximately 10% of patients are asymptomatic at presentation, and the tumor may be detected incidentally following trauma, or it may be detected by the patient's sexual partner.

B. Signs: A testicular mass or diffuse enlargement is found in the majority of cases. The mass is typically firm and nontender, and the epididymis should be easily separable from it. A hydrocele may accompany the testicular tumor and help to camouflage it. Transillumination of the scrotum can help to distinguish between these entities.

Palpation of the abdomen may reveal bulky ret-

roperitoneal disease; assessment of supraclavicular, scalene, and inguinal nodes should be performed. Gynecomastia is present in 5% of all germ cell tumors but may be present in 30–50% of Sertoli and Leydig cell tumors. Its cause seems to be related to multiple complex hormonal interactions involving testosterone, estrone, estradiol, prolactin, and hCG (Stepanas et al, 1978). Hemoptysis may be seen in advanced pulmonary disease.

C. Laboratory Findings and Tumor Markers: Anemia may be detected in advanced disease. Liver function tests may be elevated in the presence of hepatic metastases. Renal function may be diminished (elevated serum creatinine) if ureteral obstruction secondary to bulky retroperitoneal disease is present. The assessment of renal function (creatinine clearance) is mandatory in patients with advanced disease who require chemotherapy.

Several biochemical markers are of importance in the diagnosis and management of testicular carcinoma, including AFP, hCG, and LDH. Alpha-fetoprotein is a glycoprotein with a molecular mass of 70,000 daltons and a half-life of 4–6 days. Although present in fetal serum in high levels, beyond the age of 1 year it is present only in trace amounts. While present to varying degrees in many NSGCTs (Table 24–2), it is never found in seminomas.

Human chorionic gonadotropin is a glycoprotein with a molecular mass of 38,000 daltons and a half-life of 24 h. It is composed of 2 subunits: alpha and beta. The alpha subunit is similar to the alpha subunits of luteinizing hormone (LH), follicle-stimulating hormone (FSH), and thyroid-stimulating hormone (TSH). The beta subunit conveys the activity to each of these hormones and allows for a highly sensitive and specific radioimmunoassay in the determination of hCG levels. A normal man should not have significant levels of beta-hCG. While more commonly elevated in NSGCTs, hCG levels may be elevated in up to 7% of seminomas.

Lactic acid dehydrogenase is a cellular enzyme with a molecular mass of 134,000 daltons that has 5 isoenzymes; it is normally found in muscle (smooth, cardiac, skeletal), liver, kidney, and brain. Elevation of total serum LDH and in particular isoenzyme-I was shown to correlate with tumor burden in NSGCTs by Boyle and Samuels (1977). LDH may also be elevated in seminoma (Stanton et al, 1983).

Table 24–2. Incidence of elevated tumor markers by histologic type in testis cancer.

	hCG (%)	AFP (%)
Seminoma	7	0
Teratoma	25	38
Teratocarcinoma	57	64
Embryonal	60	70
Choriocarcinoma	100	0

Other markers have been described for testis cancer, including placental alkaline phosphatase (PLAP) and gamma-glutamyl transpeptidase (GGT). These markers, however, have not contributed as much to the management of patients as those mentioned previously.

D. Imaging: The primary testicular tumor can be rapidly and accurately assessed by scrotal ultrasonography. This technique can determine whether the mass is truly intratesticular, can be used to distinguish the tumor from epididymal pathology, and may also facilitate testicular examination in the presence of a hydrocele.

Once the diagnosis of testicular cancer has been established by inguinal orchiectomy, careful clinical staging of disease is mandatory. Chest radiographs (posteroanterior and lateral) and computed tomography (CT scan) of the abdomen and pelvis are used to assess the 2 most common sites of metastatic spread, namely, the lungs and retroperitoneum. The role of CT scanning of the chest remains controversial because of its decreased specificity. Of note is the fact that routine chest x-rays detect 85–90% of pulmonary metastases. Pedal lymphangiography (LAG) is rarely used owing to its invasiveness as well as low specificity, although it may be warranted in patients undergoing a surveillance protocol (see section on treatment).

Differential Diagnosis

An incorrect diagnosis is made at the initial examination in up to 25% of patients with testicular tumors and may result in delay in treatment or a suboptimal surgical approach (scrotal incision) for exploration. Epididymitis or epididymoorchitis is the most common misdiagnosis in patients with testis cancer. Early epididymitis should reveal an enlarged, tender epididymis that is clearly separable from the testis. In advanced stages, the inflammation may spread to the testis and result in an enlarged, tender, and indurated testis and epididymis. A history of acute onset of symptoms including fever, urethral discharge, and irritative voiding symptoms may make the diagnosis of epididymitis more likely. Ultrasonography may identify the enlarged epididymis as the cause of the scrotal mass.

Hydrocele is the second most common misdiagnosis. Transillumination of the scrotum may readily distinguish between a translucent, fluid-filled hydrocele and a solid testicular tumor. Since 5–10% of testicular tumors may be associated with hydroceles, however, if the testis cannot be adequately examined a scrotal ultrasound examination is mandatory. Aspiration of the hydrocele should be avoided because positive cytologic results have been reported in hydroceles associated with testicular tumors (Orecklin, 1974).

Other diagnoses to be considered include spermatocele, a cystic mass most commonly found extending from the head of the epididymis; hematocele associated with trauma; granulomatous orchitis, most commonly resulting from tuberculosis and associated with beading of the vas deferens; and varicocele, which is engorgement of the pampiniform plexus of veins in the spermatic cord and should disappear when the patient is in the supine position.

Although most intratesticular masses are malignant, one benign lesion, an epidermoid cyst, may be seen on rare occasions. Usually these cysts are very small benign nodules located just underneath the tunica albuginea; however, on occasion they can be large. The diagnosis is usually made following inguinal orchiectomy; as frozen sections, the larger lesions are often difficult to distinguish from teratoma.

Treatment

Inguinal exploration with cross-clamping of the spermatic cord vasculature and delivery of the testis into the field is the mainstay of exploration for a possible testis tumor. If cancer cannot be excluded by examination of the testis, radical orchiectomy is warranted. Scrotal approaches and open testicular biopsies should be avoided. Further therapy depends on the histologic characteristics of the tumor as well as the clinical stage.

A. Low-Stage Seminoma (I, II-A): Seminoma is exquisitely radiosensitive. Ninety-five percent of all stage A seminomas are cured with radical orchiectomy and retroperitoneal irradiation (usually 2500–3000 cGy). This low dose of radiation is usually well tolerated, with minimal, if any, gastrointestinal side effects.

Low-volume retroperitoneal disease also can be treated effectively with retroperitoneal irradiation with an average 5-year survival rate of 87%. Prophylactic mediastinal radiation is no longer employed because this may cause considerable myelosuppression and thus compromise the patient's ability to receive chemotherapy if required. Chemotherapy should be used as salvage therapy for patients who relapse following irradiation.

B. High-Stage Seminoma (II-B, III): Patients with bulky seminoma and any seminoma associated with an elevated AFP should receive primary chemotherapy. Seminomas are also sensitive to platinum-based regimens, as are their NSGCT counterparts. Some of the successful regimens include cisplatin, etoposide, and bleomycin (PEB); vinblastine, cyclophosphamide, dactinomycin, bleomycin, and cisplatin (VAB-6); and cisplatin and etoposide. All seminomas receive low-risk chemotherapy regimens, which currently consist of cisplatin and etoposide (4 cycles) or 3 cycles of PEB.

Ninety percent of patients with stage III disease achieve a complete response with chemotherapy. Residual retroperitoneal masses following chemotherapy are often fibrosis (90%) unless the mass is well circumscribed and in excess of 3 cm, under which circumstances approximately 40% of patients harbor residual seminoma. In such cases surgical excision is warranted (Stanton et al, 1985; Motzer et al, 1987).

C. Low-Stage Nonseminomatous Germ Cell Tumors: Standard treatment for stage A disease in the United States has included retroperitoneal lymph node dissection (RPLND). However, because three-fourths of patients with clinical stage A disease are cured by orchiectomy alone and the morbidity of RPLND is not negligible, other alternatives have been explored. These options include surveillance and modified RPLND.

Surveillance in stage A NSGCT was proposed because, as mentioned previously, 75% of patients with clinical stage A disease have, in fact, pathologic stage A disease. In addition, infertility related to disruption of sympathetic nerve fibers is common following RPLND. Clinical staging has been markedly improved in the presence of CT scanning and LAG. And finally, effective chemotherapy regimens have been developed for relapse. Patients are considered candidates for surveillance if the tumor is an NSGCT confined within the tunica albuginea, the tumor does not demonstrate vascular invasion, tumor markers normalize after orchiectomy, radiographic imaging shows no evidence of disease (chest x-ray [CXR], CT), and the patient is considered reliable.

Surveillance should be considered an active process on the part of both the physician and the patient. Patients are followed monthly for the first 2 years and bimonthly in the third year. Tumor markers are obtained at each visit, and CXR and CT scans are obtained every 3–4 months. Follow-up continues beyond the initial 3 years. The majority of relapses occur, however, within the first 8–10 months. With rare exceptions, patients who relapse can be cured by chemotherapy or surgery, or both.

Retroperitoneal lymph node dissection has been the preferred treatment of low-stage NSGCTs in the United States until recently. A thoracoabdominal or midline transabdominal approach may be used, and all nodal tissue between the ureters from the renal vessels to the bifurcation of the common iliac vessels is removed. Patients with negative nodes or N1 disease do not require adjuvant therapy, whereas the recommendation for those with N2 disease is to receive 2 cycles of chemotherapy because their relapse rate approaches 50%.

While effective in surgically staging and potentially curing a subset of patients, RPLND is associated with significant morbidity, especially with respect to fertility in young men. With a standard RPLND, sympathetic nerve fibers are disrupted, resulting in loss of seminal emission. Currently a modified RPLND has been developed that preserves ejaculation in up to 90% of patients. By modifying the dissection below the level of the inferior mesenteric artery to include only the nodal tissue ipsilateral to

the tumor, important sympathetic fibers from the contralateral side are preserved, thus maintaining ejaculation (Lange, Narayan, and Fraley, 1984; Pizzocaro, Salvioni, Zanoni, 1985).

D. High-Stage Nonseminomatous Germ Cell Tumors: Patients with bulky retroperitoneal disease (> 3-cm nodes or 3 or more 1-cm cuts on CT scan) or metastatic NSGCT are treated with primary platinum-based combination chemotherapy following orchiectomy. If tumor markers normalize and a residual mass is apparent on imaging studies, resection of that mass is mandatory, because 20% of the time it will harbor residual cancer, 40% of the time it will be teratoma, and 40% of the time it will be fibrosis (Figure 24–2). In patients with residual cancer in the resected tissue, the histologic picture is usually embryonal cell carcinoma, but malignant teratoma is seen in less than 5% of cases. Malignant teratoma is unresponsive to chemotherapy, and only 15% of patients survive following surgical resection. If tumor markers fail to normalize following primary chemother-

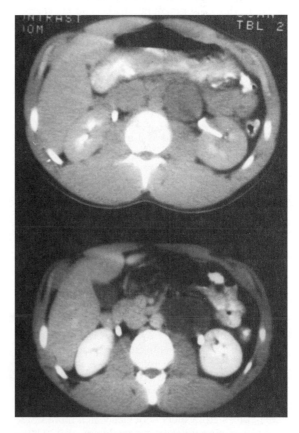

Figure 24–2. Upper: Computed tomography scan of patient with bulky retroperitoneal mass following radical orchiectomy for embryonal carcinoma. **Lower:** Residual cystic mass following chemotherapy, which was resected and found to be teratoma.

apy, salvage chemotherapy is required (cisplatin, etoposide, bleomycin, ifosfamide). Even if patients attain a complete response after chemotherapy (normal tumor markers, no mass on CT scan or CXR), some investigators advocate an RPLND because viable germ cell tumor may be seen in up to 10% of cases (Toner et al, 1990a). Such patients receive an additional 2 cycles of chemotherapy.

Although the treatment plan described cures up to 70% of patients with high-volume disease, there are patients who fail to respond. Also, the potential complications from chemotherapy including sepsis, neuropathy, renal toxicity, and death must be considered. It is thus apparent that it is important to be able to discriminate between patients who are likely to respond to standard chemotherapy (low risk) and those who may require more aggressive regimens (high risk). Bosl et al (1983), at Memorial Sloan-Kettering Cancer Center, developed a mathematic model that is useful in predicting the likelihood of attaining a complete response to standard chemotherapy. In a multivariant analysis only 3 parameters achieved statistical significance, namely, the serum LDH, the serum hCG, and the total number of sites of metastasis. The rate of decline of serum tumor markers during chemotherapy has also been used to predict response in patients with advanced disease (Toner et al, 1990b).

Follow-up Care

All patients with testicular cancer require regular follow-up care. As discussed previously, patients on a surveillance protocol require vigorous follow-up. Those who have undergone surgery (RPLND) or radiotherapy are followed at 3-month intervals for the first 2 years, then every 6 months until 5 years, and then yearly. Follow-up visits should include careful examination of the remaining testis, the abdomen, and the lymph node areas. Laboratory investigation should include AFP, hCG, and LDH levels. A CXR and an abdominal film (if an LAG was performed) should also be included at each visit.

Prognosis

Survival in testicular cancer has improved dramatically over the past several years, reflecting the continuing improvement and refinement in combination chemotherapy.

For seminoma treated by orchiectomy and radiotherapy, the 5-year disease-free survival rate is 98% for stage I and 92–94% for stage II-A in several recent series. Higher-stage disease treated by orchiectomy and primary chemotherapy has a 5-year disease-free survival rate of 35–75%, yet the lower value comes from older series in which more crude chemotherapy regimens were employed.

Survival in patients with NSGCTs treated by orchiectomy and RPLND for stage A disease ranges from 96 to 100%. For low-volume stage B disease treated with chemotherapy plus surgery, greater than 90% 5-year disease-free survival rates are attainable. Patients with bulky retroperitoneal or disseminated disease treated with primary chemotherapy followed by surgery have a 5-year disease-free survival rate of 55–80%.

Currently much work is being done to stratify patients into "high-risk" and "low-risk" groups so that treatment regimens may be modified in order to increase survival and decrease morbidity.

NON–GERM CELL TUMORS OF THE TESTIS

Approximately 5–6% of all testis tumors are non–germ cell tumors of the testis. Three types will be considered, namely, Leydig cell tumors, Sertoli cell tumors, and gonadoblastomas.

1. LEYDIG CELL TUMORS

Epidemiology & Pathology

Leydig cell tumors are the most common non–germ cell tumors of the testis and account for 1–3% of all testicular tumors. They follow a bimodal age distribution: the 5- to 9-year-old and the 25- to 35-year-old age groups. Twenty-five percent of these tumors occur in childhood. Bilaterality is seen in 5–10% of cases. The cause of these tumors is unknown; unlike germ cell tumors, there is no association with cryptorchidism.

Pathologic examination reveals a small, yellow, well-circumscribed lesion devoid of hemorrhage or necrosis. Microscopically, hexagonally shaped cells with granular, eosinophilic cytoplasm containing lipid vacuoles are seen. Reinke crystals are fusiform-shaped cytoplasmic inclusions that are pathognomonic for Leydig cells.

Clinical Findings

Prepubertal children usually present with virilization, and tumors are benign. Adults are usually asymptomatic, although gynecomastia may be present in 20–25%. Ten percent of tumors in adults are malignant. Laboratory findings include elevated serum and urinary 17-ketosteroids as well as estrogens.

Treatment & Prognosis

Radical orchiectomy is the initial treatment for Leydig cell tumors. Clinical staging is similar to that for germ cell tumors, and levels of the 17-ketosteroids can be helpful in distinguishing between benign and malignant lesions. Elevations of 10–30 times normal are typical of malignancy. RPLND is recommended for malignant lesions. Because of the rarity of these lesions, the role of chemotherapy remains to be defined. Prognosis is excellent for benign lesions, while it remains poor for patients with disseminated disease.

2. SERTOLI CELL TUMORS

Epidemiology & Pathology

Sertoli cell tumors are exceedingly rare, composing less than 1% of all testicular tumors. A bimodal age distribution is seen: 1 year old or younger and the 20- to 45-year-old age group. Approximately 10% of the lesions are malignant. Gross examination reveals a yellow or gray-white lesion with cystic components. Benign lesions are well circumscribed, while malignant lesions show ill-defined borders. Microscopically, tumors appear heterogeneous with mixed amounts of epithelial and stromal components. Sertoli cells are columnar or hexagonal cells with a large nucleus and solitary nucleolus, and contain vacuolated cytoplasm.

Clinical Findings

A testicular mass is the most common presentation. Virilization is often seen in children, and gynecomastia may be present in 30% of adults. Because of the rarity of these tumors, minimal endocrine data are available on these patients.

Treatment

Radical orchiectomy is the initial procedure of choice. In cases of malignancy, RPLND is indicated; however, the roles of chemotherapy and radiotherapy remain unclear.

3. GONADOBLASTOMAS

Epidemiology & Pathology

Gonadoblastomas comprise 0.5% of all testicular tumors and are almost exclusively seen in patients with some form of gonadal dysgenesis. The majority of these tumors occur in patients under 30 years of age, although the age distribution ranges from infancy to beyond 70 years.

Gross examination reveals a yellow or gray-white lesion that can vary in size from microscopic to greater than 20 cm and may exhibit calcifications. Microscopically, 3 cell types are seen: Sertoli cells, interstitial cells, and germ cells.

Clinical Findings

The clinical manifestations are predominantly related to the underlying gonadal dysgenesis and are discussed elsewhere in this book. It is noteworthy that four-fifths of patients with gonadoblastomas are phenotypic females. Males typically have cryptorchidism or hypospadias.

Treatment & Prognosis

Radical orchiectomy is the primary treatment of choice. In the presence of gonadal dysgenesis, a contralateral gonadectomy is recommended because the tumor tends to be bilateral in 50% of cases in this setting. Prognosis is excellent.

SECONDARY TUMORS OF THE TESTIS

Secondary tumors of the testis are rare. Three categories are considered: lymphoma, leukemia, and metastatic tumors.

1. LYMPHOMA

Epidemiology & Pathology

Lymphoma is the most common testicular tumor in a patient over the age of 50 and is the most common secondary neoplasm of the testis, accounting for 5% of all testicular tumors. It may be seen in 3 clinical settings: (1) late manifestation of widespread lymphoma; (2) initial presentation of clinically occult disease and (3) primary extranodal disease.

Gross examination reveals a bulging, gray or pink lesion with ill-defined margins. Hemorrhage and necrosis are common. Microscopically, diffuse histiocytic lymphoma is the most common type.

Clinical Findings

Painless enlargement of the testis is common. Generalized constitutional symptoms occur in one-fourth of patients. Bilateral testis involvement occurs in 50% of patients, usually asynchronously.

Treatment & Prognosis

Radical orchiectomy is indicated to make the diagnosis. Further staging and treatment should be handled in conjunction with the medical oncologist. Prognosis is related to the stage of disease. Some reports support adjuvant chemotherapy for primary testicular lymphoma, with improved survival rates of up to 93% after 44 months of follow-up (Connors et al, 1988).

2. LEUKEMIC INFILTRATION OF THE TESTIS

The testis is a common site of relapse for children with acute lymphocytic leukemia. Bilateral involvement may be present in one-half of cases. Testis biopsy rather than orchiectomy is the diagnostic procedure of choice. Bilateral testicular irradiation with 20 Gy and reinstitution of adjuvant chemotherapy constitute the treatment of choice. Prognosis remains guarded.

3. METASTATIC TUMORS

Metastasis to the testis is rare. These lesions are typically incidental findings at autopsy. The most common primary site is the prostate, followed by the lung, gastrointestinal tract, melanoma, and kidney. The typical pathologic finding is neoplastic cells in the interstitium with relative sparing of the seminiferous tubules.

EXTRAGONADAL GERM CELL TUMORS

Epidemiology & Pathology

Extragonadal germ cell tumors (EGT) are rare, accounting for approximately 3% of all germ cell tumors. Debate continues over whether these lesions originate from "burned-out" testicular primaries or originate de novo. Two theories exist as to the origin of these tumors as primary extragonadal lesions. The first theory suggests that during embryonic migration, primitive germ cells are displaced from their normal pathway and attain ectopic positions. The second theory suggests that pluripotential cells are displaced early in embryogenesis and become sequestered in ectopic sites. Our belief is that all retroperitoneal tumors have their origin from a testicular primary, whereas mediastinal germ cell tumors are truly ectopic.

The most common sites of origin in decreasing order are mediastinum, retroperitoneum, sacrococcygeal area, and pineal gland. All germ cell types may be observed. Seminoma composes more than half of the retroperitoneal and mediastinal tumors.

Clinical Findings

Clinical presentation depends on the site and volume of disease. Mediastinal lesions may present with pulmonary complaints. Retroperitoneal lesions may present with abdominal or back pain and a palpable mass. Sacrococcygeal tumors are most commonly seen in neonates and may present with a palpable mass and bowel or urinary obstruction. Pineal tumors may present with headache, visual or auditory complaints, or hypopituitarism.

Metastatic spread is to regional lymph nodes, lung, liver, bone, and brain. Metastatic workup is similar, therefore, to that of testicular germ cell tumors. A careful testicular examination is mandatory along with ultrasonography to exclude an occult testicular primary.

Treatment & Prognosis

Treatment of EGT parallels that of testicular tumors. Low-volume seminoma can be managed with radiotherapy. High-volume seminoma should receive primary chemotherapy. Prognosis parallels that of testicular seminoma. Primary chemotherapy should be employed for nonseminomatous elements with surgical excision of residual masses; however, prognosis remains poor for these patients.

TUMORS OF THE EPIDIDYMIS, PARATESTICULAR TISSUES, & SPERMATIC CORD

Primary tumors of the epididymis are rare and are most commonly benign. Adenomatoid tumors of the epididymis are the most common and typically occur in the third and fourth decade of life. They are typically asymptomatic, solid lesions that arise from any portion of the epididymis.

Leiomyomas are the second most common tumor of the epididymis. These lesions tend to be painful and are often associated with a hydrocele.

Cystadenomas are benign lesions of the epididymis that are bilateral in 30% of cases and are frequently seen in association with von Hippel-Lindau disease. Histologically these lesions are difficult to distinguish from renal cell carcinoma. Malignant lesions of the epididymis are extremely rare. In general, an inguinal approach should be used, and if frozen section confirms a benign lesion epididymectomy should be performed. If a malignant tumor is diagnosed, radical orchiectomy must be performed.

Tumors of the spermatic cord are typically benign. Lipomas of the cord account for the majority of these lesions. Of the malignant lesions, rhabdomyosarcoma is the most common, followed by leiomyosarcoma, fibrosarcoma, and liposarcoma.

Clinical diagnosis of tumors of the spermatic cord can be difficult. Differentiating between a hernia and a spermatic cord tumor may be possible only at exploration. In general, these lesions should be approached through an inguinal incision. The cord should be occluded at the internal ring and frozen sections obtained. If malignancy is diagnosed, attention should be directed toward performing wide local excision to avoid local recurrence. Staging of disease is similar to that of testicular tumors. For rhabdomyosarcoma, RPLND should be performed with adjuvant radiotherapy and chemotherapy. The value of RPLND for the other malignant spermatic cord tumors remains to be determined. Prognosis relates to the histologic status, stage, and site of disease.

TUMORS OF THE PENIS

Epidemiology & Risk Factors

Carcinoma of the penis accounts for less than 1% of cancers among males in the United States with approximately 1–2 new cases being reported per 100,000 men. There is marked variation in incidence with geographic location. In areas such as Africa and regions of South America, penile carcinoma may compose 10–20% of all malignant lesions. Penile carcinoma occurs most commonly in the sixth decade of life, although rare case reports have included children.

The one etiologic factor most commonly associated with penile carcinoma is poor hygiene. The disease is virtually unheard of in males circumcised near birth. One theory postulates that smegma accumulation under the phimotic foreskin results in chronic inflammation leading to carcinoma. A viral cause has also been suggested as a result of the association of this tumor with cervical carcinoma (Cartwright and Sinson, 1980).

Pathology

A. Precancerous Dermatologic Lesions: Leukoplakia is a rare condition that most commonly occurs in diabetic patients. A white plaque typically involving the meatus is seen. Histologic examination reveals acanthosis, hyperkeratosis, and parakeratosis. This lesion may precede or occur simultaneously with penile carcinoma.

Balanitis xerotica obliterans is a white patch originating on the prepuce or glans and usually involving the meatus. The condition is most commonly observed in middle-aged diabetic patients. Microscopic examination reveals atrophic epidermis and abnormalities in collagen deposition.

Giant condylomata acuminata are cauliflowerlike lesions arising from the prepuce or glans. The cause is believed to be viral (human papillomavirus). These lesions may be difficult to distinguish from well-differentiated squamous cell carcinoma.

B. Carcinoma in Situ (Bowen Disease, Erythroplasia of Queyrat): Bowen disease is a squamous cell carcinoma in situ typically involving the penile shaft. The lesion appears as a red plaque with encrustations.

Erythroplasia of Queyrat is a velvety, red lesion with ulcerations that usually involve the glans. Microscopic examination shows typical, hyperplastic cells in a disordered array with vacuolated cytoplasm and mitotic figures. Mikhail (1980) demonstrated that up to one-third of patients with erythroplasia of Queyrat may simultaneously have invasive carcinoma of the penis.

C. Invasive Carcinoma of the Penis: Squamous cell carcinoma composes the majority of penile cancers. It most commonly originates on the glans, with the next most common sites, in order, being the prepuce and shaft. The appearance may be papillary or ulcerative.

Verrucous carcinoma is a variant of squamous cell carcinoma composing 5–16% of penile carcinomas. This lesion is papillary in appearance and on histologic examination is noted to have a well-demarcated deep margin unlike the infiltrating margin of the typical squamous cell carcinoma.

Patterns of Spread

Invasive carcinoma of the penis begins as an ulcerative or papillary lesion, which may gradually grow to involve the entire glans or shaft of the penis. Buck's fascia represents a barrier to corporal invasion and hematogenous spread. Primary dissemination is via lymphatic channels to the femoral and iliac nodes. The prepuce and shaft skin drain into the superficial inguinal nodes (superficial to fascia lata), while the glans and corporal bodies drain to both superficial and deep inguinal nodes (deep to fascia lata). There are many cross-communications, so that penile lymphatic drainage is bilateral to both inguinal areas. Drainage from the inguinal nodes is to the pelvic nodes. Involvement of the femoral nodes may result in skin necrosis and infection or femoral vessel erosion and hemorrhage. Distant metastases are clinically apparent in less than 10% of cases and may involve lung, liver, bone, or brain.

Tumor Staging

The staging system used most commonly in the United States was proposed by Jackson (1966), as follows: In stage I, the tumor is confined to the glans or prepuce. Stage II involves the penile shaft. Stage III has operable inguinal node metastasis. In stage IV, the tumor extends beyond the penile shaft, with inoperable inguinal or distant metastases.

The TNM classification of the American Joint Committee (1996) is given in Table 24–3.

Clinical Findings

A. Symptoms: The most common complaint at

Table 24–3. TNM classification of tumors of the penis.

T—Primary tumor	
TX:	Cannot be assessed.
T0:	No evidence of primary tumor.
Tis:	Carcinoma in situ.
Ta:	Noninvasive verrucous carcinoma.
T1:	Invades subepithelial connective tissue.
T2:	Invades corpus spongiosum or cavernosum.
T3:	Invades urethra or prostate.
T4:	Invades other adjacent structures.
N—Regional lymph nodes	
NX:	Cannot be assessed.
N0:	No regional lymph node metastasis.
N1:	Metastasis in single superficial inguinal node.
N2:	Metastasis in multiple or bilateral superficial inguinal nodes.
N3:	Metastasis in deep inguinal or pelvic nodes.
M—Distant metastasis	
MX:	Cannot be assessed.
M0:	No distant metastasis.
M1:	Distant metastasis present.

Source: American Joint Committee on Cancer: *TNM Classification—Genitourinary Sites,* 1996.

presentation is the lesion itself. It may appear as an area of induration or erythema, an ulceration, a small nodule, or an exophytic growth. Phimosis may obscure the lesion and result in a delay in seeking medical attention. In fact, 15–50% of patients delay for at least 1 year in seeking medical attention. Other symptoms include pain, discharge, irritative voiding symptoms, and bleeding.

B. Signs: Lesions are typically confined to the penis at presentation. The primary lesion should be characterized with respect to size, location, and potential corporal body involvement. Careful palpation of the inguinal area is mandatory because more than 50% of patients present with enlarged inguinal nodes. This enlargement may be secondary to inflammation or metastatic spread.

C. Laboratory Findings: Laboratory evaluation is typically normal. Anemia and leukocytosis may be present in patients with long-standing disease or extensive local infection. Hypercalcemia in the absence of osseous metastases may be seen in 20% of patients and appears to correlate with volume of disease (Sklaroff and Yagoda, 1982).

D. Imaging: Metastatic workup should include CXR, bone scan, and CT scan of the abdomen and pelvis. Disseminated disease is present in less than 10% of patients at presentation.

Differential Diagnosis

In addition to the dermatologic lesions discussed previously, carcinoma of the penis must be differentiated from several infectious lesions. Syphilitic chancre may present as a painless ulceration. Serologic and darkfield examination should establish the diagnosis. Chancroid typically appears as a painful ulceration of the penis. Selective cultures for *Haemophilus ducreyi* should identify the cause. Condylomata acuminata appear as exophytic, soft, "grape cluster" lesions anywhere on the penile shaft or glans. Biopsy can distinguish this lesion from carcinoma if any doubt exists.

Treatment

A. Primary Lesion: Biopsy of the primary lesion is mandatory to establish the diagnosis of malignancy. Treatment varies depending on the pathology as well as the location of the lesion.

Carcinoma in situ may be treated conservatively in reliable patients. Fluorouracil cream application or neodymium:YAG laser treatment is effective for CIS and is preserving of the penis. Patients must come for frequent follow-up examinations to monitor response.

The goal of treatment in invasive penile carcinoma is complete excision with adequate margins. For lesions involving the prepuce, this may be accomplished by simple circumcision. For lesions involving the glans or distal shaft, partial penectomy with a 2-cm margin to decrease local recurrence has traditionally been suggested. For lesions involving the proxi-

mal shaft or when partial penectomy results in a penile stump of insufficient length for sexual function or directing the urinary stream, total penectomy with perineal urethrostomy has been recommended. Less aggressive surgical resections such as Mohs micrographic surgery and local excisions directed at penile preservation are currently being studied (Mohs et al, 1985).

B. Regional Lymph Nodes: As discussed previously, penile carcinoma spreads primarily to the inguinal lymph nodes. However, enlargement of inguinal nodes at presentation does not necessarily imply metastatic disease. In fact, up to 50% of the time this enlargement is caused by inflammation (Kossow, Hotchkiss, and Morales, 1973). Thus patients who present with enlarged inguinal nodes should undergo treatment of the primary lesion followed by a 4- to 6-week course of oral broad-spectrum antibiotics. Persistent adenopathy following antibiotic treatment should be considered to be metastatic disease, and sequential bilateral ilioinguinal node dissections should be performed. If lymphadenopathy resolves with antibiotics, observation in low-stage primary tumors (Tis, T1) is warranted. However, if lymphadenopathy resolves in higher-stage tumors, more limited lymph node samplings should be considered, such as the sen-

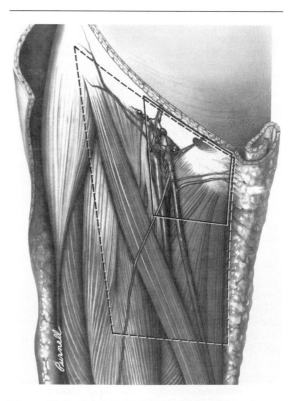

Figure 24–3. Comparison of limits of dissection of complete (dashed line) versus limited (solid line) inguinal lymphadenectomy.

tinel node biopsy described by Cabanas (1977) or a modified (limited) dissection as suggested by Catalona (1988) (Figure 24–3). If positive nodes are encountered, bilateral ilioinguinal node dissection should be performed. A decision tree for penile carcinoma is presented in Figure 24–4. Patients who initially have clinically negative nodes but later develop clinically palpable nodes should undergo a unilateral ilioinguinal node dissection.

Patients who have inoperable disease and bulky inguinal metastases are treated with chemotherapy (cisplatin and 5-fluorouracil). In some cases regional radiotherapy can provide significant palliation by delaying ulceration and infectious complications and alleviating pain.

C. Systemic Disease: Four chemotherapeutic agents demonstrate activity against penile carcinoma: bleomycin, methotrexate, cisplatin, and 5-fluorouracil. However, no long-term responders have been reported. The rarity of the disease in the United States has resulted in limited clinical trials.

Prognosis

Survival in penile carcinoma correlates with the presence or absence of nodal disease. Five-year survival rates for patients with node-negative disease range from 65 to 90%. For patients with positive inguinal nodes, this rate decreases to 30–50% and with positive iliac nodes decreases to less than 20%. In the presence of soft-tissue or bony metastases, no 5-year survivors have been reported.

Other Penile Tumors

Squamous cell carcinoma accounts for 98% of penile cancers. Sporadic cases of melanoma, basal cell carcinoma, and Paget disease have been reported. The incidence of Kaposi sarcoma of the penis is increasing with the increasing prevalence of the human immunodeficiency virus (HIV). It appears as a painful papule on the glans or shaft with bluish-purple discoloration. These lesions tend to be radiosensitive.

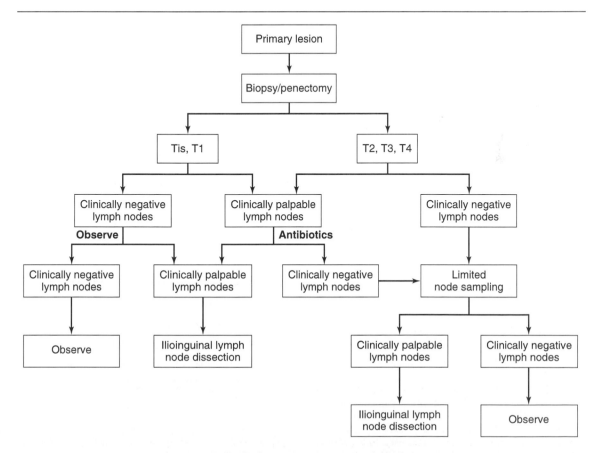

Figure 24–4. Management of penile carcinoma.

TUMORS OF THE SCROTUM

Tumors of the scrotal skin are rare. The most common benign lesion is a sebaceous cyst. Squamous cell carcinoma is the most common malignant tumor of the scrotum, although rare cases of melanoma, basal cell carcinoma, and Kaposi sarcoma have been reported. In the past, squamous cell carcinoma of the scrotum most commonly resulted from exposure to environmental carcinogens including chimney soot, tars, paraffin, and some petroleum products. Today, most cases result from poor hygiene and chronic inflammation.

Biopsy of the scrotal lesion must be performed to establish a histologic diagnosis. Wide excision with a 2-cm margin should be performed for malignant tumors. Surrounding subcutaneous tissue should be excised with the primary tumor; however, resection of the scrotal contents is rarely necessary. Primary closure using the redundant scrotal skin is usually possible. The management of inguinal nodes should be similar to that of penile cancer.

Prognosis correlates with the presence or absence of nodal involvement. In the presence of inguinal node metastasis, the 5-year survival rate is approximately 25%, while there are virtually no survivors if iliac nodes are involved.

REFERENCES

TUMORS OF THE TESTIS

American Joint Committee on Cancer: *TNM Classification—Genitourinary Sites.* 1996.

Berthelsen JG et al: Screening for carcinoma in situ of the contralateral testis in patients with germinal testicular cancer. Br Med J 1982;285:1683.

Boden G, Gibb R: Radiotherapy and testicular neoplasms. Lancet 1951;2:1195.

Bosl GJ et al: Multivariate analysis of prognostic variables in patients with metastatic testicular cancer. Cancer Res 1983;43:3403.

Boyle LE, Samuels ML: Serum LDH activity and isoenzyme patterns in nonseminomatous germinal testis tumors. Proc Am Soc Clin Oncol 1977;18:278.

Bredael JJ, Vugrin D, Whitmore WF Jr: Autopsy findings in 154 patients with germ cell tumors of the testis. Cancer 1982;50:548.

Carroll PR, Presti JC Jr: Testis cancer. Urol Clin North Am 1998;25(3). (Entire issue.)

Dixon FH, Moore RA: Tumors of the male sex organs. In: *Atlas of Tumor Pathology.* Armed Forces Institute of Pathology, 1952.

Donahue JP, Zachary JM, Magnard BR: Distribution of nodal metastases in nonseminomatous testis cancer. J Urol 1982;128:315.

Henderson BE, Ross RK, Pike MC: Epidemiology of testicular cancer. In: Skinner DG, Lieskovsky G (editors): *Diagnosis and Management of Genitourinary Cancer.* Saunders, 1988.

Lange PH, Narayan P, Fraley EE: Fertility issues following therapy for testicular cancer. Semin Urol 1984;4:264.

Mostofi FK: Testicular tumors: Epidemiologic, etiologic and pathologic features. Cancer 1973;32:1186.

Motzer R et al: Residual mass: An indication for further therapy in patients with advanced seminoma following systemic chemotherapy. J Clin Oncol 1987;5:1054.

Oliver RT: Factors contributing to delay in diagnosis of testicular tumors. Br Med J 1985;290:356.

Orecklin JR: Testicular tumor occurring with hydrocoele and positive cytologic fluid. Urology 1974;3:232.

Pizzocaro G, Salvioni R, Zanoni F: Unilateral lymphadenectomy in intraoperative stage I nonseminomatous germinal testis cancer. J Urol 1985;134:485.

Sogani PC et al: Orchiectomy alone in treatment of clinical stage I nonseminomatous germ cell tumor of the testis. J Clin Oncol 1984;2:267.

Stanton GF et al: Treatment of patient with advanced seminoma with cyclophosphamide, bleomycin, actinomycin D, vinblastine and cisplatin (VAB-6). (Abstract.) Proc Am Soc Clin Oncol 1983;2:1.

Stanton GF et al: VAB-6 as initial treatment of patients with advanced seminoma. J Clin Oncol 1985;3:336.

Stepanas A et al: Endocrine studies in testicular tumor patients with and without gynecomastia. Cancer 1978;41:369.

Teilum G: Special tumors of the ovary and testis and related extragonadal lesions. In: *Comparative Pathology and Histological Identification,* 2nd ed. Lippincott, 1976.

Toner GC et al: Adjunctive surgery after chemotherapy for nonseminomatous germ cell tumors: Recommendations for patient selection. J Clin Oncol 1990a;8:1683.

Toner GC et al: Serum tumor marker half-life during chemotherapy allows early prediction of complete response and survival in nonseminomatous germ cell tumors. Cancer Res 1990b;50:5904.

SECONDARY TUMORS OF THE TESTIS

Connors JM et al: Testicular lymphoma: Improved outcome with early brief chemotherapy. J Clin Oncol 1988;6:776.

EXTRAGONADAL GERM CELL TUMORS

Israel A et al: The results of chemotherapy for extragonadal germ-cell tumors in the cisplatin era: The

Memorial Sloan-Kettering Cancer Center experience (1975–1982). J Clin Oncol 1985;3:1073.

Jain KK et al: The treatment of extragonadal seminoma. J Clin Oncol 1984;2:820.

TUMORS OF THE EPIDIDYMIS, PARATESTICULAR TISSUES, & SPERMATIC CORD

Adrien M, Grabstald H, Whitmore WF Jr: Malignant tumors of the spermatic cord. Cancer 1969;23:525.

Farrell MA, Donnelly BJ: Malignant smooth muscle tumors of the epididymis. J Urol 1980;124:151.

Johnson DE, Harris JD, Ayala AG: Liposarcoma of spermatic cord. Urology 1978;11:190.

TUMORS OF THE PENIS

American Joint Committee on Cancer: *TNM Classification—Genitourinary Sites.* 1996.

Cabanas RM: An approach for the treatment of penile carcinoma. Cancer 1977;39:456.

Cartwright RA, Sinson JD: Carcinoma of the penis and cervix. Lancet 1980;1:97.

Catalona WJ: Modified inguinal lymphadenectomy for carcinoma of the penis with preservation of saphenous veins: Technique and preliminary results. J Urol 1988;140:306.

Jackson SM: The treatment of carcinoma of the penis. Br J Surg 1966;53:33.

Kossow JH, Hotchkiss AS, Morales PA: Carcinoma of the penis treated surgically: Analysis of 100 cases. Urology 1973;2:169.

Mikhail GR: Cancers, precancers and pseudocancer of the male genitalia: A review of clinical appearances, histopathology, and management. J Dermatol Surg Oncol 1980;6:1027.

Mohs FE et al: Microscopically controlled surgery in the treatment of carcinoma of the penis. J Urol 1985; 133:961.

Sklaroff RB, Yagoda A: Penile cancer: Natural history and therapy. In: Spiers ASD (editor): *Chemotherapy and Urological Malignancy.* Springer-Verlag, 1982.

TUMORS OF THE SCROTUM

Ray B, Whitmore WF Jr: Experience with carcinoma of the scrotum. J Urol 1977;117:741.

25 Urinary Diversion & Bladder Substitution

Peter R. Carroll, MD, & Susan Barbour, RN, MS, CETN

Selected patients with lower urinary tract cancers or severe functional or anatomic abnormalities of the bladder may require urinary diversion. Although this can be accomplished by establishing direct contact between the urinary tract and the skin surface, it is most often performed by incorporating various intestinal segments into the urinary tract. Virtually every segment of the gastrointestinal tract has been used to create urinary reservoirs or conduits. No single technique is ideal for all patients and clinical situations. A decision is based on a patient's underlying disease and its method of treatment as well as on renal function, individual anatomy, and personal preference. An ideal method of urinary diversion would most closely approximate the normal bladder: it would be nonrefluxing, low pressure, continent, and nonabsorptive.

Individual methods of urinary diversion can be categorized in various ways, such as (1) by the segment of intestine used, and (2) by whether the method provides complete continence or simply acts as a conduit carrying urine from the renal pelvis or ureter to the skin, where the urine is collected in an appliance attached to the skin surface. Continent forms of urinary diversion can be categorized further according to whether they are attached to the urethra (ie, as a bladder substitute) or are placed in the abdomen and rely on another mechanism for continence (continent urinary reservoir).

Preoperative Counseling & Preparation

All candidates for urinary diversion or bladder substitution should undergo careful preoperative counseling and preparation, including a detailed discussion of the objectives and potential complications of each method. Any potential impact of a procedure on sexual function, body image, and lifestyle should be discussed. Because they allow freedom from an external appliance, continent forms of urinary diversion or bladder substitution may be of great psychological and functional benefit to selected patients (Okada et al, 1997).

A careful history taken from the patient should note any previous abdominal or pelvic surgery, irradiation, or systemic disease. A history of intestinal resection or irradiation, renal failure, diverticulitis, regional enteritis, or ulcerative colitis would be especially important to consider when selecting a method of urinary diversion or bladder substitution. A complete blood count and measurement of serum electrolytes, urea nitrogen, and creatinine should be performed. The upper urinary tract should be imaged with intravenous urography or ultrasound to determine whether hydronephrosis, renal parenchymal scarring, or calculous disease exists. Contrast imaging of the small or large bowel or colonoscopy should be considered preoperatively for patients with a history of significant intestinal irradiation, occult bleeding, or other gastrointestinal diseases. Patients with benign bladder diseases—such as a reduced bladder capacity due to neurologic disorders or irradiation, bladder fistulas or interstitial cystitis—are occasionally considered candidates for urinary diversion or bladder substitution to manage urinary incontinence; however, with such patients, careful evaluation of bladder function and anatomy is required, as adequate urinary function can often be restored by urinary tract reconstruction, pharmacologic manipulation, or intermittent catheterization.

Patients undergo a standard mechanical and oral antibiotic bowel cleansing program beginning 1 or 2 days before surgery. Much of patients' dissatisfaction with urinary diversion can be attributed to poor stomal construction (Fitzgerald et al, 1997). The stoma site should be selected preoperatively and the patient evaluated in the lying, sitting, and standing positions. The most common site for stoma placement is along a line between the anterior superior iliac spine and umbilicus and at the lateral edge of the rectus abdominis muscle. The surface area should be flat and able to support an appliance. Bony prominences, fat folds, and scars should be avoided, as it is difficult to secure an appliance in these areas.

INTESTINAL CONDUIT URINARY DIVERSION

Ileal Conduit

Ureteroileal urinary diversion is the most common method of urinary diversion in the United States. The conduit is constructed using a segment of ileum approximately 15–20 cm proximal to the ileocecal valve (Figure 25–1). The length of the conduit varies depending on the habitus of the patient. As short a segment as possible, usually 18–20 cm, minimizes the absorptive surface of the bowel in contact with urine. Once the appropriate length of bowel is selected and isolated, the mesentery is divided proximally and distally and individual mesenteric blood

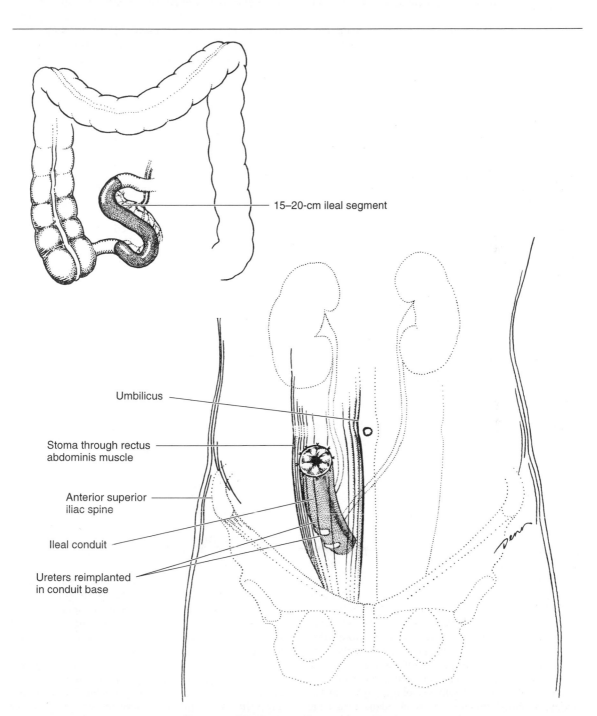

15–20-cm ileal segment

Umbilicus

Stoma through rectus
abdominis muscle

Anterior superior
iliac spine

Ileal conduit

Ureters reimplanted
in conduit base

Figure 25–1. Ileal conduit.

vessels are ligated. The bowel is divided, thus isolating the segment selected for conduit construction. The continuity of the small intestine is reestablished, allowing for normal bowel function. The conduit is usually positioned in the right lower quadrant of the abdomen in an isoperistaltic direction. The base of the conduit is closed, and the ureters are reimplanted directly on it. On occasion, ureteral stents (small-diameter, multichannel, silicone [Silastic] catheters) are placed through the ureteral anastomosis and conduit and into the renal pelvis to facilitate urinary drainage while the anastomosis is healing.

The preselected stoma site is identified and a small circle of skin and underlying fat excised. The fascia is incised in a cruciate fashion, or a small circle of it is excised. The end of the conduit is brought through the lateral aspect of the rectus abdominis muscle and anchored to the fascia, and the stoma is then formed. The stoma should protrude, without tension, approximately 1–1.5 in above the skin surface.

Jejunal Conduit

Jejunal conduit urinary diversion is used rarely, since many better alternatives are available. However, jejunal conduits have been used in cases in which there has been significant ileal and colonic disease caused by previous irradiation and inflammatory bowel disease or there has been loss of the middle and distal ureter. As is discussed later, electrolyte disturbances can occur after incorporation of intestinal segments into the urinary tract; however, these are more common when the jejunum is used for conduit construction. Approximately 40% of patients with jejunal urinary conduits develop hyponatremic, hyperkalemic, hypochloremic metabolic acidosis and azotemia. The jejunum is unable to maintain large solute gradients, so large amounts of water and solute pass through the jejunal wall. Sodium and chloride are rapidly excreted into the conduit, and potassium is passively absorbed. Aldosterone is produced, resulting in reabsorption of hydrogen and excretion of potassium into the distal tubule of the kidney and consequent acidosis and movement of potassium from the body's intracellular stores. As water is lost into the conduit, extracellular fluid volume is reduced, as is the glomerular filtration rate. The renin-angiotensin system is activated, which further stimulates aldosterone secretion. Urea may be absorbed from the jejunal lumen, which (with dehydration) contributes to azotemia.

Colon Conduit

There are several advantages to using the large bowel in construction of urinary conduits: nonrefluxing ureterointestinal anastomoses are easily performed; stomal stenosis is uncommon because of the wide diameter of the large bowel; limited absorption of electrolytes occurs; and the blood supply to the transverse and sigmoid colon is abundant. Either the transverse or the sigmoid colon can be used, allowing for placement of the conduit high or low in the abdomen, depending on the integrity and condition of the ureters. Use of the transverse colon for conduit construction is especially well suited for patients who have received extensive pelvic irradiation or when the middle and distal ureters are absent.

The blood supply of the transverse colon is based on the middle colic artery. The greater omentum is separated from the superior surface of the transverse colon, and a segment of bowel, usually 15 cm in length, is selected for the conduit (Figure 25–2). Short mesenteric incisions are made, and the colon is divided proximally and distally. Once the conduit is isolated, bowel continuity is reestablished. The proximal end of the conduit is closed and fixed in the midline posteriorly. The ureters are brought through small incisions in the posterior peritoneum and reimplanted into the base of the conduit. The stoma may be positioned on either the patient's right or his or her left side.

A sigmoid conduit is constructed in a similar manner. Great care should be taken to preserve the blood supply by carefully selecting a segment with a good blood supply and by making short mesenteric incisions. The conduit is positioned lateral to the reapproximated sigmoid colon. Ureteral reimplantation and stoma construction are completed.

The ureters can be reimplanted into the large intestine either in a way that prevents reflux or by anastomosis directly into the bowel. Ureteral reflux is prevented by constructing a short tunnel (approximately 2–3 cm in length) of bowel mucosa, through which the distal ureter runs. Frequently, this is accomplished by incising the tenia of the large bowel for a distance of 3–4 cm. The incision is carried through the muscular fibers of the bowel wall, sparing the mucosa. A small elliptic segment of mucosa is removed, and a mucosa-to-mucosa anastomosis is performed between the ureter and the mucosa of the bowel. The muscularis of the tenia is reapproximated over the ureter to create the tunnel (Figure 25–3).

CONTINENT URINARY DIVERSION & BLADDER SUBSTITUTION

General Considerations

Various procedures have been developed for construction of bladder substitutes or continent urinary reservoirs that preclude the need for an external urine collection appliance. They offer psychological and functional advantages for selected patients who require urinary diversion. Such reservoirs or bladder substitutes are composed of 3 segments: ureterointestinal (efferent limb) anastomosis, the reservoir itself, and the conduit carrying the urine from the reservoir to the surface (efferent continence mechanism). Bladder substitutes rely on the intact urethra and sphincter to provide outlet resistance and carry urine to the urethral meatus. In men and women

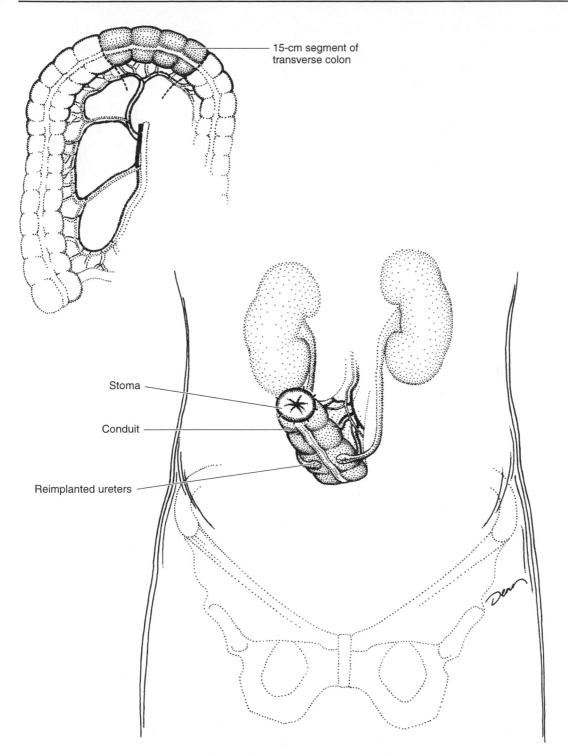

Figure 25–2. Transverse colon conduit.

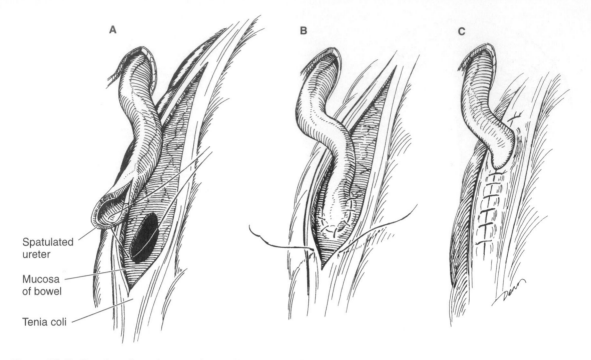

Figure 25–3. Creation of a submucosal tunnel in the wall of the colon to prevent ureteral reflux of urine. **A:** Incision in the tenia coli. **B:** Anastamosis of distal ureter to large intestine mucosa. **C:** Muscularis (tenia) approximated over ureter.

whose urethra has cancer involvement or is not functional owing to benign diseases, an efferent continence mechanism can be constructed with the appendix or short segments of tapered, intussuscepted, or reimplanted intestine.

The decision to proceed with bladder replacement is dependent on the risk of urethral recurrence and the continence of the patient. Both men and women who have low risk of urethral recurrence and who have intact external urinary sphincters should be considered for bladder replacement rather than construction of a continent urinary reservoir. The risk of urethral occurrence or recurrence in men who undergo radical cystectomy is 6.1–10.6%. Men with cancers in the prostate or at the bladder neck are more likely to have urethral disease, either initially or in a delayed fashion. Although prostatic urethral disease is a risk factor for urethral recurrence, recent evidence suggests that orthotopic diversion may be considered in those with only proximal prostatic urethral involvement (Iselin et al, 1997). Urethral recurrence may actually be lower in those who undergo bladder substitution than in those who undergo either conduit urinary diversion or construction of a continent urinary reservoir and have their urethra left in place (Freeman et al, 1996). Although orthotopic bladder replacement was once reserved for men, recent clinical and laboratory experience suggests that it may be an acceptable procedure in women as well (Stein et al, 1997). Women with blad-

der cancer whose cancers are not located at the bladder neck and have a clear urethral margin at the time of cystectomy are candidates for this procedure. Approximately 66% of women undergoing radical cystectomy for the management of bladder cancer fall into this group (Stein et al, 1995, 1998a; Stenzl et al, 1995). Women whose cancers are not located at the bladder neck should be considered for this procedure. Intraoperative inspection and frozen section assessment of the bladder neck limits the risk of urethral recurrence.

Although various segments of the gastrointestinal tract can be used, the principles for success are standard. The bowel segments should be opened and refashioned (detubularized) to interrupt the normal high-pressure contractions of the intact intestine (Hinman, 1988). A large radius is preferred, as this results in a reservoir with a larger geometric capacity and lower pressure. Continent reservoirs and bladder substitutes may be made of small intestine, large intestine, or a combination of both. Recently, there has been intense interest in bladder substitution and continent urinary diversion. It is beyond the scope of this chapter to review all techniques and minor modifications; instead, the most common techniques and the general principles of continent diversion are reviewed.

Ureterosigmoidostomy

The first direct anastomosis of the ureters into the

intact colon was performed by Smith in 1878 (Smith, 1879). Peritonitis (from fecal spillage) and pyelonephritis (resulting from ascending infection and stricturing of the ureteral anastomosis) led initially to very high surgical mortality rates. Recognizing that ascending infection from the rectum into the kidney was a major problem, surgeons developed techniques to prevent pyelonephritis, which became less common when the ureters were reimplanted into the colon in an antirefluxing fashion. Since patients will retain large amounts of urine and fecal material simultaneously in the rectum, assurance of adequate rectal sphincter function is important preoperatively. This can be ensured by instilling large-volume enemas into patients preoperatively and testing rectal continence while they perform normal daily activities. Since ammonia may be absorbed across the bowel surface, patients with liver disease who may be at an increased risk of hyperammonemic encephalopathy should not undergo this procedure. Patients who have primary diseases of the colon or have received extensive pelvic irradiation should undergo alternative forms of diversion.

The ureters are identified at or below the common iliac arteries. The overlying peritoneum is incised and the ureters are mobilized carefully to preserve their blood supply. A site low in the sigmoid is selected for ureteral reimplantation. The ureters are reimplanted separately into the respective ipsilateral tenia coli, using the antirefluxing techniques described earlier. The peritoneum is sutured over the completed ureteral anastomosis (Figure 25–4).

One particularly worrisome complication of ureterosigmoidostomy is development of adenocarcinoma at the site where the ureters have been reimplanted into the large intestine. The incidence of this problem is uncertain, but there seems to be a several thousandfold increase in its incidence in patients who have undergone ureterosigmoidostomy over individuals who have not undergone this type of surgery. The induction period varies but may be approximately 20 years; thus, the risk is especially high in young patients. Experimental studies have shown that the development of adenocarcinoma seems dependent on the presence of urine, feces, urothelium, and colonic epithelium in close approximation. All those who undergo ureterosigmoidostomy should be counseled to undergo yearly sigmoidoscopy starting 5 years after the procedure and at any time occult or gross gastrointestinal bleeding or a major change in bowel habits is noted.

Reservoirs Constructed of Small Intestine

Nils Kock was responsible for the early and ongoing development of a continent urinary reservoir fashioned entirely of small intestine (Kock et al, 1982; Nieh, 1997). Sixty to seventy centimeters of small intestine is selected for reservoir construction. The proximal and distal 15-cm segments are pre-

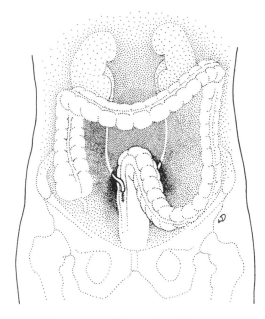

Figure 25–4. Ureterosigmoidostomy.

served for construction of nipple valves, allowing for antireflux ureteroileal anastomoses (inlet) and a continent, catheterizable abdominal stoma (outlet) (Figure 25–5). The middle 40 cm is opened along the antimesenteric border and folded into a U; the back wall is sutured together. The proximal and distal nipple valves are constructed by intussuscepting the bowel, stapling it in place, and further securing it with a mesh anchoring collar. This fixes the intussuscepted bowel segments in place and allows for high-pressure zones, which prevent ureteral reflux proximally and incontinence distally. The reservoir is closed by folding the middle segment and suturing it in place. The ureters are sutured to the proximal nipple valve. The distal nipple valve is brought to the skin as a "flush," catheterizable stoma. Revision of the nipple valve may be necessary in some patients to correct valve slippage or eversion. In men who have an intact urethra and external urinary sphincter, the distal nipple valve can be omitted and the reservoir attached directly to the urethra (Elmajian et al, 1996).

In an attempt to decrease the complication rate associated with the afferent intussuscepted antireflux nipple of the Kock ileal neobladder, Stein and colleagues (1998b) have described an innovative antireflux technique (Figure 25–6). This new reservoir, the T pouch, has several important advantages over the Kock ileal neobladder: (1) It requires a smaller segment of ileum to create the antireflux technique; (2) the serosal-lined antireflux mechanism eliminates the need for intussusception; (3) blood supply is better preserved; and (4) urine is not in contact with the implanted portion of the ileum.

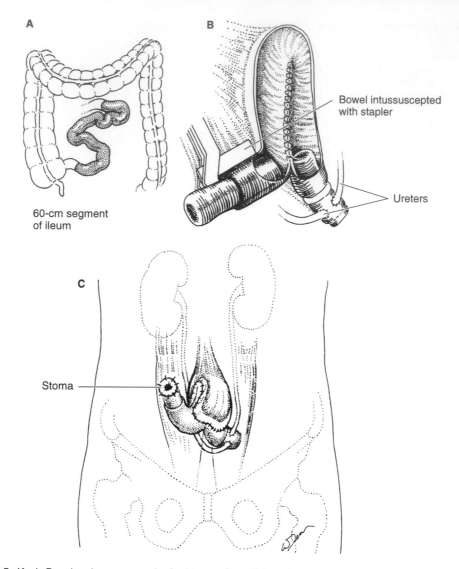

A

60-cm segment
of ileum

B

Bowel intussuscepted
with stapler

Ureters

C

Stoma

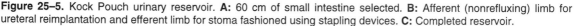

Figure 25–5. Kock Pouch urinary reservoir. **A:** 60 cm of small intestine selected. **B:** Afferent (nonrefluxing) limb for ureteral reimplantation and efferent limb for stoma fashioned using stapling devices. **C:** Completed reservoir.

Camey described a technique of bladder substitution whereby an intact segment of ileum was anastomosed directly to the urethra (Lilien and Camey, 1984). A 40-cm segment of ileum was isolated from the gastrointestinal tract, and its midpoint was anastomosed, without tension, directly to the urethra. The ureters were reimplanted into either end of the ileal segment in an antirefluxing fashion. However, failure to detubularize the ileal segment led to a high incidence of urinary incontinence compared with substitutes fashioned from detubularized small-bowel segments (Studer and Zingg, 1997; Hautmann et al, 1999). Forty- to sixty-centimeter segments of ileum can be detubularized and folded into U-, S-, or W-shaped reservoirs, which can be connected directly to

the urethra (Figure 25–7). The ureters are reimplanted directly into the small bowel wall. They may be reimplanted in a fashion to prevent urinary reflux or in a simple end-to-side fashion. The larger diameter and lower pressure of these reservoirs compared with those of nondetubularized bowel have led to better continence rates.

Reservoirs Constructed of Large Intestine

Various investigators have described using segments of the large intestine alone or combinations of large- and small-bowel segments to fashion urinary reservoirs (Lampel et al, 1996; Bihrle, 1997). Bladder substitutes have been constructed using detubu-

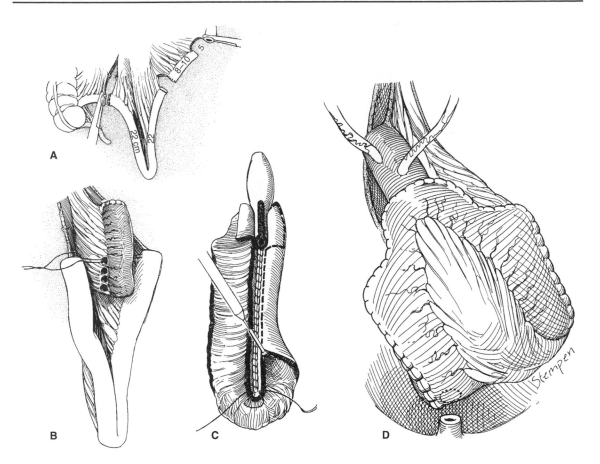

Figure 25–6. Construction of a T pouch. **A:** Two segments of small intestine are isolated; one portion will form the reservoir, and the smaller, more proximal portion will form the antireflux segment. **B:** The longer reservoir portion of the segments is folded into a V. The smaller, antireflux segment is fixed to the serosa of the reservoir portion. **C:** The antireflux segment has been opened and tapered with a stapling device. The ileal segments selected for the reservoir portion of the pouch are joined anteriorly and then opened, exposing the mucosa. As the opening reaches the ostium of the antireflux segment, the incisions are carried laterally and create wide flaps that can then be closed over the ostium to cover the tapered antireflux segment. **D:** The reservoir portion is closed.

larized bowel segments from the ileocecal region or sigmoid colon. Use of the ascending colon and terminal ileum to construct continent urinary reservoirs has gained great popularity. Cecum and ascending colon are detubularized and refashioned or augmented with small intestine to provide for a spheric reservoir. The ureters are reimplanted in a nonrefluxing fashion (Figure 25–8). The reservoir can be anastomosed directly to the urethra. In women or in men who require a urethrectomy, a continent, catheterizable stoma can be fashioned of appendix or tapered terminal ileum (Figure 25–9).

Reservoirs Constructed of Stomach

The stomach may be used for bladder augmentation or substitution. It may have some advantages over intestinal segments: Its muscular elements make ureteral reimplantation easy; it secretes chloride and hydrogen ions and therefore may be especially well suited to those with renal insufficiency; it produces little mucus and may be associated with fewer infections. A wedge of stomach is harvested, and its blood supply is based on one gastroepiploic artery. When the gastric segment is anastomosed to the urethra, a tunnel may be fashioned to increase outlet resistance and aid in continence. Alternatively, a catheterizable stoma may be fashioned of appendix.

After either gastric bladder augmentation or reservoir construction, hematuria and dysuria may result from acid secretion. Treatment with either H_2 blockers or oral alkali may be necessary to buffer urine. Distention of the gastric segment with urine could increase serum gastrin levels. However, hypergastrinemia occurs rarely; furthermore, excluding the antrum in the

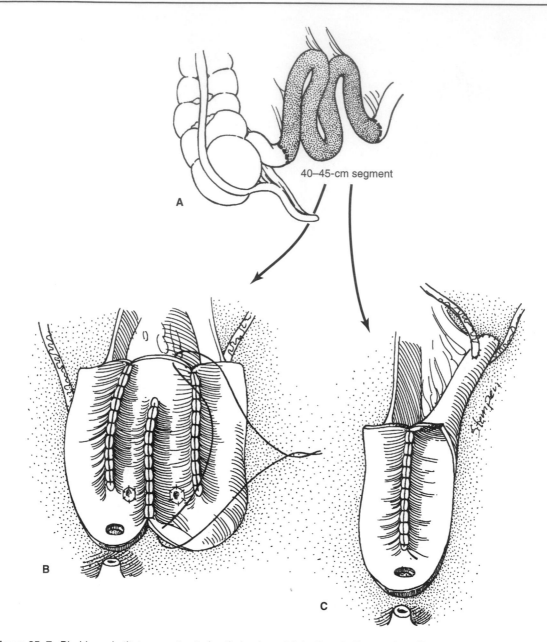

Figure 25–7. Bladder substitutes constructed entirely of small intestine. **A:** Forty to forty-five centimeters of small intestine is selected. **B:** Small intestine is opened and fashioned into a W. The ureters are reimplanted into the second and third limbs of the reservoir, and the reservoir is attached to the urethra. **C:** Small intestine is folded into a J with the most proximal portion of the segment not opened. The ureters are reimplanted into the intact ileal segment of the reservoir, and the reservoir is attached to the urethra.

gastric segment harvested decreases its likelihood further. Theoretically, in the native segment, decreased acid secretion and production of intrinsic factor could lead to protein maldigestion, iron-deficiency anemia, hypocalcemia, and vitamin B_{12} deficiency.

POSTOPERATIVE CARE

Postoperative care varies depending on the method of urinary diversion or bladder substitution. As with all patients who have undergone major abdominal surgery, early ambulation, use of intermittent compression stockings, and incentive spirometry may be

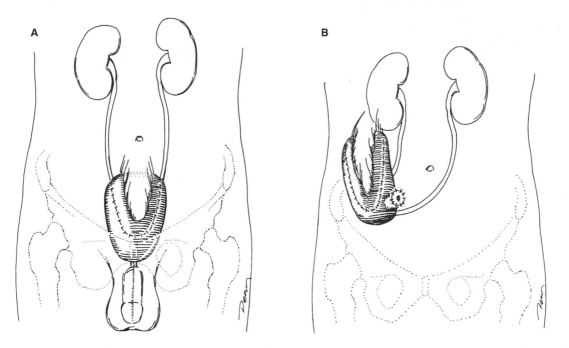

Figure 25–8. Use of the ileocecal segment to construct (**A**) a bladder substitute attached to the urethra or (**B**) a continent urinary reservoir placed in the abdomen using plicated terminal ileum as a stoma.

used to prevent pulmonary emboli or respiratory complications. Nasogastric tubes are left in place until intestinal peristalsis resumes. Serum electrolytes and creatinine should be monitored postoperatively for the development of metabolic abnormalities. If ureteral stents have been placed, they are usually removed sometime after postoperative day 5. Continent urinary reservoirs and bladder substitutes produce much mucus. They should be irrigated regularly in the early postoperative period to prevent mucus accumulation. Mucus production decreases over time, and irrigation ultimately becomes unnecessary. Upper urinary tract surveillance for hydronephrosis should be performed on a regular basis using either ultrasound or intravenous urography. An initial assessment of the upper urinary tract is made in the early postoperative period; if upper urinary tract dilation is not found, the patient undergoes repeat imaging on a yearly basis.

COMPLICATIONS

Complications occurring after urinary diversion, bladder substitution, or continent urinary diversion are generally a product of surgical technique, the underlying disease process and its treatment, the age of the patient, and the length of follow-up (Carlin, Rutchik, and Resnick, 1997; Gburek et al, 1998). Early complications, which are uncommon, include

excessive bleeding, intestinal obstruction, urinary extravasation, and infection. Late complications include metabolic disorders, stomal stenosis, pyelonephritis, and calculi.

Metabolic & Nutritional Disorders

Fluid, electrolyte, nutrient, and waste product excretion or absorption normally occurs across the intestinal wall. The extent of absorption or excretion is dependent on the concentration of these substances in the lumen or blood and on which segment of bowel is in contact with them. Metabolic abnormalities may occur when intestinal segments are interposed into the urinary tract. As pointed out previously, use of the jejunum may result in hyponatremic, hypochloremic, hyperkalemic metabolic acidosis. This syndrome is often characterized clinically by nausea, vomiting, anorexia, and muscle weakness.

The pathogenesis and nature of metabolic abnormalities occurring after incorporation of the ileum or colon into the urinary tract differ from those associated with jejunal conduits. When such segments are used, sodium and chloride are absorbed across the bowel surface. Chloride is absorbed in slight excess of sodium, resulting in a net loss of bicarbonate into the bowel lumen. Preexisting renal failure contributes to the development and severity of the disorder, as does a large bowel surface area and long contact time. Hyperchloremic acidosis is more common in patients who undergo ureterosigmoidostomy than in

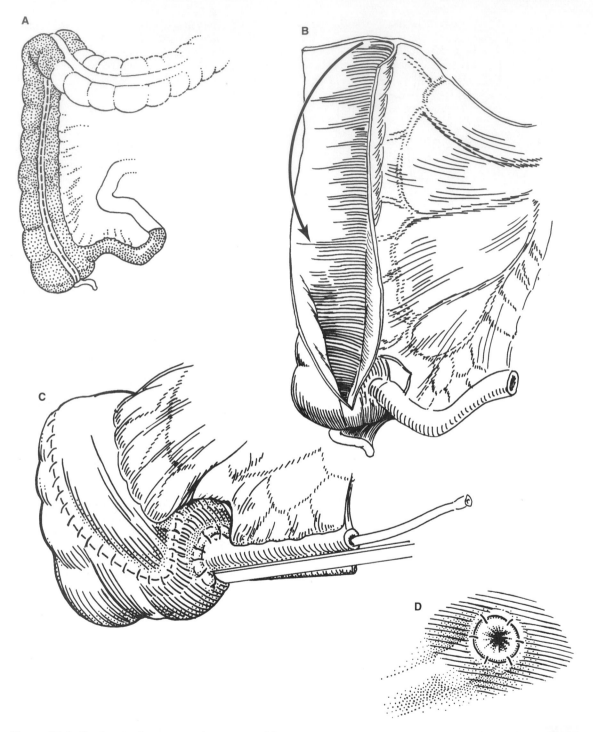

Figure 25–9. Continent urinary reservoir constructed from the ileocecal segment (**A**). **B:** Bowel detubularized. Stoma constructed by tapering the terminal ileum with intestinal stapling instrument (shown in **C**) or sutures. **D:** Completed stoma.

patients who undergo simple conduit construction using either the ileum or the colon, because of the larger surface area and longer contact time with urine associated with ureterosigmoidostomies. Hyperchloremic metabolic acidosis may manifest clinically as weakness, anorexia, vomiting, Kussmaul breathing, and coma. One potential long-term complication of chronic acidosis may be decreased bone calcium content and osteomalacia (McDougal et al, 1988; Kawakita et al, 1996).

Because patients with gastric segments incorporated into the urinary tract may lose both hydrogen and chloride, they are at risk of dehydration and - alkalosis if they suffer either diarrhea or vomiting. The resulting hyponatremic metabolic alkalosis requires treatment with intravenous salt replacement.

Bile salts are important for fat digestion and uptake of vitamins A and D. Bile salt metabolism may be altered after ileal resection (Olofsson et al, 1998). Resection of small segments of the ileum may be associated with mild malabsorption and steatorrhea owing to increased concentrations of bile salts delivered to the colon. The increased concentration of such salts leads to decreased colonic absorption of water and electrolytes. Resection of large segments of ileum may reduce bile salt reabsorption to very low levels, leading to severe fat malabsorption. Bowel transit time may be reduced further by resection of the ileocecal valve. Cholestyramine may be used to treat secretory bile salt diarrhea. If diarrhea persists, addition of agents such as loperamide that decrease bowel motility and increase transit time may be effective. Cholelithiasis may be more common after ileal resections as well.

Vitamin B_{12} deficiency may occur as a result of either gastric or ileal resection (Terai et al, 1997). Because B_{12} stores are likely to last for years, B_{12} deficiency may not become apparent for several years after intestinal surgery. B_{12} deficiency results in megaloblastic anemia and peripheral nerve paresthesias. The levels of this vitamin should be assessed routinely in patients after ileal or gastric resection, and yearly replacement is necessary in those in whom deficiency is noted.

Stoma

A good deal of patients' dissatisfaction with urinary diversion can be attributed to stomal complications. Stoma construction is especially important in procedures in which an appliance must be worn. Careful stomal construction as outlined earlier is essential (Fitzgerald et al, 1997). Stomal complications include stenosis, parastomal hernia formation, and various skin irritations or fungal infections. The likelihood of stomal stenosis increases with time. Stomal stenosis can lead to conduit elongation and upper-tract obstruction. This condition can be diagnosed relatively easily simply by catheterizing the stoma and measuring the residual urine volume. It is corrected by revision of the stoma.

Skin irritation or infections are most common in procedures in which an appliance is worn and there is prolonged contact of the skin with urine. Some patients' skin may be sensitive to adhesive agents.

Stomal or skin problems are minimized when the appliance or faceplate opening is cut to the proper size, preventing irritation of the stomal surface and prolonged skin contact with urine. The treatment of parastomal conditions is summarized in Table 25–1.

The most troublesome stomal complication of external urinary appliances is unexpected pouch leakage. This is often a result of improper application of the appliance but may be caused by poor stomal construction. With a properly constructed and located stoma, the choice of the appliance is relatively simple and is often determined by patient preference. Fac-

Table 25–1. Common peristomal skin problems and their management.[1]

Problem	Cause	Management
Fungal infections— *Candida albicans* (*Monilia*)	Urine accumulating under barrier (seen more frequently with diabetes mellitus and concurrent antibiotic use)	• Apply nystatin (Mycostatin) powder • Dry skin thoroughly (use hair dryer) • Prevent leakage under water
Allergic contact dermatitis	Sensitivity to solvents, adhesives, detergents, wafers	• Identify irritant (skin patch test) and discontinue product • Apply hydrocortisone cream (avoid prolonged use) • Avoid solvents and soaps
Mechanical trauma	• Frequent or excessive pouch changing leading to skin stripping • Pressure from belts • Overuse of adhesive strips around the faceplate of barrier	• Minimize pouch changes • Encourage gentle skin care • Consider nonadhesive pouches (used with belt) • Minimize use of sealants and adhesives
Pseudoverrucous skin lesions	• Urine contact with skin over extended time	• Ensure that the barrier and pouch are the correct size

[1]The patient should see an enterostomal therapist nurse, if available.

tors that must be taken into account when selecting an appliance include patient dexterity and preference, available resources, and stomal construction. Appliances constitute an adhesive skin barrier that attaches to the skin and a pouch that collects urine. An opening is made in the middle of the skin barrier; this opening should be of a diameter just larger than the stoma to avoid erosion of the stoma or prolonged contact of the skin with urine.

Most patients favor using disposable urinary collection appliances, although reusable ones are available. Disposable, one-piece pouches are used once. Two-piece systems allow the patient to remove the pouch, leaving the skin barrier intact. Reusable appliances are composed of a rigid or semirigid faceplate secured to the skin with adhesive. A vinyl or rubber pouch is attached to the faceplate using an O ring. These pouches are reusable and last 1 or 6 months depending on whether they are composed of vinyl or rubber, respectively. A larger collection device is often attached to the pouch at night.

Pyelonephritis & Renal Deterioration

Pyelonephritis occurs in approximately 10% of patients who have undergone urinary diversion. Treatment is based on a properly collected urine sample for culture. A urine sample should not be collected from the pouch; rather, the pouch should be removed, the stoma cleansed with an antiseptic, and a catheter advanced gently through the stoma. To minimize contamination from the stoma itself, an open-ended, large-lumen catheter can first be advanced into the conduit. A smaller lumen catheter can then be advanced through the first catheter to collect the sample. If infection has occurred in a patient with a simple conduit, the volume of residual urine within the conduit should be recorded. Obstruction and stasis of urine within the reconstructed urinary tract are risk factors for the development of infection.

Although many patients with preexisting dilation of the upper urinary tract show improvement or resolution of the dilation after urinary diversion or bladder substitution, progressive renal deterioration as manifested by hydronephrosis or deterioration in glomerular filtration rate (or both) occurs in a certain percentage of patients who undergo these procedures.

The incidence of either complication increases after 10 years. Pyelographic evidence of upper urinary tract deterioration has been noted in up to 50% of patients who have undergone urinary diversion at an early age. Recurrent upper urinary tract infection and high-pressure ureteral reflux and obstruction, usually in combination, contribute to the likelihood of renal deterioration.

Calculi

Calculi occur in approximately 8% of patients who undergo urinary diversion or bladder substitution (Cohen and Streem 1994; Terai et al, 1996). Such patients have several risk factors for the development of various calculi. Nonabsorbable staples, mesh, or suture material used to construct conduits or reservoirs may act as a nidus for stone formation. Colonization in either conduits or reservoirs is common, whereas symptomatic infection is much rarer. Certain bacteria can contribute to stone formation; some bacteria commonly found in the urinary tract, including *Proteus, Klebsiella,* and *Pseudomonas* species, produce urease, a urea-splitting enzyme that contributes to the formation of ammonia and carbon dioxide. Hydrolysis of these products results in an alkaline urine supersaturated with magnesium ammonium phosphate, calcium phosphate, and carbonate apatite crystals. Management of such infection-related stones requires stone removal, resolution of infection, and, often, use of adjunctive agents to complete stone dissolution.

The likelihood of stone formation is increased by the development of systemic acidosis, as described previously (Terai et al, 1995). Prolonged contact of the urine with the intestinal surface facilitates the exchange of chloride for bicarbonate. Bicarbonate loss results in systemic acidosis and hypercalciuria. The combination of hypercalciuria and an alkaline urine predisposes a patient to the development of calcium calculi. In addition, the terminal ileum is responsible for bile salt absorption; if this portion of the intestine is used for conduit or bladder reservoir construction, excess bile salts in the intestine may bind calcium and result in increased absorption of oxalate, which may lead to the development of oxalate-containing calculi. Excess conduit length, urine stasis, and dehydration make the development of calculi more likely.

REFERENCES

GENERAL

Carlin BI, Rutchik SD, Resnick MI: Comparison of the ileal conduit to the continent cutaneous diversion and orthotopic neobladder in patients undergoing cystectomy: A critical analysis and review of the literature. Semin Urol Oncol 1997;15:189.

Fitzgerald J et al: Stomal construction, complications, and reconstruction. Urol Clin North Am 1997;24:729.

Goldwasser B, Webster GD: Continent urinary diversion. J Urol 1985;134:227.

King LR, Stone AR, Webster GD (editors): *Bladder Reconstruction and Continent Urinary Diversion.* Year Book, 1987.

Okada Y et al: Quality of life survey of urinary diversion patients: Comparison of continent urinary diversion versus ileal conduit. Int J Urol 1997;4:26.

ILEAL CONDUIT

Bricker EM: Bladder substitution after pelvic evisceration. Surg Clin North Am 1950;30:1511.

Pitts WR, Muecke EC: A 20 year experience with ileal conduit: The fate of the kidneys. J Urol 1979;122:154.

Remigailo RV et al: Ileal conduit urinary diversion: Ten-year review. Urology 1976;7:343.

Schmidt JD et al: Complications, results and problems of ileal diversions. J Urol 1973;109:210.

Schwarz GR, Jeffs RD: Ileal conduit urinary diversion in children: Computer analysis of followup from 2 to 16 years. J Urol 1975;114:285.

Shapiro SR, Lebowitz R, Colodny AH: Fate of 90 children with ileal conduit urinary diversion a decade later. J Urol 1975;114:289.

Sullivan JW, Grabstald H, Whitmore WF: Complications of ureteroileal conduit with radical cystectomy: Review of 336 cases. J Urol 1980;124:797.

JEJUNAL CONDUIT

Golimbu M, Morales P: Jejunal conduits: Technique and complications. J Urol 1975;113:787.

COLON CONDUITS

Beckley S et al: Transverse colon conduit: A method of urinary diversion after pelvic irradiation. J Urol 1982;128:464.

Richie J, Skinner DG: Urinary diversion: The physiological rationale for nonrefluxing colonic conduits. Br J Urol 1975;47:269.

Richie JP: Sigmoid conduit urinary diversion. Urol Clin North Am 1986;13:225.

Schmidt JA, Hawtry CE, Buschbaum HJ: Transverse colon conduit: A preferred method of urinary diversion for radiation-treated pelvic malignancies. J Urol 1975;113:08.

Wilbert DM, Hohenfellner R: Colonic conduit: Preoperative requirements, operative technique, postoperative management. World J Urol 1984;2:159.

BLADDER SUBSTITUTION & CONTINENT URINARY DIVERSION

Bihrle R: The Indiana Pouch continent urinary reservoir. Urol Clin North Am 1997;24:773.

Carroll PR et al: Functional characteristics of the continent ileocecal urinary reservoir: Mechanisms of urinary continence. J Urol 1989;142:1032.

Elmajian D et al: The Kock ileal neobladder: Updated experience in 295 male patients. J Urol 1996;156:920.

Freeman JA et al: Urethral recurrence in patients with orthotopic ileal neobladders. J Urol 1996;156:1615.

Gilchrist RK, Merichs JW: Construction of a substitute bladder and urethra. Surg Clin North Am 1956;36:131.

Hautmann R et al: The ileal neobladder: Complications and functional results in 363 patients after 11 years of followup. J Urol 1999;161:422.

Hinman F Jr: Selection of intestinal segments for bladder substitution: Physical and physiological characteristics. J Urol 1988;139:519.

Iselin C et al: Does prostate transitional cell carcinoma preclude orthotopic bladder reconstruction after radical cystoprostatectomy for bladder cancer? J Urol 1997;158:2123.

Kock NG et al: Urinary diversion via a continent ileal reservoir: Clinical results in 12 patients. J Urol 1982;128:469.

Lampel A et al: Continent diversion with the Mainz pouch. World J Urol 1996;14:85.

Lilien OM, Camey M: 25-year experience with replacement of the human bladder (Camey procedure). J Urol 1984;132:886.

Nieh P: The Kock Pouch urinary reservoir. Urol Clin North Am 1997;24:755.

Rowland RG et al: Indiana continent urinary reservoir. J Urol 1987;137:1136.

Skinner DG, Lieskovsky G, Boyd S: Continent urinary diversion. J Urol 1989;141:1323.

Stein JP et al: Indications for lower urinary tract reconstruction in women after cystectomy for bladder cancer: A pathological review of female cystectomy specimens [see comments]. J Urol 1995;154:1329.

Stein J et al: Orthoptic lower urinary tract reconstruction in women using the Kock ileal neobladder: Updated experience in 34 patients. J Urol 1997;158:400.

Stein J et al: Prospective pathologic analysis of female cystectomy specimens: Risk factors for orthotopic diversion in women. Urology 1998a;51:951.

Stein J et al: The T Pouch: An orthotopic ileal neobladder incorporating a serosal lined ileal antireflux technique. J Urol 1998b;159:1836.

Stenzl A et al: The risk of urethral tumors in female bladder cancer: Can the urethra be used for orthotopic reconstruction of the lower urinary tract? J Urol 1995;153(3 Pt 2):950.

Studer U, Zingg E: Ileal orthotopic bladder substitutes. Urol Clin North Am 1997;24:781.

URETEROSIGMOIDOSTOMY

Bristol JB, Williamson RCN: Ureterosigmoidostomy and colon carcinogenesis. Science 1981;214:851.

Crissey MM, Steele GD, Gittes RF: Rat model for carcinogenesis in ureterosigmoidostomy. Science 1980; 207:1079.

Gittes RF: Carcinogenesis in ureterosigmoidostomy. Urol Clin North Am 1986;13:201.

Hinman F, Weyrauch HM Jr: A critical study of the different principles of surgery which have been used in uretero-intestinal implantation. Trans Am Assoc Genitourin Surg 1936;9:15.

Leadbetter WF, Clarke BG: Five years' experience with uretero-enterostomy by the "combined" technique. J Urol 1955;3:67.

Smith T: An account of an unsuccessful attempt to treat extroversion of the bladder by a new operation. St Barth Hosp Rep 1879;15:29.

Spirnak JP, Caldamone AA: Ureterosigmoidostomy. Urol Clin North Am 1986;13:285.

GASTRIC BLADDER

Nguyen DH, Mitchell, ME: Gastric bladder reconstruction. Urol Clin North Am 1991;18:649.

COMPLICATIONS

Bloom DA, Grossman HB, Konnak JW: Stomal construction and reconstruction. Urol Clin North Am 1986;13:275.

Carlin BI, Rutchik SD, Resnick MI: Comparison of the ileal conduit to the continent cutaneous diversion and orthotopic neobladder in patients undergoing cystectomy: A critical analysis and review of the literature. Semin Urol Oncol 1997;15:189.

Cohen T, Streem S: Minimally invasive endourologic management of calculi in continent urinary reservoirs. Urology 1994;43:865.

Dretler SP: The pathogenesis of urinary tract calculi occurring after ileal conduit diversion: 1. Clinical study. 2. Conduit study. 3. Prevention. J Urol 1973;109:204.

Filmer RB, Spencer JR: Malignancies in bladder augmentation and intestinal conduits. J Urol 1990;143:671.

Gburek B et al: Comparison of Studer ileal neobladder and ileal conduit urinary diversion with respect to perioperative outcome and late complications. J Urol 1998;160:721.

Hall MC, Koch MO, McDougal WS: Metabolic consequences of urinary diversion through intestinal segments. Urol Clin North Am 1991;18:25.

Kawakita M et al: Bone demineralization following urinary intestinal diversion assessed by urinary pyridium cross-links and dual energy x-ray absorptiometry. J Urol 1996;156:355.

Koch MO, McDougal WS: The pathophysiology of hy-

perchloremic metabolic acidosis after urinary diversion through intestinal segments. Surgery 1985;98:561.

Kosko JW, Kursh ED, Resnick MI: Metabolic complications of urologic intestinal substitutes. Urol Clin North Am 1986;13:193.

Madsen PO: The etiology of hyperchloremic acidosis following ureterointestinal anastomosis: An experimental study. J Urol 1964;92:448.

McDougal WS et al: Boney demineralization following intestinal diversion. J Urol 1988;140:853.

Olofsson G et al: Bile acid malabsorption after continent urinary diversion with an ileal reservoir. J Urol 1998;160:724.

Stamey TA: The pathogenesis and implications of the electrolyte imbalance in ureterosigmoidostomy. Surg Gynecol Obstet 1956;103:736.

Stein R et al: Long-term metabolic effects in patients with urinary diversion. World J Urol 1998;16:292.

Steiner MS, Morton RA: Nutritional and gastrointestinal complications of the use of bowel segments in the lower urinary tract. Urol Clin North Am 1991;18:725.

Tanagho EA: A case against incorporation of bowel into the closed urinary system. J Urol 1975;113:796.

Terai A et al: Effect of urinary intestinal diversion on urinary risk factors for urolithiasis. J Urol 1995;153:37.

Terai A et al: Urinary calculi as a late complication of the Indiana continent urinary diversion: Comparison with the Kock pouch procedure. J Urol 1996;155:66.

Terai A et al: Vitamin B12 deficiency in patients with urinary intestinal diversion. Int J Urol 1997;4:21.

OSTOMY CARE

Borglund E, Nordstrom G, Nyman CR: Classification of peristomal skin changes in patients with urostomy. J Am Acad Dermatol 1988;19:623.

Fitzgerald J et al: Stomal construction, complications, and reconstruction. Urol Clin North Am 1997;24:729.

Johnson DE, Smith DB: Urinary diversions. In: Smith DB, Johnson DE (editors): *Ostomy Care and the Cancer Patient: Surgical and Clinical Considerations.* Grune & Stratton, 1986.

Maidl L: Stomal and peristomal skin complications with urostomies. Urol Nurs 1990;10:17.

Nordstrom GM, Borglund E, Nyman CR: Local status of the urinary stoma: The relationship to peristomal skin complications. Scand J Urol Nephrol 1990;24:117.

Tucker SB, Smith DB: Dermatologic conditions complicating ostomy care. In: Smith DB, Johnson DE (editors): *Ostomy Care and the Cancer Patient: Surgical and Clinical Considerations.* Grune & Stratton, 1986.

Urologic Laser Surgery

26

J. Stuart Wolf, Jr., MD

Despite Einstein's elucidation of the concept of stimulated emission of radiation in 1917, the first functional laser was not created until 1960. Lasers first were used in urology in the late 1960s. Since then, there has been progressive development of urologic laser applications.

In this chapter I start by reviewing the principles of laser therapy, including the basic physics of laser function and laser-tissue interactions. Next, I outline safety aspects of the laser. Finally, I describe lasers currently used in urology and the various urologic applications of laser therapy.

PRINCIPLES OF LASER THERAPY

Basic Laser Physics

The acronym laser stands for light amplification by stimulated emission of radiation. The outermost electrons of most atoms are in the resting state (E_0). By the addition of external energy, the electrons can be raised to the next higher energy level (E_1) and, with increasing amounts of energy, to even higher states (E_n). When the electron spontaneously returns to its resting level (E_0), the atom emits a photon with energy and wavelength that is characteristic of the emitting atom. Stimulated emission occurs when one of the emitted photons strikes another atom that is already at a higher energy state. The first photon continues on, and the second atom releases an additional photon that has the same wavelength, is in the same phase, and travels in the same direction as the first photon (Figure 26–1). These processes occur in the active medium of the laser. The active medium may be gas (eg, carbon dioxide), liquid (eg, coumarin dye), solid (eg, neodymium ions in Nd:YAG), or a semiconductor, as in diode lasers. The active medium is contained space within the laser resonator. In its simplest form, a laser resonator consists of two parallel mirrors. One is completely reflective and the other transmits a variable amount of the laser light, reflecting the rest back into the laser resonator. Reflection by the mirrors produces rapid buildup of energy as the photons travel back and forth in parallel within

the laser resonator and continue to participate in stimulated emissions (Figure 26–2).

The initiating energy pumped into the active medium may be optical, chemical, or electrical. For many medical lasers, electricity is converted to optical energy with a bright light, which then stimulates the active medium. Lasers operate in continuous or pulsed mode. In continuous mode, the initiating energy is continually pumped into the active medium, and a fraction of the stimulated emissions is continually released from the laser resonator. Pulsing can be achieved by one of two mechanisms. In flashlamp pulsed lasers, noncoherent light from an arc source is briefly pulsed into the active medium to produce the pulses of laser light. In a Q-switched laser, energy is continually pumped into an active medium but is released only intermittently by means of a series of rotating mirrors or switches in the laser resonator. Q-switching can produce pulses with extremely high peak power.

Once the laser light is generated by the laser resonator, the final step in the process is transmission of the laser beam to the target. For lasers such as the CO_2 laser, which cannot be transmitted through quartz fibers, a series of reflective mirrors on an articulated arm are used to deliver the energy. Laser light with wavelengths of 400–2900 nm can be transmitted through a quartz glass fiber. Laser energy is conducted through the optical fiber by internal reflection. As long as the laser fiber is not bent beyond a certain radius of curvature, photons striking the side walls of the fiber are internally reflected and continue on down through the fiber. If the fiber is bent excessively, laser energy will no longer strike the fiber wall at the critical angle and will escape. Because of these internal reflections and other optical properties, the laser beam exiting the fiber diverges slightly (ie, photons are not traveling exactly in parallel). For a perfectly maintained 600-µm fiber, the angle of divergence is about 17 degrees. Laser energy can be further concentrated by using a contact tip. This tip at the end of a laser fiber concentrates the energy at the end of the instrument. A somewhat opaque coating provides the tip with variable ability

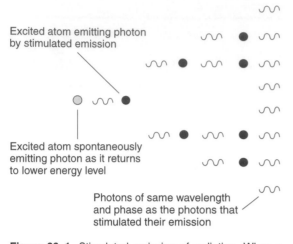

Figure 26–1. Stimulated emission of radiation. When a photon released by the spontaneous decay of an atom from an excited state to a lower energy state strikes another excited atom, an additional photon is released (stimulated emission). This second photon has the same wavelength and phase as the first and travels with it in parallel. Cascades of stimulated emission occur in a laser resonator to produce a laser beam.

to absorb the laser energy, so that extreme heating of the tip can be mixed with a degree of transmission of the laser beam beyond the tip.

Laser Characteristics

As opposed to the light from an incandescent bulb, laser light is monochromatic (same wavelength), coherent (all waves traveling in phase), and nondivergent (always in parallel). Optical principles dictate

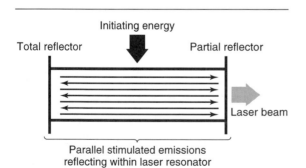

Figure 26–2. Simplified laser resonator. One of the parallel mirrors is completely reflective and the other transmits a variable amount of the laser light, reflecting the rest back into the laser resonator. Reflection by the mirrors produces rapid buildup of energy as the photons travel back and forth in parallel within the laser resonator and continue to participate in stimulated emissions.

that a laser beam always has some small degree of actual divergence, which varies with the laser wavelength and size of the exit aperture from the laser resonator. The power of a laser is expressed in watts (W), and the energy is measured in joules (J). A laser with the power of 1 W operated for 1 s delivers 1 J of energy. The power density of the laser beam is expressed in watts per square centimeter, where square centimeter is the area of the beam at the target surface. Laser power density thus varies with the inverse of the square of the radius of the spot size (assuming application to the target in a perfect circle). Since the laser beam exiting a quartz fiber is slightly divergent, the spot size increases as the fiber tip is pulled away from the target. Spot size is therefore dependent on the shape, size, and divergence of the laser beam as it exits the fiber; the laser incident angle and the surface geometry of the target; and the distance of the fiber tip from the target. These geometric relationships are important when considering the clinical effect of "free-beam" laser application.

Laser-Tissue Interactions

Laser light encountering tissue can undergo reflection, scattering, transmission, or absorption. Only the absorbed photons participate in the therapeutic effect of the laser. The primary effect of most medical lasers is photothermal (Figure 26–3). The absorbed photons raise the temperature of the absorbing substance. At temperatures above 45 °C, enzyme damage occurs and the integrity of cell membranes is challenged. Some proteins may begin to denature with long exposure, but protein denaturation and coagulation predominantly occur with temperatures above 60 °C. Once the temperature reaches 100 °C, tissue water boils off, producing cell rupture, dehydration, and tissue shrinkage. Once all of the water in a target tissue has been vaporized, the temperature begins to climb again. Above approximately 150 °C, carbonization occurs. The black, carbonized material is a universal photon absorber, so there is a sharp increase in temperature leading to complete vaporization of tissue if laser exposure is continued. The depth of penetration of a laser beam is that distance in tissue through which the laser deposits 90% of its initial energy. The depth of penetration is determined by both laser and tissue characteristics.

The primary laser characteristic affecting laser-tissue interactions is the wavelength of the laser photons. Laser energy of different wavelengths is absorbed variably by different materials. Pulse width and interval are also important, in that a pulse with a short width (duration "on") and a long interval between pulses might allow the tissue to cool down before the next pulse arrives (depending on the thermal relaxation time of the tissue). The final parameter of importance is power density, which is controlled by spot size when the other operational parameters of the laser are held constant.

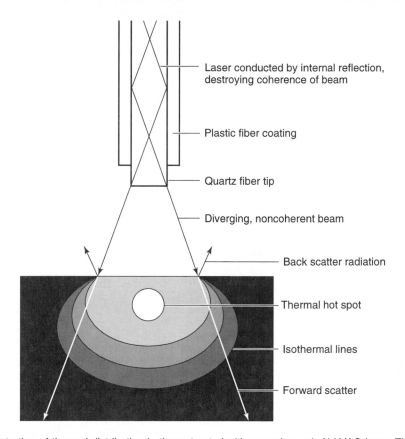

Figure 26–3. Illustration of thermal distribution in tissue treated with an endoscopic Nd:YAG laser. The beam diverges as it exits the fiber tip. Maximum heating is somewhat below the tissue surface because some surface heat is lost to the irrigating fluid. Photons not absorbed at the spot of application continue on to create photothermal effects that decrease in magnitude with increasing distance from the irradiated spot. The exact distribution of the thermal effect primarily depends on the power density and the effect achieved at the laser application spot. If surface carbonization occurs then much of the energy is absorbed by the carbonized fragments. Less energy passes deeper into the tissue than it would if only coagulation had occurred at the site of maximum power density. (Modified and reproduced, with permission, from Marchesini R et al: Lasers Surg Med 1985;5:75 and Halldorsson TH et al: Lasers Surg Med 1981;1:253.)

The tissue is critical in laser-tissue interactions because various tissues have different absorption coefficients for photons of different wavelengths. Important tissue characteristics in this regard include color, hemoglobin content, and chemical composition. In addition, increased circulation or use of fluid irrigation may carry thermal energy away from the site of laser application, thereby reducing tissue heating. Insight into the choice of laser for a given use is provided in Figure 26–4, which illustrates the relationship of laser wavelength to absorption by hemoglobin and water. A laser such as Nd:YAG, with a wavelength of 1064 nm, is poorly absorbed by both water and hemoglobin and affects primarily protein. The depth of penetration of the Nd:YAG laser is 3–5 mm. If low powers are used, then the primary effect is coagulation, because the high temperatures necessary for water vaporization are not achieved. The potassium titanyl phosphate

(KTP) laser, whose wavelength of 532 nm is absorbed well by hemoglobin but not by water, penetrates deeply (like the Nd:YAG) in white, poorly vascularized tissue but is absorbed closer to the surface in pigmented, stained, or well-vascularized tissue. The addition of exogenous chromophores (agents that impart color to the tissue) can also selectively increase a tissue's absorption of laser energy.

Even a laser wavelength that is poorly absorbed by a certain tissue can create vaporization if sufficient power density is applied. For example, the Nd:YAG laser, if applied directly to tissue with a small spot size, will impart enough energy to boil tissue water. If carbonization occurs, absorption is almost complete and high temperatures with a marked increase in the degree of vaporization can be achieved. Power density is altered by both the power of the laser beam and the spot size. During clinical use with the laser

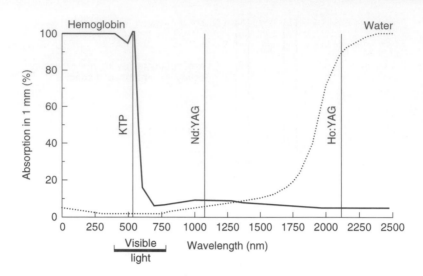

Figure 26–4. Relationship of laser wavelength to absorption by hemoglobin and water. KTP = potassium titanyl phosphate. (Modified with permission from Stein BS, Kendall AR: Urology 1984;23:405.)

set to constant power output, the physician can immediately alter the effects of the laser on tissue by changing the spot size, with a smaller spot size (ie, closer to the tissue) tending more toward tissue vaporization and a larger spot size (ie, farther away from tissue) tending toward coagulation.

Laser-tissue interactions also can be characterized by nonthermal processes. The process most familiar to a urologist is that of photoacoustic disruption. When a laser lithotripsy device such as the pulsed dye laser is applied to a calculus, the energy is absorbed by the stone surface to create high temperatures, which induce formation of a plasma bubble. When this bubble collapses, shock waves are produced that result in stone fragmentation. Photoablation occurs when narrow laser beams with extremely high power density directly break down the chemical bonds in tissue without significantly increasing temperature. Finally, photochemical processes involve the activation of chemical species such as hematoporphyrin derivatives (a photosensitizer for tumor treatment).

LASER SAFETY

Potential Dangers

The eye is especially susceptible to laser injury because even minor trauma to the optical surfaces of the eye can create significant morbidity, and also because the lens of the eye may focus laser light on the retina (Table 26–1). The eyes of all health care personnel in the room, as well of the patient, are at risk during a laser procedure and constitute the primary reason for consideration of laser safety. Exposed skin and organs in the operating room also are at risk. Because of its

photothermal effect, laser energy can produce combustion if inflammable materials are near the operative site. Additionally, the laser plume that is created during such procedures as ablation of condylomata with the CO_2 laser may contain viral particles that can be infectious to health care personnel.

Laser Equipment

Lasers that operate in a low power range, such as the diode laser used for the common laser pointer, producing a 610- to 650-nm-wavelength red beam with a power of 2–5 mW, may not require any safety precautions since the normal reflex mechanism to close one's eyes is sufficient to prevent injury. Most medical lasers, however, are of high enough power that additional precautions need to be taken. In high-powered lasers a visible or audible alert is required when the laser is activated. A laser device operating at a wavelength out of the visible range should contain a low-power aiming beam of visible light (eg, a diode laser, helium-neon gas laser, or incandescent light) so that the laser can be exactly targeted before the laser beam is activated. The laser unit itself should also have a key-operated switch and should be operated only by trained personnel.

Adjunctive Equipment

Protective eyewear must be worn by all persons present in the controlled laser area. For practical purposes, the laser area includes the entire operating room during laser surgery. The lenses of the protective eyewear should transmit as much visible light as possible. For lasers, such as the KTP laser, that operate in visible light range, this requires an optical coating that blocks out a narrow range of wave-

Table 26–1. Ocular effects of lasers.

Range	Wavelength	Activity	Tissue Injury
Ultraviolet	< 380 nm	Absorbed by lens or cornea	Cataracts or photokeratitis
Visible	380–780 nm	Penetrates to retina	Chemical or thermal damage
Infrared A	780–1400 nm	Penetrates to retina	Thermal damage
Infrared B	1400–3000 nm	Absorbed by lens	Cataracts
Infrared C	> 3000 nm	Absorbed by cornea	Photokeratitis

lengths. Laser protective eyewear is less problematic visually for lasers operating in the nonvisible light range. The windows of the operating room where the laser is being used are covered, the doors to the room are closed, and clear signs indicating that a laser is in use are posted. Extra laser glasses should be placed next to the warning sign for personnel entering the room. In operative cases where a laser plume containing particles might be produced, a plume evacuator should be on the operative field. As much as possible, equipment used at the operative site should have a dark matte finish with curved surfaces. This will minimize the possibility of reflection of laser light that might occur with flat or shiny surfaces.

Organizational Measures

A laser safety officer or committee is responsible for overseeing training and other safety issues for medical lasers in the hospital. Physicians utilizing the laser must document training for each specific laser wavelength that they use. The technician or other staff member operating the laser unit also must undergo training. A laser log should be maintained, and all laser devices should have regular maintenance and safety checks.

CLINICAL LASERS IN UROLOGY

Carbon Dioxide (CO$_2$) Laser

The CO$_2$ laser beam has a 10,600-nm wavelength (infrared) and is delivered in continuous mode. This wavelength is strongly absorbed by water and other cell components. The depth of penetration in all tissues is 0.1 mm or less. Because the CO$_2$ wavelength cannot be transmitted through quartz glass fibers, the energy must be delivered by a series of mirrors on an articulating arm, which precludes endoscopic use with current instruments. With the high degree of absorption of CO$_2$ laser energy at the tissue surface, virtually instant vaporization is produced, below which there is only a narrow zone of thermal coagulation. Soft tissue vaporization is the primary application of the CO$_2$ laser. A laser plume is generated by rapid vaporization, so an assistant should maintain suction near the operative site with a plume evacuator to prevent airborne transmission of infectious particles.

Nd:YAG Laser

The continuous-mode Nd:YAG laser, operating at a wavelength of 1064 nm, is poorly absorbed by both water and hemoglobin, so that the depth of penetration is 3–5 mm. Although tissue vaporization can be achieved through the use of high power density, the primary use for the Nd:YAG laser is tissue coagulation. The coagulated tissue provides excellent hemostasis, and the tissue is resorbed gradually over the course of weeks to months.

KTP Laser

The KTP laser is also known as the frequency-doubled Nd:YAG, since it utilizes a KTP crystal to double the frequency of a Nd:YAG laser. This produces a visible green light with a wavelength of 532 nm. Laser energy at this wavelength is absorbed well by hemoglobin, but not by water, so a KTP laser can be used effectively for tissue ablation during endoscopic procedures.

Argon Laser

The beam from an argon gas laser contains several wavelengths between 488 and 514 nm (visible blue-green light). The energy is absorbed by hemoglobin and the depth of penetration in pigmented tissue is 1–2 mm (similar to the KTP laser). Because the argon laser is limited in its power output, urologic use is restricted to small strictures or bladder tumors.

Tunable Pulsed Dye Laser

Dye lasers are tunable because the type of dye can be changed to produce a different wavelength in the active medium, or a prism placed within a laser resonator containing a dye that produces a broad spectral band with excitation can be turned so that only selected wavelengths are reflected along the axis of the laser resonator. The pulses of the tunable pulsed dye laser are produced by flashing intense light into the active medium (flashlamp). A laser of this type that is familiar to urologists uses coumarin green dye as the active media laser, which produces a visible green beam of 504-nm wavelength. The coumarin pulsed dye laser has widespread application for laser lithotripsy. A variety of rhodamine dyes also have been used as the active media in pulsed dye lasers for lithotripsy.

Energy at the 504-nm wavelength produced by the coumarin pulsed dye laser is absorbed by most urinary calculi, but it falls in between the major absorption bands of hemoglobin. Pulsed dye laser lithotripsy is performed with devices that produce pulses of 0.5–2 ms duration, with an energy of 50–140 mJ per pulse. The frequency of pulses is varied between 1 and 20 Hz (1–20 times per s). Because of the short pulse duration and because the energy is not well absorbed by hemoglobin, significant thermal damage to the urothelium does not occur during lithotripsy. The critical temperature to achieve tissue coagulation is not achieved during a single pulse, and the interval allows dissipation of the thermal effects before the next pulse. When the energy is absorbed by an appropriately colored stone surface, however, a laser plasma is created and the calculi are fragmented by the subsequent shock waves. Cystine calculi do not absorb this laser wavelength well, although the addition of colored dyes to the irrigating fluid can be used to enhance the formation of the plasma bubble in such cases. Additionally, hard stones such as calcium oxalate monohydrate may not fragment well. Nonetheless, the safety of the pulsed dye laser is an important advantage of this device over many other intracorporeal lithotriptors.

The pulsed dye laser can be fitted with an automatic stone-detection device. If the laser beam is absorbed by a stone, there is both an acoustic effect (the shock wave) and production by the laser-induced plasma of optical energy of characteristic wavelengths. Detectors are fitted to the laser lithotripsy device, so that operation of the dye laser is continued only if both the acoustic and plasma signals are detected. If the appropriate feedback is not received, the laser pulse is truncated. This process is already being used for lithotripsy of biliary stones, and further work in this area might eventually produce an instrument that allows blind (without the need for ureteroscopic visualization) intracorporeal destruction of urinary calculi.

Alexandrite Laser

With a wavelength of 755 nm (visible red light), an energy output of 30–80 mJ, and pulse duration of 150–800 ns, lithotripsy with the alexandrite pulsed laser is achieved with a plasma-induced shock wave as with the pulsed dye laser. The alexandrite laser is generally more effective on darker stones because of poor absorption of photons at this wavelength by pale stones. It is also a fairly safe laser, but fiber problems limit the power and reduce the efficacy of the alexandrite laser for lithotripsy.

Q-Switched Nd:YAG laser

Pulsing of the Q-switched Nd:YAG laser is achieved through Q-switching. The device theoretically can fragment all stones through a photoacoustic effect that is not dependent on color. With the initial Q-switched Nd:YAG device, high powers could not be delivered without damaging the fiber tip. Specially designed fibers or the use of additives to the irrigation fluid have improved the situation, but failures are still noted with hard calculi, as with the pulsed dye laser. Optomechanical couplers also can be used to generate shock waves at the fiber tip, but they are unwieldy.

Ho:YAG Laser

In the Ho:YAG laser the YAG crystal is doped with holmium atoms rather than with neodymium. The Ho:YAG laser delivers a wavelength of 2100 nm (infrared) in pulsed mode. Because of the high absorption of this wavelength by water, its use in a fluid environment requires that the tip of the fiber be placed in contact mode. The penetration depth in tissue is 0.5 mm or less. The laser has excellent ablative and cutting properties for soft tissue uses (eg, strictures and tumors). The Ho:YAG laser can be used for lithotripsy as well, with a mechanism that appears to combine photothermal ablation at the stone surface, literally vaporizing portions of the stone, with a degree of photoacoustic effect (as in the other lithotripsy lasers). It is effective on all stones, regardless of color. Because of its high absorption by water, the Ho:YAG laser is safe if discharged more than 1 mm away from the urothelium in a fluid environment. If placed in contact with the urothelium, however, effective tissue cutting ensues. Lithotripsy applications require power in the range of 5–10 W (300 μs pulse duration, 0.5–1 J/pulse, 5–12 Hz), but to achieve large-volume tissue ablation, devices capable of delivering 60–80 W are required. Experimental work involving an automatic stone-detection device similar to that described for the pulsed dye laser has been reported.

Diode Lasers

Diode lasers use semiconductors to produce the laser beam. These lasers are very small compared with other medical lasers. Although power output is somewhat limited, a therapeutic medical dye laser can be housed in a small tabletop unit. Diode lasers currently used in urology include those emitting wavelengths of 810–830 nm that are used for interstitial tissue coagulation and laser tissue welding.

CLINICAL APPLICATIONS OF LASERS IN UROLOGY
(Table 26–2)

External Genitalia

Destruction of widespread but superficial lesions of the external genitalia, such as condyloma acuminata or carcinoma in situ, are an excellent application of the CO_2 laser. Complete ablation of superficial tissue combined with a shallow depth of coagulation facilitates effective treatment with less scarring than might occur with scalpel dissection, cryotherapy, or electrocautery because damage to the deeper dermal

Table 26–2. Clinical applications of lasers in urology.

Laser	Wavelength (nm)	Penetration Depth (mm)	Uses
CO_2	10,600	≤ 0.1	External genitalia, distal urethra, tissue welding
Nd:YAG	1064	3–5	External genitalia, urethra, prostate, bladder, ureter/kidney, tissue welding
KTP	532	1–3	Urethra, prostate, bladder, ureter/kidney, tissue welding
Argon	488–514	2–4	Urethra, bladder, ureter/kidney
Coumarin green pulsed dye	504	2–4	Calculi
Alexandrite	755	2–4	Calculi
Q-switched Nd:YAG	1064	3–5	Calculi
Ho:YAG	2100	≤ 0.5	External genitalia, urethra, prostate, bladder, ureter/kidney, calculi
Diode	Variable	Variable	Photodynamic therapy, prostate, tissue welding

layers can be minimized. The CO_2 laser energy is usually delivered with a hand piece on an articulating arm, since this wavelength cannot be carried by quartz fibers. The CO_2 laser beam is focused by a lens at a point in front of the hand piece. Moving the hand piece in and out to focus or defocus the laser beam results in pinpoint or wide application, respectively. Pinpoint application produces a more rapid and complete ablation of a small area, whereas wide application produces a slower ablation with a larger band of coagulation beneath the ablated surface (although this coagulation zone is still small compared with that produced by lasers such as the Nd:YAG). As successive layers of the condyloma or carcinoma in situ lesion are treated, the carbonized surface can be removed with a moistened sponge to expose deeper layers. Treatment of condyloma acuminata and carcinoma in situ requires ablation of only the epithelial layer. Bleeding is minimal until the deeper layers of the dermis are reached; treatment into or beyond this layer is unnecessary and is associated with poorer healing and scarring. Analgesics are usually not required after superficial treatment, but an antibacterial cream may be desirable.

Although CO_2 laser treatment of condyloma acuminata is very effective for removing visible lesions, the CO_2 laser is no better than any other treatment at eradicating the viral genome that is the source of the disease. For carcinoma in situ of the penis, laser therapy is considered a second-line treatment after topical application of 5-fluorouracil cream. The CO_2 laser is generally applied to areas of visible carcinoma in situ, while the cream may be applied more broadly to treat disease that is not grossly apparent. In its role as second-line therapy, however, the laser is effective in eliminating resistant lesions.

For small, localized, invasive carcinomas of the penis, laser therapy may be an alternative to partial or complete penectomy. The CO_2 laser does not penetrate deeply enough to eradicate disease penetrating into the dermis, so the Nd:YAG laser can be applied in

this situation. The beam is applied widely with a lower-power density to achieve coagulation without vaporization or carbonization. The application of iced saline may assist in cooling the superficial tissues and preventing carbonization, which reduces effective depth of penetration of the laser because of increased energy absorption by the carbonized material. The goal of treatment is to produce a localized but well-demarcated third-degree-burn injury. In areas of complete dermal destruction, the lesion is painless. Healing of the wound by secondary intention may take several months. In properly selected patients, in whom the extent of invasive carcinoma is limited, Nd:YAG laser therapy offers potential cure of the cancer with less disfiguring surgery than penectomy.

The CO_2 laser has also been used to ablate the plaques of Peyronie disease before grafting of the defect in the tunica albuginea with a suitable material. Proponents suggest that CO_2 laser ablation makes possible the removal of the entire plaque without creating an excessively large defect in the tunica albuginea. The Nd:YAG laser also can be used for this purpose.

Urethra

Lesions of the urethra involving the fossa navicularis or meatus, including balanitis xerotica obliterans, meatal stenosis, condyloma, or strictures, may be treated with the CO_2 laser in much the same way as superficial penile lesions. Use of a nasal speculum or a metal bougie helps expose the lesion for laser application. Pinpoint application of the laser with complete ablation of tissue and minimal coagulative effect makes the CO_2 laser very useful in this situation, where electrocautery might be associated with iatrogenic injury and subsequent scarring in these delicate areas. For condyloma or strictures more proximal within the urethra, it is not known if lasers offer a significant advantage over electrocautery or cold-knife incision techniques. Since a quartz glass fiber must be used to carry the laser energy through the transurethral endoscope, the CO_2 laser cannot be used, and lasers such as the Nd:YAG, Ho:YAG, argon, or KTP are applied. To reduce the coagulative effect of these lasers and maximize their ablative properties, some urologists advocate direct application of the fibers in contact mode or the use of chiseled sapphire contact tips. With such techniques it is possible to ablate the entire circumference of a urethral stricture or bladder neck contracture. Transurethral incision of bladder neck contractures or the prostate may be effectively performed as well. Although single-modality studies have shown quite favorable results with these laser applications, comparison studies generally have failed to show significant advantages of laser therapy over electrocautery or cold incision techniques for lesions proximal to the fossa navicularis.

Prostate

Over the past decade a number of techniques have evolved for laser treatment of benign prostatic hyperplasia. The first of these to achieve popularity was the side-firing coagulation technique. The poorly absorbed Nd:YAG laser wavelength allows deep penetration of coagulative energy into the prostate when applied at a right angle to the urethral lumen; fibers are used that direct the laser beam sideways, either with a metal reflector or with an angled cleaving of the end of the fiber. The energy is applied in multiple wide spots to achieve a number of zones of coagulation surrounding the prostatic urethra. The coagulated tissue is slowly absorbed over the next few weeks to months, resulting in a tissue defect and relief of bladder outlet obstruction. The energy can be applied either with a free beam technique or by using a transurethral balloon that fills and compresses the prostatic urethra, through which the side-firing laser is passed back and forth in the center of the balloon. The former procedure is guided visually through a cystoscope, and the latter is monitored by using transrectal ultrasonography.

A number of clinical studies have addressed the effectiveness of side-firing coagulation prostatectomy. In general, the results show subjective and objective responses that approach but do not equal those following standard electrocautery transurethral resection of the prostate (TURP). Bleeding and transurethral resection syndrome are uncommon in patients undergoing side-firing laser prostatectomy, however. Hospital stay is usually short, and the treatment is generally perceived as less invasive than TURP. Because the tissue is not removed at the time of the procedure, and may even temporarily swell postoperatively, relief of symptoms by side-firing laser prostatectomy may be delayed for several weeks, and prolonged catheterization or recatheterization may be required. Delayed bleeding and sloughing of tissue can be bothersome to the patient. Retreatment rates for persistent obstruction also are higher after side-firing laser prostatectomy than after TURP.

To improve upon the delayed response noted with the coagulation technique, many urologists have approached laser prostatectomy with contact vaporization techniques. Here, the Nd:YAG energy is applied directly to the surface of the prostate under endoscopic control, either by placing a durable side-firing fiber directly on the prostatic urethral lumen and dragging it along to create a trough of ablated tissue, or by using contact laser tips to achieve high heating and ablation of prostatic tissue. The KTP laser, especially with the addition of fluorescein dye, which acts as a chromophore to enhance absorption of the KTP wavelength, may also be used for vaporization techniques in the prostate. Unfortunately, prostate laser vaporization procedures are more time consuming than either TURP or side-firing laser coagulation of the prostate. Bleeding is greater with the contact vaporization prostatectomy than with the coagulation prostatectomy, although it is still minimal compared with TURP. It appears that prolonged catheterization is avoided with vaporization techniques, but patients still may suffer irritative voiding symptoms for several weeks postoperatively.

More recently, investigators have described interstitial laser coagulation of the prostate. With this technique, cystoscopically directed laser fibers are pushed beyond the urethral mucosa into the substance of the prostate. Coagulation is thus produced below the surface of the urethral lumen, producing an eventual coagulation defect similar to that with side-firing laser coagulation prostatectomy, but without damaging the urethral mucosa. It is hoped that sparing of the urethral lining results in fewer problems with postoperative bleeding, obstruction, and irritative voiding symptoms. The Nd:YAG laser wavelength was the initial choice for this application because of its excellent coagulative properties. Use of frosted or diffusing tips allows radiation of the energy in all directions and creation of a sphere or ellipse of coagulated tissue that is slowly resorbed. Even more recently, devices involving a diode laser operating at 830 nm have been applied. For this application, a small tabletop laser diode unit can supply sufficient power. Long-term results in terms of relief of the symptoms of prostatism with the newest interstitial laser coagulation techniques are sparse but encouraging. The problems with prolonged catheterization, as with side-firing coagulation prostatectomy, appear to have been reduced but not eliminated. Postoperative bleeding and irritative voiding symptoms are minimal.

Finally, the powerful cutting properties of the Ho:YAG laser have made possible the development of laser resection prostatectomy techniques. The Ho:YAG laser is used cystoscopically in contact mode to create several incisions along the prostatic urethra, extending from the bladder neck to the verumontanum. The laser fiber is then applied in an ante-grade technique to lift a segment of prostatic tissue off the underlying capsule. With progressive sweeps of the laser, the segment is eventually released into the bladder lumen. An endoscopic morcellator is then used to grasp and discharge the resected prostatic pieces, which are considerably larger than the chips from TURP. Although bleeding is not completely eliminated with laser resection of the prostate, it does appear to be less than that with TURP. Moreover, almost all of the laser energy is absorbed by the water or used in ablation of tissue, so there is minimal energy deposition in the remaining prostatic tissue that might lead to postoperative swelling and obstruction or to irritative voiding symptoms. At this time, only early series have been reported. With continued experience and development of new incision patterns and tissue removal techniques, laser resection of the prostate may become an attractive alternative to TURP.

Bladder

Lasers have been used for the treatment of bladder hemangioma, a use for which the Nd:YAG laser appears particularly well suited. Lasers have also been described occasionally for the management of hemorrhagic cystitis and interstitial cystitis. The most common use of laser therapy in the bladder is for superficial transitional cell carcinoma. Superficial bladder cancer is often a recurrent disease, creating morbidity owing to the frequent resections required for its control. In patients with biopsy-proved superficial bladder cancer, laser therapy for recurrences can minimize the morbidity of repeated treatments. The Nd:YAG laser wavelength allows excellent coagulation of the lesions as well as treatment of the underlying tissue layers. Small lesions can be coagulated completely with a single application of the Nd:YAG laser beam in noncontact mode, whereas larger lesions require initial coagulation of all visible tumor followed by physical dislodgment of the coagulated material with the tip of the fiber or cystoscope to expose deeper layers of the papillary tumor. Repeat coagulation is then applied until the tumor base is coagulated. Treatment of large tumors may be facilitated by the use of a laser with a more ablative wavelength, such as the KTP or Ho:YAG laser.

Laser therapy for bladder tumors has several specific advantages. Bleeding is almost nonexistent with this technique, and bladder tumors can be safely laser-coagulated in patients on anticoagulant therapy. In a cooperative patient, treatment may be performed without formal anesthesia. Multiple tumors are often difficult to address with electrocautery techniques because of loss of visualization owing to bleeding and the released products of electrocautery, and laser therapy in this situation is often easier. A Foley catheter is usually not required postoperatively because of the minimal bleeding. Finally, intravesical immunotherapy can be administered very soon after laser therapy since there is a minimum of raw exposed surface of the bladder wall. A disadvantage of laser therapy is that histologic samples are not obtained unless an ablative laser is used to cut off a piece of the tumor, or unless cold cup biopsies or electrocautery resection are used adjunctively (which obviate many of the advantages of the laser). Additionally, Nd:YAG laser coagulation is a time-consuming process for large tumors.

The Nd:YAG laser penetrates 3–5 mm into the bladder wall when directed to maximize coagulation. The Nd:YAG laser should be applied with the bladder only partially full to minimize thinning of the bladder wall and the risk of bladder perforation or even damage to an adjacent viscus. In patients thought to have thin bladders, either because of appearance or history of multiple resections, laser therapy should be applied cautiously. Although Nd:YAG laser therapy for superficial bladder cancer was initially thought to be associated with fewer tumor recurrences than electrocautery resection, comparative clinical series have failed to support this contention. Lasers are therefore useful for the treatment of superficial bladder cancer predominantly as a way to minimize the morbidity of multiple tumor resections and to provide safe treatment of patients receiving anticoagulant therapy.

Lasers can also be used to assist in the diagnosis of bladder carcinoma. Certain endogenous molecules (fluorophores) fluoresce when stimulated with photons of a specific wavelength. Laser-induced autofluorescence is being investigated for the detection of bladder cancer. Monochromatic laser light with a wavelength of 280–480 nm is directed to the area of interest through a flexible quartz fiber. The cells then emit fluorescence with a variety of spectra, which are detected either by the same fiber used for excitation or by separate detection fibers. A spectrometer is used to separate out the spectral emissions and measure their relative intensity. The likelihood of neoplastic changes is determined by the ratio of the intensities of various spectra. Laser-induced autofluorescence diagnosis of bladder carcinoma is a new field of study that is not yet ready for routine application, but the technique bears hope for the eventual development of a device that allows localization of neoplastic urothelium when gross morphologic changes are not apparent.

Ureter and Kidney

Transitional cell carcinoma of the upper urinary tract can be approached with the laser in much the same way as superficial bladder tumors. As an alternative to the standard therapy of nephroureterectomy, endoscopic management of upper tract urothelial tumors is considered primarily in patients with a solitary kidney, significant medical renal disease, or bilateral upper tract tumors. Endoscopic management may also be appropriate in selected patients with small, low-grade upper tract urothelial tumors even in the presence of bilateral functioning kidneys if the patient is at poor medical risk for major surgery or strongly wishes to avoid nephroureterectomy. As in the bladder, the Nd:YAG laser is useful because of its coagulative properties. In the small confines of the ureter, however, the Ho:YAG laser may be more applicable because pinpoint destruction of tissue can be achieved without undesired coagulation effects outside the intended field. Additionally, when dealing with a larger tumor, the progression of tissue removal by the repeated process of Nd:YAG laser coagulation followed by physical removal of the coagulated tissue is very slow. In this situation, the ablative ability of the Ho:YAG laser is advantageous. When using the Ho:YAG laser for urothelial tumors, the tumor may be completely ablated or it may be cut into pieces for subsequent removal with physical techniques. It is important not to make the resected pieces too large, as they may be difficult to remove from the upper tract.

The use of lasers for upper tract urothelial tumors has several advantages over electrocoagulation. For ureteral tumors, electrocoagulation is often technically difficult or inadequate because of the small working space. The lasers offer a clean and controlled alternative. When approaching upper tract tumors in the kidney endoscopically through a large-caliber percutaneous route, traditional electrocautery resectoscopes can be applied if the tumor is accessible; in this setting the laser probably offers little advantage. If a ureteroscopic approach is taken to renal pelvic tumors, however, then the same advantages of the laser as for ureteral use apply.

The use of lasers for ureteral strictures has also been described. The most commonly used lasers have been Nd:YAG (applied in contact mode) and Ho:YAG. As in the setting of urethral strictures, laser incision is most likely to have an advantage over electrocautery incision techniques in situations where delicate precision is required, such as in pediatric ureters, strictures close to vascular or delicate structures (ureteroenteric or midureteral strictures), or infundibular stenosis of the kidney.

Control of parenchymal bleeding during partial nephrectomy or wedge resection for renal tumor can be problematic and often requires clamping of the renal artery. In some situations, however, ischemia to the kidney is undesirable and hemostatic maneuvers must be performed on perfused parenchyma. Ablative lasers such as the KTP and Ho:YAG can be used to initially resect the renal mass. Application of Nd:YAG energy may then be used to achieve coagulation. Although clean and efficient, these laser techniques may not offer a significant advantage over the traditional techniques of blunt parenchymal incision, suturing of bleeding vessels, and application of a hemostatic sponge.

Urinary Calculi

Urinary calculi occur in the bladder, ureter, and kidney. For bladder stones, electrohydraulic lithotripsy is most frequently used as the energy modality if endoscopic therapy is chosen. The uncontrolled nature of the shock wave emanating from the tip of the electrohydraulic lithotrite can create mucosal bladder injury, which produces bleeding that may limit visibility. Use of the Ho:YAG laser with a side-firing probe (similar to that used during Nd:YAG laser coagulation of the prostate) appears to be effective in removing even large bladder stones rapidly and with minimal trauma.

Laser lithotripsy techniques find their most frequent use in the treatment of ureteral calculi. The flexible laser fibers with a diameter of 200–360 μm are an excellent choice for intracorporeal lithotripsy through a flexible ureteroscope (which usually has a working channel only 1000 μm in diameter). For calculi impacted in the ureter, absolute precision during lithotripsy is required. The first laser used extensively for ureteral calculi was the tunable pulse dye laser (coumarin green dye, 504-nm wavelength). The extreme safety of this device led to its popularity. Migration of stone fragments can be a problem because of the shock wave mechanism of pulsed dye laser lithotripsy, but this can be addressed with the use of baskets specifically designed for laser lithotripsy. Additionally, harder stones may not fragment well with the pulsed dye laser, and cystine stones are resistant because of poor absorption of the 504-nm wavelength.

The pulsed Ho:YAG laser, with its combined photothermal and photoacoustic mechanism, is effective on all stones regardless of color. Compared with the pulsed dye laser, little forward propulsion of stone fragments is noted. When applied properly (ie, > 1 mm from the ureteral wall), the Ho:YAG laser is safe. If placed in contact with the ureteral wall, however, significant damage can occur. Despite this technical consideration, many urologists now prefer the Ho:YAG laser to the pulsed dye laser because of its great effectiveness, even when using the very thin, 200-μm fiber.

As an alternative to ureteral laser lithotripsy, small (1.9F, ~ 600 μm) electrohydraulic lithotrites are effective and also can be used through a flexible endoscope. The potential for ureteral injury with electrohydraulic lithotripsy is great, however, and treatment conditions often degrade significantly during prolonged treatment because of mucosal bleeding. Although randomized comparisons are lacking, it is likely that laser lithotripsy techniques offer the urologist a greater margin of safety and more effective procedures, albeit at greater equipment costs.

For urinary calculi in the kidney that are approached endoscopically, rather than with extracorporeal shock wave lithotripsy, the advantages of laser therapy over flexible electrohydraulic lithotripsy are less pronounced. Bleeding from the urothelium of the kidney during electrohydraulic lithotripsy is less troublesome than that during ureteral lithotripsy, although problems still may develop during prolonged procedures or with inaccurate positioning of the electrohydraulic lithotrite. When performing flexible nephroscopy through a percutaneous approach, irrigation through the large-caliber flexible endoscope (16F) can be generous, and a moderate amount of mucosal bleeding can be overcome to maintain visualization. If the renal calculus is being addressed in a retrograde fashion using a flexible ureteroscope (7.5–9.5F), then irrigation volume is minimal and the relatively atraumatic effect of the properly applied laser lithotrite may provide more of an advantage over electrohydraulic lithotripsy.

As with many of the laser procedures described in this chapter, comparisons with nonlaser techniques are important because of the generally high cost of lasers. Both the pulsed dye laser and Ho:YAG lasers currently cost in the range of $100,000. There are low-power Ho:YAG units that cost half as much that are useful for lithotripsy and very small volume soft tissue applications but not for moderate to large soft tissue use. In comparison, electrohydraulic lithotripsy units cost less than $20,000. The probes for electrohydraulic lithotripsy are disposable, compared with the reusable laser fibers, but their cost is minimal ($300 for a 1.9F lithotrite) relative to the difference in cost between laser and electrohydraulic base units. The choice of flexible lithotrite must be made considering these financial issues.

Photodynamic Therapy

Photodynamic therapy for superficial bladder carcinoma utilizes photochemical rather than photothermal effects of lasers. Photosensitizers are substances that render tissues more susceptible to light-induced changes. Tissue destruction during photodynamic therapy occurs when sufficient light energy is absorbed by a photosensitizer to cause an incompletely understood photooxidative process that damages proteins and nucleic acids in the cell. The cells die as a result of the accumulated injury. Clinically useful photosensitizers are selectively retained by tumor cells so that neoplastic cells rather than normal cells are preferentially destroyed by photodynamic therapy.

The most common photosensitizers for photodynamic therapy are members of the porphyrin family. A synthetic porphyrin mixture derived from bovine hemoglobin called hematoporphyrin derivative was first used. Other photosensitizers include porfimer sodium, benzoporphyrin derivative, and 5-aminolevulinic acid. 5-Aminolevulinic acid is unique in that it is a precursor of the endogenous photosensitizer protoporphyrin IX. Although the clinically used photosensitizers are concentrated by neoplastic tissue, enough remains systemically that cutaneous photosensitivity is a significant limiting problem with photodynamic therapy. Patients are sensitive to natural or intense artificial light for 4–6 weeks after administration of the photosensitizer.

Currently, photodynamic therapy is used for patients with superficial bladder carcinoma that has been refractory to intravesical chemotherapy or immunotherapy. The treatment is administered with a laser wavelength specific for each photosensitizer (ie, 630-nm red laser light from an argon pumped dye laser for the photosensitizer porfimer sodium). Several days after intravenous administration of the photosensitizer, the patient is taken to the operating room under general or regional anesthesia. Saline or water is instilled into the bladder so that it is filled but not overdistended. The light is delivered via a spherically tipped laser fiber that is placed in the middle of the bladder through a cystoscope. Transcutaneous ultrasound is used to monitor the procedure. The laser is activated long enough to deliver a dose that is calculated based on the basis of various dosimetry algorithms.

Voiding dysfunction after photodynamic therapy is common. Most patients have urinary frequency and urgency, dysuria, and hematuria. More severe but unusual side effects include bladder contracture and ureteral obstruction. Even with careful instructions to avoid sunlight or intense artificial light, many patients experience cutaneous photosensitivity reactions.

Although complete tumor regression has been reported in 40–60% of patients undergoing photodynamic therapy for superficial bladder cell carcinoma, the inconvenience associated with the photosensitizer and the high level of patient morbidity have resulted in limited enthusiasm for this technique. The adverse effects of photodynamic therapy occur because photosensitizers are not as selective for neoplastic tissue as had initially been hoped. Development of new photosensitizers and dosimetry algorithms may reduce the incidence of adverse effects and make photodynamic therapy a more appealing treatment for recurrent superficial bladder carcinoma.

Laser Tissue Welding

Welding or soldering of tissue by lasers is a technique of joining tissue together through photothermal processes. Laser energy can elevate the temperature of approximated tissue edges and thermally remodel the tissue proteins. Collagen fibers interdigitate, and essentially a biologic glue is created from the fused and cross-linked mass of denatured tissue. This mass acts as a temporary bridge until normal healing processes occur. In urology, laser tissue welding has been used clinically for hypospadias repair and vasovasostomy. Originally applied to native tissue, laser tissue welding techniques now include the use of chromophores (substances that impart color to tissues, increasing their capacity to absorb photons of a certain wavelength) and protein solders. The chromophores provide concentration of the photothermal effect in the tissue or solder bearing the chromophore. The protein solder, especially when mixed with the chromophore, selectively absorbs the laser energy so that the photothermal denaturing is limited to the solder, which melts down and bonds the tissue edges together. Damage to the native tissue is minimized. Laser-welded wounds in general have excellent strength and antileak characteristics compared with sutured wounds. The primary difficulty is one of technique; exact application of the solder and laser energy is required for good clinical results. Moreover, the temperature dependence of the photothermal process is difficult to gauge clinically. A visual change in the solder or tissue is usually used as a surrogate for the temperature change that indicates the end point of laser application. Devices currently being introduced use infrared sensors and computer control of laser output to control welding temperature and may provide for more reproducible laser tissue welding.

REFERENCES

GENERAL REFERENCES

Anson K et al: The role of lasers in urology. Br J Urol 1994;73:225.

Bhatta KM: Lasers in urology. Lasers Surg Med 1995;16:312.

Erhard MJ, Bagley DH: Urologic applications of the holmium laser: Preliminary experience. J Endourol 1995;9:383.

Hofstetter AG (editor): *Lasers in Urological Surgery.* Springer-Verlag, 1995.

Smith JA Jr, Stein BS, Benson RC Jr (editors): *Lasers in Urologic Surgery,* 3rd ed. Mosby, 1994.

Web Science Resources: Tutorial on laser physics. http://members.aol.com/WSRNet/tut/ut1.htm

EXTERNAL GENITALIA

Gerber GS: Carcinoma in situ of the penis. J Urol 1994; 151:829.

Lassus J et al: Carbon dioxide (CO_2)-laser therapy cures macroscopic lesions, but viral genome is not eradicated in men with therapy-resistant HPV infection. Sex Transm Dis 1994;21:297.

Sakkas G et al: Laser treatment in urology: Our experience with neodymium:YAG and carbon dioxide lasers. Int Urol Nephrol 1995;27:405.

URETHRA

Biyani CS, Cornford PA, Powell CS: Use of the holmium:YAG laser for urethral stricture under topical anesthesia. Int Urol Nephrol 1997;29:331.

Hrebinko RL: Circumferential laser vaporization for severe meatal stenosis secondary to balanitis xerotica obliterans. J Urol 1996;156:1735.

Niesel T et al: Alternative endoscopic management in the treatment of urethral strictures. J Endourol 1995;9:31.

Perkash I: Ablation of urethral strictures using contact chisel crystal firing neodymium:YAG laser. J Urol 1997;157:809.

PROSTATE

Arai Y et al: Interstitial laser coagulation for management of benign prostatic hyperplasia: A Japanese experience. J Urol 1998;159:1961.

de la Rosette JJ et al: Interstitial laser coagulation in the treatment of benign prostatic hyperplasia using a diode-laser system with temperature feedback. Br J Urol 1997;80:433.

Fournier GRJ et al: Nd:YAG laser transurethral evaporation of the prostate (TUEP) for urinary retention. Lasers Surg Med 1996;19:480.

Furuya S et al: Transurethral balloon laser thermotherapy for urinary retention in patients with benign prostatic hyperplasia who are at high surgical risk. Int J Urol 1997;4:265.

Gilling PJ et al: Holmium laser resection of the prostate versus neodymium:yttrium-aluminum-garnet visual laser ablation of the prostate: A randomized prospective comparison of two techniques for laser prostatectomy. Urology 1998;51:573.

Jepsen JV, Bruskewitz RC: Recent developments in the surgical management of benign prostatic hyperplasia. Urology 1998;51(4A Suppl):23.

Kabalin JN, Bite G, Doll S: Neodymium:YAG laser coagulation prostatectomy: 3 years of experience with 227 patients. J Urol 1996;155:181.

Kabalin JN et al: Prospective multicenter ProLase II clinical trial of neodymium:yttrium-aluminum-garnet laser prostatectomy. Urology 1997;50:63.

Langley SE, Gallegos CR, Moisey CU: A prospective randomized trial evaluating endoscopic Nd:YAG laser prostate ablation with or without potassium titanyl phosphate (KTP) laser bladder neck incision. Br J Urol 1997;80:880.

Mackey MJ et al: The results of holmium laser resection of the prostate. Br J Urol 1998;81:518.

Malek RS, Barrett DM, Kuntzman RS: High-power potassium-titanyl-phosphate (KTP/532) laser vaporization prostatectomy: 24 hours later. Urology 1998; 51:254.

BLADDER

Anidjar M et al: Laser induced autofluorescence diagnosis of bladder tumors: Dependence on the excitation wavelength. J Urol 1996;156:1590.

Das A, Gilling P, Fraundorfer M: Holmium laser resection of bladder tumors (HoLRBT). Techn Urol 1998;4:12.

Kardos R, Magasi P, Karsza A: Nd-Yag laser treatment of bladder tumours. Int Urol Nephrol 1994;26:317.

Koenig F et al: Autofluorescence guided biopsy for the early diagnosis of bladder carcinoma. J Urol 1998; 159:1871.

Ravi R: Endoscopic neodymium:YAG laser of radiation-induced hemorrhagic cystitis. Lasers Surg Med 1994;14:83.

Smith JAJ: Surgical management of superficial bladder cancer (stages Ta/T1/CIS). Semin Surg Oncol 1997; 13:328.

URETER AND KIDNEY

Elliott DS et al: Long-term follow-up of endoscopically treated upper urinary tract transitional cell carcinoma. Urology 1996;47:819.

Gerber GS, Lyon ES: Endourological management of upper tract urothelial tumors. J Urol 1993;150:2.

Kaufman RPJ, Carson CC: Ureteroscopic management of transitional cell carcinoma of the ureter using the neodymium:YAG laser. Lasers Surg Med 1993;13: 625.

Knipper A et al: The holmium-YAG-laser as a new cutting instrument in the ureter. Invest Urol 1994;5:233.

Merguerian PA, Seremetis G: Laser-assisted partial nephrectomy in children. J Pediatr Surg 1994;29:934.

Stratmann U et al: The interaction of laser energy with ureter tissues in a long-term investigation. Scan Microsc 1995;9:805.

Tawfiek ER, Bagley DH: Upper-tract transitional cell carcinoma. Urology 1997;50:321.

URINARY CALCULI

Adams DH: Holmium:YAG laser and pulsed dye laser: A cost comparison. Lasers Surg Med 1997;21:29.

Benizri E et al: Comparison of 2 pulsed lasers for lithotripsy of ureteral calculi: Report on 154 patients. J Urol 1993;150:1803.

Gould DL: Holmium:YAG laser and its use in the treatment of urolithiasis: Our first 160 cases. J Endourol 1998;12:23.

Grasso M: Experience with the holmium laser as an endoscopic lithotrite. Urology 1996;48:199.

Grasso M, Bagley DH: Endoscopic pulsed-dye laser lithotripsy: 159 consecutive cases. J Endourol 1994;8: 25.

Huang S, Patel H, Bellman GC: Cost effectiveness in electrohydraulic lithotripsy vs Candela pulse-dye laser in management of the distal ureteral stone. J Endourol 1998;12:237.

Pearle MS et al: Safety and efficacy of the Alexandrite laser for the treatment of renal and ureteral calculi. Urology 1998;51:33.

Razvi HA et al: Intracorporeal lithotripsy with the holmium:YAG laser. J Urol 1996;156:912.

Rink K, Delacretaz G, Salathe RP: Fragmentation process of current laser lithotriptors. Lasers Surg Med 1995; 16:134.

Teichman JM et al: Holmium:YAG lithotripsy yields smaller fragments than lithoclast, pulsed dye laser or electrohydraulic lithotripsy. J Urol 1998;159:17.

Teichman JM et al: Holmium:yttrium-aluminum-garnet laser cystolithotripsy of large bladder calculi. Urology 1997;50:44.

PHOTODYNAMIC THERAPY

Datta SN et al: Effect of photodynamic therapy in combination with mitomycin C on a mitomycin-resistant bladder cancer cell line. Br J Cancer 1997;76:312.

Manyak MJ: Practical aspects of photodynamic therapy for superficial bladder carcinoma. Techn Urol 1995; 1:84.

Nseyo UO: Photodynamic therapy in the management of bladder cancer. J Clin Laser Med Surg 1996;14:271.

Nseyo UO et al: Photodynamic therapy using porfimer sodium as an alternative to cystectomy in patients with refractory transitional cell carcinoma in situ of the bladder. Bladder Photofrin Study Group. J Urol 1998;160:39.

Wyld L et al: Cell cycle phase influences tumour cell sensitivity to aminolaevulinic acid-induced photodynamic therapy in vitro. Br J Cancer 1998;78:50.

Xiao Z et al: Biodistribution of Photofrin II and 5-aminolevulinic acid-induced protoporphyrin IX in normal rat bladder and bladder tumor models: Implications for photodynamic therapy. Photochem Photobiol 1998;67:573.

LASER TISSUE WELDING

Kirsch AJ: Laser tissue soldering: State of the art. Contemp Urol 1997;9:41.

Kirsch AJ et al: Hypospadias repair by laser tissue soldering: Intraoperative results and follow-up in 30 children. Urology 1996;48:616.

Scherr DS, Poppas DP: Laser tissue welding. Urol Clin N Am 1998;25:123.

Seaman EK et al: Results of laser tissue soldering in vasovasostomy and epididymovasostomy: Experience in the rat animal model. J Urol 1997;158:642.

27 Chemotherapy of Urologic Tumors

Eric J. Small, MD

The use of chemotherapy and biologic therapy in the treatment of malignant tumors of the genitourinary system serves as a paradigm for a multidisciplinary approach to cancer. The careful integration of surgical and chemotherapeutic treatments has resulted in impressive advances in the management of urologic cancer. By definition, surgical interventions are directed at local management of urologic tumors, whereas chemotherapy and biologic therapy are systemic in nature. While there is no question that there are times in the natural history of genitourinary tumor when only one therapeutic method is required, a multidisciplinary approach is always called for. This chapter details the importance of a joint surgical-medical approach to patients with urologic cancer. A practicing urologist should collaborate closely with an oncologist and should feel comfortable speaking with patients about the uses, risks, and benefits of chemotherapy.

PRINCIPLES OF SYSTEMIC THERAPY

A. Clinical Uses of Chemotherapy and Immunotherapy: Systemic therapy is indicated in the treatment of disseminated cancer when either cure or palliation is the goal. Additionally, chemotherapy may be used as part of a multimodality treatment plan in an effort to improve both local and distant control of the tumor. An understanding of the goals and limitations of systemic therapy in each of these settings is essential to its effective use.

1. Curative intent of metastatic disease—In considering the role of potentially curative chemotherapy or biologic therapy in patients with metastatic disease, several factors must be taken into account. The first is the responsiveness of the tumor. Responsiveness is generally defined by the observed partial, complete, and overall responses. It is important to note that a complete response implies complete resolution of abnormal serum tumor markers, if any, and complete radiographic resolution of any abnormalities. This makes the assessment of neoplasms with frequent bony metastases such as prostate cancer, renal cell car-

cinoma, and transitional cell carcinoma difficult, as a persistently abnormal bone scan does not necessarily imply residual cancer. Patients in whom the only site of disease is bone generally must be considered nonassessable by conventional measures, and if available, surrogate markers of response (such as prostate-specific antigen) are required.

If cure is the intent with systemic therapy, the relevant response criterion to consider is the percentage of patients achieving a complete response. This number is less than 10% in patients with metastatic renal cell carcinoma and hormone-refractory prostate cancer, 25% or less in patients with metastatic transitional cell carcinoma, and up to 80% in patients with metastatic germ cell malignancies. Under some circumstances, however (for example, in post-chemotherapy residual masses in patients with germ cell carcinoma), an apparent partial response can be converted into a complete response with judicious resection (see section A. 3.)

The second feature to consider in treating patients with potentially curative systemic therapy is the anticipated toxicity of such therapy. In general, higher levels of toxicity are acceptable if a cure can be achieved, although care must be exercised to avoid a "cure worse than the disease." This is particularly true in the case of fairly toxic therapies such as interleukin-2 or bone marrow transplantation. These treatments can result in apparent cures of approximately 10% and 20%, respectively, of patients with metastatic renal cell carcinoma or refractory germ cell tumors. Patients undergoing these rigorous therapies must be carefully selected and must be as fully informed as possible about potential toxicities.

2. Treatment of patients with incurable metastatic cancer—When the goal of systemic therapy is palliation of symptoms rather than cure, the toxicity of the treatment to be offered must be balanced against the cancer-related symptoms the patient is experiencing, and in general, more toxic therapies are not indicated. Nonetheless, an understanding of the potential capabilities of systemic therapy must be understood because even in otherwise incurable disease there may be a role for systemic therapy if there is a likelihood that the patient's life can be prolonged with its use.

3. Systemic therapy used in conjunction with surgery: adjuvant and neoadjuvant therapy—Systemic therapy administered after a patient has been rendered free of disease surgically is termed **adjuvant therapy.** Several important criteria must be met if adjuvant therapy is to be used outside of a research setting. First, an assessment must be undertaken of known risk factors predictive of relapse or development of distant metastases. Patients at low risk of relapse generally should not receive adjuvant therapy because they are unlikely to derive a benefit and will be unnecessarily exposed to the toxicity of therapy. Second, the proposed therapy must have been shown to decrease the rate of relapse and increase the disease-free interval (and, it is hoped, survival) in a randomized, phase III trial. Finally, because patients who are being treated with adjuvant therapy are free of disease and presumably asymptomatic, toxicity must be kept at a minimum. This opens the way to a tailored approach in which patients with high-risk disease, as determined by pathologic review of the surgical specimen, are treated in order to decrease the risk of micrometastatic disease.

By contrast, neoadjuvant therapy is administered before definitive surgical resection. Here, the potential advantages include early therapy of micrometastatic disease and tumor debulking to allow a more complete resection. Patients with known metastatic disease generally do not exhibit high enough response rates to systemic therapy to warrant surgery following chemotherapy, with the clear exception of patients with germ cell tumors. Whether or not patients with metastatic renal cell carcinoma who exhibit a partial response to systemic therapy may benefit from resection of residual masses is not known. As with adjuvant therapy, the proposed therapy must have been demonstrated to impact favorably on rate of relapse, disease-free interval, and survival in a randomized phase III trial.

B. Chemotherapeutic Agents and Their Toxicity: The usefulness of antineoplastic agents lies in their therapeutic index, or preferential toxicity to malignant cells over normal, nonmalignant cells. The mechanism of action of most chemotherapeutic drugs is based on their toxicity to rapidly dividing cells. Thus, in general, malignancies that have relatively rapid growth, such as germ cell tumors, are relatively chemosensitive, whereas slower growing neoplasms such as prostate cancer and renal cell carcinoma are less sensitive. Toxicity from chemotherapeutic agents is seen primarily in normal, nonmalignant cells that are also rapidly dividing, such as hematopoietic cells in the bone marrow, gastrointestinal mucosa, and hair follicles, and is manifested in cytopenias, mucositis, and alopecia. Other common toxicities observed with agents frequently used in the treatment of genitourinary malignancies include nephrotoxicity, neurotoxicity, hemorrhagic cystitis, pulmonary fibrosis, and cardiotoxicity. Table 27–1 summarizes the spectrum of activity and primary toxicities of commonly used chemotherapeutic agents.

The development of chemotherapy drug resistance remains an important clinical problem in the field of oncology. Malignant cells develop resistance in a variety of ways, including the induction of transport pumps, which actively pump the drug out of the cell and through increased activity of enzymes necessary to inactivate the particular chemotherapeutic agent. While there are several experimental methods of circumventing these mechanisms of drug resistance, one practical approach to this problem is the use of multiagent chemotherapy. Increased tumor cell killing is achieved by exposing neoplastic cells to multiple agents with different mechanisms of action. Furthermore, this approach allows the selection of agents with nonoverlapping toxicity profiles.

The use of increased dose intensity (higher doses of a drug administered over the same time period) as a means of overcoming drug resistance remains experimental in urologic malignancies with one clear exception. A subset of patients with chemotherapy-refractory germ cell tumors appear to be curable with high-dose chemotherapy and autologous bone marrow transplant support (see the section Germ Cell Malignancies, following).

C. Biologic Agents and Their Toxicity: Whereas chemotherapy is based on direct cytotoxicity, biologic therapy can be broadly considered to consist of treatment with agents that augment or diminish biologic phenomena normally observed in malignant cells. For the purposes of this chapter, two types of biologic therapy are considered: immunotherapy and growth-factor-related therapy. Immunotherapy is an important component of the therapy of urologic malignancies, particularly of superficial bladder carcinoma and renal cell carcinoma. Immunotherapy is designed to either elicit or augment an immune response in the patient in order to stop tumor growth or enhance tumor killing. In contrast to chemotherapy, the target of immunotherapy is not necessarily rapidly dividing cells but rather cells that can be recognized as foreign by the host. Most immunotherapeutic agents that are currently in use are fairly nonspecific. This is reflected in systemic toxicity in the form of constitutional symptoms such as fever, malaise, fatigue, myalgias, and arthralgias, as well as cutaneous toxicity. In very high doses (of IL-2, for example), toxicity may include severe vascular leak syndrome with hypotension, pulmonary edema, and renal insufficiency.

Specific biologic agents used in the therapy of urologic malignancies include bacille Calmette-Guérin (BCG), interferon-alpha, and interleukin-2. The use of BCG for the treatment of superficial bladder cancer is based on the premise that local BCG in-

Table 27–1. Commonly used antineoplastic agents in urologic oncology, and their toxicity.

Agent	Activity	Common Toxicities
Cisplatin	Bladder cancer, germ cell tumors, prostate cancer	Renal insufficiency, peripheral neuropathy, auditory toxicity, myelosuppression[1]
Carboplatin	Bladder cancer, germ cell tumors	Myelosuppression
Bleomycin	Germ cell tumors	Fever, chills, pulmonary fibrosis
Doxorubicin	Bladder cancer, prostate cancer	Myelosuppression, mucositis, cardiomyopathy
Etoposide (VP-16)	Germ cell tumors, prostate cancer[2]	Myelosuppression
5-Fluorouracil	Renal cell carcinoma, bladder cancer, prostate cancer	Mucositis, diarrhea, myelosuppression
Floxuridine (FUdR)	Renal cell carcinoma	Mucositis, diarrhea
Methotrexate	Germ cell tumors, bladder cancer	Mucositis, myelosuppression, renal toxicity
Ifosfamide	Germ cell tumors	Myelosuppression, neurologic (CNS) toxicity, cystitis
Vinblastine	Renal cell carcinoma, bladder cancer, germ cell tumors, prostate cancer[2]	Peripheral, autonomic neuropathy; myelosuppression
Estramustine	Prostate cancer	Nausea, thromboembolic events
Paclitaxel (Taxol)	Bladder cancer, germ cell tumors, prostate cancer[2]	Myelosuppression, neuropathy
Docetaxel (Taxotere)	Bladder cancer, germ cell tumors, prostate cancer	Myelosuppression, neuropathy
Gemcitabine (Gemzar)	Bladder cancer	Myelosuppression
Interferon-alpha	Renal cell carcinoma	Flulike symptoms, myelosuppression
Interleukin-2	Renal cell carcinoma	Flulike symptoms, hypotension, renal toxicity, hepatic toxicity, neurologic (CNS) toxicity, respiratory distress, dermatologic symptoms, sepsis

[1] Because of recent advances in the treatment of chemotherapy-induced nausea and vomiting, even the most emetogenic agents, such as cisplatin, have virtually no associated nausea and vomiting.
[2] In combination with estramustine.

stillation will result in a local immune response causing tumor cell kill. Interferons and interleukins are cytokines that are normally produced in the body as mediators of immune response. The exogenous administration of these agents can result in an enhanced immune response and tumor regression. Direct cytotoxicity or antiproliferative effects also appear to be mechanisms by which interferon-alpha, in particular, is active. Table 27–1 summarizes the spectrum of activity and primary toxicities of commonly used immunotherapeutic agents. Experimental immunologic approaches being evaluated include the development of vaccines for renal cell carcinoma and prostate cancer.

Growth factor manipulation is a novel and exciting element of antineoplastic therapy. The use of exogenous growth factors such as G-CSF, GM-CSF, thrombopoietin, and erythropoietin, which are normally involved in hematopoiesis, has allowed more dose-intensive therapy to be delivered. When bone marrow suppression occurs as a consequence of therapy, use of these agents has the potential for abrogating toxicity.

A completely different kind of interaction with growth factors has been observed with the experimental agent suramin, which has been used in the treatment of hormone-refractory prostate cancer. While the exact mechanisms of action of this drug are not fully understood, suramin appears to bind to and inhibit a variety of polypeptide growth factors such as fibroblast growth factor (FGF) that appear to be important in the growth and proliferation of prostate cancer cells.

D. Unique Features of Genitourinary Malignancies: The systemic therapy of urologic malignancies offers unique challenges to the practitioner. Renal insufficiency due to obstructive uropathy from local extension of the tumor or postsurgical or postradiotherapy changes is not infrequent and may alter antineoplastic drug clearance. In patients with renal cell carcinoma, previous nephrectomy also may impact on drug clearance. Furthermore, the common use of the nephrotoxic chemotherapeutic agent cisplatin in the treatment of urologic malignancies (most prominently, in bladder and testicular neoplasms) may further diminish renal function. Careful attention must be paid, therefore, to renal function throughout the course of systemic therapy, with appropriate dose adjustments made. Dosing adjustments also must be considered in patients who have undergone cystectomy because ileal conduits or neobladders have the capacity to resorb chemotherapeutic agents that are excreted in the urine in active form (most notably, methotrexate).

Frequent local extension in the pelvis presents additional unique problems. Patients with previous pelvic radiotherapy have markedly diminished bone marrow reserves, which may limit the use of myelosuppressive drugs. Furthermore, local pelvic relapses have the potential to be symptomatic and painful. Particularly in patients who have already received radiotherapy, systemic therapy may be important for palliation.

GERM CELL MALIGNANCIES

A.   Overview: The evolution of therapy for germ cell tumors (GCT) has been deliberate and thoughtful, and has resulted in cures of 80–85% of men with GCT, serving as a model for the treatment of curable cancers. Nonetheless, challenges in the management of GCT remain. Because of their young age, patients who have been cured are at risk of delayed, treatment-induced toxicity. Furthermore, an 80–85% cure rate also implies that 15–20% of patients with GCT will not be cured and ultimately will succumb to their disease. An understanding of staging and risk assessment is crucial if (1) patients with good risk features are not to be overtreated and exposed to undue toxic risks, and (2) patients with poor risk features are to receive adequate (curative) therapy.

The most common multiagent chemotherapy regimen for the treatment of GCT is a 3-drug combination consisting of cisplatin, etoposide, and bleomycin (PEB). The treatment is repeated every 21 days. One cycle consists of cisplatin 20 mg/m^2 IV d 1–5, etoposide 100 mg/m^2 IV d 1–5, and bleomycin, 30 units IV, d 2, 9, and 16. Frequently the first 5 days of treatment require hospitalization. The deletion of bleomycin from this regimen results in the PE regimen.

B.   Use of Chemotherapy for Patients With Stage I and II Disease: The standard of care for patients with stage I GCT remains orchiectomy followed by retroperitoneal lymphadenectomy (nonseminoma), radiation therapy (seminoma), or in selected patients, careful surveillance. The use of chemotherapy in stage I GCT in lieu of lymphadenectomy or irradiation remains investigational despite encouraging early results.

Patients with stage II nonseminomatous microscopic disease identified at lymphadenectomy (stage IIA) or patients with low-volume clinical stage II disease (stage IIB) who have undergone retroperitoneal lymphadenectomy may benefit from 2 cycles of adjuvant PE or PEB chemotherapy. The use of adjuvant therapy results in a 96% long-term disease-free survival. While the relapse rate for patients who do not receive adjuvant therapy approaches 40%, the vast majority of relapsing patients can also be cured with either 3 or 4 cycles of chemotherapy, yielding an identical long-term survival rate. The decision about adjuvant chemotherapy after lymphadenectomy must be individualized. Patients at high risk for relapse may choose to undergo 2 cycles of chemotherapy at that point in order to avoid the possibility of 3–4 cycles in the future.

C.   Use of Chemotherapy in Patients With Advanced Disease: Patients with advanced GCT should be treated with systemic therapy after completion of their orchiectomy. This group includes some stage IIB nonseminomatous tumors and all stage IIC or higher tumors, both seminomas and nonseminomas. A variety of chemotherapy regimens will result in approximately 80% of patients with advanced GCT achieving a complete response and 70% achieving long-term apparent cures (good prognosis). By the same token, however, 20–30% of patients have a poor prognosis and will still ultimately die from their disease. Studies of pretreatment clinical characteristics have sought to identify prognostic features that can be prospectively used to segregate this diverse group of advanced GCT patients into poor- and good-prognostic subsets.

A common classification system has been developed. In this system, good- and intermediate-prognosis patients with nonseminomatous GCT have a testis or retroperitoneal primary tumor, no nonpulmonary visceral metastases, and low serum tumor markers. Intermediate-prognosis patients are the same as good-prognosis patients but have intermediate serum tumor markers. Poor-prognosis patients have a mediastinal primary tumor or nonpulmonary visceral metastases (liver, bone, brain) or high levels of serum tumor markers. Five-year overall survival for the good-, intermediate-, and poor-prognosis categories with current regimens is 92%, 80%, and 48%, respectively. By definition, seminomas are never in the poor-prognosis category. Seminomas are segregated into good-prognosis cases (any primary site, but no nonpulmonary visceral metastases), with an 86% 5-year survival, and intermediate-prognosis cases (any primary site but with the presence of nonpulmonary visceral metastases), with a 72% 5-year survival.

Because it is not likely that the extraordinarily high cure rate for good-prognosis patients can be improved upon, most efforts in the treatment of these patients have been aimed at optimizing treatment with less toxic regimens that will have equal efficacy. Trials evaluating (1) the elimination of bleomycin, (2) a reduction in the number of chemotherapy cycles administered, or (3) the substitution of carboplatin for cisplatin have been undertaken.

The outlook for poor-prognosis patients is grim, with only 38–62% of patients achieving a complete response. Thus, whereas the major concern in good-prognosis patients has been the reduction of toxicity, the major objective of clinical investigation in poor-prognosis patients has been to improve efficacy, with less concern for reducing toxicity. Clinical trials in poor-prognosis patients have by and large relied on one or both of two approaches. The first has been to exploit agents that have been demonstrated to be efficacious in the salvage setting, and the second has been to evaluate the role of dose escalation.

There is a lack of consensus regarding the optimal management of high-risk GCT. Every effort should be made to enroll and treat patients with poor-prognosis GCT in clinical trials.

Currently acceptable regimens for good-prognosis patients are fairly well defined and include 3 cycles of PEB or 4 cycles of PE; by contrast, optimal therapy for poor-prognosis patients continues to be investigated; 4 cycles of PEB are used in many centers.

D. Adjunctive Surgery and "Salvage" Therapy: Postchemotherapy adjunctive surgery must be integrated into the treatment plan of patients with advanced germ cell tumors. Between 10% and 20% of patients with nonseminomatous tumors have residual masses after systemic therapy, and up to 80% of patients with seminomas have residual radiographic abnormalities. The role of adjunctive surgery in patients with GCT with post-chemotherapy residual masses has been reviewed. Except in rare circumstances, adjunctive surgery is not indicated in the presence of persistently elevated serum tumor markers. Adjunctive surgery usually can be undertaken safely within 1–2 months of completion of chemotherapy. It must be noted, however, that all patients who have received bleomycin, whether or not there is clinical evidence of pulmonary fibrosis, are at risk of development of oxygen-related pulmonary toxicity. The anesthesiologist must be made aware of the patient's previous exposure to bleomycin and every effort taken to maintain the FiO_2 as low as possible throughout the surgical procedure. Patients who are found to have active carcinoma in their resected specimens are frequently treated with 2 additional cycles of chemotherapy, although compelling evidence supporting this procedure is still forthcoming.

While approximately 80% of patients with germ cell tumors can currently be cured with platinum-based therapy, 20% ultimately die of their disease, either because a complete response is not achieved with induction therapy or because they relapse after becoming disease-free with primary therapy. Before the initiation of salvage therapy, the diagnosis of relapsed or primary, refractory GCT must be clearly established. In particular, falsely elevated human chorionic gonadotropin or alpha-fetoprotein values and false-positive radiographic studies of the chest due to previous bleomycin use must be ruled out. Persistent or slowly growing masses, particularly in the absence of serologic progression, may represent benign teratoma. Therapies based on ifosfamide and high-dose chemotherapy with autologous bone marrow transplant provide a salvage rate of approximately 25% in patients with relapsed or refractory germ cell tumors.

ADVANCED TRANSITIONAL CELL CARCINOMA OF THE UROEPITHELIUM

A. Nonmetastatic Disease: The development of effective chemotherapy regimens for the treatment of metastatic transitional cell carcinoma (TCC) has resulted in more widespread use of these regimens in combination with other modes for the treatment of locally advanced but nonmetastatic disease. In bulky inoperable invasive bladder tumors (T3b, T4, N+), chemotherapy has been used as a means of cytoreduction in order to make surgery possible. Chemotherapy before surgery, termed **neoadjuvant therapy,** has also been used in muscle-invasive cancers that *are* resectable, in an effort to treat micrometastatic disease before cystectomy. It must be borne in mind that the pathologic complete response rate in the bladder after neoadjuvant chemotherapy is probably in the 30–40% range; therefore, definitive surgical resection after chemotherapy is usually required. A European trial has failed to show an advantage of neoadjuvant therapy. Results of a major US intergroup trial are anticipated in the near future.

Other investigators believe that adjuvant therapy administered *after* radical cystectomy should be the means of treating patients with invasive bladder cancer at risk for relapse. Adjuvant trials generally have been used to treat only patients found to have pathologic T3 and T4 lesions. Several small randomized trials have shown a benefit to various adjuvant chemotherapy regimens; a large randomized multi-institution trial remains to be done.

Chemotherapy in combination with radiation therapy has been advocated by some as a bladder-preserving approach for muscle-invasive tumors. Patients are usually treated with 2 cycles of chemotherapy, followed by radiation therapy and concomitant cisplatin as a radiosensitizer. If follow-up cystoscopy reveals no cancer, consolidative multiagent systemic chemotherapy is administered. This approach appears to be particularly useful for smaller, lower-stage tumors, While longer follow-up is required, it appears that approximately 30–50% of patients can attain long-term disease-free status with a functional bladder with this approach.

B. Metastatic Disease: The development of successful therapy of metastatic bladder TCC has been based on the use of cisplatin. Two common cisplatin-based regimens are in wide use: (1) cisplatin, methotrexate, and vinblastine (CMV) and (2) the same drugs in a slightly different schedule and dose along with doxorubicin (Adriamycin), in a regimen known as MVAC. These regimens result in overall response rates of approximately 50–60% and complete remission rates in the 20–35% range. Median overall survival for patients with metastatic disease treated with these regimens is in the 8- to 14-month range. Despite early promise, however, long-term survival after MVAC remains in the single digits.

While CMV and MVAC have not been directly compared, their efficacy is probably similar.

Both CMV and MVAC are intensive regimens, with myelosuppression occurring commonly. The use of hematopoietic growth factors has made it easier to administer full doses on schedule, although this improvement in dose intensity does not appear to translate into a clinical benefit.

Recently, several novel agents have been shown to have activity against transitional cell carcinoma, including carboplatin, paclitaxel (Taxol), and gemcitabine. Paclitaxel and gemcitabine have impressive single-agent activity. Doublet combinations such as cisplatin-gemcitabine and carboplatin-paclitaxel are being investigated. Early results suggest that these new combinations are less toxic than MVAC, but efficacy comparisons await completion of randomized trials.

RENAL CELL CARCINOMA

The treatment of metastatic renal cell carcinoma remains largely unsatisfactory. The general lack of active agents and the excessive toxicity of many of the agents that exhibit some activity have contributed to the absence of adjuvant or neoadjuvant trials. The only such trial used adjuvant interferon-alpha for patients considered at high risk for relapse after nephrectomy and failed to show an advantage of the adjuvant therapy. Prenephrectomy systemic therapy remains experimental and cannot be advocated at this time.

Metastatic renal cell carcinoma is relatively resistant to chemotherapy. Response proportions of 10–20% have been observed with vinblastine when it is used as a single agent. Development of resistance to vinblastine is common, however, and may be due to the fact that renal cell carcinomas frequently overexpress the multiple drug resistance (MDR-1) gene. The MDR-1 gene product is a transmembrane glycoprotein (p glycoprotein) that actively pumps a variety of chemotherapeutic agents, including vinblastine, out of the cell. Some investigators have found that floxuridine (FUdR) given as a 2-week infusion every 4 weeks is well tolerated and appears to have a response rate of 20–25%.

Renal cell carcinoma is one of very few neoplasms that clearly are responsive to biologic response modifiers. Interferon-alpha has limited but reproducible activity in renal cell carcinoma. While initial response rates of 30% were reported, more recent large studies have suggested a response rate of less than 15% to single-agent interferon-alpha. Furthermore, considerable toxicities consisting of fever, chills, myalgias, and malaise are common, even though tolerance to some of these side effects may be developed over several months. The toxicities associated with interferon-alpha must be weighed against the potential benefits of the drug.

Interleukin-2 (IL-2) has been extensively studied in patients with metastatic renal cell carcinoma. The activity of IL-2 is mediated in part by its activation and promotion of growth of T cells, B cells, and natural killer cells. While IL-2 has been studied in combination with a variety of other modes of immunotherapy, including use of lymphokine-activated killer (LAK) cells or tumor-infiltrating lymphocytes, the efficacy of these combinations is not superior to that of IL-2 alone. Responses to high-dose IL-2 are observed in 15–25% of patients. Additionally, a unique feature of IL-2 is the 8–10% durable complete remission rate. These remissions may translate into cure for a highly selected group of patients. The toxicity of IL-2 therapy is substantial and requires careful screening of potential candidates to minimize the incidence of fatal toxicity. Fever, chills, hypotension, and capillary leak syndrome occur with therapy with high-dose IL-2. Treatment frequently requires the use of an intensive care unit because hypotension is severe, often requiring pressor support. Patients with brain or spinal cord metastases should not be treated with IL-2 because of peritumoral edema, and patients with renal, pulmonary, or coronary artery disease are ineligible because of the risks of azotemia, respiratory distress, and myocardial ischemia, respectively. Patients who have been treated with IL-2 have an increased risk of infection, particularly staphylococcal infections.

Although the toxicities of IL-2 are considerable, selected patients may be cured with this form of immunotherapy. The use of low-dose subcutaneous injections of IL-2 has been explored, and several trials have reported encouraging results. Combination regimens such as (1) IL-2 plus interferon-alpha or (2) 5-fluorouracil or FUdR plus interferon-alpha or IL-2 also show some promise. Other biologic response modifiers that may be less toxic than IL-2, including autolymphocyte therapy and vaccines, are currently being tested.

Despite strong opinions on both sides of the issue, it is not known whether patients with metastatic disease benefit from nephrectomy before systemic therapy. Until ongoing cooperative group trials that are addressing this question are completed, pretreatment nephrectomies cannot be advocated other than in a protocol setting.

HORMONE-REFRACTORY PROSTATE CANCER

The systemic therapy of patients with metastatic prostate cancer in whom hormonal therapy has failed has been disappointing. It must be pointed out that 15–30% of patients who have had progressive disease despite therapy with combined androgen blockade have a fall in prostate-specific antigen (PSA) when their antiandrogen is discontinued. This maneuver is mandated, therefore, before initiating other systemic therapy. Furthermore, second-line hormonal maneuvers such as adrenal androgen deprivation with ketoconazole clearly have activity and, particularly in asymptomatic patients, should be considered. As noted previously, the evaluation of responses in patients with bone disease only is difficult at best. The use of the PSA in this setting has been fairly extensively evaluated, and it appears to be a reasonable end-point surrogate. Thus, a brisk and significant (> 50%) fall in PSA appears to be predictive of longer survival for the patient. Despite this fact, it must be borne in mind that the median survival after the diagnosis of hormone-refractory prostate cancer (HRPC) is 40–60 weeks, and no agent or combination of agents has yet been shown to have an impact on overall survival. HRPC remains incurable.

Several agents or combinations of agents show promise in the therapy of HRPC. Not only can a significant decline in PSA be demonstrated in some patients, but also objective responses in patients with soft-tissue disease have been observed. Furthermore, considerable palliation of pain is often possible with chemotherapy in patients in whom narcotics or corticosteroids have failed and irradiation is not an option. Mitoxantrone, an anthracycline with a relatively broad spectrum of activity against human tumors, was recently approved in combination with prednisone for the treatment of progressive HRPC. Twenty-nine percent of those treated with the combination experienced decreased pain, compared with 12% receiving prednisone alone. In addition, there were greater improvements in quality-of-life measures. The toxicity of the treatment was mild in both groups; fewer than 2% of patients had infectious episodes. Median survival for both groups was approximately 1 year. Mitoxantrone has modest albeit definable activity in HRPC, although it probably does not significantly prolong survival.

Estramustine is an oral drug originally developed to target hormonally responsive cancers. However, more recent laboratory studies suggest that estramus-

Table 27–2. Selected chemotherapy regimens used in advanced prostate cancer.

Treatment	n	50% PSA Response (%)
Mitoxantrone + prednisone	80	33
Vinblastine + estramustine	25	46
Etoposide + estramustine	42	57
Etoposide + vinorelbine + estramustine	25	56
Paclitaxel + estramustine	32	58
Docetaxel + estramustine	21	62
Cyclophosphamide + doxorubicin	35	46
Ketoconazole + doxorubicin	38	55

tine probably affects the function of microtubules, structural nuclear proteins, and the nuclear matrix. Because of its effects on microtubules, estramustine in lower doses has been investigated in combination with other antimicrotubule agents such as vinblastine, etoposide, and the taxanes. Most of these studies have reported PSA response rates of 40–60%, and toxicity is generally acceptable.

Regimens other than mitoxantrone-prednisone and estramustine combinations may have utility against HRPC. Most of these programs incorporate doxorubicin or cyclophosphamide into the treatment scheme (Table 27–2).

The above observations suggest that chemotherapy has a palliative role to play in the management of some patients with HRPC. Patients with adequate bone marrow function and performance status but a significant tumor burden or rapidly progressive disease are candidates for cytotoxic treatment, although currently available data do not identify one regimen as superior. Future randomized studies will be necessary to compare these various treatment programs and to determine if improvements in survival can be obtained in addition to symptomatic benefit. Needless to say, because no therapy has a proven survival advantage, all patients with HRPC should be considered candidates for appropriate clinical trials.

REFERENCES

Bajorin DF, Bosl GJ: Bleomycin in germ cell tumor therapy: Not all regimens are created equal. (Editorial.) J Clin Oncol 1997;15:1717.

Beyer J et al: High-dose chemotherapy as salvage treatment in germ cell tumors: A multivariate analysis of prognostic factors. J Clin Oncol 1996;14:2638.

Beyer J et al: Long term survival of patients with recurrent or refractory germ cell tumors after high dose chemotherapy. Cancer 1997;79:161.

Garrow GC, Johnson DH: Treatment of "good risk" metastatic testicular cancer. Semin Oncol 1992;19:159.

Harker WG et al: Cisplatin, methotrexate, and vinblastine (CMV): An effective chemotherapy regimen for metastatic transitional cell carcinoma of the urinary tract. A Northern California Oncology Group study. J Clin Oncol 1985;3:1463.

Hruchesky WJM et al: Circadian-shaped infusions of floxuridine for progressive metastatic renal cell carcinoma. J Clin Oncol 1990;8:1504.

International Germ Cell Cancer Collaborative Group: International Germ Cell Consensus Classification: A prognostic factor-based staging system for metastatic germ cell cancers. J Clin Oncol 1997;15:594.

Kelly WK et al: Prostate-specific antigen as a measure of disease outcome in metastatic hormone-refractory prostate cancer. J Clin Oncol 1993;11:1566.

Oh WK, Kantoff PW: Management of hormone refractory prostate cancer: Current standards and future prospects. J Urol 1998;160:1220.

Parkinson DR, Sznol M: High-dose interleukin-2 in the therapy of metastatic renal cell carcinoma. Semin Oncol 1995;22:61.

Pienta KJ et al: Phase II evaluation of oral estramustine and oral etoposide in hormone refractory adenocarcinoma of the prostate. J Clin Oncol 1994;12:2005.

Pont J et al: Adjuvant chemotherapy for high-risk clinical stage I nonseminomatous testicular germ cell cancer: Long-term results of a prospective trial. J Clin Oncol 1996;14:441.

Small EJ, Srinivas S: The antiandrogen withdrawal syndrome: Experience in a large cohort of unselected patients with advanced prostate cancer. Cancer 1995;76:1428.

Small EJ, Vogelzang NJ. Second-line hormonal therapy for advanced prostate cancer: A shifting paradigm. J Clin Oncol 1997;15:382.

Stadler WM, Vogelzang NJ: Low-dose interleukin-2 in the treatment of metastatic renal cell carcinoma. Semin Oncol 1995;22:67.

Sternberg SN et al: Methotrexate, vinblastine, doxorubicin, and cisplatin for advanced transitional cell carcinoma of the urothelium: Efficacy and patterns of response and relapse. Cancer 1989;64:2448.

Tannock I et al: Chemotherapy with mitoxantrone plus prednisone or prednisone alone for symptomatic hormone-resistant prostate cancer: A Canadian randomized study with palliative end points. J Clin Oncol 1996;14:1756.

Vaughn DJ et al: Paclitaxel plus carboplatin in advanced carcinoma of the urothelium: An active and tolerable outpatient regimen. J Clin Oncol 1998;16:255.

Williams SD et al: Immediate adjuvant chemotherapy versus observation with treatment at relapse in pathologic stage II testicular cancer. N Engl J Med 1987;317:1433.

Williams SD et al: Treatment of disseminated germ cell tumors with cisplatin, bleomycin, and either vinblastine or etoposide. N Engl J Med 1987;316:1435.

Yagoda A, Abi-Rached B, Petrylak D: Chemotherapy for advanced renal cell carcinoma: 1983–1993. Semin Oncol 1995;22:42.

28

Radiotherapy of Urologic Tumors

Joycelyn L. Speight, MD, PhD, and Mack Roach III, MD

The primary management of genitourologic malignant diseases has been tied to the use of radiation for more than 100 years. In 1895 Roentgen described x-rays; by 1899 a patient with skin cancer was cured with radiation; and within 10 years, radiation was used to treat prostate cancer (Perez, 1998). Radiotherapy became a mainstay of treatment for bladder and testicular cancers and later prostate cancer as supervoltage sources became available. Although chemotherapy and aggressive surgery have supplanted some of the uses of radiotherapy in urologic cancers, radiation continues to play a major role in the management of carcinomas of the penis, urethra, prostate, and bladder. In this chapter we review general principles and the indications for using radiation as a component in the primary management of urologic malignant diseases. The role of radiation as an agent of palliation has been well documented elsewhere and is excluded from this review. Because of the paucity of prospective randomized trials, many of the conclusions reflect the authors' evaluation of phase II data.

GENERAL PRINCIPLES OF RADIOTHERAPY

Mechanisms of Cytotoxicity

The effects of radiation on tumor and surrounding normal tissues are thought to be mediated primarily through the induction of unrepaired double-strand breaks in DNA (Hall, 1988). It is believed that approximately two-thirds of the biologic effects are due to an indirect action via water free radicals and that such action may be modified by chemical sensitizers or protectors. Excited electron species generated in the presence of oxygen form peroxide radicals, which fix chemical lesions and result in the generation of either repairable or nonrepairable DNA double-strand breaks. The other one-third of biological effects are generated via direct electron damage to DNA. High linear energy transfer radiation (including neurons and heavy-charged particles) is associated with less DNA damage repair and directly induced DNA damage. Classically, the expression of

radiation damage is not seen until the target cells enter mitosis (Thames, Peters, and Ang, 1989). Differentiated normal tissues with low mitotic activity, such as the heart and spinal cord, tend to express the effects of radiation much later than cells from more kinetically active tissues, such as the epithelial cells lining the rectum, bladder, or urethra. However, differentiated normal tissues with low mitotic activity are more sensitive to the use of high dose per fraction or high linear energy transfer radiotherapy. In organs in which the functional stromal cells are postmitotic, such as muscle cells and neurons, the damage is expressed by slowly dividing support cells such as endothelial cells.

In addition to the classic mechanism described above, radiation has been shown to induce programmed cell death (apoptosis) (Allan, 1992). Of particular interest is the study by Sklar (1993), which documented that androgen-independent human prostate cancer cells activate a genetic program of apoptotic cell death in response to exposure to ionizing radiation, in a dose-dependent fashion. Results from Zietman et al (1997) suggest that it is better to achieve maximal androgen suppression before starting radiation treatment.

Radiation Sensitivity & Tolerance

Table 28–1 summarizes the classic radiation tolerances that have been assigned to the normal tissues of interest during conventional fractionated radiotherapy for tumors arising from the urinary tract (Rubin, Constine, and Williams, 1998). The term **conventional fractionation** generally refers to the delivery of single daily doses of from 180 cGy (1.8 Gy) to 200 cGy (2.0 Gy). The gray unit is equal to 100 rads. When used alone, cumulative doses of at least 65 Gy are necessary for local control of gross disease (adenocarcinomas, transitional cell carcinomas, and squamous carcinomas) arising from the prostate, bladder, urethra, or ureters. When used prophylactically for presumed microscopic disease (lymph nodes) or postoperatively,

Table 28–1. Whole-organ radiation tolerances for fractionated radiotherapy of urologic tumors.

Organ	TD5/5[a] (cGy)	TD5/50[b] (cGy)	Clinical End Point
Testes	100	200	Sterility
Kidney	2000	3000	Nephrosclerosis
Intestine	5000	6000	Ulcer
Colon	5500	6500	Ulcer
Bladder	6500	7500	Ulcer
Rectum	6000	8000	Ulcer
Urethra	6500	8000	Stricture

Modified from Rubin P, Constine LS, Nelson DF: Late effects of cancer treatment: Radiation and drug toxicity. In: Perez CA, Brady LW (editors): *Principles and Practice of Radiation Oncology,* 3rd ed. Lippincott-Raven, 1998.
[a]TD 5/5 = the dose associated with a 5% risk for the occurrence of the clinical end point noted at 5 years.
[b]TD 5/50 = the dose associated with a 50% risk for the occurrence of the clinical end point noted at 5 years.

doses of 45–50 Gy are generally sufficient. For testicular seminomas, doses of 25 Gy are usually adequate.

Total dose, dose per fraction, and volume of normal tissue irradiated are the major risk factors for radiation-induced complications. The presence of a number of comorbid conditions such as previous surgery, diabetes, inflammatory bowel diseases, or old age are also associated with an increased risk of radiation-induced complications. Accurate estimates of the "true tolerance" of surrounding normal tissues have been hampered until recently by our inability to reconstruct the actual relationship between normal tissue doses and volumes in 3 dimensions. Early reports assumed that organ movement and day-to-day treatment setup error had an insignificant impact on the doses of radiation delivered to surrounding normal tissues. Recent studies have demonstrated that these assumptions are inaccurate and probably result in an underestimate of the true tolerance of surrounding normal tissues to radiation (Ten Haken et al, 1991; Rosenthal et al, 1993).

A method of calculating complication probabilities for inhomogeneously irradiated tissues, such as occurs in 3-dimensional conformal radiation therapy (3-DCRT), has been popularized at Memorial Sloan Kettering Cancer Center (Kutcher et al, 1991; Lyman and Wolbarst, 1987). These probabilities provide a means to make a comparison of the relative toxicity associated with different treatment plans. When used in conjunction with isodose distributions and dose-volume histograms, this method may allow a relative evaluation of the risk of normal tissue toxicity associated with a particular treatment plan. An alternative method has been proposed by Roach et al (1996). The critical volume tolerance method uses known tolerance levels as an end point and is based on the theory that each type of normal body tissue toxicity occurs when a critical dose-volume relationship is exceeded. The critical volume is the smallest volume of the dose-limiting tissue that can receive a dose without unacceptable toxicity.

Dose per Fraction Considerations

The impact of dose per fraction on chronic genitourinary toxicity is probably more critical than the total dose, volume, or time (Rubin and Cassert, 1968). The nominal standard dose equation of Ellis (1969) represented an early attempt to provide practical quantitative guidelines for adjusting total dose for time, fraction size, and normal tissue tolerance. More recently, the linear quadratic equation (L-Q equation) has been adopted by many clinical investigators as the most useful model for comparing various dose and fractionation schemes (Fowler, 1984). This equation can be written as follows:

$$\text{Effect} = E = n(\alpha d + \beta d), \text{ where } d = \text{Dose per fraction}$$
$$\alpha = \text{Nonrepairable effects}$$
$$\beta = \text{Repairable effects}$$
$$n = \text{Number of identical fractions}$$

For comparing 2 different fractionation schemes, assuming a similar overall treatment time, the L-Q equation also can be written as follows:

$$D_2/D_1 = (1 + d_1 \beta/\alpha)/(1 + d_2\beta/\alpha)$$
$$D = \text{Total dose and } D_1 = n_1 d_1$$
$$d = \text{Dose/fraction}$$

For most clinical circumstances, it is assumed that the α/β ratio for late-reacting normal tissues such as the bladder or rectum is 3. For early-responding normal tissues and for tumor, it is assumed that the α/β ratio is 10.

Altered Fractionation Schedules

Radiobiologic modeling using the α/β ratios as described previously has been used to develop "altered fractionation schedules" to improve the therapeutic ratio between efficacy and toxicity. **Accelerated hyperfractionation** is the most frequently used altered fractionation schedule. With accelerated hyperfractionation, more than one treatment is given per day with a minimum of 6 h between treatments, using a decreased dose per fraction. Overall, the total treatment dose is increased and the treatment time is reduced. The objective of this treatment is to reduce tumor repopulation. Since most radiation-induced damage is repaired within 6 h, the use of multiple treatments per day in theory should allow greater doses of radiation to be given over a shorter period of time, reducing the opportunity for tumor repopulation. Using α/β modeling, the late effects predicted using 1.2 Gy fractions twice daily (separated by 6 h) to 69.6 Gy would be expected to be equivalent to those using conventional fractionation to 58 Gy. In contrast, early-responding tissues such as the epithelium of the bladder would be expected to respond as though they had been treated with a dose of 65 Gy using conventional fractionation. This model predicts an increase in acute effects, including tumor response, but a decrease in late effects, such as fibrosis.

Hypofractionation involves the use of larger than conventional fraction sizes. Using α/β modeling, a fractionation scheme using 3.0-Gy fractions would require a dose reduction to 51 Gy to yield similar late effects. This would result in an effect on early-responding tissues and tumor equivalent to 55 Gy by conventional fractionation. Such an approach results in nearly a 10% reduction in the total dose to the tumor without sparing late complications (assuming that the values chosen for the α/β ratio are correct for normal tissues and for tumors).

Clinical use of altered fractionation schemes in the management of urologic tumors has been limited (Vanuystel et al, 1986; Forman et al, 1993; Edsmyr et al, 1985). Preliminary results with hyperfractionation for prostate tumors have been mixed (Vanuystel et al, 1986; Forman et al, 1993). In the series by Vanuystel and colleagues, rectal complications appeared to be more frequent than expected; however, the interfraction time interval was probably insufficient to allow full repair of radiation-induced damage to surrounding normal tissues. In a more recent series from Wayne State University, acceptable toxicity was reported among the first 20 patients treated with 1.3 Gy twice daily to 78 Gy (Forman et al, 1993). In a prospective randomized trial, hyperfractionated radiotherapy resulted in an improvement in survival for patients with bladder cancer (Edsmyr et al, 1985).

Brachytherapy

The term **brachytherapy** refers to a treatment technique that places radioactive sources in close proximity to or directly into the tumor. Brachytherapy can be classified as either interstitial or intracavity. Interstitial brachytherapy involves the placement of radioactive needles, afterloaded needles or catheters, or radioac-

tive seeds directly into the prostate, bladder, penis, or periurethral soft tissues. Intracavitary brachytherapy includes placement of radioactive catheters into a lumen or orifice such as in the urethra to treat urethral and penile tumors. Seeds are used for permanent implants, while needles or catheters are used for temporary implants. High dose rate brachytherapy refers to the delivery of moderately high doses of radiation over a relatively short period of time (minutes). High dose rate brachytherapy is usually delivered over 2 or more treatment sessions to reduce the risk of late complications. Low dose rate brachytherapy is usually delivered in a continuous fashion over days to weeks via temporary or permanent implants, respectively. Figure 28–1 depicts an example of a transrectal ultrasound-based iodine-125 permanent interstitial implant of the prostate. Figure 28–2 shows an example of intracavitary brachytherapy for a urethral tumor in a female patient.

SPECIFIC UROLOGIC SITES

Prostate Cancer

A. Conventional Treatment: Conventional external-beam irradiation (XRT) has been used in this country for treating prostate cancer for more than 25 years (Bagshaw, Cox, and Ray, 1988). In the 1970s and 1980s, definitive prostate radiation was delivered to the whole pelvis by using the "4-field box" technique, followed by a "cone down" prostate boost, popularized by Bagshaw and coworkers from Stanford University. The placement of the treatment fields was based on bony anatomic landmarks, but this technique resulted in inadequate coverage of the target volume in nearly one-third of patients. Computed tomography (CT) and retrograde urethrography have improved our ability to localize and reconstruct pelvic anatomy, allowing more accurate design of treatment portals (Perez, 1998; Roach et al, 1993a; Ten-Haken et al, 1991).

A number of retrospective and prospective studies support the efficacy of radiation therapy in the management of localized prostate cancer (Bagshaw, Cox, and Ray, 1988; Leibel, Hanks, and Kramer, 1984). Based on these studies, the local control rate following XRT has been estimated to be between 70% and 90%. The end points of these studies were based primarily on a clinical assessment of "local control." These end points are now known to underestimate the true incidence of local failures because of the presence of occult cancer in clinically controlled patients. Many patients once thought to be controlled locally, according to physical examination, do in fact have persistent disease when assessed by prostate-specific antigen (PSA) or biopsy, or both. Table 28–2 summarizes the incidence of positive biopsies following XRT, reported in selected series. Although the post-treatment PSA is more sensitive, it is a less

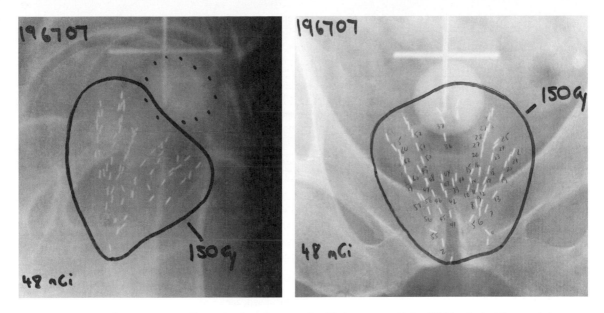

Figure 28–1. Brachytherapy. Example of an ultrasound-guided permanent interstitial implant of the prostate.

specific end point for treatment failure than is biopsy, because distant failures can contribute to a rising level (Crook et al, 1993). PSA has been accepted as a valid end point for the assessment of disease status, but it has not been validated as a predictor of disease-specific survival (DSS).

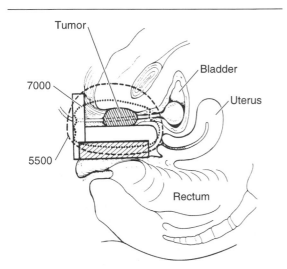

Figure 28–2. Example of intraluminal brachytherapy for urethral cancer. (Reproduced with permission from Sailer SL, Shipley WU, Wang CC: Carcinoma of the female urethra: A review of results with radiation therapy. J Urol 1988;140:1.)

Tables 28–3 and 28–4 summarize patient characteristics and treatment outcomes for selected surgical and conventional radiotherapy series. It should be kept in mind, however, that patients treated with surgery tend to have lower Gleason scores and T stages, and many surgical series excluded lymph node-positive patients. When matched for pretreatment PSA, freedom from biochemical relapse at 5 years is not significantly different, suggesting similar efficacy for surgery and XRT in the management of prostate cancer. There is a trend, however, for surgically treated patients to have a slightly higher freedom from biochemical failure. This could be explained in part by the better parameters for surgical patients at the outset.

One shortcoming of the previous comparison is that there are different definitions of biochemical failure following surgery and radiotherapy. Furthermore, contemporary series use stricter definitions of PSA failure than earlier series did. The radiotherapy series included in Table 28–5 used a definition of PSA failure that was more rigorous than the Consensus Conference definition, which requires 3 consecutive PSA increases as the most reliable indicator of biochemical failure (Horowitz et al, 1995; ASTRO Consensus Statement, 1997).

Some of the factors contributing to the risk of local failure following XRT are summarized in Table 28–6. Recent studies have demonstrated that traditional techniques were associated with inadequate coverage of the target volume in 20 to 41% of patients treated (Ten Haken et al, 1989, 1991; Roach et al, 1993a). Early series also routinely used total

Table 28–2. Incidence of positive biopsy results after external-beam irradiation in selected series.

First Author (y)	Stages (%) (A/B1/B2/C)	Positive Biopsies (%)	Comments
Nachtsheim (1978)	10/24/66	52[a]	How were patients selected?
Leach (1982)	11/7/14/68	About 65	Local control = 96%, but 10-y NED survival is about 57%; + Bx makes no difference.
Cox (1983)	0/0/100	About 19[b]	+ Bx makes no difference.
Freiha (1984)	2/3/47/48	61[a] (0–74)	89% positive if abnormal exam.
Schellhammer (1987)	10/6/51/34	33[b] (25–41)	+ Bx predictive for local and distant failure.
Scardino (1988)	16/40/18/26	32	+ Bx predictive for local failure.
Kabalin (1989)	11/11/44/22 (11% stage D)	93	How were patients selected?
Dugan (1991)	0/0/0/100	38[c]	Patients without clinical evidence of recurrent disease.
Crook (1993)	19/24/36/21	21	100 consecutive patients.

Modified and reproduced, with permission, from Scardino PT, Wheeler TM: Local control of prostate cancer with radiotherapy: Frequency and prognostic significance of positive results of postirradiation prostate biopsy. NCI Monogr 1988;7:95.
NED, no evidence of disease.
[a]At 18 months or longer.
[b]At 15–18 months.
[c]At longer than 1 year, more than 24 months post-treatment, and without endocrine therapy.

doses in the range of 65 to 70 Gy because it was believed that this dose was sufficient and close to the maximum dose allowable by the surrounding normal tissues (Hanks, Martz, and Diamond, 1988). Further contributing to the data regarding biochemical relapse is the fact that many of the patients had disease that was underestimated by physical examination, so they were incurable at the time of diagnosis (Partin et al, 1993b; Roach et al, 1994c).

An analysis of the long-term results from approximately 1500 men treated with XRT alone between 1980 and 1992 in one of 4 phase III randomized trails conducted by the Radiation Therapy Oncology Group (RTOG) has been completed (Roach et al, 1999). In a more recent multivariate analysis, Gleason score, clinical stage, and pathologic node status were correlated with overall survival and DSS. By combining patient groups with similar risk for DSS, 4 distinct prognostic subgroups have been defined with varying risk of death due to prostate cancer (Roach et al, 1998). Table 28–7 summarizes the 5-, 10-, and 15-year DSS for each subgroup. These results are likely to be among the most reliable for assessing the impact of XRT alone on DSS, and thus a guideline for treatment recommendations. These outcome data are likely to represent a worst-case scenario, since the vast majority of these patients were treated before PSA screening. In addition, the patients for whom PSA levels were available had levels in the range of 20 to 30 ng/mL. Classifying patients into one of these prognostic subgroups at diagnosis should reduce the likelihood that underestimating the extent of disease will be a major problem.

Table 28–8 summarizes the results of 3 randomized trials comparing the outcome for patients treated with XRT plus total androgen blockade versus treatment with XRT alone. These studies suggest a survival benefit for patients with high-risk disease (groups 3 and 4) who are treated with long-term adjuvant hormone therapy. The induction of apoptosis by ionizing radiation may be the biological basis of the synergism between radiation and androgen ablation, which induces apoptosis through a different mechanism. The combination of total androgen suppression and radiation then results in a dual mechanism of cell killing. It seems reasonable that this would lead to enhanced cell killing in a heterogeneous tumor population containing both androgen-dependent and androgen-independent cells. In turn, it would lead to the improved outcome seen in certain groups of patients who are treated with radiation and hormonal therapy.

B. Three-Dimensional Conformal Radiotherapy: The technical problems mentioned in Table 28–6 have been addressed in a number of centers by the use of CT-assisted localization and reconstruction of the pelvic anatomy. 3-DCRT is a sophisticated approach for delivering high doses of radiation that conform to the target volume of interest while sparing more of the surrounding normal tissues than is possible using conventional techniques (Roach, Pickett, and Phillips, 1993; Vijayakumar et al, 1993; Sandler et al, 1993; Soffen et al, 1991; Roach et al, 1993b; Roach, Rosenthal, and Hunter, 1993; Leibel et al, 1994a,b). Figure 28–3 is an example of a lateral simulation used to deliver 3-DCRT. Figure 28–4 is a computer generated solid surface reconstruction of the left lateral field. The dose distribution associated with this technique is shown in Figure 28–5, and a dose-volume histogram comparing the advantages of this technique

Table 28–3. Surgical series: Pathologic stage and outcome.

Series	Patients, n (%)		PSA NED, % (5/10 y)	Clinical NED, % (5/10 y)	10-y Cause-Specific Survival
Partin et al (1993a) Johns Hopkins	770				
Organ confined	356	(37)	97/85		
Focal capsular penetration	194	(20)	90/82		
ECE, low grade (< 7)	189	(20)	88/54		
ECE, high grade (≥ 7)	79	(8)	68/42		
Seminal vesicle involvement	66	(7)	47/43		
Lymph node involvement	71	(8)	15/0		
Stein et al (1992b) UCLA	230[a]		75/40		91
Confined	115	(50)	91/85	87.5	96
+ Capsule	82	(36)	79/62	62.5	90
+ Seminal vesicles	33	(14)	≤ 58/[b]	60.0	≤ 63[b]
Trapasso et al (1994) UCLA	601[a]		86/[c]	93 vs 78	98/94
Organ confined	293	(49)	92/	(Post- vs	99
Capsule or margin involvement	215	(36)	74/	pre-1987)	91
+ Seminal vesicles[b]	93	(15)	56/		89
Catalona and Smith (1994) Washington Univ.	925		[d]		
Organ confined	590	(64)	91/71		
+ Margins or ECE	227	(25)	73/58		
Seminal vesicle involvement	86	(9)	32/< 20		
Lymph node involvement	22	(2)	0/0		
Zietman et al (1994) Mass. General Hosp. & Boston Univ.	62		[e]		
Organ confined	30	(48)	75/		
Specimen confined	36	(58)	65/		
+ Margins	26	(42)	25/		
Seminal vesicles involved	12	(19)	0/		
Zincke et al (1994) Mayo Clinic	3170		70/52[f]		
Organ confined	1497	(47)			
ECE	1339	(42)			
+ Margins	770	(24)			
Seminal vesicle involvement	NS				
Lymph node involvement	334	(11)			
Paulson (1994) Duke	895		613[a, g]		
Organ confined	451	(50)	85/72	95/80	90
Specimen confined	219	(25)	50/40	80/70	90
+ Margins	225	(25)	45/36	63/49	65
Seminal vesicle involvement	NS				
Lymph node involvement	39	(4)			
D'Amico et al (1995) Univ. of Penn.	327		[f/h]		
Organ confined	199	(61)	< 90/		
ECE	121	(37)			
Established			< 70/		
Micro			< 90/		
+ Margins	98	(30)	< 50/		
Seminal vesicle involvement	36	(11)	< 10/		
Lymph node involvement	Excluded		—		

Reproduced from Roach and Wallner (1998).
ECE = Extracapsular extension; NED = no evidence of disease; NS = not specified; PSA = prostate-specific antigen.
[a]Excludes node-positive patients.
[b]Excludes patients with longer follow-up and excludes patients with detectable PSA postoperatively.
[c]PSA > 0.4 ng/mL.
[d]PSA > 0.6 ng/mL.
[e]"Undetectable" by Yang assay.
[f]PSA failure > 0.2 ng/mL.
[g]PSA > 0.5 ng/mL.
[h]Estimates at 30 mo.

over a standard technique is shown in Figure 28–6. Compared with a standard technique (using a 4-field box and a bilateral arc boost), 3-DCRT is associated with nearly a 30% reduction in the dose received by 50% of the rectum (Roach, Pickett, and Phillips, 1993). The advantages provided by using improved imaging modality and treatment planning have resulted in the adoption of 3-DCRT by major centers as the new standard of care (Leibel et al, 1994a,b; Roach et al, 1994a,b; Sandler et al, 1992; Vijayakumar et al,

Table 28–4. Selected conventional radiotherapy series and outcome by clinical stage.

Series	Patients, n (%)	PSA NED, % (5/10 y)	Clinical NED, % (5/10 y)	10-y Cause-Specific Survival
Kaplan, Cox, and Bagshaw (1993) Stanford	117	[a]		
T1	44 (38)	≈ 48/—	≈ 75/—	
T2	35 (30)	≈ 60/—	≈ 70/—	
T3–4	37 (31)	≈ 15/—	≈ 20/—	
Stamey, Ferrari, and Schmid (1993) Stanford	113	20[b]		
T1	14 (12)	—/43		
T2	49 (43)	—/20		
T3	33 (29)	—/21		
N1	17 (15)	0		
Schellhammer et al (1993) Eastern Virginia[c]	311			
T1	40 (13)	65/35	75/65	
T2a	29 (9)	42/20	60/40	
T2b	112 (36)	50/20	60/35	
T3	130 (42)	30/10	40/25	
Hanks et al (1994) Fox Chase	39	/≈ 38 +[c,d]	—/72	
T1b	—	or	—	
T2a	—	26 +	—	
T2b	—	(< 1.5 ng/mL)	—	
Hancock et al (1994) Stanford	110	[e]		
T1	—	72.2		
T2	—	37.3		
T3	—	28.1		
T4/N1	—	11.1		
Zagars and Pollack (1995) MD Anderson[f]	269		87/70	
T1a	18 (7)	—		
T1b	57 (21)	—		
T1c	47 (18)	—		
T2a	42 (16)	—		
T2b	81 (30)	—		
T2c	24 (9)	—		
Kuban et al (1995) Eastern Virginia	395	[c]		
T1b	27 (7)	72/35	82/66	93
T2a	60 (15)	63/18	79/57	83
T2b/2c	62 (17)	60/21	73/48	78
T3/4	246 (62)	34/11	47/29	50
Zietman et al (1995) Mass Gen. Hosp.	1044	[g]		
T1–T2a	220 (21)	66/47		
T2b–c	284 (27)	51/29		
T3–4	540 (52)	42/18		
Roach et al (1996a)	490	[a]		
T1b–c	90 (18)	60/—		
T2	272 (56)	50/—		
T3–4	128 (26)	30/—		

Reproduced from Roach and Wallner (1998).
NED = no evidence of disease; PSA = prostate-specific antigen.
[a]At 4 years.
[b]9 years' average duration of follow-up.
[c]PSA failure defined as > 4 ng/mL.
[d]9 to 13 years.
[e]12.4 years' average duration of follow-up.
[f]PSA rising.
[g]PSA > 1 ng/mL.

1991). Because 3-DCRT methods administer radiation to smaller volumes of normal tissue, they have the benefit of decreased side effects. This may in turn permit increased doses of radiation to be given and theoretically lead to improved local control. Data from the Fox Chase Cancer Center, University of California–San Francisco, Memorial Sloan Kettering Cancer Center, and MD Anderson Cancer Center suggest that PSA responses improve with the use of higher doses of radiation in some subsets of patients (Hanks et al, 1996a; Roach et al, 1996a,b; Zelefsky et al, 1998; Pollack and Zagars, 1997) (Table 28–9). Early results from these studies suggest that 10% increases in dose may improve local control rates by as much as 20%.

Table 28–5. Biochemical failure from selected surgical or radiotherapy series.

Pretreatment PSA	Surgical Aver. % (range)[a]	XRT Aver. % (range)[b]	Surgical b-NED 5 y[a]	XRT b-NED 5 y[b]	Comment
0–4	26 (15–43)	21 (11–33)	85–95	80–86	Patients treated with surgery usually
4.1–10	41 (35–52)	30 (27–32)	55–93	42–67	were not node-positive and tended to
10–20	26 (16–32)	21 (18–22)	56	30–75	have lower-grade and lower-stage
> 20	13 (6–20)	35 (18–50)	—	45	tumors than those treated with XRT.

Modified from Roach and Wallner (1998).
b-NED = no evidence of disease based on biochemical failure; PSA = prostate-specific antigen; XRT = external-beam radiotherapy.
[a]Most series exclude node-positive patients and PSA failures > 0.2–0.6.
[b]Clinical staging includes only node-positive and T3–T4 patients and PSA failures > 1.0–4.0 or rising.

The ability to administer higher radiation doses is limited by normal tissue toxicity. Table 28–10 summarizes some recent prospective trials examining dose escalation. Two prospective randomized studies have demonstrated no difference in acute toxicity in patients with localized disease who were treated with 3-DCRT versus conventional radiotherapy (Tait et al, 1997; Pollack et al, 1996). More important, in follow-up studies to these 2 trials, chronic rectal toxicity was reduced in patients treated with conformal radiotherapy. Of note is the fact that in the MD Anderson study, higher doses were given to the patients receiving 3-DCRT (78 Gy versus 70 Gy) (Dearnaley et al, 1999; Nguyen, Pollack, and Zagars, 1998). No significant difference in local control or overall survival has been seen so far, but the follow-up is short. Currently, a phase I/II RTOG dose-escalation trial is under way to determine the maximum tolerated dose of radiation that can be delivered to the prostate gland and surrounding tissues using 3-DCRT. Preliminary results show lower than expected late toxicity compared with historical experience, which suggests that

Table 28–6. Issues in risk of local failure following external-beam irradiation.

Explanations for the high local failure rate:
1. Inadequate target definitions.
   a. Field sizes too small or inferior border too high.
   b. Seminal vesicles not covered.
2. Inadequate doses of radiation.
   a. Doses limited by the belief that 65–70 Gy is sufficient for cure.
   b. Dose limited by technical difficulties and normal tissue tolerances.
3. Understanding of patients: patients with metastatic disease.

Solutions for the problems discussed:
1. Adequate target definitions: field designed conformally using 3-dimensional reconstructions of CT-based tumor volumes and urethrograms.
2. Adequate dose: higher doses of radiation to improve local control rate.
3. Better prestaging of patients: use of pretreatment PSA and Gleason score.

Ct = computed tomography; PSA = prostate-specific antigen.

the administration of doses approaching 8000 cGy is feasible (Michalski et al, 1998).

C. Brachytherapy: Alternative forms of radiation for the treatment of prostate cancer are growing in popularity. The most common of these alternative forms of radiation is brachytherapy. The major theoretic advantages of this form of radiation are the ability to deliver a very high dose of radiation to a localized area and a decreased number of treatment visits. The use of modern-era imaging techniques for visualizing the placement of radioactive seeds has obviated the need for open surgical procedures. Recent series have used CT or transrectal ultrasound-guided closed techniques (Fuks et al, 1991; Gottesman et al, 1991; Kuban, El-Mahdi, and Schellhammer, 1989; Patel et al, 1990; Marinelli et al, 1992; Wallner et al, 1993). In the 1980s a transrectal ultrasound-guided approach was adopted and refined by Blasko and colleagues at the Northwest Tumor Institute in Seattle (Blasko, Ragde, and Schumacher, 1987). They have reported higher post-treatment potency rates, reduced urinary complications and costs, and greater convenience compared with surgery (Blasko, Grimm, and Ragde, 1993). Permanent implants usually involve lower dose rates and a higher total dose. An example of an ultrasound-based iodine-125 permanent seed implant of the prostate, performed at our institution, is shown in Figure 28–1.

The failure rates reported in a number of older studies suggested that the permanent implants are less effective than XRT. More recent series suggest that the results of permanent implants may be improved with the use of either transrectal ultrasound- or CT-based guidance (Wallner et al, 1993). Table 28–11 summarizes 5 studies that compared outcomes in patients treated with seed implants or XRT with or without radical prostatectomy. Four of the studies suggested that low-risk patients (stage ≤ T2a, PSA ≤ 10 ng/mL, GS ≤ 6) treated with seed implants had PSA outcomes that were not statistically different from those treated with XRT. However, intermediate- and high-risk patients (PSA > 10, GS > 7) treated with radical prostatectomy or radiotherapy had better outcomes than those treated with implant alone (Seung et al, 1998; D'Amico et al,

Table 28–7. Disease-specific survival by risk groups: Radiation Therapy Oncology Group randomized trials, radiotherapy alone (1975–1992).

Group[a]	Deaths/No.	5-Year (%)[b]	10-Year (%)[b]	15-Year (%)[b]
1	63/474	97 (95–99)	85 (81–89)	71 (61–81)
2	69/335	91 (88–94)	75 (69–81)	59 (49–69)
3	89/336	82 (78–86)	60 (52–68)	38 (21–55)
4	138/314	66 (60–72)	34 (26–42)	28 (19–37)

Modified from Roach et al (1998).
[a]Group 1 = patients with a Gleason score (GS) = 2–5, any T stage, or T1–2Nx and GS = 6; group 2 = stage T3Nx, GS = 6, or any T stage, N+, GS = 6, or T1–2Nx, Gs = 7; group 3 = T3Nx, GS = 7, or any T stage, N+, GS = 7, or T1–2Nx, GS = 8–10; group 4 = T3Nx, GS = 8–10, or any T stage, N+, GS = 8–10.
[b]95% confidence intervals in parentheses.

1998; Brachman and Beyers, 1998; King et al, 1998; Zelefsky et al, 1999). King et al (1998) found that patients treated with seed implants fared better than those treated with XRT, but the patients treated with XRT in this series were high risk and received only 66 Gy.

Currently at the University of California–San Francisco and most other centers, intermediate- and high-risk patients (groups 3 and 4, Table 28–7) are treated with a combination of XRT and interstitial implant. This practice is supported by the results of Ragde et al (1998). In this retrospective study, the patients at highest risk, as defined by Gleason score, PSA level, and T stage, had slightly better outcomes when treated with XRT and implant than did patients at lower risk who were treated with implant alone. The patients with more aggressive disease would be expected to fare worse. Of note is the fact that there was a trend toward improved 10-year disease-free survival for the higher-risk patients when compared with lower-risk patients (group 2 versus group 1; $P = .09$); overall survival for the two groups was not significantly different (Ragde et al, 1998). Although proponents of prostate brachytherapy commonly believe that the morbidity associated with interstitial brachytherapy is less than that associated with 3-DCRT, the results of the Memorial Sloan Kettering study put this belief into question.

The results of these comparative studies suggest that brachytherapy alone is a reasonable treatment option for low-risk patients with organ-confined disease or with minimal extracapsular extension. Because of the rapid dose fall-off, if brachytherapy is used to treat high-risk patients or those with significant risk of extraprostatic disease, it should be given in conjunction with XRT to ensure adequate coverage of periprostatic tissues for the treatment of microscopic disease.

There has also been increased interest in temporary or high dose rate implants. Temporary implants have the advantage of decreasing radiation exposure to hospital personnel and the ability to compensate for less than optimal needle placement. Temporary implants may be more effective for some patient groups, but they are generally associated with higher morbidity and require hospitalization during the implant. Iridium-192 is the only widely used isotope for temporary prostate implants. Thus far, the number of patients, the number of series, and the duration of follow-up make solid conclusions about the relative merits of high dose rate implants difficult. Based on the available data, there is reason to believe that this treatment approach, in the hands of experts, should be an acceptable treatment option.

D. Neutrons, Protons, and Heavy-Charged Particles: Eradication of tumor by radiation is be-

Table 28–8. Randomized trials: Comparing androgen blockade + XRT versus XRT alone[a]

First Author (Year)	Type of Study	Major Conclusions
Pilepich et al (1998)	Neoadjuvant CAB 2 mo before and during XRT vs XRT alone	8 y experimental vs control: local control, 63% vs 51% ($P = .002$); distant failure, 34% vs 48% ($P = .03$); NED, 35% vs 23% ($P < .002$); survival 51% vs 43% ($P = .22$)
Laverdiere et al (1997)	XRT vs neoadjuvant CAB (3 mo) followed by XRT vs neoadjuvant + adjuvant CAB (10.5 mo) + XRT	Positive biopsy rates at 24 mo: XRT alone 65% vs neoadjuvant 3 mo 30% vs neoadjuvant 3 mo + 6.5 mo = 5%. Follow-up too short to evaluate survival.
Bolla et al (1997)	Phase III EORTC trial comparing neoadjuvant 1 mo, then LHRH 3 y with XRT vs XRT alone	Experimental to control arm: local control 97% vs 77% ($P < .001$); DFS = 85% vs 48% ($P < .001$); overall survival = 79% vs 62%, ($P = .001$).

CAB = combined androgen blockade; XRT = radiotherapy; DFS = disease-free survival; EORTC = European Organization for Research and Treatment of Cancer; LHRH = luteinizing hormone-releasing hormone; NED = no evidence of disease.
[a]Based on data from studies listed.

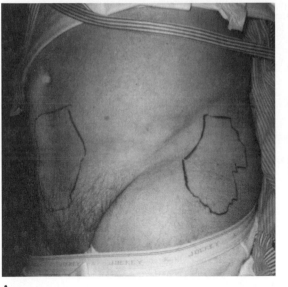

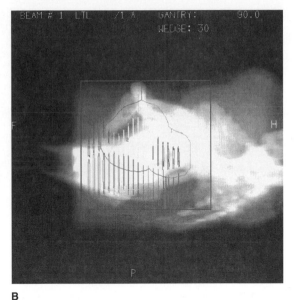

A   B

Figure 28–3. Example of a 7-field conformal external-beam irradiation technique for the treatment of prostate cancer. **A:** View of patient with skin markings. **B:** Verification film with overlay to confirm the location of the femoral heads and pubic symphysis. The prostate and seminal vesicles are also outlined.

lieved to be dose dependent. Unfortunately, the dose beyond which no additional benefit is likely is unknown (Hanks et al, 1985, 1996b, 1997). 3-DCRT has 3 interrelated goals: (1) more accurate tumor targeting, (2) the safe delivery of higher doses of radia-

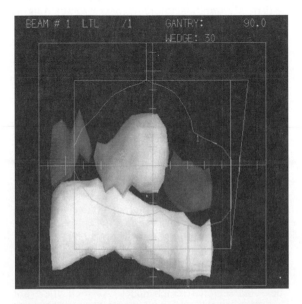

Figure 28–4. Solid surface reconstruction of a left lateral plan showing the rectum, prostate, seminal vesicles, and bulb of the penis.

tion to the tumor, and (3) diminishing of the normal tissue toxicity associated with high-dose radiation. Particle beam radiation is an alternative form of XRT. This class of radiation involves the use of heavy particles (eg, neutrons), charged particles (eg, protons), or heavy-charged particles (eg, neon) (Krieger et al, 1989; Duttenhaver et al, 1983). It is believed that the different physical characteristics and energies will permit the delivery of higher equivalent doses of radiation without increasing toxicity. The theoretic advantage of the use of protons is the more conformal dose distribution associated with this type of radiation (Lee et al, 1984). A prospective randomized trial from Massachusetts General Hospital (Shipley et al, 1995) showed a significant improvement in local control but no improvement in disease-free, relapse-free, or overall survival in patients with high-grade tumors treated with mixed photon and proton beam irradiation. However, there was no benefit to other subsets of patients, and the 5-year actuarial rates of rectal bleeding were significantly higher ($P = .002$) with mixed beam treatment. These outcomes are consistent with observations of a dose response for freedom from biochemical relapse in high-grade prostate cancer reported by other investigators (Roach et al, 1996b; Fiveash et al, 1998; Pollack et al, 1997). Results from Loma Linda University Medical Center showed 4-year freedom from PSA relapse comparable to that for surgery and 3-DCRT and lower toxicity rates than those reported at Massachusetts General Hospital (Rossi et al, 1998).

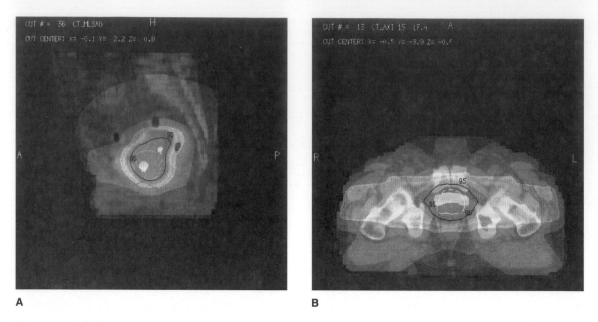

A   B

Figure 28–5. Sagittal (**A**) and axial (**B**) dose distributions superimposed on a computed tomography series from a patient undergoing 7-field conformal radiotherapy.

Closer inspection reveals that the 3-DCRT series used for comparison had the highest reported complication rate among centers performing conformal radiotherapy. However, initial reports from a multi-institutional phase I/II trial (RTOG 9406) have since shown that similar doses can be delivered with 3-DCRT with much lower complication rates (Michalski et al, 1998).

The attractiveness of neutron-based radiotherapy relates to the relative lack of oxygen dependence and resistance to the repair of sublethal radiation-induced damage (Hall, 1988). RTOG 7704 compared outcomes following treatment with high-dose photons versus high-dose photons and neutrons. At 10 years, statistically significant improvement was noted in local control (58% versus 70%; $P = .04$) and overall survival (26% versus 46%; $P = .04$) (Laramore et al, 1993). In a more recent prospective randomized trial reported by Russell et al (1994), fast neutrons were associated with a lower clinical local failure rate and a lower incidence of PSA failures compared with x-ray therapy.

Heavy-charged particles are thought to have the advantages of both neutrons and protons. Early studies using this technology have been encouraging, but the series are small, follow-up is relatively short, and this equipment has limited availability. Longer follow-up studies will be required to assess the impact of these alternative types of radiation on long-term survival.

E. Postoperative Radiotherapy: The objective of postoperative radiotherapy is to improve local-regional control by eliminating microscopic residual tumor in the surgical bed, periprostatic tissues, and regional lymph nodes. As such, there are several indications for the use of adjuvant radiation, including (1) positive surgical margins, (2) seminal vesicle involvement, (3) lymph node involvement,

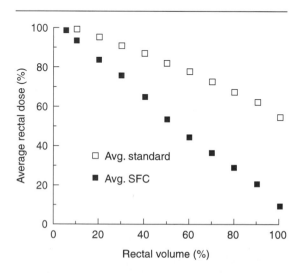

Figure 28–6. The average rectal dose-volume relationships of treatment by a standard technique consisting of a 4-field box plus bilateral 120-degree arc boosts, compared with therapy using a 3-dimensionally based 6-field conformal technique with partial transmission blocks.

Table 28–9. Retrospective studies demonstrating a dose response with radiotherapy.

First Author (Year)	Design	Subgroups	Comments
Hanks (1996a)	Retrospective study from Fox Chase Cancer Center	PSA > 10 ng/mL	Patients treated by means of a 4-field conformal technique.
Roach (1996b)	Retrospective study of 50 patients	Gleason score 8–10	Doses > 71.5 Gy improve outcomes.
Zelefsky (1998)	Retrospective study from Memorial Sloan Kettering	Favorable intermediate- and high-risk groups	Intermediate- and high-risk patients did better with higher doses.
Pollack (1997)	Retrospective study from MD Anderson	Essentially all groups	Dose response better at > 67 Gy.
Fiveash (1998)	Retrospective multi-institutional study	Gleason score 8–10	Higher doses yielded better results for patients with T1–T2.
Lyons (1998)	Retrospective study from Cleveland Clinic	Essentially all groups	Doses > 71.5 Gy associated with better results.

PSA, prostate-specific antigen.

(4) extracapsular extension, (5) increasing PSA, and (6) biopsy-proven recurrence. The presence of any of these variables is associated with a higher incidence of local recurrence (Anscher and Prosnitz, 1991; Ohori et al, 1995; Rogers et al, 1998). Several early series examining the effect of post-prostatectomy radiation suggest that adjuvant XRT appears to reduce the incidence of local recurrence in patients with postsurgical microscopic residual tumor after radical prostatectomy (Anscher, Robertson, and Prosnitz, 1995; Link, Freiha, and Stamey, 1991; Partin et al, 1993a; Schild et al, 1994; Stein et al, 1992a; Voges et al, 1992; Wu et al, 1995; Zietman et al, 1993; Freeman et al, 1993). Patients who are treated before clinically manifesting a local recurrence appear to have improved disease-free survival, time to distant metastasis (Anscher and Prosnitz, 1991; Kaplan and Bagshaw, 1992), and freedom from biochemical relapse compared with patients undergoing salvage treatment. Only 50% of such patients are successfully treated for biopsy-proven recurrence at 3 years (Rogers et al, 1998). The impact of postoperative radiation on survival outcomes remains unproved, but it seems reasonable to assume that patients who have no other disease away from the pelvis would benefit from adjuvant treatment.

Higher complication rates associated with postoperative radiotherapy appear to have been the consequence of older treatment techniques. More contemporary series suggest that, with modern equipment and planning, the incidence of complications is quite low (Presti et al, 1996).

Local treatment to the postresection bed is commonly delivered by using a 4-field box technique, bilateral 120-degree arcs, or more sophisticated techniques such as 3-DCRT (as described for primary treatment). The doses of radiation used typically range from as low as 45 to 68 Gy, depending on the risk of residual disease and the type of treatment chosen. For high-risk patients the standard minimum tumor dose at our center, for recurrences or positive margins, is approximately 70 Gy, with higher doses reserved for the occasional patient with gross recurrent disease.

F. Complications of Radiotherapy for Prostate Cancer: Most patients experience urinary fre-

Table 28–10. Three-dimensional conformal radiotherapy (3-DCRT): Prospective trials.

First Author (Year)	Institution(s)	Type of study	Conclusions
Pollack (1996)	MD Anderson	Single institution, phase III	No differences in acute toxicity
Nguyen (1998)	MD Anderson	Single institution, phase III	Reduced late effects
Tait (1997)	Royal Marsden	Phase III	No differences in acute toxicity
Dearnaley (1999)	Royal Marsden	Phase III	Associated with reduced late rectal complications
Zelefsky (1998)	Memorial Sloan Kettering	Single institution, phase I–II dose escalation	Based on historical controls, better than expected tolerance to higher doses
Michalski (1998)	Radiation Therapy Oncology Group	Multicenter, phase I–II dose escalation	Based on historical controls, better than expected tolerance to higher doses

Table 28–11. Selected series comparing implants with conventional XRT with or without surgery.

First Author (Year)	No. of Patients	Details	Conclusions
Seung (1998)	XRT = 187	Patients treated with XRT from UCSF who were thought to have been candidates for BT compared with literature	Wide range of results overlapping with XRT results.
D'Amico (1998)	BT = 66 XRT = 766 RP = 888	Radical retropubic prostatectomy at University of Penn., XRT at the Joint Center	Outcome was similar for low-risk patients regardless of treatment type; high-risk and intermediate-risk patients did worse with BT.
King (1998)	BT = 63 XRT = 85 RP = 73	Comparison of results from patients with T1/2 disease treated at Yale University	XRT patients did worse than RP or BT. Mean XRT dose 66 Gy, 42% GS ≥ 7 and PSA > 10 in 42% vs 22% and 24%, respectively, for BT and RPN0.
Brachman (1998)	XRT = 933 BT = 669	Retrospective study of patients from one multiphysician practice	Patients with GS ≥ 7 or PSA > 10 ng/mL did significantly better with XRT than BT.
Zelefsky (1998)	XRT = 743 BT = 245	Retrospective single-institution analysis of early-stage patients treated at Memorial Sloan Kettering	Excellent freedom from BcR for XRT and BT. Higher urinary toxicity with BT.

XRT = external-beam Radiotherapy; BT = permanent prostate brachytherapy; RP = radical prostatectomy; BcR = biochemical relapse; PSA = prostate-specific antigen.

quency and dysuria during the course of their treatment. Patients receiving whole-pelvic irradiation may develop mild diarrhea (Roach, Rosenthal, and Hunter, 1993). Mild, self-limited rectal bleeding occurs in approximately 10% of patients and is dose and volume related. Urinary incontinence appears to be related to previous transurethral resection of the prostate. Hematuria and ureteral strictures occur in less than 7% of patients (Rubin, Constine and Williams, 1998; Anscher and Prosnitz, 1991; Shultheiss, Hanks, and Hunt, 1995; Roach, Pickett, and Weil, 1996; Dearnaley et al, 1999; Nguyen, Pollack, and Zagars, 1998). Fecal incontinence is uncommon, but rectal urgency due to reduction in rectal distensibility may occur in 10% of patients (Litwin, 1994).

Loss of erectile function is the most worrisome, the most common, and the most permanent sequela of radiotherapy. Impotence is reported in up to 35 to 40% of patients who were potent before treatment. These rates were previously thought to be lower after brachytherapy than after XRT (DeLaney, Shipley, and O'Leary, 1985; Reddy, Mebust, and Weigel, 1990; Roach and Wallner, 1998). However, more recent data show the 5-year likelihood of post-treatment impotence to be equal for 3-DCRT and iodine-125 implant (Zelefsky et al, 1999). As assessed by self-reported responses, 80% of patients maintain potency at 15 to 20 months after treatment (Chinn, Holland, and Crownover, 1995). However, these patients experience decreased frequency and quality of intercourse, and most note a decrease in the volume of ejaculate. Potency diminishes further with time owing to aging and late radiation-induced normal tissue injury (Roach, Chinn, and Holland, 1996; Chinn, Holland, and Crownover, 1995).

Acute urinary toxicity associated with brachyther-

apy is more common and longer lasting than that seen with 3-DCRT. The incidence of strictures is also higher. Acute obstruction occurs in up to 20% of patients, and incontinence occurs in as many as 50% if they have had a previous transurethral resection of the prostate. The frequency of rectal toxicity is the same as or less than that with 3-DCRT (Zelefsky et al, 1999).

Cancer of the Urinary Bladder

A. Definitive XRT Irradiation: In the United States, surgery is the most frequently used primary treatment for carcinoma of the urinary bladder. Typically, urologists refer for definitive radiotherapy only patients who are poor surgical candidates; therefore, it is not surprising that most retrospective series report lower survival rates for patients treated with radiotherapy than for those treated with surgery. No modern prospective randomized trials comparing definitive radiotherapy with surgery have been completed. In contrast, XRT is the most common definitive primary treatment used initially to treat carcinoma of the urinary bladder in Canada and in Great Britain (Parsons and Zlotecki, 1998).

The Edinburgh series is among the largest to evaluate the efficacy of definitive radiotherapy alone in an unbiased fashion. Based on this series, the complete response rate to definitive XRT alone for all T stages is 45%, and the 5-year local control rate is 25% for T1–T3 and 16% for T4 (Duncan and Quilty, 1986; Quilty et al, 1986). Response and local control rates are higher with high-grade lesions, but the survival rate is lower because of a greater risk of distant metastases (Parsons and Zlotecki, 1998; Duncan and Quilty, 1986; Quilty et al, 1986; Quilty and Duncan, 1986). Several variables appear to influence local control, freedom from distant failure, and survival in patients treated with radiotherapy. In addition to T stage, which defines the depth of tumor invasion, other major prognostic factors that influence complete response rate and survival following radiotherapy include **tumor grade,** pretreatment hemoglobin levels, presence or absence of residual disease following transurethral resection of the bladder, and radiographically detected ureteral obstruction (Parsons and Zlotecki, 1998; Shipley et al, 1987; Cole et al, 1992; Pollack and Zagars, 1996; Quilty and Duncan, 1986). Multivariate analyses from MD Anderson have shown that the most important independent prognostic variable in predicting outcome was a complete response to treatment (Pollack, Zagars and Swanson, 1994; Pollack and Zagars, 1996).

Local-regional control may also depend on treatment duration. Local control is worse for patients treated with split-course radiotherapy. No change in local control rates has been found for patients treated with a continuous course in 44 days or less or in 45–74 days (De Neve, Lybeert, and Goor, 1995). Trials examining alternative fractionation schedules have shown survival benefits at 10 years.

The XRT techniques used to treat bladder cancer are similar to those used for prostate cancer. Definitive treatment usually begins with whole-pelvic irradiation with 15–25 mV x-rays via a 4-field box. The superior border is placed either at the L5-S1 interspace or at the middle of the sacroiliac joint. The inferior border is usually placed at the bottom of the obturator foramen unless there is extension into the prostate, in which case the inferior border may be placed as low as the lower border of the ischial tuberosities. The lateral fields extend to 1.5–2.0 cm beyond the true pelvis. The anterior border is placed just in front of the bladder with margin, and the posterior-lateral border is 2.0–3.0 cm behind the bladder and includes the presacral nodes. A 3-field technique, including an anteroposterior and opposed lateral fields, is occasionally used either initially or for the cone down boost.

The initial portals for patients being treated definitively are generally reduced after 4500–5000 cGy, and the reduced volume is continued to a final dose of 6480–6840 cGy. The final reduced volume is generally designed so that at least a portion of the uninvolved bladder is partially spared the full dose. Patients receiving preoperative radiotherapy are commonly treated to 3000 cGy (over 2 weeks), but doses as low as 2000 cGy (over 1 week) or as high as 4500–5000 cGy are occasionally used (Parsons and Zlotecki, 1998). Radiotherapy alone may be considered for favorable patients, defined as those with papillary tumors, tumors that have been completely resected, and tumors not associated with hydronephrosis. However, because of the numerous studies showing improved outcomes, combined radiation and chemotherapy have replaced radiotherapy alone for bladder-sparing treatment in most centers.

B. Combined Therapy (Chemotherapy and Radiation Therapy): The efficacy of combined chemoradiation for organ preservation in patients with localized disease has been substantiated in several reports. Overall survival is comparable to that for similar-stage patients managed with radical cystectomy. Kaufman et al (1993) reported on 53 patients with T2–T4 lesions treated with chemoradiation in a phase II bladder preservation trial. After complete transurethral resection of tumor, all patients received 2 cycles of cisplatin, methotrexate, and vinblastine with whole-pelvic irradiation to 40 Gy. Complete responders or patients who were not suitable surgical candidates received an additional cycle of cisplatin and a cone down boost, for a total dose of 68.4 Gy. Patients who failed to have a complete response underwent radical cystectomy. At 2 years' median follow-up, 45% of patients were alive without evidence of disease. More than 50% of patients had successful bladder preservation.

The largest reported series using combined modality treatment originated from the University Hospital of Earlangen (Dunst et al, 1994) and showed 5-year overall survival rates comparable to those reported in surgical series. In this series, the volume of residual tumor after transurethral resection was identified as the most important prognostic factor; 5-year overall survival rates in patients with a complete response or microscopic or gross residual tumor were 81%, 53%, and 31%, respectively. An earlier multivariate analysis from Massachusetts General Hospital (Itoku and Stein, 1992) showed that tumor stage and the absence of associated carcinoma in situ are predictive for complete response to treatment. A phase II RTOG trial (8802) also showed that bladder preservation can be achieved in many patients with combined chemoradiation, with survival rates comparable to those seen with historical surgical controls (Tester et al, 1996). However, a more recently completed phase III trial (RTOG 8903) showed no improvement in complete response rates or 5-year actuarial survival rates with neoadjuvant methotrexate/cisplatin/vinblastine chemotherapy when compared with concurrent chemoradiation with single-agent cisplatin (Shipley et al, 1998). The 3-year actuarial survival was 83%, with a 73% chance of being alive with a native bladder (Zietman et al, 1998). Taken together, these data and those from earlier studies (Goodman et al, 1981; Shipley et al, 1985) suggest that concurrent chemoradiation with a cisplatin-based regimen is an acceptable treatment option for *some* patients; neoadjuvant chemotherapy offers no additional benefit. Since only those patients who have a complete response to initial treatment are likely to experience sustained local control, careful patient selection based on prognostic factors is critical to achieve organ preservation without a compromise in survival.

D. Post- and Preoperative Radiotherapy: The value of preoperative radiotherapy followed by surgery is controversial (Parsons and Zlotecki, 1998; Bloom et al, 1982; Goodman et al, 1981; Shipley et al, 1987). Several prospective randomized trials have compared preoperative radiotherapy and surgery with radiotherapy alone. Unfortunately, most of these studies suffered from problems including small sample size, poor-quality radiotherapy, and selection bias. Nonetheless, no apparent survival difference was validated in any of these studies. However, a meta-analysis of the trials suggested a 10% survival advantage for preoperative radiation (Bloom et al, 1982; Sell et al, 1991; Parsons and Zlotecki, 1998; Blackard and Byar, 1972; Anderstrom et al, 1983; Slack, Bross, and Prout, 1977).

In a review article, Parsons and Million (1988) made a strong argument in favor of preoperative radiotherapy. They noted that most studies comparing preoperative radiation and surgery with surgery alone were in fact comparing patients staged clinically (and thus understaged) with patients staged pathologically; such a bias would obscure the benefits resulting from preoperative irradiation. These authors further noted that preoperative radiotherapy resulted in a reduction in T stage and T stage plus N stage in 75 and 50% of patients, respectively. In addition, 30–40% of patients were reported to have no identifiable tumor on pathologic inspection of the surgical specimen. Finally, the authors concluded that preoperative radiation followed by cystectomy was superior to surgery alone (Parsons and Million, 1988, 1989). Figure 28–7 summarizes the results of their analysis. A more recent trial from MD Anderson identified a subset of patients who might benefit from radiotherapy with a decrease in the incidence of

pelvic recurrence. However, no difference in overall survival was seen (Cole et al, 1995).

Postoperative radiotherapy is not a favored approach for managing bladder cancer. The impression of a higher rate of pelvic recurrence (compared with using preoperative irradiation) and a higher incidence of post-treatment complications has tended to discourage investigators from pursuing this approach (Parsons and Zlotecki, 1998).

E. Brachytherapy and Intraoperative Electron-Beam Therapy: Brachytherapy can also be used to manage localized carcinoma of the bladder (Parsons and Zlotecki, 1998; Van der Werf-Messing et al, 1981, 1983; Matsumoto et al, 1981). Van der Werf-Messing pioneered the use of a radium needle implantation–based technique. She reported 5-year bladder relapse rates of 18 and 23% for T1 and T2 lesions, respectively (Van der Werf-Messing et al, 1981, 1983). There is limited experience in the use of intraoperative radiotherapy. Matsumoto et al (1981) reported a 91% local control rate at 5 years when T1 or T2 lesions were treated by electron-beam radiotherapy followed by XRT.

F. Complications: Acute and long-term complications following definitive radiotherapy for carcinoma of the urinary bladder are usually mild (Parsons and Zlotecki, 1998). Acute toxicities include diarrhea and cystitis; nausea is uncommon. Chronic bladder discomfort or dysfunction occurs in approximately 10% of patients. Reduction of the bladder capacity is the major cause of dysfunction. Chronic, moderately severe rectal and small-bowel injuries are reported in 3–4% and 1–2%, respectively, of patients receiving high-dose radiotherapy (Parsons and

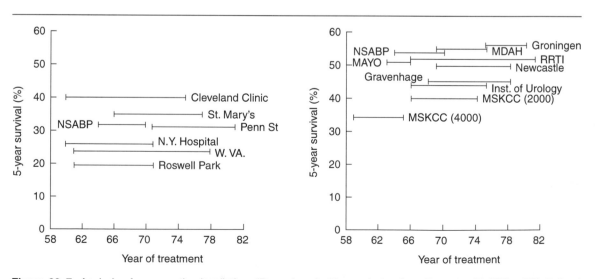

Figure 28–7. Analysis of preoperative irradiation. (Reproduced with permission from Parsons JT, Million RR: Role of planned preoperative irradiation in the management of clinical stage B2-C (T3) bladder carcinoma in the 1980s. Semin Surg Oncol 1989;5:255.)

Zlotecki, 1998). The mortality rate associated with definitive radiotherapy is reported to be approximately 1%.

Testicular Cancer

A. Radiotherapy Treatment: The role of postorchiectomy irradiation of the para-aortic and ipsilateral pelvic lymph nodes in the management of stage I seminoma is widely accepted. Figures 28–8 and 28–9 show the incidence and location of nodal metastases in early-stage left- and right-sided testicular tumors. Because only 15% of patients harbor occult nodal disease, several studies have focused on whether or not nodal irradiation is necessary. Available data from surveillance and adjuvant radiotherapy studies suggest that DSS rates are 97–99% with either management choice, making surveillance appear to be a viable treatment option (Warde et al, 1995, 1997; Miki et al, 1998; Coleman et al, 1998). Prognostic factors for relapse have been identified. They include histology, tunica invasion, small-vessel invasion, spermatic cord involvement, and epididymal involvement. On multivariate analysis, only age ≤ 34 years at diagnosis and tumor size > 6 cm predicted progression on surveillance (Warde et al, 1995; Warde and Gospodarowicz, 1998).

In a recent report on the 15 years' experience at the Royal College of Radiologists, relapse rates for surveillance patients were significantly higher than those for radiation patients (15% versus 4%; *P* < .05). There was, however, no significant difference in survival outcome between groups (Coleman et al, 1998). Over a 5-year follow-up period, surveillance programs are estimated to cost 40% more than postoperative radiotherapy (Sharda, Kinsella, and Ritter, 1996). A course of postoperative surveillance requires close, regular monitoring, with serum marker studies and CT scans at 3- to 6-month intervals. Because of the long natural history of seminoma, both physician and patient must be committed to a course of at least 10–15 years (Coleman et al, 1998). Both the psychological and financial costs of "waiting for something to happen" must be considered.

Doses of 25 Gy are considered to be sufficient for the control of microscopic disease (Thomas, 1990). Higher doses are not associated with an increase in cause-specific survival but are associated with increased normal tissue toxicity (Hamilton et al, 1986; Lai et al, 1994; Thomas, 1985; Zagars and Babaian, 1987; Fossa, Aass, and Kaaluhus, 1989).

Most patients who relapse do so in the retroperitoneum; only 0.5–3% relapse in the pelvis (Thomas, 1985). Preliminary results from a prospective study by Sultanem et al (1998) showed an overall survival rate of 97% and an actuarial DSS rate of 100% in patients treated with postorchiectomy radiation to the para-aortic nodes only. When available, results of cooperative trials from the European Organization for Research

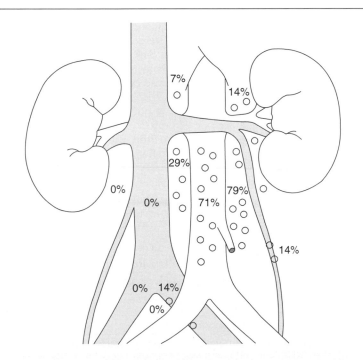

Figure 28–8. Incidence and location of lymph nodes at risk for an early-stage left-sided testicular seminoma. (Adapted from Donohue, JP et al. Distribution of nodal nets in nonseminomatous testis cancer. J Urol 1982;126:315.)

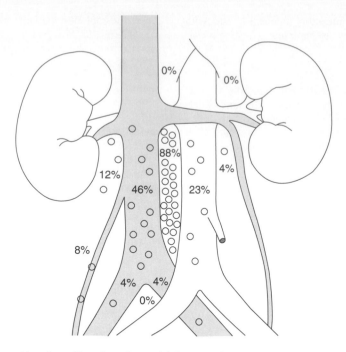

Figure 28–9. Incidence and location of lymph nodes at risk for an early stage right-sided testicular seminoma. (Adapted from Donohue, JP et al. Distribution of nodal nets in nonseminomatous testis cancer. J Urol 1982;126:315.)

and Treatment of Cancer (EORTC) comparing para-aortic radiation only with pelvic plus para-aortic radiation may further confirm these results.

The efficacy of single-agent chemotherapy in the control of advanced-stage disease and the salvage of relapsed patients has prompted the exploration of chemotherapy alone as the initial adjuvant treatment for stage I seminoma. In one such study, at 51 months' follow-up, 99% of patients remained disease free (Oliver et al, 1994). However, the length of follow-up and the limited numbers of series preclude this approach from currently being considered the standard of care.

Management of stages IIA and IIB with radiotherapy is similar to that of stage I. Relapse rates are < 5%, and salvage chemotherapy with cisplatin-containing regimens yield DSS rates of 95–100% (Warde and Gospodarowicz, 1998). In the presence of bulky disease (IIC) and locally advanced disease, chemotherapy is the initial treatment of choice. Relapse rates can be 35% or higher, with DSS rates of 85–90% after chemotherapy salvage (Warde and Gospodarowicz, 1998; Horowich and Dearnaley, 1992).

Prophylactic mediastinal and supraclavicular irradiation is no longer recommended by most authori-

Table 28–12. Summary of radiotherapy guidelines for seminomas.

Stage	Post-XRT Relapses (%)	Recommended Volume Irradiated	Dose Recommended (Gy)
Stage I–IIA (< 2 cm)	2–4	Para-aortic and ipsilateral renal hilar nodes	25
Stage IIB (2–5 cm) (Nonpalpable)	4	Ipsilateral pelvic and para-aortic nodes	25–35
Stage IIC (5–10 cm)	10	(Chemotherapy alone)	25–35
Stage IID (> 10 cm)	50	(Chemotherapy alone)	

Modified and reproduced, with permission, from Rorth BJ et al and the Danish Testicular Cancer Group. Surveillance alone versus radiotherapy after orchiectomy for clinical stage I nonseminomatous testicular cancer. J Clin Oncol 1991; 9:1543.
XRT = external-beam irradiation.

ties (Thomas and Williams, 1998; Rorth et al, 1991). The International Consensus Conference in Leeds in 1989 recommended the omission of inguinoscrotal irradiation, even if scrotal interference has occurred (Thomas and Williams, 1998). A summary of radiotherapy and management guidelines for treating seminomas is shown in Table 28–12.

Several series demonstrated that the administration of adjuvant radiotherapy for nonseminomatous tumors was both highly effective in reducing nodal failures and relatively safe. Although retroperitoneal irradiation prevented retroperitoneal relapse, 15% of stage I patients with nonseminomatous tumors subsequently required chemotherapy because of moderate relapse rates, even for early disease, in other sites (Rorth et al, 1991). Chemotherapy salvage results in long-term survival rates approaching 80–100% for patients with a good or intermediate prognosis (Rorth, 1992). This kind of data plus the limitations that extended-field irradiation places on chemotherapy tolerance led to the discontinuation of prophylactic irradiation for nonseminomatous tumors (Thomas and Williams, 1998).

B. Complications of Radiotherapy: Acute complications associated with low-dose para-aortic irradiation are mild, consisting primarily of nausea and slight skin reddening and a transient reduction in spermatogenesis (Thomas and Williams, 1998). Late complications are uncommon but include impaired contralateral spermatogenesis, second malignancies, and an increased risk of gastrointestinal complications (peptic ulcer disease, hemorrhagic gastritis, intestinal obstruction) (Thomas and Williams, 1998). Fifty percent of men with seminoma have some degree of impaired spermatogenesis before treatment, making the absolute effects of radiation somewhat difficult to assess. Significant though temporary reduction in sperm counts can result from scatter radiation to the contralateral testis. However, fertility is usually restored within 2–3 years after treatment. Careful shielding can reduce the dose to the contralateral testis to 1–2% of the prescribed dose (Shapiro, Kinsella, and Makuch, 1985).

The risk of major gastrointestinal complications appears to be dose related, with an incidence of 0%, 2%, and 6% for < 25 Gy, 25–35 Gy, and 40–45 Gy, respectively (Coia and Hanks, 1988). Some studies have reported that, within the first 10 years after treatment, radiotherapy is associated with a small but measurable increase in the risk of secondary leukemia and solid tumors, primarily in the bladder, lungs, and gastrointestinal tract. Other studies have failed to demonstrate any increase in risk (Chao et al, 1995). A risk ratio of 2.5 for malignancies of the lung and bladder has been reported; it is probably also increased for gastrointestinal primary tumors, but this is less well documented (Thomas and Williams, 1998).

Carcinomas of the Kidney, Renal Pelvis, & Ureter

Surgery is the primary treatment for renal cell carcinoma. Two prospective randomized trials of postoperative radiotherapy did not demonstrate any survival advantage for patients treated with adjuvant radiation. It may be reasonable to use radiotherapy as the initial management in patients who have inoperable tumors or are unsuitable surgical candidates or for treatment of possible surgical margins. Several series suggest that radiotherapy is of value in the postoperative setting for carcinomas of the kidney, particularly when they are high grade and accompanied by invasion beyond the primary tumor into fat or nodes (Brookland and Richter, 1985; Babaian, Johnson, and Chan, 1980; Brady and Manning, 1981).

Retrospective data suggest that radiotherapy may increase local control when used in the adjuvant setting in patients with locally advanced (T3, T4) carcinoma of the renal pelvis or ureter or in lymph node-positive disease (Brookland and Richter, 1985).

Cancer of the Female Urethra

Both XRT and brachytherapy appear to be comparable alternatives to surgical resection of urethral cancers. Early lesions in the distal one-third or anterior urethra may be treated with brachytherapy alone or with combined XRT and interstitial implants. Radiation alone is associated with high local control rates, cure rates of 80–90%, and an overall 5-year survival in excess of 65%. For larger lesions, or lesions that extend into surrounding structures, some authorities recommend that intracavity implantation be preceded by a course of XRT, including prophylactic irradiation of the inguinal, external iliac and the hypogastric nodes (Grigsby, 1998b; Sailer, Shipley, and Wang, 1988). An example of an intracavitary technique for a urethral tumor is shown in Figure 28–2.

Lesions involving the posterior urethra or the entire urethra often extend to the bladder, have a high incidence of nodal development, and are generally managed with preoperative radiotherapy and exenteration. More advanced lesions are associated with a local control rate of 20–30% and a correspondingly low 5-year survival rate (Grigsby, 1998b). Combined treatment with radiotherapy and surgery yields slightly better survival (Klein et al, 1983). Aggressive combined-modality local and regional therapy is indicated for these patients to have any chance of cure. Grigsby (1998a) reported that no patients with a primary lesion greater than 4 cm survived 5 years unless treated with exenterative surgery and radiation. Neoadjuvant combined-modality therapy has been used with favorable early results (Sailer, Shipley, and Wang, 1988; Johnson et al, 1989).

Complications of radiotherapy are common but generally transient. Urethral strictures are the most frequently reported complication. Urinary incontinence, cystitis, and vaginal stenosis occur occasionally, while fistulas and small-bowel obstruction due to radiation or tumor are less common.

Cancer of the Penis & Male Urethra

Surgery is the primary management for penile cancer. Although surgery alone is quite effective, for many men (particularly those who are potent) neither a partial nor a total penectomy is considered a desirable therapeutic choice. No randomized studies comparing surgery with radiation therapy have been completed. The potential for organ preservation with the use of radiation alone and the high rate of successful surgical salvage of radiation failures has led a number of investigators to recommend primary irradiation as a preferred treatment for the early-stage cancers (Sagerman et al, 1984; Krieg and Luk, 1981; Kaushal and Sharma, 1987). As a rule, radiotherapy is not recommended for lesions greater than 4 cm (Chao and Perez, 1998; Almgard and Edsmyr, 1973).

Both XRT and brachytherapy have been used to treat penile lesions. Precancerous lesions and very small lesions can be treated with orthovoltage or low-energy electron beams because both forms of radiation result in a relatively superficial dose distribution. Radioactive molds that are placed over the penis and worn by the patient are best suited for extensive superficial penile lesions. Larger, more penetrating lesions of the shaft of the penis or distal urethra are frequently managed with interstitial implants following XRT. Prophylactic lymph node irradiation for patients with negative nodes but advanced lesions or poorly differentiated lesions is logical but unproved.

Local control rates of 80–100% for early-stage lesions and 60% for locally advanced lesions treated with 50–60 Gy have been reported (Chao and Perez, 1998). The primary nodal drainage areas for patients with early primary tumors of the penis frequently are watched and managed with surgical "salvage" as needed. Radiation of clinically negative nodes is a standard component of definitive radiotherapeutic management and results in 95% local control rates. Twenty percent of patients who do not receive prophylactic nodal irradiation will develop nodal metastases (Ekstrom and Edsmyr, 1958). Palpable nodes are managed with postoperative radiation, which significantly improves local control.

Most urethral cancers are treated surgically, but distal urethral lesions are treated equally well with radiotherapy. Primary lesions involving the distal male urethra can be managed in a manner similar to that described for the female urethra (Chao and Perez, 1998; Krieg and Luk, 1981; Heysek et al, 1985; Srinivas and Khan, 1988). Lesions of the prostatic urethra can be managed in a manner similar to that for prostate cancer. Patients with urethral tumors seem to have a higher risk of systemic failure and a lower 5-year survival rate—approximately 55% and 15% for distal and proximal urethral tumors, respec-

Table 28–13. Summary of primary sites and roles for external-beam irradiation.

Primary Site	Definitive Irradiation Alone	Prophylactic Lymphatic Irradiation	Adjuvant Irradiation Following Surgery
Prostate	+++/++	+/−	+++ Positive margins following prostatectomy
Bladder	++	+	+/−
Kidney	−	+/−	+/−
Renal pelvis	−	+/−	+/−
Ureter	−	+/−	+/−
Testis seminoma	−	+++	−
Testis non-seminoma	−	−	−
Penis	+++[a]	+/−	+++
Urethra (male)	+++[a]	+/−	++
Urethra (female)	+++[a]	+/−	++

+++ = Highly effective; ++ = effective; + = effective–marginally effective; +/− = unknown; − = not indicated.
[a]Refers to early lesions.

tively (Heysek et al, 1985). Neoadjuvant chemotherapy followed by radiotherapy, with surgery reserved for salvage, has been proposed as a future strategy for more advanced lesions (Husein, Benedetto, and Sridhar, 1990; Eisenberger, 1992). A phase I/II trial is under way under the direction of the Southwest Oncology Group; the results may allow us to assess the merits of this approach.

Urethral strictures are the most common long-term major complication occurring in up to 50% of patients (Krieg and Luk, 1981). These are easily managed with urethral dilation. The risk of forming a urethral stricture is dependent on the treatment technique and doses used. Soft-tissue necrosis is an uncommon complication. Nearly 90% of patients maintain potency after radiotherapy (Krieg and Luk, 1981).

CONCLUSION

Table 28–13 provides a brief summary of the role for XRT in the management of urologic malignancies. Despite the lack of scientifically rigorous studies, the available data suggest that a close working relationship between the urologist and the radiation oncologist is likely to ensure that patients with urologic tumors have the maximum probability of being rendered free of cancer.

REFERENCES

GENERAL PRINCIPLES

Allan DJ: Radiation-induced apoptosis: Its role in a MADCaT (mitosis-apoptosis-differentiation-calcium toxicity) scheme of cytotoxicity mechanisms. Int J Radiat Biol 1992;2:145.

Edsmyr F et al: Irradiation therapy with multiple small fractions per day in urinary bladder cancer. Radiother Oncol 1985;4:197.

Ellis F: Dose, time and fractionation: A clinical hypothesis. Clin Radiol 1969;20:1.

Forman JD et al: Preliminary results of a hyperfractionated dose escalation study for locally advanced adenocarcinoma of the prostate. Radiother Oncol 1993;27:203.

Fowler JF: What next in fractionated radiotherapy? Br J Cancer 1984;49(Suppl VI):285.

Hall EJ: *Radiobiology for the Radiologist.* 3rd ed. Lippincott, 1988.

Kutcher GJ et al: Histogram reduction method for calculating complication probabilities for three-dimensional treatment planning evaluations. Int J Radiat Oncol Biol Phys 1991;21:137.

Lyman J, Wolbarst AB: Optimization of radiation Therapy. III: A method of assessing complication probabilities from dose-volume histogram. Int J Radiat Oncol Biol Phys 1987;13:103.

Perez CA: Prostate. In: Perez CA, Brady LW (editors): *Principles and Practice of Radiation Oncology,* 3rd ed. Lippincott-Raven, 1998.

Roach M, Pickett B, Weil M: The "Critical Volume Tolerance Method" for estimating the limits of dose escalation during three-dimensional conformal radiotherapy for prostate cancer. Int J Radiat Oncol Biol Phys 1996;35:1019.

Rosenthal SA et al: Immobilization improves the reproducibility of patient positioning during six-field conformal radiation therapy for prostate cancer. Int J Radiat Oncol Biol Phys 1993;27:921.

Rubin P, Casarett GW: *Clinical Radiation Pathology,* vol. 1, p. 423–470. Saunders, 1968.

Rubin P, Constine LS, Williams JP: Late effects of cancer treatment: Radiation and drug toxicity. In: Perez CA, Brady LW (editors): *Principles and Practice of Radiation Oncology,* 3rd ed. Lippincott-Raven, 1998.

Sklar G: Combined anti-tumor effect of suramin plus irradiation in human prostate cancer cells. The role of apoptosis. J Urol 1993;150:1526.

Ten Haken RK et al: Treatment planning issues related to prostate movement in response to differential filling of the rectum and bladder. Int J Radiat Oncol Biol Phys 1991;20:1317.

Thames HD, Peters LJ, Ang KK: Time-dose considerations for nomal tissue tolerance. In: Vaeth JM, Meyer JL (editors): *Radiation Tolerance of Normal Tissues,* vol. 23, p. 113–130. Karger, 1989.

Vanuystel L et al: Radiotherapy in multiple fractions per day for prostatic carcinoma: Late complications. Int J Radiat Oncol Biol Phys 1986;12:1589.

Zietman AL et al: The effects of androgen deprivation and radiation therapy on androgen-sensitive murine tumor: An in vitro and in vivo study. Cancer J Sci Am 1997;3:31.

PROSTATE CANCER

Anscher MS, Prosnitz LR: Multivariate analysis of factors predicting relapse after radical prostatecomy: possible indications for postoperative radiotherapy. Int J Radiat Oncol Biol Phys 1991;21:941.

Anscher MS, Robertson CN, Prosnitz LR: Adjuvant radiotherapy for pathologic stage T3/4 adenocarcinoma of the prostate: Ten-year update. Int J Radiat Oncol Biol Phys 1995;33:37.

ASTRO Consensus Statement: Guidelines for PSA following radiation therapy. Int J Radiat Oncol Biol Phys 1997;37:1035.

Bagshaw MA, Cox RS, Ray GR: Status of prostate cancer at Stanford University. NCI Monogr 1988;7:47.

Benk VT et al: Late rectal bleeding following 75.6 cGE by proton radiation as boost therapy to stage T3–4 prostate cancer irradiated on a phase III trial: The significance, in the anterior rectum, of both fractional volume treated and total dose received. Proceedings of the 34nd Annual ASTRO Meeting. Int J Radiat Oncol Biol Phys 1992;24:148.

Blasko JC, Grimm P, Ragde H: Brachytherapy and organ preservation in the management of carcinoma of the prostate. Semin Radiat Oncol 1993;3:240.

Blasko JC, Ragde H, Schumacher D: Transperineal percutaneous iodine-125 implantation for prostatic carcinoma using transrectal ultrasound and template guidance. Endo Hypertherm Oncol 1987;3:131.

Bolla M et al: Improved survival in patients with locally advanced prostate cancer treated with radiotherapy and goserelin. N Engl J Med 1997;337:295.

Brachman D, Beyers D: PSA failure-free survival following brachytherapy of external beam irradiation for T1/T2 prostate tumors in 1600 patients: Results from a single practice. Proceedings of the American Society for Therapeutic Radiology and Oncology, 40th Annual Meeting. Int J Radiat Oncol Biol Phys 1998 (Suppl);42:131.

Catalona WJ, Smith DS: 5 year tumor recurrence after anatomical radical prostatectomy for prostate cancer. J Urol 1994;152:1837.

Chinn DM, Holland J, Crownover RL: Potency following high dose 3-D conformal radiotherapy and the impact of prior major urologic surgical procedures in patients treated for prostate cancer. Int J Radiat Oncol Biol Phys 1995;33:15.

Cox JD, Kline RW: Do prostatic biopsies 12 months or more after external irradiation for adenocarcinoma, stage III, predict long term survival? Int J Radiat Oncol Biol Phys 1983;9:299.

Crook J et al: Clinical relevance of trans-rectal ultrasound, biopsy, and serum prostate-specific antigen following external beam radiotherapy for carcinoma of the prostate. Int J Radiat Oncol Biol Phys 1993;27:31.

D'Amico AV et al: Biochemical outcome after radical prostatectomy, external beam radiotherapy or interstitial radiation therapy for clinically localized prostate cancer. JAMA 1998;280:969.

D'Amico AV et al: A multivariate analysis of clinical and pathological factors which predict for prostate specific antigen failure after radical prostatectomy for prostate cancer. Proc Am Urol Assoc 1995;153: 430A.

Dearnaley DP et al: Reduction of radiation proctitus by conformal radiotherapy techniques in prostate cancer: A randomized trial. Lancet 1999;353:267.

DeLaney TF, Shipley WU, O'Leary MP: Preoperative irradiation and 125-iodine implantation for patients with localized carcinoma of the prostate. Int J Radiat Oncol Biol Phys 1985;12:1779.

Dugan TC et al: Biopsy after external beam radiation therapy for adenocarcinoma of the prostate: Correlation with histological grade and current prostate specific antigen. J Urol 1991;146:1313.

Duttenhaver JR et al: Protons or megavoltage x-rays as boost therapy for patients irradiated for localized prostatic carcinoma: An early phase I/II comparison. Cancer 1983;51:1599.

Fiveash JB et al: 3D conformal radiation therapy (3DCRT) for high grade prostate cancer: A multi-institutional review. Proceedings of the American Society for Therapeutic Radiology and Oncology, 40th Annual Meeting. Int J Radiat Oncol Biol Phys 1998 (Suppl);42:143.

Freeman JA et al: Radical retropubic prostatectomy and postoperative adjuvant radiation for pathologic stage C (PCN0) prostate cancer from 1976 to 1989: Intermediate findings. J. Urol 1993;149:1029.

Freiha FS, Bagshaw MA: Carcinoma of the prostate: Results of post-irradiation biopsy. Prostate 1984;5:19.

Fuks Z et al: The effect of local control on metastatic dissemination in carcinoma of the prostate: Long-term results in patients treated with 125-I implantation. Int J Radiat Oncol Biol Phys 1991;31:537.

Gottesman JE et al: Failure of open radioactive 125 iodine implantation to control localized prostate cancer: A study of 41 patients. J Urol 1991;146:1317.

Hall EJ: *Radiobiology for the Radiologist.* 3rd ed. Lippincott, 1988.

Hancock SL et al: Biochemical control of prostate cancer and kinetics of prostate specific antigen in a cohort of patients treated by external beam irradiation. Int J Radiat Oncol Biol Phys 1994;30(Suppl 1):217.

Hanks GE, Martz KL, Diamond JJ: The effect of dose on local control of prostate cancer. Int J Radiat Oncol Biol Phys 1988;5:1299.

Hanks GE et al: Optimization of conformal radiation treatment of prostate cancer: Report of a dose escalation study. Int J Radiat Oncol Biol Phys 1997;37: 543.

Hanks GE et al: Conformal technique dose escalation for prostate cancer: Biochemical evidence of improved cancer control with higher doses in patients with pretreatment prostate specific antigen > 10 ng/ml. Int J Radiat Oncol Biol Phys 1996a;35:861.

Hanks GE et al: Dose escalation in the conformal treatment of prostate cancer: Optimization is made possible by understanding the dose responses for control of cancer and late morbidity. Int J Radiat Oncol Biol Phys 1996b;36(Suppl 1):77.

Hanks GE et al: PSA confirmation of cure at 10 years of T1b, T2, NO, MO prostate protocol 7706 with external beam irradiation. Int J Radiat Oncol Biol Phys 1994;30:289.

Hanks GE et al: Prostatic specific antigen confirmation of long term cure of prostate cancer treated by external beam radiation in the RTOG. Int J Radiat Oncol Biol Phys 1993;27(Suppl 1):192.

Hanks GE et al: ASTRO 1984 Presidential Address. Optimizing the radiation treatment and outcome of prostate cancer. Int J Radiat Oncol Biol Phys 1985; 11:1235.

Horowitz E et al: Assessing the variability of outcome for patients with localized prostate irradiation using different definitions of biochemical failure. Int J Radiat Oncol Biol Phys 1995;31:226.

Kabalin JN et al: Identification of residual cancer in the prostate following radiation therapy: Role of transrectal ultrasound guided biopsy and prostate specific antigen. J Urol 1989;142:326.

Kaplan ID, Bagshaw MA: Serum prostate-specific antigen after post-prostatectomy radiotherapy. Urology 1992;39:401.

Kaplan ID, Cox RS, Bagshaw MA: Prostate-specific antigen after external beam radiotherapy for prostatic cancer: Followup. J Urol 1993;149:519.

King CR et al: Definitive therapy for stage T1/T2 prostate carcinoma: PSA-based comparision between surgery, external beam and implant radiotherapy. J Brachyther Int 1998;14:169.

Krieger JN et al: Fast neutron radiotherapy for locally advanced prostate cancer. Urology 1989;34:1.

Kuban DA, El-Mahdi AM, Schellhammer PF: I-125 interstitial implantation for prostate cancer: What have we learned 10 years later? Cancer 1989;63:2415.

Kuban DA et al: Potential benefit of improved local tumor control in patients with prostate carcinoma. Cancer 1995;75:2373.

Laramore GE et al: Fast Neutron therapy for locally advanced prostate cancer. Am J Clin Oncol 1993;16: 174.

Laramore GE et al: Fast Neutron radiotherapy for locally advanced prostate cancer: Result of an RTOG randomized study. Int J Radiat Oncol Biol Phys 1985;11:1621.

Laverdière J et al: Beneficial effect of hormonal therapy administered prior and following external beam radiation therapy in localized prostate cancer. Int J Radiat Oncol Biol Phys 1997;37:247.

Lawton CA et al: Evaluation of significant late morbidity from external beam irradiation for adenocarcinoma of the prostate (analysis from RTOG studies 7506 and 7706). Proceedings of the 32nd Annual ASTRO Meeting. Abstract 144. Int J Radiat Oncol Biol Phys 1990;19(Suppl 1):1190.

Leach GE et al: Radiotherapy for prostatic carcinoma: Post-irradiation prostatic biopsy and recurrence patterns with long-term followup. J Urol 1982;128:505.

Lee M et al: A comparison of proton and megavoltage X-ray treatment planning for prostate cancer. Radiother Oncol 1984;33:239.

Leibel SA, Hanks GE, Kramer S: Patterns of care outcome studies: Result of the national practice in adenocarcinoma of the prostate. Int J Radiat Oncol Biol Phys 1984;10:401.

Leibel SA et al: Three-dimensional conformal radiation therapy in localized carcinoma of the prostate: Interim report of a phase I dose escalation study. J of Urol 1994a;25:1792.

Leibel SA et al: Three-dimensional conformal radiation therapy in locally advanced carcinoma of the prostate:

Preliminary results of a phase I dose escalation study. Int J Radiat Oncol Biol Phys 1994b;28:55.

Link P, Freiha FS, Stamey TA: Adjuvant radiation therapy in patients with detectable prostate specific antigen following radical prostatectomy. J Urol 1991;145:532.

Litwin MS: Measuring health related quality of life in men with prostate cancer. J Urol 1994;152:1882.

Lyons JA, Kupelian PA: Importance of radiation dose in the treatment of stage T1–T2 adenocarcinoma of the prostate. Proceedings of the American Society for Therapeutic Radiology and Oncology, 40th Annual Meeting. Int J Radiat Oncol Biol Phys 1998(Suppl); 42:308.

Marinelli D et al: Followup prostate biopsy in patients with carcinoma of the prostate treated by 192 iridium template irradiation plus supplemental external beam radiation. J Urol 1992;147:922.

Michalski JM et al: Preliminary report of toxicity following 3-D radiation therapy for prostate cancer on 3DOG/RTOG 9406. Proceedings of the American Society for Therapeutic Radiology and Oncology, 40th Annual Meeting. Int J Radiat Oncol Biol Phys 1998(Suppl);42:142.

Nachtsheim DA et al: Latent residual tumor following external radiotherapy for prostate cancer. J Urol 1978;120:312.

Nguyen LN, Pollack A, Zagars ZK: Late effects after radiotherapy for prostate cancer in a randomized dose-response study: Results of a self-assessment. Urology 1998;51:991.

Ohori M et al: Prognostic significance of positive surgical margins in radical prostatectomy specimens. J Urol 1995;154:1818.

Partin AW et al: Serum PSA after anatomic radical prostatectomy: The Johns Hopkins experience after 10 years. Urol Clin North Am 1993a;20:713.

Partin AW et al: The use of prostate specific antigen, clinical stage and Gleason score to predict pathologic stage in men with localized prostate cancer. J Urol 1993b;150:110.

Patel J et al: Late results of combined iodine-125 and external beam radiotherapy in carcinoma of prostate. Urology 1990;36:27.

Paulson DF: Impact of radical prostatectomy in the management of clinically localized disease. J Urol 1994: 152:1826.

Perez CA: Prostate. In: Perez CA, Brady LW (editors): *Principles and Practice of Radiation Oncology,* 3rd ed. Lippincott-Raven, 1998.

Pilepich MV et al: Phase III Radiation Therapy Oncology Group (RTOG) trial 86-10 of androgen deprivation before and during radiotherapy in locally advanced carcinoma of the prostate. Proceedings of the American Society for Therapeutic Radiology and Oncology, 40th Annual Meeting. Int J Radiat Oncol Biol Phys 1998(Suppl);42:105.

Pisansky TM et al: Prostate-specific antigen as a pretherapy prognostic factor in patients treated with radiation therapy for clinically localized prostate cancer. J Clin Oncol 1993;11:2158.

Pollack A, Zagars G: External beam radiotherapy dose-response of prostate cancer. Int J Radiat Oncol Bio Phys 1997;39:192.

Pollack A et al: Conventional vs. conformal radiotherapy for prostate cancer: Preliminary results of dosimetry and acute toxicity. Int J Radiat Oncol Biol Phys 1996; 3:4555.

Presti JC et al: Effect of adjuvant radiation therapy on urodynamic parameters following radical retropubic prostatectomy. Radiat Oncol Invest 1996;4:192.

Prestidge BR, Kaplan I, Bagshaw MA: The clinical significance of a positive post-irradiation prostatic biopsy without distant metastases. Proceedings of the 33rd Annual ASTRO Meeting. Abstract 72. Int J Radiat Oncol Biol Phys 1991;21(Suppl 1):152.

Ragde H et al: Cancer Ten-year disease free survival after transperineal sonography-guided iodine-125 brachytherapy with or without 45-gray external beam irradiation in the treatment of patients with clinically localized, low Gleason grade prostate cancer. Cancer 1998;83:989.

Reddy EK, Mebust WK, Weigel JW: Iodine-125 implantation in localized prostatic cancer. Endo Hypertherm Oncol 1990;6:239.

Rehman J et al: The timing of adjuvant radiotherapy (RT) after radical prostatectomy and its relationship to pathologic stage and systemic recurrence. Annual Meeting of the American Urological Association, May 14–19, 1994. J Urol 1994.

Ritter MA et al: Prostate-specific antigen as predictor of radiotherapy response and patterns of failure in localized prostate cancer. J Clin Oncol 1992;10:1208.

Roach M: Equations for predicting the pathologic stage of men with localized prostate cancer using the preoperative prostate specific antigen (PSA) and Gleason score. J Urol 1993;150:1923.

Roach M, Chinn DM, Holland J: A pilot survey of sexual function and quality of life following 3-D conformal radiotherapy for clinically localized prostate cancer. Int J Radiat Oncol Biol Phys 1996;35:869.

Roach M, Pickett B, Phillips TL: An analysis of the advantages as well as the physical and clinical limitations of three-dimensionally (3-D) based co-planar conformal external beam irradiation (XRT) in the treatment of localized prostate cancer. In: Minet P (editor): *Three-Dimensional Treatment Planning.* Liege, 1993.

Roach M, Pickett B, Weil M. The "Critical Volume Tolerance Method" for estimating the limits of dose escalation during three-dimensional conformal radiotherapy for prostate cancer. Int J Radiat Oncol Biol Phys 1996;35:1019.

Roach M, Rosenthal S, Hunter D: 100 consecutive patients treated for clinically localized prostate cancer by six field conformal radiotherapy: Acute toxicity and lessons learned from the UCSF/Davis experience. Radiology 1993;189:183.

Roach M, Wallner K: Prostate cancer. In: Leibel SA, Phillips TL (editors): *Textbook of Radiation Oncology.* Saunders, 1998.

Roach M et al: Long-term survival after radiotherapy alone: Radiation therapy oncology group prostate cancer trials. J Urol 1999;161:864.

Roach M et al: Prognostic subgroups predict disease specific survival for men treated with radiotherapy alone on radiation therapy oncology group (RTOG) prostate cancer trials. Proceedings of the American Society of Clinical Oncology, 34th Annual Meeting. Proceedings of the American Society for Clinical Oncology 1998;17:312a.

Roach M et al: 501 men irradiated for clinically localized prostate cancer (1987–1995): Preliminary analysis of experience at UCSF and affiliated facilities. Int J Radiat Oncol Biol Phys 1996a;36(Suppl 1):248.

Roach M et al: Radiotherapy (XRT) for high grade (HG) clinically localized adenocarcinoma of the prostate (CAP). J Urol 1996b;156:1719.

Roach M et al: Bilateral arcs using "averaged beam's eye views": A simplified technique for delivering 3-D based conformal radiotherapy. Med Dosimetry 1994a; 19:159.

Roach M et al: Defining treatment margins for 3-D based six field conformal (SFC) irradiation of localized prostate cancer. Int J Radiat Oncol Biol Phys 1994b;28:267.

Roach M et al: Predicting the risk of lymph node involvement using the pre-treatment prostate specific antigen and Gleason score in men with clinically localized prostate cancer. Int J Radiat Oncol Biol Phys 1994c;28:33.

Roach M et al: The role of the urethrogram during simulation for localized prostate cancer. Int J Radiat Oncol Biol Phys 1993a;25:299.

Roach M et al: Treatment of 100 consecutive patients by using six-field conformal radiation therapy: Acute and short term toxicity. Radiology 1993b;189(Suppl): 183.

Rogers R et al: Radiation therapy for the management of biopsy-proven, local recurrence following radical prostatectomy. J Urol 1998;160:1748.

Rossi CJ et al: Particle beam radiation therapy in prostate cancer: Is there an advantage? Semin Radiat Oncol 1998;8:115.

Rubin P, Constine LS, Williams JP: Late effects of cancer treatment: Radiation and drug toxicity. In: Perez CA, Brady LW (editors): *Principles and Practice of Radiation Oncology,* 3rd ed. Lippincott-Raven, 1998.

Russell KJ et al: Photon versus neutron external beam radiotherapy in the treatment of locally advanced prostate cancer: Results of a randomized prospective trial. Int J Radiat Oncol Biol Phys 1994;28:47.

Russell KJ et al: Prostate specific antigen in the management of patients with localized adenocarcinoma of the prostate treated with primary radiation therapy. J Urol 1991;146:1046.

Sandler H et al: 3D conformal radiotherapy for the treatment of prostate cancer: Low risk of chronic rectal morbidity observed in a large series of patients. Proceedings of the 35th ASTRO Meeting. Int J Radiat Oncol Biol Phys 1993;27(Suppl 1):135.

Sandler HM et al: Dose escalation for stage C (T3) prostate cancer: Minimal rectal toxicity observed using conformal radiotherapy. Radiother Oncol 1992; 23:54.

Scardino PT, Wheeler TM: Local control of prostate cancer with radiotherapy: Frequency and prognostic significance of positive results of postirradiation prostate biopsy. NCI Monogr 1988;7:95.

Schellhammer PF et al: Prostate specific antigen to determine progression free survival after radiation therapy. Urology 1993;42:13.

Schellhammer PF et al: Prostate biopsy after definitive treatment by interstitial 125-iodine implant or external beam radiation therapy. J Urol 1987;37:897.

Schild SE et al: Radiotherapy for isolated increases in serum prostate-specific antigen levels after radical prostatectomy. Mayo Clin Proc 1994;69:613.

Seung SK et al: External beam radiotherapy in men who would have been candidates for I-125 implantation monotherapy. Cancer J Sci Am 1998;4:168.

Shipley WU et al: Advanced prostate cancer: The results of a randomized comparative trial of high dose irradiation boosting with conformal protons compared with conventional dose irradiation using photons alone. Int J Radiat Oncol Biol Phys 1995;32:3.

Shultheiss TE, Hanks GE, Hunt MA: Incidence of and factors related to late complications in conformal and conventional radiation treatment of cancer of the prostate. Int J Radiat Oncol Biol Phys 1995;32:643.

Smit WG et al: Late radiation damage in prostate cancer patients treated by high dose external radiotherapy in relation to rectal dose. Int J Radiat Oncol Biol Phys 1990;18:23.

Soffen EM et al: Decreased acute morbidity with conformal static field radiation therapy treatment of early prostate cancer as compared to non-conformal techniques. Proceedings of the 33nd Annual ASTRO Meeting. Abstract 71. Int J Radiat Oncol Biol Phys 1991;21(Suppl 1):152.

Stamey TX, Ferrari MK, Schmid HS: The value of serial prostate specific antigen determinations 5 years after radiotherapy: Steeply increasing values characterize 80% of patients. J Urol 1993;50:1856.

Stein A et al: Adjuvant radiotherapy in patients with post-radical prostatectomy with tumor extending through capsule or positive seminal vesicles. Urology 1992a;39:59.

Stein A et al: Prostate specific antigen levels after radical prostatectomy in patients with organ confined and locally extensive prostate cancer. J Urol 1992b;147:942.

Tait DM et al: Acute toxicity in pelvic radiotherapy; A randomized trial of conformal versus conventional treatment. Radiother Oncol 1997;42:121.

Ten Haken RK et al: Treatment planning issues related to prostate movement in response to differential filling of the rectum and bladder. Int J Radiat Oncol Biol Phys 1991;20:1317.

Ten Haken RK et al: Boost treatment of the prostate using shaped, fixed fields. Int J Radiat Oncol Biol Phys 1989;6:193.

Trapasso JG et al: The incidence and significance of detectable levels of serum after radical prostatectomy. J Urol 1994;152:1821.

Vijayakumar S et al: Acute toxicity during external-beam radiotherapy for localized prostate cancer: Comparison of different techniques. Int J Radiat Oncol Biol Phys 1993;25:359.

Vijayakumar S et al: Beams eye view-based photon radiotherapy. Int J Radiat Oncol Biol Phys 1991;21: 1575.

Voges GE et al: Morphologic analysis of surgical margins with positive findings in prostatectomy for adenocarcinoma of the prostate. Cancer 1992;69:520.

Wallner K et al: PSA response after transperineal I-125 prostate implantation. Int J Radiat Oncol Biol Phys 1993;27(Suppl 1):228.

Wu JJ et al: The efficacy of postprostatectomy radiotherapy in patients with an isolated elevation of serum prostate-specific antigen. Int J Radiat Oncol Biol Phys 1995;32:317.

Zagars GK, Pollack A: Radiation therapy for T1 and T2 prostate cancer: Prostate-specific antigen and disease outcome. Urology 1995;45:476.

Zagars GK, von Eschenbach AC: Prostate-specific antigen: An important marker for prostate cancer treated by external beam radiation. Cancer 1993;72:538.

Zelefsky MJ et al: Comparison of the 5-year outcome and morbidity of three-dimensional conformal radiotherapy versus transperianal permanent iodine-125 implantation for early stage prostate cancer. J Clin Oncol 1999;17:517.

Zelefsky MJ et al: Three-dimensional conformal radiotherapy and dose escalation: Where do we stand? Semin Radiat Oncol 1998;8;107.

Zietman AL et al: The treatment of prostate cancer by conventional radiation therapy: An analysis of long term outcome. Int J Radiat Oncol Biol Phys 1995;32: 287.

Zietman AL et al: Radical prostatectomy for adenocarcinoma of the prostate: The influence of pre-operative and pathologic findings on biochemical disease free outcome. Urology 1994;43:828.

Zietman AL et al: Adjuvant irradiation after radical prostatectomy for adenocarcinoma of prostate: Analysis of freedom from PSA failure. Urology 1993;42: 292.

Zincke H et al: Long term (15 years) results after radical prostatectomy for clinically localized (staged T2c or lower) prostate cancer. J Urol 1994;152:1850.

BLADDER CANCER

Anderstrom C et al: A prospective randomized study of preoperative irradiation with cystectomy or cystectomy alone for invasive bladder carcinoma. Eur Urol 1983;9:142.

Blackard CE, Byar DP: Veterans Administration Cooperative Urological Research Group: Results of a clinical trial of surgery and radiation in stage II and III carcinoma of the bladder. J Urol 1972;108:875.

Bloom HJG et al: Treatment of T3 bladder cancer: Controlled trial of pre-operative radiotherapy and radical cystectomy versus radical radiotherapy. Br J Urol 1982;54:136.

Cole DJ et al: Local control of muscle invasive bladder cancer: Pre-operative radiotherapy and cystectomy versus cystectomy alone. Int J Radiat Oncol Biol Phys 1995;32:331.

Cole DJ et al: A pilot study of accelerated fractionation in the radiotherapy of invasive carcinoma of the bladder. Br J Radiol 1992;65:792.

De Neve W, Lybeert ML, Goor C: Radiotherapy for T2 and T3 carcinoma of the bladder: The influence of overall treatment time. Radiother Oncol 1995;26:183.

Duncan W, Quilty PM: The results of a series of 963 patients with transitional cell carcinoma of the bladder primarily treated by radical megavoltage x-ray therapy. Radiother Oncol 1986;7:299.

Dunst J et al: Organ-sparing treatment of advanced bladder cancer: A 10 year experience. Int J Radiat Oncol Biol Phys 1994;30:261.

Goodman GB et al: Conservation of bladder function in patients with invasive bladder cancer treated by definitive irradiation and selective cystectomy. Int J Radiat Oncol Biol Phys 1981;7:569.

Itoku KA, Stein BS. Superficial bladder cancer. Hematol Oncol Clin North Am 1992;6:99.

Kaufman DS et al: Selective bladder preservation by combination treatment of invasive bladder cancer. N Engl J Med 1993;329:1377.

Matsumoto K et al: Clinical evaluation of intraoperative radiotherapy for carcinoma of the urinary bladder. Cancer 1981;47:509.

Parsons JT, Million RR: Role of planned preoperative irradiation in the management of clinical stage B2-C (T3) bladder carcinoma in the 1980s. Semin Surg Oncol 1989;5:255.

Parsons JT, Million RR: Planned preoperative irradiation in the management of clinical stage B2-C (T3) bladder carcinoma. Int J Radiat Oncol Biol Phys 1988;14:797.

Parsons JT, Zlotecki RA: Bladder. In: Perez CA, Brady LW (editors): *Principles and Practice of Radiation Oncology,* 3rd cd. Lippincott Raven, 1998.

Pollack A, Zagars GZ: Radiotherapy for stage T3b transitional cell carcinoma of the bladder. Semin Urol Oncol 1996;14:86.

Pollack A, Zagars G, Swanson D: Muscle-invasive bladder cancer treated with external beam radiotherapy: Prognostic factors. Int J Radiat Oncol Biol Phys 1994;30:267.

Quilty PM, Duncan W: Primary radical radiotherapy for T3 transitional carcinoma of the bladder: An analysis of survival and control. Int J Radiat Oncol Biol Phys 1986;12:861.

Quilty PM et al: Results of surgery following radical radiotherapy for invasive bladder cancer. Br J Urol 1986;58:396.

Radwin HM: Radiotherapy and bladder cancer: A critical review. J Urol 1980;124:43.

Sell A et al: Treatment of advanced Bladder cancer category T2, T3 and T4a. A randomized multicenter study of preoperative irradiation and cystectomy versus radical irradiation and early salvage cystectomy for residual tumor. DAVECA protocol 8201. Danish Vesical Cancer Group. Scand J Urol Nephrol 1991(Suppl); 138:193.

Shipley WU et al: Phase III trial of neoadjuvant chemotherapy in patients with invasive bladder cancer treated with selective bladder preservation by combined radiation therapy and chemotherapy: Initial results of radiation therapy oncology group 89-03. J Clin Oncol 1998;16:3576.

Shipley WU et al: The importance of initial transurethral surgery and other significant prognostic factors for improved survival with full-dose irradiation. Cancer 1987;60:514.

Shipley WU et al: Full-dose irradiation for patients with invasive bladder carcinoma: Clinical and histologic factors prognostic of improved survival. J Urol 1985; 134:679.

Slack NH, Bross IDJ, Prout GR: Five year folowup of results of a collaborative study of therapies for carcinoma of the bladder. J Surg Oncol 1977;9:393.

Tester W et al: Neoadjuvant combined modality program with selective organ preservation for invasive bladder cancer: Results of Radiation Therapy Oncology Group phase II trial 8802. J Clin Oncol 1996;14: 119.

Van der Werf-Messing BHP et al: Cancer of the urinary

bladder category T2, T3 (NxMo) treated by interstitial radium implant: Second report. Int J Radiat Oncol Biol Phys 1983;9:481.

Van der Werf-Messing BHP et al: Carcinoma of the urinary bladder (category T1NxMo) treated either by radium implant or transurethral resection only. Int J Radiat Oncol Biol Phys 1981;7:299.

Warde P, Gospodarowicz MK: New approaches in the use of radiation therapy in the treatment of infiltrative transitional-cell cancer of the bladder. World J Urol 1997;15:125.

Zietman A et al: A phase I/II trial of transurethral surgery combined with concurrent cisplatin, 5-fluorouracil and twice daily radiation followed by selective bladder preservation in operable patients with muscle invading bladder cancer. J Urol 1998;160:1673.

TESTICULAR CANCER

Chao CK et al: Secondary malignancy among seminoma patients treated with adjuvant radiation therapy. Int J Radiat Oncol Biol Phys 1995;33:831.

Coia LR, Hanks GE: Complications from large field intermediate dose infradiaphragmatic radiation: An analysis of the Patterns of Care outcome studies for Hodgkin's disease and Seminoma. Int J Radiat Oncol Biol Phys 1988;15:29.

Coleman JM et al: The management and clinical course of testicular seminoma: 15 years' experience at a single institution. Clin Oncol 1998;10:237.

Fossa SD, Aass N, Kaaluhus O: Radiotherapy for testicular seminoma stage. I: Treatment results and long term post-irradiation morbidity in 365 patients. Int J Radiat Oncol Biol Phys 1989;16:383.

Hamilton C et al: Radiotherapy for stage I seminoma testis: Results of treatment and complications. Radiother Oncol 1986;6:115.

Horowich A, Dearnaley DP: Treatment of seminoma. Semin Oncol 1992;19:171.

Lai PP et al: Radiation therapy for stage I and IIA testicular seminoma. Int J Radiat Oncol Biol Phys 1994;28:373.

Miki T et al: Long-term results of adjuvant irradiation or surveillance for stage I testicular seminoma. Int J Urol 1998;5:357.

Oliver RTD et al: Pilot studies of 2 and 1 course carboplatin as adjuvant for stage I seminoma: Should it be tested in a randomized trial against radiotherapy? Int J Radiat Oncol Biol Phys 1994;29:3.

Rorth BJ et al and the Danish Testicular Cancer Group: Surveillance alone versus radiotherapy after orchiectomy for clinical stage I nonseminomatous testicular cancer. J Clin Oncol 1991;9:1543.

Rorth M: Therapeutic alternatives in clinical stage I non-seminomatous disease. Semin Oncol 1992;19:190.

Shapiro E, Kinsella TI, Makuch RW: Effects of fractionated irradiation on endocrine aspects of testicular function. J Clin Oncol 1985;3:1232.

Sharda NN, Kinsella TI, Ritter MA: Adjuvant radiation versus observation: A cost analysis of alternate management schemes in early stage testicular seminoma. J Clin Oncol 1996;14:2933.

Sultanem K et al: Para-aortic irradiation only appears to be adequate treatment for patients with stage I semi-

noma of the testis. Int J Radiat Oncol Biol Phys 1998;40:455.

Thomas GM: Consensus statement on the investigation and management of testicular seminoma. In: Newling DW, Jones WG (editors): *Prostate Cancer and Testicular Cancer* (EORTC Genitourinary Group Monograph 7). Wiley-Liss, 1990.

Thomas GM: Controversies in the management of testicular seminoma. Cancer 1985;55:2298.

Thomas GM, Williams SD: Testis. In: Perez CA, Brady LW (editors): *Principles and Practice of Radiation Oncology,* 3rd ed. Lippincott-Raven, 1998.

Warde P, Gospodarowicz M: Management of stage II seminoma. J Clin Oncol 1998;16:290.

Warde P et al: Prognostic factors for relapse in stage I testicular seminoma treated with surveillance. J Urol 1997;157:1705.

Warde P et al: Stage I testicular seminoma: Results of adjuvant irradiation and surveillance. J Clin Oncol 1995;13:2255.

Zagars GK, Babaian RJ: The role of radiation in stage II testicular seminoma. Int J Radiat Oncol Biol Phys 1987;13:163.

CANCER OF THE KIDNEY, RENAL PELVIS, & URETER

Babaian RJ, Johnson DE, Chan RC: Combination nephroureterectomy and postoperative radiotherapy for infiltrative ureteral carcinoma. Int J Radiat Oncol Biol Phys 1980;6:1229.

Brady LW, Manning DM: The role of radiation therapy in primary carcinoma of the ureter. In: Berman H (editor): *The Ureter,* 2nd ed. Springer-Verlag, 1981.

Brookland RK, Richter MP: The postoperative irradiation of transitional cell carcinoma of the renal pelvis and ureter. J Urol 1985;133:952.

Michalski JM: Kidney, Renal pelvis and ureter. In: Perez CA, Brady LW (editors): *Principles and Practice of Radiation Oncology,* 3rd ed. Lippincott-Raven, 1998.

CANCER OF THE FEMALE URETHRA

Grigsby PW: Carcinoma of the urethra in women. Int J Radiat Oncol Biol Phys 1998a;41:535.

Grigsby PW: Female urethra. In: Perez CA, Brady LW (editors): *Principles and Practice of Radiation Oncology,* 3rd ed. Lippincott-Raven, 1998b.

Johnson DW et al: Low dose combined chemotherapy/radiotherapy in the management of locally advanced urethral squamous cell carcinoma. J Urol 1989;141:615.

Klein FA et al: Inferior pubic rami resection with en bloc radical excision for invasive proximal urethral carcinoma. Cancer 1983;51:1238.

Sailer SL, Shipley WU, Wang CC: Carcinoma of the female urethra: A review of results with radiation therapy. J Urol 1988;140:1.

CANCER OF THE PENIS & MALE URETHRA

Almgard LE, Edsmyr F: Radiotherapy in treatment of patients with carcinoma of the penis. Scand J Urol Nephrol 1973;7:1.

Chao KS, Perez CA. Penis and male urethra. In: Perez CA, Brady LW (editors): *Principles and Practice of Radiation Oncology,* 3rd ed. Lippincott-Raven, 1998.

Eisenberger MA: Chemotherapy for carcinomas of the penis and urethra. Urol Clin North Am 1992;2:333.

Ekstrom T, Edsmyr F: Cancer of the penis: A clinical study of 229 cases. Acta Chir Scand 1958;15:25.

Heysek RV et al: Carcinoma of the male urethra. J Urol 1985;134:753.

Husein AM, Benedetto P, Sridhar KS: Chemotherapy with cisplatin and 5-fluorouracil for penile and urethral squamous cell carcinomas. Cancer 1990;65:433.

Kaushal V, Sharma SC: Carcinoma of the penis. A 12-year review. Acta Oncol 1987;26:413.

Krieg RM, Luk KH: Carcinoma of the penis: Review of cases treated by surgery and radiation therapy 1960–1970. Urology 1981;18:149.

Sagerman RH et al: External beam irradiation of carcinoma of the penis. Radiology 1984;152:183.

Srinivas V, Khan SA: Male urethral cancer: A review. Int Urol Nephrol 1988;20:61.

29

Neuropathic Bladder Disorders

Emil A. Tanagho, MD, & Tom F. Lue, MD

The urinary bladder is probably the only visceral smooth-muscle organ that is under complete voluntary control from the cerebral cortex. Normal bladder function requires coordinated interaction of sensory and motor components of both the somatic and autonomic nervous systems. Recent advances in the understanding of neural pathways and neurotransmitters have shown that most levels of the nervous system are involved in the regulation of voiding function. Therefore, many neurologic diseases cause changes in bladder function: multiple sclerosis, spinal injury, cerebrovascular disease, Parkinson disease, diabetes mellitus, meningomyelocele, and amyotrophic lateral sclerosis. Injury to the sacral roots or pelvic plexus from spinal surgery, herniation of an intervertebral disk, or pelvic surgery (hysterectomy, abdominoperineal resection) can also cause neuropathic bladder.

Significant bladder dysfunction can evolve for reasons not readily clear, possibly because of poor voiding habits developed in childhood or because of degenerative changes in peripheral tissue and nerve endings caused by aging, inflammation, or anxiety disorders. All can disrupt efficient reflex coordination between sphincter and bladder, and with time, this leads to symptomatic dysfunction.

NORMAL VESICAL FUNCTION

ANATOMY & PHYSIOLOGY

The Bladder Unit

The bladder wall is composed of a syncytium of smooth-muscle fibers that run in various directions; near the internal meatus, however, 3 layers are distinguishable: a middle circular layer and inner and outer longitudinal layers. In females the outer layer extends down the entire length of the urethra, while in males it ends at the apex of the prostate. The muscle fibers become circular and spirally oriented around the urethra and thus function as the smooth-muscle sphincter. The middle circular layer ends at the internal meatus of the bladder and is most developed anteriorly. The inner layer remains longitudinally oriented and reaches the distal end of the urethra in females and the apex of the prostate in males. The convergence of these muscle fibers forms a thickened bladder neck, which functions as the internal sphincter.

The normal bladder is able to distend gradually to a capacity of 400–500 mL without appreciable increase in intravesical pressure because of its spheric shape. When the sensation of fullness is transmitted to the sacral cord, the motor arc of the reflex causes a powerful and sustained detrusor contraction and urination if voluntary control is lacking (as in infants). As myelinization of the central nervous system progresses, the young child is able to suppress the sacral reflex so that he or she can urinate when it is appropriate.

The functional features of the bladder include (1) a normal capacity of 400–500 mL, (2) a sensation of fullness, (3) the ability to accommodate various volumes without a change in intraluminal pressure, (4) the ability to initiate and sustain a contraction until the bladder is empty, and (5) voluntary initiation or inhibition of voiding despite the involuntary nature of the organ.

The Sphincteric Unit

In both males and females, there are 2 sphincteric elements: (1) an internal involuntary smooth-muscle sphincter at the bladder neck, and (2) an external voluntary striated-muscle sphincter from the prostate to the membranous urethra in males and at the mid urethra in females.

The bladder neck sphincter is a condensation of smooth muscle of the detrusor. This area is rich in sympathetic innervation. Active contraction of the bladder neck region occurs simultaneously with seminal emission, just before ejaculation. In the filling phase, the bladder neck remains closed to provide a continence mechanism. It opens during both spontaneous contraction and contraction induced by stimulation of the pelvic nerve, indicating that it can be pulled open by contraction of the longitudinal muscles.

The external sphincter is composed of slow-twitch, small muscle fibers located between the fascial layers of the urogenital diaphragm. This voluntary sphincter maintains a constant tonus and is the primary continence mechanism. While the resting tone is maintained by the slow-twitch intrinsic muscle, it can be voluntarily increased by contraction of the striated muscles of the pelvic floor (eg, levator ani), which contain both fast- and slow-twitch fibers. The levator muscles also contribute indirectly to continence through support of the bladder base. Weakness of the pelvic floor may impair the efficiency of the closure mechanism of the otherwise normal bladder and sphincteric units. During abdominal straining, the diaphragm and abdominal muscles contract, and the increased abdominal pressure is transmitted to add to the intravesical pressure. A reflex contraction of the pelvic musculature together with transmitted abdominal pressure helps to close the urethra and prevent stress incontinence.

Relaxation of the sphincter is mostly a voluntary act without which voiding is normally inhibited. Failure to initiate sphincteric relaxation is a mechanism of urinary retention often seen in children with dyssynergic voiding. In infancy, the detrusor behaves in an uninhibited fashion. As the central nervous system matures, children learn to suppress or enhance the micturition reflex through voluntary contraction or relaxation of the pelvic musculature.

The Ureterovesical Junction

The function of the ureterovesical junction is to prevent backflow of urine from the bladder to the upper urinary tract. Longitudinal muscle from the ureter contributes to the makeup of the trigone. Stretching of the trigone has an occlusive effect on the ureteral openings. During normal detrusor contraction, the increased pull on the ureters prevents reflux of urine. Conversely, the combination of detrusor hypertrophy and trigonal stretch owing to residual urine can significantly obstruct the flow of urine from the ureters into the bladder.

INNERVATION & NEUROPHYSIOLOGY

Nerve Supply

The lower urinary tract receives afferent and efferent innervation from both the autonomic and somatic nervous systems. The parasympathetic innervation originates in the second to fourth sacral segments and projects to the pelvic plexus. The cholinergic postganglionic fibers supply both the bladder and sphincter. The sympathetic nerves originate at T10–L2. The noradrenergic postganglionic fibers from the hypogastric

or pelvic plexus innervate the smooth muscles of the bladder base, internal sphincter, and proximal urethra. Somatic motor innervation originates in S2–3 and travels to the external urethral sphincter via the pudendal nerve. Some motor neurons to the tonic small muscle fibers of the striated sphincter may also project through the pelvic nerve (Gosling and Dixon, 1990).

There are both somatic and visceral afferents from the bladder and urethra. The somatic afferent is carried by the pudendal nerve, while the visceral afferent projects through the sympathetic and parasympathetic nerves to their respective spinal areas. During bladder filling, the sensation of fullness is perceived by the receptors located in the muscle layers of the bladder wall and is carried by the myelinated sacral visceral afferents. The bladder mucosa and submucosa are also innervated by unmyelinated sacral afferents that are normally silent but can be activated during inflammation (Janig and Koltzenburg, 1993). On the other hand, the thoracolumbar visceral afferents may transmit discomfort and pain (Janig and Koltzenburg, 1993).

The Micturition Reflex

Intact reflex pathways via the spinal cord and the pons are required for normal micturition. Afferents from the bladder are essential for the activation of the sacral center, which then causes detrusor contraction, bladder neck opening, and sphincteric relaxation. The pontine center, through its connection with the sacral center, may send either excitatory or inhibitory impulses to regulate the micturition reflex. Electrical or chemical stimulation of the neurons in the medial pontine micturition center generates contraction of the detrusor and relaxation of the external sphincter. Disruption of pontine control, as in upper spinal cord injury, leads to contraction of the detrusor without sphincteric relaxation (detrusor-sphincter dyssynergia).

In pathologic conditions affecting the urethra (eg, urethritis or prostatitis) or the bladder (eg, cystitis or obstructive hypertrophy), uninhibited detrusor contraction may occur because of facilitation of the micturition reflex (Figure 29–1).

The Storage Function

The external sphincter plays an important role in urine storage. The afferents from pelvic and pudendal nerves activate both the sacral and lateral pontine center; this enhances sphincteric contraction while suppressing the parasympathetic impulse to the detrusor. Voluntary tightening of the sphincter can also inhibit the urge to urinate. In addition, activation of sympathetic nerves increases urethral resistance and facilitates bladder storage (Figure 29–2).

Cerebral (Suprapontine) Control

Although micturition and urine storage are primarily functions of the autonomic nervous system, these are under voluntary control from suprapontine cerebral centers, so that other groups of muscles (arm, leg,

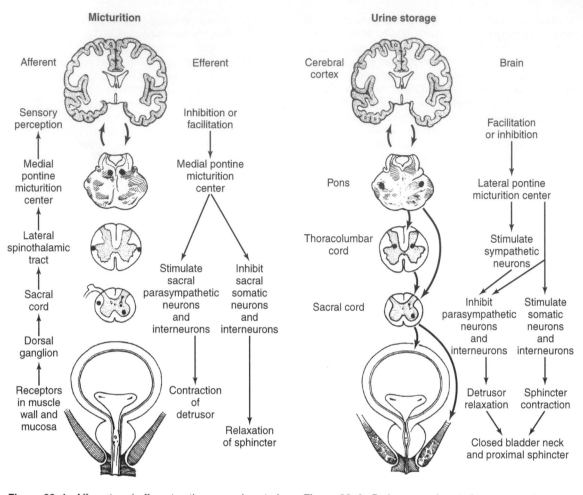

Figure 29–1. Afferent and efferent pathways and central nervous system centers involved in micturition.

Figure 29–2. Pathways and central nervous system centers involved in urine storage.

hand, bulbocavernosus) can be integrated to assist in urination at the appropriate time and place. Cerebral lesions (eg, from tumor, Parkinson disease, vascular accident) are known to affect the perception of bladder sensation and result in voiding dysfunction.

Neurotransmitters & Receptors

In parasympathetic innervation, acetylcholine and nicotinic receptors mediate pre- to postganglionic transmission, while acetylcholine and M_2 muscarinic receptors mediate the postganglionic neuron–smooth-muscle transmission. In some species, adenosine triphosphate (ATP) is released with acetylcholine and acts on purinoceptors (P_2) in the smooth-muscle cell. In sympathetic nerves, noradrenaline can act on the beta-2-adrenoreceptors to relax the detrusor or the alpha-1 receptors to contract the bladder neck and the external sphincter.

In addition, many neuropeptides, which usually colocalize with the classic transmitters, are also found in the genitourinary tract. Neuropeptide Y, encephalin, and vasoactive intestinal polypeptide (VIP) are found in cholinergic postganglionic neurons, while calcitonin gene-related peptide (CGRP), VIP, substance P, cholecystokinin, and encephalins are distributed in sacral visceral afferent fibers. These peptides are thought to be involved in modulation of efferent and afferent neurotransmissions.

URODYNAMIC STUDIES
(See also Chapter 30.)

Micturition

Micturition is completely under voluntary control. Detrusor response to stretch can be inhibited, permitting the bladder to accommodate larger volumes, or detrusor contraction can be initiated whether or not the bladder is full. Detrusor contraction is usually preceded by relaxation of the pelvic floor musculature, including the voluntary sphincter around the urethra. This appreciably reduces the efficiency of urethral closure and also leads to a drop in the vesical base, further minimizing urethral resistance.

Next, the trigone contracts, exerting increased pull on the ureterovesical junction and thus increasing ureteral occlusion. This prevents vesicoureteral reflux during the period of high intravesical pressure that develops with voiding. It also pulls the posterior portion of the bladder neck open, leading to its funneling. Only then do the detrusor fibers of the bladder contract, and intravesical pressure begins to rise. Because the vesical longitudinal muscles insert into the urethra, their contraction along with that of the trigone tends to pull the internal meatus of the bladder open, further contributing to funneling of the vesical outlet. The increased hydrostatic pressure (30–40 cm of water) exerted by the detrusor is directed down the urethra. The urethral counterpressure drops reciprocally, and voiding ensues. The detrusor maintains its contraction until the bladder is completely empty.

When the bladder is empty, the detrusor muscle relaxes, and the bladder neck is allowed to close; urethral and perineal muscle tone return to normal. Finally, the trigone resumes its normal tone. The urinary stream can also be interrupted by voluntary contraction of the external sphincter. The detrusor muscle then relaxes by reciprocal reflex action, and the bladder neck closes.

Urodynamic studies are techniques used to obtain graphic recordings of activity in the urinary bladder, urethral sphincter, and pelvic musculature. The 3 current methods involve use of gas or water to transfer pressure to a transducer housed near a polygraph or use of a transducer-tipped catheter to transfer pressure recordings directly to a polygraph. All the techniques have limitations, with gas being the least reliable of the three. Pressure recordings may be complemented by electromyography of the perineal musculature, ultrasound, or radiography (Figure 29–3).

Uroflowmetry

Uroflowmetry is without doubt the most useful of all the urodynamic tests. It is the study of the flow of urine from the urethra. Uroflowmetry is best performed separately from all other tests and, whenever possible, as a standard office screening or monitoring procedure. The normal peak flow rate for males is 20–25 mL/s and for females 20–30 mL/s. Lower flow rates suggest outlet obstruction or a weak detrusor; higher flow rates suggest bladder spasticity or excessive use of abdominal muscles to assist voiding. Intermittent flow patterns generally reflect spasticity of the sphincter or straining to overcome resistance in the urethra. The test can be very informative in assessing the functional state of the lower urinary tract. It is useful as both a diagnostic and a monitoring tool.

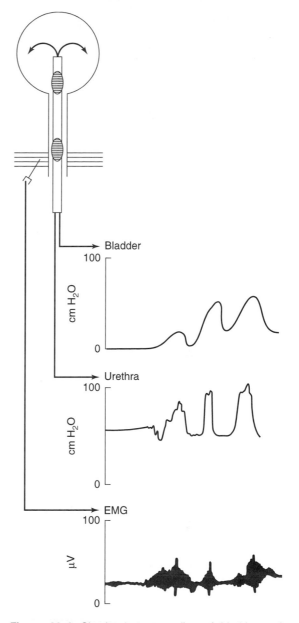

Figure 29–3. Simultaneous recording of bladder and urethral pressure as well as electromyographic recording of the external sphincter. Note the dyssynergic response. With bladder contraction there is increased activity in the external sphincter and pelvic floor, as recorded by the intraurethral pressure and electromyogram tracings.

There are a number of electronic devices for recording the flow rate. However, a patient can record the flow rate simply by averaging the volume voided over time. A maximum or peak flow can be measured by timing only the middle portion of the void, when the flow is strongest.

Cystometry

Cystometry is the urodynamic evaluation of the reservoir function of the lower urinary tract. Both gas and water cystometers have been used. Gas cystometers originally became popular because they were simpler and faster to use, but they have proved less reliable and less informative than water cystometers. Gas cystometers should be used only for initial screening; if any abnormalities are found, they should be confirmed by water cystometry.

Cystometric evaluations are performed to ascertain total bladder **capacity;** intravesical pressure during filling, up to the point at which voiding occurs (**accommodation**); bladder pressure during voiding; ability of the bladder to **contract** and sustain a contraction; the presence of premature or "**unstable**" bladder activity; the ability to perceive **fullness;** the ability to **inhibit** or **initiate** voiding; and the presence of **residual** urine after voiding. Cystometry is most informative when combined with studies of the external urethral sphincter and pelvic floor.

Normal bladder capacity is 400–500 mL. Bladder pressure during filling should remain constant up to the point of voiding. The first desire to void is generally felt when the volume reaches 150–250 mL, but detrusor filling pressure should remain unchanged until there is a definite sense of fullness at 350–450 mL, the true capacity of the bladder. Detrusor contractions before this point are considered abnormal and the result of hyperreflexic or uninhibited behavior. Normal voiding pressures in the bladder should not rise above 30 cm of water pressure. With normal voiding there should not be any residual urine, and voiding should be accomplished without straining.

Urethral Pressure Recordings

Bladder function should be focused on expelling urine rather than overcoming abnormal resistance in the urethra. High pressures in the bladder during voiding reflect abnormal resistance in the urethral outlet. Increased outlet resistance can result from benign prostatic hypertrophy, urethral stricture, bladder neck contracture, or spasm of the external urethral sphincter. Low resistance in the urethral outlet generally reflects compromised function of the sphincter mechanism. Recording of urethral pressures with the bladder at rest as well as during contraction helps determine the presence of functional or anatomic disorders. It also helps assess the sphincteric integrity of the urethral musculature.

Electromyography

With electromyography, the activity of the striated urethral muscles can be monitored without obstructing the urethral lumen. In the normal urethra, activity increases slightly as the bladder fills and falls precipitously just before voiding begins. Denervation results in an overall decrease in activity as well as production of denervation potentials. An overall increase in activity reflects a state of hyperreflexia. The disadvantages of the technique are dependence on accurate needle position and a tendency to record artifacts. The technique does provide a sensitive study of urethral and pelvic muscle behavior.

ABNORMAL VESICAL FUNCTION

CLASSIFICATION OF NEUROPATHIC BLADDER

Attempts have been made over the years to classify bladder dysfunction due to neural injury. The traditional classification was according to neurologic deficit. Thus, the terms motor, spastic, upper motor neuron, reflexic, and uninhibited were used to describe dysfunction found with injury above the spinal cord micturition center. Coordination between the bladder and the sphincter was considered either balanced or unbalanced. The terms flaccid, atonic, areflexic, and sensory were used to describe loss of ability of the bladder to contract owing to injury of the pelvic nerves or the spinal micturition center. Dysfunction with both types of features was described as mixed.

Descriptions of neuromuscular dysfunction of the lower urinary tract should be individualized because no 2 neural injuries (no matter how similar) result in the same type of dysfunction. The standardization committee for the International Continence Society has attempted to create a functional classification that is easy to understand and provides a simple basis for therapy (Table 29–1).

1. NEUROPATHIC BLADDER DUE TO LESIONS ABOVE THE SACRAL MICTURITION CENTER

Most lesions above the level of the cord where the micturition center is located will cause bladder spasticity. Sacral reflex arcs remain intact, but loss of inhibition from higher centers results in spastic bladder and sphincter behavior on the segmental level. The degree of spasticity varies between the bladder and sphincter, from lesion to lesion, and from patient to patient with similar lesions. Common lesions found above the brain stem that affect voiding include dementia, vascular accidents, multiple sclerosis, tumors, and inflammatory disorders such as encephalitis or meningitis. These lesions can produce a wide range of functional changes, including precipitate urge, frequency, residual urine, retention of urine, recurrent urinary tract infections, and gross inconti-

Table 29–1. Various classifications of neuropathic bladder.

International Continence Society
Detrusor: Normal (N), hyperreflexic (+), hyporeflexic (−)
Striated sphincter: Normal (N), hyperactive (+),
  incompetent (−)
Sensation: Normal (N), hypersensitive (+),
  hyposensitive (−)
Bors and Comarr
Sensory neuron lesion
Motor neuron lesion (balanced or unbalanced)
Sensory-motor neuron lesion
  Upper motor neuron lesion
  Lower motor neuron lesion
  Mixed upper and lower motor neuron lesion
Nesbit, Lapides, and Baum
Sensory neuron lesion
Motor neuron lesion
Unihibited bladder
Reflex bladder
Autonomous bladder
Krane
Detrusor hyperreflexia
  Coordinated sphincters
  Striated muscle dyssynergia
  Smooth muscle dyssynergia
Detrusor areflexia
  Coordinated sphincters
  Nonrelaxing striated sphincter
  Denervated striated sphincter
  Nonrelaxing smooth sphincter
Wain, Benson, and Raezer
Failure to empty
Failure to store

nence. Symptoms range from mild to disabling. Obviously, incontinence is especially troublesome. If the lesion is above the pontine micturition center, detrusor–striated sphincter dyssynergia usually does not occur. However, leakage may occur because the need to void cannot be felt or because the sphincter becomes more relaxed and can no longer inhibit spontaneous voiding.

Lesions of the internal capsule include vascular accidents and Parkinson disease. Both spastic and semiflaccid voiding disorders are found with these lesions.

Spinal cord injury can be the result of trauma, herniated intervertebral disk, vascular lesions, multiple sclerosis, tumor, syringomyelia, or myelitis, or it may be iatrogenic. Traumatic spinal cord lesions are of greatest clinical concern. Partial or complete injuries may cause equally severe genitourinary dysfunction. Sphincter spasticity and voiding dyssynergia can lead to detrusor hypertrophy, high voiding pressures, ureteral reflux, or ureteral obstruction. With time, renal function may become compromised. If infection is combined with back pressure on the kidney, loss of renal function can be particularly rapid.

Spinal cord injuries at the cervical level are often associated with a condition known as **autonomic dysreflexia.** Because the lesions occur above the sympathetic outflow from the cord, hypertensive blood pressure fluctuations, bradycardia, and sweating can be triggered by insertion of a catheter, mild overdistention of the bladder with filling, or dyssynergic voiding.

In summary, the spastic neuropathic bladder is typified by (1) reduced capacity, (2) involuntary detrusor contractions, (3) high intravesical voiding pressures, (4) marked hypertrophy of the bladder wall, (5) spasticity of the pelvic striated muscle, and (6) autonomic dysreflexia in cervical cord lesions.

2. NEUROPATHIC BLADDER DUE TO LESIONS AT OR BELOW THE SACRAL MICTURITION CENTER

Injury to the Detrusor Motor Nucleus

The most common cause of flaccid neuropathic bladder is injury to the spinal cord at the micturition center, S2–4. Other causes of anterior horn cell damage include infection due to poliovirus or herpes zoster and iatrogenic factors such as radiation or surgery. Herniated disks can injure the micturition center but more commonly affect the cauda equina or sacral nerve roots. Myelodysplasias could also be grouped here, but the mechanism is actually failure in the development or organization of the anterior horn cells. Lesions in this region of the cord are often incomplete, with the result commonly being a mixture of spastic behavior with weakened muscle contractility. Mild trabeculation of the bladder may occur. External sphincter and perineal muscle tone are diminished. Urinary incontinence usually does not occur in these cases because of the compensatory increase in bladder storage. Because pressure in the bladder is low, little outlet resistance is needed to provide continence. Evacuation of the bladder may be accomplished by straining, but with variable success.

Injury to the Afferent Feedback Pathways

Flaccid neuropathic bladder also results from a variety of neuropathies, including diabetes mellitus, tabes dorsalis, pernicious anemia, and posterior spinal cord lesions. Here the mechanism is not injury of the detrusor motor nucleus but a loss of sensory input to the detrusor nucleus or a change in motor behavior due to loss of neurotransmission in the dorsal horns of the cord. The end result is the same. Loss of perception of bladder filling permits overstretching of the detrusor. Atony of the detrusor results in weak, inefficient contractility. Capacity is increased and residual urine significant.

In summary, the flaccid neuropathic bladder is typified by (1) large capacity, (2) lack of voluntary detrusor contractions, (3) low intravesical pressure, (4) mild trabeculation (hypertrophy) of the bladder wall, and (5) decreased tone of the external sphincter.

Injury Causing Poor Detrusor Distensibility

Another cause of atonic neuropathic bladder is peripheral nerve injury. This category includes injury caused by radical surgical procedures such as low anterior resection of the colon or Wertheim hysterectomy. This type of dysfunction has been referred to as autonomous because the smooth muscle remains active but there is no central reflex to organize muscle activity. The end result is a bladder that stores poorly owing to failure to accommodate with filling. There is a rather steep pressure rise in the bladder with filling due to hypertonicity in the detrusor wall.

Radiation therapy can result in denervation of the detrusor or the sphincter. More commonly, it damages the detrusor, resulting in fibrosis and loss of distensibility. Other inflammatory causes of injury to the detrusor include chronic infection, interstitial cystitis, and carcinoma in situ. These lesions produce a fibrotic bladder wall that, for obvious reasons, distends poorly.

Selective Injury to the External Sphincter

Pelvic fracture often tears the nerves to the external sphincter. Selective denervation of the external sphincter muscle, with incontinence, can follow if the bladder neck is not sufficiently competent. Radical surgery in the perineum is highly unlikely to damage the motor innervation to the urethra, although sensory innervation of the external sphincter can be affected.

SPINAL SHOCK & RECOVERY OF VESICAL FUNCTION AFTER SPINAL CORD INJURY

Immediately following severe injury to the spinal cord or conus medullaris, regardless of level, there is a stage of flaccid paralysis, with numbness below the level of the injury. The smooth muscle of the detrusor and rectum is affected. The result is detrusor overfilling to the point of overflow incontinence and rectal impaction.

Spinal shock may last from a few weeks to 6 months (usually 2–3 months). Reflex response in striated muscle is usually present from the time of injury but is suppressed. With time, the reflex excitability of striated muscle progresses until a spastic state is achieved. Smooth muscle is much slower to develop this hyperreflex activity and, unlike striated muscle, loses spontaneous response after the injury. Urinary retention is the rule, therefore, in the early months following injury.

Urodynamic studies are indicated periodically to monitor the progressive return of reflex behavior. In the early recovery stages, a few weak contractions of the bladder may be found. Later, in injuries above the micturition center, more significant reflex activity will be found. Low pressure storage can be managed via intermittent catheterization. High pressure storage should be addressed early to avoid problems with the upper urinary tract.

A seldom used but valuable test is instillation of ice water. A strong detrusor contraction in response to filling with cold saline (3.3 °C [38 °F]) is one of the first indications of return of detrusor reflex activity. This test is of value in differentiating upper from lower motor neuron lesions early in the recovery phase.

Activity of the bladder after the spinal shock phase depends on the site of injury and extent of the neural lesion. With upper motor neuron (suprasegmental) lesion, there is obvious evidence of spasticity toward the end of the spinal shock phase (eg, spontaneous spasms in the extremities, spontaneous leakage of urine or stool, and, possibly, the return of some sensation). A plan of management can be made at this time. A few patients will retain the ability to empty the bladder reflexively by using trigger techniques, ie, by tapping or scratching the skin above the pubis or external genitalia. More often, detrusor hyperreflexia must be suppressed by anticholinergic medication to prevent incontinence. Evacuation of urine can then be accomplished by intermittent catheterization. Although incomplete lesions are more amenable to this approach than complete lesions, 70% of complete lesions ultimately can be managed using this program. Patients who cannot be managed in this way can be evaluated for sphincterotomy, dorsal rhizotomy, diversion, augmentation, or a pacemaker procedure.

In cases of lower motor neuron (segmental or infrasegmental) lesions, it is difficult to distinguish spinal shock from the end result of the injury. Spontaneous detrusor activity cannot be elicited on urodynamic evaluation. If the bladder is allowed to fill, overflow incontinence will occur. Striated muscle reflexes will be suppressed or absent. The bladder may be partially emptied by the Credé maneuver (ie, by manually pushing on the abdomen above the pubic symphysis) or, preferably, by intermittent catheterization.

DIAGNOSIS OF NEUROPATHIC BLADDER

The diagnosis of a neuropathic bladder disorder depends on a complete history and physical (including neurologic) examination, as well as use of radiologic studies (voiding cystourethrography, excretory urography, computed tomography scanning, magnetic resonance imaging, when necessary); urologic studies (cystoscopy, ultrasound); urodynamic studies (cystometry, urethral pressure recordings, uroflowmetry); and neurologic studies (electromyography, evoked potentials). Patients should be reevaluated often as recovery progresses.

1. SPASTIC NEUROPATHIC BLADDER

Spastic neuropathic bladder results from partial or extensive neural damage above the conus medullaris (T12). The bladder functions on the level of segmental reflexes, without efficient regulation from higher brain centers.

Clinical Findings

A. Symptoms: The severity of symptoms depends on the site and extent of the lesion as well as the length of time from injury. Symptoms include involuntary urination, which is often frequent, spontaneous, scant, and triggered by spasms in the lower extremities. A true sensation of fullness is lacking, although vague lower abdominal sensations due to stretch of the overlying peritoneum may be felt. The major nonurologic symptoms are those of spastic paralysis and objective sensory deficits.

B. Signs: A complete neurologic examination is most important. The sensory level of the injury needs to be established, followed by assessment of the anal, bulbocavernosal, knee, ankle, and toe reflexes. These reflexes vary in degree of hyperreflexia on a scale of 1–4. Levator muscle tone and anal tone should be gauged separately, also on a scale of 1–4. Bladder volumes in established lesions are usually less than 300 mL (not infrequently, < 150 mL) and cannot be detected by abdominal percussion. Ultrasound can be a useful, rapid means of determining detrusor capacity. Voiding often can be triggered by stimulation of the skin of the abdomen, thigh, or genitalia, often with spasm of the lower extremities.

With high thoracic and cervical lesions, distention of the bladder (due to a plugged catheter or during cystometry or cystoscopy) can trigger a series of responses, including hypertension, bradycardia, headache, piloerection, and sweating. This phenomenon is known as **autonomic dysreflexia.** It is triggered by pelvic autonomic afferent activity (overdistention of bowel or bladder, erection) and somatic afferent activity (ejaculation, spasm of lower extremities, insertion of a catheter, dilation of the external urethral sphincter). The headache can be severe and the hypertension life-threatening. Treatment must be immediate. Inserting a catheter and leaving the catheter on open drainage usually quickly reverses the dysreflexia.

C. Laboratory Findings: Virtually all patients experience one or more urinary tract infections during the recovery phase of spinal shock. This is due to the necessity of catheter drainage, either intermittent or continuous. Urinary stasis, prolonged immobilization, and urinary tract infections predispose to stone formation. Renal function may be normal or impaired, depending on the efficacy of treatment and the absence of complications (hydronephrosis, pyelonephritis, calculosis). Red blood cells (erythrocytes) in the urine may reflect a number of abnormalities. Uremia will result if complications are not addressed appropriately and the patient is not checked at regular intervals. In this era of medicine and with this group of patients, renal failure should not occur.

D. X-Ray Findings: Periodic excretory urograms and retrograde cystograms are essential because complications are common. A trabeculated bladder of small capacity is typical of this type of neuropathic dysfunction. The bladder neck may be dilated. The kidneys may show evidence of pyelonephritic scarring, hydronephrosis, or stone disease. The ureters may be dilated from obstruction or reflux. A voiding film often clearly outlines a narrowed zone created by the spastic sphincter but may also identify a strictured segment of the urethra. Most, if not all, of these features can be detected with ultrasound. Magnetic resonance imaging is especially useful for the sagittal view it offers of the bladder neck and posterior urethral zones.

E. Instrumental Examination: Cystoscopy and panendoscopy help assess the integrity of the urethra and identify stricture sites. The bladder shows variable degrees of trabeculation, occasionally with diverticula. Bladder capacity, stones, competency of the ureteral orifices, changes secondary to chronic infection or indwelling catheters, and the integrity of the bladder neck and external urethral sphincter can be assessed.

F. Urodynamic Studies: Combined recording of bladder and urethral sphincter activity during filling will reveal a low-volume bladder with spastic dyssynergy of the external sphincter (Figure 29–4). High voiding pressures in the bladder are not unusual. Ureteral reflux or obstruction is more likely if voiding pressures exceed 40 cm of water. A high resting pressure is noted in the external sphincter on the urethral pressure profile, and labile spastic behavior is noted during filling and voiding. Various auras replace a true sense of bladder filling, eg, sweating, vague abdominal discomfort, spasm of the lower extremities. Movement of a catheter in the urethra can trigger detrusor contraction and voiding.

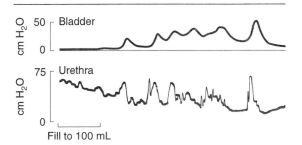

Figure 29–4. Spinal cord injury at T12. Simultaneous recording of intravesical and urethral pressure with bladder filling. Note the rise in intravesical pressure associated with unstable activity of the external sphincter, as reflected on the urethral pressure tracing.

2. MILDLY SPASTIC NEUROMUSCULAR DYSFUNCTION

Incomplete lesions of the cerebral cortex, pyramidal tracts, or spinal cord may weaken, but not abolish, cerebral restraint. The patient may have frequency and nocturia or urinary incontinence due to precipitous urge or voiding. Common causes include brain tumors, Parkinson disease, multiple sclerosis, dementias, cerebrovascular accidents, prolapsed disks, or partial spinal injury.

In many cases, the cause is unclear. The hyperreflexic behavior often seems to be associated with a peripheral abnormality (eg, prostatitis, benign prostatic hypertrophy, urethritis) or follows pelvic surgery (eg, anterior colporrhaphy, anteroposterior tumor resection). Symptoms are commonly associated with psychological factors.

Clinical Findings

A. Symptoms: Frequency, nocturia, and urgency are the principal symptoms. Hesitancy, intermittency, double voiding, and residual urine are also common. Incontinence may vary from pre- or postvoiding dribbling to complete voiding that the patient does not recognize or cannot inhibit once started.

B. Signs: The degree of voiding dysfunction does not parallel neurologic deficits. Slight physical disabilities can be associated with gross disturbances in bladder function, and the reverse is also true. However, it is always important to check lower extremity and perineal reflexes for evidence of hyperreflexia. Sensory or motor deficits may also be detected in the lumbar or sacral segments.

C. X-Ray Findings: In the early stages, radiologically evident change is minimal for the most part in both the lower and upper urinary tracts. Low bladder volume and mild trabeculation of the bladder are usually evident.

D. Instrumental Examination: Cystoscopy and urethroscopy are generally unremarkable. Mild detrusor and sphincter irritability and diminished capacity can be demonstrated.

E. Urodynamic Studies: The behavior patterns of the sphincter and bladder are similar to those of the previous group but on a milder scale. Uninhibited detrusor activity evident urodynamically may not be associated with the same symptom pattern on the clinical level. The patient occasionally perceives a sense of urgency and the need to void. However, these sensations may not be present, and the patient may complain of the actual leakage as the main inconvenience. Morphologic changes in the bladder are slight, with changes in the upper urinary tract occurring rarely and late because of lower pressures in the bladder.

3. FLACCID (ATONIC) BLADDER

Direct injury to the peripheral innervation of the bladder or sacral cord segments S2–4 results in flaccid paralysis of the urinary bladder. Characteristically, the capacity is large, intravesical pressure low, and involuntary contractions absent. Because smooth muscle is intrinsically active, fine trabeculations in the bladder may be seen. Common causes of this type of bladder behavior are trauma, tumors, tabes dorsalis, and congenital anomalies (eg, spina bifida, meningomyelocele).

Clinical Findings

A. Symptoms: The patient experiences flaccid paralysis and loss of sensation affecting the muscles and dermatomes below the level of injury. The principal urinary symptom is retention with overflow incontinence. Male patients lose their erections. Surprisingly, despite weakness in the striated sphincter, neither bowel nor urinary incontinence is a major factor. Storage pressures within the bladder remain below the outlet resistance.

B. Signs: Neurologic changes are typically lower motor neuron. Extremity reflexes are hypoactive or absent. Sensation is diminished or absent. It is important to check sensation over the penis (S2) and perianal region (S2–3) for evidence of a mixed or partial injury. Anal tone (S2) should be compared with levator tone (S3–4), again for evidence of a mixed injury.

Similarly, sensation over the outside of the foot (S2), sole of the foot (S2–3), and large toe (S3) should be compared for evidence of mixed injury. Occasionally, extremity findings do not parallel those of the perineum, with the pattern being absent sensation and tone in the feet but partial tone or sensation in the perineum. This is especially true in patients who have spina bifida or meningomyelocele.

C. Laboratory Findings: Repeated urinalysis at regular intervals is no less important in this group than in others. Infection with white blood cells (leukocytes) and bacteria may occur because of the need for bladder catheterization. Advanced renal change is unusual because bladder storage is under low pressure, but chronic renal failure secondary to pyelonephritis, hydronephrosis, or calculus formation is still possible.

D. X-Ray Findings: A plain film of the abdomen may reveal fracture of the lumbar spine or extensive spina bifida. Calcific shadows compatible with urinary stone may be seen. Excretory urograms should be performed initially to check for calculus, hydronephrosis, pyelonephritic scarring, or ureteral obstruction secondary to an overdistended bladder. A cystogram may detect morphologic changes in the detrusor (it is usually large and smooth-walled); vesicoureteral reflux may be present. Checks on the integrity of both the lower and upper urinary tracts can subsequently be made using ultrasound.

E. Instrumental Examination: Visual inspection is performed to rule out pathologic changes (eg, bladder stones, urethral stricture, or ureteral reflux or obstruction).

Cystoscopy and urethroscopy performed some months or weeks after the injury will confirm the laxity and areflexia of the sphincter and pelvic floor; the bladder neck is usually funneled and open and the bladder should be large and smooth-walled. The integrity of the ureteral orifices should be normal. Fine trabeculation may be evident.

F. Urodynamic Studies: The urethral pressure profile reflects low smooth and striated sphincter tone. Bladder filling pressures are low; detrusor contractions are weak or absent; voiding is accomplished by straining or by the Credé maneuver, if at all; and there is a large volume of residual urine. Awareness of filling is markedly diminished and usually results from stretch on the peritoneum or abdominal distention.

G. Denervation Hypersensitivity: This test is classically performed by giving bethanechol chloride (Urecholine) 15 mg subcutaneously. A cystometrogram is performed after 20 min, and the results are compared with the findings obtained before the bethanechol was given. If the results are positive, a rise in filling pressure of more than 15 cm of water is noted, with a shift in the filling curve to the left; the same behavior in the bladder is noted only at a lower filling volume and slightly higher pressure. A finding of no change on filling reflects myogenic damage to the detrusor. A more physiologic way to perform the test is to fill the bladder to about half its capacity, administer urecholine, and monitor for change in storage pressure. The ice water test also checks for detrusor hypersensitivity.

Bethanechol does not facilitate a detrusor contraction; it can only increase tone in the detrusor wall, which in turn might trigger the voiding reflex. The test is not a check on the integrity of the voiding reflex but demonstrates denervation hypersensitivity in flaccid bladders and differentiates this condition from myogenic damage.

The test is not applicable in patients with reduced bladder capacity, decreased compliance (ie, sharp rise in detrusor filling pressure), or forceful contractions of the detrusor.

DIFFERENTIAL DIAGNOSIS OF NEUROPATHIC BLADDER

The diagnosis of neuropathic bladder is usually obvious from the history and physical examination. Neural impairment is evidenced by abnormal sacral reflex activity and decreased perineal sensation. Some disorders with which neuropathic bladder may be confused are cystitis, chronic urethritis, vesical irritation secondary to psychic disturbance, myogenic damage, interstitial cystitis, cystocele, and infravesical obstruction.

Cystitis

Inflammation of the bladder, both nonspecific and tuberculous, causes frequency of urination and urgency, even to the point of incontinence. Infections secondary to residual urine caused by neuropathic behavioral disturbance should be ruled out.

The urodynamics of the inflamed bladder are similar to those of the uninhibited neuropathic bladder. However, with inflammation, symptoms disappear after definitive antibiotic therapy, and the urodynamic behavior reverts to normal. If symptoms persist or infections return repeatedly, a neuropathic behavioral abnormality should be considered (eg, multiple sclerosis or even idiopathic detrusor-sphincter dysfunction).

Chronic Urethritis

Symptoms of frequency, nocturia, and burning on urination may be due to chronic inflammation of the urethra not necessarily associated with infection. Urethroscopy will reveal signs of urethral inflammation most prominently in the region of the external sphincter. The urodynamics will show an irritable urethral sphincter zone with labile, spastic tendencies. The cause is unknown but is thought to be long-standing inefficiency of the sphincter, perhaps complicated by superimposed serious acute infection.

Vesical Irritation Secondary to Psychic Disturbance

Anxious, tense individuals or those with pathologic psychological fixation on the perineum may present a long history of periodic bouts of urinary frequency or perineal or pelvic pain. The clinical picture and urodynamic findings are similar to those described previously for chronic urethritis. Often, however, if the patient's anxieties can be allayed, the symptoms subside. The underlying problem is one of excessive pelvic muscle tension and inefficient sphincter behavior.

Interstitial Cystitis

Interstitial cystitis is poorly understood and commonly overdiagnosed and may be confused with chronic urethritis. The typical patient is a woman over 40 years of age, with symptoms of frequency, nocturia, urgency, and suprapubic pain. The symptoms are brought on by bladder distention. Capacity is limited (often < 100 mL in the most symptomatic and disabled patients). Urinalysis is normal, and there is no residual urine. Urodynamic studies show a hypertonic, poorly compliant bladder. Distention of the bladder with cystoscopy produces bleeding from petechial hemorrhages and fissuring in the mucosa. The condition represents an end-stage inflammatory process of unknown cause in the detrusor. Severe symptoms are usually relieved only through bladder augmentation.

Cystocele

Relaxation of the pelvic floor following childbirth may cause some frequency, nocturia, and stress incontinence. Residual urine may be present and predispose to infection. Loss of urine occurs with lifting, standing, or coughing.

Pelvic examination usually reveals relaxation of the anterior vaginal wall and descent of the urethra and bladder when the patient strains to void. Cystoscopy shows similar findings. Urodynamic studies show definite improvement in sphincter tone when the bladder is held in the proper supported position, as compared with the nonsupported position.

Infravesical Obstruction

Urethral strictures, benign or malignant enlargement of the prostate gland, and congenital urethral valves all can produce significant obstruction of the urinary outlet. Hypertrophy (ie, trabeculation) of the detrusor develops, and residual urine can accumulate. Uninhibited detrusor activity is often found at this stage and resembles that of the spastic neuropathic bladder.

If decompensation occurs, the vesical wall becomes attenuated and atonic, and capacity may be markedly increased. Overflow incontinence may develop. The behavior of the bladder is similar to that of the flaccid neuropathic bladder.

If the difficulty is nonneuropathic, the anal sphincter tone is normal and the bulbocavernosus reflex intact. Peripheral sensation, voluntary muscle contraction, and limb reflexes should also be normal. Cystoscopy and urethroscopy reveal the local lesion causing obstruction. Once the obstruction is relieved, bladder function improves but may never return to normal.

TREATMENT OF NEUROPATHIC BLADDER

The treatment of any form of neuropathic bladder is guided by the need to restore low pressure activity to the bladder. In doing so, renal function is preserved, continence restored, and infection more readily controlled. Reflex evacuation may develop if detrusor integrity is protected and trigger techniques are practiced.

1. SPINAL SHOCK

Following severe injury to the spinal cord, the bladder becomes atonic. With suprasegmental spinal

injuries, the bladder gradually recovers its contractile capabilities within months. A spastic state evolves, the degree of which varies from patient to patient according to level of injury. Injuries to the sacral cord, if complete enough, may leave the bladder permanently flaccid. More often, however, these lesions are partial, and a mixed degree of detrusor-sphincter spasticity is found along with a variable degree of weakness.

During the spinal shock stage, some type of bladder drainage must be instituted immediately and maintained. Chronic overdistention can damage the detrusor smooth muscle and limit functional recovery of the bladder. Intermittent catheterization using strict aseptic technique has proved to be the best form of management. This avoids urinary tract infection as well as the complications of an indwelling catheter (eg, urethral stricture, abscess, erosions, stones).

If a Foley catheter becomes necessary, a few principles need to be followed. The catheter should not be larger than 16F and preferably should be made of silicon, and it should be taped to the abdomen. Taping the catheter to the leg puts unnecessary stress on the penoscrotal junction and bulbous urethra (ie, the curves in the urethra), and this can lead to stricture formation. The catheter should be changed with sterile procedure every 2–3 weeks.

Some urologists advocate the use of suprapubic cystostomy rather than a urethral catheter to avoid the risks associated with permanent indwelling catheters. Certainly, whenever catheter-related complications occur, the physician should not hesitate in resorting to cystostomy drainage.

Irrigation of the bladder with antibiotic solutions, use of systemic antibiotics, or covering the tip of the meatus with antibiotic creams does not significantly lower the long-term risk of bladder infection. Keeping the meatus lubricated does help avoid meatal stricturing, however.

As peripheral reflex excitability gradually returns, urodynamic evaluation should be performed. A cystogram is needed to rule out reflux. The urodynamic study should be repeated every 3 months as long as spasticity is improving and then annually to check for complications of the upper urinary tract.

To control infection, a fluid intake of at least 2–3 L/d should be maintained (100–200 mL/h) if at all possible. This reduces stasis and decreases the concentration of calcium in the urine. Renal and ureteral drainage are enhanced by moving the patient frequently, with ambulation in a wheelchair as soon as possible, and even by raising the head of the bed. These measures improve ureteral transport of urine, reduce stasis, and lower the risk of infection.

Additional measures aid in prophylaxis for calculus formation (eg, reduction of intake of calcium and oxalate and elimination of vitamin D in the diet).

2. SPECIFIC TYPES OF NEUROPATHIC BLADDER

Once a neuropathic voiding disorder is established, regardless of cause, the following steps should be taken to attain optimum function.

Spastic Neuropathic Bladder

A. Patient With Reasonable Bladder Capacity: To consider a bladder rehabilitated to a functional state, a patient should be able to go 2–3 h between voiding and not be incontinent during this interval. Voiding is initiated using trigger techniques—tapping the abdomen suprapubically, tugging on the pubic hair, squeezing the penis, or scratching the skin of the lower abdomen, genitalia, or thighs. Patients can accomplish this on their own unless they are high quadriplegics with no upper limb function.

Some patients in this category can empty the bladder completely but are incontinent due to inconvenient triggering of the voiding reflex. They may be helped by low-dose anticholinergic medication or by neural stimulation.

B. Patient With Markedly Diminished Functional Vesical Capacity: If the functional capacity of the bladder is under 100 mL, involuntary voiding can occur as often as every 15 min. Satisfactory training of the bladder cannot be achieved, and alternative measures must be taken. First, the possibility that reduced functional bladder capacity is due to a large residual volume of urine must be ruled out. One of the following treatment regimens can then be administered.

1. A permanent indwelling catheter with or without anticholinergic medication.

2. A condom catheter and a leg bag in males if residual urine volumes are small and the patient does not have bladder pressures above 40 cm of water on urodynamic evaluation. If either of these parameters is found, the upper urinary tract is considered at risk from obstruction or reflux.

3. Performance of a sphincterotomy in males. It is possible to turn the bladder into a urinary conduit by surgically eliminating all outlet resistance from the bladder. This option should be used only when other options have failed, as it is irreversible. Patients having this procedure are usually suffering from more serious sequelae of a highly spastic bladder (ie, upper urinary tract dilatation, recurrent urinary tract infections, or marked autonomic dysreflexia).

4. Conversion of the spastic bladder to a flaccid bladder through sacral rhizotomy. Complete surgical section or percutaneous heat fulguration of the S3 and S4 roots is necessary. Chemical rhizotomy is unreliable, as spasticity usually returns after 6–9 months. These procedures may cause loss of reflex erections, and the decision to perform them should be weighed accordingly. They can relieve spasticity, lower intravesical pressures, increase bladder storage, and decrease the risk of damage to the upper urinary tract.

The bladder would then be managed as a flaccid bladder (see below).

5. Neurostimulation of the sacral nerve roots to accomplish bladder evacuation (see section following).

6. Urinary diversion for irreversible, progressive upper urinary tract deterioration. A variety of procedures are available, including the standard ileal conduit, cutaneous ureterostomies, transureteroureterostomy, or nonrefluxing urinary reservoir (eg, Mainz pouch, Koch pouch, or one of several other continent diversions designed to protect the upper urinary tract and kidneys).

7. In females with a spastic bladder, one does not have the option of performing a sphincterotomy. If pharmacologic methods are unsuccessful, surgical conversion to a flaccid, low-pressure system or a urinary diversion should be considered.

C. Parasympatholytic Drugs: Because of the chronic nature of the neuropathic bladder, patients are not always willing to tolerate the side effects of parasympatholytic drugs. Several drugs in this category can be alternated to reduce the side effects of either drug. They also may be useful when given with skeletal muscle relaxants. Dosages must be individualized. Commonly used drugs and dosages are as follows: oxybutynin chloride (Ditropan), 5 mg 2–3 times daily; Ditropan XL, once daily; dicyclomine hydrochloride (Bentyl), 80 mg in 4 equally divided doses daily; methantheline bromide (Banthine), 50–100 mg every 6 h; and propantheline bromide (Pro-Banthine), 15 mg 30 min before meals and 30 mg at bedtime and Tolterodine (Detrol), 2 mg 2 times daily. These drugs may not be effective if incontinence is the result of uninhibited sphincter relaxation or compliance changes in the bladder wall.

D. Neurostimulation (Bladder Pacemaker): Neuroprosthetics are becoming an established alternative to managing selective neuropathic bladder disorders. Patients are evaluated for a bladder pacemaker primarily by urodynamic monitoring of bladder and sphincter responses to trial stimulation of the various sacral nerve roots. Selective blocks are then prepared to the right and left pudendal nerves. If voiding is produced, patients are considered suitable for a neuroprosthesis. Other factors such as detrusor storage capability, sphincter competence, age, kidney function, and overall neurologic and psychological status are also taken into consideration.

Electrodes are implanted on the motor (ventral) nerve roots of those sacral nerves that will produce detrusor contraction on stimulation (always S3, occasionally S4). Steps are then taken to reduce sphincter hyperreflexia by selectively dividing the sensory (dorsal) component of these same sacral nerve roots and selective branches of the pudendal nerves. The electrodes are connected to a subcutaneous receiver that can be controlled from outside the body. Bladder or bowel evacuation or continence can then be controlled selectively by the external transmitter.

There are 3 overall goals in the management of the bladder in spastic upper motor neuron lesions—preservation of renal function, continence, and evacuation. The first 2 are accomplished by reducing intravesical pressures. This step protects the integrity of the upper urinary tract and restores continence by increasing storage capacity. Both can be achieved by combining neurostimulation of the sphincter with selective sacral neurotomies. This approach preserves sphincter integrity and avoids the need for drugs. Other options include complete bladder denervation or bladder augmentation.

The third goal, restoration of controlled evacuation, eliminates the need for catheters and associated risk of infection. This is the most difficult goal to achieve, and patients need to be carefully evaluated for their suitability.

Flaccid Neuropathic Bladder

If the neurologic lesion completely destroys the micturition center, volitional voiding cannot be accomplished without manual suprapubic pressure, ie, the Credé maneuver. Bladder evacuation can be accomplished by straining, using the abdominal and diaphragmatic muscles to raise intra-abdominal pressures. Partial injuries to the lower spinal cord (T10–11) result in a spastic bladder and a weak or weakly spastic sphincter. Incontinence can then result from spontaneous detrusor contraction.

A. Bladder Training and Care: In partial lower motor neuron injury, voiding should be tried every 2 h by the clock to avoid embarrassing leakage. This helps protect the bladder from overdistention due to a buildup of residual urine.

B. Intermittent Catheterization: Any patient with adequate bladder capacity can benefit from regular intermittent catheter drainage every 3–6 h. This technique eliminates residual urine, helps prevent infection, avoids incontinence, and protects against damage to the upper urinary tract. It simulates normal voiding and is easily learned and adapted by patients. It is an extremely satisfactory solution to the problems of the flaccid neuropathic bladder. A clean technique is used rather than the inconvenient, expensive, sterile technique. Urinary tract infections are infrequent, but if they occur, a prophylactic antibiotic can be given once daily. The method is contraindicated if ureteral reflux is present, unless the reflux is mild and the bladder emptied frequently.

C. Surgery: Transurethral resection is indicated for hypertrophy of the bladder neck or an enlarged prostate, either of which may cause obstruction of the bladder outlet and retention of residual urine. It also may be performed in some male patients to weaken the outlet resistance of the bladder to permit voiding by the Credé maneuver or abdominal straining.

Complete urinary incontinence due to sphincter incompetence can be managed by implanting an artificial sphincter. Bladder pressure should be low, however, for this to be successful. Bladder neck reconstruction also may be considered as a way to increase outlet resistance.

Incontinence in this group of patients can be treated with drugs or neurostimulation if it results from mild bladder spasticity.

D. Parasympathomimetic Drugs: The stable derivatives of acetylcholine are at times of value in assisting the evacuation of the bladder. Although they *do not* initiate or effect bladder contraction, they do provide increased bladder tonus. They may be helpful in symptomatic treatment of the milder types of flaccid neuropathic bladder. Drugs may be tried empirically, but usefulness is best gauged during urodynamic evaluation. If filling pressure or resting tonus is increased after bethanechol chloride (Urecholine) is administered, evacuation of the bladder through trigger reflexes or straining should be more effective. The drug then should be clinically helpful.

Bethanechol chloride is the drug of choice. It is given orally, 25–50 mg every 6–8 h. In special situations (eg, urodynamic study or immediately following operation), it may be given subcutaneously, 5–10 mg every 6–8 h.

Neuropathic Bladder Associated With Spina Bifida

Spina bifida is incomplete formation of the neural arch at various levels of the spine. The defect is recognized at birth and closed immediately to prevent infection. The scarring that results can entrap and tether nerves in the cauda equina. With failure of the neural arch to close, there is failure of anterior horn cell development and organization. The end result is a mixed type of neuropathic defect. Roughly two-thirds of patients have a spastic bladder with weakness in the feet and toes. About one-third have a flaccid bladder. Often, there is a greater degree of flaccidity in the pelvic floor than in the detrusor.

The goals of therapy are to control incontinence and preserve renal function.

A. Conservative Treatment: Clean intermittent catheterization is the best management. Parents can be taught to do this for the child, and eventually the child can take over this function. Frequency should be determined by the storage capacity of the bladder and the fluid intake, usually every 3–6 h. An anticholinergic drug may be required to mediate bladder spasticity and improve storage function in order to control incontinence.

1. Mild symptoms—If there is occasional dribbling or some residual urine associated with lack of desire to void, the patient should try to void every 2 h when awake. Manual suprapubic pressure enhances the efficiency of emptying. An external condom catheter or a small pad can be worn to protect against small-volume losses of urine.

2. More severe symptoms—If urinary incontinence is associated with residual urine or if ureteral reflux is found, the following steps should be taken:

a. Hypotonic bladder—If reflux has been demonstrated, intermittent self-catheterization 4–6 times a day may protect the upper urinary tract from deterioration and the consequences of pyelonephritis. Ureteral reimplantation can be considered for bilateral reflux or a transureteroureterostomy for single-sided reflux if all other considerations are favorable. Intermittent catheterization should then be reinstituted.

b. Hypertonic bladder—The problem with patients in this category is more serious because the bladder is spastic with reduced capacity and the sphincter is hypotonic. Virtually constant dribbling can result. The cystogram will reveal heavy trabeculation of the bladder, often with reflux and advanced hydroureteronephrosis. Anticholinergic medication should be given, and an indwelling catheter should be inserted for several months. Once upper urinary tract dilatation has improved and the bladder has been restored to a more spheric shape, intermittent catheterization may be reinstituted. With time and care, many of these children develop a more balanced type of bladder behavior. Continence may be gained without compromising the upper urinary tract.

Most of these patients will not require urinary diversion if they are carefully followed up and if the parents actively participate in their care.

B. Surgical Treatment: If the bladder is of the spastic type with diminished capacity, there are several surgical options short of actual urinary diversion. Sacral nerve block during urodynamic evaluation helps in determining whether sacral nerve root section would be beneficial. This helps in cases of spastic bladder but not in cases of poorly compliant, fibrotic bladder. Sectioning the S3 nerves reduces intravesical pressures, improves storage, and reduces the risk of reflux or obstruction of the ureters.

For the patient with a mildly spastic bladder and reasonable storage capacity (> 200 mL), urinary incontinence might be controlled via electrostimulation of the pelvic floor. Many of these patients have intact nerves to the sphincter. These can be stimulated to enhance sphincter tone and inhibit voiding. If the bladder has a limited capacity with poor compliance and poor contractility, augmentation cystoplasty followed by intermittent self-catheterization is the treatment of choice.

If the refluxing patient suffers recurrent fever (equivalent to pyelonephritis) despite the presence of an indwelling catheter or if incontinence cannot be controlled because of poor detrusor compliance, urinary diversion must be considered. Nonrefluxing continent reservoirs offer the most favorable long-term outlook for preservation of the upper urinary tract.

3. CONTROL OF URINARY INCONTINENCE

In the Hospital

Urinary incontinence is one of the most distressing aspects of neurovesical dysfunction, especially when the bladder has otherwise adequate function. The problem is minimized in men who are hospitalized because supervision is available, bathrooms are nearby, and a bedside urinal is always available. Women have a greater problem because they must use a bedpan or may require an indwelling catheter. Catheters have associated risks and do not always control leakage associated with spastic bladder. No simple, satisfactory solution to this problem has been devised for women.

After Discharge

After discharge from the hospital, most men with spastic bladders rely on a condom catheter for protection against leakage and for practical urine collection. The only exception is patients who are predictably dry between catheterizations. The condom catheter attaches to the penis without pressure and has a conduit to a leg bag. The adhesives are nonirritating and long-lasting. Problems involved in keeping these catheters in place are limited to noncircumcised patients and those with large suprapubic fat pads that shorten the length of the shaft of the penis. Circumcision or placement of a penile prosthesis will correct for these limitations.

Urethral compression by means of a Cunningham clamp is occasionally preferred by patients. This protects only against low-pressure leakage, however, and if it is applied too tightly, a urethral diverticulum may develop.

Other types of external collection devices are available (McGuire urinal, Texas catheter), but with advancements in adhesive glues for condom catheters and use of penile prostheses, the other methods are being used less frequently.

Neurostimulation

Extensive research continues to be conducted on methods of restoring complete voluntary control over the storage and evacuation functions of the bladder. Sacral and pudendal nerve anatomy has been determined, so that surgical exposure of these nerves and their branches is possible. An electrode can be placed for selective stimulation of the bladder, levator, and urethral or anal sphincters. A number of possibilities exist for neurostimulation or rhizotomy, but only a few are practical. Urodynamic evaluation of bladder function following a nerve block or during neurostimulation can help determine the therapeutic value of these treatments.

Single or multiple electrodes can be placed on selected nerves and coupled to a subcutaneous receiver. The desired function (continence or evacuation) can be selected. Usually, one or the other is needed in any one patient. Much will change in this approach as technologic advances become adapted to the increased understanding of bladder physiology. Striking successes are also being seen with electroevacuation in highly selected patients.

COMPLICATIONS OF NEUROPATHIC BLADDER

The principal complications of the neuropathic bladder are recurrent urinary tract infection, hydronephrosis secondary to ureteral reflux or obstruction, and stone formation. The primary factors contributing to these complications are the presence of residual urine, sustained high intravesical pressures, and immobilization, respectively.

Incontinence in neuropathic disorders may be passive, as in flaccid lesions when outlet resistance is compromised, or may be the result of uninhibited detrusor contractions, as in spastic lesions.

Infection

Infection is virtually inevitable with the neuropathic bladder state. During the stage of spinal shock that follows cord injury, the bladder must be emptied by catheterization. Sterile intermittent catheterization is recommended at this stage, but for practical purposes or for the sake of convenience, a Foley catheter is often left indwelling. Chronic catheter drainage guarantees infection regardless of any preventive measures taken.

The upper urinary tract is usually protected from infection by the integrity of the ureterovesical junction. If this becomes incompetent, infected urine will reflux up to the kidneys. Decompensation of the ureterovesical junction results from the high intravesical pressures generated by the spastic bladder. It is most important that these cases be treated aggressively with an intensive program of self-catheterization and anticholinergic medication. The Credé maneuver should not be used.

A number of infective complications can result from the presence of a chronically indwelling Foley catheter. These include cystitis and periurethritis resulting from mechanical irritation. A periurethral abscess may follow, with formation of a fistula via eventual rupture of the abscess through the perineal skin. Drainage may also take place through the urethra, with the end result being a urethral diverticulum. Infection may travel up into the prostatic ducts (prostatitis) or seminal vesicles (seminal vesiculitis) and along the vas into the epididymis (epididymitis).

A. Treatment of Pyelonephritis: Episodic renal infection should be treated aggressively with appropriate antibiotics to prevent renal loss. The source and cause of infection should be eliminated if possible.

B. Treatment of Epididymitis: This condition is a complication of either dyssynergic voiding or an indwelling catheter. Treatment consists of appropriate antibiotics, bed rest, and scrotal elevation. The indwelling catheter should be removed or replaced with a suprapubic catheter. Preferred long-term management is to place the patient on an intermittent self-catheterization program. Rarely, ligation of the vas is required.

Hydronephrosis

Two mechanisms lead to back pressure on the kidney. Early, the effect of trigonal stretch secondary to residual urine and detrusor hypertonicity becomes compounded by evolving trigonal hypertrophy. The combination causes abnormal pull on the ureterovesical junction, with increased resistance to the passage of urine. A "functional" obstruction results, which leads to progressive ureteral dilatation and back pressure on the kidney. At this stage, this condition can be relieved by continuous catheter drainage or by combined intermittent catheter drainage and use of anticholinergics.

A delayed consequence of trigonal hypertrophy and detrusor spasticity is reflux due to decompensation of the ureterovesical junction. The causative factor appears to be a combination of high intravesical pressure and trabeculation of the bladder wall. The increased stiffness of the ureterovesical junction weakens its valvelike function, slowly eroding its ability to prevent reflux of urine during forceful bladder contractions.

When ureteral reflux is detected by cystography, previous methods of bladder care must be radically adjusted. An indwelling catheter may manage the problem temporarily. However, if the reflux persists after a reasonable period of drainage, antireflux surgery must be considered. In addition, measures to reduce high intravesical pressure are needed (bladder augmentation, sacral rhizotomy, transurethral resection of the bladder outlet, or sphincterotomy). Progressive hydronephrosis may require nephrostomy. Urinary diversion is a last resort, which should be avoidable if the patient is followed regularly.

Calculus

A number of factors contribute to stone formation in the bladder and kidneys. Bed rest and inactivity cause demineralization of the skeleton, mobilization of calcium, and subsequent hypercalciuria. Recumbency and inadequate fluid intake both contribute to urinary stasis, possibly with increased concentration of urinary calcium. Catheterization of the neurogenic bladder may introduce bacteria. Subsequent infection is usually due to a urea-splitting organism, which causes the urine to become alkaline, with reduced solubility of calcium and phosphate.

A. Bladder Stones: Because these stones are usually soft, they can be crushed and will wash out through a cystoscope sheath. Occasionally, they are large and need to be removed via a suprapubic cystotomy.

B. Ureteral Stones: Virtually all ureteral stones can now be removed by antegrade or retrograde retrieval methods or by extracorporeal shock wave lithotripsy (ESWL).

C. Renal Stones: In a patient with neurogenic bladder, kidney stones generally are the result of infection; if the infection in untreated, the stones become the source of persistent renal infection and eventual renal loss. Most of the stones in the renal pelvis can be removed by either a percutaneous endoscopic procedure or ESWL. Occasionally, a large staghorn stone may require open surgery.

Renal Amyloidosis

Secondary amyloidosis of the kidney is a common cause of death in patients with neuropathic bladder. It is a result of chronic debilitation in patients with difficult decubitus ulcers and poorly controlled infection. Fortunately, due to better medical care, this is an uncommon finding today.

Sexual Dysfunction

Men who have suffered traumatic cord or cauda equina lesions experience varying degrees of sexual dysfunction. Those with upper motor lesions fare well, with the majority having reflexogenic erectile capability. Dangerous elevations in blood pressure can occur with erections in patients with high thoracic or cervical lesions. Problems of quality of erection or premature detumescence are found with all levels of injury. Patients with lower motor lesions are, as a rule, impotent, unless the lesion is incomplete. There is a high degree of variability in the sexual capabilities of patients with all levels of spinal injury. Fortunately, sexual function can be restored to most patients by oral sildenafil, transurethral medications, a vacuum erection device, intracavernous injection, or a penile prosthesis.

Often, patients with spinal injury lose the ability to ejaculate even with preservation of functional erections. This is a result of lost coordination between reflexes normally synchronized through higher center regulation. Patients may have the capability to ejaculate after an erection but are either unable to trigger this sexual event or are unable to trigger it in proper sequence. Techniques using vibratory stimulation of the penis or transrectal electrical stimulation have been developed to accomplish semen collection in patients with "functional infertility."

Autonomic Dysreflexia

Autonomic dysreflexia is sympathetically mediated reflex behavior triggered by sacral afferent feedback to the spinal cord. The phenomenon is seen in patients with cord lesions above the sympathetic outflow from the cord. As a rule, it occurs in rather spastic lesions above T1 but on occasion in lesions of mild spasticity or those as low as T5. Symptoms include dramatic elevations in systolic or diastolic blood pressure (or both), increased pulse pressure, sweating, bradycardia, headache, and piloerection. Symptoms are brought on by overdistention of the bladder. Immediate catheterization is indicated and usually brings about prompt lowering of blood pressure. Oral nifedipine (20 mg) has been shown to alleviate this syndrome when given 30 min before cystoscopy (Dykstra, Sidi, and Anderson, 1987) or electroejaculation (Steinberger et al, 1990). The acute hemodynamic effect can be managed with a parenteral ganglionic blocking agent or alpha-adrenergic blockers (Barrett and Wein, 1987). Sphincterotomy and peripheral rhizotomy have been used by some to prevent recurring autonomic dysreflexia.

PROGNOSIS

The greater threat to the patient with a neuropathic bladder is progressive renal damage (pyelonephritis, calculosis, and hydronephrosis). Advances in the management of the neuropathic bladder, together with better follow-up of patients at regular intervals, have substantially improved the outlook for long-term survival.

REFERENCES

Andersson KE: The overactive bladder: Pharmacologic basis of drug treatment. Urology 1997;50(6A Suppl): 74.

Artibani W: Diagnosis and significance of idiopathic overactive bladder. Urology 1997;50(6A Suppl):25.

Barrett D, Wein AJ: Voiding dysfunction: Diagnosis, classification and management. In: Gillenwater JY et al (editors): *Adult and Pediatric Urology.* Year Book Medical, 1987.

Barrington FJF: The component reflexes of micturition in the cat. Brain 1941;64:239.

Bauer SB: Neurogenic bladder dysfunction. Pediatr Clin North Am 1987;34:1121.

Bauer SB et al: The unrecognized neuropathic bladder of infancy. J Urol 1989;142:589.

Bazeed MA et al: Histochemical study of urethral striated musculature in the dog. J Urol 1982;128:406.

Bosch J, Groen J: Sacral (S3) segmental nerve stimulation as a treatment for urge incontinence in patients with detrusor instability: Results of chronic electrical stimulation using an implantable neural prosthesis. J Urol 1995;154:504.

Brading AF: A myogenic basis for the overactive bladder. Urology 1997;50(6A Suppl):57.

Bradley WE: Cerebrocortical innervation of the urinary bladder. Tohoku J Exp Med 1980;131:7.

Brindley GS: The sacral anterior root stimulator as a means of managing the bladder in patients with spinal cord lesions. Baillieres Clin Neurol 1995;4:1.

Buyse G et al: Intravesical oxybutinin for neurogenic bladder dysfunction: Less systemic side effects due to reduced first pass metabolism. J Urol 1998;160:892.

Churchill BM et al: Biological response of bladders rendered continent by insertion of artificial sphincter. J Urol 1987;138:1116.

Crowe R, Burnstock G, Light JK: Adrenergic innervation of the striated muscle of the intrinsic external urethral sphincter from patients with lower motor spinal cord lesion. J Urol 1989;141:47.

Crowe R, Burnstock G, Light JK: Spinal cord lesions at different levels affect either the adrenergic or vasoactive intestinal polypeptide–immunoreactive nerves in the human urethra. J Urol 1988;140:1412.

Cruz F: Desensitization of bladder sensory fibers by the intravesical capsaicin or capsaicin analogs. A new strategy for treatment of urge incontinence in patients with spinal detrusor hyperreflexia or bladder hypersensitivity disorders. Int Urogynecol J Pelvic Floor Dysfunct 1998;9:214.

De Groat WC: Anatomy of the central neural pathways controlling the lower urinary tract. Eur Urol 1998;34 (Suppl 1):2.

De Groat WC: A neurologic basis for the overactive bladder. Urology 1997;50(6A Suppl):36.

DeGroat WC et al: Neural control of micturition: the role of neuropeptides. J Auton Nerv Syst 1986;(Suppl 369).

Donker PJ, Droes JT, VanUlden BM: Anatomy of the musculature and innervation of the bladder and the urethra. In: Williams DI, Chisolm GD (editors): Scientific Foundations of Urology. Year Book, 1976.

Duel BP, Gonzalez R, Barthold JS: Alternative techniques for augmentation cystoplasty. J Urol 1998; 159:998.

Dykstra D, Sidi AA, and Anderson LL: The effect of nifedipine on cystoscopy induced autonomic hyperreflexia in patients with high spinal cord injuries. J Urol 1987;138:1155.

Dykstra DD et al: Effects of botulinum A toxin on detrusor-sphincter dyssynergia in spinal cord injury patients. J Urol 1988;139:919.

Enhorning G: Simultaneous recording of intraurethral and intravesical pressure. Acta Chir Scand [Suppl] 1961;276:1.

Fowler CJ: Investigation of the neurogenic bladder. J Neurol Neurosurg Psychiatry 1996;60:6.

Ghoniem GM et al: Bladder compliance in meningomyelocele children. J Urol 1989;141:1404.

Gosling JA, Dixon JS: Anatomy of the bladder and urethra. In: Chisholm GP, Fair WR (editors): Scientific Foundations of Urology. Year Book Medical, 1990.

Gosling JA, Dixon JS, Lendon RG: The autonomic innervation of the human male and female bladder neck and proximal urethra. J Urol 1977;118:302.

Gosling JA et al: A comparative study of the human external sphincter and periurethral levator ani muscles. Br J Urol 1981;53:35.

Gosling JA et al: Decrease in the autonomic innervation of human detrusor muscle in outflow obstruction. J Urol 1986;136:501.

Hackler RH: A 25-year prospective mortality study in the spinal cord injured patient: Comparison with the long-term living paraplegic. J Urol 1977;117:486.

Hackler RH, Hall MK, Zampieri TA: Bladder hypocompliance in the spinal cord injury population. J Urol 1989;141:1390.

Jackson S: The patient with an overactive bladder—symptoms and quality-of-life issues. Urology 1997; 50(6A Suppl):18.

Janig W, Koltzenburg M: Pain arising from the urogenital tract. In: Maggi CA (editor): Nervous Control of the Urogenital System. Harwood Academic Publishers, 1993.

Jayanthi VR et al: The nonneurogenic neurogenic bladder of early infancy. J Urol 1997;158(3 Pt 2):1281.

Joseph DB et al: Clean, intermittent catheterization of infants with neurogenic bladder. Pediatrics 1989;84:78.

Klück P: The autonomic innervation of the human urinary bladder, bladder neck and urethra: A histochemical study. Anat Rec 1980;198:439.

Krane RJ, Siroky MB: Classification of neurourologic disorders. In: Krane RJ, Siroky MB (editors): Clinical Neurourology. Little, Brown, 1979.

Léger L, Hernandez-Nicaise ML: The cat locus coeruleus: Light and electron microscopic study of the neuronal somata. Anat Embryol 1980;159:181.

Lepor H et al: Muscarinic cholinergic receptors in the normal and neurogenic human bladder. J Urol 1989; 142:869.

Light JK, Beric A, Wise PG: Predictive criteria for failed sphincterotomy in spinal cord injury patients. J Urol 1987;138:1201.

McGuire EJ, Cespedes RD, O'Connell HE: Leak-point pressures. Urol Clin North Am 1996;23:253.

McGuire EJ, Rossier AB: Treatment of acute autonomic dysreflexia. J Urol 1983;129:1185.

McGuire EJ, Savastano JA: Long-term follow-up of spinal cord injury patients managed by intermittent catheterization. J Urol 1983;219:775.

McLorie GA et al: Determinants of hydronephrosis and renal injury in patients with myelomeningocele. J Urol 1988;140:1289.

Mollard P, Mouriquand P, Joubert P: Urethral lengthening for neurogenic urinary incontinence (Kropp's procedure): Results of 16 cases. J Urol 1990;143:95.

Nickell K, Boone TB: Peripheral neuropathy and peripheral nerve injury. Urol Clin North Am 1996;23:491.

Pengelly A: Effect of prolonged bladder distention on detrusor function. Urol Clin North Am 1979;6:279.

Rivas DA, Figueroa TE, Chancellor MB: Bladder autoaugmentation. Tech Urol 1995;1:181.

Rudy DC, Awad SA, Downie JW: External sphincter dyssynergia: An abnormal continence reflex. J Urol 1988;140:105.

Satoh K: Descending projection of the nucleus tegmentis laterodorsalis to the spinal cord. Neurosci Lett 1978; 8:9.

Satoh K: Localization of the micturition center at dorsolateral pontine tegmentum of the rat. Neurosci Lett 1978;8:27.

Schmidt RA: Advances in genitourinary neurostimulation. Neurosurgery 1986;19:1041.

Sidi AA, Reinberg Y, Gonzalez R: Comparison of artificial sphincter implantation and bladder neck reconstruction in patients with neurogenic urinary incontinence. J Urol 1987;138:1120.

Smith AR, Hosker GL, Warrell DW: The role of partial denervation of the pelvic floor in the aetiology of genitourinary prolapse and stress incontinence of urine. A neurophysiological study. Br J Obstet Gynaecol 1989;96:24.

Smith AR, Hosker GL, Warrell DW: The role of pudendal nerve damage in the aetiology of genuine stress incontinence in women. Br J Obstet Gynaecol 1989; 96:29.

Snyder SH: Brain peptides as neurotransmitters. Science 1980;209:976.

Speakman MJ et al: Bladder outflow obstruction: A cause of denervation supersensitivity. J Urol 1987; 138:1461.

Steers WD, De Groat WC: Effect of bladder outlet obstruction on micturition reflex pathways in the rat. J Urol 1988;140:864.

Steinberger RE et al: Nifedipine pretreatment for autonomic dysreflexia during electroejaculation. Urology 1990;36:228.

Stone AR: Neurourologic evaluation and urologic management of spinal dysraphism. Neurosurg Clin North Am 1995;6:269.

Sullivan MP, Comiter CV, Yalla SV: Micturitional urethral pressure profilometry. Urol Clin North Am 1996; 23:263.

Tanagho EA, Schmidt RA: Electrical stimulation in the clinical management of the neurogenic bladder. J Urol 1988;140:1331.

Tanagho EA, Schmidt RA, Orvis BR: Neural stimulation for control of voiding dysfunction: A preliminary report in 22 patients with serious neuropathic voiding disorders. J Urol 1989;142:340.

Thomas TM, Karran OD, Meade TW: Management of urinary incontinence in patients with multiple sclerosis. J R Coll Gen Pract 1981;31:296.

Torrens MJ, Griffith HB: Management of the uninhibited bladder by selective sacral neurectomy. J Neurosurg 1976;44:176.

Van Kerrebroeck PE: The role of electrical stimulation in voiding dysfunction. Eur Urol 1998;34(Suppl 1):27.

Vorstman B et al: Nerve crossover techniques for urinary bladder reinnervation: Animal and human cadaver studies. J Urol 1987;137:1043.

Watanabe T, Rivas DA, Chancellor MB: Urodynamics of spinal cord injury. Urol Clin North Am 1996;23: 459.

Woodside JR, McGuire EJ: Detrusor hypertonicity as a late complication of a Wertheim hysterectomy. J Urol 1982;127:1143.

30

Urodynamic Studies

Emil A. Tanagho, MD

Urodynamic study is an important part of the evaluation of patients with voiding dysfunctions—dysuria, urinary incontinence, neuropathic disorders, etc. Formerly, the examiner simply observed the act of voiding, noting the strength of the urinary stream and drawing inferences about the possibility of obstruction of the bladder outlet. In the 1950s, it became possible to observe the lower urinary tract by fluoroscopy during the act of voiding; and in the 1960s, the principles of hydrodynamics were applied to lower urinary tract physiology. The field of urodynamics now has clinical applications in evaluating voiding problems resulting from lower urinary tract disease.

The nomenclature of the tests used in urodynamic studies is not yet settled, and the meanings of urodynamic terms are sometimes overlapping or confusing. In spite of these difficulties, urodynamic tests are extremely valuable. Symptoms elicited by the history or by physical, endoscopic, or even radiographic examination often must be investigated further by urodynamic tests so that therapy can be devised that is based on an understanding of the altered physiology of the lower urinary tract.

As is true of many high-technology testing procedures (eg, electrocardiography, electroencephalography), urodynamic tests have the greatest clinical validity when their interpretation is left to the treating physician, who should either supervise the study or be responsible for correlating all of the findings with personal clinical observations.

FUNCTIONS RELEVANT TO URODYNAMICS & TESTS APPLICABLE TO EACH

Urodynamic study of the lower urinary tract can provide useful clinical information about the function of the urinary bladder, the sphincteric mechanism, and the voiding pattern itself.

Bladder function has been classically studied by cystography and active motion fluoroscopy. Urody-namic studies use cystometry. Conventional radiographic studies and urodynamic studies can, of course, be usefully combined.

Sphincteric function depends on 2 elements: the smooth muscle sphincter and the voluntary sphincter. The activity of both elements can be recorded urodynamically by pressure measurements; the activity of the voluntary sphincter also can be recorded by electromyography.

The act of voiding is a function of the interaction between bladder and sphincter, and the result is the **flow rate.** The flow rate is one major aspect of the total function of the lower urinary tract. It is generally recorded in milliliters per second as well as by total urine volume voided. The simultaneous recording of bladder activity (by intraluminal pressure measurements), sphincteric activity (by electromyography or pressure measurements), and flow rate reveals interrelationships among the 3 elements. Each measurement may give useful information about the normality or abnormality of one specific aspect of lower urinary tract function. A more complete picture is provided by integrating all 3 lower tract elements in a simultaneously recorded comparative manner. This comprehensive approach may involve synchronous recordings of variable pressures, flow rate, volume voided, and electrical activity of skeletal musculature around the urinary sphincter (electromyography), along with fluoroscopic imaging of the lower urinary tract. The multiple pressures to be recorded are quite variable and usually include intravesical pressure, intraurethral pressure at several levels, intra-abdominal pressure, and anal sphincteric pressure as a function of muscular activity of the pelvic floor.

The techniques of urodynamic study must be tailored to the needs of specific patients. Each method has advantages and limitations depending on the requirements of the study. In one patient, results of a single test might be sufficient to establish the diagnosis and suggest appropriate therapy; in another, many more studies might be necessary.

PHYSIOLOGIC & HYDRODYNAMIC CONSIDERATIONS

URINARY FLOW RATE

Because urinary flow rate is the product of detrusor action against outlet resistance, a variation from the normal flow rate might reflect dysfunction of either. The normal flow rate from a full bladder is about 20–25 mL/s in men and 25–30 mL/s in women. These variations are directly related to the volume voided and the person's age. Obstruction should be suspected in any adult voiding with a full bladder at a rate of less than 15 mL/s. A flow rate less than 10 mL/s is considered definite evidence of obstruction. Occasionally, one encounters "supervoiders" with flow rates far above the normal range. This may signify low outlet resistance but is of less concern clinically than obstruction.

Outlet Resistance

Outlet resistance is the primary determinant of flow rate and varies according to mechanical or functional factors. Functionally, outlet resistance is primarily related to sphincteric activity, which is controlled by both the smooth sphincter and the voluntary sphincter. The smooth sphincter is rarely overactive in women; we have never seen an example of it in any of our urodynamic evaluations. Overactivity of the smooth sphincter is rarely seen in men also but it may occur in association with hypertrophy of the bladder neck due to neurogenic dysfunction or distal obstruction. However, such cases must be critically evaluated before this conclusion is reached.

Increased voluntary sphincteric activity is not uncommon. It is often neglected as a primary underlying cause of increased sphincteric resistance. It is manifested either as lack of relaxation or as actual overactivity during voiding. The normal voluntary sphincter provides adequate resistance, along with the smooth sphincter, to prevent escape of urine from the bladder; if the voluntary sphincter does not relax during detrusor contraction, partial functional obstruction occurs. Overactivity of the sphincter, resulting in increased outlet resistance, is usually a neuropathic phenomenon. However, it can also be functional, resulting from irritative phenomena such as infection or other factors—chemical, bacterial, hormonal, or, even more commonly and often not appreciated, psychological.

Mechanical Factors

Mechanical factors resulting in obstruction to urine flow are the easiest to identify by conventional methods. In women, they may take the form of cysto-

celes, urethral kinks, or, most commonly, iatrogenic scarring, fibrosis, and compression from previous vaginal or periurethral operative procedures. Mechanical factors in men are well known to all urologists; the classic form is benign prostatic hypertrophy. Urethral stricture from various causes and posterior urethral valves are other common causes of urinary obstruction in men, and there are many others.

Normal voiding with a normal flow rate is the product of both detrusor activity and outlet resistance. A high intravesical pressure resulting from detrusor contraction is not necessary to initiate voiding, because outlet resistance has usually dropped to a minimum. Sphincteric relaxation usually precedes detrusor contraction by a few seconds, and when relaxation is maximal, detrusor activity starts and is sustained until the bladder is empty.

Variations in Normal Flow Rate

The sequence just described is not essential for normal flow rates. The flow rate may be normal in the absence of any detrusor contraction if sphincteric relaxation is assisted by increased intra-abdominal pressure from straining. Persons with weak outlet resistance and weak sphincteric control can achieve a normal flow rate by complete voluntary sphincteric relaxation without detrusor contraction or straining. A normal flow rate can be achieved in spite of increased sphincteric activity or lack of complete relaxation if detrusor contraction is increased to overcome outlet resistance.

Because a normal flow rate can be achieved in spite of abnormalities of one or more of the mechanisms involved, recording the flow rate alone does not provide insight into the precise mechanisms by which it occurs. Distinction between patterns of flow can be difficult. For practical purposes, if the flow rate is adequate and the recorded pattern and configuration of the flow curve are normal, these variations may not be clinically significant except in rare cases.

Nomenclature

The study of urinary flow rate itself is usually called **uroflowmetry.** The flow rate is generally identified as **maximum flow rate, average flow rate, flow time, maximum flow time** (the time elapsed before maximum flow rate is reached), and **total flow time** (the aggregate of flow time if the flow has been interrupted by periods of no voiding) (Figure 30–1). The **flow rate pattern** is characterized as continuous or intermittent, etc.

Pattern Measurement of Flow Rate

A normal flow pattern is represented by a bell-shaped curve (Figure 30–1). However, the curve is rarely completely smooth; it may vary within limits and still be normal. Flow rate can be determined by measuring a 5-s collection at the peak of flow and di-

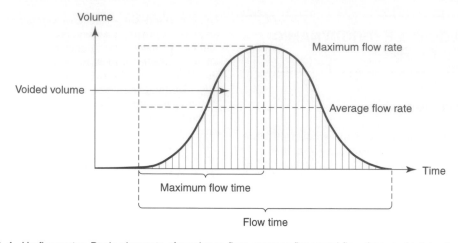

Figure 30–1. Uroflowmetry. Basic elements of maximum flow, average flow, total flow time, and total volume voided.

viding the amount obtained by 5 to arrive at the average rate per second. This rough estimate is useful, especially if the flow rate is normal and the values are above 20 mL/s. Peak urine flow can also be measured quite easily with a peakometer—a device employing a color indicator strip that, when impregnated with urine, shows maximum flow rate by changes in color against a predetermined scale. The Drake uroflowmeter is a plastic container with several chambers into which the patient voids; the maximum flow rate is determined by noting how many chambers contain urine.

In modern practice, the flow rate is more often recorded electronically: The patient voids into a container on top of a measuring device that is connected to a transducer, the weight being converted to volume and recorded on a chart in milliliters per second.

Figure 30–2 is an example of such a recording from a normal man. The general bell-shaped curve is quite clear, and the tracing shows all of the values discussed previously: total flow time, maximum flow time, maximum flow rate, average flow rate, and total volume voided. Occasional "supervoiders" can exceed the limits of the chart, but this is usually not of clinical concern (Figure 30–3). A possible variation in the bell appearance is seen in Figure 30–4.

The overall appearance of the flow curve may disclose unsuspected abnormalities. In Figure 30–5, for example, flow time is greatly prolonged. Maximum flow rate may not be low, but the average flow rate is very low—though the maximum flow rate is at one point within the normal range. Such fluctuation in flow rate is most commonly related to variations in voluntary sphincteric activity. In Figure 30–6, this

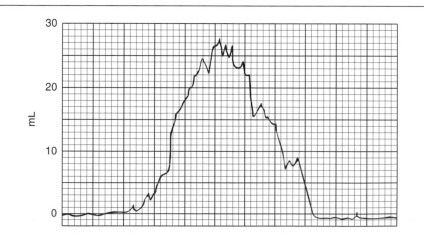

Figure 30–2. Classic normal flow rate, with peak of about 30 mL/s and average of about 20 mL/s. On the horizontal scale, one large square equals 5 s.

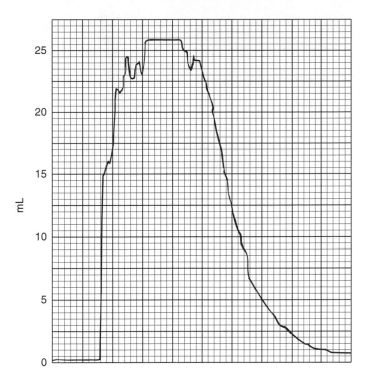

Figure 30–3. Flow rate of "supervoider." Maximum flow rate exceeds limits of chart. Tracing shows fast buildup and complete bladder emptying of large volume of urine in very short period. On the horizontal scale, one large square equals 5 s.

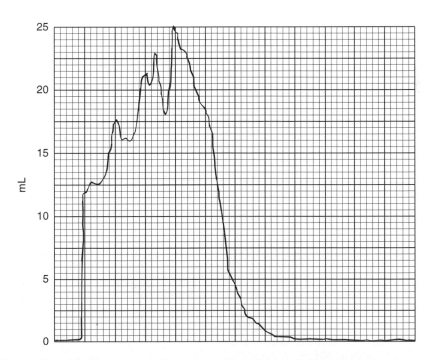

Figure 30–4. Normal flow rate with some variation in appearance of curve. Note rapid pressure rise but progressive increase to maximum, followed by a sharp drop. There is also fluctuation in ascending limb of tracing. On the horizontal scale, one large square equals 5 s.

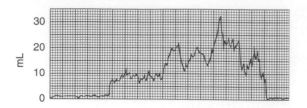

Figure 30–5. Rather low flow rate (not exceeding 10 mL/s), yet at one point the peak reaches 30–32 mL/s. Note again fluctuation in flow. On the horizontal scale, one large square equals 5 s.

pattern is extreme: Maximum flow rate never exceeds 15 mL/s, and average flow rate is about 10 mL/s, which is indicative of obstruction. (Again, this fluctuation in pattern probably reflects sphincteric hyperactivity.)

The flow rate pattern reveals a great deal about the forces involved. For example, if the patient is voiding without the aid of detrusor contractions—primarily by straining—this can be easily deduced from the pattern of the flow rate. Figure 30–7 shows an example of intermittent voiding, primarily by straining, with no detrusor activity and at a rate that sometimes does not reach the usual peaks. With experience, one becomes expert at detecting the mechanisms underlying abnormalities in flow rate. For example, in Figure 30–5, the maximum flow rate is in the normal range, the average flow rate is slightly low, and the curve has a general bell pattern, yet brief partial intermittent obstructions to flow can be readily interpreted as due to overactivity of the voluntary sphincter, a mild form of detrusor/sphincter dyssynergia (see discussion following).

Flow rates in mechanical obstruction are totally different, classically in the range of 5–6 mL/s; flow

time is greatly prolonged, and there is sustained low flow with minimal variation (Figure 30–8). Figure 30–9 is a striking example of a curve for a patient with benign prostatic hypertrophy. No simultaneous studies are needed with such a pattern, since the pattern is obviously one of mechanical obstruction.

Reduced flow rate in the absence of mechanical obstruction is due to some impairment of sphincteric or detrusor activity. This is seen in a variety of conditions, eg, normal detrusor contraction with no associated sphincteric relaxation and normal detrusor contraction with sphincteric overactivity, which is more serious. These 2 entities are commonly referred to as **detrusor/sphincter dyssynergia.** If with detrusor contraction the sphincter does not relax and open up or (worse) if it becomes overactive, urine flow is obstructed, ie, flow rate is reduced and of abnormal pattern. Reduced flow rate may occur even with increased detrusor activity if the latter is not adequate to overcome sphincteric resistance.

So many variations are possible in the shape of the flow curve—no matter how accurately the flow is recorded or how often the study is repeated to confirm abnormal findings—that it is beneficial to relate it to simultaneous recordings, such as of bladder pressure, pelvic floor electromyography, urethral pressure profile, or simply cinefluoroscopy. Nevertheless, by itself it can be one of the most valuable urodynamic studies undertaken to evaluate a specific type of voiding dysfunction. Flowmetry not only is of diagnostic value but also is valuable in follow-up studies and in deciding on treatment. In some cases, however, flowmetry alone does not provide enough data about the abnormality in the voiding mechanism. More information must then be obtained by evaluation of bladder function.

BLADDER FUNCTION

The basic factors of normal bladder function are bladder capacity, accommodation, sensation, contractility, voluntary control, and response to drugs. All of them can be evaluated by cystometry. If all are within the normal range, bladder physiology can be assumed to be normal. Every evaluation of every factor has its own implication and, before a definitive conclusion is reached, must be examined in the light of associated manifestations and findings.

Capacity, Accommodation, & Sensation

Cystometry can be done by either of 2 basic methods: (1) allowing physiologic filling of the bladder with secreted urine and continuously recording the intravesical pressure throughout a voiding cycle (starting the recording when the patient's bladder is empty and continuing it until the bladder has been filled—at which time the patient is asked to uri-

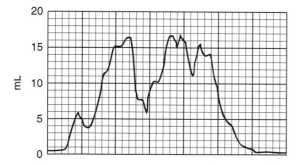

Figure 30–6. Very low flow rate of short duration and small volume. Note that maximum flow is not above 15 mL/s; however, flow average is less than 10 mL/s, and flow is almost completely interrupted in middle. On the horizontal scale, one large square equals 5 s.

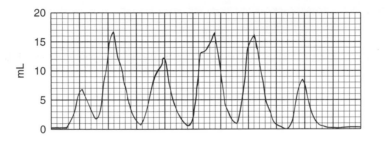

Figure 30–7. Classic flow rate due to abdominal straining with no detrusor activity. See effect of spurts of urine with complete interruption between them; patient cannot sustain increased intra-abdominal pressure. On the horizontal scale, one large square equals 5 s.

nate—and voiding begins) or (2) by filling the bladder with water and recording the intravesical pressure against the volume of water introduced into the bladder. (Gas cystometry is now being used in some laboratories as a substitute for water cystometry. However, the results are so unreliable that the technique should be used only for preliminary screening. If gas cystometry reveals any abnormality, the results must be confirmed by water cystometry.)

With the first (physiologic filling) method, the assessment of bladder function is based on voided volume (assuming that the presence of residual urine has been ruled out). The second method permits accurate determination of the volume distending the bladder and of the pressures at each level of filling, yet it has inherent defects: fluid is introduced rather than naturally secreted, and bladder filling occurs more rapidly than it normally does.

The cystometrogram (Figure 30–10) is obtained during the phase of bladder filling; the volume of fluid in the bladder is plotted against the intravesical pressure to show bladder wall compliance to filling. The normal cystometric curve shows a fairly constant low intravesical pressure until the bladder nears capacity, then a moderate rise until capacity is reached, and then a sharp rise as voiding is initiated. Nor-

mally, the sensation of fullness is first perceived when the bladder contains 100–200 mL of fluid and strongly felt as the bladder nears capacity; the desire to void occurs when the bladder is full (normal capacity, 400–500 mL). However, the bladder has a power of accommodation, ie, it can maintain an almost constant intraluminal pressure throughout its filling phase regardless of the volume of fluid present, and this directly influences compliance. As the bladder progressively accommodates larger volumes with no change in intraluminal pressure, the compliance values become higher (Compliance = Volume/Pressure) (Figure 30–10).

Contractility & Voluntary Control

The bladder normally shows no evidence of contractility or activity during the filling phase. However, once it is filled to capacity and the patient perceives the desire to urinate and consciously allows urination to proceed, strong bladder contractions occur and are sustained until the bladder is empty. The patient can of course consciously inhibit detrusor contraction. Both of these aspects of voluntary detrusor control must be assessed during cystometric study in order to rule out uninhibited bladder activity and to determine whether

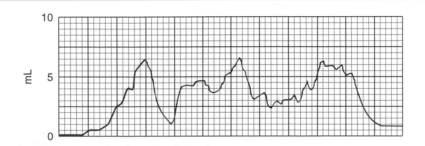

Figure 30–8. Flow rate in a case of urinary obstruction showing very low average flow rate (not above 5 or 6 mL/s). Prolonged duration of flow is associated with incomplete emptying. On the horizontal scale, one large square equals 5 s.

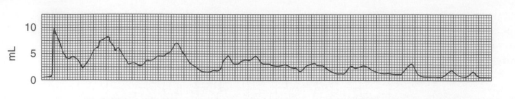

Figure 30–9. Classic low flow rate of bladder outlet obstruction (benign prostatic hypertrophy), markedly prolonged flow time, and fluctuation due to attempt at improving flow by increasing intra-abdominal pressure. On the horizontal scale, one large square equals 5 s.

the patient can inhibit urination with a full bladder and initiate urination when asked to do so. The latter is occasionally difficult to verify clinically because of conscious inhibition by a patient who may be embarrassed by the unnatural circumstances.

Responses to Drugs

Drugs are being used with increasing frequency in the evaluation of detrusor function. They can help to diagnose underlying neuropathy and to determine whether drug treatment might be of value in individual cases. Study of the relationship of bladder capacity to intravesical pressure and bladder contractility gives a rough evaluation of the patient's bladder function. Low intravesical pressure with normal bladder capacity might not be significant, whereas low pressure with a very large capacity might imply sensory loss or flaccid lower motor neuron lesion, a chronically distended bladder, or a large bladder due to myogenic damage. High pressure (usually associated with reduced capacity) that rises rapidly with bladder filling is most commonly due to inflammation, enuresis, or reduced bladder capacity. However, uninhibited bladder activity during this high-pressure filling phase might indicate neuropathic bladder or an upper motor neuron lesion.

The parasympathetic drug bethanechol chloride (Urecholine) is often used to assess bladder muscle function in patients with low bladder pressure associated with lack of detrusor contraction. No response to bethanechol suggests myogenic damage; a normal response indicates a bladder of large capacity with normal musculature; and an exaggerated response indicates a lower motor neuron lesion. The test has so many variables that it must be done meticulously to give reliable results.

Testing with anticholinergic drugs or muscle depressants may be helpful in the evaluation of uninhibited detrusor contraction or increased bladder tonus and low compliance. The information thus obtained can be useful in choosing drugs for treatment.

Recording of Intravesical Pressure

Intravesical pressure can be measured directly from the vesical cavity, either by a suprapubic approach or via a transurethral catheter. The pressure

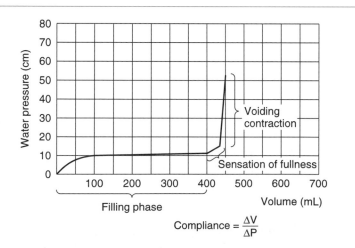

$$Compliance = \frac{\Delta V}{\Delta P}$$

Figure 30–10. Cystometrogram of patient with normal bladder capacity. Note stable intravesical pressure during filling phase; slight rise at end of filling phase, indicating bladder capacity perceived as sense of fullness; and sharp rise at end (voiding contraction).

inside the bladder is actually a function of both intra-abdominal and intravesical pressure. Thus, true detrusor pressure is the pressure recorded from the bladder cavity (intravesical pressure) minus intra-abdominal pressure. The point is important because variations in intra-abdominal pressure may alter the recorded intravesical pressure, and if the recorded intravesical pressure is mistakenly considered to reflect only detrusor pressure and not increased intra-abdominal pressure due to straining as well, erroneous conclusions may be reached.

In clinical practice, it is not necessary to measure intra-abdominal pressure, since abdominal wall contraction can be observed during the course of cystometry. A notation in the patient's chart serves to distinguish true detrusor contraction from possible overlap or increase in intra-abdominal pressure. When necessary—ie, in case of uncertainty and in order to be absolutely accurate—intra-abdominal pressure should be recorded simultaneously with intravesical pressure, since there is no other way to determine the true detrusor pressure. Intra-abdominal pressure is usually recorded by a small balloon catheter inserted high in the rectum and connected to a separate transducer.

The most valuable part of the cystometric study is the determination of voiding activity or voiding contraction. The characteristics of intravesical pressure can be quite significant. Normally, voiding contractions are not high (20–40 cm of water); this magnitude of intravesical pressure is generally adequate to deliver a normal flow rate of 20–30 mL/s and completely empty the bladder if it is well sustained. A higher voiding pressure is indicative of possible increase in outlet resistance yet denotes an overactive, healthy detrusor musculature. Figure 30–11 shows a normal flow rate associated with normal detrusor contraction at a magnitude of 20 cm of water that is well sustained and of short duration and results in complete bladder emptying.

The quality of bladder pressure can also be informative, even without simultaneous recording of flow rate. In such cases, however, it is preferable to record flow rate under normal circumstances. A well-sustained detrusor contraction, high at initiation and sustained at normal values, is seen in Figure 30–12. In Figure 30–13, the voiding pressure is too high—there is an element of sphincteric dyssynergia triggering variations in voiding pressures and flow rate. Simul-

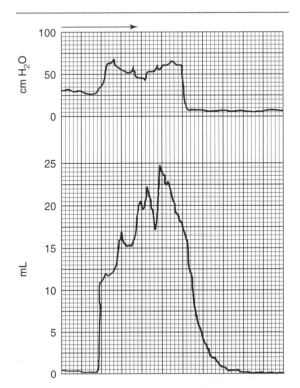

Figure 30–11. Simultaneous recording of voiding contraction and resulting flow rate. Note normal range of intravesical pressure during voiding phase as well as adequate normal flow rate (shown in Figure 30–4). On the horizontal scale, one large square equals 5 s.

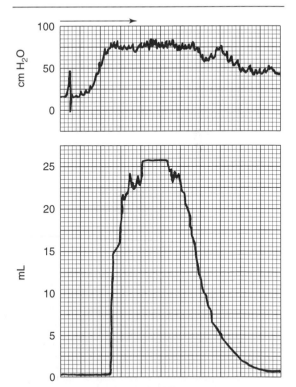

Figure 30–12. Recording of bladder pressure simultaneously with flow rate. Note slightly higher intravesical pressure with high flow rate, which, at its maximum, is that of a supervoider (see Figure 30–3). On the horizontal scale, one large square equals 5 s.

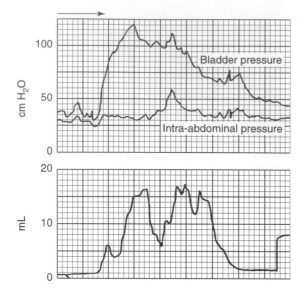

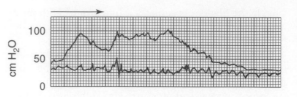

Figure 30–15. Simultaneous recording of 2 measurements—intravesical pressure (**top**) and intra-abdominal pressure (**bottom**)—on a single channel. The difference between the two can be clearly seen as pure detrusor contraction.

Figure 30–13. Simultaneous recording of flow rate and intra-abdominal pressure; intravesical pressure overlap in top recording. Note very high voiding pressure. However, flow rate is relatively low, with some interruption most likely due to sphincteric overactivity. On the horizontal scale, one large square equals 5 s.

taneous recording of bladder and intra-abdominal pressures would provide more information. As suggested previously, recording the intravesical pressure alone does not give as much information as may be required, and increased intra-abdominal pressure might be mistaken for detrusor action. This situation is illustrated in Figure 30–14. The bladder pressure

appears to indicate good detrusor function; nevertheless, simultaneous recording of intra-abdominal pressure makes it clear that all of the apparent changes in vesical intraluminal pressure in fact represent variations in intra-abdominal pressure.

Figure 30–15 shows the 2 pressures recorded on the same chart, on the same channel, by having the writing pen share the time between 2 transducers—one recording intra-abdominal pressure; the other, intravesical pressure.

A. Pathologic Changes in Bladder Capacity:
The bladder capacity is normally 400–500 mL, but it can be reduced or increased in a variety of disorders and lesions (Table 30–1). Some common causes of reduced bladder capacity are enuresis, urinary tract infection, contracted bladder, upper motor neuron lesion, and defunctionalized bladder. Reduced capacity also may occur in association with incontinence and in postsurgical bladder. Increased bladder capacity is not uncommon in women who have trained themselves to retain large volumes of urine. Bladder capacity is increased also in sensory neuropathic disorders, lower motor neuron lesions, and chronic obstruction from myogenic damage. It is important to relate bladder capacity to the intravesical pressure (Table 30–2). Slight variations in bladder capacity with no change in bladder pressure might be of less

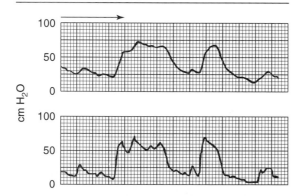

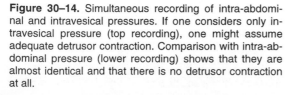

Figure 30–14. Simultaneous recording of intra-abdominal and intravesical pressures. If one considers only intravesical pressure (top recording), one might assume adequate detrusor contraction. Comparison with intra-abdominal pressure (lower recording) shows that they are almost identical and that there is no detrusor contraction at all.

Table 30–1. Causes of reduced or increased bladder capacity. (Normal capacity in adults is 400–500 mL.)

Causes of reduced bladder capacity
Enuresis or incontinence
Bladder infections
Bladder contracture due to fibrosis (from tuberculosis, interstitial cystitis, etc)
Upper motor neuron lesions
Defunctionalized bladder
Postsurgical bladder
Causes of increased bladder capacity
Sensory neuropathic disorders
Lower motor neuron lesions
Megacystis (congenital)
Chronic urinary tract obstruction

Table 30–2. Relationship between intravesical pressure and capacity in various diseases.

Low intravesical pressure
Normal capacity
Large capacity
  Sensory deficits (diabetes mellitus, tabes dorsalis)
  Flaccid lower motor neuron lesions
  Large bladder (due to repeated stretching)
High intravesical pressure
Rapidly rising
  Reduced capacity
  Inflammation
  Enuresis
Uninhibited contraction
  Uninhibited neurogenic bladder
  Upper motor neuron lesions

Table 30–3. Variations in detrusor contractility in various diseases.

Normal contractions
Normal volume
Well-sustained contractions
Absent or weak contractions
Sensory neuropathic disorders
Conscious inhibition of contractions
Lower motor neuron lesions
Uninhibited contractions
Upper motor neuron lesions
Cerebrovascular lesions

significance than the reverse. What is usually of greatest significance is the bladder with reduced capacity associated with normal pressure or, more important, with increased pressure, or the bladder with large capacity associated with decreased pressure.

B. Pathologic Changes in Accommodation: Accommodation reflects intravesical pressure in response to filling. In a bladder with normal power of accommodation—in which case the micturition center of the spinal cord is controlled by the central nervous system—intravesical pressure does not vary with progressive bladder filling until capacity is reached; in other words, when compliance is reduced, there will be a progressive increase in intravesical pressure and loss of accommodation. This usually occurs at smaller volumes and with reduced capacity. The patient being studied by cystometry can always note the presence or absence of a sensation of fullness. One normally does not sense volumes in the bladder but only changes in pressure.

C. Pathologic Changes in Sensation: A slight rise in intravesical pressure on cystometry signifies that the bladder is full to normal capacity and that the patient is perceiving it. This sign is usually absent in pure sensory neuropathy and in mixed sensory and motor loss. (Other sensations can be tested for in different ways; see Chapter 29.)

D. Pathologic Changes in Contractility: The bladder is normally capable of sustaining contraction until it is empty. Absence of residual urine after voiding usually denotes well-sustained contractions. Neuropathic dysfunction is usually associated with residual urine of variable amount depending on the type of dysfunction. Significant outlet resistance—mechanical or functional—is also a cause of residual urine.

Cystometric study may disclose complete absence of detrusor contractility due to motor or sensory deficits or conscious inhibition of detrusor activity (Table 30–3). Detrusor hyperactivity is shown as uninhibited activity, usually due to interruption of the neural connection between spinal cord centers and the higher midbrain and cortical centers.

An integrated picture of bladder capacity, intravesical pressure, and contractility is useful for general assessment of the basic physiologic mechanisms of the bladder. Low intravesical pressure in a patient with normal bladder capacity may have no clinical significance, whereas low pressure with a very large capacity may signify sensory loss or a flaccid lower motor neuron lesion, a chronically distended bladder, or a large bladder due to myogenic damage. High pressure (usually associated with reduced capacity) that rises rapidly with bladder filling is most commonly associated with inflammation, enuresis, or reduced bladder capacity. However, uninhibited activity during the interval of rising pressure that occurs with bladder filling may indicate a neurogenic bladder or an upper motor neuron lesion.

SPHINCTERIC FUNCTION

Urinary sphincteric function can be evaluated either by recording the electromyographic activity of the voluntary component of the sphincteric mechanism or by recording the activity of both smooth and voluntary components by measuring the intraurethral pressure of the sphincteric unit. The latter method is called **pressure profile measurement (profilometry)**.

Profilometry

The urethral pressure profile is determined by recording the pressure in the urethra at every level of the sphincteric unit from the internal meatus to the end of the sphincteric segment. Profilometry has been performed by gas or water perfusion techniques, but these methods have serious limitations. Gas profilometry requires a very high flow rate (120–150 mL/min) and is neither accurate, consistent, nor sensitive; it should no longer be used. Water profilometry, which requires a flow rate of about 2 mL/min, gives fairly accurate results. It may be used for screening patients with incontinence or functional obstruction, but it is not very sensitive and only provides information about total urethral pressure. The membrane catheter and microtransducer techniques of profilometry described in the following sections provide much more accurate and detailed information.

A. Membrane Catheter Technique: Membrane catheters used for recording pressure profiles usually have several channels, so that several measurements can be obtained simultaneously. My group's current membrane catheter has 4 lumens and an outside diameter of 7F. Two of the 4 lumens are open at the end, one for bladder filling and the other for recording bladder pressure; the other 2 lumens, which are situated 7 and 8 cm from the catheter tip, are covered by a thin membrane with a small chamber underneath (Figure 30–16). The space under the membrane and the lumen connected to it are filled with fluid, free of any gas, and connected to a pressure transducer. The pressure under this membrane should be zero at the level of the transducer so that it can register any pressure applied to the membrane whatever its level at any time. The catheter also has radiopaque markers at 1-cm intervals starting at the tip, with a heavier marker every 5 cm; it also has a special marker showing the site of each membrane. The markers permit fluoroscopic visualization of the catheter and the membrane levels during the entire study.

B. Microtransducer Technique: The results of microtransducer profilometry are as accurate as those obtained with the membrane catheter. Two microtransducers can be mounted on the same catheter, one at the tip for recording of bladder pressure and the other about 5–7 cm from the tip to record the urethral pressure profile as the catheter is gradually withdrawn from the bladder cavity to below the sphincteric segment.

Electromyographic Study of Sphincteric Function

Electromyography alone gives useful information about sphincteric function, but it is most valuable when done in conjunction with cystometry. There are several techniques for electromyographic studies of the urinary sphincter; either surface electrodes or needle electrodes are used. Surface electrode recordings can be obtained either from the lumen of the urethra in the region of the voluntary sphincter or, preferably, from the anal sphincter by using an anal plug electrode. Recording via needle electrodes can be obtained from the anal sphincter, from the bulk of the musculature of the pelvic floor, or from the external sphincter itself, though in the latter case the placement is difficult and the accuracy of the results is questionable.

Direct needle electromyography of the urethral sphincter provides the most accurate information. Because the technique is difficult, however, simpler approaches are generally used. The anal sphincter is readily accessible for electromyographic testing, and testing of any area of the pelvic floor musculature generally reflects the overall electrical activity of the pelvic floor, including the external sphincter. Electromyography is not simple, and the assistance of an experienced electromyographer is probably essential. Electromyographic study makes use of the electrical

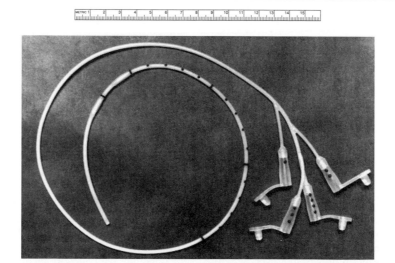

Figure 30–16. Membrane catheter showing radiopaque markers. Note 2 membrane chambers for urethral pressure measurements and 4 separate channels—2 channels for urethral pressure recording, one for bladder pressure recording, and one for bladder filling—each of which is connected to a separate ending. (Reproduced, with permission, from Tanagho EA, Jonas U: Membrane catheter: Effective for recording pressure in lower urinary tract. Urology 1977;10:173.)

activity that is constantly present within the pelvic floor and external urinary sphincter at rest and that increases progressively with bladder filling. If the bladder contracts for voiding, electrical activity ceases completely, permitting free flow of urine, and is resumed at the termination of detrusor contraction to secure closure of the bladder outlet (Figure 30–17). Electromyography is important in showing this effect and, along with bladder pressure measurement, can pinpoint the exact time of detrusor contraction. Persistence of electromyographic activity during the phase of detrusor contraction for voiding—or, even worse, its overactivity during that phase—interferes with the voiding mechanism and leads to incoordination between detrusor and sphincter (**detrusor/sphincter dyssynergia**). During the interval of detrusor contraction, increased electromyographic activity interferes with the free flow of urine, as can be shown by simultaneous recording of flow rate.

Electromyographic recording shows only the activity of the voluntary component of the urinary sphincteric mechanism and the overall activity of the pelvic floor. More information is gained when the electromyogram is recorded simultaneously with detrusor pressure or flow rate. However, this method gives no information about the smooth component of the urinary sphincter.

Pressure Measurement for Evaluation of Sphincteric Function

Perfusion profilometry, usually performed with the patient supine and with an empty bladder, provides a simple pressure profile that allows determination of the maximum pressure within the urethra. This is adequate for screening patients with incontinence or functional obstruction. However, in order to determine the maximum closure pressure (see section following), the bladder pressure must be recorded si-multaneously with the urethral pressure profile. Such simultaneous recording is not possible with perfusion profilometry.

The membrane catheter and microtransducer techniques of profilometry, because they use multichannel recording, routinely provide much more detailed information; at least 4 distinct sets of measurements can be obtained from the simplest pressure profile made using the membrane catheter or microtransducer (Figure 30–18): (1) the maximum pressure exerted around the sphincteric segment, (2) the net closure pressure of the urethra, (3) the distribution of this closure pressure along the entire length of the sphincter, and (4) the exact functional length of the sphincteric unit and its relation to the anatomic length.

A. Total Pressure: The urethral pressure profile recording shows the pressure directly recorded within the urethral lumen along the entire length of the urethra from internal to external meatus. From this measurement, the maximum pressure exerted around the sphincteric segment can be determined.

B. Closure Pressure: The urethral closure pressure is the difference between intravesical pressure (bladder pressure) and urethral pressure, ie, the net closure pressure. The **maximum closure pressure** is the most important measurement in evaluating the activity of the sphincteric unit and its responses to various factors.

C. Distribution of Closure Pressure: As the catheter is withdrawn down the urethra, the closure pressure at various levels along the entire length of the sphincteric segment is recorded.

D. Functional Length of Sphincteric Unit: The functional length of the sphincteric unit is the portion with positive closure pressure, ie, where urethral pressure is greater than bladder pressure. The distinction between anatomic length and functional length is important. Regardless of the anatomic length, the effectiveness of the urethral sphincter

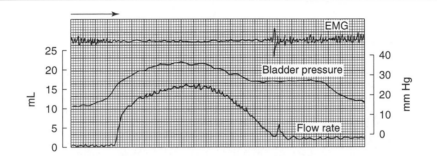

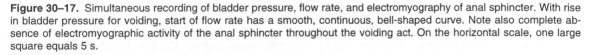

Figure 30–17. Simultaneous recording of bladder pressure, flow rate, and electromyography of anal sphincter. With rise in bladder pressure for voiding, start of flow rate has a smooth, continuous, bell-shaped curve. Note also complete absence of electromyographic activity of the anal sphincter throughout the voiding act. On the horizontal scale, one large square equals 5 s.

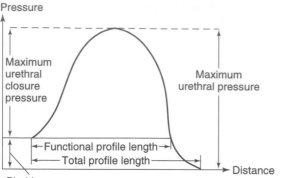

Figure 30–18. Urethral pressure profile and its components. Note functional length, anatomic length, and the shape of the profile, with maximum closure pressure in the middle segment of the urethra rather than at the level of the internal meatus. (Reproduced, with permission, from Bradley W: Cystometry and sphincter electromyography. Mayo Clin Proc 1976;329:335.)

may be limited to a shorter segment. In women, the pressure is normally rather low at the level of the internal meatus but builds up gradually until it reaches its maximum in the mid urethra, where the voluntary sphincter is concentrated; it slowly drops until it is at its lowest at the external meatus. On the basis of these measurements, it is clear that the anatomic and functional lengths of the normal urethra in women are about the same and that the maximum closure pressure is at about the center of the urethra—not at the level of the internal meatus. In men, the pressure profile is slightly different: the functional length is longer, and the maximum closure pressure builds up in the prostatic segment, reaches a peak in the membranous urethra, and drops as it reaches the level of the bulbous urethra (Figure 30–19). The entire functional length in men is about 6–7 cm; in women, it is about 4 cm.

Dynamic Changes in Pressure Profile

The usefulness of the pressure profile is enhanced if the examiner notes the sphincteric responses to various physiologic stimuli: (1) postural changes (supine, sitting, standing), (2) changes in intra-abdominal pressure (sharp increase with coughing; sustained increase with bearing down), (3) voluntary contractions of the pelvic floor musculature to assess activity of the voluntary sphincter, and (4) bladder filling. The latter test consists of making baseline recordings with both an empty bladder and a full bladder and comparing these recordings with recordings made under conditions of stress (coughing, bearing down) and during voluntary contraction with an empty bladder and a full bladder.

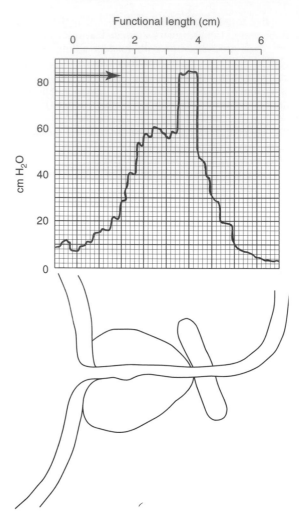

Figure 30–19. Normal male urethral pressure profile showing progressive rise throughout prostatic segment and peak being reached in membranous urethra. (Reproduced, with permission, from Tanagho EA: Membrane and microtransducer catheters: Their effectiveness for profilometry of the lower urinary tract. Urol Clin North Am 1979;6:110.)

A simple pressure profile is informative but does not provide data that will delineate and identify specific sites of sphincteric dysfunction. The advantage of using a membrane catheter or microtransducer is that the pressure profile can be expanded by slowing the rate of withdrawal of the catheter and speeding up the motion of the recording paper. Since the catheter can be held at different levels for any length of time, other tests can be made and their effects monitored. Response to stress (particularly when standing), response to bladder distention, response to changes in position, the effects of drugs, and the effects of nerve stimulation can all be evaluated if needed. Bladder filling nor-

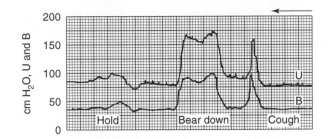

Figure 30–20. Simultaneous recording of intraurethral (U) and intravesical (B) pressures and their responses to coughing and bearing down. Rise in intravesical pressure as a result of increase in intra-abdominal pressure is associated with simultaneous rise in intraurethral pressure, maintaining a constant closure pressure.

mally leads to increase in tonus of the sphincteric element, with some rise in closure pressure, especially when bladder filling approaches maximum capacity. Stress from coughing or straining also normally results in sustained or increased closure pressure (Figure 30–20). When the patient stands up, closure pressure is usually substantially increased (Figure 30–21). Testing for activity of the voluntary sphincter by the hold maneuver (asking the patient to actively contract the perineal muscles) produces a significant rise in urethral pressure (Figure 30–22). When the effects of all of these responses are recorded concomitantly with intravesical pressure, the data can be interrelated and the exact closure pressure at any given time can be ascertained.

The response to stress with the patient standing usually should be recorded also. Especially in cases of stress incontinence, weakness of the sphincteric mechanism may not be apparent with the patient sitting or supine but becomes clear when the patient stands up.

The effectiveness of drugs in increasing or reducing the urethral pressure profile can be tested also. For example, phenoxybenzamine (Regitine) can be administered and the urethral pressure profile recorded; a drop in pressure indicates that alpha blockers may be an ef-fective means of decreasing urethral resistance, with obvious implications for the management of urinary obstruction. Anticholinergic drugs such as propantheline bromide can be tested for possible use as detrusor depressants. Detrusor activity can be investigated by administering bethanechol chloride (Urecholine) and simultaneously recording bladder and urethral pressures.

Characteristics of Normal Pressure Profile (Figure 30–23)

The basic features of the ideal pressure profile are not easily defined. In women, the normal urethral pressure profile has a peak of 100–120 cm of water, and the closure pressure is in the range of 90–100 cm of water. Closure pressure is lowest at the level of the internal meatus, gradually builds up in the proximal 0.5 cm, and reaches its maximum about 1 cm below the internal meatus. It is sustained for another 2 cm and then starts to drop in the distal urethra. The functional length of a normal adult female urethra is about 4 cm. The response to stress with coughing and bearing down is sustained or augmented closure pressure.

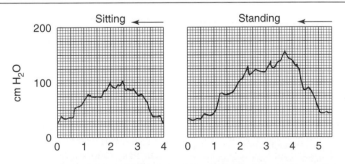

Figure 30–21. Urethral pressure profile of normal woman in sitting and standing positions. Note marked improvement in closure pressure (in both functional length and magnitude) when patient stands up. (Reproduced, with permission, from Tanagho EA: Urodynamics of female urinary incontinence with emphasis on stress incontinence. J Urol 1979;122:200.)

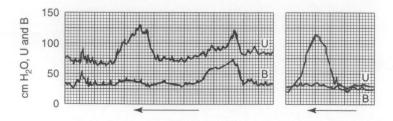

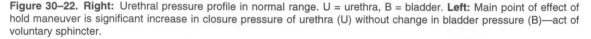

Figure 30–22. Right: Urethral pressure profile in normal range. U = urethra, B = bladder. **Left:** Main point of effect of hold maneuver is significant increase in closure pressure of urethra (U) without change in bladder pressure (B)—act of voluntary sphincter.

Standing up also increases this pressure, with maximum rise in the mid segment. Nervous stimulation is rarely tested in normal people, but sacral root stimulation can reveal the closure pressure in the voluntary element of the sphincteric segment of the urethra.

Pressure Profile in Pathologic Conditions

A. Urinary Stress Incontinence: The classic pressure changes noted in this type of incontinence are as follows:

1. Low urethral closure pressure.
2. Short urethral functional length at the expense of the proximal segment.
3. Weak responses to stress.
4. Loss of urethral closure pressure with bladder filling.
5. Fall in closure pressure on assuming the upright position.
6. Weak responses to stress in the upright position.

B. Urinary Urge Incontinence: The most per-

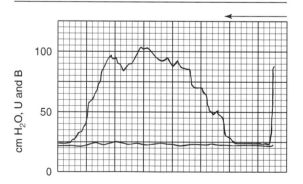

Figure 30–23. Recording of normal female urethral pressure profile, showing basic features and actual values, including anatomic as well as functional length. U = urethra, B = bladder. (Reproduced, with permission, from Tanagho EA: Membrane and microtransducer catheters: Their effectiveness for profilometry of the lower urinary tract. Urol Clin North Am 1979;6:110.)

tinent pressure changes in urinary urge incontinence are normal or high closure pressures with normal responses to stress, normal responses to bladder filling, and normal responses when the patient stands up. Urge incontinence can result from any of the following mechanisms (Figure 30–24):

1. Detrusor hyperirritability, with active detrusor contractions overcoming urethral resistance and leading to urine leakage.
2. The exact reverse, ie, a constant detrusor pressure with no evidence of detrusor instability but with urethral instability in that urethral pressure becomes less than bladder pressure, so that urine leakage occurs without any detrusor contraction.
3. A combination of the 2 preceding mechanisms (the most common form), ie, some drop in closure pressure and some rise in bladder pressure. In such cases, the drop in urethral pressure is often the initiating factor.

C. Combination of Stress and Urge Incontinence: In this common clinical condition, profilometry is used to determine the magnitude of each component, ie, whether the incontinence is primarily urge, primarily stress, or both equally. As a guide to treatment, profilometric studies sometimes show that stress incontinence precipitates urge incontinence. The stress elements initiate urine leakage in the proximal urethra, exciting detrusor response and sphincteric relaxation and ending with complete urine leakage. Once the stress components are corrected, the urge element disappears. This combination cannot be detected clinically.

D. Postprostatectomy Incontinence: After prostatectomy, there is usually no positive pressure in the entire prostatic fossa, minimal closure pressure at the apex of the prostate, and normal or greater than normal pressure within the voluntary sphincteric segment of the membranous urethra. It is the functional length of the sphincteric segment above the genitourinary diaphragm that determines the degree of incontinence; the magnitude of closure pressure in the voluntary sphincteric segment has no bearing on the patient's symptoms. High pressure is almost always

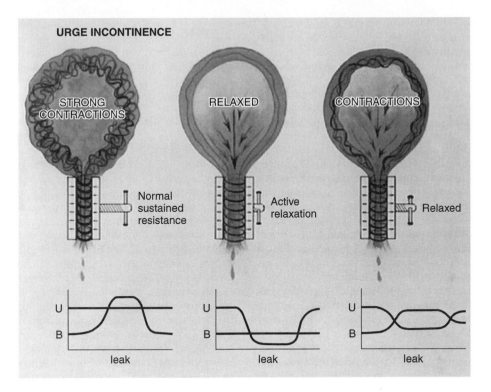

URGE INCONTINENCE

Figure 30–24. Three mechanisms of urinary urge incontinence. **Left:** Normal sphincter activity exceeded by hyperactive detrusor. **Center:** Normal detrusor, without any overactivity, yet unstable urethra with marked drop in urethral pressure leading to leakage. **Right:** Most common combination—some rise in intravesical pressure due to detrusor hyperirritability associated with drop in urethral pressure due to sphincteric relaxation. U = urethra, B = bladder.

recorded within the voluntary sphincter despite the common belief that what someone termed "iatrogenically induced incontinence" is due to damage to the voluntary sphincter—which is definitely not the case.

E. Detrusor/Sphincter Dyssynergia: In this situation, findings of cystometric studies are normal at the filling phase, with possible closure pressure above average. However, the pathologic entity becomes clear when the patient attempts to void: Detrusor contraction is associated with a simultaneous increase in urethral closure pressure instead of a drop in pressure. This is a direct effect of overactivity of the voluntary component, leading to obstructive voiding or low flow rate and frequent interruption of voiding. This phenomenon is commonly seen in patients with supraspinal lesions. It can be encountered in several other conditions as well.

VALUE OF SIMULTANEOUS RECORDINGS

Measurement of each of the physiologic variables described previously gives useful clinical information. A rise in intravesical pressure has greater signif-

icance when related to intra-abdominal pressure. The urine flow rate is more significant if recorded in conjunction with the total volume voided as well as with evidence of detrusor contraction. The urethral pressure profile is more significant when related to bladder pressure and to variations in intra-abdominal pressure and voluntary muscular activity. And for greatest clinical usefulness, all data must be recorded simultaneously so that the investigator can analyze the activity involved in each sequence.

At a minimum, a proper urodynamic study should include recordings of intravesical pressure and intra-abdominal pressure (true detrusor pressure is intravesical pressure minus intra-abdominal pressure), urethral pressure or electromyography, flow rate, and, if possible, voided volume. For a complete study, the following are necessary: intra-abdominal pressure, intravesical pressure, urethral sphincteric pressure at various (usually 2) levels, flow rate, voided volume, anal sphincteric pressure (as a function of pelvic floor activity), and electromyography of the anal or urethral striated sphincter. These physiologic data are recorded with the patient quiet as well as during activity (ie, voluntary increase in intra-abdominal pressure, changes in the state of bladder filling, voluntary contraction of perineal muscles, or—more comprehensively—an entire voiding act starting from an empty bladder; continuing through complete filling of the bladder, and initiation of voiding; and ending when the bladder is empty).

The data derived from urodynamic studies are descriptive of urinary tract function. Simultaneous visualization of the lower urinary tract as multiple recordings are made gives more precise information about the pathologic changes underlying the symptoms. By means of cinefluoroscopy, the examiner can observe the configuration of the bladder, bladder base, and bladder outlet during bladder filling (usually with radiopaque medium). The information obtained can then be correlated with the level of catheters, with pressure recordings, and with changes in pelvic floor support during voiding. Combined cinefluoroscopy and pressure measurements thus represent the ultimate in urodynamic studies.

A model of such a urodynamic laboratory has been developed at the University of California School of Medicine (San Francisco). As shown in Figure 30–25, the patient sits in a specially designed toilet chair over a device for collecting urine and measuring flow rate. The patient faces the x-ray tube that receives the image of the bladder and bladder outlet, which is projected on a fluoroscopic screen. The pressure-recording catheters are connected to a set of transducers that are in turn connected to a

polygraph recording machine, on top of which a television camera is mounted. On a separate television monitor, the image of the pressure recording is combined with the image from the fluoroscopic monitor. A permanent record can be obtained on videotape or motion picture film.

Such studies are recorded on a polygraph chart as well as on motion picture film or videotape. Sound usually can be added to the film or videotape to provide the history, the examiner's observations and instructions during the study, and a spoken version of pressure measurements so that they can be followed from outside the examination room.

Several machines are available for recording urodynamic studies. Some of them are simple, limited to one or two channels; more complex machines may have as many as 8 channels. Each type is designed to meet a particular need of the investigator or institution. The needs in private practice are quite different from those of a large institution or referral center for complex urologic problems, especially neuropathic dysfunctions. In our laboratory, my colleagues and I have developed a series of pressure-recording units ranging from a single-channel instrument to a 4-channel instrument. Every channel is capable of recording 2 sets of measurements, so that the single-channel machine represents in reality 2 channels and the 4-channel machine represents 8 channels. Pressure recordings are obtained with an 8-channel machine (Figure 30–26). Six

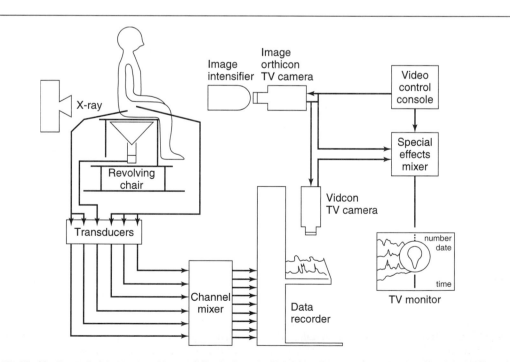

Figure 30–25. Urodynamic laboratory with specially designed toilet chair; patient sits between x-ray tube and image intensifier. A television camera records the fluoroscopic image, and a second camera picks up recordings from a polygraph machine to be projected onto one television monitor, photographed, and recorded on videotape.

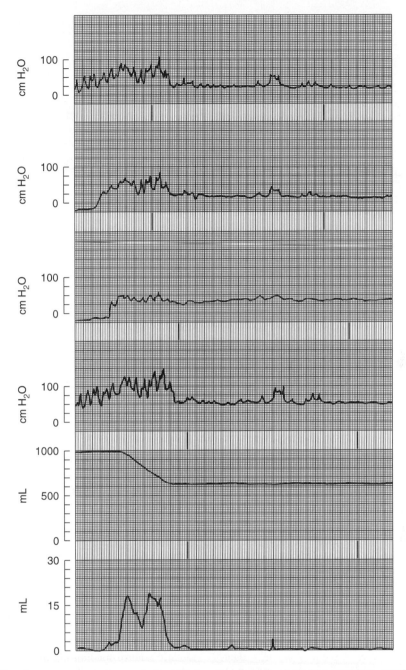

Figure 30–26. Simultaneous pressure recordings, showing (top to bottom) bladder pressure, proximal urethral pressure, midurethral pressure, intra-abdominal pressure, total volume voided, and flow rate. On the horizontal scale, one large square equals 5 s.

such channels are used to record bladder pressure, 2 urethral pressures, rectal pressure, flow rate, and total volume voided, and 2 additional channels are used to record anal sphincteric pressure and electromyogram (not shown). Because every channel can be used to record 2 sets of measurements simultaneously, the in-vestigator can record intra-abdominal pressure and bladder pressure overlapped (so that the net detrusor pressure is recorded) and anal sphincteric pressure and midurethral pressure in such a way that the reflection of each on the other is also readily seen (Figure 30–27).

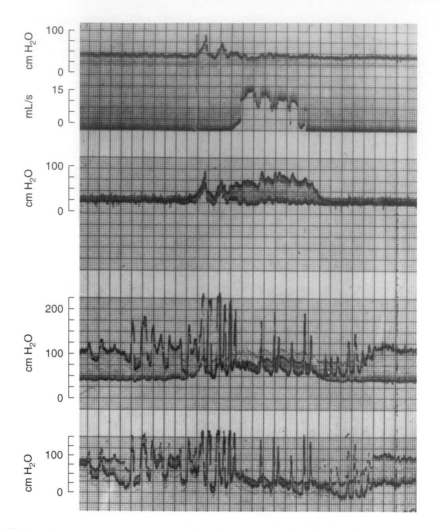

Figure 30–27. Eight sets of measurements recorded on 4-channel unit, in which each pen is writing 2 records. **Top channel:** Flow rate and intra-abdominal pressure. **Second channel:** Combination of bladder pressure and intra-abdominal pressure, the difference between the two showing true detrusor contraction pressure. **Third channel:** Combination of bladder pressure and maximum urethral pressure, the difference between the two showing urethral closure pressure. **Bottom channel:** Anal sphincteric pressure and midurethral pressure as a function of overall perineal activity. Any combination can be set on such a machine.

The complete recording machine contains 4 data-transmission channels attached to transducers; plotters to record the volume infused into the bladder, the volume voided, and the flow rate; devices for visual and auditory monitoring of data; and a variable-speed pump for infusing fluids into the bladder, with an automatic control for limiting the total volume infused (between 25 and 1000 mL, depending on the patient's age and bladder capacity). The recording machine is portable, ie, it can be rolled anywhere, and it can be attached to the cinefluoroscopic machine if this is desired.

REFERENCES

URETHRA & BLADDER

Abrams P: Lower urinary tract symptoms in women: Who to investigate and how. Br J Urol 1997;80(Suppl 1):43.

Abrams P: Managing lower urinary tract symptoms in older men. Br Med J 1995;310:1113.

Abrams P: Objective evaluation of bladder outlet obstruction. Br J Urol 1995;76(Suppl 1):11.

Andersen JT, Bradley WE: Urethral pressure profilometry: Assessment of urethral function by combined intraurethral pressure and EMG recording. Urol Int 1978;33:40.

Artibani W: Diagnosis and significance of idiopathic overactive bladder. Urology 1997;50(6A Suppl):25.

Awad SA et al: Urethral pressure profile in female stress incontinence. J Urol 1978;120:475.

Bazeed MA et al: Histochemical study of urethral striated musculature in the dog. J Urol 1982;128:406.

Beck RP, McCormick S, Nordstrom L: Intraurethral-intravesical cough-pressure spike differences in 267 patients surgically cured of genuine stress incontinence of urine. Obstet Gynecol 1988;72:302.

Berger Y et al: Urodynamic findings in Parkinson's disease. J Urol 1987;138:836.

Bruschini H, Schmidt RA, Tanagho EA: Effect of urethral stretch on urethral pressure profile. Invest Urol 1977;15:107.

Bruskewitz R, Raz S: Urethral pressure profile using microtip catheter in females. Urology 1979;14:303.

Bump RC, Fantl JA, Hurt WG: Dynamic urethral pressure profilometry pressure transmission ratio determinations after continence surgery: Understanding the mechanism of success, failure, and complications. Obstet Gynecol 1988;72:870.

Cardenas DD et al: Residual urine volumes in patients with spinal cord injury: Measurement with a portable ultrasound instrument. Arch Phys Med Rehabil 1988; 69:514.

Churchill BM, Gilmour RF, Williot P: Urodynamics. Pediatr Clin North Am 1987;34:1133.

Coolsaet B: Bladder compliance and detrusor activity during the collection phase. Neurourol Urodynam 1985;4:263.

DeGroat WC: A neurologic basis for the overactive bladder. Urology 1997;50(6A Suppl):36.

Desai P: Bladder pressure studies combined with micturating cystourethrography. Radiography 1985;52:2.

Desmond AD, Ramayya GR: The adaptation of urethral pressure profiles to detect sphincter incompetence and sphincter obstruction using a microcomputer. J Urol 1987;137:457.

Diokno AC et al: Clinical and cystometric characteristics of continent and incontinent noninstitutionalized elderly. J Urol 1988;140:567.

Dørflinger T et al: Urodynamic and histological correlates of benign prostatic hyperplasia. J Urol 1988;140: 1487.

Fantl JA et al: Urinary incontinence in community-dwelling women: Clinical, urodynamic, and severity characteristics. Am J Obstet Gynecol 1990;162:946.

Fidas A et al: Prevalence of spina bifida occulta in patients with functional disorders of the lower urinary tract and its relation to urodynamic and neurophysiological measurements. Br Med J 1989;298:357.

Finkbeiner AE: Is bethanechol chloride clinically effective in promoting bladder emptying? A literature review. J Urol 1985;134:443.

Gilmour RF et al: Analysis of the urethral pressure profile using a mechanical model. Invest Urol 1980;18: 54.

Glen ES, Eadie A, Rowan D: Urethral closure pressure profile measurements in female urinary incontinence. Acta Urol Belg 1984;52:174.

Gosling JA et al: A comparative study of the human external sphincter and periurethral levator ani muscles. Br J Urol 1981;53:35.

Graber P, Laurent G, Tanagho EA: Effect of abdominal pressure rise on the urethral profile: An experimental study on dogs. Invest Urol 1974;12:57.

Griffiths DJ, Versi E: Urethral function. Curr Opin Obstet Gynecol 1996;8:372.

Henriksson L, Andersson K-E, Ulmsten U: The urethral pressure profiles in continent and stress-incontinent women. Scand J Urol Nephrol 1979;13:5.

Henriksson L, Aspelin P, Ulmsten U: Combined urethrocystometry and cinefluorography in continent and incontinent women. Radiology 1979;130:607.

Holmes DM, Plevnik S, Stanton SL: Bladder neck electrical conductivity in female urinary urgency and urge incontinence. Br J Obstet Gynaecol 1989;96:816.

Jepsen JV, Bruskewitz RC: Comprehensive patient evaluation for benign prostatic hyperplasia. Urology 1998; 51(4A Suppl):13.

Jonas U, Klotter HJ: Study of three urethral pressure recording devices: Theoretical considerations. Urol Res 1978;6:119.

Jones KW, Schoenberg HW: Comparison of the incidence of bladder hyperreflexia in patients with benign prostatic hypertrophy and age-matched female controls. J Urol 1985;133:425.

Karram MM et al: Urodynamic changes following hormonal replacement therapy in women with premature ovarian failure. Obstet Gynecol 1989;74:208.

Kelly MJ, Roskamp D, Leach GE: Transurethral incision of the prostate: A preoperative and postoperative analysis of symptoms and urodynamic findings. J Urol 1989;142:1507.

Khan Z, Mieza M, Leiter E: Role of detrusor hyperreflexia (bladder instability in primary enuresis). Proc Int Continence Soc 1984;14:107.

Kim YH, Kattan MW, Boone TB: Bladder leak point pressure: The measure for sphincterotomy success in spinal cord injured patients with external detrusor-sphincter dyssynergia. J Urol 1998;159:493.

Koefoot RB Jr, Webster GD: Urodynamic evaluation in women with frequency, urgency symptoms. Urology 1983;21:648.

Koelbl H, Bernaschek G: A new method for sonographic urethrocystography and simultaneous pressure-flow measurements. Obstet Gynecol 1989;74:417.

Langer R et al: Detrusor instability following colposuspension for urinary stress incontinence. Br J Obstet Gynaecol 1988;95:607.

Lim CS, Abrams P: The Abrams-Griffiths nomogram. World J Urol 1995;13:34.

Lose G: Urethral pressure measurement. Acta Obstet Gynecol Scand Suppl 1997;166:39.

Lytton B, Green DF: Urodynamic studies in patients undergoing bladder replacement surgery. J Urol 1989; 141:1394.

Manoliu RA: Voiding cystourethrography with synchronous measurements of pressures and flow in the diagnosis of subvesical obstruction in men: A radiological view. J Urol 1987;137:1196.

McGuire EJ: The role of urodynamic investigation in the assessment of benign prostatic hypertrophy. J Urol 1992;148:1133.

McGuire EJ, Cespedes RD, O'Connell HE: Leak-point pressures. Urol Clin North Am 1996;23:253.

Nielsen KT et al: Symptom analysis and uroflowmetry 7 years after transurethral resection of the prostate. J Urol 1989;142:1251.

Nørgaard JP et al: Standardization and definitions in lower urinary tract dysfunction in children. International Children's Continence Society. Br J Urol 1998; 81(Suppl 3):1.

Ouslander J et al: Clinical versus urodynamic diagnosis in an incontinent geriatric female population. J Urol 1987;137:68.

Ouslander J et al: Simple versus multichannel cystometry in the evaluation of bladder function in an incontinent geriatric population. J Urol 1988;140:1482.

Saxton HM: Urodynamics: The appropriate modality for the investigation of frequency, urgency, incontinence, and voiding difficulties. Radiology 1990;175: 307.

Schafer W: Analysis of bladder-outlet function with the linearized passive urethral resistance relation, linPURR, and a disease-specific approach for grading obstruction: From complex to simple. World J Urol 1995;13:47.

Schafer W: Principles and clinical application of advanced urodynamic analysis of voiding function. Urol Clin North Am 1990;17:553.

Schmidt RA, Tanagho EA: Urethral syndrome or urinary tract infection? Urology 1981;18:424.

Schmidt RA, Witherow R, Tanagho EA: Recording urethral pressure profile. Urology 1977;10:390.

Schmidt RA et al: Urethral pressure profilometry with membrane catheter compared with perfusion catheter systems. Urol Int 1978;33:345.

Snyder JA, Lipsitz DU: Evaluation of female urinary incontinence. Urol Clin North Am 1991;18:197.

Starer P, Libow L: Cystometric evaluation of bladder dysfunction in elderly diabetic patients. Arch Intern Med 1990;150:810.

Styles RA et al: Long-term monitoring of bladder pressure in chronic retention of urine: The relationship between detrusor activity and upper tract dilatation. J Urol 1988;140:330.

Sullivan MP, Comiter CV, Yalla SV: Micturitional urethral pressure profilometry. Urol Clin North Am 1996; 23:263.

Tanagho EA: Interpretation of the physiology of micturition. In: Hinman F Jr (editor): Hydrodynamics. Thomas, 1971.

Tanagho EA: Membrane and microtransducer catheters: Their effectiveness for profilometry of the lower urinary tract. Urol Clin North Am 1979;6:110.

Tanagho EA: Neurophysiology of urinary incontinence. In: Cantor EB (editor): Female Urinary Stress Incontinence. Thomas, 1979.

Tanagho EA: Urinary stress incontinence. Urol Arch (Belgrade) 1977;8:17.

Tanagho EA: Urodynamics of female urinary incontinence with emphasis on stress incontinence. J Urol 1979;122:200.

Tanagho EA: Vesicourethral dynamics. In: Lutzeyer W, Melchior H (editors): Urodynamics. Springer-Verlag, 1974.

Tanagho EA, Jones U: Membrane catheter: Effective for recording pressure in lower urinary tract. Urology 1977;10:173.

Tanagho EA, Meyers FH, Smith DR: Urethral resistance: Its components and implications. 2. Striated muscle component. Invest Urol 1969;7:136.

Tanagho EA, Miller ER: Functional considerations of urethral sphincteric dynamics. J Urol 1973;109:273.

Turner WH, Brading AF: Smooth muscle of the bladder in the normal and the diseased state: Pathophysiology, diagnosis and treatment. Pharmacol Ther 1997;75:77.

van Geelen JM et al: The clinical and urodynamic effects of anterior vaginal repair and Burch colposuspension. Am J Obstet Gynecol 1988;159:137.

Versi E: Discriminant analysis of urethral pressure profilometry data for the diagnosis of genuine stress incontinence. Br J Obstet Gynaecol 1990;97:251.

Wang SC, McGuire EJ, Bloom DA: A bladder pressure management system for myelodysplasia: Clinical outcome. J Urol 1988;140:1499.

Woodside JR, McGuire EJ: A simple inexpensive urodynamic catheter. J Urol 1979;122:788.

Yalla SV et al: Striated sphincter participation in distal passive urinary continence mechanisms: Studies in male subjects deprived of proximal sphincter mechanism. J Urol 1979;122:655.

Zerin JM, Lebowitz RL, Bauer SB: Descent of the bladder neck: A urographic finding in denervation of the urethral sphincter in children with myelodysplasia. Radiology 1990;174:833.

URINARY FLOW

Gleason DM, Bottaccini MR: Urodynamic norms in female voiding. 2. Flow modulation zone and voiding dysfunction. J Urol 1982;127:495.

Griffiths D: Basics of pressure-flow studies. World J Urol 1995;13:30.

Griffiths DJ: Pressure-flow studies of micturition. Urol Clin North Am 1996;23:279.

Jensen KM-E, Jørgensen JB, Mogensen P: Relationship between uroflowmetry and prostatism. Proc Int Continence Soc 1985;15:134.

Jørgensen JB, Jensen KM: Uroflowmetry. Urol Clin North Am 1996;23:237.

Jørgensen JB, Jensen KM-E, Mogensen P: Uroflowmetry in asymptomatic elderly males. Proc Int Continence Soc 1985;15:136.

Mainprize TC, Drutz HP: Accuracy of total bladder volume and residual urine measurements: Comparison between real-time ultrasonography and catheterization. Am J Obstet Gynecol 1989;160:1013.

Meyhoff HH, Gleason DM, Bottaccini MR: The effects of transurethral resection on the urodynamics of prostatism. J Urol 1989;142:785.

Nording J: A clinical view of pressure-flow studies. World J Urol 1995;13:70.

Siroky MB: Interpretation of urinary flow rates. Urol Clin North Am 1990;17:537.

Siroky MB, Olsson CA, Krane RJ: The flow rate nomogram. 2. Clinical correlation. J Urol 1980;23:208.

Stubbs AJ, Resnic MI: Office uroflowmetry using maximum flow rate purge meter. J Urol 1979;122:62.

Tanagho EA, McCurry E: Pressure and flow rate as related to lumen caliber and entrance configuration. J Urol 1971;105:583.

van Mastrigt R, Kranse M: Analysis of pressure-flow data in terms of computer-derived urethral resistance parameters. World J Urol 1995;13:40.

ELECTROMYOGRAPHY

Colstrup H et al: Urethral sphincter EMG activity registered with surface electrodes in the vagina. Neurourol Urodynam 1985;4:15.

DiBenedetto M, Yalla SV: Electrodiagnosis of striated urethral sphincter dysfunction. J Urol 1979;122:361.

Girard R et al: Anal and urethral sphincter electromyography in spinal cord injured patients. Paraplegia 1978; 16:244.

King DG, Teague CT: Choice of electrode in electromyography of external urethral and anal sphincter. J Urol 1980;124:75.

Koyanagi T et al: Experience with electromyography of the external urethral sphincter in spinal cord injury patients. J Urol 1982;127:272.

Nielsen KK et al: A comparative study of various electrodes in electromyography of the striated urethral and anal sphincter in children. Br J Urol 1985;57:557.

Petrican P, Sawan MA: Design of a miniaturized ultrasonic bladder volume monitor and subsequent preliminary evaluation on 41 enuretic patients. IEEE Trans Rehabil Eng 1998;6:66.

Siroky MB: Electromyography of the perineal floor. Urol Clin North Am 1996;23:299.

URODYNAMIC TESTING

Barrent DM, Wein AJ: Flow evaluation and simultaneous external sphincter electromyography in clinical urodynamics. J Urol 1981;125:538.

Bauer SB et al: Predictive value of urodynamic evaluation in newborns with myelodysplasia. JAMA 1984; 252:650.

Blaivas JG: Multichannel urodynamic studies. Urology 1984;23:421.

Blaivas JG: Multichannel urodynamic studies in men with benign prostatic hyperplasia: Indications and interpretation. Urol Clin North Am 1990;17:543.

Blaivas JG: Urodynamics: Second generation. J Urol 1983;129:783.

Blaivas JG, Fischer DM: Combined radiographic and urodynamic monitoring: Advances in technique. J Urol 1981;125:693.

Blaivas JG, Salinas JM, Katz GP: The role of urodynamic testing in the evaluation of subtle neurologic lesions. Neurourol Urodynam 1985;4:211.

Gerber GS: The role of urodynamic study in the evaluation and management of men with lower urinary tract symptoms secondary to benign prostatic hyperplasia. Urology 1996;48:668.

Giacobini S et al: To the ICS Committee for Standardization of the Terminology in Urodynamics: A possible contribution to define urethral functionality. Proc Int Continence Soc 1985;15:201.

Kulseng-Hanssen S: Reliability and validity of stationary cystometry, stationary cysto-urethrometry and ambulatory cysto-urethro-vaginometry. Acta Obstet Gynecol Scand Suppl 1997;166:33.

Massey A, Abrams P: Urodynamics of the female lower urinary tract. Urol Clin North Am 1985;12:231.

McGuire EJ: Observations of part-time urodynamicist. J Urol 1983;129:102.

McGuire EJ, Woodside JR: Diagnostic advantages of fluoroscopic monitoring during urodynamic evaluation. J Urol 1981;125:830.

O'Donnell PD: Pitfalls of urodynamic testing. Urol Clin North Am 1991;18:257.

Penders L, De Leval J: Simultaneous urethrocystometry and hyperactive bladders: A manometric differential diagnosis. Neurourol Urodynam 1985;4:89.

Sand PK, Bowen LW, Ostergaard DR: Uninhibited urethral relaxation: An unusual cause of incontinence. Proc Int Continence Soc 1985;15:117.

Schafer W: Urethral resistance? Urodynamic concepts of physiological and pathological bladder outlet function during voiding. Neurourol Urodynam 1985;4:161.

Shulman Y, Brown J: Pressure flow-analysis of micturition: A reappraisal. Urology 1982;19:450.

Siroky MB: Urodynamic assessment of detrusor denervation and areflexia. World J Urol 1984;2:181.

Sutherst JR, Brown MC: Comparison of single and multichannel cystometry in diagnosing bladder instability. Br Med J 1984;288:1720.

Tanagho EA: Membrane and microtransducer catheters: Their effectiveness for profilometry of the lower urinary tract. Urol Clin North Am 1979;6:110.

Throff JW: Mechanism of urinary continency: Animal model to study urethral responses to stress conditions. J Urol 1982;127:1202.

Turner-Warwick R, Brown AD: A urodynamic evaluation of urinary incontinence in the female and its treatment. Urol Clin North Am 1979;6:203.

Turner-Warwick R, Milroy E: A reappraisal of the value of routine urological procedures in the assessment of urodynamic function. Urol Clin North Am 1979;6:63.

van Waalwijk van Doorn ES et al: Ambulatory urodynamics: Extramural testing of the lower and upper urinary tract by Holter monitoring of cystometrogram, uroflowmetry, and renal pelvic pressures. Urol Clin North Am 1996;23:345.

Vardi Y, Ginesin Y, Levin DR: Preoperative evaluation of prostatic size by urethral pressure profilometry. Eur Urol 1985;11:257.

Wein AJ et al: Effects of bethanechol chloride on urodynamic parameters in normal women and in women with significant residual urine volumes. J Urol 1980; 124:397.

31

Urinary Incontinence

Emil A. Tanagho, MD

Urinary incontinence is a major health issue that affects an estimated 10 million patients to some degree. Approximately 50% of all nursing home residents and between 15 and 30% of women over age 65 in retirement communities suffer from urinary incontinence. In excess of $15–20 billion is spent on this problem annually.

PATHOPHYSIOLOGY

Elderly patients frequently accept urinary incontinence as a sign of aging and fail to seek help. In fact, it is a manifestation of an underlying disease; occasionally it is transient and resolves spontaneously, but most often it is chronic and progressive. Transient incontinence may occur after childbirth or may be associated with an acute bladder infection. Chronic urinary incontinence can result from a multitude of causes and can be classified under these main headings:

- Anatomic or genuine urinary stress incontinence
- Urge incontinence
- Neuropathic incontinence
- Congenital incontinence
- False (overflow) incontinence
- Post-traumatic or iatrogenic incontinence
- Fistulous incontinence.

Each entity listed has its own basic mechanism, although a combination of more than one of the varieties of incontinence is not uncommon.

A. Anatomic (Genuine Stress Incontinence): Anatomic incontinence is primarily the result of hypermobility of the vesicourethral segment owing to pelvic floor weakness. Its basic features are an essentially intact sphincteric mechanism, a weak pelvic floor support, and an anatomic abnormality. It is easily demonstrable radiologically, and restoration of the anatomy restores function.

B. True Urge Incontinence: The basic features of true urge incontinence are detrusor instability with a normal sphincteric component, normal anatomy, and no neuropathy. Sphincteric instability is less common.

Leakage occurs with either detrusor instability and spontaneous contraction or, less commonly, with sphincteric instability and relaxation.

C. Neuropathic Incontinence: Neuropathic incontinence varies, depending on the nerve lesion. The neuropathy is usually identifiable. The incontinence can be active (detrusor hyperreflexia) or passive (sphincteric atony) or, occasionally, a combination of the two.

D. Congenital Incontinence: The causes of congenital incontinence are ectopic ureters, duplicate or single system, with epispadias, exstrophy, or cloacal malformation.

E. False (Overflow) Incontinence: False incontinence is usually the result of an obstructive or neuropathic lesion. It is not true incontinence.

F. Traumatic Incontinence: Traumatic incontinence is associated with a fractured pelvis or with surgical damage to the sphincter during bladder neck resection or extensive internal urethrotomy; it also may result from failure of urethral diverticulectomy or repair of erosion of an artificial sphincter.

G. Fistulous Communication: The fistula can be ureteral, vesical, or urethral. Most of the time, the cause is iatrogenic, from either pelvic or vaginal surgery.

This chapter discusses the most common and significant disorders: urinary stress incontinence and neuropathic incontinence.

Urinary incontinence is the involuntary loss of urine when the intravesical pressure exceeds maximal urethral pressure. Under resting conditions continence is effected by an adequate urethral tone, which is the result of smooth and striated muscle activity, tension of the fibroelastic elements in the urethral wall, and the cushioning effect of the soft, compressible, submucosal vascular bed (Figure 31–1).

The major contribution to urethral resistance comes from the smooth and striated muscle components (Figures 31–2 and 31–3). In experimental animals, as well as in humans, the striated external sphincter provides about 50% of static urethral resistance, while smooth muscle is primarily responsible for proximal urethral closure pressure (Figure 31–4).

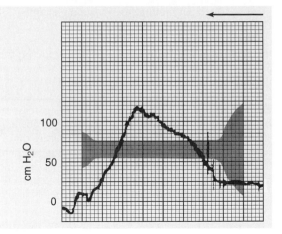

Figure 31–1. Urethral pressure profile in a normal female. Closure pressure at the level of the internal meatus is very low; the pressure rises progressively to reach its maximum at approximately the middle third of the urethra—the site of maximal condensation of striated muscle.

The rise in pressure in the mid urethra results from the combined function of the smooth musculature and the striated muscle fibers around it. To maintain continence under stress conditions, the striated urethral sphincter has to resist a raised bladder pressure owing to intra-abdominal pressure increase (Figures 31–5 and 31–6). The activity of the external sphincter helped by the pelvic floor provides for this increased urethral resistance. Involuntary loss of urine with increased intra-abdominal pressure, in the absence of detrusor contraction, is usually labeled stress incontinence. When loss of urine is associated with increased intravesical pressure owing to detrusor contraction, it is commonly referred to as urge incontinence.

Genuine stress incontinence is invariably associated with weakness of the pelvic floor support, permitting hypermobility of the vesicourethral segments, which in turn impairs the efficiency of the sphincteric musculature. The increase in intraurethral pressure observed during coughing results mainly from contraction of the voluntary muscles with sphincteric action. Part of the rise is passive (ie, by direct transmission), but a significant component is active (ie, caused by reflex musculature contraction).

URINARY STRESS INCONTINENCE

Often seen in women after middle age (with repeated pregnancies and vaginal deliveries), urinary stress incontinence is usually a result of weakness of the pelvic floor and poor support of the vesicourethral sphincteric unit. Urethral closure pressure normally responds to bladder filling; a change in position; or stressful events such as coughing, sneezing, and bearing down. The sphincteric mechanism has its own ca-

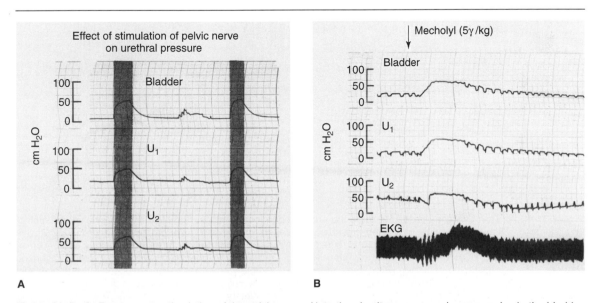

Figure 31–2. A: Response to stimulation of the pelvic nerve. Note the simultaneous, equal pressure rise in the bladder, proximal urethra (U_1), and mid urethra (U_2). **B:** Vesical and sphincteric responses to an injection of the parasympathetic drug methacholine chloride. Note again the simultaneous rise in pressure at the bladder, proximal urethra (U_1), and mid urethra (U_2).

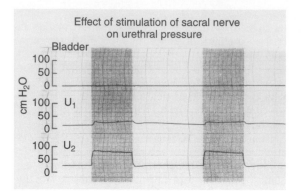

Figure 31–3. Response of the striated component to stimulation of the sacral nerves. Note that the bladder pressure does not change and the proximal urethral pressure (U_1) rises only slightly, but that the increase in midurethral pressure (U_2) is sharp and sustained.

pacity to augment urethral resistance under stress reflexively and thus to prevent leakage.

The urethral pressure profile is a good measure of the activity of the external sphincter. A static profile demonstrates the resting tonus of both components of the sphincteric mechanism (see Figure 31–1); a dynamic profile gives the responses of these sphincteric elements to various activities, such as an increase in bladder volume, assumption of the upright position (Figure 31–7), the prolonged stress of bearing down, or the sudden stress of coughing and sneezing (Figure 31–8). Normally, the urethral closure pressure—the net difference between the intraurethral and intravesical pressures—is maintained or augmented during stress.

Anatomy

In genuine stress incontinence, the assumption is that the intrinsic structure of the sphincter itself is in-

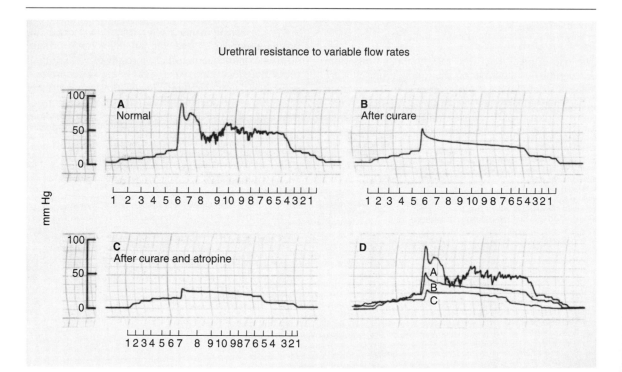

Figure 31–4. A: The resistance needed to force the urethra open, overcoming both voluntary and involuntary sphincteric elements. With progressively increasing pressure, the urethra opens at the **critical opening pressure** (in this recording, about 85 mm Hg). Once the urethra is forced open, the resistance to flow drops precipitously and becomes sustained at the level of **sustained urethral resistance** (in this recording, roughly 50 mm Hg). **B:** A similar recording obtained after administration of curare, which completely blocks voluntary sphincteric responses. Note the appreciable drop in both critical opening pressure and sustained resistance. **C:** Recording after administration of both curare and atropine (a combination that eliminates the activity of smooth and voluntary sphincteric elements). The critical opening pressure drops markedly and is now equal to the sustained resistance; both are very low. **D:** An overlap of the 3 recordings shows the contribution of each muscular element: The voluntary component contributes roughly 50% of the total resistance, while the smooth component contributes the other 50%. The minimal residual resistance is a function of the collagen elastic element of the urethral wall; this collagen element has no sphincteric significance.

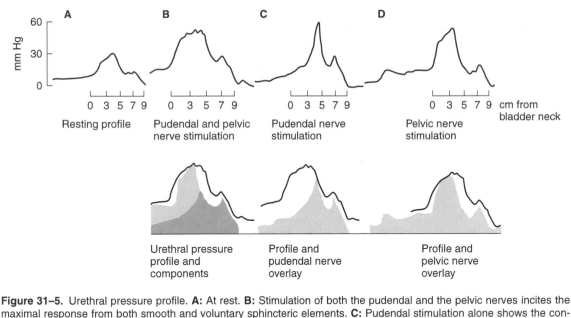

Figure 31–5. Urethral pressure profile. **A:** At rest. **B:** Stimulation of both the pudendal and the pelvic nerves incites the maximal response from both smooth and voluntary sphincteric elements. **C:** Pudendal stimulation alone shows the contribution of the voluntary component. **D:** Pelvic nerve stimulation shows the response of the smooth-muscle component alone. **Bottom tracings:** Total maximal pressure profile obtained by stimulation of pelvic and pudendal nerves shown by overlapping the profile of simultaneous stimulation of both nerves. The contribution and anatomic distribution of each element are clearly seen. Their summation results in the overall total responses recorded in **B** above.

tact and normal. However, it loses efficiency because of excessive mobility and loss of support. Thus, the anatomic feature of genuine stress incontinence is consistently that of hypermobility or a lowering of the position of the vesicourethral segment (or a combination of the two factors) (Figure 31–9).

The relationships among the urethra, the bladder base, and various bony points have been the object of much study. For many years the posterior vesicourethral angle has been considered a key factor indicating the presence of anatomic stress incontinence. Some authors, however, have emphasized the axis of inclination, ie, the angle between the urethral line and the vertical plane. Other investigators stress bony landmarks in the pelvis in their descriptions of the relationship of the bladder base and the vesicourethral junction to the sacrococcygeal inferior pubic point (Figure 31–10).

These descriptions illustrate that abnormal anatomic position and excessive mobility are essential elements in the diagnosis of genuine anatomic stress incontinence. To evaluate this aspect of incontinence, I recommend a simplified cystographic study (a lateral cystogram with a urethral catheter in place) to define the vesicourethral segment clearly. With the patient lying on the flat x-ray table, a lateral film is obtained, first at rest to determine the position of the vesicourethral segment in relation to the pubic bone and then with straining to ascertain its degree of mobility (Figures 31–11 and 31–12). Normally, the vesi-

courethral junction is opposite the lower third of the pubic bone and moves 0.5–1.5 cm with straining. It should be emphasized, however, that cystography is not the means of diagnosing stress incontinence. This demonstration of abnormal position or excessive mobility of the vesicourethral segment is helpful in confirming the cause of existing urinary incontinence. Some authors like to classify urinary incontinence in various stages. Stages I and II depend on the degree of hypermobility and usually relate to the amount of urinary leakage. Stage III, which most often is not associated with hypermobility, is usually due to intrinsic sphincteric damage—most often iatrogenic.

Urodynamic Characteristics of Stress Incontinence

A. Pressure Profile: As would be expected, patients have a low urethral pressure profile with reduced closure pressure. This factor varies with the severity of the sphincteric impairment as a result of the excessive mobility: The pressure profile might be low-normal when weakness is minimal or it might be quite significant when mobility is severe. Not infrequently, however, this weakness of the pressure profile is not demonstrable when the bladder is partially full. It characteristically becomes more significant when the bladder has been distended (Figure 31–13). Also, the pressure profile may appear normal when the patient is in the resting (sitting) position; when he

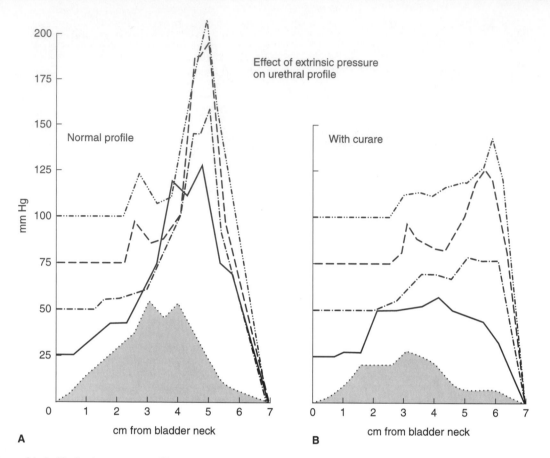

Figure 31–6. Urethral pressure profile at rest and after subjecting an experimental animal to progressively increasing extrinsic pressure applied around the abdomen—not involving any muscular activity. **A:** Extrinsic pressure was increased by 25–mm Hg increments. Note the sharp increase in urethral closure pressure with each increment, marked after 25 and 50 mm Hg, less so after 75 and 100 mm Hg. The increase in urethral closure pressure is far higher than the increase in extrinsic pressure, which denotes not simple transmitted pressure but active muscular function. **B:** Curare administration demonstrates that much of the rise in closure pressure recorded in **A** results from the activity of the voluntary sphincter, which is lost after blockade by curare.

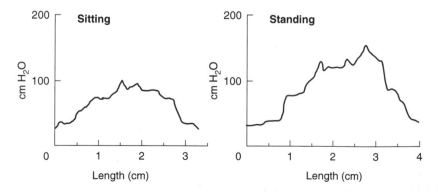

Figure 31–7. Urethral pressure profile with patient in sitting and upright positions. Approximately a 50% increase in urethral closure pressure occurs when the patient assumes the upright position. Urethral functional length is well sustained.

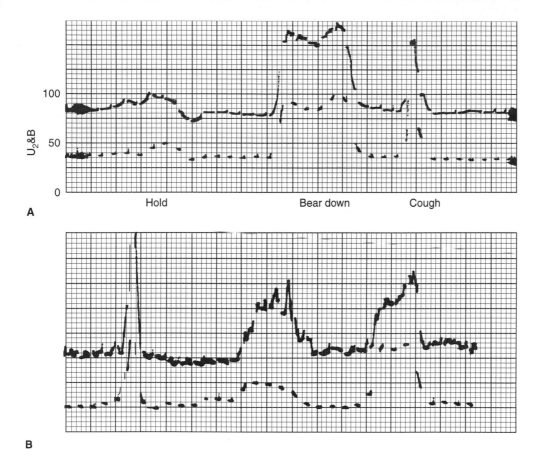

Figure 31–8. A: Intravesical and urethral pressure responses to the stresses of coughing, bearing down, and the hold maneuver. Note the sharp increase in intra-abdominal pressure reflected in intravesical pressure with coughing and the simultaneous greater increase in urethral pressure. The response is similar with bearing down. Closure pressure is maintained and even augmented during these periods of stress. The hold maneuver (recording membrane is in the proximal urethra) produces a minimal response in closure pressure of the proximal urethra. **B:** Recording comparable to that in **A,** but the membrane is in the mid urethra. Note again the sustained closure pressure as a result of coughing and bearing down and the marked pressure increase in the midurethral segment with the hold maneuver.

or she assumes the upright position in the dynamic pressure profile, the weakness becomes more apparent (Figure 31–14).

B. Functional Urethral Length: The anatomic length of the urethra is usually maintained, yet the functional length is invariably shorter. The loss is in the proximal urethral segment (Figure 31–15). Although it might not look funneled on the cystogram, this segment has very low closure efficiency, or none at all, and its pressure is almost equal to intravesical pressure. The functional shortening might be minimal or it might involve more than one-half of the length of the urethra. It is important to note that the functional length, like the pressure profile, might appear normal when the bladder is partially full or the patient is in the sitting position.

C. Response to Stress: With the sustained stress of bearing down or the sudden stress of coughing or sneezing, the net urethral closure pressure is reduced, depending on the degree of sphincteric weakness. In severe urinary stress incontinence, any strain or increase in intravesical pressure leads to negative closure pressure and urinary leakage (Figure 31–16).

D. Voluntary Increase in Urethral Closure Pressure: Patients with mild stress incontinence might be capable of activating their external sphincter maximally and generating a high urethral closure pressure. However, with progression of the anatomic problem and hypermobility, this voluntary increase progressively diminishes; depending on the severity of the weakness and inefficiency of the external sphincter, this weakness becomes more readily apparent.

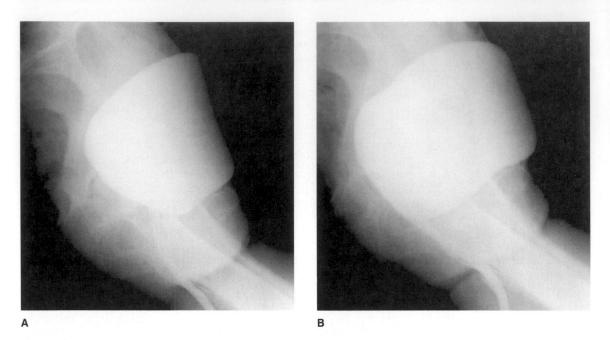

A   B

Figure 31–9. Lateral cystograms in a 53-year-old woman with stress incontinence. **A:** Preoperative, relaxed. Note slightly low-lying vesicourethral junction. The posterior vesicourethral angle is near normal. **B:** With straining, excessive downward and posterior mobility of the vesicourethral segment is shown. Posterior angle almost disappears.

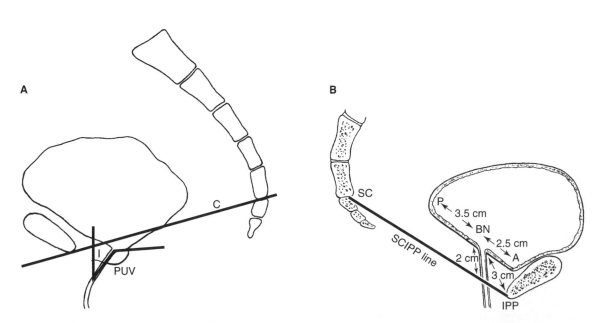

Figure 31–10. Diagrammatic representation of (**A**) the angles considered when assessing adequacy of bladder support (posterior vesicourethral angle; angle of inclination) and (**B**) the "SCIPP line" (sacrococcygeal inferior pubic point) and its relationship to the bladder base and the vesicourethral segment as a reference to adequate pelvic support.

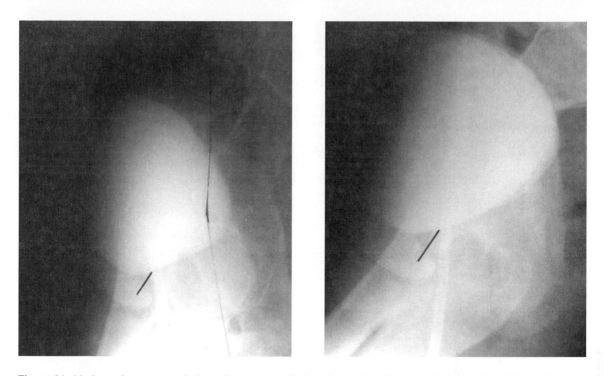

Figure 31–11. Lateral cystograms in 2 continent women in the relaxed state. A perpendicular line from the anterior vesicourethral angle over the long axis of the pubic bone crosses the bone near the junction of the middle and lower thirds.

E. Response to Bladder Distention and Change in Position: It must be emphasized that, although the features described might be normal in the resting position with minimal bladder filling, all of them can become aggravated with a full bladder or the upright position. In testing these patients urodynamically one must ascertain the changes that occur with a full bladder and the assumption of the upright position (Figures 31–14 and 31–17).

Diagnosis

A detailed history is important, including the degree of leakage; its relation to activity, position, and state of bladder fullness; the timing of its onset; and the course of its progression. Knowledge of past surgical and obstetric history, medications taken, dietary habits, and systemic diseases (eg, diabetes) can be helpful in the diagnosis. Whether the incontinence is purely stress or purely urge or a combination of the two can be assessed, as can its degree—minimal, moderate, severe, or complete.

Physical examination is essential. The pelvic examination demonstrates laxity of pelvic support, presence of any degree of prolapse, cystocele, rectocele, and mobility of the anterior vaginal wall. A neurologic examination should be done if neuropathy is suspected. Cystographic study for demonstration of the anatomic abnormality is important, as is urodynamic study to confirm the classic features of urinary incontinence and determine its cause. The goals of cystographic and urodynamic study are, first, to demonstrate the anatomic abnormality and its extent and, second, to assess the activity of the sphincteric mechanism and hence the potential for improvement by correcting the anatomic abnormality. In recurrent cases, repeated previous surgeries may have caused so much intrinsic damage to the sphincteric musculature that simple suspension cannot provide satisfactory results. Indirect evidence of the degree of sphincteric weakness can be obtained by measurement of what is called the **leak pressure** (ie, by measuring the intra-abdominal pressure through a rectal transducer during the Valsalva maneuver and noting at what pressure the first leakage of urine occurs). A low reading indicates a severe degree of sphincteric weakness.

Treatment

The principal treatment of urinary stress incontinence is proper suspension and support of the vesicourethral segment in a normal position. The rationalization is that, in genuine stress incontinence, the intrinsic sphincteric mechanism is intact but its efficiency is impaired because of excessive mobility in the abnormal position. Once the position is restored, the sphincteric mechanism usually regains its function.

There are numerous approaches to restoring the

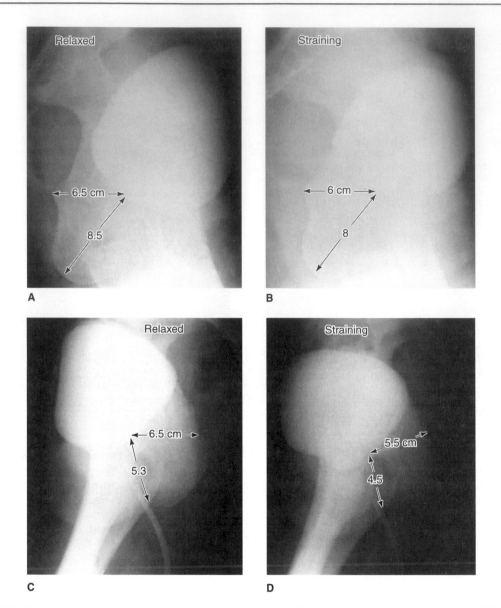

Figure 31–12. Lateral cystograms in two young continent women. **A:** Relaxed state, 28-year-old woman. **B:** With straining, the vesicourethral segment is displaced 0.5 cm downward and posteriorly. **C:** Relaxed state, 34-year-old woman. **D:** With straining, the vesicourethral segment is displaced 0.8 cm downward and 1 cm posteriorly.

normal position and providing adequate support—some vaginal, others suprapubic. The suprapubic approach was popularized by the classic Marshall-Marchetti-Krantz (MMK) retropubic suspension described in 1949, in which periurethral tissue is attached to the back of the pubic symphysis. A modification was introduced by Burch in 1961, in which the anterior vaginal wall is fixed to Cooper's ligament. Many urologic surgeons today have found that the latter technique, with modifications, provides the most lasting results (Figures 31–18 and 31–19).

The vaginal suspension has various forms; in some, the tissue is gathered behind the bladder neck (eg, the Kelly procedure), while others rely on sutures in the paravaginal tissues that are passed bluntly to the suprapubic area by a needle to be tied over the rectus sheath. This technique was originally described by Pereyra in 1959 and subsequently was modified—in 1973 by Stamey, who added endoscopic confirmation of suture placement and the degree of compression, and in 1981 by Raz. Most of these techniques have a high initial success rate;

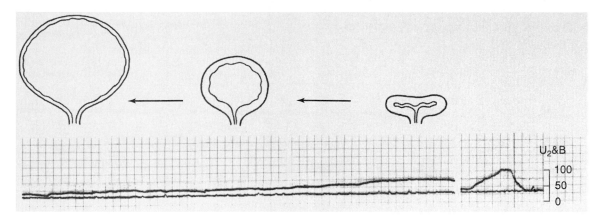

Figure 31–13. Urethral pressure profile with minimally filled bladder. Bladder pressure remains constant, but urethral pressure drops progressively. Closure pressure becomes minimal at the end of bladder filling.

however, there is some concern about the long-term results. Hence, the retropubic approach remains the recommended procedure.

With excessive sphincteric damage and intrinsic weakness, suspension alone might not be adequate and sling procedures are advised. Of the various techniques and materials, the most popular uses a strip of the anterior rectus sheath, first reported by McGuire. Raz advocates the vaginal wall sling, in which an island of the anterior vaginal wall is mobilized and used to support the vesicourethral segment. More recently, in instances of significant intrinsic sphincteric damage, local injection of bulking material such as polytetra fluoro-ethylene (Teflon), or preferably collagen, is used to increase the bladder outlet resistance to help in patients in whom mobility is not excessive and whose primary problem is intrinsic sphincteric weakness.

NEUROPATHIC INCONTINENCE

Neuropathic incontinence can be broken down into 2 broad classifications: active and passive. **Active neuropathic incontinence** is found in patients who have a spastic lesion but in whom the sphincteric mechanism, although not under voluntary control, still exerts adequate closure pressure. The presence of a hyperreflexive detrusor with uninhibited contractions increases the intravesical pressure. When intravesical pressure exceeds sphincteric pressure, there is a leakage of urine (Figure 31–20). Active incontinence is most often associated with suprasegmental, or upper motor neuron, lesions.

Passive neuropathic incontinence occurs when

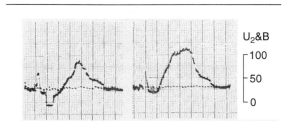

Figure 31–14. Urethral pressure profile in moderately severe stress incontinence: closure pressure with patient in the sitting position with half-distended bladder, then after the upright position is assumed. Note that closure pressure is close to 75 cm H_2O with the patient in the sitting position but decreases to approximately 25 cm H_2O with the upright position. Note also the marked shortening of functional urethral length once the upright position is assumed.

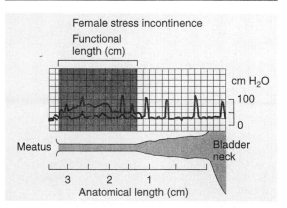

Figure 31–15. Urethral pressure profile in a female patient with moderate urinary stress incontinence. Note the relatively low closure pressure, the short functional urethral length, and the loss of closure pressure of the proximal 1.5 cm of urethra.

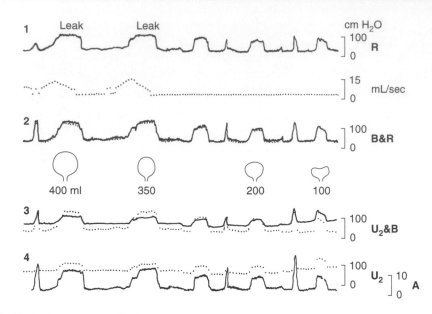

Figure 31–16. Urethral pressure profile in moderate stress incontinence. Note that, with the bladder relatively empty, closure pressure is close to the normal range. At the start of bladder filling, resting pressure is again normal; as filling progresses, bladder pressure remains stable and urethral closure pressure decreases progressively to a minimum with full bladder distention.

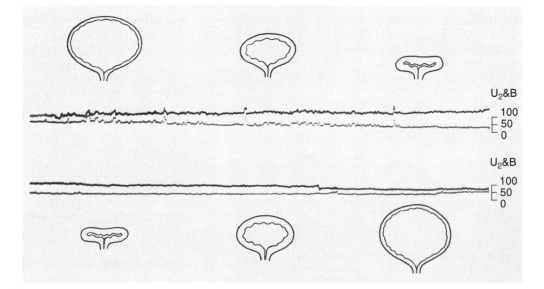

Figure 31–17. Effect of bladder filling and emptying on urethral pressure. **Top:** Effect of progressive filling, which leads to a gradual drop in urethral pressure. At the end of filling, urethral closure pressure is only a fraction of the relatively normal initial closure pressure. **Bottom:** At the start, the bladder is full. With gradual emptying, note the progressive buildup in urethral resistance and closure pressure.

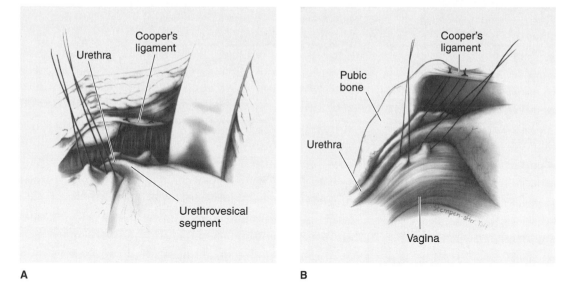

Figure 31–18. A: Diagrammatic depiction of the retropubic space after mobilization of the anterior vaginal wall and placement of sutures, 2 on either side and far from the midline laterally. Distal sutures are opposite the mid urethra, while proximal sutures are at the end of the vesicourethral junction. Sutures are attached to Cooper's ligament. **B:** Side view of suture placement with one side tied. The anterior vaginal wall acts as a broad sling, supporting and lifting the vesicourethral segment. The urethra is free in the retropubic space.

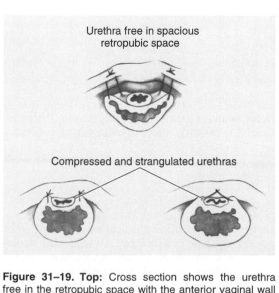

Figure 31–19. Top: Cross section shows the urethra free in the retropubic space with the anterior vaginal wall lifting and supporting it. **Bottom:** The urethra is compressed and strangulated against the pubic bone when vaginal sutures are applied close to the urethra and fixed to the symphysis pubis.

the sphincteric mechanism is weakened or completely lacking. Even without abnormally high intravesical pressure, any increase in intra-abdominal pressure results in urinary leakage. Passive incontinence is most often associated with lesions involving the micturition center or more distal lesions.

The more common classification of neurogenic incontinence is based on an evaluation of the functions of the lower urinary tract: incontinence owing to failure of the reservoir or to failure of retention.

A. Failure of Reservoir Function: Loss of reservoir function in the contractile or contracted bladder can be caused by poor compliance in the detrusor muscle. Intravesical pressure rises with minimal bladder filling, exceeding the outlet resistance and causing urinary leakage. In contrast to the classification of active incontinence associated with suprasegmental lesions, failure of reservoir function may be found in patients who have meningomyelocele who exhibit other lower motor neuron lesions. Although these patients may have partial lesions with significant striated sphincteric activity, offering some degree of resistance, early loss of bladder compliance increases intravesical pressure with minimal bladder filling, overcoming what outlet resistance there is. These patients, once recognized, must be managed aggressively because they often have a significant back-pressure effect in the upper urinary tract, which can lead to early deterioration and possible vesicoureteral reflux or lower ureteral obstruction.

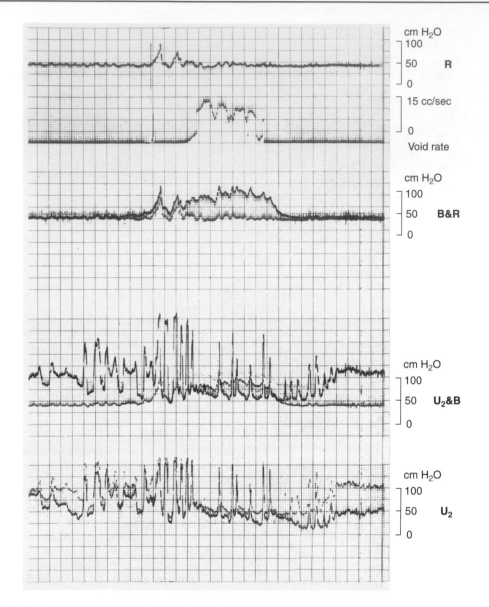

Figure 31–20. Urodynamic recording in a patient with evidence of detrusor/sphincter dyssynergia, showing spontaneous activity in the bladder associated with a burst of activity in the external sphincter interrupting voiding. This represents a classic demonstration of upper motor neuron dysfunction leading to urinary incontinence as a result of detrusor hyperactivity or hyperreflexia.

B. Failure of Retention Function: Complete lesions of the sacral segment or the cauda equina result in a total loss of smooth and striated sphincteric activity. The external sphincter offers minimal resistance. Most patients experiencing such failure can retain some volume, because the bladder musculature becomes atonic and lax and intravesical pressure remains low, but any increase in intravesical pressure can cause leakage, and the bladder never reaches full capacity. Consequently, the integrity of the upper urinary tract is not endangered, as in cases of reservoir failure. It must

be stressed, however, that most cases involve the loss of some components, with the patient retaining some activity. For example, if a patient were to retain some activity in the internal sphincter but experience a complete loss of the striated sphincter, the entire pelvic floor would become flaccid and atonic.

Diagnosis

Diagnostic evaluation of neuropathic urinary incontinence determines whether the condition arises from detrusor or sphincteric dysfunction, or from a combination of the two. In exceptional cases, such as patients with multiple sclerosis with spinal stenosis or those with disk problems in addition to partial traumatic damage to the spinal cord, the neuropathy is less clear.

A complete urologic and neurologic history should be taken, followed by radiographic evaluation to determine the integrity of the upper urinary tract, the status of the reservoir, and the state of the sphincteric mechanism. Intravenous pyelography, cystourethrography, and cinefluoroscopy are also recommended. The following are valuable in determining the underlying cause of incontinence:

1. Bladder responses to progressive filling
2. Sphincteric pressure profile and its response to progressive filling and the initiation of voiding
3. The presence of detrusor hyperreflexia and uninhibited activity (in patients with hyperreflexia)
4. Electromyographic studies of the striated urinary sphincter
5. In selected patients, response to neurostimulation of the sacral roots and pudendal nerve, with or without blocking and measurement of latencies.

Differentiation among incontinence caused by uninhibited detrusor contractions, detrusor hyperreflexia, and poor bladder compliance is a straightforward process. Significant findings include sphincteric weakness, precipitous sphincteric relaxation, and decrease in pressure, as well as a lack of electromyographic activity of the pelvic floor musculature and external sphincter. The proper diagnosis can be achieved by establishing the integrity of the sacral root reflex arc by neurostimulation of the sacral roots, with simultaneous recording of intravesical and intraurethral pressures at the levels of the internal and the external sphincter. One must be alert to the possibility of overlapping causes, and the responses of the external sphincter and pelvic floor musculature to active contraction, progressive bladder filling, and sacral root stimulation can be informative. The extent of one cause relative to another (for example, sphincteric weakness versus detrusor hyperreflexia) should be taken into account, and management should be directed toward the predominating cause of incontinence.

Treatment

Although diagnosis of the causes of incontinence is relatively easy, management is generally difficult. The rehabilitation of the neuropathic condition and the alleviation of the potentially damaging sequelae must be the guiding principles of management. Choices must be made according to the severity and potential progression of the lesion and the integrity of the system. Especially in the previously mentioned cases of patients with spinal cord injury and meningomyelocele,

early treatment provides the best chance of preserving the integrity of the entire urinary system.

A. Conservative Management:

1. Failure of reservoir function—Adequate reservoir function can be restored, allowing patients to maintain dryness for 2–4 h, with successful pharmacologic manipulation to suppress the detrusor hyperreflexia. The response to pharmacologic agents depends on the initial functional bladder capacity, extent of spasticity and hyperreflexia, lack of compliance owing to collagen deposition, and mural changes in the bladder wall. For this reason, an understanding of the function and capacity of the bladder and the role of detrusor hyperreflexia is essential to the conservative management of reservoir dysfunction.

There are 3 categories of pharmacologic agents for the treatment of reservoir dysfunction: Anticholinergic drugs are used primarily to treat detrusor hyperreflexia and uninhibited contractions. Oxybutynin (Ditropan), a tertiary amine anticholinergic drug with antispasmodic action, is the most commonly used, with a dosage of 5 mg 2–4 times a day, depending on the patient's tolerance and responses. Possible side effects include dry mouth, drowsiness, palpitations, and occasional nausea, and patients must be careful to stay below their threshold of tolerance. Oxybutynin is contraindicated in patients with high intraocular pressure. Tolterodine tartrate (Detrol), a new antimuscarinic agent, is effective in reducing detrusor hyperactivity with fewer side effects than oxybutynin.

Propantheline bromide (Pro-Banthine), although often less effective than oxybutynin, can be a useful supplement to oxybutynin and is better tolerated by some patients. The usual dosage is 15 mg 2–3 times a day, with perhaps a larger dose at bedtime. Side effects include dry mouth, visual disturbances, and increased intraocular pressure.

Imipramine hydrochloride (Tofranil), a tricyclic antidepressant with a strong anticholinergic, antimuscarinic action, has a significant effect on detrusor hyperreflexia. The usual dosage is 25 mg 2–4 times daily. Side effects include dry mouth, constipation, blurred vision, and drowsiness.

Antihistaminic drugs antagonize the histamine-mediated release of acetylcholine to produce an anticholinergic effect. Chlorpheniramine maleate can be taken alone in the long-acting 8-mg capsules or tablets orally twice a day or in combination with 75 mg of phenylpropanolamine hydrochloride (Ornade Spansules). The latter produces an anticholinergic effect on the detrusor as well as alpha-receptor stimulation to improve outlet resistance.

Musculotropic relaxants depress smooth-muscle activity directly. Flavoxate hydrochloride (Urispas, 200 mg), the most common, is taken 3–4 times daily by mouth.

2. Failure of retention mechanism—Intermittent catheterization is the first line of conservative management in these patients. Although such patients have very low outlet resistance, their bladder atonia permits some retention. Most of the time, catheterization every 4–6 h enables them to avoid leakage. When catheterization is not possible and the increase in intravesical pressure becomes excessive, the patient can wear minimal protection.

Pharmacologic manipulation is less successful. Ephedrine sulfate and phentermine (Ionamin) have a stimulating effect on both alpha and beta receptors, which increases urethral sphincteric smooth-muscle activity and partially relaxes the detrusor muscle. The former is usually given in 30- to 60-mg doses 3–4 times daily orally; the latter is usually given in a 15-mg dose 2–3 times daily orally.

B. Surgical Management:

1. Sphincterotomy–In spastic hyperreflexive situations in male patients, this operation is performed to eliminate outlet resistance so that, with an external appliance or condom catheter, the bladder will remain empty. Although many consider this procedure the easiest way to preserve the upper urinary tract, it is clearly not rehabilitative and might interfere with other treatments.

2. Bladder augmentation–In patients with poor compliance owing to mural changes and chronic hypertrophy, this procedure improves reservoir function. If the sphincteric mechanism is adequate, detubularized bowel segments can be used in patients in whom the bladder will not expand even under anesthesia. Usually patients have to rely on intermittent catheterization postoperatively, but they regain continence and the upper urinary tract is preserved.

3. Artificial sphincter–In patients with severe sphincteric damage and a low-pressure, large-capacity bladder, this device can be useful. In males it is applied around the bulbous urethra. When the device is deflated, the patient can void either by detrusor contraction (if some capability is preserved) or by straining and the Valsalva maneuver. A complete sphincterotomy can be done first. Intermittent catheterization is hazardous in patients with a urethral cuff and is rarely necessary.

4. Continent urinary diversion–This method should be considered only with progressively deteriorating upper urinary tract function, and even then a simple conduit is preferable. Approaches to be condemned are denervation of the bladder through cystolysis or transvesical transection and resuturing and denervation of the bladder base through phenol or alcohol injection. In the long term, these methods have been complete failures.

5. Neurostimulation–In selected patients with detrusor hyperreflexia, stimulation of the sacral roots has effectively suppressed the hyperactivity, relying on the known reflex response of the detrusor muscle to stimulate the somatic component of the sacral plexus (which aborts and inhibits detrusor contractility). If such patients with spinal cord injury, meningomyelocele, multiple sclerosis, and other neuropathies show significant improvement after temporary testing, a permanent electrode can be placed over the most responsive root, usually S_3.

6. Dorsal rhizotomy–Complete dorsal rhizotomy of S_2–S_4 extra- or intradurally effectively eliminates detrusor hyperreflexia and increases bladder capacity. Increases have been seen from a capacity of 150 or 200 mL to one of 600–800 mL. In patients with suprasegmental lesions and spastic upper motor neuron lesions, sacral root electrode implantation promotes detrusor contraction and bladder evacuation (the so-called bladder pacemaker).

REFERENCES

Abrams P et al: The standardisation of terminology of lower urinary tract function. The International Continence Society Committee on Standardisation of Terminology. Scand J Urol Nephrol 1988;114:5.

Appell RA: Electrical stimulation for the treatment of urinary incontinence. Urology 1998;51(2A Suppl):24.

Bates CP, Whiteside CG, Turner-Warwick R: Synchronous cine-pressure-flowcysto-urethrography with special reference to stress and urge incontinence. Br J Urol 1970;42:714.

Bernstein IT: The pelvic floor muscles: Muscle thickness in healthy and urinary-incontinent women measured by perineal ultrasonography with reference to the effect of pelvic floor training. Estrogen receptor studies. Neurourol Urodyn 1997;16:237.

Burch JC: Cooper's ligament urethrovesical suspension for stress incontinence: Nine years' experience—results, complications, technique. Am J Obstet Gynecol 1968;100:764.

Burch JC: Urethrovaginal fixation to Cooper's ligament for correction of stress incontinence, cystocele, and prolapse. Am J Obstet Gynecol 1961;81:281.

Cardozo LD, Stanton SL: Genuine stress incontinence and detrusor instability: A review of 200 patients. Br J Obstet Gynaecol 1980;87:184.

Carey MP, Dwyer PL: Position and mobility of the urethrovesical junction in continent and in stress incontinent women before and after successful surgery. Aust N Z J Obstet Gynaecol 1991;31:279.

Chai TC, Steers WD: Neurophysiology of micturition and continence in women. Int Urogynecol J Pelvic Floor Dysfunct 1997;8:85.

Chye PLH: Clinical Handbook for the Management of Incontinence. Society for Continence, Singapore, 1994.

DeGroat WC: A neurologic basis for the overactive bladder. Urology 1997;50(6A Suppl):36.

DeLancey JO: The pathophysiology of stress urinary incontinence in women and its implications for surgical treatment. World J Urol 1997;15:268.

DeLancey JO: Structural aspects of the extrinsic continence mechanism. Obstet Gynecol 1988;72:296.

Denny-Brown D, Robertson GE: On the physiology of micturition. Brain 1933;56:149.

Diokno AC et al: Prevalence of urinary incontinence and other urological symptoms in the noninstitutionalized elderly. J Urol 1986;136:1022.

Eastham JA et al: Risk factors for urinary incontinence after radical prostatectomy. J Urol 1996;156:1707.

Elbadawi A: Functional anatomy of the organs of micturition. Urol Clin North Am 1996;23:177.

Enhorning G: Simultaneous recording of intravesical and intraurethral pressure. Acta Chir Scand 1967;30:309.

Fantl JA et al: Efficacy of bladder training in older women with urinary incontinence. JAMA 1991;265:609.

Fantl JA et al: Urinary incontinence in community-dwelling women: clinical, urodynamic and severity characteristics. Am J Obstet Gynecol 1990;162:946.

Ghoniem GM, Hassouna M: Alternatives for the pharmacologic management of urge and stress urinary incontinence in the elderly. J Wound Ostomy Continence Nurs 1997;24:311.

Gosling J: Structure of the lower urinary tract and pelvic floor. Clin Obstet Gynaecol 1985;2:285.

Hodgkinson CP, Stanton SL: Retropubic urethropexy or colposuspension. In: Stanton SL, Tanagho EA (editors): Surgery of Female Incontinence. Springer-Verlag, 1980.

Hu TW: Impact of urinary incontinence on health-care costs. J Am Geriatr Soc 1990;38:292.

Hutch JA: A new theory of the anatomy of the internal urinary sphincter and the physiology of micturition. 5. The base plate and stress incontinence. Obstet Gynecol 1967;30:309.

Jones JA, Mitchell ME, Rink RC: Improved results using a modification of the Young-Dees-Leadbetter bladder neck repair. Br J Urol 1993;71:555.

Leach GE et al: For better or worse, managing incontinence by the book. Contemp Urol (Nov) 1993;16.

Litwiller SE et al: Post-prostatectomy incontinence and the artificial urinary sphincter: A long-term study of patient satisfaction and criteria for success. J Urol 1996;156:1975.

Lockhart JL et al: Periurethral polytetrafluoroethylene injection following urethral reconstruction in female patients with urinary incontinence. J Urol 1988;140:51.

Marshall VV, Marchetti AA, Krantz KE: The correction of stress incontinence by simple vesicourethral suspension. Surg Gynecol Obstet 1949;88:509.

McGuire EJ, Cespedes RD: Proper diagnosis: A must before surgery for stress incontinence. J Endourol 1996;10:201.

McGuire EJ, English SF: Periurethral collagen injection for male and female sphincteric incontinence: Indications, techniques, and result. World J Urol 1997;15:306.

McGuire EJ, Savastano JA: Stress incontinence and detrusor instability/urge incontinence. Neurourol Urodynam 1985;4:313.

McGuire EJ et al: Clinical assessment of urethral sphincter function. J Urol 1993;150:1452.

McGuire EJ et al: Experience with pubovaginal slings for urinary incontinence at the University of Michigan. J Urol 1987;138:525.

Mostwin JL: Current concepts of female pelvic anatomy and physiology. Urol Clin North Am 1991;18:175.

Mostwin JL et al: Anatomic goals in the correction of female stress urinary incontinence. J Endourol 1996;10:207.

Mouritsen L, Lose G, Glavind K: Assessment of women with urinary incontinence. Acta Obstet Gynecol Scand 1998;77:361.

Noll LE, Hutch JA: The SCIPP line: An aid in interpreting the voiding lateral cystourethrogram. Obstet Gynecol 1969;33:680.

The Overactive Bladder: From Basic Science to Clinical Management Consensus Conference. Proceedings. London, England, June 29, 1997. Urology 1997;50 (6A Suppl):1.

Payne CK: Epidemiology, pathophysiology, and evaluation of urinary incontinence and overactive bladder. Urology 1998;51(2A Suppl):3.

Pereyra AJ: A simplified surgical procedure for the correction of stress incontinence in women. West J Surg Obstet Gynecol 1959;67:223.

Pereyra AJ, Lebherz TB: The modified Pereyra procedure. In: Buschbaum HJ, Schmidt JD (editors): Gynecologic and Obstetric Urology, 2nd ed. Saunders, 1982.

Petros PE, Ulmsten U: Bladder instability in women: A premature activation of the micturition reflex. Neurourol Urodynam 1993;12:235.

Petros PE, Ulmsten U: An integral theory and its method for the diagnosis and management of female urinary incontinence. Scand J Urol Nephrol 1993;[Suppl]:153:1.

Petros PE, Ulmsten U: Urge incontinence history is an accurate predictor of urge incontinence. Acta Obstet Gynecol Scand 1992;71:537.

Raz S: Modified bladder neck suspension for female stress incontinence. Urology 1981;17:82.

Raz S: Vaginal surgery for stress incontinence. J Am Geriatr Soc 1990;38:348.

Raz S et al: Vaginal wall sling. J Urol 1989;141:43.

Rijkhoff NJ et al: Urinary bladder control by electrical stimulation: Review of electrical stimulation techniques in spinal cord injury. Neurourol Urodyn 1997;16:39.

Robinson D: Urinary incontinence in the elderly: A growing problem that needs attention. Curr Opin Obstet Gynecol 1997;9:285.

Sampselle CM, DeLancey JO: Anatomy of female incontinence. J Wound Ostomy Continence Nurs 1998;25:63.

Sarver R, Govier FE: Pubovaginal slings: Past, present and future. Int Urogynecol J Pelvic Floor Dysfunct 1997;8:358.

Smith ARB, Hosker GL, Warrell DW: The role of partial denervation of the pelvic floor in the aetiology of genitourinary prolapse and stress incontinence of urine: A neurophysiological study. Br J Obstet Gynaecol 1989;96:24.

Stage P, Fischer-Rasmussen W, Iversen HR: The value of colpo-cysto-urethrography in female stress and urge incontinence and following operation. Acta Obstet Gynecol Scand 1986;65:401.

Stamey TA: Endoscopic suspension of the vesical neck for urinary incontinence. Surg Gynecol Obstet 1973; 136:547.

Stamey TA: Endoscopic suspension of the vesical neck for urinary incontinence in females: Report on 203 consecutive patients. Ann Surg 1980;192:465.

Stanton SL: Surgical treatment of sphincteric incontinence in women. World J Urol 1997;15:272.

Stanton SL et al: Clinical and urodynamic factors of failed incontinence surgery in the female. Obstet Gynecol 1978;51:515

Su TH et al: Prospective comparison of laparoscopic and traditional colposuspensions in the treatment of genuine stress incontinence. Acta Obstet Gynecol Scand 1997;76:576.

Summitt RL Jr, Bent AE, Ostergard DR: The pathophysiology of genuine stress incontinence. Int Urogynecol J 1990;1:12.

Tanagho EA: The anatomy and physiology of micturition. Clin Obstet Gynaecol 1978;5:3.

Tanagho EA: Colpocystourethropexy, the way we do it. J Urol 1976;116:751.

Tanagho EA: Simplified cystography in stress incontinence. Br J Urol 1974;74:295.

Tanagho EA: Urodynamics of female urinary incontinence with emphasis on stress incontinence. J Urol 1979;122:200.

Tanagho EA, Smith DR: Clinical evaluation of a surgical technique for the correction of complete urinary incontinence. J Urol 1972;107:402.

Tanagho EA, Stoller ML: Urodynamics: Uroflowmetry and female voiding patterns. In: Ostergard D, Bent AE (editors): *Urogynecology and Urodynamics: Theory and Practice,* 3rd ed. Williams & Wilkins, 1991.

Thunedborg P, Fischer-Rasmussen W, Jensen SB: Stress urinary incontinence and posterior bladder suspension defects: Results of vaginal repair versus Burch colposuspension. Acta Obstet Gynecol Scand 1990;69:55.

Turner-Warwick R: Observations of the function and dysfunction of the sphincter and detrusor mechanisms. Urol Clin North Am 1979;6:13.

Ulmsten U: Some reflections and hypotheses on the pathophysiology of female urinary incontinence. Acta Obstet Gynecol Scand Suppl 1997;166:3.

Ulmsten U, Asmussen M, Lindstrom KA: A new technique for simultaneous urethrocystometry and measurements of the urethral pressure profile. Urol Int 1977;32:88.

Vancaillie TG: Laparoscopic colposuspension and pelvic floor repair. Curr Opin Obstet Gynecol 1997;9:244.

Weber AM, Walters MD: Anterior vaginal prolapse: Review of anatomy and techniques of surgical repair. Obstet Gynecol 1997;89:311.

Wein AJ: Pharmacologic treatment of incontinence. J Am Geriatr Soc 1990;38:317.

Weiss BD: Diagnostic evaluation of urinary incontinence in geriatric patients. Am Fam Physician 1998; 57:2688.

Zacharin RF: *Pelvic Floor Anatomy and the Surgery of Pulsion Enterocele.* Springer-Verlag, 1985.

Zacharin RF: The suspensory mechanism of the female urethra. J Anat 1963;97:423.

Disorders of the Adrenal Glands

32

J. Blake Tyrrell, MD

Disorders of the adrenal glands result in classic endocrine syndromes such as Cushing syndrome, hyperaldosteronism, and pheochromocytoma (Figure 32–1). In addition, tumors of the adrenals may present with abdominal pain or as an abdominal mass. The diagnosis of these disorders requires careful endocrine evaluation, and in many patients, adrenal imaging studies are required to define adrenal anatomy.

There are, in addition to functioning tumors and hyperplasias of the adrenal cortex and medulla and nonfunctioning malignant tumors, other, often benign types of involvement of the adrenal glands. These enter into the differential diagnosis of adrenal lesions.

DISEASES OF THE ADRENAL CORTEX

CUSHING SYNDROME

Cushing syndrome is the clinical disorder caused by overproduction of cortisol. Most cases (80%) are due to bilateral adrenocortical hyperplasia stimulated by overproduction of pituitary adrenocorticotropic hormone (corticotropin, ACTH), known as Cushing disease. About 10% of cases are due to the ectopic production of ACTH from nonpituitary tumors. Ectopic ACTH production occurs most frequently in small-cell lung carcinoma; other tumors producing ACTH include carcinoids (lung, thymic, gastrointestinal tract), islet cell tumors of the pancreas, medullary thyroid carcinoma, pheochromocytoma, and small-cell carcinoma of the prostate. Adrenal adenoma is the cause in 5% of cases and carcinoma in 5%. In children, adrenocortical carcinoma is the most common cause of Cushing syndrome.

Pathophysiology

Overproduction of cortisol by adrenocortical tissue

leads to a catabolic state. This causes liberation from muscle tissue of amino acids, which are transformed into glucose and glycogen in the liver by gluconeogenesis. The resulting weakened protein structures (muscle and elastic tissue) cause a protuberant abdomen and poor wound healing, generalized muscle weakness, and marked osteoporosis, which is made worse by excessive loss of calcium in the urine.

In addition, glucose is transformed largely into fat and appears in characteristic sites such as the abdomen, supraclavicular fat pads, and cheeks. There is a tendency to diabetes, with an elevated fasting plasma glucose level in 20% of cases and diabetic glucose tolerance curve in 80%.

The cortisol excess also suppresses the immune mechanisms, which makes these patients susceptible to repeated infection. Inhibition of fibroblast function by excess cortisol further interferes with wound healing and host defenses against infection.

Hypertension is present in 90% of cases. Although the aldosterone level is not usually elevated, cortisol itself exerts a hypertensive effect when present in excessive amounts, as does 11-deoxycorticosterone. The hypertension may be accompanied by manifestation of mineralocorticoid excess (hypokalemia and alkalosis), especially in patients with the ectopic ACTH syndrome or adrenocortical carcinoma.

Pathology

The cells in adrenal hyperplasia resemble those of the zona fasciculata of the normal adrenal cortex. Frank adenocarcinoma reveals pleomorphism and invasion of the capsule, the vascular system, or both (Figure 32–2). Local invasion may occur, and metastases are common to the liver, lungs, bone, or brain. Histologic differentiation between adenoma and adenocarcinoma is frequently difficult.

In the presence of adenoma or malignant tumor, atrophy of the cortices of both adrenals occurs because the main secretory product of the tumor is cortisol, which inhibits the pituitary secretion of ACTH. Thus, although the tumor continues to grow, the contralateral adrenal cortex undergoes atrophy.

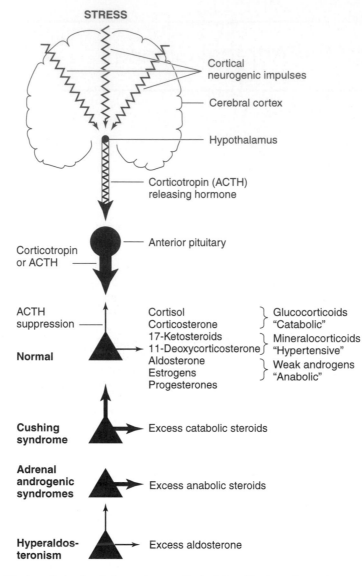

Figure 32–1. The hypothalamic-pituitary-adrenocortical relationships in various adrenocortical syndromes.

Clinical Findings

A. Symptoms and Signs: (Figures 32–3 and 32–4.) The presence of at least 3 of the following strongly suggests Cushing syndrome:

1. Obesity (with sparing of the extremities), moon face, and fat pads of the supraclavicular and dorsocervical areas (buffalo hump). The abnormal distribution of fat is more characteristic of the disease than is the actual amount of weight gain.
2. Striae (red and depressed) over the abdomen and thighs. Poor healing of minor wounds and lower-extremity ulcers may be present.
3. Hypertension (almost always present).

4. Proximal myopathy with marked weakness, especially in the quadriceps femoris, making unaided rising from a chair difficult.
5. Emotional lability, irritability, difficulty in sleeping, and sometimes psychotic personality.
6. Osteoporosis (common), with back pain from compression fractures of the lumbar vertebrae as well as rib fractures.
7. In 80% of cases, post-prandial hyperglycemia is present, and in 20% there is an elevated fasting plasma glucose level.
8. To a variable extent, there are features of adrenal androgen excess in women with Cushing syndrome; these are absent in the case of adenoma, most severe with carcinoma, and present to an in-

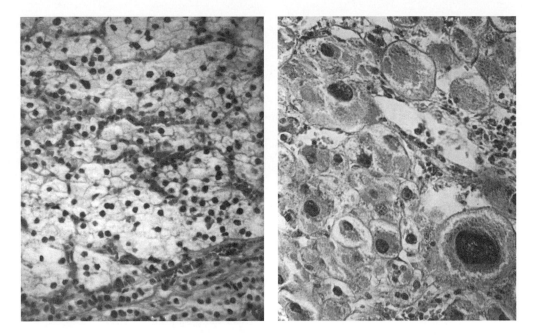

Figure 32–2. **Left:** Histologic appearance of a typical benign adenoma of the adrenal cortex made up of a large number of identical cells from the zona fasciculata removed from a 39-year-old woman with Cushing syndrome. **Right:** Section of an adenocarcinoma removed from a 36-year-old woman with metastatic adenocarcinoma showing significant pleomorphism of the cells. Invasion of a large vein is not shown in this micrograph. Note that benign adenomas will occasionally have this appearance but without invasion of the bloodstream. (Reproduced, with permission, from Forsham PH: The adrenal cortex. In: Williams RH [editor]: *Textbook of Endocrinology,* 4th ed. Saunders, 1968.)

termediate degree with Cushing disease. They consist of recession of the hairline, hirsutism, small breasts, and generalized muscular overdevelopment, with deepening of the voice.

On the basis of the foregoing clinical findings alone, it is not possible to differentiate those patients with ACTH excess causing bilateral adrenocortical hyperplasia from those with unilateral adenoma or adenocarcinoma.

The most rapid onset is noted in cases caused by ectopic ACTH-producing tumor with high glucocorticoid output or those due to adrenocortical carcinoma. In the case of adrenocortical carcinoma, the tumor may be palpable.

B. Laboratory Findings: The leukocyte count may be elevated to the range of 12,000–20,000/μL, usually with fewer than 20% lymphocytes. Eosinophils are few in number or absent. Polycythemia is present in over half the cases, with the hemoglobin ranging from 14 to 16 g/dL. Anemia, however, may occur in patients with malignant tumors ectopically secreting ACTH.

Blood chemical analyses may show an increase in serum Na^+ and CO_2 levels and a decrease in serum K^+ levels. Hyperglycemia may occur.

1. Specific tests for Cushing syndrome–

The following tests are performed to determine whether the patient has Cushing syndrome or is an anxious individual with elevated plasma levels of cortisol.

a. 24-h urinary cortisol level–Urine cortisol is measured in a 24-h urine collection by high-performance liquid chromatography (normal range, 10–50 μg/24 h), and urine creatinine is also measured to ensure completeness of the collection. A urine cortisol value more than 2-fold elevated is typical of Cushing syndrome. False-positive elevations can occur in acute illness, depression, and alcoholism. However, obesity does not raise the level of urinary free cortisol above normal.

b. Suppression of ACTH and plasma cortisol by dexamethasone–Dexamethasone in low doses is used to assess the feedback suppression of ACTH and cortisol production by glucocorticoids. If dexamethasone is given at 11 PM, ACTH is suppressed in normal persons but not in those with Cushing syndrome. Dexamethasone is useful because it has 30 times the potency of cortisol as an ACTH suppressant and it is not measured in current plasma or urine cortisol methods.

The procedure is to give 1 mg of dexamethasone by mouth at 11 PM and to draw blood at 8–9:00 AM for measurement of plasma cortisol. If the level is be-

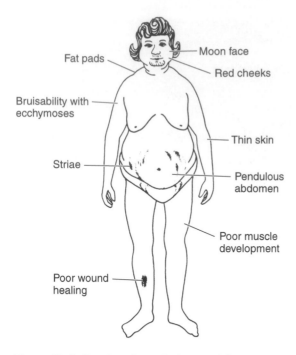

Figure 32–3. Drawing of a typical case of Cushing syndrome showing the principal clinical features. (Reproduced, with permission, from Forsham PH: The adrenal cortex. In: Williams RH [editor]: *Textbook of Endocrinology,* 4th ed. Saunders, 1968.)

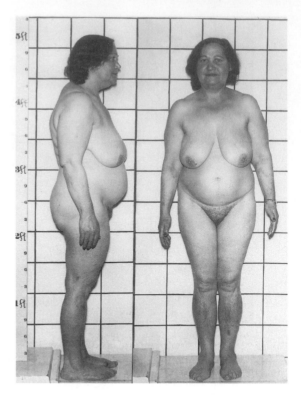

Figure 32–4. A patient with Cushing disease. Note the red moon face, receding hairline, buffalo hump over the seventh vertebra, protuberant abdomen, and inappropriately thin arms and legs.

low 5 μg/dL (normal is 5–20 μg/dL), Cushing syndrome can be ruled out. If the value is above 10 μg/dL, Cushing syndrome is present (Figure 32–5). A level in the range of 5–10 μg/dL is equivocal, and the test should be repeated or the urine cortisol may be measured.

Women taking birth control pills have high plasma cortisol levels because, as in pregnancy, the estrogen stimulates production of the cortisol-binding globulin. The pills must be withheld for at least 3 weeks before the dexamethasone suppression test. Other conditions causing false-positive responses are acute illness, depression, and alcoholism. Also, about 15% of obese patients do not suppress cortisol with this test.

2. Specific tests for differentiation of causes of Cushing syndrome–The various causes of Cushing syndrome can be determined with great accuracy (95% of cases).

a. Plasma ACTH level–If the diagnosis of Cushing syndrome has been established, this test will differentiate ACTH-dependent causes (Cushing disease and the ectopic ACTH syndrome) from adrenal tumors, which are ACTH-independent. ACTH is currently measured by a sensitive immunoradiometric assay (IRMA) (normal range, 10–50 pg/mL). Patients with Cushing disease have ACTH levels that range from 10 to 200 pg/mL; in the ectopic ACTH syndrome, levels are usually greater than 200 pg/mL; and patients with adrenal tumors have suppressed ACTH levels (< 5 pg/mL with the IRMA ACTH assay) and thus are easily differentiated.

b. Plasma androgen levels–In patients with adrenal adenomas, androgen levels are normal or low, and in adrenocortical carcinoma these levels are often markedly elevated.

C. X-Ray Findings and Special Examinations:

1. Localization of source of ACTH excess–When tests suggest Cushing disease or the ectopic ACTH syndrome and an elevated plasma level of ACTH is present, the source of ACTH must be identified. Because the great majority of these patients have Cushing disease and because most of the patients with ectopic ACTH secretion have an obvious malignancy, the first step is to perform pituitary magnetic resonance imaging (MRI). These are positive in 50–60% of patients with Cushing disease; in the remainder, the diagnosis should be established by the sampling of ACTH levels in the venous drainage of the anterior pituitary, ie, the cavernous sinuses and inferior petrosal sinuses. If the MRI and venous sam-

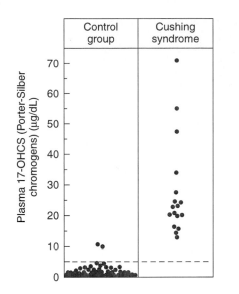

Figure 32–5. Results of the dexamethasone suppression test in obese individuals and patients with Cushing syndrome. See text for procedure. 17-OHCS = 17-hydroxycorticosteroids. (Reproduced, with permission, from Pavlatos FC, Smilo RP, Forsham PH: A rapid screening test for Cushing's syndrome. JAMA 1975;193:720.)

pling do not reveal a pituitary source of ACTH, computed tomography (CT) scans of the chest and abdomen are used to localize an ectopic tumor.

2. Localization of adrenal lesions–Patients with Cushing syndrome with suspected adrenal tumors and suppressed ACTH levels should undergo a CT scan of the abdomen with 3-mm sections through the adrenals. Adrenal tumors causing Cushing syndrome are virtually always greater than 3 cm in diameter (Figure 32–6) and are therefore easily visualized. Adenomas are usually 3–6 cm in diameter; carcinomas are usually greater than 5 cm in diameter and are frequently locally invasive or metastatic to the liver and lungs at the time of diagnosis. In patients with adrenal tumors, the contralateral adrenal is suppressed and therefore appears atrophic or normal on CT scan. The finding of bilateral adrenal enlargement is typical of Cushing disease or the ectopic ACTH syndrome. Ultrasound or MRI may also be used for adrenal localization, although these techniques do not appear to offer significant advantage over CT scans.

Complications

Hypertension may lead to cardiac failure or stroke. Diabetes may be a problem but is usually mild. Intractable skin or systemic infections are common. Compression fractures of osteoporotic vertebrae and rib fractures may develop. Renal stones are not uncommon as a result of bone resorption. Psychosis is

not uncommon; it usually subsides after successful surgery.

Treatment

A. Cushing Disease: A pituitary microadenoma, which is the most common cause of bilateral adrenocortical hyperplasia, must be located and removed surgically. **Transsphenoidal resection** performed by an experienced neurosurgeon is the method of choice. Success is reported in over 80% of cases, and in most instances the endocrine functions of the pituitary gland are preserved.

B. Ectopic ACTH Syndrome: The treatment of these patients is difficult because most have an advanced malignancy and severe hypercortisolism. Removal of the primary tumor is clearly the therapy of choice; however, curative resection is limited to the few patients with benign tumors such as bronchial carcinoids. Patients with residual or metastatic tumors should be managed first with adrenal inhibitors, and if that is not successful, bilateral adrenalectomy should be considered.

At present, it is best to perform bilateral adrenalectomy via a laparoscopic approach. One adrenal is removed by a flank approach, the patient is then turned, and the contralateral adrenal is removed. The procedure does not reduce anesthesia or surgical time, but it decreases morbidity and length of hospital stay.

C. Total Bilateral Adrenalectomy: Total bilateral adrenalectomy is indicated in patients with Cushing disease in whom the pituitary tumor is not resectable and in whom radiotherapy and medical therapy fail to control the cortisol excess. Bilateral adrenalectomy is also indicated in patients with ectopic ACTH syndrome who have life-threatening hypercortisolism that cannot be controlled by inhibitors of adrenal secretion.

1. Preoperative preparation–Because removal of the source of excessive cortisol will inevitably lead to temporary or permanent adrenal insufficiency, it is of the utmost importance to administer cortisol preoperatively and to continue substitution therapy after surgery to control Addison disease. In the postoperative period, the dose is tapered downward until oral medication provides sufficient control.

2. Postoperative status–The patient feels moderately well following removal of the source of excess ACTH or adrenalectomy or while receiving a high dose of hydrocortisone in excess of the usual daily output of approximately 20 mg. When dosage approaches the maximum normal physiologic output, the patient may complain of nausea, abdominal pain, and extreme weakness with the steroid withdrawal syndrome. Thus, it is important to reduce the steroid substitution gradually over a period of several days. On the day of operation, 200 mg of cortisol is given; the dosage is then reduced gradually on successive

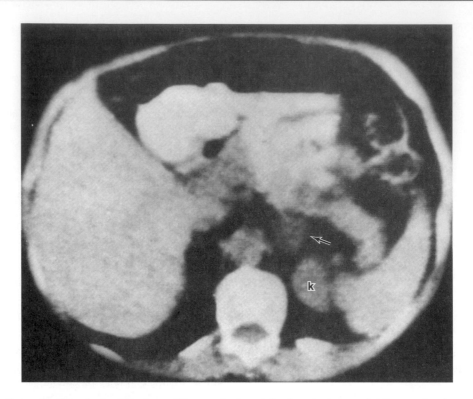

Figure 32–6. Localization of adrenal lesions. CT scan of a 3-cm left adrenal adenoma (white arrow) anteromedial to the left kidney (k). (Reproduced, with permission, from Korobkin MT et al: Am J Roentgenol 1979;132:231.)

days (150, 100, 80, 60, and 40 mg) until a maintenance dosage of 20–30 mg cortisol combined with 0.1 mg fludrocortisone is reached.

D. Adrenal Adenoma and Adenocarcinoma: Virtually all adrenal adenomas and smaller adrenal carcinomas are now removed laparoscopically, again allowing decreased hospital stay and more rapid recovery from surgery. Adrenal carcinomas that are large (greater than 8–10 cm) are likely to be metastatic or locally invasive. Thus, if there is evidence of invasion of adjacent structures or invasion of the adrenal or renal veins or the vena cava, these tumors are best approached by a traditional abdominal or flank incision.

1. Preoperative preparation–Preoperative preparation is the same as that for bilateral hyperplasia, since, in this case, the remaining adrenal gland will be atrophic and thus the patient will be hypoadrenal.

2. Postoperative treatment and follow-up–Cortisol is administered perioperatively in the doses described above and then tapered to a replacement dose of 20–30 mg per day. Hydrocortisone is given orally in a dosage of 10 mg 3 times daily initially and reduced within 2–3 weeks to 10 mg daily given at 7 or 8 AM. Substitution therapy may be necessary for 6 months to 2 years depending on the rate of recovery of the residual gland. Mineralocorticoid therapy is rarely necessary, since the atrophic adrenal usually produces sufficient aldosterone. Patients with adrenocortical carcinoma are usually not cured by surgery and require additional therapy.

E. Medical Therapy: There is no effective method of inhibiting ACTH secretion; however, adrenal hypersecretion can be controlled in many patients by inhibitors of adrenal cortisol secretion. Medical therapy is indicated in patients who either cannot undergo surgery (eg, because of debility, recent myocardial infarction) or in those who have had unsuccessful resection of their pituitary, ectopic, or adrenal tumor.

Ketoconazole is the current drug of choice; it blocks cortisol secretion by inhibiting P450c11 and P450scc. The total dose required is 800–1600 mg/d given in 2 divided doses. Side effects are adrenal insufficiency, abnormal liver function tests, and hepatotoxicity in a few patients.

Metyrapone may be used alone or may be added if ketoconazole alone is unsuccessful in normalizing cortisol levels. The usual dosage is 1–4 g daily given in 4 divided doses.

Aminoglutethimide and trilostane also inhibit adrenal secretion, but they are uncommonly used at present.

Mitotane (o,p'-DDD) is both an inhibitor of adrenal secretion and a cytotoxic agent that damages adrenocortical cells. It is used almost exclusively in patients with residual adrenocortical carcinoma, in whom it helps to reduce cortisol hypersecretion. The usual dosage is 6–12 g/daily in 3–4 divided doses. About 70% of patients achieve a reduction in steroid secretion and 35% achieve a reduction in tumor size; however, there is no convincing evidence that the drug prolongs survival. Side effects occur in 80% of patients and include nausea, vomiting, diarrhea, depression, and somnolence.

Prognosis

Treatment of hypercortisolism usually leads to disappearance of symptoms and many signs within days to weeks, but osteoporosis usually persists in adults, whereas hypertension and diabetes often improve. Cushing disease treated by pituitary adenomectomy has an excellent early prognosis, and long-term follow-up shows a recurrence rate of about 10%. Patients with the ectopic ACTH syndrome and malignant tumors in general have a poor prognosis; these patients usually die within several months of diagnosis. Patients with benign lesions may be cured by resection of the tumor. Removal of an adrenal adenoma offers an excellent prognosis; and these patients are cured by unilateral adrenalectomy.

The outlook for patients with adrenocortical carcinoma is poor. The antineoplastic drug mitotane (*o,p'*-DDD; Lysodren) given in doses of up to 6–12 g orally daily reduces the symptoms and signs of Cushing syndrome but does little to prolong survival. Radiotherapy and chemotherapy are not successful in these patients.

ADRENAL ANDROGENIC SYNDROMES

Adrenal androgenic syndromes are more common in females. Congenital bilateral adrenal hyperplasia and tumors, both benign and malignant, may be observed. They are all caused by excessive secretion of adrenal androgens. In contrast to Cushing syndrome, which is protein catabolic, the androgenic syndromes are anabolic. In untreated cases, there is a marked recession of the hairline, increased beard growth, and excessive growth of pubic and sexual hair in general in both sexes. In males, there is enlargement of the penis, usually with atrophic testes; in females, enlargement of the clitoris occurs, with atrophy of the breasts and amenorrhea (Figure 32–7). Muscle mass increases and fat content decreases, leading to a powerful but trim figure. The voice becomes deeper, particularly in females; this condition is irreversible, because it is due to enlargement of the larynx. In both sexes there may be increased physical sexual aggressiveness and libido.

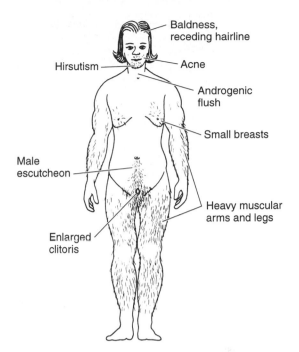

Figure 32–7. Clinical features of a full-blown case of virilism in a female with adrenogenital syndrome. (Reproduced, with permission, from Forsham PH: The adrenal cortex. In: Williams RH [editor]: *Textbook of Endocrinology,* 4th ed. Saunders, 1968.)

1. CONGENITAL BILATERAL ADRENAL ANDROGENIC HYPERPLASIA

Pathophysiology

A congenital defect in certain adrenal enzymes results in the production of abnormal steroids, causing **pseudohermaphroditism** in females and **macrogenitosomia** in males. The enzyme defect is associated with excess androgen production in utero. In females, the müllerian duct structures (eg, ovaries, uterus, and vagina) develop normally, but the excess androgen exerts a masculinizing effect on the urogenital sinus and genital tubercle, so that the vagina is connected to the urethra, which, in turn, opens at the base of the enlarged clitoris. The labia are often hypertrophied. Externally, the appearance is that of severe hypospadias with cryptorchidism.

The adrenal cortex secretes mostly anabolic and androgenic steroids, leading to various degrees of cortisol deficiency depending on the nature of the enzyme block. This increases the secretion of ACTH, which causes hyperplasia of both adrenal cortices. The cortices continue to secrete large amounts of inappropriate anabolic, androgenic, or hypertensive steroids. Absence or reduction of the usual tissue concentration of various enzymes accounts for blocks in the adrenocortical synthetic pathways.

A **block at P450scc** leads to the rare congenital lipoid adrenal hyperplasia with complete absence of any steroidal hormone production; the infant will die at an early age unless full substitution therapy is given for life.

A **block at 3β-hydroxydehydrogenase/isomerase enzyme** prevents formation of progesterone, aldosterone, and cortisol. Dehydroepiandrosterone (DHEA) is produced in excess. This uncommon syndrome is characterized by adrenal insufficiency and male pseudohermaphroditism, with females showing unusual sexual development with hirsutism.

A **block at P450c21,** which is the most common cause of congenital adrenal hyperplasia, does not allow for the transformation of 17α-hydroxyprogesterone to cortisol. This common deficiency occurs in 2 forms: the salt-losing variety, with low to absent aldosterone, and the more frequent non-salt-losing type. Infants present with adrenal insufficiency and ambiguous genitalia; older children develop pseudoprecocious puberty and accelerated growth and skeletal maturation.

A **block at P450c17** with lack of 17-hydroxylase occurs mostly in females and may not be discovered until puberty. Findings include low cortisol levels with high ACTH levels, primary amenorrhea, and sexual infantilism, as neither the glucocorticoids nor the sex steroids are produced in adequate amounts. Rarely, there is male pseudohermaphroditism. Hypertension due to excess mineralocorticoids, notably 11-deoxycorticosterone, is characteristically present.

A **block at P450c11** with lack of 11-hydroxylase prevents formation of cortisol and corticosterone and thus leads to overproduction of adrenal androgens and 11-deoxycorticosterone. Patients usually have clinical features of mild androgen excess with hypertension and hypokalemia.

A **block at P450aldo** results in the inability to produce aldosterone in the zona glomerulosa; these patients present with isolated mineralocorticoid deficiency with hypotension and hyperkalemia.

Clinical Findings

A. Symptoms and Signs: In newborn girls, the appearance of the external genitalia resembles severe hypospadias with cryptorchidism. Infant boys may appear quite normal at birth. The earlier in intrauterine life the fetus has been exposed to excess androgen, the more marked the anomalies.

In untreated cases, hirsutism, excess muscle mass, and, eventually, amenorrhea are the rule. Breast development is poor. In males, growth of the phallus is excessive. The testes are often atrophic because of inhibition of gonadotropin secretion by the elevated androgens. On rare occasions, hyperplastic adrenocortical rests in the testes make them large and firm. In most instances, there is aspermia after puberty.

In both males and females with androgenic hyperplasia, the growth rate is initially increased, so that they are taller than their classmates. At about age 9–10 years, premature fusion of the epiphyses caused by excess androgen causes termination of growth, so that these patients are short as adults.

B. Laboratory Findings: Urinary 17-ketosteroid levels are higher than normal for sex and age, and plasma anchostenedione, DHEA, DHEA-S, and testosterone are elevated. Plasma ACTH is also elevated, and in patients with the most common defect (ie, 21-hydroxylase deficiency), plasma 17α-hydroxyprogesterone is markedly elevated. Chromosome studies are normal.

C. X-Ray Findings: X-rays show acceleration of bone age.

D. CT Scans: Scans usually show the hypertrophied adrenals.

E. Urologic Evaluation: This is indicated to define the anatomic abnormalities.

Differential Diagnosis

A number of congenital anomalies that affect the development of the external genitalia resemble adrenal androgenic syndrome. These include (1) severe hypospadias with cryptorchidism, (2) female pseudohermaphroditism of the nonadrenal type (caused by administration of androgens or progestational compounds during the pregnancy), (3) male pseudohermaphroditism, and (4) true hermaphroditism. These children show no hormonal abnormalities, and bone age and maturation are not accelerated.

Treatment

It is imperative to make the diagnosis early. Treatment of the underlying cause is medical, with the goal of suppressing excessive ACTH secretion, thus minimizing excess androgenicity. This is accomplished by adrenal replacement with cortisol or prednisone in doses sufficient to suppress adrenal androgen production and therefore prevent virilization and rapid skeletal growth. In patients with mineralocorticoid deficiency, fludrocortisone (0.05–0.3 mg, depending on severity and age) together with good salt intake is necessary to stabilize blood pressure and body weight.

After puberty, the vaginal opening can be surgically separated from the urethra and opened in the normal position on the perineum. Judicious administration of estrogens or birth control pills feminizes the figure in pseudohermaphrodites and improves their psyche considerably.

Prognosis

If the condition is recognized early and ACTH suppression is begun even before surgical repair of the genital anomaly, the outlook for normal linear growth and development is excellent. Delay in treatment inevitably results in stunted growth. In some female pseudohermaphrodites, menses begin after treatment, and conception and childbirth can occur when the anatomic abnormalities are minimal or have been surgically repaired.

2. ADRENOCORTICAL TUMORS

Adrenocortical tumors producing androgens are most frequently carcinomas; however, a few benign adenomas have been reported. Most of the carcinomas also hypersecrete other hormones (ie, cortisol or 11-deoxycorticosterone), and thus the clinical presentation is variable. Female patients present with androgen excess, which may be severe enough to cause virilization; many of these patients also have Cushing syndrome and mineralocorticoid excess (hypertension and hypokalemia). In adult males excess androgens may cause no clinical manifestations, and diagnosis in these patients may be delayed until there is abdominal pain or an abdominal mass. These patients may also present with Cushing syndrome and mineralocorticoid excess.

The tumor can be located by CT scan, which is also used to define the extent of tumor spread (see Figure 32–6). Local invasion and distant spread to the liver and lungs are common at the time of diagnosis. The primary therapy is surgical resection of the adrenal tumor, as discussed above; however, surgical cure is rare. These patients are subsequently treated with mitotane and other adrenal inhibitors, as discussed in the section on Cushing syndrome.

THE HYPERTENSIVE, HYPOKALEMIC SYNDROME (PRIMARY ALDOSTERONISM)

Excessive production of aldosterone, due mostly to aldosteronoma or to spontaneous bilateral hyperplasia of the zona glomerulosa of the adrenal cortex, leads to the combination of hypertension, hypokalemia, nocturia, and polyuria. A syndrome resembling nephrogenic diabetes insipidus may occur as a result of reversible damage to the renal collecting tubules. The alkalosis may produce tetany.

Pathophysiology

Excessive aldosterone, acting on most cell membranes in the body, produces typical changes in the distal renal tubule and the small bowel that lead to urinary potassium loss together with increased renal sodium reabsorption and hydrogen ion secretion. This results in potassium depletion, metabolic alkalosis, increased plasma sodium concentration, and hypervolemia. With low serum levels of potassium, the concentrating ability of the kidney is lowered and the tubules no longer respond to the administration of vasopressin by increased reabsorption of water. Finally, impairment of insulin release secondary to po-

tassium depletion increases carbohydrate intolerance in about 50% of cases.

Plasma renin and, secondarily, plasma angiotensin are depressed by excess aldosterone as a result of blood volume expansion (Figure 32–8). Early in the course of excess aldosterone production, there may be hypertension with a normal serum potassium level. Later, the potassium level will be low as well, and this suggests the diagnosis.

Clinical Findings

A. Symptoms and Signs: Hypertension is usually the presenting manifestation, and the accompanying hypokalemia suggests mineralocorticoid excess. Headaches are common, nocturia is invariably present, and rare episodes of paralysis occur with very low serum potassium levels. Numbness and tingling of the extremities are related to alkalosis that may lead to tetany. Hypertension is of varying severity.

Ophthalmoscopic examination usually shows normal vessels inconsistent with the degree of hypertension. Unless acute heart failure is present, there is no edema.

B. Laboratory Findings: Before the tests outlined below are done, one must ascertain that the patient is not taking oral contraceptives or other estrogen preparations, since these may increase renin and angiotensin levels and therefore aldosterone levels, thus raising the blood pressure artificially. Withdrawal of these medications for 1 week is mandatory. Diuretics must also be discontinued, since they lower blood volume and induce secondary aldosteronism

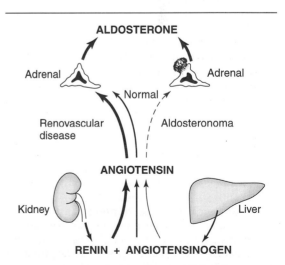

Figure 32–8. The angiotensin-aldosterone relationships in a case of aldosteronoma and hypertension due to renal vascular disease. (Reproduced, with permission, from Forsham PH: The adrenal cortex. In: Williams RH [editor]: *Textbook of Endocrinology,* 4th ed. Saunders, 1968.)

and hypokalemia. Also, if the patient is following a salt-restricted diet, aldosterone is normally elevated.

Before serum electrolytes are measured, the patient receives a loading dose of 6 g of salt for at least 2 days. This will furnish exchangeable sodium in the distal tubule and allow potassium to exchange with sodium, thus clearly revealing the low serum potassium level and electrolyte imbalance. Later, serum potassium must also be replenished, because a very low level of this ion may artificially decrease the secretory rate of aldosterone.

In true aldosterone excess, serum sodium is slightly elevated and CO_2 increased, whereas serum potassium is very low, eg, 3 mEq/L or less. Urine and serum potassium determinations while the patient is receiving good sodium replacement provide a screening test. Potassium wasting is considered to be established if the urinary potassium level is greater than 30 mEq/L/24 h but the serum potassium level is low (3 mEq/L or less).

Definitive diagnosis rests on demonstration of an elevated urine or plasma aldosterone level. The initial step is to obtain simultaneous plasma aldosterone and plasma renin levels. If the aldosterone is elevated and the renin is suppressed with a ratio of greater than 20:1, the diagnosis is established. Further confirmation can be obtained by demonstrating an elevated aldosterone level in a 24-h urine sample.

C. Localization: A thin-section CT scan is the initial procedure and will localize an adenoma in approximately 90% of patients (Figure 32–9). If no adenoma is visualized, adrenal vein sampling of aldosterone and cortisol will correctly differentiate adenoma from hyperplasia in virtually all cases.

Differential Diagnosis

Secondary hyperaldosteronism may accompany renovascular hypertension. An abdominal bruit suggests this condition initially. This too is associated with hypokalemic alkalosis; however, the renin level is elevated rather than suppressed.

Essential hypertension does not cause changes in the electrolyte pattern. Definitive tests for hyperaldosteronism show negative results.

Treatment

A. Aldosteronoma: If the site of the tumor has been established, only the affected adrenal need be removed. Again, the procedure of choice is laparoscopic unilateral adrenalectomy.

B. Bilateral Nodular Hyperplasia: Most authorities do not recommend resection of both adrenals, since the fall in blood pressure is only temporary and electrolyte imbalance may continue. Medical treatment is recommended.

C. Medical Treatment: If surgery must be postponed, if the hypertension is mild in an older person, or if bilateral hyperplasia is the cause, one may treat medically with spironolactone (Aldactone),

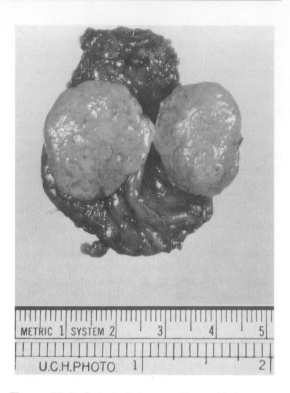

Figure 32–9. A typical canary-yellow aldosteronoma associated with the syndrome of hypertension, hypokalemia, and alkalosis. Note the relatively small size of this tumor compared with other types of adrenocortical tumors.

25–50 mg orally 4 times daily. Amiloride, a potassium-sparing diuretic, may be given in doses of up to 20–40 mg per day. Other antihypertensive agents may also be necessary.

Prognosis

Following removal of an adrenal adenoma, the hypokalemia resolves. Seventy percent of patients become normotensive and 50% show some lowering of hypertension. Bilateral nodular hyperplasia is not amenable to surgical treatment, and the results of medical treatment are only fair.

DISEASES OF THE ADRENAL MEDULLA

PHEOCHROMOCYTOMA

Pheochromocytoma, derived from the neural crest, is one of the surgically curable hypertensive syndromes. There is no sex predilection. Pheochromocytoma accounts for fewer than 1% of cases of hypertension, but it is readily diagnosed if the possibility is kept in mind. It usually occurs spontaneously, but 10% of cases occur in patients with other disorders such as neurofibromatosis or familial syndromes such as multiple endocrine neoplasia type II or von Hippel-Lindau disease. The tumor is bilateral or extra-adrenal in 10% of cases in adults and in an even greater percentage in children and is then most often familial.

Clinical Findings

A. Symptoms and Signs: Hypertension is both systolic and diastolic. Hypertension may be either sustained and indistinguishable from ordinary blood pressure elevation, or paroxysmal, coming on for variable lengths of time and then subsiding to normal levels. Such attacks are usually precipitated by trigger mechanisms of various sorts, eg, emotional upsets or straining at stool.

Headache is a frequent complaint and is commensurate in severity with the degree of hypertension. Increased sweating without appropriate causes such as exertion or environmental heat resembles the phenomenon seen during menopause and may be accompanied by flushing or blanching. Tachycardia with palpitations occurs mainly as a consequence of epinephrine rather than norepinephrine excess. Postural hypotension is a frequent finding, as a result of diminished plasma volume.

Profound weakness may occur after an attack of hypertension. Weight loss is common.

Decreased gastrointestinal motility occurs, leading to nausea and vomiting and constipation. This effect is a direct pharmacologic consequence of excessive circulating catecholamines. Episodes of psychic instability verging on hysteria are frequent and are probably due to increased concentrations of catecholamines and other neurotransmitters in the brain, although circulating catecholamines, unlike some of their precursors, penetrate the blood-brain barrier to only a limited extent.

B. Biochemical Diagnosis: The choice of biochemical test and whether to measure plasma or urine values remain controversial, but certain principles are clear: (1) Screening the hypertensive population is not recommended because of the low incidence of pheochromocytoma (about 0.1%). (2) Regardless of the test chosen, specific methodology is essential, and thus methods using high-performance liquid chromatography, radioimmunoassay, or radioenzymatic assays should be selected. Older colorimetric or fluorometric methods are still in use in many laboratories and should be avoided because of frequent interference by drugs and diet. (3) Patients with pheochromocytoma who have sustained hypertension usually have clearly elevated catecholamines or metabolites in both urine and plasma. More than 80% of these patients

have urine values 2 times greater than normal and total plasma catecholamine (Epi + Norepi) above 2000 ng/L. Levels of this magnitude are unusual in patients without pheochromocytoma except in acute major illness. (4) Patients with only episodic hypertension may have normal random plasma catecholamine levels and normal 24-h urine values. Evaluation of these patients must be directed to obtaining plasma catecholamine during an episode or having the patient collect timed urine values (eg, 2–4 h) from the onset of an episode. (5) Suppression or stimulation tests are not recommended except in the rare instances when the diagnosis cannot be established by routine procedures.

1. Urinary measurements–Urine measurements are the traditional diagnostic procedure. Normal values are shown in Table 32–1, and recent series in patients with pheochromocytoma are summarized in Table 32–2. These data suggest that measurements of metanephrines or catecholamine are more useful than measurement of vanillylmandelic acid, since more than 80% of patients have values that were elevated more than 2 times. Simultaneous measurement of urine catecholamines and either metanephrines or vanillylmandelic acid yields elevated values in virtually all patients with pheochromocytoma, and if both values are greater than 2-fold elevated, pheochromocytoma is likely. False-positive elevations occur in as many as 10% of hypertensive patients; however, these are usually less than 50% above normal and are usually normal on repeat measurement. Patients with only episodic symptoms or episodic hypertension should be studied with shorter urine collections if 24-h studies are normal.

2. Plasma catecholamines–These values, when measured by specific methods, are elevated in most patients with pheochromocytoma; however, the frequency of false-positive values limits diagnostic utility. Thus, in patients with pheochromocytoma and sustained hypertension, 85% have plasma catecholamine values above 2000 ng/L. When patients with only paroxysmal hypertension are included, however, only 75% have values above 2000 ng/L. Values between 600 and 2000 ng/mL are commonly obtained in stressed or anxious patients without pheochromocytoma. This is especially true if samples are obtained by

Table 32–1. Catecholamines in urine and plasma.[a]

Urine
 Norepinephrine: 10–100 µg/24 h
 Epinephrine: Up to 20 µg/24 h
 Normetanephrine and metanephrine: < 1.5 mg/24 h
 Vanillylmandelic acid (VMA): 2–9 mg/24 h
Plasma
 Norepinephrine: 100–200 pg/mL
 Epinephrine: 30–50 pg/mL

[a]The values listed represent the means of the normal ranges, which vary for each laboratory.

Table 32–2. 24-h urine measurements in patients with pheochromocytoma.[a]

	Normal No. (%)	1–2X Elevated No. (%)	> 2X Elevated No. (%)
VMA (n = 384)	41 (11)	86 (22)	257 (67)
MN (n = 271)	12 (5)	33 (12)	226 (83)
UFC (n = 319)	14 (4)	30 (10)	275 (86)

[a]Reprinted with permission from Stein PP, Black HR: A simplified diagnostic approach to pheochromocytoma. Medicine 1991;70:46.

venipuncture without prior placement of an intravenous line with the patient supine for 30 min. Plasma catecholamine measurements do have a role, though, because markedly elevated levels during an episode may be diagnostic; conversely, the finding of normal values during episodes of severe hypertension essentially excludes the diagnosis.

Tumor Localization

Pheochromocytomas are intra-abdominal in 98% of cases, and 90% are intra-adrenal (10% are bilateral, especially in familial syndromes). Extra-adrenal pheochromocytomas are usually within the abdomen and are located along the sympathetic chain, the periaortic areas, and at the bifurcation of the aorta. The tumors may also arise from the bladder. Extra-abdominal pheochromocytomas occur in posterior mediastinum, rarely in the heart or pericardium and rarely in the neck. Tumors less than 2 cm in diameter are rare, and most are greater than 3 cm (Figure 32–10). Thus, the vast majority of pheochromocytomas are larger than the lower limits of resolution of current imaging techniques.

A. CT Scans: CT is currently the initial imaging procedure of choice; with current technology, it demonstrates virtually all intra-abdominal tumors and the majority of those that are extra-adrenal. Small tumors in the abdomen, pelvis, and chest may be obscured by surrounding structures. CT is not useful in determining whether an adrenal mass is in fact a pheochromocytoma (ie, if the adrenal mass is found coincidentally or the catechol determinations are equivocal, the adrenal mass could be a nonfunctioning adenoma). In this case, MRI or metaiodobenzylguanidine (MIBG) techniques may be useful.

B. MRI: The accuracy of detecting pheochromocytoma with MRI is as good as that obtained with CT, but the cost is greater at most institutions. MRI has the advantage of greater diagnostic specificity in that T2-weighted images or those obtained with gadolinium enhancement show greater signal intensity of the pheochromocytoma (compared with liver) than that obtained with adrenal adenomas. Limited data suggest that MRI may be superior to CT in localizing extra-adrenal tumors.

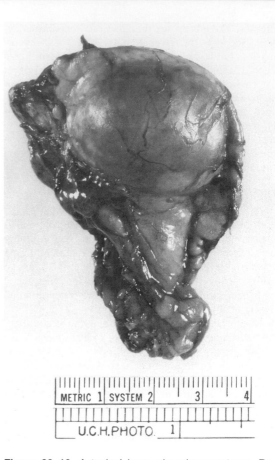

Figure 32–10. A typical large pheochromocytoma. Removal was followed by complete remission of hypertension.

C. MIBG Scanning: Radionuclide scanning with MIBG has assumed a prominent role in the localization of pheochromocytomas. The compound is taken up by pheochromocytomas, ganglioneuromas, neuroblastomas, and other neural crest tumors as well as some carcinoids. MIBG scans are positive in 85–90% of patients with pheochromocytomas, which limits their usefulness as a screening procedure. The procedure is extremely useful, however, since false-positive results are rare and a positive scan in the presence of elevated catechols is diagnostic. In addition, MIBG scans have great utility in the localization of (1) small lesions, (2) extra-adrenal lesions, (3) bilateral lesions, and (4) metastatic deposits in patients with malignant tumors.

Diagnostic Strategy

Patients in whom there is a high index of clinical suspicion and those who have greater than a 2-fold elevation of urine catechols should undergo an adrenal CT scan. If the CT scan reveals a unilateral tumor and the contralateral tumor adrenal is normal, the diagnosis is established. Patients with familial syndromes and those in whom cancer is suspected should undergo MIBG scanning to determine the extent of disease. If the adrenal CT is negative, MIBG scanning or MRI of the chest and abdomen is indicated to localize the tumor. This approach localizes virtually all tumors.

If the clinical suspicion is low and urine catechols are normal, imaging procedures are not indicated. However, it is not infrequent that patients at low risk on the basis of clinical manifestations have persisting mild elevations of catecholamines. In this situation, a single negative adrenal imaging procedure should suffice to terminate the evaluation, and the patient may be followed clinically and reevaluated if appropriate.

Therapy

A. Preoperative Management: Once the diagnosis of pheochromocytoma is established, the patient should be prepared for surgery to reduce the incidence of intraoperative complications and postoperative hypotension. The greatest experience is with the long-acting alpha-adrenergic blocker phenoxybenzamine, and its use has minimized surgical mortality and morbidity. The initial dosage is 10 mg twice daily, and patients may require hospitalization for bed rest and intravenous fluids to overcome the initially increased orthostatic hypotension that occurs in most patients. The dose may then be titrated upward every 2–3 days over several weeks until the blood pressure is less than 160/90 mm Hg and symptoms are abolished. Doses in the range of 100–200 mg/d are routinely used; however, no data are available that establish the superiority of these dosage levels. Higher doses of phenoxybenzamine are not associated with a higher risk of postoperative hypotension. Beta blockers are generally unnecessary unless tachycardia and arrhythmias are present, and these occur most frequently in the minority of patients with epinephrine hypersecretion.

Metyrosine (alpha-methylparatyrosine), an inhibitor of catecholamine synthesis, is also useful for preoperative management although current experience is limited. Initial dosage is 250 mg every 6 h, and total daily dosages of 2–4 g are required. Preoperative treatment for 1–2 weeks appears to be sufficient to prevent operative complications. Metyrosine can be used in conjunction with alpha blockers.

Successful preoperative management with prazosin, calcium channel blockers, and labetolol has been reported in a few cases.

B. Surgery: Surgery is the mainstay of therapy for pheochromocytoma; it requires adequate preoperative control of symptoms and hypertension with alpha blockers or metyrosine. Intraoperatively, hypertension is controlled with nitroprusside, and antiarrhythmics are used as needed. Adequate volume replacement is essential and in conjunction with preoperative medical therapy prevents postoperative hypotension.

If CT and MIBG show only a solitary adrenal lesion in patients with sporadic disease, a unilateral laparoscopic approach may be used. Bilateral or malignant disease requires a transabdominal approach, and even if total resection is not feasible, debulking of tumor mass facilitates subsequent medical management of catecholamine excess.

Malignant Pheochromocytoma

The incidence of cancer in pheochromocytoma has been traditionally estimated to be in the range of 10%, although recent series describe a higher incidence. Thus, all patients should undergo serial follow-up to detect early recurrences. Patients with known metastatic disease should undergo surgical debulking of accessible disease. Catecholamine excess can be controlled in most patients with alpha blockade, metyrosine, or both. Despite encouraging reports of chemotherapy or ^{131}I-MIBG therapy, it appears that only a minority of patients have sustained remissions.

Prognosis

In general, the prognosis is good. With better understanding of the disease, surgical deaths are now rare. Blood pressure falls to normal levels in most patients with benign tumors. Patients with cancer have persisting hypertension and require the multiple therapies described above.

NEUROBLASTOMA

Neuroblastomas (Figure 32–11) are of neural crest origin and may therefore develop from any portion of the sympathetic chain. Most arise in the retroperitoneum, and 45% involve the adrenal gland. The latter offer the poorest prognosis. In childhood, neuroblastoma is the third most common neoplastic disease after leukemia and brain tumors. Most are encountered in the first 2½ years of life, but a few are seen as late as the sixth decade, when they seem to be less aggressive. Mancini et al (1982) found 24 examples of more than one case of neuroblastoma in a family. In 5 cases, bilateral tumors were discovered in identical twins, which suggests the hereditary nature of the disease. Abnormalities of muscle and heart and hemihypertrophy have been observed in association with neuroblastoma.

Metastases spread through both the bloodstream and lymphatics. Common sites in children include the skull and long bones, regional lymph nodes, liver, and lungs. Local invasion is common. In infants, who enjoy the best prognosis, metastases are usually limited to the liver and subcutaneous fat.

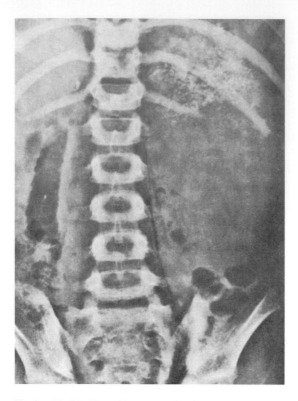

Figure 32–11. Neuroblastoma of adrenal gland. Plain film, child age 7 years, showing large mass occupying left flank. Punctate calcification in upper portion is typical of neuroblastoma.

The following staging of neuroblastoma is generally accepted:

Stage A: Tumors confined to the stricture of origin.

Stage B: Tumors extending in continuity beyond the organ but not crossing the midline. Ipsilateral lymph nodes may be involved.

Stage C: Tumors extending in continuity beyond the midline. Regional lymph nodes may be involved.

Stage D: Remote disease involving skeletal organs, soft tissues, and distant lymph node groups.

Stage E: Stage A or B tumors locally but with distant metastases.

Clinical Findings

A. Symptoms: An abdominal mass is usually noted by parents, the physician, or the patient. About 70% of patients have metastases when first seen. Symptoms relating to metastases include fever, malaise, bone pain, failure to thrive, and constipation or diarrhea.

B. Signs: A flank mass is usually palpable and may even be visible; it often extends across the midline. The tumor is usually nodular and fixed, since it tends to be locally invasive. Evidence of metastases may be noted: ocular proptosis from metastases to the skull, enlarged nodular liver, or a mass in bone. Hypertension is often found.

C. Laboratory Findings: Anemia is common. Urinalysis and renal function are normal. Because 70% of neuroblastomas elaborate increased levels of norepinephrine and epinephrine, urinary vanillylmandelic acid and homovanillic acid levels should be measured. Serial estimations of these substances during definitive treatment can be used as tumor markers. A return to normal levels is encouraging, while rising levels imply residual or progressive tumor. Bone marrow aspiration may reveal tumor cells.

D. X-Ray Findings: Plain radiographs may show a mass and displacement of the kidneys or other organs. CT scans are used to define tumor size, vascular invasion (eg, of the vena cava), local tumor spread, and distant metastases. Further evaluation includes CT of the chest to determine whether lung metastases are present and a bone scan to define skeletal metastases. Many of these tumors take up ^{131}I-MIBG; thus this test can be used for staging.

Differential Diagnosis

Nephroblastoma (Wilms tumor) is also a disease of childhood. Intravenous urograms show the caliceal distortion characteristic of an intrinsic renal tumor; no such distortion is shown in neuroblastoma, which merely displaces the kidney. Urinary catecholamines are normal with Wilms tumor but are usually elevated in neuroblastoma. Urinary lactic dehydrogenase may be increased with Wilms tumor but is normal with neuroblastoma. Sonography and CT are useful in characterizing the lesion and demonstrating its renal origin.

Hydronephrosis may also occur as a flank mass but is ordinarily neither hard nor nodular. Evidence of urinary infection is common. Hydronephrosis is often bilateral, in which case renal function is depressed.

Polycystic renal disease usually presents with palpable masses in both flanks. Renal function is impaired, and imaging studies establish the diagnosis.

Neonatal adrenal hemorrhage may be confused with neuroblastoma. These infants have a palpable upper quadrant mass, are apt to be jaundiced, and have increased serum bilirubin and a low hematocrit. CT is very useful in demonstrating the cystic nature of the lesion. Neuroblastomas cause the excretion of large amounts of catecholamines (eg, vanillylmandelic acid).

Treatment

Surgical excision of a tumor should be followed by radiotherapy to the tumor bed. If the tumor is very large or is deemed unresectable, preoperative x-ray therapy should be given, followed by surgical excision. In disseminated disease, chemotherapy must be given. Useful drugs include cyclophosphamide (Cytoxan), vincristine (Oncovin), and dacarbazine.

Prognosis

About 90% of patients who die of the disease do so within 14 months following initiation of treatment. Infants have the best prognosis; their 2-year survival rate approaches 60%, and if the tumor is confined to the primary site with or without adjacent regional spread, the cure rate is about 80%. Less than 10% of children age 2 or older are cured. When the disease is disseminated, few cures are obtained.

In a few infants, spontaneous maturation of neuroblastoma to ganglioneuroma has been observed. It is thought by some that x-ray treatment and chemotherapy can also accomplish this.

Serial estimation of urinary catecholamines following therapy usually indicates the presence of residual tumor.

REFERENCES

GENERAL

Doppman JL et al: Differentiation of adrenal masses by magnetic resonance imaging. Surgery 1987;102:1018.

Findling JW, Aron DC, Tyrrell JB: Glucocorticoids and adrenal androgens. In: Greenspan FS, Strewfer GJ (editors): *Basic and Clinical Endocrinology,* 5th ed. Appleton and Lange, 1997.

James VHT (editor): *The Adrenal Gland,* 2nd ed. Raven Press, 1992.

Miller WL, Tyrrell JB: The adrenal cortex. In: Felig P et al (editors): *Endocrinology and Metabolism,* 3rd ed. McGraw-Hill, 1995.

Orth DN, Kovacs WJ: The adrenal cortex. In: Wilson JD et al (editors): *Williams Textbook of Endocrinology,* 9th ed. Saunders, 1998.

Ross NS, Aron DC: Hormonal evaluation of the patient with an incidentally discovered adrenal mass. N Engl J Med 1990;323:1401.

Smith CD, Weber CJ, Amerson JR: Laparoscopic adrenalectomy: New gold standard. World J Surg 1999;23:389.

Winfield HN et al: Laparoscopic adrenalectomy: The preferred choice? A comparision to open adrenalectomy. J Urol 1998;160:325.

CUSHING SYNDROME & ADRENOCORTICAL TUMORS

Aron DC, Findling JW, Tyrrell JB: Cushing's disease. Endocrinol Metab Clin North Am 1987;16:705.

Atkinson AB: The treatment of Cushing's syndrome. Clin Endocrinol 1991;34:507.

Benecke R et al: Plasma level monitoring of mitotane (*o,p'*-DDD) and its metabolite (*o,p'*-DDE) during long-term treatment of Cushing's disease with low doses. Eur J Clin Pharmacol 1991;41:259.

Bloom LS, Libertino JA: Surgical management of Cushing's syndrome. Urol Clin North Am 1989;16:547.

Brennan MF: Adrenocortical carcinoma. CA Cancer J Clin 1987;37:348.

Crapo L: Cushing's syndrome: A review of diagnostic tests. Metabolism 1979;28:955.

Decker RA et al: Eastern Cooperative Oncology Group Study 1879: Mitotane and Adriamycin in patients with advanced adrenocortical carcinoma. Surgery 1991;110:1006.

Doherty GM et al: Time to recovery of the hypothal-
amic-pituitary-adrenal axis after curative resection of adrenal tumors in patients with Cushing's syndrome. Surgery 1990;108:1085.

Dwyer AJ et al: Pituitary adenomas in patients with Cushing's disease: Initial experience with Gd-DTPA-enhanced MR imaging. Radiology 1987;163:421.

Findling JW, Tyrrell JB: Occult ectopic secretion of corticotropin. Arch Intern Med 1986;146:929.

Flack MR et al: Urine free cortisol in the high-dose dexamethasone suppression test for the differential diagnosis of the Cushing syndrome. Ann Intern Med 1992;116:211.

Grus JR, Nelson DH: ACTH-producing pituitary tumors. Endocrinol Metab Clin North Am 1991;20:319.

Hamper UM et al: Primary adrenocortical carcinoma: Sonographic evaluation with clinical and pathologic correlation in 26 patients. Am J Roentgenol 1987; 148:915.

Howlett TA et al: Megavoltage pituitary irradiation in the management of Cushing's disease and Nelson's syndrome: Long-term follow-up. Clin Endocrinol 1989; 31:309.

Hutter AM, Kayhoe DE: Adrenal cortical carcinoma: Clinical features of 138 patients. Am J Med 1966;41:572.

Jex RK et al: Ectopic ACTH syndrome: Diagnostic and therapeutic aspects. Am J Surg 1985;149:276.

Jones KL: The Cushing syndromes. Pediatr Clin North Am 1990;37:1313.

Kaye TB, Crapo L: The Cushing's syndrome: An update on diagnostic tests. Ann Intern Med 1990;112:434.

Luton J-P et al: Clinical features of adrenocortical carcinoma, prognostic factors, and the effect of mitotane therapy. N Engl J Med 1990;322:1195.

Mampalam TJ, Tyrrell JB, Wilson CB: Transsphenoidal microsurgery for Cushing's disease. Ann Intern Med 1988;109:487.

Oldfield EH et al: Petrosal sinus sampling with and without corticotropin-releasing hormone for the differential diagnosis of Cushing's syndrome. N Engl J Med 1991;325:897.

Pojunas KW et al: Pituitary and adrenal CT of Cushing's syndrome. Am J Roentgenol 1986;146:1235.

Sheeler LR: Cushing's syndrome. Urol Clin North Am 1989;16:447.

Sonino N et al: Prolonged treatment of Cushing's disease by ketoconazole. J Clin Endocrinol Metab 1985; 61:718.

Styne DM et al: Treatment of Cushing's disease in childhood and adolescence by transsphenoidal microadenomectomy. N Engl J Med 1984;B310:889.

Tabarin A et al: Use of ketoconazole in the treatment of Cushing's disease and ectopic ACTH syndrome. Clin Endocrinol 1991;34:63.

Trainer PJ, Grossman A: The diagnosis and differential diagnosis of Cushing's syndrome. Clin Endocrinol 1991;34:317.

Tyrrell JB et al: An overnight high-dose dexamethasone suppression test: Rapid differential diagnosis of Cushing's syndrome. Ann Intern Med 1986;104:180.

Watson RGK et al: Results of adrenal surgery for Cushing's syndrome: 10 years' experience. World J Surg 1986;10:531.

Zeiger MA et al: Primary bilateral adrenocortical causes of Cushing's syndrome. Surgery 1991;110:1106.

ADRENAL ANDROGENIC SYNDROMES

Cumming DC et al: Treatment of hirsutism with spironolactone. JAMA 1982;247:1295.

Ehrmann DA, Rosenfield RL: Hirsutism: Beyond the steroidogenic block. N Engl J Med 1990;323:909.

Killeen AA et al: Prevalence of nonclassical congenital adrenal hyperplasia among women self-referred for electrolytic treatment of hirsutism. Am J Med Genet 1992;42:197.

Longcope C: Adrenal and gonadal androgen secretion in normal females. Clin Endocrinol Metab 1986;15:213.

Marshburn PB, Carr BR: Hirsutism and virilization. A systematic approach to benign and potentially serious causes. Postgrad Med 1995;97:99.

Masiakos PT, Flynn CE, Donahoe PK: Masculinizing and feminizing syndromes caused by functioning tumors. Semin Pediatr Surg 1997;6:147.

McKenna TJ: Pathogenesis and treatment of polycystic ovary syndrome. N Engl J Med 1988;318:558.

Mendonca BB et al: Clinical, hormonal and pathological findings in a comparative study of adrenocortical neoplasms in childhood and adulthood. J Urol 1995;154:2004.

Miller WL: Genetics, diagnosis, and management of 21-hydroxylase deficiency. J Clin Endocrinol Metab 1994;78:241.

Miller WL: Congenital adrenal hyperplasias. Endocrinol Metab Clin North Am 1991;20:721.

Moltz L, Schwartz U: Gonadal and adrenal androgen secretion in hirsute females. Clin Endocrinol Metab 1986;15:229.

Sciarra F, Tosti-Croce C, Toscano V: Androgen-secreting adrenal tumors. Minerva Endocrinologica 1995;20:63.

Siegel SF et al: ACTH stimulation tests and plasma dehydroepiandrosterone sulfate levels in women with hirsutism. N Engl J Med 1990;323:849.

HYPERALDOSTERONISM

Baxter JD et al: The endocrinology of hypertension. In: Felig P et al (editors): *Endocrinology and Metabolism,* 3rd ed. McGraw-Hill, 1995.

Biglieri EG: The spectrum of mineralocorticoid hypertension. Hypertension 1991;18:251.

Dye NV et al: Unilateral adrenal hyperplasia as a cause of primary aldosteronism. South Med J 1989;82:82.

Ganguly A: Primary aldosteronism. N Engl J Med 1998; 339:1828.

Gomez-Sanchez CE: Primary aldosteronism and its variants. Cardiovasc Res 1998;37:8.

Gordon RD: Primary aldosteronism. J Endocrinol Invest 1995;18:495.

Gordon RD et al: High incidence of primary aldosteronism in 199 patients referred with hypertension. Clin Exp Pharmacol Physiol 1994;21:315.

Ikeda DM et al: The detection of adrenal tumors and hyperplasia in patients with primary aldosteronism: Comparison of scintigraphy, CT, and MR imaging. Am J Roentgenol 1989;153:301.

Irony I et al: Correctable subsets of primary aldosteronism: Primary adrenal hyperplasia and renin responsive adenoma. Am J Hypertens 1990;3:576.

Kater CE et al: Stimulation and suppression of the mineralocorticoid hormones in normal subjects and adrenocortical disorders. Endocr Rev 1989;11:149.

Schalekamp MA, Wenting GJ, Man in't Veld AJ: Pathogenesis of mineralocorticoid hypertension. Clin Endocrinol Metab 1981;10:397.

Siren J et al: Laparoscopic adrenalectomy for primary aldosteronism. Surg Laparosc Endosc 1999;9:9.

Vallotton MB: Primary aldosteronism. Part I. Diagnosis of primary hyperaldosteronism. Clin Endocinol 1996; 45:47.

Vallotton MB: Primary aldosteronism. Part II. Differential diagnosis of primary hyperaldosteronism and pseudoaldosteronism. Clin Endocrinol 1996;45:53.

Young WF Jr et al: Primary aldosteronism: Adrenal venous sampling. Surgery 1996;120:913.

Young WF Jr, Hogana MJ: Renin-independent hypermineralocorticoidism. Trends Endocrinol Metab 1994;5: 97.

PHEOCHROMOCYTOMAS & RELATED TUMORS

Averbuch SD et al: Malignant pheochromocytoma: Effective treatment with a combination of cyclophosphamide, vincristine, and dacabazine. Ann Intern Med 1988;109:267.

Bouloux PMG, Fakeeh M: Investigation of phaeochromocytoma. Clin Endocrinol 1995;43:657.

Bravo EL: Plasma or urinary metanephrines for the diagnosis of pheochromocytoma? That is the question. Ann Intern Med 1996;125:331.

Bravo EL: Pheochromocytoma: New concepts and future trends. Kidney Int 1991;40:544.

Caty MG et al: Current diagnosis and treatment of pheochromocytoma in children: Experience with 22 consecutive tumors in 14 patients. Arch Surg 1990; 125:978.

Chevinsky AH, Minton JP, Falko JM: Metastatic pheochromocytoma associated with multiple endocrine neoplasia syndrome type II. Arch Surg 1990; 125:935.

Francis IR, Korobkin M: Pheochromocytoma. Radiol Clin North Am 1996;34:1101.

Golub MS, Tuck ML: Diagnostic and therapeutic strategies in pheochromocytoma. The Endocrinologist 1992;2:101.

Heron et al: The urinary metanephrine-to-creatinine ratio for the diagnosis of pheochromocytoma. Ann Intern Med 1996;125:300.

Hoefnagel CA et al: Radionuclide diagnosis and therapy of neural crest tumors using iodine-131 metaiodobenzylguanidine. J Nucl Med 1987;28:308.

Joris JL et al: Hemodynamic changes and catecholamine release during laparoscopic adrenalectomy for pheochromocytoma. Anesth Analg 1999;88:16.

Kebebew E, Duk Q-Y: Benign and malignant pheochromocytoma. Diagnosis, treatment and follow-up. Surg Oncol Clin North Am 1998;7:765.

Lenders JWM et al: Plasma metanephrines in the diagnosis of pheochromocytoma. Ann Intern Med 1995; 123:101.

Loh K-C et al: The treatment of malignant pheochromocytoma with iodine-131 metaiodobenzylguanidine (^{131}1-MIBG): A comprehensive review of 116 reported patients. J Endocrinol Invest 1997;20:648.

Malone MJ et al: Preoperative and surgical management of pheochromocytoma. Urol Clin North Am 1989;16: 567.

Peaston RT, Lennard TWJ, Lai LC: Overnight excretion of urinary catecholamines and metabolites in the detection of pheochromocytoma. J Clin Endocrinol Metab 1996;81:1379.

Perry RR et al: Surgical management of pheochromocytoma with the use of metyrosine. Ann Surg 1990; 212:621.

Plunin P: Recent advances in pheochromocytoma diagnosis and imaging. Adv Nephrol 1988;17:275.

Proye C et al: High incidence of malignant pheochromocytoma in a surgical unit. 26 cases out of 100 patients operated from 1971 to 1991. J Endocrinol Invest 1992;15:651.

Shapiro B et al: Iodine-131 metaiodobenzylguanidine for the locating of suspected pheochromocytoma. Endocrinol Metab Clin North Am 1989;18:443.

Sheps SG, Jiang N-S, Klee GG: Diagnostic evaluation of pheochromocytoma. Endocrinol Metab Clin North Am 1988;17:397.

Sheps SG et al: Recent developments in the diagnosis and treatment of pheochromocytoma. Mayo Clin Proc 1990;65:88.

Stein PP, Black HR: A simplified diagnostic approach to pheochromocytoma: A review of the literature and report of one institution's experience. Medicine 1991; 70:46.

Swensen T et al: Use of ^{131}I-MIBG scintigraphy in the evaluation of suspected pheochromocytoma. Mayo Clin Proc 1985;60:299.

Whalen RK, Althausen AF, Daniels GH: Extra-adrenal pheochromocytoma. J Urol 1992;147:1.

Young WF: Pheochromocytoma: 1926–1993. Trends Endocrinol Metab 1993;4:122.

NEUROBLASTOMA

Evans AE, D'Angio GJ, Randolph J: A proposed staging for children with neuroblastoma. Cancer 1979;27:374.

Evans AE et al: Prognostic factors in neuroblastoma. Cancer 1987;59:1853.

Evans AE et al: A review of 17 IV-S neuroblastoma patients at the Children's Hospital of Philadelphia. Cancer 1980;45:833.

Forman HP et al: Congenital neuroblastoma: Evaluation with multimodality imaging. Radiology 1990;175:365.

Hann H-WL et al: Biologic differences between neuroblastoma stages IV-S and IV: Measurement of serum ferritin and E-rosette inhibition in 30 children. N Engl J Med 1981;305:425.

Kushner BH, Cheung NK: Neuroblastoma. Pediatr Ann 1988;17:269.

Lopez R, Karakousis C, Rao U: Treatment of adult neuroblastoma. Cancer 1980;45:840.

Mancini AF et al: Neuroblastoma in a pair of identical twins. Med Pediatr Oncol 1982;10:45.

Reynolds CP et al: Catecholamine fluorescence and tissue culture morphology: Technics in the diagnosis of neuroblastoma. Am J Clin Pathol 1981;75:275.

Rogers LE, Lyon GM Jr, Porter FS: Spot test for vanillylmandelic acid and other guaiacols in urine of patients with neuroblastoma. Am J Clin Pathol 1972;58:383.

Smith EI, Castleberry RP: Neuroblastoma. Curr Prob Surg 1990;27:573.

CONGENITAL ANOMALIES OF THE KIDNEYS

Congenital anomalies occur more frequently in the kidney than in any other organ. Some cause no difficulty, but many (eg, hypoplasia, polycystic kidneys) cause impairment of renal function. It has been noted that children with a gross deformity of an external ear associated with ipsilateral maldevelopment of the facial bones are apt to have a congenital abnormality of the kidney (eg, ectopy, hypoplasia) on the same side as the visible deformity. Lateral displacement of the nipples has been observed in association with bilateral renal hypoplasia.

A significant incidence of renal agenesis, ectopy, malrotation, and duplication has been observed in association with congenital scoliosis and kyphosis. Unilateral agenesis, hypoplasia, and dysplasia are often seen in association with supralevator imperforate anus.

For a better understanding of these congenital abnormalities, see the discussion of the embryology and development of the kidney in Chapter 2.

AGENESIS

Bilateral renal agenesis is extremely rare; no more than 400 cases have been reported. The children do not survive. The condition does not appear to have any predisposing factors. Prenatal suspicion of the anomaly exists when oligohydramnios is present on fetal ultrasound examination. Pulmonary hypoplasia and facial deformities (Potter facies) are usually present. Abdominal ultrasound examination usually establishes the diagnosis.

One kidney may be absent. In some cases, this may be because the ureteral bud (from the wolffian duct) failed to develop or, if it did develop, did not reach the metanephros (adult kidney). Without a drainage system, the metanephric mass undergoes atrophy. The ureter is absent on the side of the unformed kidney in 50% of cases, although a blind ureteral duct may be found. (See Chapter 2.)

Renal agenesis causes no symptoms; it is usually found by accident on abdominal or renal imaging. It is not an easy diagnosis to establish even though on inspection of the bladder the ureteral ridge is absent and no orifice is visualized, for the kidney could be present but be drained by a ureter whose opening is ectopic (into the urethra, seminal vesicle, or vagina). If definitive diagnosis seems essential, midstream angiography, renal venography, isotope studies, ultrasonography, and computed tomography (CT) should establish the diagnosis.

There appears to be an increased incidence of infection, hydronephrosis, and stones in the contralateral organ. Other congenital anomalies associated with this defect include cardiac, vertebral column, and anal anomalies as well as anomalies of the long bones, hands, and genitalia.

HYPOPLASIA

Hypoplasia implies a small kidney. The total renal mass may be divided in an unequal manner, in which case one kidney is small and the other correspondingly larger than normal. Some of these congenitally small kidneys prove, on pathologic examination, to be dysplastic. Unilateral or bilateral hypoplasia has been observed in infants suffering from fetal alcohol syndrome, and renal anomalies have been reported in infants with in utero cocaine exposure (Rosenstein, Wheeler, and Heid, 1990).

Differentiation from acquired atrophy is difficult. Atrophic pyelonephritis usually reveals typical distortion of the calyces. Vesicoureteral reflux in infants may cause a dwarfed kidney even in the absence of infection. Stenosis of the renal artery leads to shrinkage of the kidney.

Such kidneys have small renal arteries and branches and are associated with hypertension, which is relieved by nephrectomy. Selective renal venography is helpful in differentiating between a congenitally absent kidney and one that is small and nonvisualized. A major side effect of the administration of cisplatin is shrinkage of the kidneys as revealed by serial radioisotope scans.

SUPERNUMERARY KIDNEYS

The presence of a third kidney is very rare; the presence of 4 separate kidneys in one individual has been reported only once. The anomaly must not be confused with duplication (or triplication) of the renal pelvis in one kidney, which is not uncommon (N'Guessan and Stephens, 1983).

DYSPLASIA & MULTICYSTIC KIDNEY

Renal dysplasia has protean manifestations. Multicystic kidney of the newborn is usually unilateral, nonhereditary, and characterized by an irregularly lobulated mass of cysts; the ureter is usually absent or atretic. It may develop because of faulty union of the nephron and the collecting system. At most, only a few embryonic glomeruli and tubules are observed. The only finding is the discovery of an irregular mass in the flank. Nothing is shown on urography, but in an occasional case, some radiopaque fluid may be noted. If the cystic kidney is large, its mate is usually normal. However, when the cystic organ is small, the contralateral kidney is apt to be abnormal. The cystic nature of the lesion may be revealed by sonography, and the diagnosis can be established in utero. If the physician feels that the proper diagnosis has been made, no treatment is necessary. If there is doubt about the diagnosis, nephrectomy is considered the procedure of choice. Dimmick et al (1989) noted neoplastic changes in multicystic renal dysplasia.

Multicystic kidney is often associated with contralateral renal and ureteral abnormalities. Contralateral ureteropelvic junction obstruction is one of the common problems noted. Diagnostic evaluation of both kidneys is required to establish the overall status of anomalous development.

Dysplasia of the renal parenchyma is also seen in association with ureteral obstruction or reflux that was probably present early in pregnancy. It is relatively common as a segmental renal lesion involving the upper pole of a duplicated kidney whose ureter is obstructed by a congenital ureterocele. It may also be found in urinary tracts severely obstructed by posterior urethral valves; in this instance, the lesion may be bilateral.

Microscopically, the renal parenchyma is "disorganized." Tubular and glomerular cysts may be noted; these elements are fetal in type. Islands of metaplastic cartilage are often seen. The common denominator seems to be fetal obstruction.

ADULT POLYCYSTIC KIDNEY DISEASE (See also p 600.)

Adult polycystic kidney disease is an autosomal dominant hereditary condition and almost always bilateral (95% of cases). The disease encountered in infants is different from that seen in adults, although the literature reports a small number of infants with the adult type. The former is an autosomal recessive disease in which life expectancy is short, whereas that diagnosed in adulthood is autosomal dominant; symptoms ordinarily do not appear until after age 40. Cysts of the liver, spleen, and pancreas may be noted in association with both forms. The kidneys are larger than normal and are studded with cysts of various sizes.

Etiology & Pathogenesis

The evidence suggests that the cysts occur because of defects in the development of the collecting and uriniferous tubules and in the mechanism of their joining. Blind secretory tubules that are connected to functioning glomeruli become cystic. As the cysts enlarge, they compress adjacent parenchyma, destroy it by ischemia, and occlude normal tubules. The result is progressive functional impairment.

Pathology

Grossly, the kidneys are usually much enlarged. Their surfaces are studded with cysts of various sizes (Figure 33–1). On section, the cysts are found to be scattered throughout the parenchyma. Calcification is rare. The fluid in the cyst is usually amber-colored but may be hemorrhagic.

Microscopically, the lining of the cysts consists of a single layer of cells. The renal parenchyma may show peritubular fibrosis and evidence of secondary infection. There appears to be a reduction in the number of glomeruli, some of which may be hyalinized. Renal arteriolar thickening is a prominent finding in adults.

Clinical Findings

A. Symptoms: Pain over one or both kidneys may occur because of the drag on the vascular pedicles by the heavy kidneys, from obstruction or infection, or from hemorrhage into a cyst. Gross or microscopic total hematuria is not uncommon and may be severe; the cause for this is not clear. Colic may occur if blood clots or stones are passed. The patient may notice an abdominal mass.

Infection (chills, fever, renal pain) commonly complicates polycystic disease. Symptoms of vesical irritability may be the first complaint. When renal in-

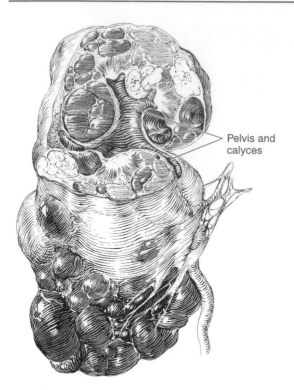

Pelvis and calyces

Figure 33–1. Polycystic kidney. Multiple cysts deep in the parenchyma and on the surface. Note distortion of the calyces by the cysts.

sufficiency ensues, headache, nausea and vomiting, weakness, and loss of weight occur.

B. Signs: One or both kidneys are usually palpable. They may feel nodular. If infected, they may be tender. Hypertension is found in 60–70% of these patients. Evidence of cardiac enlargement is then noted.

Fever may be present if pyelonephritis exists or if cysts have become infected. In the stage of uremia, anemia and loss of weight may be evident. Ophthalmoscopic examination may show changes typical of moderate or severe hypertension.

C. Laboratory Findings: Anemia may be noted, caused either by chronic loss of blood or, more commonly, by the hematopoietic depression accompanying uremia. Proteinuria and microscopic (if not gross) hematuria are the rule. Pyuria and bacteriuria are common.

Progressive loss of concentrating power occurs. Renal clearance tests show varying degrees of renal impairment. About a third of patients with polycystic kidney disease are uremic when first seen.

D. X-Ray Findings: Both renal shadows are usually enlarged on a plain film of the abdomen, even as much as 5 times normal size. Kidneys more than 16 cm in length are suspect.

Excretory infusion urograms with tomography are helpful to establish the diagnosis. Tomography re-

veals multiple lucencies representing cysts. On tomograms or on retrograde urograms, the renal masses are usually enlarged and the caliceal pattern is quite bizarre (spider deformity). The calyces are broadened and flattened, enlarged, and often curved, as they tend to hug the periphery of adjacent cysts (Figure 33–2). Often the changes are only slight or may even be absent on one side, leading to the erroneous diagnosis of tumor of the other kidney.

If cysts are infected, perinephritis may obscure the renal and even the psoas shadows.

Angiography reveals bending of small vessels around the cysts and the "negative" shadows (nonvascular) of the cysts (Figure 33–2).

E. CT Scanning: CT is an excellent noninvasive technique used to establish the diagnosis of polycystic disease. The multiple thin-walled cysts filled with fluid and the large renal size make this imaging method extremely accurate (95%) for diagnosis.

F. Isotope Studies: Photoscans (see Chapter 10) reveal multiple "cold" avascular spots in large renal shadows.

G. Ultrasonography: Sonography appears to be superior to both excretory urography and isotope scanning in diagnosis of polycystic disorders.

H. Instrumental Examination: Cystoscopy may show evidence of cystitis, in which case the urine will contain abnormal elements. Bleeding from a ureteral orifice may be noted. Ureteral catheterization and retrograde urograms are rarely indicated.

Differential Diagnosis

Bilateral hydronephrosis (on the basis of congenital or acquired ureteral obstruction) may present bilateral flank masses and signs of impairment of renal function, but urography and ultrasonography show changes quite different from those of the polycystic kidney.

Bilateral renal tumor is rare but may mimic polycystic kidney disease perfectly on urography. Differentiation of a unilateral tumor may be quite difficult if one of the polycystic kidneys shows little or no distortion on urography. However, tumors are usually localized to one portion of the kidney, whereas cysts are quite diffusely distributed. The total renal function should be normal with unilateral tumor but is usually depressed in patients with polycystic kidney disease. Computed tomography or renal angiography may be needed at times to differentiate between the two conditions (Figure 33–2). Photoscans or sonograms may also prove helpful in differentiation.

In **von Hippel-Lindau disease** (angiomatous cerebellar cyst, angiomatosis of the retina, and tumors or cysts of the pancreas), multiple bilateral cysts or adenocarcinomas of both kidneys may develop. Urograms or nephrotomograms may suggest polycystic kidney disease. The presence of other stigmas should

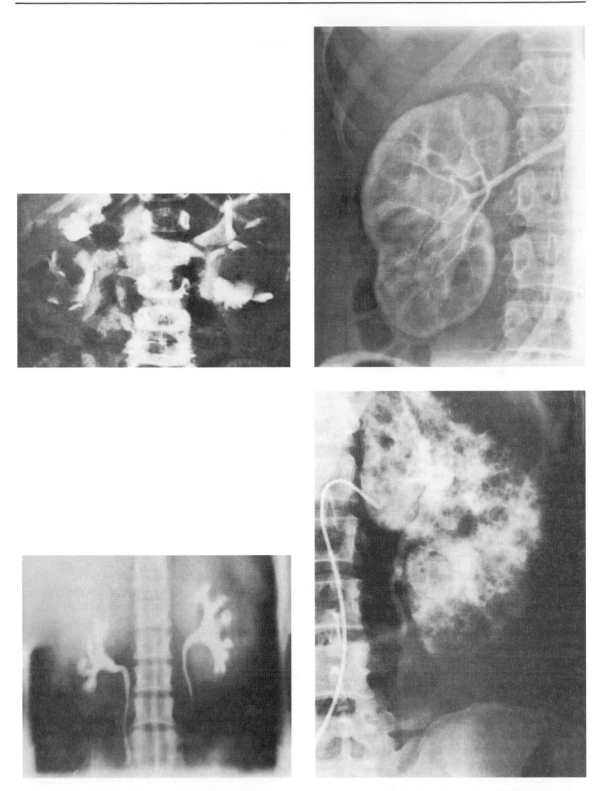

Figure 33–2. Polycystic kidneys. **Upper left:** Excretory urogram in a child, showing elongation, broadening, and bending of the calyces around cysts. Good renal function. **Upper right:** Angiogram of right kidney, showing "negative" shadows of cysts. **Lower left:** Angionephrotomogram showing kidneys of essentially normal size. All infundibula on left and infundibulum of right upper calyx are widened, suggesting polycystic kidneys. **Lower right:** Nephrogram phase of left selective angiogram (same patient) showing multiple small negative shadows representing the cysts.

make the diagnosis. CT, angiography, sonography, or scintiphotography should be definitive.

Tuberous sclerosis (convulsive seizures, mental retardation, and adenoma sebaceum) is typified by hamartomatous tumors often involving the skin, brain, retinas, bones, liver, heart, and kidneys (see Chapter 22). The renal lesions are usually multiple and bilateral and microscopically are angiomyolipomas. Urograms obtained during the stage of uremia are apt to suggest polycystic disease; the presence of other stigmas and use of CT or sonography should make the differentiation.

A **simple cyst** (see section following) is usually unilateral and single; total renal function should be normal. Urograms usually show a single lesion (Figure 33–3), whereas polycystic kidney disease is bilateral and has multiple filling defects.

Complications

For reasons that are not clear, pyelonephritis is a common complication of polycystic kidney disease. It may be asymptomatic; pus cells in the urine may be few or absent. Stained smears or quantitative cultures make the diagnosis. A gallium-67 citrate scan will definitely reveal the sites of infection, including abscess.

Infection of cysts is associated with pain and tenderness over the kidney and a febrile response. The differential diagnosis between infection of cysts and pyelonephritis may be difficult, but here again a gallium scan will prove helpful.

In rare instances, gross hematuria may be so brisk and persistent as to endanger life.

Treatment

Except for unusual complications, the treatment is conservative and supportive.

A. General Measures: The patient should be placed on a low-protein diet (0.5–0.75 g/kg/d of protein) and fluids forced to 3000 mL or more per day. Physical activity may be permitted within reason, but strenuous exercise is contraindicated. When the patient is in the state of absolute renal insufficiency, one should treat as for uremia from any cause. Hypertension should be controlled. Hemodialysis may be indicated.

B. Surgery: There is no evidence that excision or decompression of cysts improves renal function. If a large cyst is found to be compressing the upper ureter, causing obstruction and further embarrassing renal function, it should be resected or aspirated. When the degree of renal insufficiency becomes life-threatening, chronic dialysis or renal transplantation should be considered.

C. Treatment of Complications: Pyelonephritis must be rigorously treated to prevent further renal damage. Infection of cysts requires surgical drainage. If bleeding from one kidney is so severe that exsanguination is possible, nephrectomy or embolization

of the renal or, preferably, the segmental artery must be considered as a lifesaving measure.

Concomitant diseases (eg, tumor, obstructing stone) may require definitive surgical treatment.

Prognosis

When the disease affects children, it has a very poor prognosis. The large group presenting clinical signs and symptoms after age 35–40 has a somewhat more favorable prognosis. Although there is wide variation, these patients usually do not live longer than 5 or 10 years after the diagnosis is made unless dialysis is made available or renal transplantation is done.

SIMPLE (SOLITARY) CYST

Simple cyst (Figures 33–3 and 33–4) of the kidney is usually unilateral and single but may be multiple and multilocular and, more rarely, bilateral. It differs from polycystic kidneys both clinically and pathologically.

Etiology & Pathogenesis

Whether simple cyst is congenital or acquired is not clear. Its origin may be similar to that of polycystic kidneys, ie, the difference may be merely one of degree. On the other hand, simple cysts have been produced in animals by causing tubular obstruction and local ischemia; this suggests that the lesion can be acquired.

As a simple cyst grows, it compresses and thereby may destroy renal parenchyma, but rarely does it destroy so much renal tissue that renal function is impaired. A solitary cyst may be placed in such a position as to compress the ureter, causing progressive hydronephrosis. Infection may complicate the picture.

Feiner, Katz, and Gallo (1981) have noticed that acquired cystic disease of the kidney is commonly observed as an effect of chronic dialysis. The spontaneous regression of cysts has occasionally been noted.

Pathology

Simple cysts usually involve the lower pole of the kidney. Those that produce symptoms average about 10 cm in diameter, but a few are large enough to fill the entire flank. They usually contain a clear amber fluid. Their walls are quite thin, and the cysts are "blue-domed" in appearance. Calcification of the sac is occasionally seen. About 5% contain hemorrhagic fluid, and possibly one-half of these have papillary cancers on their walls.

Simple cysts are usually superficial but may be deeply situated. When a cyst is situated deep in the kidney, the cyst wall is adjacent to the epithelial lining of the pelvis or calyces, from which it may be

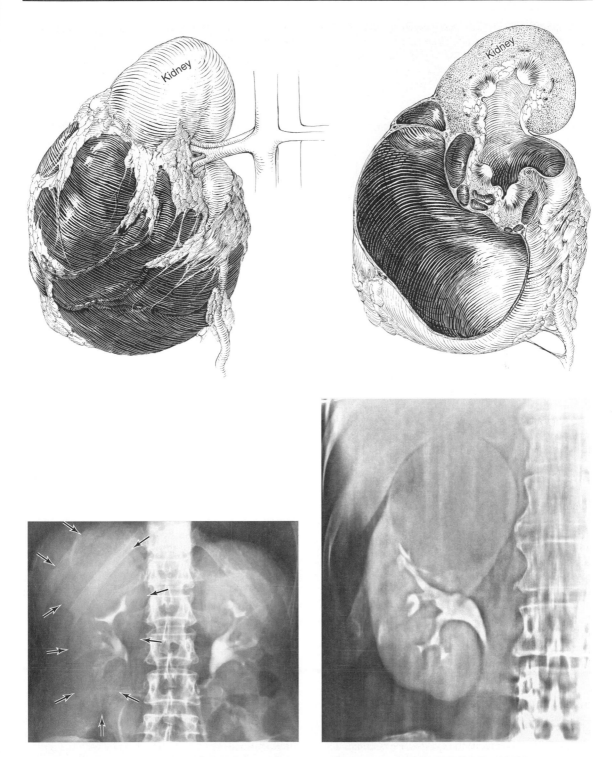

Figure 33–3. Simple cyst. **Upper left:** Large cyst displacing lower pole laterally. **Upper right:** Section of kidney showing one large and a few small cysts. **Lower left:** Excretory urogram showing soft-tissue mass in upper pole of right kidney. Elongation and distortion of upper calyces by cyst. **Lower right:** Infusion nephrotomogram showing large cyst in upper renal pole distorting upper calyces and dislocating upper portion of kidney laterally.

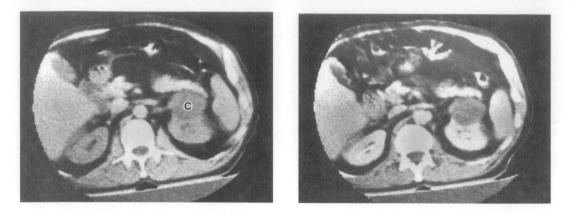

Figure 33–4. Left renal cyst. **Left:** Computed tomography (CT) scan shows a homogeneous low-density mass (C) arising from anterior border of left kidney just posterior to tail of the pancreas. The CT attenuation value was similar to that of water, indicating a simple renal cyst. **Right:** After intravenous injection of contrast material, the mass did not increase in attenuation value, adding further confirmatory evidence of its benign cystic nature.

separated only with great difficulty. Cysts do not communicate with the renal pelvis (Figure 33–3). Microscopic examination of the cyst wall shows heavy fibrosis and hyalinization; areas of calcification may be seen. The adjacent renal tissue is compressed and fibrosed. A number of cases of simple cysts have been reported in children. However, large cysts are rare in children; the presence of cancer must therefore be ruled out.

Multilocular renal cysts may be confused with tumor on urography. Sonography usually makes the diagnosis. Occasionally, CT and magnetic resonance imaging (MRI) may be necessary.

Clinical Findings

A. Symptoms: Pain in the flank or back, usually intermittent and dull, is not uncommon. If bleeding suddenly distends the cyst wall, pain may come on abruptly and be severe. Gastrointestinal symptoms are occasionally noted and may suggest peptic ulcer or gallbladder disease. The patient may discover a mass in the abdomen, although cysts of this size are unusual. If the cyst becomes infected, the patient usually complains of pain in the flank, malaise, and fever.

B. Signs: Physical examination is usually normal, although occasionally a mass in the region of the kidney may be palpated or percussed. Tenderness in the flank may be noted if the cyst becomes infected.

C. Laboratory Findings: Urinalysis is usually normal. Microscopic hematuria is rare. Renal function tests are normal unless the cysts are multiple and bilateral (rare). Even in the face of extensive destruction of one kidney, compensatory hypertrophy of the other kidney will maintain normal total function.

D. X-Ray Findings: An expansion of a portion of the kidney shadow or a mass superimposed on it can usually be seen on a plain film of the abdomen. The axis of the kidney may be abnormal because of rotation due to the weight or position of the cyst. Streaks of calcium can sometimes be seen in the border of the mass.

Excretory urograms establish the presumptive diagnosis of cyst. On a film taken 1–2 min after infusion of radiopaque fluid, the vascularized parenchyma becomes white while the space-occupying cyst does not because it is avascular. The urographic series shows changes compatible with a mass. One or more calyces or the renal pelvis usually are indented or bent around the cyst; these are often broadened and flattened or even obliterated (Figures 33–3 and 33–5). Oblique and lateral films may prove helpful. If a mass occupies the lower pole of the kidney, the upper part of the ureter may be displaced toward the spine. The kidney itself may be rotated. The psoas muscle may be seen through the radiolucent cyst fluid.

If the routine urogram fails to opacify the parenchyma significantly, infusion nephrotomography should be done to increase the contrast between vascular renal tissue and the cyst (Figure 33–3). Occasionally, a renal parenchymal tumor may be relatively avascular and thus be confused with a cyst. In a few instances, carcinoma may grow on the cyst wall (Ljungberg et al, 1990). Because of these phenomena, further steps in differential diagnosis should be performed.

E. CT Scanning: CT appears to be the most accurate means of differentiating renal cyst and tumor (Figure 33–4). Cysts have an attenuation approximating that of water, whereas the density of tumors is similar to that of normal parenchyma. Parenchyma is made more dense with the intravenous injection of radiopaque fluid, but a cyst remains unaffected. The

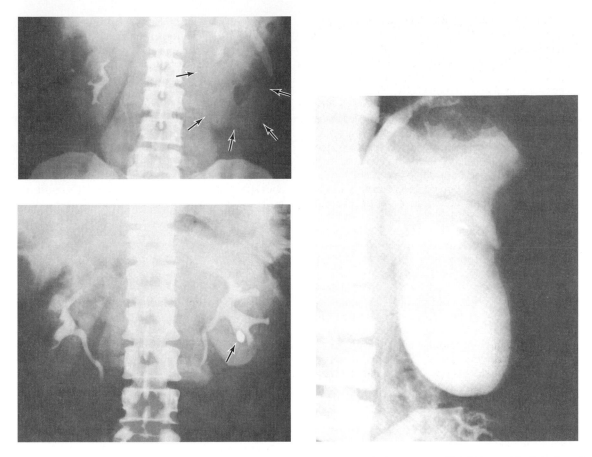

Figure 33–5. Upper left: Excretory urogram showing large smooth mass in lower pole of left kidney with distortion of calyces. **Right:** Cyst punctured and radiopaque fluid instilled. Cyst is smooth-walled; iophendylate then instilled. **Lower left:** Excretory urogram 3 months later; iophendylate occupies what is left of cyst in the lower medial calyx (arrow). Urogram normal.

wall of a cyst is sharply demarcated from the renal parenchyma; a tumor is not. The wall of a cyst is thin; that of a tumor is not. CT may well supplant cyst puncture in the differentiation of cyst and tumor in many cases.

F. Renal Ultrasonography: Renal ultrasonography is a noninvasive diagnostic technique that in a high percentage of cases differentiates between a cyst and a solid mass. If findings on ultrasonography are also compatible with a cyst, a needle can be introduced into the cyst under ultrasonographic control and the cyst can be aspirated.

G. Isotope Scanning: A rectilinear scan clearly delineates the mass but does not differentiate cyst from tumor. The technetium scan, made with the camera, reveals that the mass is indeed avascular (see Chapter 10).

H. Percutaneous Cyst Aspiration With Cystography: If the studies listed leave some doubt about the differentiation between cyst and tumor, as-

piration may be done. (See Treatment, following, and p. 137.)

Differential Diagnosis

Carcinoma of the kidney also occupies space but tends to lie more deeply in the organ and therefore causes more distortion of the calyces. Hematuria is common with tumor, rare with cyst. If a solid tumor overlies the psoas muscle, the edge of the muscle is obliterated on the plain film; it can be seen through a cyst, however. Evidence of metastases (ie, loss of weight and strength, palpable supraclavicular nodes, chest film showing metastatic nodules), erythrocytosis, hypercalcemia, and increased sedimentation rate suggest cancer. It must be remembered, however, that the walls of a simple cyst may undergo cancerous degeneration. If the renal vein is occluded by cancer, the excretory urogram may be visualized only faintly or not at all. Sonography, CT scan, or MRI should be almost definitive in differential diagnosis. Angiography or nephrotomography may reveal "pooling" of the medium in the highly vascularized tumor, whereas the density of a cyst is not affected (Figure 33–6). It is wise to assume that all space-occupying lesions of the kidneys are cancers until proved otherwise.

Polycystic kidney disease is almost always bilateral, as shown by urography (Figure 33–2). Diffuse caliceal and pelvic distortion is the rule. Simple cyst is usually solitary and unilateral. Polycystic kidney disease is usually accompanied by impaired renal function and hypertension; simple cyst is not.

Renal carbuncle is a rare disease. A history of skin infection a few weeks before the onset of fever and local pain may be obtained. Urograms may show changes similar to those of cyst or tumor, but the renal outline as well as the edge of the psoas muscle may be obscured because of perinephritis. The kidney may be fixed; this can be demonstrated by comparing the position of the kidney when the patient is supine and upright. Angiography demonstrates an avascular lesion. A gallium-67 scan demonstrates the inflammatory nature of the lesion, but an infected simple cyst might have a similar appearance.

Hydronephrosis may present the same symptoms and signs as simple cyst, but the urograms are quite different. Cyst causes calyceal distortion; with hydronephrosis, dilatation of the calyces and pelvis due to an obstruction is present. Acute or subacute hydronephrosis usually produces more local pain because of increased intrapelvic pressure and is more apt to be complicated by infection.

Extrarenal tumor (eg, adrenal, mixed retroperitoneal sarcoma) may displace a kidney, but rarely does it invade it and distort its calyces.

If an echinococcal cyst of the kidney does not communicate with the renal pelvis, it may be difficult to differentiate from solitary cyst, for no scoleces or hooklets will be present in the urine. The wall of a hydatid cyst often reveals calcification on x-ray examination (Figure 15–5). A skin sensitivity test (Casoni) for hydatid disease may prove helpful.

Complications
(Rare)

Spontaneous infection in a simple cyst is rare, but when it occurs, it is difficult to differentiate from carbuncle. Hemorrhage into the cyst sometimes occurs. If sudden, it causes severe pain. The bleeding may come from a complicating carcinoma arising on the wall of the cyst.

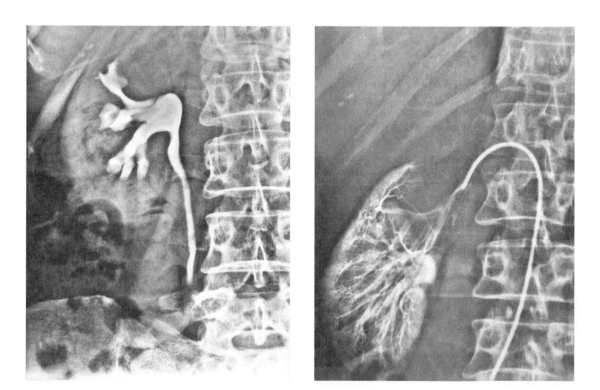

Figure 33–6. Diagnosis of simple renal cyst. **Left:** Excretory urogram showing lateral and inferior displacement and distortion of upper calyx, right kidney. Differential diagnosis: Cyst versus tumor. **Right:** Same patient. Selective femoral angiogram showing a completely avascular mass typical of cyst.

Hydronephrosis may develop if a cyst of the lower pole impinges on the ureter. This in itself may cause pain from back pressure of urine in the renal pelvis. This obstruction may lead to renal infection.

Treatment

A. Specific Measures:

1. If excretory urography, nephrotomography, renal sonography, CT, or MRI does not lead to a definitive diagnosis, renal angiography or needle aspiration of the cyst may be necessary. Should aspiration be necessary, it can be done under sonographic guidance. The recovery of clear fluid is characteristic of a benign cyst, which should be confirmed by cytologic evaluation. In some centers, contrast radiopaque fluid is injected into the cyst after aspiration for a more thorough evaluation of the cyst wall. A smooth cyst wall, free of irregularities, supports the presence of a benign cyst. To decrease the chance of reaccumulation of fluid, 3 mL of iophendylate is instilled into the cavity before the radiopaque fluid is removed.

If the aspirate contains blood, surgical exploration should be considered, because the chances are great that the growth is cancerous.

2. If the diagnosis can be clearly established, one should consider leaving the cyst alone, since it is rare for a cyst to harm the kidney. Sonography is useful in follow-up of patients with cysts.

B. Treatment of Complications:
If the cyst becomes infected, intensive antimicrobial therapy should be instituted, although Muther and Bennett (1980) found that antimicrobial drugs attained very low concentrations in the cyst fluid. Therefore, percutaneous drainage is often required. Surgical excision of the extrarenal portion of the cyst wall and drainage are curative when percutaneous drainage fails.

If hydronephrosis is present, excision of the obstructing cyst will relieve the ureteral obstruction.

Pyelonephritis in the involved kidney should suggest urinary stasis secondary to impaired ureteral drainage. Removal of the cyst and consequent relief of urinary back pressure make antimicrobial therapy more effective.

Prognosis

Simple cysts can be diagnosed with great accuracy using sonography and CT. Yearly sonography is recommended as a method of following the cyst for changes in size, configuration, and internal consistency. CT may be done if changes suggest carcinoma, and aspiration may then be performed if necessary to establish a diagnosis. Most cysts cause little difficulty.

RENAL FUSION

About 1 in 1000 individuals has some type of renal fusion, the most common being the horseshoe kidney. The fused renal mass almost always contains 2 excretory systems and therefore 2 ureters. The renal tissue may be divided equally between the 2 flanks, or the entire mass may be on one side. Even in the latter case, the 2 ureters open at their proper places in the bladder.

Etiology & Pathogenesis

It appears that this fusion of the 2 metanephroi occurs early in embryologic life, when the kidneys lie low in the pelvis. For this reason, they seldom ascend to the high position that normal kidneys assume. They may even remain in the true pelvis. Under these circumstances, such a kidney may derive its blood supply from many vessels in the area (eg, aorta, iliacs).

In patients with both ectopia and fusion, 78% have extraurologic anomalies and 65% exhibit other genitourinary defects.

Pathology
(Figure 33–7)

Because the renal masses fuse early, normal rotation cannot occur; therefore, each pelvis lies on the anterior surface of its organ. Thus, the ureter must ride over the isthmus of a horseshoe kidney or traverse the anterior surface of the fused kidney. Some degree of ureteral compression may arise from this or from obstruction by one or more aberrant blood vessels. The incidence of hydronephrosis and, therefore, infection is high. Vesicoureteral reflux has frequently been noted in association with fusion.

In horseshoe kidney, the isthmus usually joins the lower poles of each kidney; each renal mass lies lower than normal. The axes of these masses are vertical, whereas the axes of normal kidneys are oblique to the spine, because they lie along the edges of the psoas muscles.

On rare occasions, the 2 nephric masses are fused into one mass containing 2 pelves and 2 ureters. The mass may lie in the midline in order to open into the bladder at the proper point (crossed renal ectopy with fusion).

Clinical Findings

A. Symptoms: Most patients with fused kidneys have no symptoms. Some, however, develop ureteral obstruction. Gastrointestinal symptoms (renodigestive reflex) mimicking peptic ulcer, cholelithiasis, or appendicitis may be noted. Infection is apt to occur if ureteral obstruction and hydronephrosis or calculus develops.

B. Signs: Physical examination is usually negative unless the abnormally placed renal mass can be felt. With horseshoe kidney, it may be possible to palpate a mass over the lower lumbar spine (the isthmus). In the case of crossed ectopy, a mass may be felt in the flank or lower abdomen.

C. Laboratory Findings: Urinalysis is normal unless there is infection. Renal function is normal unless disease coexists in each of the fused renal masses.

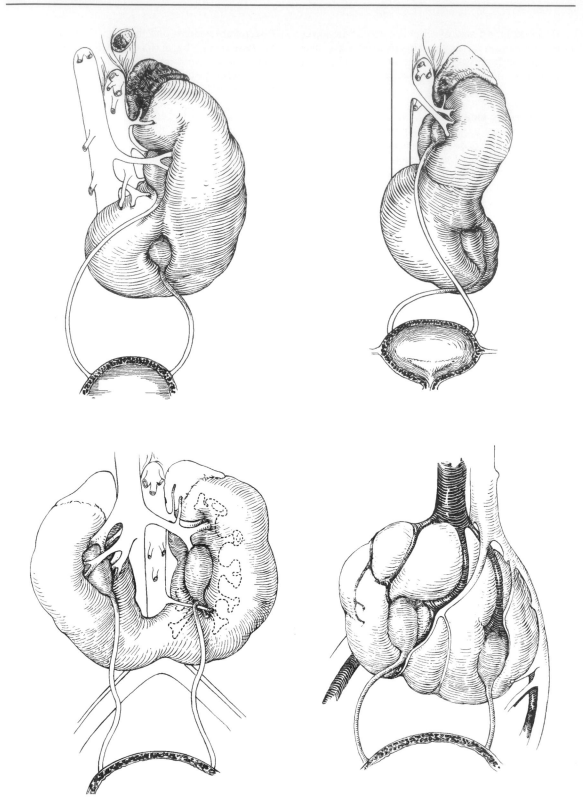

Figure 33–7. Renal fusion. **Upper left:** Crossed renal ectopy with fusion. The renal mass lies in the left flank. The right ureter must cross over the midline. **Upper right:** Example of "sigmoid" kidney. **Lower left:** Horseshoe kidney. Pelves are anterior. Note aberrant artery obstructing left ureter and the low position of renal mass. **Lower right:** Pelvic kidney. Pelves are placed anteriorly. Note aberrant blood supply.

D. X-Ray Findings: In the case of horseshoe kidney, the axes of the 2 kidneys, if visible on a plain film, are parallel to the spine. At times the isthmus can be identified. The plain film may also reveal a large soft-tissue mass in one flank yet not show a renal shadow on the other side (Figure 33–8).

Excretory urograms establish the diagnosis if the renal parenchyma has been maintained. The increased density of the renal tissue may make the position or configuration of the kidney more distinct. Urograms also visualize the pelvis and ureters.

1. With horseshoe kidney, the renal pelves lie on the anterior surfaces of their kidney masses, whereas the normal kidney has its pelvis lying mesial to it. The most valuable clue to the diagnosis of horseshoe kidney is the presence of calyces in the region of the lower pole that point medially and lie medial to the ureter (Figures 33–7 and 33–8).

2. Crossed renal ectopy with fusion shows 2 pelves and 2 ureters. One ureter must cross the midline in order to empty into the bladder at the proper point (Figures 33–7 and 33–8).

3. A cake or lump kidney may lie in the pelvis (fused pelvis kidney), but again its ureters and pelves will be shown (Figures 33–7 and 33–8). It may compress the dome of the bladder.

CT clearly outlines the renal mass but is seldom necessary for diagnosis. With pelvic fused kidney or one lying in the flank, the plain film taken with ureteral catheters in place gives the first hint of the diagnosis. Retrograde urograms show the position of the pelves and demonstrate changes compatible with infection or obstruction (Figure 33–9). Renal scanning delineates the renal mass and its contour (see Chapter 10), as does sonography.

Differential Diagnosis

Separate kidneys that fail to undergo normal rotation may be confused with horseshoe kidney. They lie along the edges of the psoas muscles, whereas the poles of a horseshoe kidney lie parallel to the spine and the lower poles are placed on the psoas muscles. The calyces in the region of the isthmus of a horseshoe kidney point medially and lie close to the spine.

The diagnosis of fused or lump kidney may be missed on excretory urograms if one of the ureters is markedly obstructed, so that a portion of the kidney, pelvis, and ureter fails to visualize. Infusion urograms or retrograde urograms demonstrate both excretory tracts in the renal mass.

Complications

Fused kidneys are prone to ureteral obstruction because of a high incidence of aberrant renal vessels and the necessity for one or both ureters to arch around or over the renal tissue. Hydronephrosis, stone, and infection, therefore, are common.

A large fused kidney occupying the concavity of the sacrum may cause dystocia.

Treatment

No treatment is necessary unless obstruction or infection is present. Drainage of a horseshoe kidney may be improved by dividing its isthmus. If one pole of a horseshoe is badly damaged, it may require surgical resection.

Prognosis

In most cases, the outlook is excellent. If ureteral obstruction and infection occur, renal drainage must be improved by surgical means so that antimicrobial therapy will be effective.

ECTOPIC KIDNEY

Congenital ectopic kidney usually causes no symptoms unless complications such as ureteral obstruction or infection develop.

Simple Ectopy

Simple congenital ectopy usually refers to a low kidney on the proper side that failed to ascend normally. It may lie over the pelvic brim or in the pelvis. Rarely, it may be found in the chest (Figure 33–9) (Kirshenbaum, Puri, and Rao, 1981). It takes its blood supply from adjacent vessels, and its ureter is short. It is prone to ureteral obstruction and infection, which may lead to pain or fever. At times such a kidney may be palpable, leading to an erroneous presumptive diagnosis (eg, cancer of the bowel, appendiceal abscess).

Excretory urograms (Figure 33–9) reveal the true position of the kidney. Hydronephrosis, if present, is evident. There is no redundancy of the ureter, as is the case with nephroptosis or acquired ectopy (eg, displacement by large suprarenal tumor).

Obstruction and infection may complicate simple ectopy and should be treated by appropriate means.

Crossed Ectopy Without Fusion

In crossed ectopy without fusion, the kidney lies on the opposite side of the body but is not attached to its normally placed mate. Unless 2 distinct renal shadows can be seen, it may be difficult to differentiate this condition from crossed ectopy with fusion (Figure 33–7). Sonography, angiography, or CT should make the distinction.

ABNORMAL ROTATION

Normally, when the kidney ascends to the lumbar region, the pelvis lies on its anterior surface. Later, the pelvis comes to lie mesially. Such rotation may fail to occur, although this seldom leads to renal disease. Urography demonstrates the abnormal position.

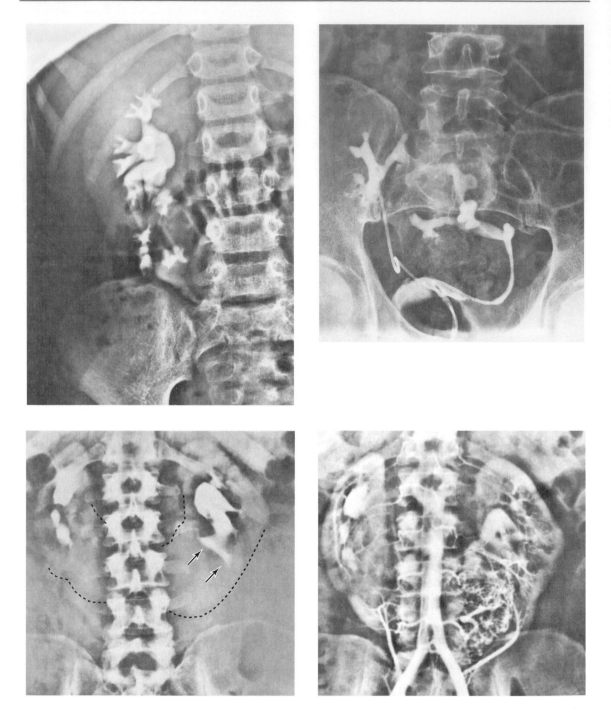

Figure 33–8. Renal fusion. **Upper left:** Excretory urogram showing fused renal masses on the right side. Both kidneys are normal. Crossed renal ectopy. **Upper right:** Retrograde urogram showing pelvic kidney. **Lower left:** Excretory urogram showing horseshoe kidney with expansion of left side of isthmus and compression of lower left calyceal system. **Lower right:** Angiogram on same patient. Hypervascular mass in left side of isthmus typical of adenocarcinoma.

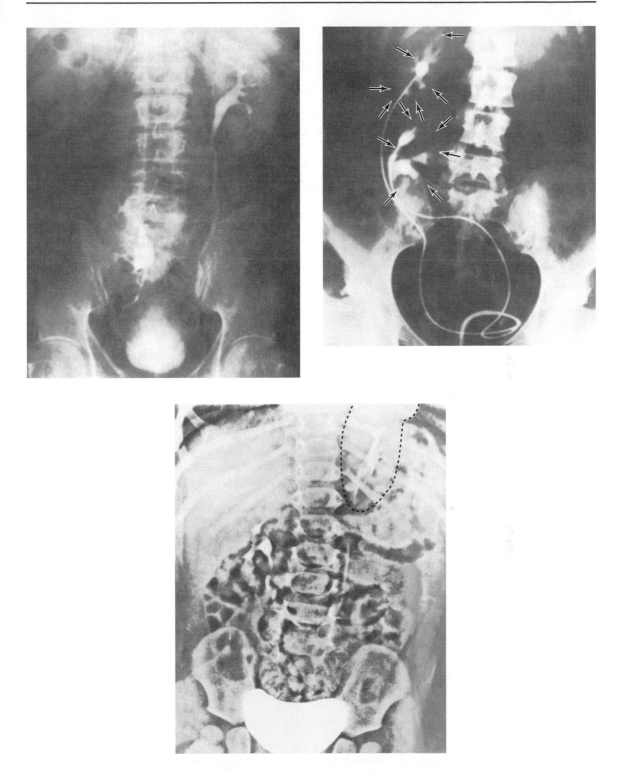

Figure 33–9. Renal ectopy. **Upper left:** Excretory urogram showing congenital ectopy, right kidney. **Upper right:** Retrograde urogram showing crossed renal ectopy. In this film, the differentiation between fusion and nonfusion cannot be made. **Bottom:** Left kidney, ectopic in the chest.

MEDULLARY SPONGE KIDNEY
(Cystic Dilatation of the Renal Collecting Tubules)

Medullary sponge kidney is a congenital autosomal recessive defect characterized by widening of the distal collecting tubules. It is usually bilateral, affecting all of the papillae, but it may be unilateral. At times, only one papilla is involved. Cystic dilatation of the tubules is often present also. Infection and calculi are occasionally seen as a result of urinary stasis in the tubules. It is believed that medullary sponge kidney is related to polycystic kidney disease. Its occasional association with hemihypertrophy of the body has been noted.

The only symptoms are those arising from infection and stone formation. The diagnosis is made on the basis of excretory urograms (Figure 33–10). The pelvis and calyces are normal, but dilated (streaked) tubules are seen just lateral to them; many of the dilated tubules contain round masses of radiopaque material (the cystic dilatation). If stones are present, a plain film will reveal small, round calculi in the pyramidal regions just beyond the calyces. Retrograde urograms often do not reveal the lesion unless the mouths of the collecting ducts are widely dilated.

The differential diagnosis includes tuberculosis, healed papillary necrosis, and nephrocalcinosis. Tuberculosis is usually unilateral, and urography shows ulceration of calyces; tubercle bacilli are found on bacteriologic study. Papillary necrosis may be complicated by calcification in the healed stage but may be distinguished by its typical calyceal deformity, the presence of infection, and, usually, impaired renal function. The tubular and parenchymal calcification seen in nephrocalcinosis is more diffuse than that seen with sponge kidney (Figure 17–3); the symptoms and signs of primary hyperparathyroidism or renal tubular acidosis may be found.

There is no treatment for medullary sponge kidney. Therapy is directed toward the complications (eg, pyelonephritis and renal calculi). Only a small percentage of people with sponge kidney develop complications. The overall prognosis is good. A few patients may pass small stones occasionally.

ABNORMALITIES OF RENAL VESSELS

A single renal artery is noted in 75–85% of individuals and a single renal vein in an even higher percentage. Aberrant veins and, especially, arteries occur. An aberrant artery passing to the lower pole of the kidney

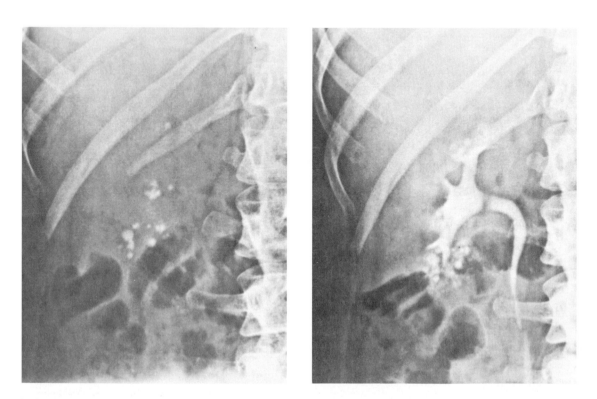

Figure 33–10. Medullary sponge kidneys. **Left:** Plain film of right kidney showing multiple small stones in its mid portion. **Right:** Excretory urogram showing relationship of calculi to calyces. Typically, the calyces are large; the stones are located in the dilated collecting tubules.

or crossing an infundibulum can cause obstruction and hydronephrosis. These causes of obstruction can be diagnosed on angiography or spiral CT.

ACQUIRED LESIONS OF THE KIDNEYS

ANEURYSM OF THE RENAL ARTERY

Aneurysm of the renal artery usually results from degenerative arterial disease that weakens the wall of the artery so that intravascular pressure may balloon it out. It is most commonly caused by arteriosclerosis or polyarteritis nodosa, but it may develop secondary to trauma or syphilis. Well over 300 cases have been reported. Congenital aneurysm has been recorded. Most cases represent an incidental finding on angiography.

Aneurysmal dilatation has no deleterious effect on the kidney unless the mass compresses the renal artery, in which case some renal ischemia and, therefore, atrophy are to be expected. A true aneurysm may rupture, producing a false aneurysm. This is especially likely to occur during pregnancy. The extravasated blood in the retroperitoneal space finally becomes encapsulated by a fibrous covering as organization occurs. An aneurysm may involve a small artery within the renal parenchyma. It may rupture into the renal pelvis or a calyx.

Most aneurysms cause no symptoms unless they rupture, in which case there may be severe flank pain and even shock. If an aneurysm ruptures into the renal pelvis, marked hematuria occurs. The common cause of death is severe hemorrhage from rupture of the aneurysm. Hypertension is not usually present. A bruit should be sought over the costovertebral angle or over the renal artery anteriorly. If spontaneous or traumatic rupture has occurred, a mass may be palpated in the flank.

A plain film of the abdomen may show an intrarenal or extrarenal ringlike calcification (Figure 33–11). Urograms may be normal or reveal renal atrophy. Some impairment of renal function may be noted if compression or partial obstruction of the renal artery has developed. Aortography delineates the aneurysm. Sonography and CT scanning may prove helpful.

The differential diagnosis of rupture of an aneurysm and injury to the kidney is difficult unless a history or evidence of trauma is obtained. A hydronephrotic kidney may present a mass, but urography clarifies the issue.

Because a significant number of noncalcified and large calcified aneurysms rupture spontaneously, the presence of such a lesion is an indication for operation, particularly during pregnancy. The repair of ex-

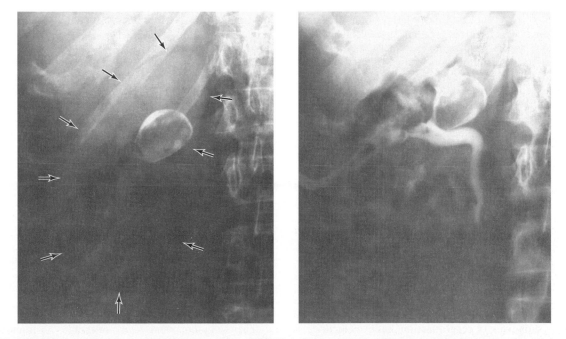

Figure 33–11. Intrarenal aneurysm of renal artery. **Left:** Plain film showing calcified structure over right renal shadow. **Right:** Excretory urogram relating calcific mass to pelvis and upper calyx. (Courtesy of CD King.)

trarenal aneurysms may be considered, but complications (eg, thrombosis) are not uncommon. If an intrarenal aneurysm is situated in one pole, heminephrectomy may be feasible. If it is in the center of the organ, however, nephrectomy is required. Therapeutic occlusion of an aneurysm by intra-arterial injection of autologous muscle tissue has been reported. Those few patients with hypertension may become normotensive following definitive surgery.

RENAL INFARCTS

Renal infarcts are caused by arterial occlusion. The major causes are subacute infective endocarditis, atrial or ventricular thrombi, arteriosclerosis, polyarteritis nodosa, and trauma. A thrombotic process in the abdominal aorta may gradually extend upward to occlude the renal artery. Renal infarcts may be unilateral or bilateral.

If smaller arteries or arterioles become obstructed, the tissue receiving blood from such a vessel will first become swollen and then undergo necrosis and fibrosis. Multiple infarcts are the rule. If the main renal artery becomes occluded, the entire kidney will react in kind. The kidney may become functionless and atrophic, therefore, as it undergoes necrosis and fibrosis.

Partial renal infarction is a silent disease, but it can result in flank pain and microscopic or gross hematuria. Sudden and complete infarction may cause renal or chest pain and at times gross or microscopic hematuria. Proteinuria and leukocytosis are found. "Epitheluria," representing sloughing of renal tubular cells, has been noted. Tenderness over the flank may be elicited. The kidney is not significantly enlarged by arterial occlusion. Serum aspartate aminotransferase (glutamic-oxaloacetic transaminase, AST [SGOT]) and lactate dehydrogenase levels will be elevated for 1 or 2 days after the incident.

Excretory urograms may fail to visualize a portion of the kidney with partial infarction; with complete infarction, none of the radiopaque fluid is excreted. If complete renal infarction is suspected, a radioisotope renogram should be performed. A completely infarcted kidney shows little or no radioactivity. A similar picture is seen on CT scans performed after injection of radiopaque contrast medium. Even though complete loss of measurable function has occurred, renal circulation may be restored spontaneously in rare instances.

Renal angiography or CT makes the definitive diagnosis. A dynamic technetium scan will reveal no perfusion of the affected renal vasculature.

During the acute phase, infarction may mimic ureteral stone. With stone the excretory urogram may also show lack of renal function, but even so there is usually enough medium in the tubules for a "nephrogram" to be obtained (Figure 17–3). This will not oc-

cur with complete infarction. Evidence of a cardiac or vascular lesion is helpful in arriving at a proper diagnosis.

The complications are related to those arising from the primary cardiovascular disease, including emboli to other organs. In a few cases, hypertension may develop a few days or weeks after the infarction. It may later subside.

While emergency surgical intervention has been done, it has become clear that anticoagulation therapy is the treatment of choice. It has been shown that an infusion of streptokinase may dissolve the embolus. Renal function returns in most cases.

THROMBOSIS OF THE RENAL VEIN

Thrombosis of the renal vein is rare in adults. It is frequently unilateral and usually associated with membranous glomerulonephritis and nephrotic syndrome. Invasion of the renal vein by tumor or retroperitoneal disease can be the cause. Thrombosis of the renal vein may occur as a complication of severe dehydration and hemoconcentration in children with severe diarrhea from ileocolitis. The thrombosis may extend from the vena cava into the peripheral venules or may originate in the peripheral veins and propagate to the main renal vein. The severe passive congestion that develops causes the kidney to swell and become engorged. Degeneration of the nephrons ensues. There is usually flank pain, and hematuria may be noted. A large, tender mass is often felt in the flank. Thrombocytopenia may be noted. The urine contains albumin and red cells. In the acute stage, urograms show poor or absent secretion of the radiopaque material in a large kidney. Stretching and thinning of the calyceal infundibula may be noted. Clots in the pelvis may cause filling defects. Later, the kidney may undergo atrophy. Urograms may then show notching of the upper ureter caused by dilated collateral veins.

Ultrasonography shows the thrombus in the vena cava in 50% of cases. The involved organ is enlarged. CT scan is also a valuable diagnostic tool; visualization of the thrombus can be noted in a high percentage of cases. Recently, MRI has proved to be a very sensitive diagnostic tool. Renal angiography reveals stretching and bowing of small arterioles. In the nephrographic phase, the pyramids may become quite dense. Late films may show venous collaterals. Venacavography or, preferably, selective renal venography demonstrates the thrombus in the renal vein (Figure 33–12) and, at times, in the vena cava. If washout from the vein gives poor filling, filling may be enhanced by an injection of epinephrine into the renal artery.

The symptoms and signs resemble obstruction from a ureteral calculus. The presence of a stone in the ureter should be obvious; some degree of dilata-

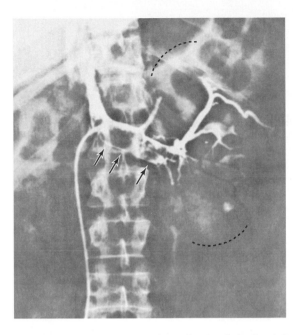

Figure 33–12. Thrombosis of renal vein. Selective left renal venogram showing almost complete occlusion of vein. Veins to lower pole failed to fill. Note large size of kidney.

tion of the ureter and pelvis also should be expected. Clot obstruction in the ureter must be differentiated from an obstructing calculus.

While thrombectomy and even nephrectomy have been recommended in the past, it has become increasingly clear that medical treatment is usually efficacious. The use of heparin anticoagulation in the acute phase and warfarin chronically offers satisfactory resolution of the problems in most patients. In infants and children, it is essential to correct fluid and electrolyte problems and administer anticoagulants. Fibrinolytic therapy has also been successful (Bromberg and Firlit, 1990). Renal function is usually fully recovered.

ARTERIOVENOUS FISTULA

Arteriovenous fistula may be congenital (25%) or acquired. A number of these fistulas have been reported following needle biopsy of the kidney or trauma to the kidney. A few have occurred following nephrectomy secondary to suture or ligature occlusion of the pedicle. These require surgical repair. A few have been recognized in association with adenocarcinoma of the kidney.

A thrill can often be palpated and a murmur heard both anteriorly and posteriorly. In cases with a wide communication, the systolic blood pressure is ele-

vated and a widened pulse pressure is noted. Renal angiography or isotopic scan establishes the diagnosis. CT scan, sonography, and, recently, duplex ultrasound with color flow are particularly helpful. Arteriovenous fistula involving the renal artery and vein requires surgical repair or nephrectomy. Most, however, can be occluded by embolization, balloon, or steel coil. Those that develop secondary to renal biopsy tend to heal spontaneously.

ARTERIOVENOUS ANEURYSM

About 100 instances of this lesion have been reported (Figure 33–13). Most follow trauma. Hypertension is to be expected and is associated with high-output cardiac failure. A bruit is usually present. Nephrectomy is usually indicated.

RENOALIMENTARY FISTULA

Over 100 instances of renoalimentary fistula have been reported. They usually involve the stomach, duodenum, or adjacent colon, although fistula formation with the esophagus, small bowel, appendix, and rectum has been reported.

The underlying cause is usually a pyonephrotic kidney or renal cell carcinoma that becomes adherent to a portion of the alimentary tract and then ruptures spon-

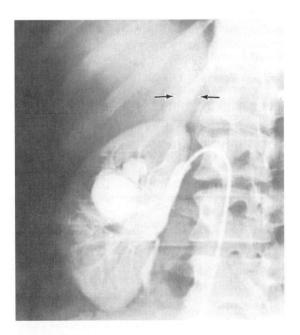

Figure 33–13. Arteriovenous aneurysm. Selective renal angiogram. Note aneurysm in center of kidney, with prompt filling of the vena cava (shown by arrows).

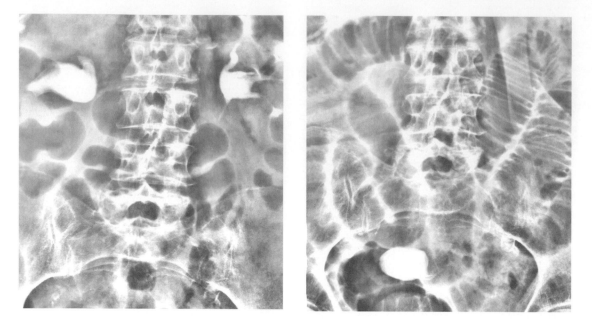

Figure 33–14. Nephroduodenal fistula and small-bowel obstruction from renal staghorn calculus. **Left:** Excretory urogram showing nonfunction of right kidney; staghorn stone. **Right:** Patient presented with symptoms and signs of bowel obstruction 4 years later. Plain film showing dilated loops of small bowel down to a point just proximal to ileocecal valve. Obstruction due to stone extruded into duodenum. (Courtesy of CD King.)

taneously, thus creating a fistula (Figure 33–14). A few cases following trauma have been reported. The patient is apt to suffer symptoms and signs of acute pyelonephritis. Urography may show radiopaque material escaping into the gastrointestinal tract. Gastrointestinal series may also reveal the connection with the kidney. The treatment is nephrectomy with closure of the opening into the gut.

RENOBRONCHIAL FISTULA

Nephrobronchial fistulas are rare (Borum, 1997). They are caused by rupture of an infected, calculous kidney through the diaphragm.

REFERENCES

CONGENITAL ANOMALIES

General

Donohue RE, Fauver HE: Unilateral absence of the vas deferens: A useful clinical sign. JAMA 1989;261:1180.

Elder JS et al: Evaluation of fetal renal function: Unreliability of fetal urinary electrolytes. J Urol 1990;144:574.

Johnson CE et al: The accuracy of antenatal ultrasonography in identifying renal abnormalities. Am J Dis Child 1992;146:1181.

Leads from the MMWR. Renal agenesis surveillance: United States. JAMA 1988;260:3114.

Mandell J et al: Human fetal compensatory renal growth. J Urol 1993;150:790.

Mandell J et al: Structural genitourinary defects detected in utero. Radiology 1991;178:193.

Patten RM et al: The fetal genitourinary tract. Radiol Clin North Am 1990;28:115.

Sanders RC: Prenatal ultrasonic detection of anomalies with a lethal or disastrous outcome. Radiol Clin North Am 1990;28:163.

Scott JE, Renwick M: Urological anomalies in the Northern Region Fetal Abnormality Survey. Arch Dis Child 1993;68(1 Spec No):22.

Sheih CP et al: Renal abnormalities in schoolchildren. Pediatrics 1989;84:1086.

Agenesis

Acien P et al: Renal agenesis in association with malformation of the female genital tract. Am J Obstet Gynecol 1991;165:1368.

Hill LM, Rivello D: Role of transvaginal sonography in the diagnosis of bilateral renal agenesis. Am J Perinatol 1991;8:395.

Ouden van den D et al: Diagnosis and management of seminal vesicle cysts associated with ipsilateral renal agenesis: A pooled analysis of 52 cases. Eur Urol 1998;33:433.

Robson WL, Leung AK, Rogers RC: Unilateral renal agenesis. Adv Pediatr 1995;42:575.

Sanders RC: Prenatal ultrasonic detection of anomalies with a lethal or disastrous outcome. Radiol Clin North Am 1990;28:163.

Sheih CP et al: Cystic dilatations within the pelvis in patients with ipsilateral renal agenesis or dysplasia. J Urol 1990;144:324.

Hypoplasia

Rosenstein BJ, Wheeler JS, Heid PL: Congenital renal abnormalities in infants with in utero cocaine exposure. J Urol 1990;144:110.

Saborio P, Scheinman J: Genetic renal disease. Curr Opin Pediatr 1998;10:174.

Sheih CP et al: Cystic dilatations within the pelvis in patients with ipsilateral renal agenesis or dysplasia. J Urol 1990;144:324.

Supernumerary Kidneys

N'Guessan GH, Stephens FD: Supernumerary kidney. J Urol 1983;130:649.

Dysplasia & Multicystic Kidney

Atiyeh B, Husmann D, Baum M: Contralateral renal abnormalities in patients with renal agenesis and noncystic renal dysplasia. Pediatrics 1993;91:812.

Carey PO, Howards SS: Multicystic dysplastic kidneys and diagnostic confusion on renal scan. J Urol 1988;139:83.

Corrales JG, Elder JS: Segmental multicystic kidney and ipsilateral duplication anomalies. J Urol 1996;155:1398.

Dimmick JE et al: Wilms tumorlet, nodular renal blastema and multicystic renal dysplasia. J Urol 1989;142:484.

Pinto E, Guignard JP: Renal masses in the neonate. Biol Neonate 1995;68:175.

Sanders RC, Nussbaum AR, Solez K: Renal dysplasia: Sonographic findings. Radiology 1988;167:623.

Strife JL et al: Multicystic dysplastic kidney in children: US follow-up. Radiology 1993;186:785.

Polycystic Kidneys

Eckardt KU et al: Erythropoietin in polycystic kidneys. J Clin Invest 1989;84:1160.

Levine E et al: Current concepts and controversies in imaging of renal cystic diseases. Urol Clin North Am 1997;24:523.

MacDermot KD et al: Prenatal diagnosis of autosomal dominant polycystic kidney disease PKD1 presenting in utero and prognosis for very early onset disease. J Med Genet 1998;35:13.

Maher ER, Kaelin WG Jr: von Hippel-Lindau disease. Medicine (Baltimore) 1997;76:381.

Martinez JR, Grantham JJ: Polycystic kidney disease: Etiology, pathogenesis, and treatment. Dis Mon 1995;41:693.

McHugo JM et al: Pre-natal diagnosis of adult polycystic kidney disease. Br J Radiol 1988;61:1072.

Reichard EAP, Roubidoux MA, Dunnick NR: Renal neoplasms in patients with renal cystic diseases. Abdom Imaging 1998;23:237.

Romanowski CA, Cavallin LI: Tuberous sclerosis, von Hippel-Lindau disease, Sturge-Weber syndrome. Hosp Med 1998;59:226.

Thomsen HS et al: Renal cystic diseases. Eur Radiol 1997;7:1267.

Vinocur L et al: Follow-up studies of multicystic dysplastic kidneys. Radiology 1988;167:311.

Watson ML, Macnicol AM, Wright AF: Adult polycystic kidney disease. Br Med J 1990;300:62.

Simple Cyst

Eilenberg SS et al: Renal masses: Evaluation with gradient-echo Gd-DTPA-enhanced dynamic MR imaging. Radiology 1990;176:333.

Feiner HD, Katz LA, Gallo GR: Acquired cystic disease of kidney in chronic dialysis patients. Urology 1981;17:260.

Ljungberg B et al: Renal cell carcinoma in a renal cyst: A case report and review of the literature. J Urol 1990;143:797.

Muther RS, Bennett WM: Concentration of antibiotics in simple renal cysts. J Urol 1980;124:596.

Sandler CM, Raval B, David CL: Computed tomography of the kidney. Urol Clin North Am 1985;12:657.

Renal Fusion

Dalla Palma L et al: Radiological anatomy of the kidney revisited. Br J Radiol 1990;63:680.

Decter RM: Renal duplication and fusion anomalies. Pediatr Clin North Am 1997;44:1323.

Hendron WH, Donahoe PK, Pfister RC: Crossed renal ectopia in children. Urology 1976;7:135.

Pitts WR Jr, Muecke EC: Horseshoe kidneys: A 40-year experience. J Urol 1975;113:743.

Ectopic Kidney

Bolton DM, Stoller ML: Pseudo-crossed renal ectopia secondary to ureteropelvic junction obstruction. J Urol 1995;153:397.

Hertz M et al: Crossed renal ectopia: Clinical and radiological findings in 22 cases. Clin Radiol 1977;28:339.

Kirshenbaum AS, Puri HC, Rao BR: Congenital intrathoracic kidney. J Urol 1981;125:412.

Medullary Sponge Kidney

Ginalski JM, Portmann L, Jaeger P: Does medullary sponge kidney cause nephrolithiasis? AJR 1990;155:299.

Indridason OS, Thomas L, Berkoben M: Medullary sponge kidney associated with congenital hemihypertrophy. J Am Soc Nephrol 1996;7:1123.

Kaver I et al: Segmental medullary sponge kidney mimicking a renal mass. J Urol 1989;141:1181.

Nunley JR, Sica DA, Smith V: Medullary sponge kidney and staghorn calculi. Urol Int 1990;45:118.

ACQUIRED LESIONS

Aneurysm of the Renal Artery

Cinat M, Yoon P, Wilson SE: Management of renal artery aneurysms. Semin Vasc Surg 1996;9:236.

Cooper GG, Atkinson AB, Barros D'Sa AA: Simultaneous aortic and renal artery reconstruction. Br J Surg 1990;77:194.

Dayton B et al: Ruptured renal artery aneurysm in a pregnant uninephric patient: Successful ex vivo repair and autotransplantation. Surgery 1990;107:708.

Fick GM et al: Causes of death in autosomal dominant polycystic kidney disease. J Am Soc Nephrol 1995;5:2048.

Helenon O et al: Renovascular disease: Doppler ultrasound. Semin Ultrasound CT MR 1997;18:136.

Jebara VA et al: Renal artery pseudoaneurysm after blunt abdominal trauma. J Vasc Surg 1998;27:362.

Renal Infarcts

Bartolozzi C, Neri E, Caramella D: CT in vascular pathologies. Eur Radiol 1998;8:679.

Gasparini M, Hofmann R, Stoller M: Renal artery embolism: Clinical features and therapeutic options. J Urol 1992;147:567.

Reznik VM et al: Successful fibrinolytic treatment of arterial thrombosis and hypertension in a cocaine-exposed neonate. Pediatrics 1989;84:735.

Skinner RE et al: Recovery of function in a solitary kidney after intra-arterial thrombolytic therapy. J Urol 1989;141:108.

Thrombosis of the Renal Vein

Brill PW et al: Adrenal hemorrhage and renal vein thrombosis in the newborn: MR imaging. Radiology 1989;170:95.

Bromberg WD, Firlit CF: Fibrinolytic therapy for renal vein thrombosis in the child. J Urol 1990;143:86.

Hibbert J et al: The ultrasound appearances of neonatal renal vein thrombosis. Br J Radiol 1997;70:1191.

Laplante S et al: Renal vein thrombosis in children: Evidence of early flow recovery with Doppler US. Radiology 1993;189:37.

Witz M et al: Renal vein occlusion: A review. J Urol 1996;155:1173.

Arteriovenous Fistula

Crotty KL, Orihuela E, Warren MM: Recent advances in the diagnosis and treatment of renal arteriovenous malformations and fistulas. J Urol 1993;150:1355.

Fogazzi GB, Moriggi M, Fontanella U: Spontaneous renal arteriovenous fistula as a cause of haematuria. Nephrol Dial Transplant 1997;12:350.

Morton MJ, Charboneau JW: Arteriovenous fistula after biopsy of renal transplant: Detection and monitoring with color flow and duplex ultrasonography. Mayo Clin Proc 1989;64:531.

Novick AC: Management of renovascular disease: A surgical perspective. Circulation 1991;83:1167.

Renoalimentary Fistula

Bissada NK, Cole AT, Fried FA: Reno-alimentary fistula: An unusual urological problem. J Urol 1973;110:273.

Schwartz DT et al: Pyeloduodenal fistula due to tuberculosis. J Urol 1970;104:373.

Tan SM, The CH, Tan PK: Duodeno-ureteric fistula secondary to chronic duodenal ulceration. Ann Acad Med Singapore 1997;26:850.

Renobronchial Fistula

Borum ML: An unusual case of nephrobronchial and nephrocolonic fistula complication xanthogranulomatous pyelonephritis. Urology 1997;50:443.

Diagnosis of Medical Renal Diseases

34

Flavio G. Vincenti, MD, & William J.C. Amend, Jr., MD

The medical renal diseases are those that involve principally the parenchyma of the kidneys. Many of the symptoms and signs of urinary tract disease are common to both medical and surgical diseases of the kidneys and other urologic organs. Hematuria, proteinuria, pyuria, oliguria, polyuria, pain, renal insufficiency with azotemia, acidosis, anemia, electrolyte abnormalities, hypertension, and auditory and ocular involvement may occur in a wide variety of disorders affecting any portion of the parenchyma of the kidney, the blood vessels, or the excretory tract.

Every effort must be made to rule out nonsurgical disease of the urinary tract before resorting to diagnostic or therapeutic procedures that may prove to be unnecessary or dangerous.

A complete medical history and physical examination, a thorough examination of the urine, and blood chemistry examinations as indicated are essential initial steps in the workup of any patient.

History

A. Family History: The family history may reveal disease of genetic origin, eg, tubular metabolic anomalies, polycystic kidneys, unusual types of nephritis, or vascular or coagulation defects that may be essential clues to the diagnosis.

B. Past History: The past history should cover infections, injuries, and exposure to toxic agents, anticoagulants, or drugs that may produce toxic or sensitivity reactions, including blood dyscrasias. A history of diabetes, hypertensive disease, and autoimmune disease may be obtained. The inquiry must also elicit symptoms of uremia, debilitation, and the vascular complications of chronic renal disease.

Physical Examination

One must look for such physical signs as pallor, edema, hypertension, retinopathy, and stigmas of congenital and hereditary disease (eg, enlarged kidneys in polycystic disease).

Urinalysis

Examination of the urine is the essential part of the investigation.

A. Proteinuria: Proteinuria of any significant degree (2–4+) is suggestive of medical renal disease (parenchymal involvement). Proteinuria should be interpreted with consideration of the urine specific gravity, since a proteinuria of 1+ in a dilute urine may indicate a considerable protein loss. Formed elements present in the urine additionally establish the diagnosis. Significant proteinuria occurs in immune-mediated glomerular diseases or metabolic disorders with glomerular involvement such as diabetes mellitus. Interstitial nephritis, polycystic kidneys, and other tubular disorders are not associated with significant proteinuria.

B. Erythrocyte Casts: When red blood cell (erythrocyte) casts are not present, microscopic hematuria may or may not be of glomerular origin. Phase contrast microscope study may reveal dysmorphic changes in the erythrocytes present in the urine in patients with parenchymal renal disorders.

C. Fatty Casts and Oval Fat Bodies: Tubular cells showing fatty changes occur in degenerative diseases of the kidney (nephrosis, glomerulonephritis, autoimmune disease, amyloidosis, and damage due to toxins such as mercury).

D. Other Findings: The presence of abnormal urinary chemical constituents may be the only indication of a metabolic disorder involving the kidneys. These disorders include diabetes mellitus, renal glycosuria, aminoacidurias (including cystinuria), oxaluria, gout, hyperparathyroidism, hemoglobinuria, and myoglobinuria.

Examination of the Kidneys & Urinary Tract

Roentgenographic, sonographic, and radioisotopic studies provide information about the size, structure, blood supply, and function of the kidneys and urinary tract.

Renal Biopsy

Renal biopsy is a valuable diagnostic procedure that also serves as a guide to rational treatment. The technique has become well established, frequently providing sufficient tissue for light and electron microscopy and for immunofluorescence examination. Absolute contraindications for percutaneous kidney biopsy include the anatomic presence of only one kidney; severe malfunction of one kidney even though function is adequate in the other; bleeding diathesis; the presence of hemangioma, tumor, or large cysts; abscess or infection; hydronephrosis; and an uncooperative patient. Relative contraindications include severe hypertension, uremia, severe arteriosclerosis, and unusual difficulty in doing a biopsy due to obesity, anasarca, or inability of the patient to lie flat.

Clinical indications for renal biopsy, in addition to the necessity for establishing a diagnosis, include the need to determine prognosis, to follow progression of a lesion and response to treatment, to confirm the presence of a generalized disease (autoimmune disorder, amyloidosis, sarcoidosis), and to diagnose renal dysfunction in a transplanted kidney.

GLOMERULONEPHRITIS

Information obtained from experimentally induced glomerular disease in animals and from correlations with evidence derived by modern methods of examination of tissue obtained by biopsy and at necropsy has provided new concepts of glomerulonephritis.

The clinical manifestations of renal disease are apt to consist only of varying degrees of hematuria, excretion of characteristic formed elements in the urine, proteinuria, and renal insufficiency and its complications. Excluding diabetes, immunologic renal diseases are the most common cause of proteinuria and the nephrotic syndrome.

Alterations in glomerular architecture as observed in tissue examined by light microscopy are also apt to be minimal, nonspecific, and difficult to interpret. For these reasons, specific diagnoses of renal disease require targeted immune fluorescent techniques for demonstrating a variety of antigens, antibodies, and complement fractions. Electron microscopy has complemented these immunologic methods. The combination of light microscopy, immunofluorescence staining for antibodies and immune mediators, and electron microscopy has led to new concepts of the origins and pathogenesis of glomerular disease. Tissue analysis can be complemented by serologic studies of immunoglobulins, complement, and other mediators of inflammation.

The two important humoral mechanisms leading to deposition of antibodies within the glomerulus are based on the location of the antigen, whether fixed within the kidney or present in soluble form in circulation. The fixed antigens are either a natural structural element of the glomerulus or foreign materials that have been trapped within the glomerulus for a variety of immunologic or physiochemical reasons. The best examples of the fixed natural antigens are those associated with the glomerular basement membrane. These antigens lead to antibody binding that is evenly distributed in the glomerular basement membrane and causes characteristic linear immunoglobulin (IgG) deposition, as determined in immunofluorescence studies. This process represents 10% of cases of immune-mediated glomerular disease and is referred to as anti-GBM (glomerular basement membrane) disease. However, most patients with glomerular immune deposits have discontinuous immune aggregates caused by antibody binding to native renal cell antigens or to antigens trapped within the glomerulus. In addition, immune complexes formed in the circulation can deposit and accumulate in the glomerular basement membrane and the mesangium. Once antibodies combined with antigens are formed and deposited in the kidney, a number of immune mediator pathways are activated and cause tissue injury.

A group of immune-mediated nephritides characterized by necrotizing and crescentic architecture and rapid progression are referred to as pauci-immune glomerular nephritides because, while antibodies may contribute to the pathogenesis of the disease, they are rarely demonstrated within the glomeruli. These diseases include Wegener granulomatosis and other forms of microscopic vasculitis. In these diseases, antineutrophil cytoplasmic antibodies (ANCA) react with antigens in the cytoplasm of neutrophils and monocytes. Two types of ANCA have been characterized on the basis of their localization: c-ANCA is found in a diffuse granular cytoplasmic pattern, and p-ANCA has a perinuclear staining pattern. The c-ANCA reaction is specific for Wegener granulomatosis.

Although in most instances of immune-mediated glomerular diseases, the role of antibody is of major importance, cellular immune processes are likely to be stimulated and contribute in different ways in the various forms of glomerulonephritides.

The current classification of glomerulonephritis is based on the mechanism, the presence, and the localization of immune aggregates in the glomeruli.

I. **Immunologic Mechanisms Likely**
   A. **Subepithelial Immune Deposits:**
      Glomerulonephritis associated with postinfectious glomerulonephritis such as poststreptococcal glomerulonephritis
      Membranous nephropathy idiopathic or secondary to other causes such as systemic lupus erythematosus, cancer, gold penicillamine
   B. **Subendothelial Immune Deposits:**
      Glomerulonephritis associated with systemic lupus erythematosus, type I membranoproliferative glomerulonephritis, glomerulonephritis associated with hepatitis C infection, bacterial endocarditis, and shunt nephritis

C. **Mesangial Immune Deposits**
   IgA nephropathy, Schönlein-Henoch purpura
D. **Anti-GBM Disease**
   Diffuse linear deposition of immunoglobulin
II. **Immunologic Mechanisms Not Clearly Established**
   Minimal change nephropathy
   Focal glomerulosclerosis
   Hemolytic-uremic syndrome and thrombotic thrombocytopenic purpura
   ANCA-associated disease, Wegener granulomatosis, and small-vessel vasculitis
   Type II membranoproliferative glomerulonephritis (dense deposit disease)

1. POST-STREPTOCOCCAL GLOMERULONEPHRITIS

Essentials of Diagnosis

- History of streptococcal infection.
- Malaise, headache, anorexia, low-grade fever.
- Mild generalized edema, mild hypertension, retinal hemorrhages.
- Gross hematuria; protein, erythrocyte casts, granular and hyaline casts, white blood cells (leukocytes), and renal epithelial cells in urine.
- Elevated antistreptolysin O titer, hypocomplementemia.

General Considerations

Glomerulonephritis is a disease affecting both kidneys. In most cases recovery from the acute stage is complete, but progressive involvement may destroy renal tissue leading to renal insufficiency. Acute glomerulonephritis is most common in children aged 3–10 years, although 5% or more of initial attacks occur in adults over age 50. By far the most common cause is an antecedent infection of the pharynx and tonsils or of the skin with group A β-hemolytic streptococci, certain strains of which are nephritogenic. Nephritis occurs in 10–15% of children and young adults who have clinically evident infection with a nephritogenic strain. In children under age 6, pyoderma (impetigo) is the most common antecedent; in older children and young adults, pharyngitis is a common antecedent and skin infection a rare antecedent. Rarely, nephritis may follow infection due to pneumococci, staphylococci, some bacilli and viruses, or *Plasmodium malariae* and exposure to some drugs.

The pathogenesis of the glomerular lesion has been further elucidated by the use of new immunologic techniques (immunofluorescence) and electron microscopy. A likely sequel to infection by nephritogenic strains of β-hemolytic streptococci is injury to the mesangial cells in the intercapillary space. The glomerulus may then become more easily damaged by antigen-antibody complexes developing from the immune response to the streptococcal infection. Complement is deposited in association with IgG or alone in a granular pattern on the epithelial side of the basement membrane and occasionally in subendothelial sites as well.

Gross examination of the involved kidney shows only punctate hemorrhages throughout the cortex. Microscopically, the primary alteration is in the glomeruli, which show proliferation and swelling of the mesangial and endothelial cells of the capillary tuft. The proliferation of capsular epithelium produces a thickened crescent about the tuft, and in the space between the capsule and the tuft there are collections of leukocytes, erythrocytes, and exudate. Edema of the interstitial tissue and cloudy swelling of the tubular epithelium are common. As the disease progresses, the kidneys may enlarge. The typical histologic findings in glomerulitis are enlarging crescents that become hyalinized and converted into scar tissue and obstruct the circulation through the glomerulus. Degenerative changes occur in the tubules, with fatty degeneration, necrosis, and ultimately scarring of the nephron. Arteriolar thickening and obliteration become prominent.

Clinical Findings

A. Symptoms and Signs: Often the disease is mild, and there may be no reason to suspect renal involvement unless the urine is examined. In severe cases, about 2 weeks after the acute streptococcal infection, the patient develops headache, malaise, mild fever, puffiness around the eyes and face, flank pain, and oliguria. Hematuria is usually noted as "bloody" or, if the urine is acid, as "brown" or "coffee-colored." Respiratory difficulty with shortness of breath may occur as a result of salt and water retention and circulatory congestion. There may be moderate tachycardia and moderate to marked elevation of blood pressure. Tenderness in the costovertebral angle is common.

B. Laboratory Findings: The diagnosis is confirmed by examination of the urine, which may be grossly bloody or coffee-colored (acid hematin) or may show only microscopic hematuria. In addition, the urine contains protein (1–3+) and casts. Hyaline and granular casts are commonly found in large numbers, but the classic sign of glomerulitis, the erythrocyte cast, is found only occasionally in the urinary sediment. The erythrocyte cast resembles a blood clot formed in the lumen of a renal tubule; it is usually of small caliber, is intensely orange or red, and, under high power with proper lighting, may show the mosaic pattern of the packed erythrocytes held together by the clot of fibrin and plasma protein.

With the impairment of renal function (decrease in glomerular filtration rate and blood flow) and with oliguria, plasma or serum urea nitrogen and creatinine become elevated, the levels varying with the severity of the renal lesion. The sedimentation rate is rapid. A mild normochromic anemia may result from fluid retention and dilution. Infection of the throat with nephritogenic streptococci is frequently followed by increasing antistreptolysin O titers in the serum, whereas high titers are usually not demonstrable following skin infections. Production of antibody against streptococcal deoxyribonuclease B (anti-DNase B) is more regularly observed following both throat and skin infections. Serum complement levels are usually low.

Confirmation of diagnosis is made by examination of the urine, although the history and clinical findings in typical cases leave little doubt. The finding of erythrocytes in a cast is proof that erythrocytes were present in the renal tubules and did not arise from elsewhere in the genitourinary tract.

Treatment

There is no specific treatment. Eradication of infection, prevention of overhydration and hypertension, and prompt treatment of complications such as hypertensive encephalopathy and heart failure require careful observation and management.

Prognosis

Most patients with the acute disease recover completely; 5–20% show progressive renal damage. If oliguria, heart failure, or hypertensive encephalopathy is severe, death may occur during the acute attack. Even with severe acute disease, however, recovery is the rule, particularly in children.

2. IgA NEPHROPATHY

Primary hematuria (idiopathic benign and recurrent hematuria, Berger disease) is now known to be an immune complex glomerulopathy in which deposition of IgA and occasionally IgG or IgM with C3 and fibrin-related antigens occurs in a granular pattern in the mesangium of the glomerulus. The associated light microscope findings are variable and range from normal to extensive crescentic glomerulonephritis.

Recurrent macroscopic and microscopic hematuria and mild proteinuria are usually the only manifestations of renal disease. Most patients with IgA nephropathy are between the ages of 16 and 35 years at the time of diagnosis. The disease occurs much more frequently in males than females and is the most common cause of glomerular nephritis in Asians. While most patients continue to have episodes of gross hematuria or microscopic hematuria, the renal function is likely to remain stable. However, approximately 30% of patients will have progressive renal dysfunction and develop end-stage renal disease. Clinical features that indicate a poor prognosis include male sex, older age at onset of disease, the presence of nephrotic-range proteinuria, and hypertension.

There is no satisfactory therapy for IgA nephropathy. The role of immunosuppressive drugs such as steroids and cytotoxic agents is not clear, and there have been few rigorously performed controlled trials. Mycophenolate mofetil, a de novo purine synthesis inhibitor, has been reported to induce a remission in anecdotal case reports. A more intriguing approach is the use of omega-3 fatty acids (fish oils) to delay progression of the renal disease. A large prospective randomized placebo-controlled trial in patients with IgA nephropathy using 12 g of omega-3 fatty acids has shown that fish oils probably can reduce the deterioration of renal function and the number of patients developing end-stage renal disease.

3. ANTIGLOMERULAR BASEMENT MEMBRANE NEPHRITIS (Goodpasture Syndrome)

The patient usually gives a history of recent hemoptysis and often of malaise, anorexia, and headache. The clinical syndrome is that of a severe acute glomerulonephritis, which may be accompanied by diffuse hemorrhagic inflammation of the lungs. The urine shows gross or microscopic hematuria, and laboratory findings of severely suppressed renal function are usually evident. Biopsy shows glomerular crescents, glomerular adhesions, and inflammatory infiltration interstitially. Electron microscope examination shows an increase in basement membrane material and deposition of fibrin beneath the capillary endothelium. In some cases, circulating antibody against glomerular basement membrane can be identified. IgG, C3, and, often, other components of the classic complement pathway can be demonstrated as linear deposits on the basement membranes of the glomeruli and the lung. Antiglomerular basement membrane antibody also reacts with lung basement membrane.

Large doses of corticosteroids in combination with immunosuppressive therapy may be useful. Plasmapheresis to remove circulating antibody has been reported to be effective in some patients. Transplantation should be delayed until circulating antiglomerular basement antibodies have disappeared.

A number of patients present with rapidly progressive renal failure and on kidney biopsy have crescenteric glomerulonephritis. However, these patients do not show any immune deposits or antibody deposition by immunofluorescence studies and are diagnosed as having pauci-immune idiopathic rapidly progressive glomerulonephritis. Many of these patients are serologically ANCA-positive. High-dose prednisone pulse therapy and cytotoxic agents may result in prolonged remission.

NEPHROTIC SYNDROME

Essentials of Diagnosis

- Edema.
- Proteinuria > 3.5 g/d.

- Hypoalbuminemia < 3 g/dL.
- Hyperlipidemia: Cholesterol > 300 mg/100 mL.
- Lipiduria: Free fat, oval fat bodies, fatty casts.

General Considerations

Because treatment and prognosis vary with the cause of nephrotic syndrome (nephrosis), renal biopsy and appropriate examination of an adequate tissue specimen are important. Light microscopy, electron microscopy, and immunofluorescence identification of immune mechanisms provide critical information for identification of most causes of nephrosis.

Glomerular diseases associated with nephrosis include the following:

A. Minimal Glomerular Lesions: Minimal-change nephropathy (lipoid nephrosis) accounts for about 20% of cases of nephrosis in adults. No abnormality is visible by examination of biopsy material with the light microscope. With the electron microscope, alterations of the glomerular basement membrane, with swelling and vacuolization and loss of organization of foot processes of the epithelial cells (foot process disease) are evident. There is no evidence of immune disease by immunofluorescence studies. The response to treatment with corticosteroids is good, but for patients who have frequent relapses with steroids or are steroid-resistant, a course of cyclophosphamide or chlorambucil usually induces a prolonged remission since patients who do not respond to these agents may show a favorable response with cyclosporine. Renal function remains stable.

B. Focal Glomerulosclerosis: Focal glomerulosclerosis is the second most common cause of nephrotic syndrome in children and an increasing cause of the nephrotic syndrome in adults. The diagnosis is based on light microscope findings of segmental hyalinosis and sclerosis associated with effacement of the foot processes on electron microscopy. Focal glomerulosclerosis is frequently idiopathic but can be associated with human immunodeficiency virus infection and heroin use. A secondary form of focal glomerulosclerosis without the diffuse changes in foot processes may occur in patients with a solitary kidney, hyperfiltration syndromes, and reflux nephropathy. The response of the idiopathic form of focal glomerulosclerosis to therapy is suboptimal. Prolonged corticosteroid therapy produces remission in approximately 40% of patients. Over a 10-year period, approximately 50% of patients will develop chronic renal failure. Focal glomerulosclerosis has a recurrence rate of 25% after transplantation.

C. Membranous Nephropathy: (About 25–27% of cases.) Examination of biopsy material with the light microscope shows thickening of the glomerular cells but no cellular proliferation. With the electron microscope, irregular lumpy deposits appear between the basement membrane and the epithelial cells, and new basement membrane material protrudes from the glomerular basement membrane as spikes or domes. Immunofluorescence studies show diffuse granular deposits of immunoglobulins (especially IgG) and complement (C3 component). As the membrane thickens, glomeruli become sclerosed and hyalinized.

The pathogenesis of most cases of membranous nephropathy in humans is unclear. Several mechanisms have been suggested. The first mechanism may involve glomerular trapping of circulating immune complexes. The source of the antigen could be derived from normal tissues or from exogenous sources such as the hepatitis B or C viruses or exposure to heavy metals or organic solvents. Second, this lesion may arise from circulating antibody binding with an intrinsic glomerular antigen. Third, a circulating antibody may bind to an antigen previously planted in the glomerulus because of a biochemical or electrostatic affinity to the glomerular basement membrane.

There is considerable controversy regarding the effectiveness of therapy with steroids or immunosuppressive agents or both in membranous nephropathy. Therapy should be reserved for patients at high risk of progressive renal failure with the following criteria: proteinuria > 10, hypertension, and elevated serum creatine.

D. Membranoproliferative Glomerulonephritis—Type I: Light microscopy shows thickening of glomerular capillaries, accompanied by mesangial proliferation and obliteration of glomeruli. With the electron microscope, subendothelial deposits and growth of mesangium into capillary walls are demonstrable. Immunofluorescence studies show the presence of the C3 component of complement and, rarely, the presence of immunoglobulins. The most common cause of membranoproliferative glomerulonephritis type I is chronic hepatitis C virus infection. This condition is usually associated with high levels of IgG/IgM cryoimmunoglobulins with normal or slightly reduced levels of complement. There is no known effective treatment, but patients with hepatitis C infection may benefit from prolonged interferon therapy.

E. Membranoproliferative Glomerulonephritis—Type II: Type II is characterized by dense deposits visible by electron microscopy and lack of findings by immunofluorescence studies. Treatment is unsatisfactory, and there is a high rate of recurrence after kidney transplantation.

F. Miscellaneous Diseases: A large number of metabolic, autoimmune, infectious, and neoplastic diseases and reactions to drugs and other toxic substances can produce glomerular disease. These include diabetic glomerulopathy, systemic lupus erythematosus, ANCA-positive renal disease (including Wegener granulomatosis), amyloid disease, multiple myeloma, lymphomas, carcinomas, syphilis, reaction to toxins, reaction to drugs (eg, trimethadione), and exposure to heavy metals.

Two recent glomerular lesions have been described that are found in patients with a nephrotic syndrome: fibrillary and immunotactoid glomerular nephritis. The lesions of fibrillary glomerulonephritis are characterized by randomly oriented fibril deposits 10–30 nm in diameter located within the mesangium and capillary wall. Immunotactoid glomerulopathy is characterized by deposits of microtubular structures of 18–19 nm and has been associated with lympho-proliferative disorders. The deposits in both diseases are Congo red–negative. Treatment of fibrillary and immunotactoid glomerulopathies is generally unsatisfactory.

Clinical Findings

A. Symptoms and Signs: Edema may appear insidiously and increase slowly; often it appears suddenly and accumulates rapidly. As fluid collects in the serous cavities, the abdomen becomes protuberant, and the patient may complain of anorexia and become short of breath. Symptoms other than those related to the mechanical effects of edema and serous sac fluid accumulation are not remarkable.

On physical examination, massive edema is apparent. Signs of hydrothorax and ascites are common. Pallor is often accentuated by the edema, and striae commonly appear in the stretched skin of the extremities.

B. Laboratory Findings: The urine contains large amounts of protein, 4–10 g or more per 24 h. The sediment contains casts, including the characteristic fatty and waxy varieties; renal tubular cells, some of which contain fatty droplets (oval fat bodies); and variable numbers of erythrocytes. A mild normochromic anemia is common, but anemia may be more severe if renal damage is great. Nitrogen retention varies with the severity of impairment of renal function. The plasma is often lipemic, and the blood cholesterol is usually greatly elevated. Plasma protein is greatly reduced. The albumin fraction may fall to less than 2 g/dL or even below 1 g/dL. Serum complement is usually low in active disease. The serum electrolyte concentrations are often normal, although the serum sodium may be slightly low; total serum calcium may be low, in keeping with the degree of hypoalbuminemia and decrease in the protein-bound calcium moiety. During edema-forming periods, urinary sodium excretion is very low and urinary aldosterone excretion is elevated. If renal insufficiency (see preceding discussion) is present, the blood and urine findings are usually altered accordingly.

Renal biopsy is essential to confirm the diagnosis and to indicate prognosis.

Differential Diagnosis

The nephrotic syndrome (nephrosis) may be associated with a variety of renal diseases, including primary glomerular disease, collagen-vascular diseases (eg, disseminated lupus erythematosus, polyarteritis), diabetic nephropathy, amyloid disease, thrombosis of the renal vein, myxedema, multiple myeloma, malaria, syphilis, reaction to toxins or heavy metals, reactions to drugs, and constrictive pericarditis.

Treatment

An adequate diet with restricted sodium intake (0.5–1 g/d) and prompt treatment of intercurrent infection are the basis of therapy. Diuretics may be given but are often only partially effective. Salt-free albumin and other oncotic agents are of little help, and their effects are transient. Other measures may be added as required.

The corticosteroids have been shown to be of value in treating nephrotic syndrome in children and in adults when the underlying disease is minimal glomerular lesion (lipoid nephrosis), focal segmental glomerulosclerosis, systemic lupus erythematosus, or proliferative and crescentic glomerulonephritis. These drugs are less often effective in the treatment of membranous disease and membranoproliferative lesions of the glomerulus. They are of little or no value in amyloidosis or renal vein thrombosis and are contraindicated in diabetic nephropathy.

Immunosuppressive drugs (eg, alkylating agents, cyclophosphamide, chlorambucil, azathioprine) have been used in the treatment of nephrotic syndrome. Encouraging early results have been reported in children and adults with proliferative or membranous lesions and with systemic lupus erythematosus. Those with minimal lesions refractory to corticosteroid therapy did no better when immunosuppressive agents were added. Improvement was noted in the glomerular changes and renal function in many patients responding well to treatment. It is not known what percentage of patients can be expected to benefit from these drugs.

Both the corticosteroids and the cytotoxic agents are commonly associated with serious side effects. At present, this form of therapy should be employed only by those experienced in treating nephrotic syndrome in patients in whom the disease has proved refractory to well-established treatment regimens.

Reduction in proteinuria and improvement in nephrotic edema have been reported using low-protein diets and angiotensin-converting enzyme (ACE) inhibitors. Most recently, studies have shown some improvements with lipid-lowering drugs.

Prognosis

The course and prognosis depend on the basic disease responsible for nephrotic syndrome. In most children with nephrosis (probably secondary to minimal change nephropathy), the disease appears to run a rather benign course when properly treated and to leave insignificant sequelae. Of the remaining children, most go inexorably into the terminal state with renal insufficiency. Adults with nephrosis fare less well. Hypertension, heavy proteinuria, and renal dysfunction are poor prognosticators.

RENAL INVOLVEMENT IN COLLAGEN DISEASES

The collagen diseases often produce symptoms and signs of renal disease indistinguishable from those of acute or chronic glomerulonephritis. Although it may not be accurate to classify all of these disorders as collagen diseases, acute disseminated lupus erythematosus, polyarteritis nodosa, scleroderma, Wegener granulomatosis, and thrombotic thrombocytopenic purpura have been implicated as causes of a syndrome resembling glomerulonephritis. In about one-third to one-half of cases, the urine sediment is diagnostic, containing erythrocytes and erythrocyte casts; renal tubular cells, including some filled with fat droplets; and waxy and granular broad casts. The presence of these formed elements is indicative of active glomerular and tubular disease with extensive focal destruction of nephrons. The symptoms and signs of the primary disease, involving extrarenal findings (eg, pulmonary or ear, nose, or throat changes with Wegener granulomatosis; dermatologic abnormalities, or carditis with systemic lupus erythematosus; dysphagia with scleroderma), and a variety of new tests of autoimmune disease as well as the presence of ANCA help to differentiate the form of collagen disease present. When collagen disease involves the kidneys, complete recovery from the disease is not likely to occur, although steroid and immunosuppressive drugs (alone or in combination) may be effective for long-term amelioration.

DISEASES OF THE RENAL TUBULES & INTERSTITIUM

1. INTERSTITIAL NEPHRITIS

Acute interstitial diseases are usually due to sensitivity to drugs, including antibiotics (penicillin, sulfonamides), nonsteroidal anti-inflammatory drugs, and phenytoin. The hallmark of acute interstitial nephritis is the infiltration of inflammatory cells in the interstitium. A typical presentation is a rapid deterioration in renal function associated with a recent introduction of a new drug. The finding of eosinophils in the urine sediment is very suggestive of allergic interstitial nephritis. Recovery may be complete, especially if the offending drug is withdrawn. A short course with corticosteroids may hasten the recovery of renal function.

Chronic interstitial nephritis is characterized by focal or diffuse interstitial fibrosis accompanied by infiltration, with inflammatory cells ultimately associated with extensive atrophy of renal tubules. It represents a nonspecific reaction to a variety of causes: analgesic abuse, lead and cadmium toxicity, nephrocalcinosis, urate nephropathy, radiation nephritis, sarcoidosis, Balkan nephritis, and some instances of obstructive uropathy. There are a few cases in which antitubular basement membrane antibodies have been identified. Systemic lupus erythematosus occasionally has a predominant pattern of interstitial nephritis instead of glomerulonephritis.

2. ANALGESIC NEPHROPATHY

Long-term ingestion of nonsteroidal analgesic and noninflammatory drugs and fulminating urinary tract selection in the presence of diabetes mellitus are the 2 principal causes of renal papillary necrosis. Analgesic nephropathy typically occurs in a middle-aged woman with chronic and recurrent headaches or a patient with chronic arthritis who habitually consumes large amounts of the drugs. Phenacetin was implicated initially, but with elimination of phenacetin from the mixtures, the incidence of analgesic nephropathy has not decreased. The ensuing damage to the kidneys usually is detected late, after renal insufficiency has developed. Careful history taking or the detection of analgesic metabolites in the urine can lead to this diagnosis.

The kidney lesion is pathologically nonspecific, consisting of peritubular and perivascular inflammation with degenerative changes of the tubular cells (chronic interstitial nephritis). There are no glomerular changes. Renal papillary necrosis extending into the medulla may involve many papillae.

Hematuria is a common presenting complaint. Renal colic occurs when necrotic renal papillae slough away. Polyuria may be prominent. Signs of acidosis (hyperpnea), dehydration, and pallor of anemia are common. Infection is a frequent complication. The history of excessive use of analgesics may be concealed by the patient.

The urine usually is remarkable only for the presence of blood and small amounts of protein. Elevated blood urea nitrogen and creatinine and the electrolyte changes characteristic of renal failure are typically present. Urinary concentrating impairments are usually present. Urograms show cavities and ring shadows typical of areas of destruction of papillae.

Treatment consists of withholding analgesics containing phenacetin and aspirin. Renal failure and infection are treated as outlined elsewhere in this chapter.

3. URIC ACID NEPHROPATHY

Crystals of urate produce an interstitial inflammatory reaction. Urate may precipitate out in acid urine in the calyces to form uric acid stones. Patients with myeloproliferative disease under treatment may develop hyperuricemia and are subject to occlusion of the upper urinary tract by uric acid crystals. Alkalinization of the urine and a liberal fluid intake help prevent crystal formation. Allopurinol is a useful drug to prevent hyperuricemia and hyperuricosuria. Recently, it has been suggested that many instances considered to be chronic "gouty nephropathy" are instead related to chronic lead renal injury and not due to primary uric acid depositions.

4. OBSTRUCTIVE UROPATHY

Interstitial nephritis due to obstruction may not be associated with infection. Tubular conservation of salt and water is impaired. Following relief of obstruction, diuresis may be massive and may require vigorous but judicious replacement of water and electrolytes.

5. MYELOMATOSIS

Features of myelomatosis that contribute to renal disease include proteinuria (including filtrable Bence Jones protein and κ and λ chains) with precipitation in the tubules leading to accumulation of abnormal proteins in the tubular lumen, hypercalcemia, and occasionally an increase in viscosity of the blood associated with macroglobulinemia. A Fanconi-like syndrome may develop.

Plugging of tubules, giant cell reaction around tubules, tubular atrophy, and, occasionally, the accumulation of amyloid are evident on examination of renal tissue.

Renal failure may occur acutely or develop slowly. Hemodialysis may rescue the patient during efforts to control the myeloma with chemical agents.

HEREDITARY RENAL DISEASES

The importance of inheritance and the familial incidence of disease warrants the inclusion of a classification of hereditary renal diseases. Although relatively uncommon in the population at large, hereditary renal disease must be recognized to permit early diagnosis and treatment in other family members and to prepare the way for genetic counseling.

1. CHRONIC HEREDITARY NEPHRITIS

Evidence of the disease usually appears in childhood, with episodes of hematuria often following an upper respiratory infection. Renal insufficiency commonly develops in males but only rarely in females. Survival beyond age 40 is rare.

In many families, deafness and abnormalities of the eyes accompany the renal disease (so-called Alport disease). Another form of the disease is accompanied by polyneuropathy. Infection of the urinary tract is a common complication.

The anatomic features in some cases resemble proliferative glomerulonephritis; in others, there is thickening of the glomerular basement membrane or podocyte proliferation and thickening of Bowman's capsule. In a few cases there are fat-filled cells (foam cells) in the interstitial tissue or in the glomeruli.

Recently, kindreds have been described that have "thin-membrane disease." This condition is characterized by microscopic hematuria and, often, later progression to chronic renal failure. This, like Alport disease, may represent inherited abnormalities or deficiencies in type 4 collagen in the glomerular basement membrane.

Laboratory findings with these conditions are commensurate with existing renal function. Treatment is symptomatic.

2. CYSTIC DISEASES OF THE KIDNEY

Congenital structural anomalies of the kidney must be considered in any patient with hypertension, pyelonephritis, or renal insufficiency. The manifestations of structural renal abnormalities are related to the superimposed disease, but management and prognosis are modified by the structural anomaly. Many of these patients are at increased risk of urinary tract infection.

Polycystic Kidneys

Polycystic kidney disease is familial and often involves not only the kidney but the liver and pancreas as well. It is clear that at least 2 genetic loci can lead to autosomal dominant polycystic kidney disease.

The formation of cysts on the cortex of the kidney is thought to result from failure of union of the collecting tubules and convoluted tubules of some nephrons. Intrarenal cysts may be of a proximal or a distal luminal type, differing on analysis by their cyst electrolyte content. This is important if one or more of these cysts become infected, and an antibiotic (with varying cyst-type penetrance) is chosen. New cysts do not form, but those present enlarge and, by exerting pressure, cause destruction of adjacent tissue. Cysts may be found in the liver and pancreas. The incidence of cerebral vessel aneurysms is higher than normal.

Cases of polycystic disease are discovered during the investigation of hypertension, by diagnostic study in patients presenting with pyelonephritis or hematuria, or by investigation of families of patients with polycystic disease. At times, flank pain due to hemorrhage into a cyst calls attention to a kidney disorder. Otherwise the symptoms and signs are those commonly seen in hypertension or renal insufficiency. On physical examination, the enlarged, irregular kidneys are often easily palpable.

The urine may contain leukocytes and erythrocytes. With bleeding into the cysts, there may also be bleeding into the urinary tract. The blood chemistry findings reflect the degree of renal insufficiency. Examination by sonography, computed tomography scan, or x-ray shows the enlarged kidneys, and urography demonstrates the classic elongated calyces and renal pelves stretched over the surface of the cysts.

No specific therapy is available, and surgical interference is indicated to decompress very large cysts in patients with severe pain. Hypertension, infection, and uremia are treated in the conventional manner.

Patients with polycystic kidney disease live in reasonable comfort with slowly advancing uremia; both hemodialysis and renal transplantation extend the life of these patients. Pretransplant nephrectomy is indicated only in patients with recurrent infections of cysts, severe recurrent bleeding requiring transfusions, or markedly enlarged kidneys with persistent pain.

Cystic Disease of the Renal Medulla

Two syndromes have been recognized with increasing frequency as their diagnostic features have become better known.

Medullary cystic disease is a familial disease that may become symptomatic during adolescence. Anemia is usually the initial manifestation, but azotemia, acidosis, and hyperphosphatemia soon become evident. The urine is not remarkable, although there is often an inability to produce a concentrated urine, and renal salt wasting often occurs. Many small cysts are scattered through the renal medulla. Renal transplantation is indicated by the usual criteria for the operation.

Medullary sponge kidney is asymptomatic and is discovered by the characteristic appearance of tubular ectasia in the urogram. Enlargement of the papillae and calyces and small cavities within the pyramids are demonstrated by the contrast media in the excretory urogram. Many small calculi often occupy the cysts, and infection may be troublesome. Life expectancy is not affected, and only symptomatic therapy for ureteral impaction of a stone or for infection is required.

3. ANOMALIES OF THE PROXIMAL TUBULE

Defects of Amino Acid Reabsorption

A. Congenital Cystinuria: Increased excretion of cystine results in the formation of cystine calculi in the urinary tract. Ornithine, arginine, and lysine are also excreted in abnormally large quantities. There is

also a defect in absorption of these amino acids in the jejunum. Nonopaque stones should be examined chemically to provide a specific diagnosis.

One must maintain a high urine volume by giving a large fluid intake and maintain the urine pH above 7.0 by giving sodium bicarbonate and sodium citrate plus acetazolamide at bedtime to ensure an alkaline night urine. In refractory cases, a low-methionine (cystine precursor) diet may be necessary. Penicillamine has proved useful in some cases.

B. Aminoaciduria: Many amino acids may be poorly absorbed, resulting in unusual losses. Failure to thrive and the presence of other tubular deficits suggest the diagnosis. There is no treatment.

C. Hepatolenticular Degeneration (Wilson Disease): In this congenital familial disease, aminoaciduria and renal tubular acidosis are associated with cirrhosis of the liver and neurologic manifestations. Hepatomegaly, evidence of impaired liver function, spasticity, athetosis, emotional disturbances, and Kayser-Fleischer rings around the cornea constitute a unique syndrome. There is a decrease in synthesis of ceruloplasmin, with a deficit of plasma ceruloplasmin and an increase in free copper that may be etiologically specific.

Penicillamine is given to chelate and remove excess copper. Edathamil (EDTA) may also be used to remove copper.

Multiple Defects of Tubular Function (De Toni-Fanconi-Debre Syndrome)

Aminoaciduria, phosphaturia, glycosuria, and a variable degree of renal tubular acidosis characterize this syndrome. Osteomalacia is a prominent clinical feature; other clinical and laboratory manifestations are associated with specific tubular defects described previously.

The proximal segment of the renal tubule is replaced by a thin tubular structure constituting the swan-neck deformity. The proximal segment also is shortened to less than half the normal length.

Treatment consists of replacing cation deficits (especially potassium), correcting acidosis with bicarbonate or citrate, replacing phosphate loss with isoionic neutral phosphate (mono- and disodium salts) solution, and ensuring a liberal calcium intake. Vitamin D is usually useful, but the dose must be controlled by monitoring serum of calcium and phosphate.

Defects of Phosphorus & Calcium Reabsorption

A. Renal Hypophosphatemic Rickets (and Osteomalacia): A number of sporadic, genetically transmitted, and acquired disorders are grouped under this category and are characterized by persisting hypophosphatemia because of excessive phosphaturia and an associated metabolic bone disorder, rickets in childhood, and osteomalacia in adulthood. Response to vitamin D therapy (1,25,-dihydroxycholecalciferol, the active analog of vitamin D) is variable.

B. Pseudohypoparathyroidism: Pseudohypoparathyroidism is a heterogeneous group of hereditary diseases characterized by end-organ unresponsiveness to parathyroid hormone. As a result of excessive reabsorption of phosphorus, hyperphosphatemia and hypocalcemia occur. Symptoms include muscle cramps, fatigue, weakness, tetany, and mental retardation. The signs are those of hypocalcemia; in addition, the patients are short and round-faced and characteristically have short fourth and fifth metacarpal and metatarsal bones. The serum phosphorus level is high, serum calcium low, and serum alkaline phosphatase normal. There is no response to parathyroid hormone. Vitamin D therapy and calcium supplementation may prevent tetany.

Defects of Glucose Absorption (Renal Glycosuria)

Renal glycosuria results from an abnormally poor ability to reabsorb glucose and is present when blood glucose levels are normal. Ketosis is not present. The glucose tolerance response is usually normal. In some instances, renal glycosuria may precede the onset of true diabetes mellitus. There is no treatment for renal glycosuria.

Defects of Bicarbonate Reabsorption

Proximal renal tubular acidosis (RTA, type II) is due to a deficiency in the production of H^+ in the proximal tubule, with resultant loss of bicarbonate in the urine and decreased bicarbonate concentration in extracellular fluid. Accompanying the limitation of H^+ secretion are increased K^+ secretion into the urine and retrieval of Cl^- instead of HCO^-. The acidosis is therefore associated with hypokalemia and hyperchloremia. Transport of glucose, amino acids, phosphate, and urate may be deficient as well and may result in Fanconi syndrome.

4. ANOMALIES OF THE DISTAL TUBULE

Defects of Hydrogen Ion Secretion & Bicarbonate Reabsorption (Classic Renal Tubular Acidosis, Type I)

Failure to secrete hydrogen ion and to form ammonium ion results in loss of "fixed base" sodium, potassium, and calcium. There is also a high rate of excretion of phosphate. Vomiting, poor growth, and symptoms and signs of chronic metabolic acidosis are accompanied by weakness due to potassium deficit and bone discomfort due to osteomalacia. Nephrocalcinosis, with calcification in the medullary portions of the kidney, occurs in about one-half of cases. The urine is alkaline and contains larger than normal quantities of sodium, potassium, calcium, and phosphate. An abnormality in urinary anion gap ($U.Na^+ + U. K.^+ - U.C^-$) is noted (low), which is associated with the reduced NH_4^+ production. This abnormality differentiates this condition from type II RTA and from the metabolic acidosis seen with diarrhea. The blood chemistry findings are those of metabolic acidosis (low HCO_3^- or CO_2) with hyperchloremia, low serum calcium and phosphorus, low serum potassium, and, occasionally, low serum sodium.

Treatment consists of replacing deficits and increasing the intake of sodium, potassium, calcium, and phosphorus. Sodium and potassium should be given as bicarbonate or citrate. Additional vitamin D may be required.

Excess Potassium Secretion (Potassium "Wastage" Syndrome)

Excessive renal secretion or loss of potassium may occur in 4 situations: (1) chronic renal insufficiency with diminished H^+ secretion; (2) renal tubular acidosis and the de Toni-Fanconi syndrome, with cation loss resulting from diminished H^+ and NH_4^+ secretion; (3) hyperaldosteronism and hyperadrenocorticism; and (4) tubular secretion of potassium, the cause of which is unknown. Hypokalemia indicates that the deficit is severe. Muscle weakness, metabolic alkalosis, and polyuria and dilute urine are signs attributable to hypokalemia.

Treatment consists of correcting the primary disease and giving supplementary potassium.

Reduced Potassium Secretion

Reduced potassium secretion is noted in conditions in which extrarenal aldosterone is reduced or when intrarenal production of renin (and secondary hypoaldosteronism) occurs. The latter condition is termed RTA, type IV, and is associated with impaired H^+ and K^+ secretion in the distal tubule. Drug-induced interstitial nephritis, gout, and diabetes mellitus are clinical circumstances that may produce type IV RTA and resulting hyperkalemia and mild metabolic acidosis. Treatment is to promote kaliuresis (with loop diuretics) to prescribe potassium-binding gastrointestinal resins (Kayexalate), or to provide the patient with a mineralocorticoid, fludrocortisone acetate.

Defects of Water Absorption (Renal Diabetes Insipidus)

Nephrogenic diabetes insipidus occurs more frequently in males than females. Unresponsiveness to antidiuretic hormone is the key to differentiation from pituitary diabetes insipidus.

In addition to congenital refractoriness to antidiuretic hormone, obstructive uropathy, lithium, methoxyflurane, and demeclocycline also may render the tubule refractory to the hormone.

Symptoms are related to an inability to reabsorb water, with resultant polyuria and polydipsia. The urine volume approaches 12 L/d, and osmolality and specific gravity are low. Mental retardation, atonic bladder, and hydronephrosis occur frequently.

Treatment consists primarily of an adequate water intake. Chlorothiazide may ameliorate the diabetes; the mechanism of action is unknown, but the drug may act by increasing isosmotic reabsorption in the proximal segment of the tubule.

5. UNSPECIFIED RENAL TUBULAR ABNORMALITIES

In idiopathic hypercalciuria, decreased reabsorption of calcium predisposes to the formation of renal calculi. Serum calcium and phosphorus are normal. Urine calcium excretion is high; urine phosphorus excretion is low. Microscopic hematuria may be present. See treatment of urinary stones containing calcium.

REFERENCES

GENERAL

Agnello V, Chung RT, Kaplan LM: A role for hepatitis C virus infection in type II cryoglobulinemia. N Engl J Med 1992;327:1490.

Anaemia of chronic renal failure. (Editorial.) Lancet 1983;1:965.

Anderson RJ, Schrier RW: *Clinical Uses of Drugs in Patients With Kidney and Liver Disease.* Saunders, 1981.

Bennett WM et al: Drug prescribing in renal failure: Dosing guidelines for adults. Am J Kidney Dis 1983; 3:155.

Bodziak KA, Hammond WS, Molitoris BA: Inherited diseases of the glomerular basement membrane. Am J Kidney Dis 1994;23:605.

Brenner BM, Rector FC Jr: *The Kidney,* 3rd ed. Saunders, 1986.

Carvalho AC: Bleeding in a uremia: A clinical challenge. (Editorial.) N Engl J Med 1983;308:38.

Eschbach JW: Treatment of anemia of progressive renal failure with recombinant human erythropoietin. N Engl J Med 1989;321:158.

Fer MF et al: Cancer and the kidney: Renal complications of neoplasms. Am J Med 1981;71:704.

Heptinstall RH: *Pathology of the Kidney,* 3rd ed. Little, Brown, 1983.

Ihle BV et al: The effect of protein restriction on the progression of renal insufficiency. N Engl J Med 1989;321:1773.

Jennette CJ, Falk RJ: Diagnostic classification of anti-neutrophil cytoplasmic autoantibody-associated vasculitides. Am J Kidney Dis 1991;18:184.

Klahr S: Pathophysiology of obstructive nephropathy. Kidney Int 1983;23:414.

Klahr S et al: The progression of renal disease. N Engl J Med 1988;318:1657.

Krupp MA: Genitourinary tract. In: Krupp MA, Tierney LM Jr, Schroeder SA (editors): *Current Medical Diagnosis & Treatment 1987.* Appleton & Lange, 1987.

Madaio MP: Renal biopsy. Kidney Int 1990;38:529.

Ramuzzi G, Bertain T: Pathophysiology of progressive nephropathies. N Engl J Med 1998;339:1448.

Schrier RW (editor): *Renal and Electrolyte Disorders,* 2nd ed. Little, Brown, 1980.

URINALYSIS

Cushner HM, Copley JB: Back to basics: The urinalysis: A selected national survey and review. Am J Med Sci 1989;297:193.

Ghiggen GM: Proteinuria: Definition, mechanisms and clinical value. Child Nephrol Urol 1989;9:181.

Haber MH: *Urine Casts: Their Microscopy and Clinical Significance.* American Society of Clinical Pathologists, 1975.

Hauglustaine D et al: Detection of glomerular bleeding using a simple staining method for light microscopy. Lancet 1982;2:761.

Kamel SK et al: Urine electrolytes and osmolality: When and how to use them. Am J Nephrol 1990;10: 89.

Stamey TA, Kindrachuk RW: *Urinary Sediment and Urinalysis: A Practical Guide for the Health Professional.* Saunders, 1985.

GLOMERULONEPHRITIS

Adler SG et al: Secondary glomerular diseases. In: Brenner BM (editor): *The Kidney,* 5th ed. Saunders, 1996.

Austin HA III et al: Therapy of lupus nephritis: Controlled trial of prednisone and cytotoxic drugs. N Engl J Med 1986;314:614.

Baldwin DS: Chronic glomerulonephritis: Nonimmunologic mechanisms of progressive glomerular damage. Kidney Int 1982;21:109.

Couser WG: Mediation of immune glomerular injury. J Am Soc Nephrol 1990;1:13.

Couser WG: Rapidly progressive glomerulonephritis: Classification, pathogenetic mechanisms, and therapy. Am J Kidney Dis 1988;11:449.

Glassock RJ et al: Human immunodeficiency virus (HIV) infection and the kidney. Ann Intern Med 1990;112: 35.

Glassock RJ et al: Primary glomerular diseases. In: Brenner BM (editor): *The Kidney,* 5th ed. Saunders, 1996.

Hricak DE, Chung-Park M, Sedor FR: Glomerulonephritis. N Engl J Med 1998;339:888.

Kashtan CE, Michael AF: Hereditary nephritis. Semin Nephrol 1989;9:135.

Paolo Schena F: A retrospective analysis of the natural history of primary IgA worldwide. Am J Med 1990;89:209.

Ponticelli C: Prognosis and treatment of membranous nephropathy. Kidney Int 1986;29:927.

Tiebosch ATMG et al: Thin-basement membrane nephropathy in adults with persistent hematuria. N Engl J Med 1989;320:14.

Wilson CB: Renal response to immunologic glomerular injury. In: Brenner BM (editor): *The Kidney,* 5th ed. Saunders, 1996.

NEPHROTIC SYNDROME

Bernard DB: Extrarenal complications of the nephrotic syndrome. Kidney Int 1988;33:1184.

Bernard DB: Nephrotic syndrome: A clinical approach. Hosp Pract 1990;25:114.

Rocher L: Diabetic nephropathy. Arch Intern Med 1990; 150:26.

Schnaper HW: The immune system in minimal change nephrotic syndrome. Pediatr Nephrol 1989;3:101.

Trompter RS: Immunosuppressive therapy in the nephrotic syndrome in children. Pediatr Nephrol 1989; 3:194.

INTERSTITIAL NEPHRITIS

Carmichael J, Shankel SW: Effects of nonsteroidal anti-inflammatory drugs on prostaglandins and renal function. Am J Med 1985;78:992.

Cooper K, Bennett WM: Nephrotoxicity of common drugs used in clinical practice. Arch Intern Med 1987;147:1213.

Eknoyan G et al: Chronic tubulo-interstitial nephritis: Correlation between structural and functional findings. Kidney Int 1990;38:736.

Hart D, Lifschitz MD: Renal physiology of the prostaglandins and the effects of nonsteroidal anti-inflammatory agents on the kidney. Am J Nephrol 1987; 7:408.

Neilson EG: Pathogenesis and therapy of interstitial nephritis. Kidney Int 1989;35:1257.

Rastegar A, Kashgarian M: The clinical spectrum of tubulointerstitial nephritis. Kidney Int 1998;54:313.

Sander DP et al: Analgesic use and chronic renal disease. N Engl J Med 1989;320:1238.

Toto RD: Acute tubulointerstitial nephritis. Am J Med Sci 1990;299:392.

CYSTIC DISEASE

Fick GM, Gabow PA: Hereditary and acquired cystic disease of the kidney. Kidney Int 1994;46:951.

Gabow PA: Autosomal dominant polycystic kidney disease. Am J Kidney Dis 1993;22:511.

Perrone RD: Extrarenal manifestations of ADPKD. Kidney Int 1997;51:2022.

Welling LW, Grantham JJ: Cystic and developmental diseases of the kidney. In: Brenner BM (editor): *The Kidney,* 5th ed., Saunders, 1996.

TUBULAR DISORDERS

Adamson MD et al: Cystinosis. Semin Nephrol 1989; 9:147.

Brenner RJ et al: Incidence of radiographically evident bone disease, nephrocalcinosis, and nephrolithiasis in various types of renal tubular acidosis. N Engl J Med 1982;307:217.

Foreman JW, Roth KS: Human renal Fanconi syndrome: Then and now. Nephron 1989;51:301.

Kurtzman NA: Disorders of distal acidification. Kidney Int 1990;38:720.

Mattern WD: Renal tubular acidosis. Kidney 1982;15: 11.

Morris RC Jr: Renal tubular acidosis. (Editorial.) N Engl J Med 1981;304:418.

Morris RC, Ives HE: Inherited disorders of the renal tubule. In: Brenner BM (editor): *The Kidney,* 5th ed., Saunders, 1996.

Segal S: Disorders of renal amino acid transport. N Engl J Med 1976;294:1044.

Stanbury JB et al (editors): *The Metabolic Basis of Inherited Disease,* 5th ed. McGraw-Hill, 1983.

Oliguria; Acute Renal Failure

35

William J.C. Amend, Jr., MD, & Flavio G. Vincenti, MD

Oliguria literally means "reduced" urine volume—less than that necessary to remove endogenous solute loads that are the end products of metabolism. As long as the patient's kidney can usually concentrate urine in a normal fashion to a specific gravity of 1.035, oliguria (for that person) is present at urine volumes under 400 mL/d, or approximately 6 mL/kg body weight. On the other hand, if the kidney concentration is impaired and the patient can achieve a specific gravity of only 1.010, oliguria is present at urine volumes under 1000–1500 mL/d.

Acute renal failure is a condition in which the glomerular filtration rate is abruptly reduced, causing a sudden retention of endogenous and exogenous metabolites (urea, potassium, phosphate, sulfate, creatinine, administered drugs) that are normally cleared by the kidneys. The urine volume is usually low (under 400 mL/d). However, if renal concentrating mechanisms are impaired during acute renal failure, the daily urine volume may be normal or even high (**high-output or nonoliguric renal failure**). Rarely, there is no urine output at all (anuria) in acute renal failure.

The causes of acute renal failure are listed in Table 35–1. Prompt differentiation of the cause is important in determining appropriate therapy. Prerenal renal failure is reversible if treated promptly, but a delay in therapy may allow it to progress to a fixed, nonspecific form of intrinsic renal failure (eg, acute tubular necrosis). The other causes of acute renal failure are classified on the basis of their involvement with vascular lesions, intrarenal disorders, or postrenal disorders.

PRERENAL RENAL FAILURE

The term **prerenal** denotes inadequate renal perfusion because of reduced intravascular volume or lowered effective arterial circulation. The most common cause of this form of acute renal failure is dehydration due to renal or extrarenal fluid losses from diarrhea, vomiting, excessive use of diuretics, and so on.

Less common causes are septic shock, "third spacing" with extravascular fluid pooling (eg, pancreatitis), and excessive use of antihypertensive drugs, which causes relative or absolute depletion of intravascular fluid volume. Heart failure with reduced cardiac output also can reduce effective renal blood flow. Careful clinical assessment may identify the primary condition responsible for prerenal renal failure, but many times several conditions can coexist. In the hospital setting, these circulatory abnormalities often lead to more fixed, acute renal failure (acute tubular necrosis), since these patients often have multiple comorbid conditions.

Acute reductions in glomerular filtration rate may also be noted in patients with cirrhosis (hepatorenal failure) or in patients taking cyclosporine, tacrolimus, nonsteroidal anti-inflammatory drugs, or angiotensin-converting enzyme inhibitors. It is felt that these conditions represent significant intrarenal hemodynamic functional derangements mediated by prostaglandins and renin-angiotensin such that the glomerular capillary pressure suddenly falls. In these clinical circumstances, the urinary findings may mimic prerenal renal failure, but the patient's clinical assessment does not demonstrate the extrarenal findings seen in common prerenal conditions, as noted in the following section. Improvements in glomerular filtration rate are usually noted after drug discontinuance or, in cases of hepatorenal renal failure, with management of the liver disease or liver transplantation.

Clinical Findings

A. Symptoms and Signs: Except for rare cases with associated cardiac or "pump" failure, patients usually complain of thirst or of dizziness in the upright posture (orthostatic dizziness). There may be a history of overt fluid loss. Weight losses over hours to days quantitatively reflect the degree of dehydration.

Physical examination frequently reveals decreased skin turgor, collapsed neck veins, dry mucous membranes and axillas, and, most important, orthostatic or postural changes in blood pressure and pulse.

Table 35–1. Causes of acute renal failure.

I. **Prerenal renal failure:**
  1. Dehydration
  2. Vascular collapse due to sepsis, antihypertensive drug therapy, "third spacing"
  3. Reduced cardiac output
II. **Functional–hemodynamic:**
  1. Angiotensin-converting enzyme inhibitor drugs
  2. Nonsteroidal anti-inflammatory drugs
  3. Cyclosporine; tacrolimus
  4. Hepatorenal syndrome
III. **Vascular:**
  1. Atheroembolism
  2. Dissecting arterial aneurysms
  3. Malignant hypertension
IV. **Parenchymal (intrarenal):**
  1. Specific:
    a. Glomerulonephritis
    b. Interstitial nephritis
    c. Toxin, dye-induced
    d. Hemolytic uremic syndrome
  2. Nonspecific:
    a. Acute tubular necrosis
    b. Acute cortical necrosis
V. **Postrenal:**
  1. Calculus in patients with solitary kidney
  2. Bilateral ureteral obstruction
  3. Outlet obstruction
  4. Leak, post-traumatic

Table 35–2. Acute renal failure versus prerenal azotemia.

	Acute Renal Failure	Prerenal Azotemia
Urine osmolarlity (mOsm/L)	< 350	> 500
Urine/plasma urea	< 10	> 20
Urine/plasma creatinine	< 20	> 40
Urine Na (mEq/L)	> 40	< 20
Renal failure index* = $\dfrac{U_{Na}}{U/P_{cr}}$	> 1	< 1
$FE_{N_a} = \dfrac{U/P_{Na}}{U/P_{Cr}} \times 100$	> 1	< 1

* Excreted fraction of filtered sodium. See Espinel CH: JAMA 1976;236:579; and Miller TR et al: Ann Intern Med 1978; 89:47.

B. Laboratory Findings:

1. Urine–The urine volume is usually low. Accurate assessment may require bladder catheterization followed by hourly output measurements (which will also rule out lower urinary tract obstruction; see discussion following). High urine specific gravity (> 1.025) and urine osmolality (> 600 mOsm/kg) also are noted in this form of acute apparent renal failure. Routine urinalysis usually shows no abnormalities.

2. Urine and blood chemistries–The blood urea nitrogen-creatinine ratio, normally 10:1, is usually increased with prerenal renal failure. Other findings are set forth in Table 35–2. Because mannitol, radiocontrast dyes, and diuretics affect the delivery and tubular handling of urea, sodium, and creatinine, urine and blood chemistry tests performed after these agents have been given produce misleading results.

3. Central venous pressure–A low central venous pressure indicates hypovolemia, which may be due to blood loss or dehydration. If severe cardiac failure is the principal cause of prerenal renal failure (it is rarely the sole cause), reduced cardiac output and high central venous pressure are apparent.

4. Fluid challenge–An increase in urine output in response to a carefully administered fluid challenge is both diagnostic and therapeutic in cases of prerenal renal failure. Rapid intravenous administration of 300–500 mL of physiologic saline or 125 mL of 20% mannitol (25 g/125 mL) is the usual initial treatment. Urine output is measured over the subsequent 1–3 h. A urine volume increase of more than 50 mL/h is considered a favorable response that warrants continued intravenous infusion with physiologic solutions to restore plasma volume and correct dehydration. If the urine volume does not increase, the physician should carefully review the results of blood and urine chemistry tests, reassess the patient's fluid status, and repeat the physical examination to determine whether an additional fluid challenge (with or without furosemide) might be worthwhile.

Treatment

In states of dehydration, measured and estimated fluid losses must be rapidly corrected to treat oliguria of prerenal origin. Inadequate fluid management may cause further renal hemodynamic deterioration and eventual renal tubular ischemia (with fixed acute tubular necrosis; see discussion following). If oliguria persists in a well-hydrated patient, vasopressor drugs are indicated in an effort to correct the hypotension associated with sepsis or cardiogenic shock. Pressor agents that restore systemic blood pressure while maintaining renal blood flow and renal function are most useful. Dopamine, 1–5 µg/kg/min, gives "renal-dose" levels providing an increase in renal blood flow without systemic pressor responses. Higher doses of 5–20 µg/kg may be necessary if systemic hypotension persists after volume correction. Discontinuance of antihypertensive medications or diuretics can, by itself, cure the apparent acute renal failure resulting from prerenal conditions.

VASCULAR RENAL FAILURE

Common causes of acute renal failure due to vascular disease include atheroembolic disease, dissecting arterial aneurysms, and malignant hypertension. Atheroembolic disease is rare before age 60 and in patients who have not undergone vascular procedures or angiographic studies. Dissecting arterial aneurysms and malignant hypertension are usually clinically evident. Acute renal venous thrombosis, unless it affects both kidneys, has no deleterious effect on renal clearance function.

Rapid assessment of the arterial blood supply to the kidney requires arteriography or other renal blood flow studies (eg, magnetic resonance imaging or Doppler ultrasound). The cause of malignant hypertension may be identified on physical examination (eg, scleroderma). Primary management of the vascular process is necessary to affect the course of these forms of acute renal failure.

INTRARENAL DISEASE STATES; INTRARENAL ACUTE RENAL FAILURE

Diseases in this category can be divided into specific and nonspecific parenchymal processes.

1. SPECIFIC INTRARENAL DISEASE STATES

The most common causes of intrarenal acute renal failure are acute or rapidly progressive glomerulonephritis, acute interstitial nephritis, toxic nephropathies, and hemolytic uremic syndrome.

Clinical Findings

A. Symptoms and Signs: Usually the history shows some salient data such as sore throat or upper respiratory infection, diarrheal illness (occasionally as epidemic), use of antibiotics, or intravenous use of drugs (often illicit types). Bilateral back pain, at times severe, is occasionally noted. Gross hematuria may be present. It is unusual for pyelonephritis to present as acute renal failure unless there is (1) associated sepsis or dehydration, (2) obstruction, or (3) involvement of a solitary kidney. Systemic diseases in which acute renal failure occurs include Henoch-Schönlein purpura, systemic lupus erythematosus, and scleroderma. Human immunodeficiency virus (HIV) infection may present with acute renal failure from HIV nephropathy. The prognosis is quite poor with this condition.

B. Laboratory Findings:

1. Urine–Urinalysis discloses variably active sediments: many red and white cells and multiple types of cellular and granular casts (telescopic urine). Phase contrast microscopy usually reveals dysmorphic red cells in the urine. In allergic interstitial nephritis, eosinophils may be noted. The urine sodium concentration may range from 10 to 40 mEq/L.

2. Blood test–Components of serum complement are often diminished during deposition of immune complexes. In a few conditions, circulating immune complexes can be identified. Other tests may disclose systemic diseases such as lupus erythematosus. Thrombocytopenia and altered red cell morphologic structure are noted in peripheral blood smears in the hemolytic uremic syndrome (HUS).

3. Renal biopsy–Biopsy examination shows characteristic changes of glomerulonephritis, acute interstitial nephritis, or glomerular capillary thrombi (in HUS). There may be extensive crescents involving Bowman's space.

C. X-Ray Findings: Poor visualization on intravenous urography or radionuclide renal scans is characteristic. Routine intravenous urography should be avoided because of the risk of dye-induced renal injury. For this reason, sonography is preferable to rule out obstruction.

Treatment

Therapy is directed toward eradication of infection, removal of antigen, elimination of toxic materials and drugs, suppression of autoimmune mechanisms, removal of autoimmune antibodies, or a reduction in effector-inflammatory responses. Immunotherapy may involve drugs, anticoagulants, or the temporary use of plasmapheresis. Initiation of supportive dialysis may be required (see discussion below).

2. NONSPECIFIC INTRARENAL STATES

Nonspecific intrarenal causes of acute renal failure include acute tubular necrosis and acute cortical necrosis. The latter presents with anuria and associated intrarenal intravascular coagulation and generally has a poorer prognosis than the former. These forms of acute renal failure usually occur in hospital settings. Various morbid conditions leading to septic syndrome–like physiologic disturbances are often present.

Acute tubular necrosis was initially described by Lücke during World War II in patients suffering crush injuries and shock. Degenerative changes of the distal tubules (lower nephron nephrosis) were believed to be due to ischemia. When dialysis became available, most of these patients recovered—sometimes completely—provided intrarenal intravascular coagulation and cortical necrosis had not occurred.

Elderly patients are more prone to develop this form of oliguric acute renal failure following hypotensive episodes. It appears that exposure to some drugs (eg, prostaglandin inhibitors such as nonsteroidal anti-inflammatory agents) may increase the risk of acute tubular necrosis. Although the classic picture of lower nephron nephrosis may not develop, a similar nonspecific acute renal failure is noted in some cases of mercury (especially mercuric chloride) poisoning and following exposure to radiocontrast agents, especially in patients with diabetes mellitus or myeloma.

Clinical Findings

A. Symptoms and Signs: Usually the clinical picture is that of the associated clinical state. Dehydration and shock may be present concurrently, but the urine output and acute renal failure fail to improve following administration of intravenous fluids, in contrast to the situation in patients who have prerenal renal failure (see preceding discussion). On the other hand, there may be signs of excessive fluid retention in patients with acute renal failure following radiocontrast exposure. Symptoms of uremia per se (eg, altered mentation or gastrointestinal symptoms) are unusual in acute renal failure (in contrast to chronic renal failure).

B. Laboratory Findings: (See also Table 35–2.)

1. Urine–Although the specific gravity may be high immediately after the acute event, it usually becomes low or fixed in the 1.005–1.015 range. Urine osmolality is also low (< 450 mOsm/kg and U/P osmolal ratio < 1.5:1). Urinalysis often discloses tubular cells and granular casts; the urine may be muddy brown. If the test for occult blood is positive, one must be concerned about the presence of myoglobin as well as hemoglobin. Tests for differentiating myoglobin pigment are available.

2. Central venous pressure–This is usually normal to slightly elevated.

3. Fluid challenges–There is no increase in urine volume following intravenous administration of mannitol or physiologic saline. Occasionally following the use of furosemide or "renal doses" of dopamine (1–5 μg/kg/min), a low urine output is converted to a high fixed urine output (low-output renal failure to high-output renal failure), but there is usually no change in the rate of increase of blood urea nitrogen or creatinine.

Treatment

If there is no response to the initial fluid or mannitol challenge, the volume of administered fluid must be sharply curtailed and the amount given related to measured fluid losses (eg, urine and gastrointestinal) and estimated insensible fluid losses. An early assessment of the rate of rise of serum creatinine and blood urea nitrogen and of the concentrations of electrolytes is necessary to predict the possible use of dialysis therapy. There is some evidence that early use of hyperalimentation might be beneficial in reducing both the need for dialysis and the morbidity and mortality. With appropriate regulation of the volume of fluid administered, solutions of glucose and essential amino acids to provide 30–35 kcal/kg are used to correct or reduce the severity of the catabolic state accompanying acute tubular necrosis.

Serum or plasma potassium must be closely monitored and serial ECGs done to ensure early recognition of hyperkalemia. This condition can be treated with (1) intravenous sodium bicarbonate administration, (2) Kayexalate, 25–50 g (with sorbitol) orally or by enema, (3) intravenous glucose and insulin, and (4) intravenous calcium preparations to prevent cardiac irritability.

Peritoneal dialysis or hemodialysis should be used as necessary to avoid or correct uremia, hypokalemia, or fluid overload. Hemodialysis in patients with acute renal failure can be either intermittent or continuous (with arteriovenous or venovenous hemofiltration techniques). Vascular access is obtained with percutaneous catheters. The continuous dialysis techniques allow for easier management in many hemodynamically unstable patients in intensive care units.

Prognosis

Most cases are reversible within 7–14 days. Residual renal damage may be noted, particularly in elderly patients.

POSTRENAL ACUTE RENAL FAILURE

The conditions listed in Table 35–1 involve primarily the need for urologic diagnostic and therapeutic interventions. Following lower abdominal surgery, urethral or ureteral obstruction should be considered as a cause of acute renal failure. The causes of bilateral ureteral obstruction are (1) peritoneal or retroperitoneal neoplastic involvement, with masses or nodes; (2) retroperitoneal fibrosis; (3) calculous disease; and (4) postsurgical or traumatic interruption. With a solitary kidney, ureteral stones can produce total urinary tract obstruction and acute renal failure. Urethral or bladder neck obstruction is a frequent cause of renal failure, especially in elderly men. Post-traumatic urethral tears are discussed in Chapter 19.

Clinical Findings

A. Symptoms and Signs: Renal pain and renal tenderness often are present. If there has been an operative ureteral injury with associated urine extravasation, urine may leak through a wound. Edema from overhydration may be noted. Ileus is often present along with associated abdominal distention and vomiting.

B. Laboratory Findings: Urinalysis is usually not helpful. A large volume of urine obtained by catheterization may be both diagnostic and therapeutic for lower tract obstruction.

C. X-Ray Findings: Poor visualization on intravenous urography is characteristic. Radionuclide renal scans may show a urine leak or, in cases of obstruction, retention of the isotope in the renal pelvis. Renal scans are helpful in acute but not in chronic obstruction. Ultrasound examination often reveals a dilated upper collecting system with deformities characteristic of hydronephrosis.

D. Instrumental Examination: Cystoscopy and retrograde ureteral catheterization demonstrate ureteral obstruction.

Treatment

For further discussion of ureteral injuries, see Chapter 19.

REFERENCES

Amend WA: Pathogenesis of hepatorenal syndrome. Trans Proc 1993;25:1730.

Bonventre JV: Mechanisms of ischemic acute renal failure. Kidney Int 1993;43:1160.

Chertow GM et al: Predictors of mortality and the provision of dialysis in patients with acute tubular necrosis. J Am Soc Nephrol 1998;9:692.

Golper TA: Indications, technical considerations and strategies for renal replacement therapies in the intensive care unit. J Intensive Care Med 1992;7:310.

Klahr S, Miller SB: Acute oliguria. N Engl J Med 1998; 338:671.

Nolan CR, Anderson RJ: Hospital-acquired acute renal failure. J Am Soc Nephrol 1998;9:710.

Olivero JJ: Postsurgical acute renal failure: Which patients are at greatest risk? J Crit Illness 1994;9:673.

Rangel-Frausto MS et al: The natural history of the systemic inflammatory response syndrome (SIRS). JAMA 1995;273:117.

Singer I, Epstein M: Potential of dopamine A-1 agonists in the management of acute renal failure. Am J Kidney Dis 1998;31:743.

Thadhani R et al: Acute renal failure. N Engl J Med 1996; 334:1448.

Wish JB, Mortiz CE: Preventing radiocontrast-induced acute renal failure. J Crit Illness 1990;5:16.

36

Chronic Renal Failure & Dialysis

William J.C. Amend, Jr., MD, & Flavio G. Vincenti, MD

In chronic renal failure, reduced clearance of certain solutes principally excreted by the kidney results in their retention in the body fluids. The solutes are end products of the metabolism of substances of exogenous origin (eg, food) or endogenous origin (eg, catabolism of tissue). The most commonly used indicators of renal failure are blood urea nitrogen and serum creatinine. However, marked elevation of blood urea nitrogen can be due to nonrenal causes such as prerenal azotemia, gastrointestinal hemorrhage, or high protein intake. The clearance of creatinine can be used as a reasonable measure of glomerular filtration rate (GFR).

Renal failure may be classified as acute or chronic depending on the rapidity of onset and the subsequent course of azotemia. An analysis of the acute or chronic development of renal failure is important in understanding physiologic adaptations, disease mechanisms, and ultimate therapy. In individual cases, it is often difficult to establish the duration of renal failure. Historical clues such as preceding hypertension or radiologic findings such as small, shrunken kidneys tend to indicate a more chronic process. Certain forms of acute renal failure tend to progress to irreversible chronic renal failure. For a discussion of acute renal failure, see Chapter 35.

The incidence of severe chronic renal failure leading to end-stage renal disease is 253 cases per million population per year. These patients require chronic dialysis or renal transplantation as renal replacement therapy. The medical acceptance criteria for dialysis and transplant are strict. All age groups are affected. The severity and the rapidity of development of uremia are hard to predict. The use of dialysis and transplantation is expanding rapidly worldwide. Over 200,000 such patients in the United States are currently treated with dialysis. A trend toward increasingly older patients has been noted. At the present time, 72,000 patients have functioning kidney transplants.

Historical Background

There are various causes of progressive renal dysfunction leading to end-stage or terminal renal failure. In the 1800s, Bright described several patients who presented with edema, hematuria, and proteinuria and ended in death. Early chemical analyses of patients' sera drew attention to retained nonprotein nitrogen (NPN) compounds, and an association was made between this and the clinical findings of uremia. Although the pathologic state of uremia was well described in the intervening years, long-term survival was not achieved in substantial numbers of patients until chronic renal dialysis and renal transplantation became available after 1960–1970. Significant improvements in patient survival have been made in the past 30 years.

Etiology

A variety of disorders are associated with end-stage renal disease. Either a primary renal process (eg, glomerulonephritis, pyelonephritis, congenital hypoplasia) or a secondary one (eg, a kidney affected by a systemic process such as diabetes mellitus or lupus erythematosus) may be responsible. Superimposed physiologic alterations secondary to dehydration, infection, or hypertension often "tip the scale" and put a borderline patient into uncompensated chronic uremia.

Clinical Findings

A. Symptoms and Signs: Symptoms such as pruritus, generalized malaise, lassitude, forgetfulness, loss of libido, nausea, and easy fatigability are frequent and nonfocal complaints in this chronic disorder. There is often a strong family history of renal disease. Growth failure is a primary complaint in preadolescent patients. Symptoms of a multisystem disorder (eg, skin rashes, pericarditis, and arthritis in lupus erythematosus) may be present coincidentally. Most patients with renal failure have elevated blood pressure secondary to volume overload and overhydration. Occasionally, hyperreninemia accounts for significant hypertension. However, the blood pressure may be normal or low if patients are on a very low sodium diet or, alternatively, have marked renal salt-losing tendencies (eg, medullary cystic disease). The pulse and respiratory rates are rapid as manifestations of anemia and metabolic acidosis. Clinical findings of uremic fetor, pericarditis, neurologic findings of asterixis, altered mentation, and peripheral neuropathy are often present. Palpable kidneys suggest polycystic disease. Ophthalmoscopic examination may show hypertensive or diabetic retinopathy. Alterations involving the cornea have been associated with metabolic disease (eg, Fabry disease, cystinosis, and Alport hereditary nephritis).

B. Laboratory Findings:

1. Urine composition–The urine volume varies depending on the severity and type of renal disease. Quantitatively normal amounts of water and salt losses in urine can be associated with polycystic and interstitial forms of disease. Usually, however, urine volumes are quite low when the GFR falls below 5% of normal. Daily salt losses become more fixed, and, if they are low, a state of sodium retention occurs soon after. Proteinuria may be variable but often is not excessive when the GFR is severely reduced. Urinalysis examinations may reveal mononuclear white blood cells (leukocytes) and occasionally broad waxy casts, but usually the urinalysis is nonspecific and inactive. There is a distal acidification defect (renal tubular acidosis, type I) in patients with chronic renal failure.

2. Blood studies–Anemia is the rule, but the hematocrit may be normal in polycystic disease. Platelet dysfunction or thrombasthenia is characterized by abnormal bleeding times. Platelet counts and prothrombin content are normal.

Several abnormalities in serum electrolytes and mineral metabolism become manifest when the GFR drops below 30 mL/min. Progressive reduction of body buffer stores and an inability to excrete titrable acids result in progressive acidosis characterized by reduced serum bicarbonate and compensatory respiratory hyperventilation. The metabolic acidosis of uremia is associated with a normal anion gap, hyperchloremia, and normokalemia. Hyperkalemia is not usually seen unless the GFR is below 5 mL/min or conditions are present that predispose to an increase in serum potassium (ie, intercurrent illness associated with increased catabolism or acute acidosis). Patients with interstitial renal diseases, gouty nephropathy, or diabetic nephropathy may develop hyperchloremic metabolic acidosis with hyperkalemia (renal tubular acidosis, type IV) even when the GFR is over 30 mL/min. In these cases the acidosis and hyperkalemia are out of proportion to the degree of renal failure and are related to a decrease in renin and aldosterone secretion. Multiple factors lead to an increase in serum phosphate and a decrease in serum calcium. The hyperphosphatemia develops as a consequence of reduced phosphate clearance by the kidney. Uremic patients have a reduced appetite and thus ingest less calcium. In addition, vitamin D activity is diminished because of reduced conversion of vitamin D_2 to the active form of vitamin D_3 in the kidney. These alterations lead to secondary hyperparathyroidism with skeletal changes of both osteomalacia and osteitis fibrosa cystica. Uric acid levels are frequently elevated secondary to reduced renal excretion but rarely lead to calculi or gout during chronic uremia.

C. X-Ray Findings: Patients with reduced renal function should not be routinely subjected to contrast studies. Important diagnostic information can be obtained through the use of ultrasonography. Renal sonograms are helpful in determining renal size and cortical thickness and in localizing tissue for percutaneous renal biopsy. Bone x-rays may show retarded growth, osteomalacia (renal rickets), or osteitis fibrosa. Soft-tissue or vascular calcification may be present.

D. Renal Biopsy: Renal biopsies may not reveal much except nonspecific interstitial fibrosis and glomerulosclerosis. There may be pronounced vascular changes consisting of thickening of the media, fragmentation of elastic fibers, and intimal proliferation, which may be secondary to uremic hypertension or due to primary arteriolar nephrosclerosis. Percutaneous or open biopsies of end-stage shrunken kidneys are associated with a high morbidity rate, particularly bleeding. However, if kidney size is still normal, a renal biopsy may be diagnostic and useful. Appropriate examination by light microscopy, immunofluorescence, and electron microscopy is also indicated.

Treatment

Management should be conservative until it becomes impossible for patients to continue their customary lifestyles. Conservative management includes restriction of dietary protein (0.5 g/kg/d), potassium, and phosphorus, as well as maintenance of close sodium balance in the diet so that patients become neither sodium-expanded nor -depleted. This is best monitored by the accurate and frequent monitoring of the patient's weight. Use of bicarbonate can be helpful when moderate acidemia occurs. Anemia can be treated with recombinant erythropoietin. Prevention of possible uremic osteodystrophy and secondary hyperparathyroidism requires close attention to calcium and phosphorus balance. Phosphate-retaining antacids and calcium or vitamin D supplements may be needed to maintain the balance. Extreme care must be paid to this treatment, however, because if the $Ca \times P$ product is greater than 65 mg/dL, metastatic calcifications can occur.

A. Chronic Peritoneal Dialysis: Chronic peritoneal dialysis is used electively or when circumstances (ie, no available vascular access) prohibit chronic hemodialysis. Improved soft catheters can be used for repetitive peritoneal lavages. In comparison to hemodialysis, small molecules (such as creatinine and urea) are cleared less effectively than larger molecules (vitamin B_{12}), but excellent treatment can be accomplished. Intermittent thrice-weekly treatment

(IPPD), continuous cycler-assisted peritoneal dialysis (CCPD), or chronic ambulatory peritoneal dialysis (CAPD) is possible. With the latter, the patient performs 3–5 daily exchanges using 1–2 L of dialysate at each exchange. Bacterial contamination and peritonitis are becoming less common with improvements in technology.

B. Chronic Hemodialysis: Chronic hemodialysis using semipermeable dialysis membranes is now widely performed. Access to the vascular system is provided by an arteriovenous fistula, vascular grafts (with saphenous vein or synthetic material), or by a subclavian permcatheter (placed either surgically or with interventional radiology). These methods all allow repetitive entrance to the vascular system. The actual dialyzers may be of a parallel plate, coil, or hollow fiber type. Body solutes and excessive body fluids can be easily cleared by using dialysate fluids of known chemical composition. Newer, high-efficiency membranes (high/flux) are serving to reduce dialysis treatment time.

Treatment is intermittent—usually 3–5 h 3 times weekly. Computer modeling, using measurements of urea kinetics, has provided more precise hemodialysis prescriptions. Treatments may be given in a kidney center, a satellite unit, or the home. Very ill patients and those who for any reason cannot be trained in the use of the equipment with an assistant require treatment in a dialysis center. Home dialysis is optimal because it provides greater scheduling flexibility and is generally more comfortable and convenient for the patient, but only 30% of dialysis patients meet the medical and training requirements for this type of therapy.

More widespread use of dialytic techniques has permitted greater patient mobility. Treatment on vacations and business trips can be provided by prior arrangement.

Common problems with either type of chronic dialysis include infection, bone symptoms, technical accidents, persistent anemia, and psychological disorders. The morbidity associated with atherosclerosis often occurs with long-term treatment. It is now recognized that chronically uremic patients, despite dialysis, can develop wasting syndrome, cardiomyopathy, polyneuropathy, and secondary dialysis-amyloidosis so that kidney transplant must be urgently done. Bilateral nephrectomy should be avoided because it increases the transfusion requirements of dialysis patients as well as the attendant morbidity and mortality from the procedure. Nephrectomy in dialysis patients should be performed in cases of refractory hypertension, reflux with infection, and polycystic disease with recurrent bleeding and pain. The dialysis patient can occasionally develop acquired renal-cystic disease. Such patients need close monitoring for the development of in situ renal cell carcinoma.

Yearly costs range from an average of $25,000 for patients who receive dialysis at home to as much as $35,000–60,000 for patients treated at dialysis centers, but much of this is absorbed under HR-1 (Medicare) legislation. If the patient has no other systemic problems (eg, diabetes) the mortality rates are 8–10%/year once maintenance dialysis therapy is instituted. Despite these medical, psychological, social, and financial difficulties, most patients lead productive lives while receiving dialysis treatment.

C. Renal Transplantation: After immunosuppression techniques and genetic matching were developed, renal homotransplantation became an acceptable alternative to maintenance hemodialysis. Improved transplantation results are now noted owing to the development of newer immunosuppressant drugs. Currently employed post-transplant drugs include prednisone, azathioprine, mycophenolate mofetil, cyclosporine, and tacrolimus. In addition, monoclonal and polyclonal antibodies are used to prevent and treat rejections. The great advantage of transplantation is reestablishment of nearly normal constant body physiology and chemistry without intermittent dialysis. Diet can be less restrictive. The disadvantages include bone marrow suppression, susceptibility to infection, cushingoid body habitus, and the psychological uncertainty of the homograft's future. Most of the disadvantages of transplantation are related to the medicines given to counteract the rejection. Later problems with transplantation include recurrent disease in the transplanted kidney. Genitourinary infection appears to be of minor importance if structural urologic complications (eg, leaks) do not occur.

Nephrology centers, with close cooperation between medical and surgical staff, attempt to use these treatment alternatives of dialysis and transplantation in an integrated fashion.

For a more detailed review, see Chapter 37.

REFERENCES

Amend W: Kidney transplant revisited. (Editorial.) West J Med 1990;152:711.

Chaimovitz C: Peritoneal dialysis. Kidney Int 1994;45: 1226.

Friedman EA: End-stage renal disease therapy, an American success story. JAMA 1996;275:118.

Hakim RM, Lazarus JM: Initiation of dialysis. J Am Soc Nephrol 1995;6:1319.

Hakim RM et al: Adequacy of hemodialysis. Am J Kidney Dis 1992;20:107.

Jacobson HR: Chronic renal failure: Pathophysiology. Lancet 1991;338:419.

Khanna R, Nolph KD: The physiology of peritoneal dialysis. Am J Nephrol 1989;9:504.

Klahr S: Chronic renal failure: Management. Lancet 1991;338:423.

Rettig RA: The social contract and the treatment of permanent kidney failure. JAMA 1996;275:1123.

US Renal Data System 1997 Annual Data Report. [Excerpts.] Am J Kidney 1997;30(Suppl 1):1.

Vanholder R, Ringoir S: Evolution of renal replacement therapy by hemodialysis: A review. J Nephrol 1991;3:199.

37

Renal Transplantation

Peter N. Bretan, Jr., MD, & Michael J. Malone, MD

Renal transplantation has become the procedure of choice and the most cost-effective strategy for the management of patients with end-stage renal disease. Although major advances have been made in both dialysis and renal transplantation in the last 10 years, current knowledge firmly supports the notion that successful renal transplant is associated with a substantial improvement in quality of life and significant reduction in morbidity and mortality from end-stage renal disease (Mathur, Bretan, and Tomlanovich, 1994). Much has changed in the last 10 years, during the so-called cyclosporine era. Today more than 10,000 renal transplants are performed annually in the United States. This number is likely to increase, but more important it is hoped that the current high rate of success will continue to improve through advances in preservation and development of more specific forms of immunosuppression. More than 5500 renal transplants have been performed at the University of California, San Francisco (UCSF). A review of this experience has documented many recent advances. Much of our philosophy regarding the surgical and medical management of renal transplant candidates and patients has evolved from this experience, as well as from the experience of other large centers, and is summarized here.

Selection & Preparation of Recipients

The causes of renal failure in the United States include: diabetes, 36%; hypertension nephrosclerosis, 30%; chronic glomerulonephritis, 24%; and autosomal dominant polycystic kidney disease, 12% (Urban Institute, 1986). Renal failure patients in the pediatric age group (< 18 years of age) have congenital urologic conditions (hydronephrosis with obstruction or congenital atrophy) as the major causes (45%) of renal failure (McEnery et al, 1992). While there are no categories of patients that are deemed untransplantable, these patients will have increased morbidity and mortality post-transplantation. Today, there are few absolute contraindications to renal transplantation, other than active infection and active malig-

nant disease. Improved graft and patient survival has led to less restrictive policies regarding the determination of candidacy for renal transplant. Usually the upper age limit for consideration of transplantation is 70 years; however, all decisions must be individualized, and patients with a life expectancy of less than 5 years probably should be maintained on dialysis. Determination of transplant candidacy depends on identification of risk factors that are associated with increased mortality and graft loss. The following risk factors define high-risk patients who require specific studies or therapies to help assess candidacy.

A. Cardiac Status: Potential transplant candidates who are at high risk for coronary artery disease (CAD), such as patients with a history of CAD, older men, or diabetics, should undergo coronary arteriography (Steinmuller, 1983). Noninvasive studies such as Doppler ultrasonography are helpful, although these tests are not reliable enough to differentiate patients with surgical correctable disease from those with high mortality risk or noncorrectable lesions (Philipson et al, 1986). In the former group mortality risks can be reduced substantially if bypass surgery is successfully accomplished (Braun et al, 1983).

B. Malignant Disease: Active malignant disease is an absolute contraindication to renal transplantation. Concurrent use of immunosuppressive drugs can enhance growth of microscopic metastases. The safe waiting period for transplantation after surgical removal of solid tumors varies and depends on the grade and stage of tumor on presentation and the associated risk of subsequent metastasis. These waiting times range from a period of 1–2 years for tumors with low metastatic potential to 5–6 years for patients at high risk. Specific risks have been determined using data from the 1993 Transplant Tumor Registry (Tables 37–1, 37–2, 37–3) (Penn, 1993). The majority of recurrences after transplantation reported by Penn occur within 2 years (Figure 37–1). Transplantation can be performed safely after removal of tumor if there has been adequate follow-up to determine whether the risk of subsequent metastasis or recurrence of disease is acceptable.

Patients with renal failure who have a prostatic nod-

Table 37–1. Pretransplant tumors: Low recurrence rates.

Type	N	Recurrence Rate (%)	Deaths
Incidental Renal	59	0(0)	0
Testicular	34	1(3)	0
Cervix	59	3(5)	2
Thyroid	39	3(8)	1
Lymphoma	29	3(10)	2

Table 37–3. Pretransplant tumors: High recurrence rates.

Type	N	Recurrence Rate (%)	Deaths
Bladder	42	11(26)	4
Sarcomas	14	4(28)	2
Melanoma	20	6(30)	6
Symptomatic renal	169	51(30)	39
Nonmelanoma skin	79	49(62)	1
Myeloma	8	7(88)	7

ule, elevated prostate-specific antigen (PSA > 4.0 ng/mL), or history of low-grade prostatic cancer (stage A1) should have a sextant prostate biopsy prior to renal transplantation. Patients with a PSA greater than 10.0 ng/mL or a positive biopsy (greater than stage A1) should probably not be considered for transplant.

C. Infection: Active infection is an absolute contraindication to transplantation. For urinary tract infections, it is important to distinguish between bacterial colonization and true tissue penetration of bacteria as noted in cystitis, pyelonephritis, or prostatitis. In the former, bacteria can be adequately treated with a 3-way Foley catheter and antibiotic bladder irrigations along with systemic antibiotics before the bladder is opened during renal transplantation. When any questions arise as to the cause of recurrent urinary tract infections in a potential transplant candidate, a full urologic evaluation should be carried out prior to renal transplantation.

Patients who have the human immunodeficiency virus (HIV) are considered to have active infection, which precludes transplantation in all cases because of the subsequent development of the acquired immunodeficiency syndrome (AIDS).

D. Systemic and Metabolic Disease: Viral hepatitis (C antibody–positive and hepatitis B antigenicity) is associated with a 2- to 3-fold increase in morbidity and mortality from progressive cirrhosis. Despite these relative contraindications, transplantation may be justified if there is no biochemical evidence of hepatic dysfunction; informed consent is obtained because of the possibility of future problems. Similarly, the activity and extent of systemic diseases such as Fabry disease, cystinosis, vasculitis, systemic lupus erythematosus, amyloidosis, and oxalosis necessitate individualized and careful assessment before a final decision on transplantation is made. The basic rationale to perform a transplant is based on an overall judgment that the benefits exceed the relative risks of subsequent complications.

E. Gastrointestinal Disease: Patients with active peptic ulcer disease should be treated appropriately; complete resolution of this process should be obtained prior to transplantation. Endoscopy can be performed just before transplantation if there is suspicion of peptic ulcer disease, and if necessary, the transplant should be postponed. Lower tract abnormality, suggested by symptoms or stools positive for occult blood, may require a sodium diatrizoate (Hypaque) enema or colonoscopy to screen for inflammatory bowel disease or occult malignant disease. Close observation is maintained after transplantation if a history of diverticulitis exists.

F. Genitourinary Tract Abnormalities: Pa-

Table 37–2. Pretransplant tumors: Intermediate recurrence rates.

Type	N	Recurrence Rate (%)	Deaths
Uterus	19	2(11)	2
Wilms	61	10(16)	8
Colon	38	8(21)	5
Prostate	21	5(21)	1
Breast	64	16(25)	13

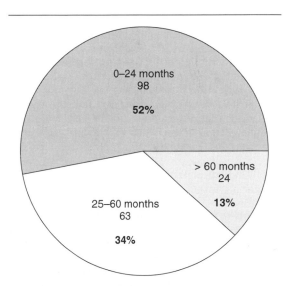

Figure 37–1. Tumor recurrences related to pretransplant treatment time. Three different waiting time periods prior to transplantation are shown, with the relative proportion of patients developing cancer recurrence after renal transplantation. Note that the longer the wait, the less likely the tumors are to recur. (Modified with permission from Penn I: The effect of immunosuppression in pre-existing cancers. Transplantation 1993;55:742.)

tients with a history of urologic dysfunction or recurrent urinary tract infections should have a voiding cystourethrogram to rule out vesicoureteral reflux and to assess lower urinary tract function. If a significant postvoid residual exists, cystourethrometry (urodynamic profile) may be required to rule out spastic bladder or bladder neck, sphincteric, and urethral obstruction. Vesicoureteral reflux greater than grade 3 (hydronephrosis) may require bilateral nephrectomy. When high-grade (> 3) reflux exists with a small noncompliant bladder, augmentation may be required to create a low-pressure urinary reservoir. Ileal conduits have been performed for urinary drainage of a renal transplant when the bladder is not repairable or usable, with acceptable results (MacGregor et al, 1986; Hatch et al, 1993); nevertheless, bladder augmentation may provide a better quality of life. For example, an internal reservoir is often preferred to an external appliance. In addition, supravesical urinary diversion in males is associated with a 20% incidence of subsequent pyocystitis. Internal continent urinary reservoirs made up of portions of stomach, ileum, and colon have been used to augment the bladder. Each method has an inherent and specific complication profile (Gold et al, 1992), and routine use has been questioned (Churchill et al, 1993). The native dilated ureter has been used to augment the bladder. The procedure of augmentation native ureterocystoplasty has been used to augment neurogenic bladders in preparation for transplantation (Koyle et al, 1994). Since nephrectomy is often required for recurrent pyelonephritis from high-grade reflux associated with neurogenic bladder, this procedure can be done instead and seems ideal for these pathologic processes, avoiding the complications that occur when the gastrointestinal tract is used.

G. Distal Urinary Obstruction: Incomplete urethral strictures or prostatic hypertrophy can be surgically corrected post-transplantation. The production of urine post-transplantation in these patients, who often have had anuric renal failure in the past, diminishes the incidence of bladder neck contracture and subsequent stenosis. In addition, although the full recovery of detrusor function after transplantation may require some time, it is expected in the majority of cases. During this interim period of adaptation, the patient can be maintained on intermittent clean straight catheterization, or with a suprapubic tube.

H. Acquired Renal Cystic Disease (ARCD) and Risk of Renal Cell Carcinoma (RCCa): Chronic renal failure has been shown to be a significant risk factor in the development of ARCD and RCCa (Sasagawa, Terasawa, and Sekino, 1992; Bretan et al, 1986). ARCD is a bilateral and premalignant state with up to 45% of cases developing in patients who have had renal failure for longer than 3 years. Of the patients who have ARCD, 20% will develop renal tumors, with an overall metastatic rate of 1–2%. Baseline ultrasonography is used to screen for RCCa pretransplantation in patients with end-stage renal disease. This screening should be carried out in those with single high-risk factors (flank pain, history of renal mass, or gross hematuria) or those with double (any 2) moderate-risk factors (ARCD with increasing size, more than 4 years of dialysis, male sex, or questionable renal mass) (Levine, 1992). Questionable renal masses should be followed periodically with radiologic screening (computed tomography is preferred), and established renal masses should be removed via radical nephrectomy.

I. Peritoneal Dialysis (PD): PD catheters can be removed in most living related transplant recipients just after completion of the transplant, during the same anesthesia. We delay removal of PD catheters in many recipients of cadaveric renal transplants, especially in those with delayed graft function or with high immunologic risk factors. If PD is required, we have performed it immediately postoperatively. After renal function has returned, the PD catheter can be removed without difficulty (1–8 weeks postoperatively, and often under local anesthesia).

J. Pretransplant Bilateral Native Kidney Nephrectomy: Native kidney nephrectomies are seldom required pretransplantation. Common indications include pyelonephritis, medically uncontrolled renin-mediated hypertension, malignant disease, and nephrotic syndrome. In selected patients, kidneys causing hypertension can be ablated using percutaneous angiographically induced embolization. Other, less common indications are extremely large polycystic kidneys and immunologically active disease. The most direct approach is through the anterior subcostal (chevron) incision, though small kidneys may be removed via a dorsal approach. For patients with bilateral high-grade vesicoureteral reflux, a thorough examination of the bladder should be conducted to assess the need for augmentation. If this is required, the procedure of choice is use of both native dilated ureters as augmentation vascularized patch grafts. The availability of synthetic erythropoietin diminishes the validity of old arguments to leave problematic and symptomatic native kidneys in situ.

K. Transplant Allograft Nephrectomy: It often is not necessary, for patients undergoing retransplantation, to remove a failed, chronically rejected but asymptomatic allograft if the contralateral side can be used as an implant site. Prognosis in the retransplant patient is strongly associated with the time period in which the primary graft was lost. If loss is secondary to rejection within 6 months of the first transplant, the success rate is greatly diminished compared with the rate in those who have lost kidneys more than 6 months after the initial transplant. Indications for allograft nephrectomy include acute rejection while on dialysis, fevers, gross hematuria, myalgias consistent with systemic inflammation and reaction, malaise, graft tenderness, infection, and uncontrolled hypertension. The subcapsular allograft nephrectomy is the safest approach to prevent iliac vessel injury.

SELECTION OF DONORS

Types of Donors

A. Living Related Donors (LRDs): The potential donor must be free of any condition that could increase the risk of any complication from the operation, diminish the function of the remaining kidney, or change their baseline quality of life. First-order LRDs continue to provide significantly higher success rates in renal transplantation than cadaveric donors. When strict policies are enforced to ensure that only medically suitable donors are selected, long-term studies of these patients (up to 45 years of follow-up) have consistently demonstrated that donation can be performed with acceptable perioperative morbidity, no renal compromise, and negligible perioperative mortality (Dunn et al, 1986; Torres, Offord, and Anderson, 1987; Bohannon, Norman, and Barry, 1987; Williams, Oler, and Jorkasky, 1986; Narkun-Burgess et al, 1993).

Current allograft half-life is more than 10 years greater for LRD transplants than for cadaveric donor transplants (13.4 versus 8.2 years) (Yuge and Burgos, 1992). Cyclosporine-treated human leukocyte antigen (HLA)-mismatched (1-haplotype) recipients of transplants from LRDs enjoy similar graft and patient survival to that of recipients of HLA-identical (2-haplotype, or haploididentical) LRD transplants (Leivestad et al, 1986). Thus LRD continues to be a valuable and important resource for transplantation not only because of the superior results, but also because of the growing shortage of cadaver organs.

B. Living-Unrelated Donors (LURDs): There has been increasing use of LURDs as an important method to circumvent the worldwide shortage of organs; published reports of 1-year graft survival in recipients of these kidneys range from 83% to 93%. However, donor selection standards are often not stated. Physicians in underdeveloped countries have used kidneys from total strangers who were paid for their donation; poor donor patient survival times (71–85% at 1 year) and graft survival times (63–82% at 1 year) are reported. In addition, there were 5 cases of HIV transmission to recipient patients in this study population (Daar and Sells, 1990). Thus overt commercialism of human organ tissues and transplantation is unacceptable. LURD should be considered only when medically and ethically appropriate. It is medically acceptable if better results can be expected compared with cadaveric renal transplantation. It is ethically appropriate if an enduring relationship between the donor and recipient exists, such as in spousal donation. Any compromise of these minimum standards regarding LURD would hurt the spirit of altruism of organ donation and would be detrimental to all aspects of renal transplantation. When these criteria are used, the results of LURD transplants continue to be superior regarding graft and patient survival to those of transplants from cadaveric donors, and are equivalent to the results in LRD transplants. The excellent physiologic quality (no preservation or ischemic injury) of these kidneys is one of the major factors responsible for these outstanding results (Wyner et al, 1993; Park et al, 1990; Pirsch, 1990).

C. Cadaver Donors: Cadaver donors should not have any generalized disease that could adversely affect renal vascular integrity or perfusion, such as chronic hypertension, diabetes, malignant disease (with significant metastatic potential), or infections (Khauli, 1986). In older donors (> 60 years of age) or in those with questionable or minimal systemic disease (eg, hypertension), a renal biopsy should be considered. A biopsy finding of significant glomerulosclerosis (> 10–20%), intimal hyperplasia, interstitial fibrosis, tubular atrophy, or evidence of disseminated intravascular coagulopathy, renders the donor suboptimal to unacceptable. Any member of a group at high risk for HIV is not an acceptable donor. Hemodynamically stable, heart-beating donors are preferred to prevent hypotension-induced oliguria and subsequent acute tubular necrosis (ATN). Young adult donors are much more resistant to ATN, and every attempt to use organs from that age group should be made. Donors between 2 and 60 years of age are associated with the highest success rates. Donors younger than 2 years of age can be successfully used if induction antibody immunotherapy is instituted in conjunction with a policy to minimize donor-recipient size differences. At UCSF we have used pediatric donor kidneys (< 2 years of age or < 14 kg) either en bloc (Bretan et al, 1992), or as single kidneys (Bretan, Banafsche, and Garovoy, 1994), with excellent results when adhering to specific immunosuppressive protocols.

Procedures for Donors

A. Donor Pretreatment: Cadaveric donor pretreatment principles are simple yet often are difficult to institute properly. The difficulty often arises in the interim period in which a ventilator-dependent "brain-dead" patient is going through the final process of aggressive neurologic management prior to being established as an irreversible, global, brain-dead patient. At this time, fluid often is restricted in order to prevent cerebral edema. In addition, the majority (74%) of patients with isolated central nervous system pathology develop diabetes insipidus (Keogh et al, 1988), causing a relative diuresis that can lead to systemic hypotension and subsequent renal shutdown. The importance of adequate hydration and volume status of donors preharvest is underscored by the great variability of recipient ATN rates worldwide (5–50%), which may reflect the fact that donor situations and pretreatment managements are not as standardized as are harvest and transplant techniques.

B. Blood Transfusion: Historically, recipient blood transfusions produced a positive effect on subsequent graft survival; however, in the postcyclosporine and synthetic erythropoietin era it is evident that the degree of benefit from donor-specific or third-party transfusions depends on the efficacy of the posttransplant immunosuppressive regimen. In our experience, pretransplant third-party blood transfusions had a positive effect on recipients treated with cyclosporine and prednisone. However, no effect was noted in the more intensively immunosuppressed sequential therapy group (Melzer and Salvatierra, 1987). Additionally, results reported by investigators from Houston demonstrated no difference in allograft success in 200 transfused compared with 100 untransfused renal recipients (Kerman, 1987; Flechner et al, 1986; Kahan, 1987).

In addition to transmitting viral hepatitis and cytomegalovirus, a blood transfusion may lead to sensitization and render less likely the chance of achieving a negative cross-match for potential transplant recipients. For this reason, blood transfusions will continue to play a minor role in future immunosuppressive protocols for living donor and cadaveric renal recipients.

C. HLA Tissue Matching: The strong positive correlation between histocompatibility matching for A, B, and DR locus antigens and allograft survival has been widely accepted for LRD renal transplants. With first-degree relatives (sibling, parent, and offspring), there is a consistent inherited homogeneity to these antigen histocompatibility complexes found on the sixth chromosome, and thus matching these loci in closely related individuals implies matching for most of the whole chromosome (haplotype).

HLA matching is more difficult in cadavers and unrelated donor populations because of the greater heterogeneity in these groups compared with living related donors. Results of matching these loci in cadaver renal transplants have been less impressive, and the clinical effects on allograft survival continue to be controversial. Single centers report both favorable (Takiff et al, 1988; Leivestad, Berger and Thorsby, 1992; Gjertson and Terasaki, 1991; Opelz, 1992) and nonsignificant (Matas et al, 1990; Hayes et al, 1993) influences on HLA (ABDR) matching. Nevertheless, it is generally accepted based on overwhelming experience that 6-antigen (6-AG)-matched kidneys have superior results compared with other, less well matched kidneys (Takemoto, Carnahan, and Terasaki, 1990). The United Network of Organ Sharing (UNOS) 6-AG-matched or zero-mismatched program reports an 87% 1-year graft survival and 13-year half-life compared with 79% graft survival and 7-year half-life in controls. In addition, there are fewer rejection episodes noted per patient with these matched recipients.

We analyzed our results with shared 6-AG and other ABDR-matched cadaveric renal recipients to determine the clinical influences of HLA matching. The outcome was determined in all cadaveric renal transplants performed (N = 1420) between January 1984 and September 1992 at UCSF in the cyclosporine era. The HLA-matched groups studied were 6-AG (57), 2-DR (133), 1-DR (418), and 0-DR (734). HLA matching had a significant inverse impact on *rejection episodes.* The mean number of rejection episodes per patient (Figure 37–2) was significantly different for the 6-AG (*P* < .008) and 2-DR (*P* < .03) groups when each was compared with the 1- and 0-DR matched groups. Overall, HLA matching had a positive and significant (*P* < .05) impact on graft survival (Figure 37–3). Thus in our experience, 6-AG-matched kidney recipients had superior graft survival (92% 1-year graft survival) and significantly fewer rejection episodes. This result supports previous reports recommending continuation of the mandatory UNOS national sharing program. DR matching had a positive graded effect on graft survival and was associated with diminution of rejection episodes; this finding also was significant but to a lesser extent. Nevertheless, DR matching should be strongly considered in the allocation of organs within a local region. On the national level, the beneficial effect of less than perfect (6-AG) matching would be offset by the increase in preservation time incurred in attempting to match these recipients with donor organs that are a long distance away.

Extracorporeal Renal Preservation

A. Simple Hypothermic Storage and Flush Solutions: Kidneys for transplantation can be stored using preservation methods of simple cold storage or continuous hypothermic pulsatile perfusion. These methods and indications have been previously described in detail (Bretan, 1989). The most commonly used method is simple cold (hypothermic) storage. In

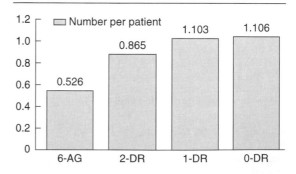

Figure 37–2. Impact of human leukocyte antigen (HLA) matching on rejection episodes. HLA matching had a significant inverse impact on subsequent rejection episodes. The mean number of rejection episodes per patient is significantly less for 6-AG (*P* < .008) and 2-DR (*P* < .03) matched groups than for the 1 + 0-DR matched groups. UCSF Renal Transplant Registry data. (N =1420 cadaver kidneys.) Time period 1984–1992.

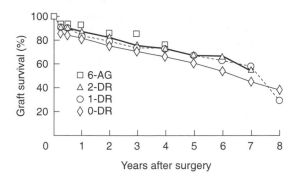

Figure 37–3. Impact of human leukocyte antigen (HLA) matching on graft survival. HLA matching had a positive and significant impact on graft survival, (*P* < .04). UCSF Renal Transplant Registry data. (N = 1420 cadaver kidneys.) Time period 1984–1992.

this method, the kidneys are removed from the donor and flushed out immediately with cold preservation solution. For most living donor kidneys, an extracellular (lactated Ringer's) solution can be used, since the total cold ischemia time (CIT) is minimal (1–3 h). Longer CITs require an intracellular solution to prevent cell swelling, which is caused by free water moving into the cells. To counteract this effect, high-osmotic solutions are used. Currently, the most popular cold storage flush solution is University of Wisconsin solution (UW-1). Since the advent of UW-1 solution, liver preservation has improved significantly. Because 80% of all organ donors are combined multiple organ donors (eg, liver, kidney and pancreas), UW-1 is now the preferred flush and storage preservation solution for abdominal organs and thus is preferred for the majority of cadaveric kidneys.

B. Pulsatile Perfusion: Pulsatile perfusion is most commonly used for kidneys of questionable viability; however, its use is limited to fewer than 20% of all kidneys because of the distribution and transportation disadvantages associated with sharing kidneys stored and the required bulky machinery needed for this technique (Barry et al, 1980; Gregg et al, 1986; Halloran and Aprile, 1987).

C. Results: Viability is consistently good with either method if the transplantation is performed prior to 24 h of CIT. With total preservation times of greater than 48 h, concerns arise because of a significant increase in the incidence of ATN and delayed renal function. Kidneys with prolonged delayed function are susceptible to undiagnosed rejection episodes, because the functional clinical renal parameters that are usually monitored in immediately functioning kidneys to assess and treat allograft rejection properly are not present. In our experience, cadaver kidneys transplanted within total preservation times of less than 24 h have significantly better graft survival (*P* < .04) than kid-

neys with CITs greater than 24 h (Figure 37–4). This experience is from the cyclosporine era of 1984–1992 and represents clinical experience with 1420 cadaver kidneys. Other major registries have validated our experience with reports that diminished graft survival is strongly associated with prolonged preservation time (Opelz, 1986). Much research progress has been made in developing and understanding new renal preservation maneuvers during simple cold storage (Bretan et al, 1991; Bretan, 1994; Bretan, Paul, and Sharma, 1993). It is hoped that continued progress not only will decrease the incidence of delayed function in suboptimally preserved kidneys, but also will translate to increased graft survival.

Donor Nephrectomy

As previously discussed, the best results in renal transplantations are obtained by using highly screened, healthy living donors. Nevertheless, there exists a chronic shortage of organs, and transplantation using cadaveric donors not only is a suitable alternative, but is the most common (> 70% of all renal transplants) method for renal transplantation in the world today.

A. Living Donors:

1. Evaluation–In addition to the rationales previously delineated, potential living donors are primarily identified on the basis of the ABO blood group compatibility, optimum HLA typing, and preliminary serologic cross-matching. The general health of the living donor is assessed, and if it is acceptable, renal function is quantified. Subsequently, excretory urography and renal arteriography are performed to assess the urologic and vascular status of the donor's kidneys. The donor is always left with the better kidney. If the kidneys are equal and symmetric, the left kidney is preferred for transplantation

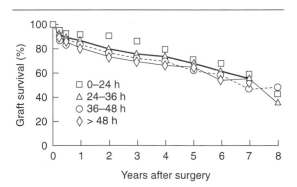

Figure 37–4. Impact of cold ischemia time (CIT) on graft survival. There was a significant (*P* < .04) increase in graft survival in kidney transplants with a total CIT of less than 24 h, compared with those with a CIT greater than 24 h. UCSF Renal Transplant Registry data. (N = 1420 cadaver kidneys.) Time period 1984–1992.

because of an associated longer renal vein. The patient is hydrated intravenously overnight preoperatively. Mannitol (up to 25–50 g) and fluid boluses are administered intraoperatively to ensure continuous diuresis.

2. Surgical technique—While multiple approaches for living donor nephrectomy have been described, the most commonly used approach is the extraperitoneal flank approach via a superior 11th or 12th rib incision (Streem and Bretan, 1992). Based on preoperative arteriography, multiple vessels are usually avoided, as most people (> 60%) have a single renal artery at least on one side. Nevertheless, bilateral multiple renal arteries are encountered, and reconstruction can be performed during hypothermic conditions (cold bench surgery) by the recipient transplant surgeon to simplify the final in situ donor-to-recipient arterial anastomosis. Reconstruction of double or triple vessels can be revascularized end-to-side to the largest artery. Smaller upper pole arteries (< 2 mm) often can be sacrificed, while the lower pole vessels cannot because of a risk to the ureteral blood supply.

B. Cadaver Donors: The donor patient is declared brain dead, usually by 2 independent physicians designated by the referring hospital. Family consent is obtained for organ donation. Since the majority (80%) of all donors are multiple organ donors, they require removal of the liver, and often the heart and pancreas, in addition to the kidneys. The retrieval is often performed by a combination of a liver and a heart procurement team. Occasionally, there is a separate renal procurement team. These principles of immediate in situ flush do not change for kidney-only donors; however, the dissection is less extensive depending on the habitus of the patient.

Technique of Transplantation

Either iliac fossa is acceptable for the transplant. However, the right external iliac vessels are more nearly horizontal with respect to each other, and this facilitates the anastomoses, making the right side the preferred choice. A lower quadrant curvilinear incision is made, and the iliac vessels are exposed through a retroperitoneal approach.

The renal-to-iliac-vein anastomosis is usually performed first, in an end-to-side fashion with 5-0 permanent monofilament. No heparin is needed. For the end-to-end arterial anastomosis, the internal iliac artery is isolated and transected. In men with a compromised bilateral internal iliac artery, such as in diabetes, the development of impotence postoperatively is common, because vascular insufficiency to the corpus cavernosum is exacerbated. Thus, patients with these risk factors should not undergo internal iliac anastomoses. Because of these factors, we prefer an end-to-side anastomosis of the renal artery to the external iliac artery.

An extravesical ureteroneocystostomy (often the

Gregoir-Lich technique) is the preferred method to reimplant the transplant ureter. This technique does not require a large vesicotomy as does the traditional Politano-Leadbetter ureteral reimplant procedure. In addition to being faster, the Lich implant procedure is associated with less obstruction.

Immediate Pretransplant & Post-Transplant Care

Preoperative and postoperative care can be divided into surgical and immunosuppressive issues. Immunosuppressive regimens are discussed in the following section.

Preoperative surgical assessment is obtained prior to the patient's pretransplant admission to the hospital for a potential cadaveric renal transplant as an extensive outpatient evaluation to determine transplant candidacy. Cardiac evaluation is necessary in many patients with end-stage renal failure; it should be performed earlier as an outpatient assessment. Central venous pressures should be kept at the high end of normal to maintain adequate preload (normal range 1–11 cm water), and urine output is replaced milliliter for milliliter. Urine outputs greater than 1 mL/kg/h are desirable, and low-dose dopamine (2–3 µg/kg/min) is used routinely. If these parameters are met and urine output is poor, other factors must be taken into consideration. Extended cold preservation or warm ischemia times predispose to ATN in the immediately postoperative period and should be anticipated. Nevertheless, technical problems also must be considered. A Doppler ultrasound study is the most convenient test; it can confirm anastomotic patency indirectly via graft blood flow and determine whether ureteral dilation is present. Fluid overload can cause pulmonary edema; this situation can be prevented if furosemide (Lasix) is given in the immediate postoperative period when central venous pressures are excessively high (> 14 cm water).

Many transplant patients have baseline ultrasound and renal scintiphotography performed in the first few days postoperatively. Information from these 2 studies is overlapping and confirmatory. Information ascertained on ultrasound includes vascular patency, presence of ureteral obstruction or hydronephrosis, lymphocele formation, and indirect evidence of rejection. Common ultrasound findings with acute rejection include graft swelling, increased vascular resistivity (resistive index > 70%), pelvi-infundibular thickening, reduced sinus fat, and prominent medullary pyramids. Renal scintiphotography using Tc-99m mercaptoacetyltriglycerine (^{99m}Tc-MAG-3) has largely supplanted the ^{131}I-orthoiodohippurate scan (O'Malley, Ziessman, and Chantarapitak, 1993). This scan gives important information on blood flow and renal function. Allograft uptake, accumulation, clearance, and excretion of isotope can be used to assess renal function and help differentiate pathologic states such as rejection, ATN, and hydronephrosis. The Bretan scale evaluates overall renal allograft function based on these specific renal isotope criteria (Zaki et al, 1990). This simple and accurate method for grading post-transplant renal function by renal isotope scan is as follows:

- Grade 0—no uptake
- Grade 1—can define kidney outline, no excretion, and no peak accumulation
- Grade 2—excretion with no peak accumulation
- Grade 3—excretion, delayed peak accumulation, and delayed clearance
- Grade 4—excretion, normal peak accumulation, and delayed clearance
- Grade 5—excretion, normal peak accumulation, and normal clearance

Increase in grade by renal scan correlated well with the subsequent clinical function of the graft. For example, a grade between 0 and 1 predicted dialysis requirements for the first week post-transplant in more than 77% of the patients (grade 2, 50%; grade 3, 19%). Grades 4 and 5 predicted no dialysis requirement for delayed function (Figure 37–5).

Transplant Immunobiology & Rejection

Transplantation antigens are glycoproteins expressed on the surface of an individual's cells. Every individual has a unique set of inherited transplant antigens—the **human leukocyte antigens (HLA)**—which are genetically encoded on chromosome 6.

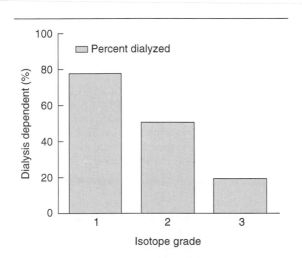

Figure 37–5. Relation between isotope grade and dialysis dependence. Bretan Scale of Renal Isotope grades on first postoperative day. The higher the grade, the less likely dialysis will be required after transplantation. (N = 138.) (Reproduced, with permission, from Zaki SK et al: A simple and accurate grading system for orthoiodohippurate renal scans in the assessment of post-transplant renal function. J Urol 1990;143:1099.)

Each parent contributes one HLA-containing chromosome to the offspring. The HLA of each parent is co-expressed in the offspring. The purpose of these antigens is to help the body recognize what is self and what is not. In this manner, bacteria and other pathogens harmful to the individual can be sensed as nonself and destroyed by the immune system. When an organ is transplanted between unrelated people (allotransplantation), that organ is recognized as nonself because of unrecognized HLA, and can be destroyed; thus, the phenomenon of rejection. In the same fashion, organs transplanted between identical twins are recognized as self and not rejected. The first successful human transplant took advantage of this premise—the kidney was transplanted between identical twins.

Three types of rejection may take place in renal transplant patients: hyperacute, acute, and chronic. Hyperacute rejection is analogous to a blood transfusion reaction, as it is a humoral response mediated by preformed recipient antibodies against the HLA expressed on the donor renal vascular endothelium. To have these preformed antibodies, the recipient must be sensitized by either a previous blood transfusion, a previous pregnancy, or a previous transplant. All potential recipients are screened for these antibodies preoperatively by placement of donor lymphocytes with recipient serum. If this cross-match is positive, ie, antibodies are present in the recipient serum against the donor HLA, transplant surgery is contraindicated. Clinically, hyperacute rejection is seen as soon as blood flow to the donor kidney is established. The graft turns from white to a mottled bluish black and should be removed immediately. Hyperacute rejection is rarely (1:1000) observed because of current sensitive cross-match screening.

Acute rejection occurs in the first weeks to months after transplant. The most common differential diagnosis includes ATN and ureteral obstruction. Interleukin-2 inhibitor (cyclosporine or tacrolimus) toxicity can occur, but it remains a diagnosis of exclusion. Approximately 25–55% of patients have an episode of acute rejection after renal transplantation, with 5–12% having 2 or more (Sutherland et al, 1993; Pirsch et al, 1992; Cecka, Cho, and Terasaki, 1992; Frey et al, 1992; Hayes, 1993). Most episodes of acute rejection can be treated successfully with immunosuppressive drugs, although in a minority of cases the graft is lost secondary to unrelenting and severe acute rejection (< 10%) (Basadonna et al, 1993; Tesi et al, 1993; Bertolatus, 1992).

The T lymphocyte is the main cell involved in this process. Receptors found on the T lymphocyte cell surface (T-cell receptor–CD3 complex) are stimulated by foreign transplantation antigens (HLA) found on allotransplants. Other cell surface antigens found on T cells are CD2, CD4, CD8, and CD25 receptors. With T-cell stimulation, a cascade of events is initiated. Intimately involved with this cascade is interleukin-1 production by donor and recipient antigen-presenting cells and interleukin-2 production by recipient T-helper-lymphocyte CD4+ cells. In this milieu, class II–stimulated CD4+ cells undergo clonal expansion. Recipient CD8+ cytotoxic cells, stimulated by foreign class I antigens, cause graft destruction in the presence of interleukin-2. Clinically, patients with acute rejection may be febrile and have tenderness over the graft; however, these signs and symptoms are often absent, and suspicion arises only because of worsening renal function. Although rejection can be diagnosed clinically in many patients, the gold standard is renal biopsy, which is performed in most patients prior to treatment of steroid-resistant acute rejection (Pozniak, Dodd, and Kelcz, 1992; Delaney et al, 1993; Olsen et al, 1989). With the advent of cyclosporine, more than 80% of cadaveric and 90% of living related allografts are functioning after 1 year (Sutherland et al, 1993; Pirsch et al, 1992; Cecka, Cho, and Terasaki, 1992; Frey et al, 1992; Hayes, 1993).

Chronic rejection is defined as a process of gradual, progressive decrease in renal function that cannot be attributed to another cause. Other causes of graft dysfunction such as acute rejection, infection, or obstruction uropathy must be excluded before this diagnosis is made. Unlike the cases of hyperacute and acute rejection, the underlying immune mechanism of chronic rejection is not well understood. Chronic rejection is the single most important cause of late graft failure, with an attrition rate of approximately 5–7% per year after the first year in cadaveric kidney recipients. Thus, although 1-year cadaveric graft survival is greater than 80%, at 5 years graft survival has dropped to 60% (Hayes, 1993; Pirsch et al, 1992; Gray and Kasiske, 1992). Factors implicated in chronic rejection include donor source, incidence and timing of acute rejection, post-transplant infections, ischemic renal injury, suboptimal immunosuppression, and noncompliance with drug therapies. There is no known treatment for chronic rejection, and many patients in the late transplant period return to dialysis treatment. Investigation of the cause, pathogenesis, and treatment of chronic rejection remains a high priority in transplant research.

Immunosuppression

As discussed, hyperacute rejection is mediated by antibodies and is rarely encountered with the use of current screening techniques (cross-matching). The exact mechanisms responsible for chronic rejection have not been elucidated, although research is increasing in this area. Immunosuppressive therapy has focused, therefore, on preventing or reversing acute rejection. Although a significant proportion of renal transplant patients have at least one episode of acute rejection despite maintenance immunosuppression, these episodes are usually reversible.

Immunosuppressive agents can be used in one of three ways: (1) as an induction agent used immedi-

ately after transplantation, (2) for maintenance immunosuppressive therapy initiated once serum creatinine has normalized, or (3) for treatment of acute rejection.

Azathioprine, a purine analog was discovered to have immunosuppressive effects in the early 1960s and, along with steroids, has been the mainstay of most immunosuppressive regimens. Azathioprine and its metabolites are incorporated into DNA and inhibit cell mitosis and proliferation. The major complication associated with this drug is bone marrow suppression exemplified by leukopenia. Other rapidly dividing cells, such as activated lymphocytes, are also susceptible. Azathioprine acts in the proliferative phase of the immune response and thus is useful for induction and maintenance immunotherapy. It is not useful as therapy for an acute rejection episode.

Corticosteroids also have been used since the early 1960s. They have a diverse array of immunosuppressive and anti-inflammatory effects, inducing inhibition of interleukin-1 release for antigen-presenting cells. Because of this, the overall effect of corticosteroids is nonspecific, and secondary complications are common, especially with prolonged high-dose therapy. Steroids are used for induction, maintenance immunosuppression, and acute rejection episodes.

Cyclosporine A was introduced into clinical use approximately in the year 1978. It was isolated from a soil fungus and was shown to have a lymphocyte-specific immunosuppressive effect. Because of its specific immunosuppressive effect, it helps decrease the therapeutic steroid dose required (steroid-sparing effect) and diminishes complications associated with nonspecific steroid immunosuppression. The drug appears to inhibit gene transcription for interleukin-2 production and other genes required for proliferation (calcineurin inhibition) and differentiation of the T lymphocyte. Cyclosporine is used for maintenance immunotherapy but is not effective in reversing acute rejection. Because of its deleterious effect on renal blood flow, cyclosporine often is not used for induction in the United States. Oral cyclosporine is usually started once serum creatinine has normalized. There are 2 oral forms, standard (Sandimmune [Novartis]) and microemulsion (Neoral [Novartis] and Sang-35 [Sang Stat Medical Corporation]). The latter has better absorption profiles, leading to an increased area-under-the-curve (AUC) pharmacokinetics and better immunosuppression. Cyclosporine revolutionized the field of solid organ transplants; 1-year cadaveric renal allograft survival increased from 50% to nearly 90% after its introduction.

Antilymphocyte/antithymocyte globulins (ALG/ATG) were developed in the early 1960s as potential immunosuppressive agents. They are xenoantibodies produced by immunizing laboratory animals with human lymphocytes. The animal sera are pooled and the polyclonal globulin fraction is purified. Undesired antibodies against platelets, neutrophils, and erythrocytes are greatly diminished by immunoabsorption techniques. Antilymphocyte/antithymocyte globulin is used both for induction and for reversing acute rejection episodes. Because of significant side effects, it is not useful for maintenance therapy.

OKT3 is a murine monoclonal antibody specific for the CD3 portion of the T-lymphocyte-receptor complex. It was developed as a specific immunosuppressive agent against T lymphocytes. OKT3 appears to modulate the T-cell-receptor complex, inhibiting the ability of lymphocytes to recognize alloantigen. Similar to ALG/ATG, OKT3 is used only for induction therapy and for acute rejection. ALG/ATG and OKT3 are effective in reversing steroid-resistant rejection.

New Antibody Immunotherapy

New DNA technology has been used to help alleviate some of the clinical problems associated with the use of both monoclonal (OKT3) and polyclonal (ALG/ATG) antilymphocyte antibodies as previously described. For example, both chimeric (basiliximab; Simulect [Novartis]) and humanized (daclizumab; Xenapac [Roche]) monoclonal antibodies have been generated against specific T-cell surface proteins (CD3 receptors). By reducing xenogenic epitomes, a decrease in development of antixenogenic antibodies and thus serum sickness is achieved. Clinical phase 3 studies show that these new monoclonal antibodies appear to decrease acute rejection without toxicity; thus they are likely to replace polyclonal antibodies currently used for sequential immunotherapy.

FK506 (tacrolimus; ProGraft [Fujisawa Healthcare, Inc]) is an immunosuppressive agent discovered recently. It has similar properties and modes of action to cyclosporine. It also suppresses interleukin-2 production from the CD4+ cells. The experience with FK506 in kidney transplant patients indicates similar efficacy to cyclosporine A. Like cyclosporine, FK506 is used for maintenance immunosuppression therapy. There is some evidence that FK506 may rescue grafts undergoing rejection when substituted for cyclosporine.

Rapamycin (sirolimus, rapamune) is another new immunosuppressive agent that blocks the effect of interleukin-2. Unlike FK506 and cyclosporine, rapamycin does not seem to be nephrotoxic. Early findings indicate that rapamycin can be combined with cyclosporine and that there may be some synergy between them. Clinical phase 1 and 2 studies have been initiated in the United States.

Mycophenolate mofetil (Cellcept [Roche]) is an antimetabolite drug that inhibits the synthesis of purines. Its effect is different from and more lymphocyte-specific than that of azathioprine. It has undergone clinical trials in the last 3–5 years. Initial results are favorable for its use in induction and maintenance immunotherapy with an associated decrease in acute rejection rate (first year post-transplantation) of almost 50%.

Current immunosuppressive regimens vary according to center preference and requirements of ongoing clinical trials. Most institutions in the United States use a combination of prednisone, an antimetabolite, with or without anti-CD3 or -CD25 antibodies for induction immunosuppression. This regimen avoids the deleterious effect of induction cyclosporine or FK506 on early graft function. At UCSF, methylprednisolone (7 mg/kg) and azathioprine (4 mg/kg) are given intraoperatively for primary first-time living related renal transplant recipients. Oral cyclosporine (5 mg/kg/12 h) or tacrolimus (0.1 mg/kg/12 h) is started the next day and titrated to therapeutic levels of 200–250 µg/L or 10–15 µg/L, respectively (HPLC assay). Cadaveric recipients with expected ATN or delayed function or with high immunogenic risk (previous transplant or Panel Reactive Antibodies [PRA] > 15%) are given either OKT3 (5 mg) intraoperatively or daclizumab (1 mg/kg) preoperatively. Patients are given these drugs until serum creatinine levels have normalized (< 2.5 mg/dL), which usually takes 5–14 days. Cyclosporine (5 mg/kg/12 h) or tacrolimus (0.1 mg/kg/12 h) is then started, and the antibody preparations are discontinued when adequate serum cyclosporine levels are achieved. Individual drug doses are gradually adjusted, and the patients are sent home on this maintenance drug combination. This protocol is called **quadruple therapy with sequential interleukin-2 inhibitor institution.** For patients undergoing acute rejection episodes, high-dose steroids, 7 mg/kg, are usually given for 3 days. If patients are unresponsive to steroids, OKT3 (5 mg) is used for 7–14 days. CD3 cell levels are monitored, and the dose is increased if the absolute count is greater than 50 cells/mm^3.

Results

Great improvements in 1-year patient and graft survival have been made in the last 3 decades. One-year patient survival has increased from approximately 50% to about 92% (Gray and Kasiske, 1992). Similarly, graft survival has paralleled this trend, with 1-year graft survival currently at 80–85% for cadaveric and greater than 90% for living related renal transplants (Sutherland et al, 1993; Pirsch et al, 1992; Cecka, Cho, and Terasaki, 1992; Frey et al, 1992; Hayes, 1993; Gray and Kasiske, 1992). However, graft attrition over a 10-year period remains high, as discussed previously, secondary to chronic rejection as well as patient death. Death with a functioning graft is the second major cause of graft loss. Most deaths after the first year are cardiovascular in origin in patients with functioning grafts (Pirsch et al, 1992; Gray and Kasiske, 1992). After 10 years, therefore, not more than 40–50% of cadaveric grafts can be expected to be functioning. The cause of long-term graft failure is uncertain. Graft loss secondary to patient noncompliance with medications has been estimated at 10%. Although late acute rejection episodes can account for some late graft failures, most grafts undergo a slow, chronic, progressive deterioration, ending in graft failure. Thus, although improved surgical techniques and better immunosuppression has had a great effect in the short term, there are improvements to be made in long-term graft survival. Only recently has chronic rejection become a major focus, since it is apparent that cyclosporine has not really affected long-term graft attrition (Pirsch et al, 1992; Hayes, 1993; Gray and Kasiske, 1992; Paul, 1993; Kuo and Monaco, 1993; Paul et al, 1993). Elucidating the mechanisms of late graft failure/chronic rejection is a current focus in transplantation research. In reviewing the progress in transplantation over the last decade, further progress seems probable.

Complications

A. Technical: Various technical complications can occur post-transplantation, including renal artery or vein occlusion, renal artery stenosis, ureteral leak or occlusion, and lymphocele.

Immediate renal artery occlusion is unusual (< 1% incidence) but may be the cause of a sudden decrease or cessation of urine output post-transplantation. In a diuresing kidney, acute cessation of urine output in the immediately postoperative period should prompt emergent reexploration once Foley catheter occlusion has been eliminated as a cause. Prompt recognition and treatment offer the only chance for graft salvage.

Delayed transplant renal artery stenosis is a well-recognized complication. The true incidence of this complication has been estimated in recent retrospective studies to range from 1.5 to 8% (Sutherland et al, 1993; Roberts et al, 1989; Macia et al, 1991). Both technical and immunologic causes have been postulated (Sutherland et al, 1993; Macia et al, 1991). Patients may present with poorly controlled hypertension, a bruit over the transplant, or gradually worsening renal function (Sutherland et al, 1993; Roberts et al, 1989). Stenosis must be considered in this scenario, although rejection or cyclosporine toxicity is more common. Diagnosis is made by renal angiogram, although duplex and color Doppler ultrasonography are useful noninvasive screening techniques with excellent reported accuracy (Pozniac, Dodd, and Kelcz, 1992). Treatment options include surgical correction and percutaneous transluminal angioplasty. Although somewhat controversial, percutaneous transluminal angioplasty is favored for small segmental or intraparenchymal stenoses and in patients who are at high risk for further surgery (Farrugia and Schwab, 1992).

Urologic complications are unusual, with a range of 2–5% in most series (Loughlin, Tilney, and Richie, 1984; Brayman et al, 1992). Specific technical complications include anastomotic leaks, ureteral or anastomotic stricture formation, ureteral obstruction, and ureterovesical disruption. Clinical signs include decreased output and graft dysfunction. Diagnosis of most complications can be made by ultrasound or renal scan. Ureterography of the renal allograft by percutaneous fine-needle puncture and antegrade catheterization also may be necessary for evaluation and formulation of corrective strategies.

Lymphocele formation is another complication seen postoperatively. This is thought to arise from lymphatic disruption during iliac artery dissection. The reported incidence is variable, ranging from 6 to 18% in several large series. Most are asymptomatic, and the majority resolve spontaneously over several months (Khauli et al, 1993). Clinical presentation may include wound swelling, ipsilateral leg edema, or graft dysfunction, depending upon which pelvic structures are being compressed. Diagnosis is made by ultrasound (Pozniak, Dodd, and Kelcz, 1992). In a recent multivariate analysis, acute rejection was implicated as the main factor in the development of symptomatic lymphoceles. The treatment of choice is marsupialization and drainage into the peritoneal cavity. Percutaneous drainage should be performed only for diagnostic purposes and is not therapeutic.

Primary acute renal failure, or ATN in the transplanted kidney, is seen in 5–40% of kidneys from cadaver donors (Cecka, Cho, and Terasaki, 1992; Delaney et al, 1993; Olsen et al, 1989). This injury is usually attributed to cold preservation ischemia or prolonged anastomotic times. Older and unstable donors are more susceptible. The diagnosis of ATN is confirmed by renal scan demonstrating good blood flow and poor tubular function and by duplex scanning to exclude other possible causes such as urinary obstruction. Treatment is expectant and supportive; ATN may take several weeks to resolve (Pozniak, Dodd, and Kelcz, 1992). Morphologically, transplant ATN differs from native kidney ATN; the former has increased interstitial infiltrates and necrotic tubular cells (Olsen et al, 1989). It is controversial whether ATN is associated with a worse long-term prognosis or predisposes to acute chronic rejection. Immunosuppressive strategies during ATN include sequential use of ALG/ATG or antitac (anti-CD25) monoclonal antibodies, followed by careful monitoring of interleukin-2 inhibitor (cyclosporine or tacrolimus) levels and biopsy to detect presence of unsuspected rejection.

B. Nontechnical: Important nontechnical complications include infection and cancer. A recent study confirmed that post-transplant infections are the second most frequent cause of death following renal transplantation (Brayman et al, 1992; Dlugosz et al, 1989). Life-threatening infections tend to occur in the first 4 months following transplantation. In the first month following renal transplantation, conventional bacterial infections of the wound, lung, and urinary tract predominate. Prophylactic antibiotics are used perioperatively and have been shown to reduce significantly the incidence of wound infections in renal transplant patients to approximately 1%

(Brayman et al, 1992; Paul et al, 1993). Trimethoprim-sulfamethoxazole (TMP-SMX) given daily has been shown to decrease the incidence of urinary tract infections and *Pneumocystis carinii* 4-fold and is used routinely at UCSF (Brayman et al, 1992). Although bladder irrigation with an antibiotic/antifungal solution has not been studied in a randomized fashion, many centers routinely use this procedure (Goodman and Hargreave, 1989). Established urinary tract infections are treated with broad-spectrum antibiotics until organism sensitivities are established. Most bacterial infections respond to antibiotic therapy, drainage, or both, as appropriate.

Opportunistic infections predominate throughout the next 2–6 months. Transplant patients are most susceptible to viruses and intracellular infectious agents because immunosuppressive agents inhibit the cellular component of the immune response. As mentioned, TMP-SMX has significantly decreased the incidence of *P. carinii*. For patients with allergies to sulfa drugs, inhaled pentamidine is an effective alternative. The major viral pathogen during this period is the cytomegalovirus (CMV), causing symptomatic disease in 35% and death in 2% of renal transplant recipients (Farrugia and Schwab, 1992). Seronegative recipients of positive donor kidneys are at the highest risk of having the symptomatic disease 50–60% (Farrugia and Schwab, 1992). The initial clinical manifestations are those of a flulike illness including fever, fatigue, malaise, myalgias, and arthralgias. If it is untreated, manifestations of site-specific disease occur; usually the respiratory, urinary, or gastrointestinal tract is affected. Common initial laboratory findings include elevated serum transaminases and an atypical lymphocytosis. Leukopenia and thrombocytopenia are also commonly seen. Cell culture currently is the most widely used method of detecting active infection. The shell-vial culture technique uses a monoclonal antibody against an early viral antigen to detect the presence of CMV. Results are often available within 24–48 h. Treatment of established CMV infection involves decreasing immunosuppressive therapy, supportive treatment such as hydration and antipyretics, and the administration of the antiviral agent ganciclovir. In infected renal transplant patients, ganciclovir decreases rates of viral shedding, alleviates symptoms, and arrests progression of CMV disease (Farrugia and Schwab, 1992). The prophylactic administration of oral acyclovir for the first 6 months post-transplantation has been shown to suppress virus infection. Prophylaxis with ganciclovir has substantially decreased the incidence of CMV when given to patients taking OKT3 at UCSF.

Another effect of immunosuppression is the increased incidence of cancer (Penn, 1987; Cockfield et al, 1993). Analysis of malignant disease occurrences since the advent of cyclosporine therapy reveals an increase in lymphoma and Kaposi sarcoma (Penn, 1987). Post-transplant lymphoproliferative disorders (PTLD) have an incidence of 2.5% in cadaveric renal allografts (Cockfield et al, 1993). Mean time of onset of PTLD with cyclosporine use was about 15 months, with 32% occurring within 4 months of allografting. Primary infection with Epstein-Barr virus at the time of transplantation seems to be a major risk factor. Patients may present with or without renal allograft involvement. By immunohistochemistry, lesions can be identified as polyclonal or monoclonal populations of B lymphocytes. A reduction or cessation of immunotherapy may allow the host immune system to bring the disease under control. Monoclonal lesions tend to have a worse prognosis, although if immunosuppression is stopped early enough, these also have been reported to regress (Cockfield et al, 1993).

REFERENCES

Barry JM et al: Comparison of intracellular flushing and cold storage to machine perfusion for human kidney preservation. J Urol 1980;123:14.

Basadonna G et al: Early versus late acute renal allograft rejection: Impact on chronic rejection. Transplantation 1993;55:993.

Bertolatus J: Clinical immunosuppressive regimens and clinical results in renal transplantation. Semin Nephrol 1992;12:332.

Bohannon LL, Norman DJ, Barry JM: Renal functional consequences of kidney donation: A long term follow-up study. Clin Transplant 1987;I:225.

Braun WE et al: The course of coronary artery disease in diabetics with and without renal allografts. Transplantation Proc 1983;15:1114.

Brayman KL et al: Analysis of infectious complications occurring after solid organ transplant. Arch Surg 1992; 127:38.

Bretan PN: Characterization of improved renal transplant preservation mechanisms using PB-2 flush solution by HPLC assay. Transplant Int (Suppl 1) 1994; 5465.

Bretan PN: Extracorporeal renal preservation. In: Novick AC (editor): *Stewart Textbook of Operative Urology.* Williams & Wilkins, 1989.

Bretan PN, Banafsche R, Garovoy M: Minimizing recipient/donor size differences improves long-term graft survival using single pediatric cadaver kidneys. Transplantation Proc 1994;26:28.

Bretan PN, Paul G, Sharma J: Improved renal preservation with PB-3 flush solution during 72 hours cold storage: Demonstration of a salutary effect on isolated mitochondrial respiration. Transplantation Proc 1993;25:3215.

Bretan PN et al: Chronic renal failure: A significant risk factor in the development of acquired renal cyst and renal cell carcinoma. Case reports and reviews of the literature. Cancer 1986;57:1871.

Bretan PN et al: Improved allograft survival using en bloc renal transplants from pediatric donors less than 14 kg: Technical and immunologic considerations. J Urol 1992;147:342A.

Bretan PN et al: Improved renal transplant preservation using PB-2 flush solution: Characterization of intracellular mechanisms by renal clearance, HPLC, 31P-MRS and EM studies. Urol Res 1991;19:73.

Cecka J, Cho Y, Terasaki P: Analysis of the UNOS scientific renal transplant registry at three years: Early events affecting transplant success. Transplantation 1992;53:59.

Churchill BM et al: Ureteral bladder augmentation. J Urol 1993;150:716.

Cockfield SM et al: Post-transplant lymphoproliferative disorder in renal allograft recipients. Transplantation 1993;56:88.

Daar AJ, Sells RA: Living nonrelated donor renal transplantation: A reappraisal. Transplant Rev 1990;4:128.

Delaney V et al: Comparison of fine-needle aspiration biopsy, Doppler ultrasound, and radionuclide scintigraphy in the diagnosis of acute allograft dysfunction in renal transplant recipients: Sensitivity, specificity, and cost analysis. Nephron 1993;63:263.

Dlugosz BA et al: Causes of death in kidney transplant recipients. Transplantation Proc 1989;21:2168.

Dunn JF et al: Living related kidney donors: A 14 year experience. Ann Surg 1986;203:637.

Farrugia E, Schwab T: Subspecialty clinics: Nephrology. Mayo Clin Proc 1992;67:879.

Flechner SM et al: Long-term results of cyclosporine therapy in recipients of mismatched living related kidneys. Transplantation Proc [Suppl 1] 1986;18:47.

Frey D et al: Sequential therapy: A prospective randomized trial of MALG versus OKT3 for prophylactic immunosuppression in cadaver renal allograft recipients. Transplantation 1992;54:50.

Gjertson DW, Terasaki PL: National allocation of cadaveric kidneys by HLA matching: Projected effect on outcome and cost. N Engl J Med 1991;324:1032.

Gold BD et al: Gastrointestinal complications of gastrocystoplasty. Arch Dis Child 1992;67:1272.

Goodman CM, Hargreave TB: Survey of antibiotic prophylaxis in European renal transplantation practice. Int J Urol Nephrol 1989;22:173.

Gray J, Kasiske B: Patient and renal allograft survival in the late posttransplant period. Semin Nephrol 1992; 12:343.

Gregg CM et al: Recovery of glomerular and tubular function in autotransplanted dog kidneys preserved by hypothermic storage or machine perfusion. Transplantation 1986;42:453.

Halloran P, Aprile M: A randomized prospective trial of cold storage versus pulsatile perfusion for cadaver kidney preservation. Transplantation 1987;43:827.

Hatch DA et al: Fate of renal allograft transplanted in patients with urinary diversion. Transplantation 1993; 56:838.

Hayes JM: The immunobiology and clinical use of current immunosuppressive therapy for renal transplantation. J Urol 1993;149:437.

Hayes JM et al: A single center experience with shared 6

Ag matched cadaver renal transplants. Transplantation 1993;55:669.

Kahan BD: Blood transfusion. (Editorial) Transpl Immunol Lett 1987;4:1.

Keogh AM et al: Pituitary function in brain stem dead organ donors: A prospective survey. Transplantation Proc 1988;20:729.

Kerman RH: To be or not to be transfused? That is the question in the cyclosporine era! Transpl Immunol Lett 1987;4:2.

Khauli RB: Current policies in renal procurement and transplantation. In: Stamey T (editor): Monographs in Urology. Medical Directions Publishing Co., Inc, Monterde, Fla., 1986.

Khauli RB et al: Post-transplant lymphoceles: A critical look into the risk factors, pathophysiology and management. J Urol 1993;150:22.

Koyle MA et al: Bladder reconstruction with the dilated ureter for renal transplantation. Transplantation Proc 1994;26:35.

Kuo P, Monaco AP: Chronic rejection and suboptimal immunosuppression. Transplantation Proc 1993;25: 2082.

Leivestad T, Berger L, Thorsby E: Beneficial effect of DR matching on cadaveric renal graft survival in Scandian transplant. Transplantation Proc 1992;24:2447.

Leivestad T et al: Renal transplants from HLA-haploididentical living-related donors: The influence of donor-specific transfusions and different immunosuppressive regimens. Transplantation 1986;42:35.

Levine E: Chronic renal failure and renal cell carcinoma in uremic acquired renal cystic disease: Incidence, detection and management. Urol Radiol 1992; 13:203.

Loughlin KR, Tilney NL, Richie JP: Urologic complications in 718 renal transplant patients. Surgery 1984; 95:297.

MacGregor P et al: Renal transplantation in end stage renal disease patients with existing urinary diversion. J Urol 1986;135:686.

Macia M et al: Posttransplant renal artery stenosis: A possible immunological phenomenon. J Urol 1991; 145:251.

Matas AJ et al: The impact of HLA matching on graft survival and on sensitization after a failed transplant. Transplantation 1990;50:599.

Mathur VS, Bretan, PN, Tomlanovich SJ: Management of ESRD-transplantation versus dialysis. In: Novick AC (editor): Current Opinion in Urology. Current Science, 1994.

McEnery PT et al: Renal transplantation in children: A report from the North American Pediatric Cooperative Study. N Engl J Med 1992;326:1727.

Melzer JS, Salvatierra O: The blood transfusion effect in cadaver donor transplantation: The University of California, San Francisco experience. Transpl Immunol Lett 1987;4:6.

Narkun-Burgess DM et al: Forty-five-year follow-up after uninephrectomy. Kidney Int 1993;43:1110.

Olsen S et al: Primary acute renal failure (acute tubular necrosis) in the transplanted kidney: Morphology and pathogenesis. Medicine 1989;68:173.

O'Malley JP, Ziessman HA, Chantarapitak N: Tc-99m MAG3 as an alternative to Tc-99m DTPA and I-131

Hippuran for renal transplant evaluation. Clin Nucl Med 1993;18:22.

Opelz G: How unusual are the University of Minnesota HLA matching results? Transplantation 1992;53:694.

Opelz G: Multicenter impact of cyclosporine on cadaver kidney graft survival. Prog Allergy 1986;38:329.

Park K et al: Single-center experience of unrelated living-donor renal transplantation in the cyclosporine era. In: Terasaki P (editor): *Clinical Transplants.* UCLA Tissue Typing Laboratory, 1990.

Parlevliet K, Schellekens P: Monoclonal antibodies in renal transplantation: A review. Transplant Int 1992; 5:234.

Paul LC: Chronic rejection of organ allografts: Magnitude of the problem. Transplantation Proc 1993;25:2024.

Paul LC et al: Diagnostic criteria for chronic rejection/accelerated graft atherosclerosis in heart and kidney transplants: Joint proposal from the fourth Alexis Carrel Conference on chronic rejection and accelerated arteriosclerosis in transplanted organs. Transplantation Proc 1993;25:2022.

Penn I: Cancers following cyclosporine therapy. Transplantation 1987;43:32.

Penn I: The effect of immunosuppression in pre-existing cancers. Transplantation 1993;55:742.

Philipson JB et al: Evaluation of cardiovascular risk for renal transplantation in diabetic patients. Am J Med 1986;81:630.

Pirsch J et al: The effect of donor age, recipient age, and HLA match on immunologic graft survival in cadaver renal transplant recipients. Transplantation 1992;53:55.

Pirsch JD: Living-unrelated renal transplantation at the University of Wisconsin. In: Terasaki P (editor): *Clinical Transplants.* UCLA Tissue Typing Laboratory, 1990.

Pozniak M, Dodd G, Kelcz F: Ultrasonographic evaluation of renal transplantation. Radiol Clin North Am 1992;30:1053.

Roberts PP et al: Transplant renal artery stenosis. Transplantation 1989;48:580.

Sasagawa I, Terasawa KI, Sekino H: Acquired cystic disease of kidney and renal cell carcinoma in hemodialysis patients. Br J Urol 1992;70:236.

Steinmuller DR: Evaluation and selection of candidates for renal transplantation. Urol Clin North Am 1983; 10:217.

Streem SB, Bretan PN: Considerations in donor nephrectomy. In: Droller MJ (editor): *Surgical Management of Urologic Disease: An Anatomic Approach.* Mosby Yearbook, 1992.

Sutherland R et al: Renal artery stenosis after renal transplantation: The impact of the hypogastric artery anastomosis. J Urol 1993;149:980.

Takemoto S, Carnahan E, Terasaki PL: Report on 604 6-Ag matched transplants. In: Terasaki P (editor): *Clinical Transplants.* UCLA Tissue Typing Laboratory, 1990.

Takiff H et al: Dominant effect of histocompatibility on ten-year kidney transplant survival. Transplantation 1988;45:410.

Tesi R et al: OKT3 for primary therapy of the first rejection episode in kidney transplants. Transplantation 1993;55:1023.

Tilney NL et al: Factors contributing to the declining mortality rate in renal transplantation. N Engl J Med 1978;299:1321.

Torres VE, Offord KP, Anderson CF: Blood pressure determinants in living-related renal allograft donors and their recipients. Kidney Int 1987;31:1383.

Urban Institute. Medicare ESRD incidence per million by primary diagnosis. The Urban Institute 1980–1986. Based on HCFA data. 1986.

Williams SL, Oler J, Jorkasky DK: Long-term renal function in kidney donors: A comparison of donors and their siblings. Ann Intern Med 1986;105:1.

Wyner LM et al: Improved success of living unrelated renal transplantation with cyclosporine immunosuppression. J Urol 1993;149:706.

Yuge J, Burgos D: Long term kidney graft survival. In: Terasaki PI, Cecka JM (editors): *Clinical Transplants.* UCLA Tissue Typing Laboratory, 1992.

Zaki SK et al: A simple and accurate grading system for orthoiodohippurate renal scans in the assessment of post-transplant renal function. J Urol 1990;143:1099.

Disorders of the Ureter & Ureteropelvic Junction

Barry A. Kogan, MD

The ureter is a complex functional conduit carrying urine from the kidneys to the bladder. Any pathologic process that interferes with this activity can cause renal abnormalities, the most common sequels being hydronephrosis (see Chapter 12) and infection. Disorders of the ureter can be classified as congenital or acquired.

CONGENITAL ANOMALIES OF THE URETER

Congenital ureteral malformations are common and range from complete absence to duplication or triplication of the ureter. They may cause severe obstruction requiring urgent attention, or they may be asymptomatic and of no clinical significance. The nomenclature can be confusing and has been standardized to prevent ambiguity (Glassberg et al, 1984).

URETERAL ATRESIA

The ureter may be absent entirely, or it may end blindly after extending only part of the way to the flank. The anomaly is caused during embryologic development, either by failure of the ureteral bud to form from the mesonephric duct or by an arrest in its development before it comes in contact with the metanephric blastema. The end result is an absent or multicystic kidney. When bilateral, this condition presents as Potter syndrome and is incompatible with life. When unilateral, the multicystic kidney is usually asymptomatic and of no clinical significance, although it can be associated with hypertension (Javadpour et al, 1970), infection (Yoshida and Sakamoto, 1986), or tumor. Contralateral vesicoureteral reflux is common, and most clinicians recommend a voiding

cystourethrogram as part of the initial workup (Selzman and Elder, 1995). There is a natural tendency of these kidneys to involute (Rottenberg, Gordon, and DeBruyn, 1997); hence, most clinicians feel observation is the best treatment. A few recommend nephrectomy owing to the small risk of neoplasia (Homsy et al, 1997).

DUPLICATION OF THE URETER

Complete or incomplete duplication of the ureter is one of the most common congenital malformations of the urinary tract. Nation (1944) found some form of duplication of the ureter in 0.9% of a series of autopsies. The condition occurs more frequently in females than in males and is often bilateral. The mode of inheritance is autosomal dominant, although the gene is of incomplete penetrance (Atwell et al, 1974).

The incomplete (Y) type of duplication is caused by branching of the ureteral bud before it reaches the metanephric blastema. In most cases, this anomaly is associated with no clinical abnormality. However, disorders of peristalsis may occur near the point of union (Figure 38–1) (O'Reilly et al, 1984). In such cases, one segment may be obstructed or dilated owing to ureteroureteral reflux. A ureteropyelostomy is effective treatment in most cases (Sole, Randall, and Arkell, 1987).

In complete duplication of the ureter, the presence of 2 ureteral buds leads to the formation of 2 totally separate ureters and 2 separate renal pelves. Because the ureter to the upper segment arises from a cephalad position on the mesonephric duct, it remains attached to the mesonephric duct longer and consequently migrates farther, ending medial and inferior to the ureter draining the lower segment (Weigert-Meyer law). Thus, the ureter draining the upper segment may migrate too far caudally and become ectopic and obstructed, while the ureter draining the lower segment may end laterally and have a short intravesical tunnel, which leads to vesicoureteral reflux

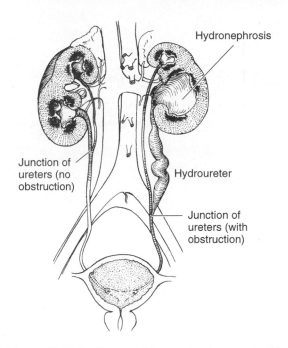

Figure 38–1. Duplication of the ureter. Incomplete (Y) type with hydronephrosis of lower pole of left kidney. Ureteroureteral (yo-yo) reflux can also occur and account for the radiographic appearance.

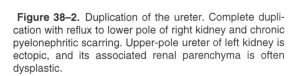

Figure 38–2. Duplication of the ureter. Complete duplication with reflux to lower pole of right kidney and chronic pyelonephritic scarring. Upper-pole ureter of left kidney is ectopic, and its associated renal parenchyma is often dysplastic.

(Figure 38–2) (Kaplan, Nasrallah, and King, 1978; Tanagho, 1976). The same general principle is noted in rare ureteral triplication (Zaontz and Maizels, 1985).

Although many patients with duplication of the ureter are asymptomatic, a common presentation is persistent or recurrent infections. In females, the ureter to the upper pole may be ectopic, with an opening distal to the external sphincter or even outside the urinary tract. Such patients have classic symptoms: incontinence characterized by constant dribbling, but a normal pattern of voiding. In males, because the mesonephric duct becomes the vas and seminal vesicles, the ectopic ureter is always proximal to the external sphincter, and associated incontinence does not occur. In recent years, prenatal ureteral ultrasonography has provided the diagnosis in many asymptomatic neonates.

Excretory urography and voiding cystourethrography have been the classic studies for detecting duplication of the ureter. The excretory urogram shows the duplication in most cases. Occasionally, one segment of the kidney functions so poorly that it is not visualized. In such cases, the diagnosis can be inferred from the displacement of the visualized calyces or ureter or from the discrepancy between the amount of renal parenchyma and the relatively small number of visualized calyces. The excretory urogram also demonstrates any pyelonephritic scarring. The voiding cys-

tourethrogram discloses vesicoureteral reflux and may demonstrate the presence of a ureterocele. At the present time, the excretory urogram has been supplanted by sonography, which usually can visualize a nonexcreting upper pole and a dilated distal ureter and can readily evaluate parenchymal thickness and the presence of bladder anomalies. Renal scanning (especially with ^{99m}Tc-dimercaptosuccinic acid) is helpful for estimating the degree of renal function in each kidney and renal segment (Carter, Malone, and Lewington, 1998) (Figure 38–3).

The treatment of reflux alone should not be influenced by the presence of ureteral duplication (Lee et al, 1991). Lower grades of reflux are generally treated medically and higher grades of reflux surgically. Because of anatomic variations, many surgical options are available (Decter, 1997). If upper-pole obstruction or ectopy is present, surgery is almost always required. Numerous operative approaches have been recommended (Belman, Filmer, and King, 1974). If renal function in one segment is very poor, heminephrectomy is the most appropriate procedure (Barrett, Malek, and Kelalis, 1975). In an effort to preserve renal parenchyma, treatment by pyeloureterostomy, ureteroureterostomy, or ureteral reimplantation is feasible (Amar, 1970; Amar, 1978; Bieri et al, 1998).

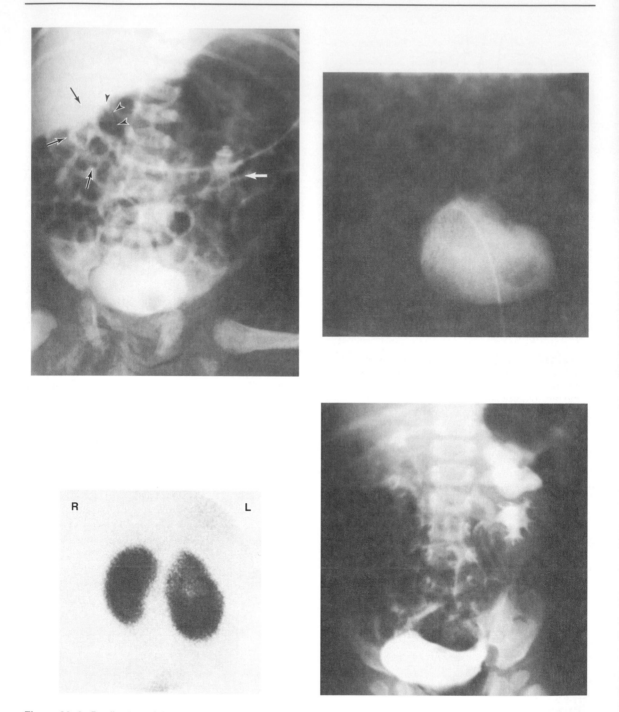

Figure 38–3. Duplication of the ureter and the ureterocele. **Upper left:** Excretory urogram shows duplication of the right kidney (arrow heads on upper pole) and visualization of only the lower pole (arrows on lower pole) of the left kidney (white arrow). There is a filling defect on the left side of the bladder. **Upper right:** Cystogram confirms the filling defect. There is no reflux. **Lower left:** Renal scan with 99mTc-dimercaptosuccinic acid shows some functioning parenchyma in upper pole to left kidney. **Lower right:** After excision of ureterocele and reimplantation of both ureters on left, repeat excretory urogram shows improved excretion of contrast medium from upper pole of left kidney.

URETEROCELE

A ureterocele is a sacculation of the terminal portion of the ureter (Figure 38–4). It may be either intravesical or ectopic; in the latter case, some portion is located at the bladder neck or in the urethra. Intravesical ureteroceles are associated most often with single ureters, whereas ectopic ureteroceles nearly always involve the upper pole of duplicated ureters. Ectopic ureteroceles are 4 times more common than intravesical ureteroceles (Snyder and Johnston, 1978). Ureterocele occurs 7 times more often in girls than in boys, and about 10% of cases are bilateral. Mild forms of ureterocele are found occasionally in adults examined for unrelated reasons.

Ureterocele has been attributed to delayed or incomplete canalization of the ureteral bud leading to an early prenatal obstruction and expansion of the ureteral bud prior to its absorption into the urogenital sinus (Tanagho, 1976). The cystic dilation forms between the superficial and deep muscle layers of the trigone. Large ureteroceles may displace the other orifices, interfere with the muscular backing of the bladder, or even obstruct the bladder outlet. There is nearly always significant hydroureteronephrosis, and a dysplastic segment of the upper pole of the kidney may be found in association with a ureterocele. Also, it has been shown that the dysplastic segment may contain nodular renal blastema and hence may be prone to neoplasia (Cromie, Engelstein, and Duckett, 1980).

Clinical findings vary considerably. Patients commonly present with infection, but bladder outlet obstruction or incontinence may be the initial complaint. Occasionally, a ureterocele may prolapse through the female urethra (Ahmed, 1984). Calculi can develop secondary to urinary stasis and are often seen in the distal ureter. Currently, many cases are diagnosed by antenatal maternal ultrasound (Gloor, Ogburn, and Matsumoto, 1996). Excretory urography (Figures 38–3 and 38–5) is usually diagnostic and may show a cystic dilatation or a filling defect in the bladder. The urogram also indicates the degree of hydronephrosis and may reveal a duplicated kidney. Again, sonography has replaced the excretory urogram in most centers. Voiding cystourethrography should always be part of the workup (Bauer and Retik, 1978). It may demonstrate reflux into the lower pole or contralateral ureter and occasionally shows eversion of the ureterocele during urination, in which case the ureterocele has the appearance of a diverticulum. Renal scanning is helpful for estimating renal function (Geringer et al, 1983).

Treatment must be individualized. Transurethral incision was used previously only in very ill children with pyohydronephrosis; however, it has been recognized as the definitive procedure in many instances, particularly in patients with intravesical ureteroceles

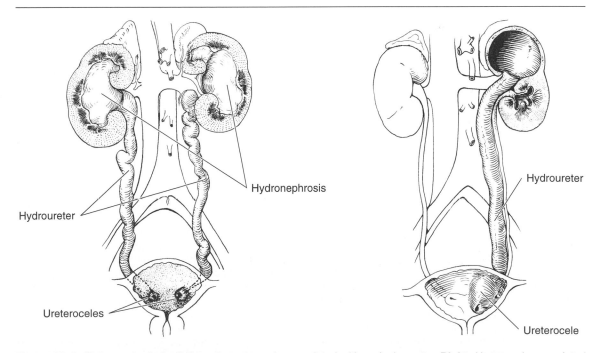

Figure 38–4. Ureterocele. **Left:** Orthotopic ureterocele associated with a single ureter. **Right:** Ureterocele associated with ureteral duplication and poor function of upper pole of kidney.

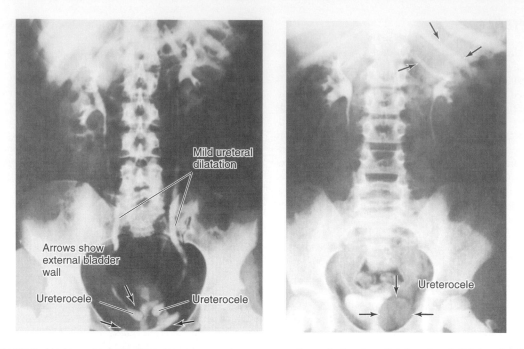

Figure 38–5. Ureterocele. **Left:** Excretory urogram in a woman shows "cobra head" deformity of distal ends of both ureters, bilateral ureteroceles causing minimal obstruction, and pressure on the bladder from the uterus. No treatment is indicated. **Right:** Excretory urogram in an 8-year-old girl shows a space-occupying lesion (left side of bladder) caused by ureterocele. Absence of calyceal system in upper portion of left kidney (arrows) implies duplication of ureters and renal pelves and a nonfunctioning upper pole (advanced hydronephrosis); the dilated ureter from that pole drains into an obstructing ureterocele and displaces the visualized ureter laterally just below the kidney.

(Blyth et al, 1993; Pfister et al, 1998). When an open operation is needed, the procedure must be chosen on the basis of the anatomic location of the ureteral meatus, the position of the ureterocele, and the degree of hydroureteronephrosis and impairment of renal function. In general, choices range from heminephrectomy and ureterectomy (Husmann et al, 1995) to excision of the ureterocele, vesical reconstruction, and ureteral reimplantation. Often, a second procedure is necessary (Caldamone, Snyder, and Duckett, 1984).

ECTOPIC URETERAL ORIFICE

Although an ectopic ureteral orifice most commonly occurs in association with ureterocele and duplication of the ureter (see preceding sections), single ectopic ureters do occur (Gotoh et al, 1983). They are caused by a delay or failure of separation of the ureteral bud from the mesonephric duct during embryologic development. The primary anomaly may be an abnormally located ureteral bud, which explains the high incidence of dysplastic kidneys associated with single ectopic ureters.

The clinical picture varies according to the sex of

the patient and the position of the ureteral opening. Boys usually do not present with incontinence, but many are seen because of epididymitis. In these cases, the ureter drains directly into the vas deferens or seminal vesicle (Umeyama et al, 1985). In girls, the ureteral orifice may be in the urethra, vagina, or perineum. Although infection may be present, particularly when the ectopic ureter allows reflux, incontinence is the rule. Continual dribbling despite normal voiding is pathognomonic. Urgency and urge incontinence may confound the diagnosis. Genital tract anomalies are often present in patients with ectopic ureteral orifices (Johnson and Perlmutter, 1980).

Sonography and voiding cystourethrography help delineate the problem. However, because an ectopic kidney may be both tiny and in an abnormal location, it may be difficult to find by ultrasound (Borer et al, 1998). During cystoscopy, the ectopic orifice in boys may be visualized directly or demonstrated by retrograde catheterization of the ejaculatory duct (Figure 38–6). The presence of a hemitrigone plus a cystic mass in the flank is presumptive evidence of an ectopic ureter. In girls, the orifice sometimes can be visualized next to the urethra by cystoscopy or vaginoscopy. If so, a retrograde ureterogram may demonstrate anatomic abnormalities (Figure 38–7). Renal scanning is

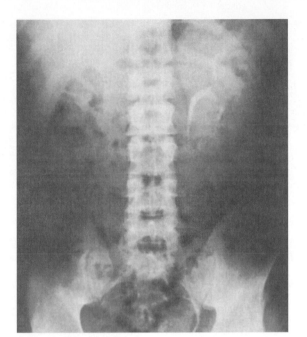

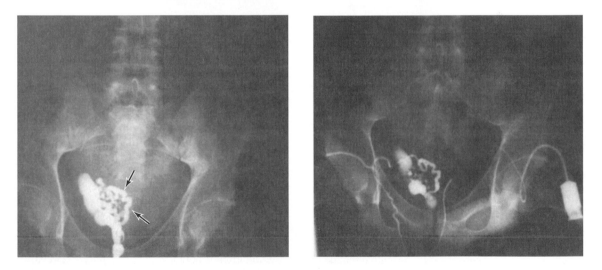

Figure 38–6. Ectopic ureter. **Top:** Excretory urogram demonstrates no right renal outline and no excretion of contrast medium on right. **Lower left:** Endoscopic injection of contrast medium into ejaculatory duct demonstrates seminal vesicle and stump of ectopic ureter (arrows). **Lower right:** Same anatomy visualized on a vasogram. (Courtesy of DW Ferguson.)

also helpful in delineating the structures and estimating relative renal function.

As in ureteroceles and duplication of the ureter, the clinical picture and the degree of renal function dictate the therapeutic approach. Surgical treatment usually involves either ureteral reimplantation or nephroureterectomy (Plaire et al, 1997). Although not true of most ureteral duplications, it is possible occasionally to reimplant only the ectopic ureter (Marshall, 1986).

ABNORMALITIES OF URETERAL POSITION

Retrocaval ureter (also called circumcaval ureter and postcaval ureter) is a rare condition in which an embryologically normal ureter becomes entrapped behind the vena cava because of abnormal development of the abdominal blood vessels. Persistence of the right subcardinal vein, as opposed to the supracardinal vein, forces the right ureter to encircle the vena cava from behind. There are 2 anatomic types

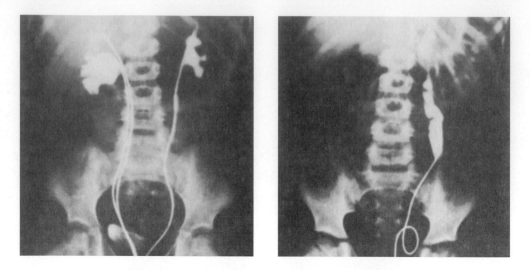

Figure 38–7. Ectopic ureter. **Left:** Cystoscopy in a 6-year-old girl with a lifelong history of urinary incontinence revealed 2 ureteral orifices on the right and one on the left; these were catheterized and urograms obtained. **Right:** Same patient. An ectopic ureteral orifice near the urethral meatus was catheterized. Retrograde urogram demonstrates second hydronephrotic renal pelvis on left. Resection of upper pole and ureter cured incontinence.

of retrocaval ureter (Kenawi and Williams, 1976). In one, the upper ureter and renal pelvis are almost horizontal as they pass behind the vena cava; there is generally no obstruction, and no therapy is needed. In the other type, the ureter descends normally to approximately the level of L3, where it curves back upward in the shape of a reverse J to pass behind and around the vena cava. Obstruction generally results.

The diagnosis of retrocaval ureter is most easily made by excretory urography. However, since sonography is usually the first test performed, the radiologist must be suspicious of the anomaly based on a dilated proximal (but not distal) ureter. A retrograde ureterogram will demonstrate the abnormality quite clearly. A simultaneous venacavogram can be obtained but is overly invasive (Figure 38–8). Currently, magnetic resonance imaging (MRI) is the best single study to delineate the anatomy clearly and noninvasively.

Surgical repair for retrocaval ureter, when indicated, consists of dividing the ureter (preferably across the dilated portion), bringing the distal ureter from behind the vena cava, and reanastomosing it to the proximal end. The procedure has been performed laparoscopically to reduce morbidity (Polascik and Chen, 1998). If the retrocaval part of the ureter is fibrotic or stenotic, the infracaval ureter is used for the anastomosis (Kumar and Bhandari, 1985).

A number of other rare anomalies of ureteral position occur. Brooks (1962) reported a retrocaval left ureter in a patient with situs inversus. Several cases of retroiliac ureter have been reported (Hanna, 1972). Treatment is similar to that described for retrocaval ureter.

OBSTRUCTION OF THE URETEROPELVIC JUNCTION

In children, primary obstruction of the ureter usually occurs at the ureteropelvic junction or the ureterovesical junction (Figure 38–9). Obstruction of the ureteropelvic junction is probably the most common congenital abnormality of the ureter. It is seen more often in boys than in girls (5:2 ratio) and, in unilateral cases, more often on the left than on the right side (5:2 ratio). Bilateral obstruction occurs in 10– 15% of cases and is especially common in infants (Johnston et al, 1977). The abnormality may occur in several members of the same family, but it shows no clear genetic pattern.

The exact cause of obstruction of the ureteropelvic junction often is not clear. Ureteral polyps and valves have been reported but are very rare (Punjani, 1983; Sant, Barbalias, and Klauber, 1985). There is almost always an angulation and kink at the junction of the dilated renal pelvis and ureter. This by itself can cause obstruction, but it is unclear whether this is primary or merely secondary to another obstructive lesion. True stenosis is found rarely; however, a thin-walled, hypoplastic proximal ureter is frequently observed. Characteristic histologic and ultrastructural changes are observed in this area and could account for abnormal peristalsis through the ureteropelvic junction and consequent interference with pelvic emptying (Hanna et al, 1976). Two other findings sometimes seen at operation are a high origin of the ureter from the renal pelvis and an abnormal relationship of the proximal ureter to a lower-pole renal artery. It is debatable whether these findings are the

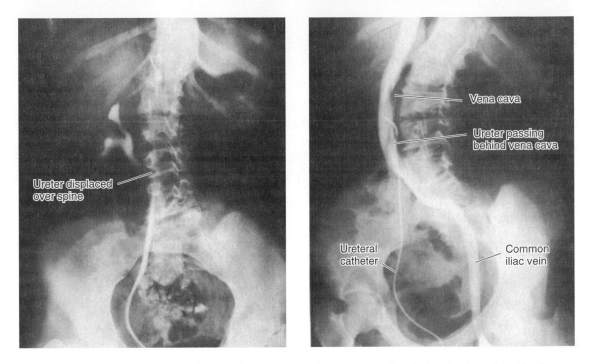

Figure 38–8. Retrocaval ureter. **Left:** Retrograde ureterogram shows upper ureter displaced onto vertebral bodies, suggesting retrocaval ureter. Note congenital deformity of spine. **Right:** Femoral venacavogram (right oblique view) shows ureter in retrocaval position.

result or the cause of pelvic dilatation, but Stephens (1982) has presented data suggesting that abnormal rotation of the renal pelvis allows the ureter to become entrapped in the blood vessels of the lower pole of the kidney, ultimately leading to obstruction. Using careful studies at the time of operation, it is possible to define whether the principal lesion is intrinsic or extrinsic (Koff et al, 1986; Johnston, 1969).

Clinical findings vary depending on the patient's age at diagnosis. Recent improvements in prenatal ultrasonography now allow the majority of cases to be diagnosed in utero (Mandell et al, 1991). Occasionally, infants present with an abdominal mass. In children, pain and vomiting are the most common symptoms; however, hematuria and urinary infection may be seen also. A few patients have complications such as calculi (Figure 38–10), trauma to the enlarged kidney, or (rarely) hypertension. Some children are completely asymptomatic.

The diagnosis is most often made by sonography. In equivocal cases, diuretic renography or (rarely) antegrade urography with pressure-flow studies are helpful (Thrall, Koff, and Keyes, 1981; Whitaker, 1973). Many surgeons consider a voiding cystourethrogram a routine part of the preoperative workup, since radiographic findings in vesicoureteral reflux may be similar to those in ureteropelvic junction obstruction. This fact is especially relevant when the ureter is well seen

or dilated (or both) below the ureteropelvic junction (Maizels, Smith, and Firlit, 1984).

Symptomatic obstruction of the ureteropelvic junction should be treated surgically. Because most cases are now detected by hydronephrosis on prenatal ultrasonography and the infants are asymptomatic, it becomes important to assess the significance of the hydronephrosis. On the one hand, early surgery may prevent future urinary tract infections, stones, or other complications; on the other hand, many of the patients could live their whole lives without experiencing a consequence of the hydronephrosis. This remains an area of considerable controversy. Early surgery is recommended for patients who have kidneys with diminished function, massive hydronephrosis, infection, or stones. Nonoperative surveillance with good follow-up is thought to be safe (Koff and Campbell, 1992), although about 25% of patients will ultimately require an operative repair for pain, urinary infection, or reduced renal function on repeat nuclear scan (Palmer et al, 1998).

Because of anatomic variations, no single procedure is sufficient for all situations in which surgery is indicated (Smart, 1979). Regardless of the technique used, all successful repairs have in common the creation of a dependent and funnel-shaped ureteropelvic junction of adequate caliber. Although preservation of the intact ureteropelvic junction is feasible in some cir-

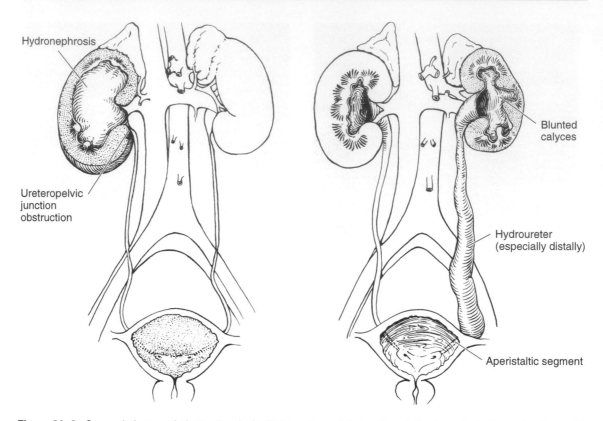

Figure 38–9. Congenital ureteral obstruction. **Left:** Right ureteropelvic junction obstruction with hydronephrosis. **Right:** Left ureterovesical junction obstruction (obstructed megaureter) with hydroureteronephrosis.

cumstances (Perlberg and Pfau, 1984), when the obstruction appears to be caused by a dyskinetic segment of proximal ureter, the most popular operation is a dismembered pyeloureteroplasty (Anderson, 1963). Dismembered pyeloureteroplasty is also favored when the proximal ureter is hooked over a lower-pole blood vessel. When there is a dilated extrarenal renal pelvis, dismembered pyeloureteroplasty can be combined with a Foley Y-V plasty to create a more funnel-shaped ureteropelvic junction (Foley, 1937). Pelvic flap procedures (Culp and DeWeerd, 1951; Scardino and Prince, 1953) are ideally suited to cases in which the ureteropelvic junction has remained in a dependent position despite significant pelvic dilatation. They also have the advantage of interfering less with the ureteral blood supply; this is particularly relevant when distal ureteral surgery (eg, ureteral reimplantation) is contemplated in the future. In most centers, the dismembered pyeloureteroplasty is the mainstay of repairs.

Both the Y-V plasty and the flap techniques are useful in managing ureteropelvic junction obstructions in horseshoe or pelvic kidneys, in which the anatomy may prevent creation of a dependent ureteropelvic junction if a dismembered technique is attempted. The use of stenting catheters and proximal diversion at the time of pyeloplasty has been the subject of debate, and the issue has not been resolved. Excellent results have been reported both with and without stents and diversions (Bejjani and Belman, 1982; Perlmutter, Kroovand, and Lai, 1980; King et al, 1984).

The prognosis is generally good, since the disease is usually unilateral and since one side is nearly always less involved in cases of bilateral disease. In several large series, the reported reoperation rate has been only 2–4%, but the postoperative radiographic appearance of the area is often disappointing. There can be marked improvement when a large extrarenal renal pelvis has prevented massive calyceal distortion; however, in most cases considerable deformity persists despite adequate drainage of the kidney. Furthermore, it is usually many years before the radiographic appearance improves (Amling et al, 1996).

The recent explosion in the field of endourology as a subspecialty of urology has encouraged use of percutaneous techniques for the repair of ureteropelvic junction obstruction in selected patients (Ramsay et al, 1984; Badlani, Eshghi, and Smith, 1986; Van Cangh et al, 1989). The technique is similar to that reported by Davis (1943) but is done entirely endoscopically. The technique may be applied ante-

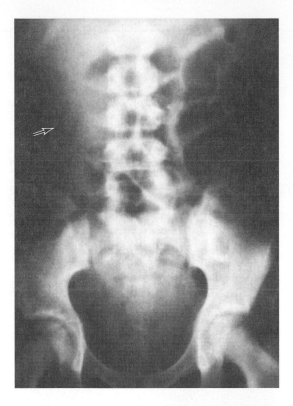
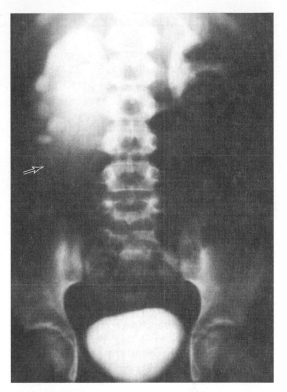
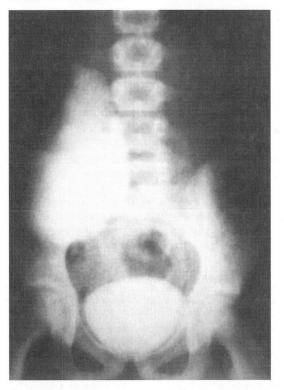

Figure 38–10. Ureteropelvic junction obstruction with calculi. **Upper left:** Plain film of abdomen shows radiopacities in region of right kidney. **Upper right:** Early film from excretory urogram demonstrates dilation of calyces on right and layering of calculi in large right renal pelvis. **Bottom:** Delayed film from excretory urogram shows a typical right ureteropelvic junction obstruction.

grade, via a nephrostomy tract, or retrograde, using either a ureteroscope (for direct vision) or an Acusize (Applied Urology, Laguna Beach, Calif.) balloon catheter with fluoroscopic visualization. In adults the procedure is clearly an option with an anticipated success rate of 80–85% and a marked reduction in morbidity (Aslan and Preminger, 1998). In children, retrograde endopyelotomy also has an 85% success rate, but this is still considerably less than 98% and the benefit in terms of reduced morbidity is less significant (Bogaert et al, 1996). An intriguing new option is laparoscopic pyeloplasty (Moore et al, 1997).

OBSTRUCTED MEGAURETER

Obstruction at the ureterovesical junction is 4 times more common in boys than in girls. It is often bilateral but usually asymmetric. The left ureter is slightly more often involved than the right. Of more consequence is the observation that the contralateral kidney is either absent or dysplastic in 10–15% of cases (Tiburcio and Lima, 1978).

The embryogenesis of the lesion is uncertain. It is clear that in most cases there is no stricture at the ureterovesical junction. At operation, a retrograde catheter or probe can usually be passed through the area of obstruction. Close observation either at operation or by fluoroscopy reveals a failure of the distal ureter to transmit the normal peristaltic wave, resulting in a functional obstruction. Moreover, on fluoroscopy, retrograde peristalsis is seen, which transmits abnormal pressures up to the kidney, resulting in the calyceal dilation out of proportion with the renal pelvic dilation. Histologic findings include an excess of circular muscle fibers and collagen in the distal ureter, which may account for the problem (Tanagho, Smith, and Guthrie, 1970). Ultrastructural studies show that this obstruction is similar in appearance to obstruction of the ureteropelvic junction.

Currently, most cases are discovered on prenatal sonography. Other symptoms are infection, fever, and abdominal pain. Hematuria is frequent and may be seen even in the absence of infection. This is presumably due to disruption of mucosal vessels in the ureter secondary to ureteral distention. Hematuria may also be a sign of calculus formation secondary to urinary stasis. Sonography usually shows the pathognomonic configuration of a dilated distal ureter, a less dilated proximal ureter, a relatively normal-appearing renal pelvis, and blunted calyces (Figure 38–11). In occasional cases, retrograde or antegrade urograms are necessary to delineate the lesion. A diuretic renogram may be helpful in delineating relative renal function, but the "washout" information does not usually correlate with prognosis.

It was previously assumed that surgery was indicated in most cases. Ureteral reimplantation with excision of the distal ureter is curative. Because of the ex-

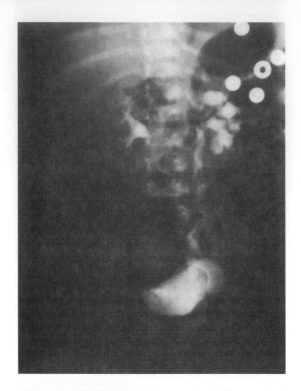

Figure 38–11. Obstructed megaureter. Follow-up study in a 9-month-old boy with unilateral hydronephrosis detected by ultrasonography in utero. Excretory urogram shows the classic configuration of a dilated distal ureter, a less dilated proximal ureter, and blunted calyces.

cessive dilation of the ureter, ureteral tapering is frequently necessary. This is usually done by excision of a portion of the ureteral wall along the antimesenteric border (Hendren, 1969); however, there are recent reports of good results obtained by folding the ureter onto itself if it is only moderately dilated (Hanna, 1982; Ehrlich, 1985). Because the ureteral muscle is generally healthy, these cases have an excellent prognosis (Peters et al, 1989). However, in recent years it has become obvious that at least 50% of cases will have spontaneous resolution. A period of observation is nearly always appropriate when the diagnosis is made in an asymptomatic patient (Baskin et al, 1994). Because of the high risk of infection, 1–2 years of prophylactic antibiotics are recommended in neonates.

UPPER URINARY TRACT DILATATION WITHOUT OBSTRUCTION

It should not be assumed that every dilated upper urinary tract is obstructed. A voiding cystourethrogram is an essential part of the evaluation, not only to rule out reflux but also to ensure that no abnormality of the lower urinary tract is responsible for the upper urinary tract dilatation. Other cases in which diagnosis may be difficult include residual dilatation in a previously obstructed system, dilatation associated with bacterial infection (presumably related to a direct effect of endotoxin on the ureteral musculature), neonatal hydronephrosis (Homsy, Williot, and Danais, 1986), and prolonged polyuria in patients with diabetes insipidus.

In such cases, the usual investigations may not provide sufficient information. A radionuclide diuretic renogram is especially helpful in distinguishing nonobstructive from obstructive dilation (Figure 38–12) (Thrall, Koff, and Keyes, 1981). Use of percutaneous renal puncture is occasionally beneficial; in the dilated system, it carries minimal risk, making antegrade urography and pressure-flow studies feasible in selected cases. Measurement of the renal pelvic pressure during infusion of saline into the renal pelvis at high rates (10 mL/min) (**the Whitaker test; see p 133**) may help differentiate nonobstructive from obstructive dilation (Wolk and Whitaker, 1982). Unfortunately, there is no true "gold standard," and these studies do not always agree; clinical judgment is the final arbiter (Lupton et al, 1985).

ACQUIRED DISEASES OF THE URETER

Nearly all acquired diseases of the ureter are obstructive in nature. Although they are seen frequently, their actual incidence is unknown. Their clinical manifestations, effects on the kidney, complications, and treatment are similar to those described previously. The lesions can be broadly categorized as either intrinsic or extrinsic.

Intrinsic Ureteral Obstruction

The most common causes of intrinsic ureteral obstruction are as follows:

(1) Ureteral stones (see Chapter 17).
(2) Transitional cell tumors of the ureter (see Chapter 21).
(3) Chronic inflammatory changes of the ureteral wall (usually due to tuberculosis or schistosomiasis) leading to contracture or insufficient peristalsis (see Chapter 15 and Figures 15–2 and 15–4).

Extrinsic Ureteral Obstruction

The following are frequent causes of extrinsic ureteral obstruction:

(1) Severe constipation, sometimes with bladder obstruction, seen primarily in children but in adult women as well.
(2) Secondary obstruction due to kinks or fibrosis

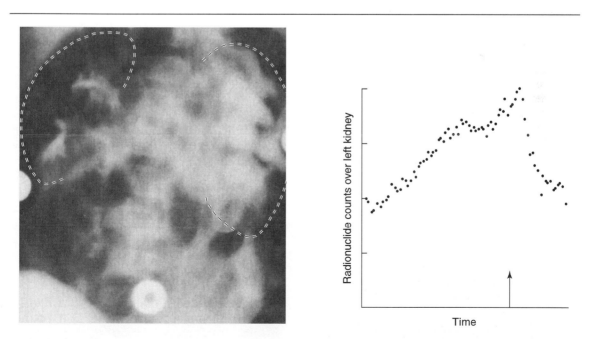

Figure 38–12. Upper urinary tract dilatation. **Left:** Three months after resection of posterior urethral valves, hydronephrosis in the right kidney has completely resolved. The left collecting system remains dilated. (Dashed lines outline kidneys.) **Right:** Radionuclide diuretic renography was performed to determine if there was secondary ureteropelvic or ureterovesical obstruction. Renogram demonstrates clear-cut "washout" of radionuclide following injection of furosemide (arrow). There is no significant obstruction.

around redundant ureters. The primary process is either distal obstruction or massive reflux.

(3) Benign gynecologic disorders such as endometriosis or right ovarian vein syndrome (Gourdie and Rogers, 1986).

(4) Local neoplastic infiltration associated with carcinoma of the cervix, bladder, or prostate (Richie, Withers, and Ehrlich, 1979).

(5) Pelvic lymphadenopathy associated with metastatic tumors.

(6) Iatrogenic ureteral injuries, primarily after extensive pelvic surgery (Figure 38–13) and also after extensive radiotherapy.

(7) Retroperitoneal fibrosis.

RETROPERITONEAL FIBROSIS
(Retroperitoneal Fasciitis, Chronic Retroperitoneal Fibroplasia, Ormond Disease)

One or both ureters may be compressed by a chronic inflammatory process that involves the retroperitoneal tissues over the lower lumbar vertebrae. This occurs primarily in adults but may be seen in children (Chan, Johnson, and McLoughlin, 1979). There are numerous causes of retroperitoneal fibrosis. Malignant diseases (most commonly Hodgkin disease, carcinoma of the breast, and carcinoma of the colon) should always be suspected and ruled out. Some medications have been implicated, most notably methysergide (Sansert), an ergot derivative used to treat migraine headaches. Rarely, inflammatory bowel disease (Siminovitch and Fazio, 1980) or an aortic aneurysm (Brock and Soloway, 1980; Peters and Cowie, 1978) is responsible. The remainder of cases are idiopathic, a condition sometimes referred to as Ormond disease.

The symptoms are nonspecific and include low back pain, malaise, anorexia, weight loss, and, in severe cases, uremia. Infection is uncommon. The diagnosis is usually made by excretory urography (Figure 38–14). There is medial deviation of the ureters with proximal dilation. A long segment of ureter is usually involved, and in some cases there is a pipestem appearance caused by aperistalsis related to the fibrosis. A retrograde ureterogram is necessary when renal function is poor and, in any case, helps to delineate the length of the affected segment of ureter. Ultrasonography is useful, not only for diagnosis but also for monitoring the response to therapy. Computed tomography (CT) scanning or MRI is essential for evaluating the retroperitoneum itself, as well as for imaging the ureters (Hricak, Higgins, and Williams, 1983).

Treatment is usually surgical, although a course of corticosteroids may be tried first if the hydronephrosis is mild (Moody and Vaughan, 1979). When the

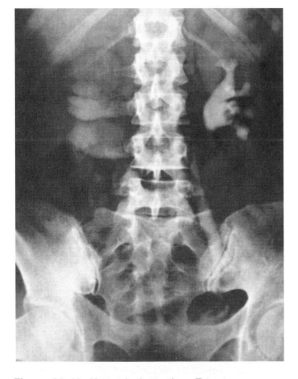

Figure 38–13. Ureteral obstruction. Excretory urogram obtained 2 weeks after Wertheim operation shows bilateral ureteral obstruction and marked hydronephrosis on right.

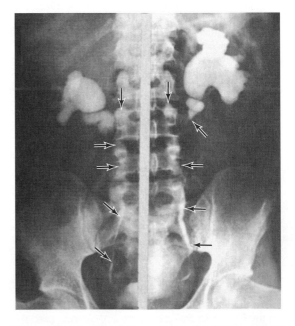

Figure 38–14. Retroperitoneal fibrosis. Right and left kidneys of same patient as shown by excretory urography. Note medial deviation of upper portions of ureters (arrows) with marked obstruction. (Courtesy of JA Hutch.)

response to corticosteroids is poor or the obstruction is severe, the ureter must be dissected surgically from the fibrous plaque. After it is freed, it should either be placed intraperitoneally or wrapped in omentum in an attempt to prevent recurrence (Lepor and Walsh, 1979). Rarely, autotransplantation is necessary (Deane, Gingell, and Pentlow, 1983). Numerous biopsies of the fibrous tissue should be obtained at the time of operation to determine whether there is a malignant tumor. Corticosteroids are sometimes used postoperatively; however, their efficacy is uncertain.

URETERAL OBSTRUCTION SECONDARY TO MALIGNANT DISEASE

Ureteral obstruction associated with widespread malignant disease was at one time a terminal event. Because therapy for malignant diseases has improved, however, urinary diversion is indicated more frequently in such cases. Diversion usually is necessary for relatively short periods of time; either the tumor is progressive, or if therapy is effective, the obstruction resolves. Thus, the goal of treatment is to leave the urinary tract intact and effect as little morbidity as possible. This can be accomplished with indwelling stents passed either retrogradely during cystoscopy (Hepperlen, Mardis, and Kammandel, 1979) or antegradely using percutaneous techniques (Elyaderani et al, 1982). Temporary percutaneous nephrostomy is a reasonable alternative, although indwelling stents are preferable for the patient (Ball et al, 1983; Andriole et al, 1984).

REFERENCES

CONGENITAL ANOMALIES

General

Glassberg KI et al: Suggested terminology for duplex systems, ectopic ureters and ureteroceles. J Urol 1984;132:1153.

Ureteral Atresia

Homsy Y et al: Wilms tumor and multicystic kidney disease. J Urol 1997;158:2256.

Javadpour N et al: Hypertension in a child caused by a multicystic kidney. J Urol 1970;104:918.

Rottenberg G, Gordon I, DeBruyn R: The natural history of the multicystic dysplastic kidney in children. Br J Radiol 1997;70:347.

Selzman A, Elder J: Contralateral vesicoureteral reflux in children with a multicystic kidney. J Urol 1995; 113:1252.

Yoshida T, Sakamoto K: Bilateral blind-ending duplex ureters. Br J Urol 1986;58:459.

Duplication of the Ureter

Amar AD: Ipsilateral ureteroureterostomy for single ureteral disease in patients with ureteral duplication: A review of 8 years of experience with 16 patients. J Urol 1978;119:472.

Amar AD: Ureteropyelostomy for relief of single ureteral obstruction in cases of ureteral duplication. Arch Surg 1970;101:379.

Atwell JD et al: Familial incidence of bifid and double ureters. Arch Dis Child 1974;49:390.

Barrett DM, Malek RS, Kelalis PP: Problems and solutions in surgical treatment of 100 consecutive ureteral duplications in children. J Urol 1975;114:126.

Belman AB, Filmer RB, King LR: Surgical management of duplication of the collecting system. J Urol 1974; 112:316.

Bieri M et al: Ipsilateral ureteroureterostomy for single ureteral reflux or obstruction in a duplicate system. J Urol 1998;159:1016.

Carter C, Malone P, Lewington V: Lower moiety heminephroureterectomy in the duplex refluxing kidney: The accuracy of isotopic scintigraphy in functional assessment. Br J Urol 1998;81:356.

Decter RM: Renal duplication and fusion anomalies. Pediatr Clin North Am 1997;44:1323.

Kaplan WE, Nasrallah P, King LR: Reflux in complete duplication in children. J Urol 1978;120:220.

Lee PH et al: Duplex reflux: A study of 105 children. J Urol 1991;146:657.

Nation EF: Duplication of the kidney and ureter: A statistical study of 230 new cases. J Urol 1944;51:456.

O'Reilly PH et al: Ureteroureteric reflux: Pathologic entity or physiological phenomenon? Br J Urol 1984; 56:159.

Sole GM, Randall J, Arkell DG: Ureteropyelostomy: A simple and effective treatment for symptomatic ureteroureteric reflux. Br J Urol 1987;60:325.

Tanagho EA: Embryologic basis for lower ureteral anomalies: A hypothesis. Urology 1976;7:451.

Zaontz MR, Maizels M: Type I ureteral triplication: An extension of the Weigert-Meyer law. J Urol 1985; 134:949.

Ureterocele

Ahmed S: Prolapsed single system ureterocele in a girl. J Urol 1984;132:1180.

Bauer SB, Retik AB: The non-obstructive ectopic ureterocele. J Urol 1978;119:804.

Blyth B et al: Endoscopic incision of ureteroceles: Intravesical versus ectopic. J Urol 1993;149:556.

Caldamone AA, Snyder HM III, Duckett JW: Ureteroceles in children: Follow-up of management with upper tract approach. J Urol 1984;131:1130.

Cromie WJ, Engelstein MS, Duckett JW Jr: Nodular renal blastema, renal dysplasia and duplicated collecting systems. J Urol 1980;123:100.

Geringer AM et al: The diagnostic approach to ectopic ureterocele and the renal duplication complex. J Urol 1983;129:539.

Gloor JM, Ogburn P, Matsumoto J: Prenatally diagnosed ureterocele presenting as fetal bladder outlet obstruction. J Perinatol 1996;16:285.

Husmann DA et al: Ureterocele associated with ureteral duplication and a nonfunctioning upper pole segment: Management by partial nephroureteroectomy alone. J Urol 1995;154:723.

Pfister C et al: The value of endoscopic treatment for ureteroceles during the neonatal period. J Urol 1998; 159:1006.

Snyder HM, Johnston JH: Orthotopic ureteroceles in children. J Urol 1978;119:543.

Tanagho EA: Embryologic basis for lower ureteral anomalies: A hypothesis. Urology 1976;7:451.

Ectopic Ureteral Orifice

Borer JG et al: A single-system ectopic ureter draining an ectopic dysplastic kidney: Delayed diagnosis in the young female with continuous urinary incontinence. Br J Urol 1998;81:474.

Gotoh T et al: Single ectopic ureter. J Urol 1983;129: 271.

Johnson DK, Perlmutter S: Single system ectopic ureteroceles. J Urol 1980;123:81.

Marshall S: Reimplantation of the dilated ectopic ureter of the duplex system as a separate unit. J Urol 1986;135:574.

Plaire JC et al: Management of ectopic ureters: Experience with the upper tract approach. J Urol 1997;158: 1245.

Umeyama T et al: Ectopic ureter presenting with epididymitis in childhood: Report of 5 cases. J Urol 1985;134:131.

Abnormalities of Ureteral Position

Brooks RJ: Left retrocaval ureter associated with situs inversus. J Urol 1962;88:484.

Hanna MK: Bilateral retroiliac artery ureters. Br J Urol 1972;44:339.

Kenawi MM, Williams DI: Circumcaval ureter: A report of 4 cases in children with a review of the literature and a new classification. Br J Urol 1976;48:183.

Kumar S, Bhandari M: Selection of operative procedure for circumcaval ureter (type I): A rational approach. Br J Urol 1985;57:399.

Polascik TJ, Chen RN: Laparoscopic ureteroureterostomy for retrocaval ureter. J Urol 1998;160:121.

Obstruction of the Ureteropelvic Junction

Amling CL et al: Renal ultrasound changes after pyeloplasty in children with ureteropelvic junction obstruction: Long-term outcome in 47 renal units. J Urol 1996;156:2020.

Anderson JC: *Hydronephrosis.* Heinemann, 1963.

Aslan P, Preminger GM: Retrograde balloon cautery incision of ureteropelvic junction obstruction. Urol Clin North Am 1998;25:295.

Badlani G, Eshghi M, Smith AD: Percutaneous surgery for ureteropelvic junction obstruction (endopyelot-

omy): Technique and early results. J Urol 1986;135: 26.

Bejjani B, Belman AB: Ureteropelvic junction obstruction in newborns and infants. J Urol 1982;128:770.

Bogaert GA et al: Efficacy of retrograde endopyelotomy in children. J Urol 1996;156:734.

Culp OS, DeWeerd JH: A pelvic flap operation for certain types of ureteropelvic obstruction. Mayo Clin Proc 1951;26:483.

Davis DM: Intubated ureterotomy: A new operation for ureteral and ureteropelvic strictures. Surg Gynecol Obstet 1943;76:513.

Foley FEB: A new plastic operation for stricture at the ureteropelvic junction. J Urol 1937;38:643.

Hanna MK et al: Ureteral structure and ultrastructure. 1. The normal human ureter. 2. Congenital ureteropelvic junction obstruction and primary obstructive megaureter. J Urol 1976;116:718, 725.

Johnston JH: The pathogenesis of hydronephrosis in children. Br J Urol 1969;41:724.

Johnston JH et al: Pelvic hydronephrosis in children: A review of 219 personal cases. J Urol 1977;117:97.

King LR et al: The case for immediate pyeloplasty in the neonate with ureteropelvic junction obstruction. J Urol 1984;132:725.

King LR et al: Initial experiences with percutaneous and transurethral ablation of postoperative ureteral strictures in children. J Urol 1984;131:1167.

Koff SA, Campbell K: Nonoperative management of unilateral neonatal hydronephrosis. J Urol 1992;148:525.

Koff SA et al: Pathophysiology of ureteropelvic junction obstruction: Experimental and clinical observations. J Urol 1986;136:336.

Maizels M, Smith CK, Firlit CF: The management of children with vesicoureteral reflux and ureteropelvic junction obstruction. J Urol 1984;131:722.

Mandell J et al: Structural genitourinary defects detected in utero. Radiology 1991;178:193.

Moore RG et al: Laparoscopic pyeloplasty: Experience with the initial 30 cases. J Urol 1997;157:459.

Palmer LS et al: Surgery versus observation for managing obstructive grade 3 to 4 unilateral hydronephrosis: A report from the Society for Fetal Urology. J Urol 1998;159:222.

Perlberg S, Pfau A: Management of ureteropelvic junction obstruction associated with lower polar vessels. Urology 1984;23:13.

Perlmutter AD, Kroovand RL, Lai Y-W: Management of ureteropelvic obstruction in the first year of life. J Urol 1980;123:535.

Punjani HM: Transitional cell papilloma of the ureter causing hydronephrosis in a child. Br J Urol 1983;55: 572.

Ramsay JWA et al: Percutaneous pyelolysis: Indications, complications and results. Br J Urol 1984;56:586.

Sant GR, Barbalias GA, Klauber GT: Congenital ureteral valves: An abnormality of ureteral embryogenesis? J Urol 1985;133:427.

Scardino PL, Prince CL: Vertical flap ureteropelvioplasty. South Med J 1953;46:325.

Smart WR: Surgical correction of hydronephrosis. In: Harrison JH et al (editors): *Campbell's Urology,* vol. 3. Saunders, 1979.

Stephens FD: Ureterovascular hydronephrosis and the "aberrant" renal vessels. J Urol 1982;128:984.

Thrall JH, Koff SA, Keyes JW Jr: Diuretic radionuclide renography and scintigraphy in the differential diagnosis of hydroureteronephrosis. Semin Nucl Med 1981;11:89.

Van Cangh PJ et al: Endoureteropyelotomy: Percutaneous treatment of ureteropelvic junction obstruction. J Urol 1989;141:1317.

Whitaker RH: Methods of assessing obstruction in dilated ureters. Br J Urol 1973;45:15.

Obstructed Megaureter

Baskin LS et al: Primary dilated megaureter: Long-term followup. J Urol 1994;152:618.

Ehrlich RM: The ureteral folding technique for megaureter surgery. J Urol 1985;134:668.

Hanna MK: Recent advances and further experience with surgical techniques for one-stage total remodeling of massively dilated ureters. Urology 1982;19:495.

Hendren WH: Operative repair of megaureter in children. J Urol 1969;101:491.

Peters CA et al: Congenital obstructed megaureter in early infancy: Diagnosis and treatment. J Urol 1989; 142:641.

Tanagho EA, Smith DR, Guthrie TH: Pathophysiology of functional ureteral obstruction. J Urol 1970;104:73.

Tiburcio MA, Lima SVC: Functionally obstructed megaureter. Braz J Urol 1978;4:36.

Upper Urinary Tract Dilatation
Without Obstruction

Homsy YL, Williot P, Danais S: Transitional neonatal hydronephrosis: Fact or fantasy? J Urol 1986;136:339.

Lupton EW et al: A comparison of diuresis renography, the Whitaker test and renal pelvic morphology in idiopathic hydronephrosis. Br J Urol 1985;57:119.

Thrall JH, Koff SA, Keyes JW Jr: Diuretic radionuclide renography and scintigraphy in the differential diagnosis of hydroureteronephrosis. Semin Nucl Med 1981;11:89.

Wolk FN, Whitaker RH: Late follow-up of dynamic evaluation of upper urinary tract obstruction. J Urol 1982;128:346.

ACQUIRED DISEASES

General

Gourdie RW, Rogers ACN: Bilateral ureteric obstruction due to endometriosis presenting with hypertension and cyclical oliguria. Br J Urol 1986;58:244.

Richie JP, Withers G, Ehrlich RM: Ureteral obstruction secondary to metastatic tumors. Surg Gynecol Obstet 1979;148:355.

Retroperitoneal Fibrosis

Brock J, Soloway MS: Retroperitoneal fibrosis and aortic aneurysm. Urology 1980;15:14.

Chan SL, Johnson HW, McLoughlin MG: Idiopathic retroperitoneal fibrosis in children. J Urol 1979;122:103.

Deane AM, Gingell JC, Pentlow BD: Idiopathic retroperitoneal fibrosis: The role of autotransplantation. Br J Urol 1983;55:254.

Hricak H, Higgins CB, Williams RD: Nuclear magnetic resonance imaging in retroperitoneal fibrosis. AJR 1983;141:35.

Lepor H, Walsh PC: Idiopathic retroperitoneal fibrosis. J Urol 1979;122:1.

Moody TE, Vaughan ED Jr: Steroids in the treatment of retroperitoneal fibrosis. J Urol 1979;121:109.

Peters JL, Cowie AG: Ureteric involvement with abdominal aortic aneurysm. Br J Urol 1978;50:313.

Siminovitch JM, Fazio VW: Ureteral obstruction secondary to Crohn's disease: A need for ureterolysis? Am J Surg 1980;139:95.

Ureteral Obstruction Secondary
to Malignant Disease

Andriole GL et al: Indwelling double-J ureteral stents for temporary and permanent urinary drainage: Experience with 87 patients. J Urol 1984;131:239.

Ball AJ et al: The indwelling ureteric stent: The Bristol experience. Br J Urol 1983;55:622.

Elyaderani MK et al: Facilitation of difficult percutaneous ureteral stent insertion. J Urol 1982;128:1173.

Hepperlen TW, Mardis HK, Kammandel H: The pigtail ureteral stent in the cancer patient. J Urol 1979;121:17.

Disorders of the Bladder, Prostate, & Seminal Vesicles

Emil A. Tanagho, MD

CONGENITAL ANOMALIES OF THE BLADDER*

EXSTROPHY

Exstrophy of the bladder is a complete ventral defect of the urogenital sinus and the overlying skeletal system (see Chapter 2). Other congenital anomalies are frequently associated with it. The lower central abdomen is occupied by the inner surface of the posterior wall of the bladder, whose mucosal edges are fused with the skin. Urine spurts onto the abdominal wall from the ureteral orifices.

The rami of the pubic bones are widely separated. The pelvic ring thus lacks rigidity, the femurs are rotated externally, and the child "waddles like a duck." Since the rectus muscles insert on the rami, they are widely separated from each other inferiorly. A hernia, made up of the exstrophic bladder and surrounding skin, is therefore present. Epispadias almost always accompanies it.

Many untreated exstrophic bladders reveal fibrosis, derangement of the muscularis mucosae, and chronic infection. These changes tend to defeat efforts to form a bladder of proper capacity. About 60 instances of adenocarcinoma developing in such bladders have been reported.

Renal infection is common, and hydronephrosis caused by ureterovesical obstruction may be found on urography. These films also reveal separation of the pubic bones.

During the last few years, there have been encouraging reports of complete reconstruction of this defect. Earlier, urinary diversion and resection of the bladder, with later repair of the epispadiac penis, was usually accomplished. With improved techniques and early surgery before the bladder deteriorates, however, good

results are being obtained with complete reconstruction. Lattimer et al (1978), pioneers in this field, followed up their 17 patients with reconstructed bladders for as long as 20 years. They reported that the quality of life of these patients was good.

Ansel (1979) performed reconstruction in 28 patients in the neonatal period in an attempt to protect the bladder from later serious changes. Half of these patients did well, and most were continent. De Maria et al (1980) found the renal function and urine cultures of their patients to be normal. Eight of their patients had complete continence, while 12 suffered from enuresis. Toguri et al (1978) reported that all of their 23 patients were continent.

Lima et al (1981) reconstructed the bladder with human dura mater to increase vesical capacity; they were successful in 8 cases. They perform osteotomy as part of the first stage and recommend that the surgery be performed when patients are 3–18 months old. Enterocystoplasty is currently the method of choice to augment bladder capacity and aid reservoir function. Mollard (1980) recommends the following steps for satisfactory repair of bladder exstrophy: (1) bladder closure with sacral osteotomy in order to close the pelvic ring at the pubic symphysis, plus lengthening of the penis; (2) antiureteral reflux procedure and bladder neck reconstruction; and (3) repair of the epispadiac penis. He completed 16 such 3-step procedures, with satisfactory results in 11. In 1983 and 1989, Jeffs and Gearhart reported results of staged reconstruction: 86% of patients who underwent primary repair were continent, and renal function was preserved in approximately 90%. Urethral and genital reconstruction have been equally successful. These are the best reported results. In small-capacity bladders, augmentation cystoplasty might be needed (Oesterling and Jeffs, 1987; Gearhart and Jeffs, 1988).

When the bladder is small, fibrotic, and inelastic, functional closure becomes inadvisable, and urinary diversion with cystectomy is the treatment of choice. Some physicians perform ureteroileocutaneous anastomosis, while others prefer to use the colon for the diversion. A continent reservoir is a current consideration and is preferable. Spence, Hoffman, and Pate

---

*Congenital vesicorectal fistulas are discussed with urethrorectal fistulas on **p 665.**

(1975) employ ureterosigmoidostomy. Turner, Ransley, and Williams (1980) noted that, although untreated newborns have normal upper urinary tracts, urinary diversion often causes hydronephrosis or pyelonephritis in these patients.

The common complication of total reconstruction is urinary incontinence, but Light and Scott (1983) reported on the implantation of an artificial sphincter in 11 patients who were still incontinent after total reconstruction. They claimed 10 perfect results. Ikeme (1981) reported on 2 patients who became pregnant after repair of bladder exstrophy; one woman had 3 successful pregnancies, and the other had one.

PERSISTENT URACHUS

Embryologically, the allantois connects the urogenital sinus with the umbilicus. Normally, the allantois is obliterated and is represented by a fibrous cord (urachus) extending from the dome of the bladder to the navel (see Chapter 2). Urachal formation is directly related to bladder descent. Lack of descent is more commonly associated with patent urachus than with bladder outlet obstruction.

Incomplete obliteration sometimes occurs. If obliteration is complete except at the superior end, a draining umbilical sinus may be noted. If it becomes infected, the drainage will be purulent. If the inferior end remains open, it will communicate with the bladder, but this does not usually produce symptoms. Rarely,

the entire tract remains patent, in which case urine drains constantly from the umbilicus. This is apt to become obvious within a few days of birth. If only the ends of the urachus seal off, a cyst of that body may form and may become quite large, presenting a low midline mass (Figure 39–1). If the cyst becomes infected, signs of general and local sepsis will develop.

Adenocarcinoma may occur in a urachal cyst, particularly at its vesical extremity, and tends to invade the tissues beneath the anterior abdominal wall. It may be seen cystoscopically. Stones may develop in a cyst of the urachus. These can be identified on a plain x-ray film.

Treatment consists of excision of the urachus, which lies on the peritoneal surface. If adenocarcinoma is present, radical resection is required.

Unless other serious congenital anomalies are present, the prognosis is good. The complication of adenocarcinoma offers a poor prognosis.

CONTRACTURE OF THE BLADDER NECK

There is considerable debate about the incidence of congenital narrowing of the bladder neck. Some feel that its presence is a common cause of vesicoureteral reflux, vesical diverticula, a bladder of large capacity, and the syndrome of irritable bladder associated with enuresis. A few observers consider this contracture a rare phenomenon and believe that the diagnosis is purely presumptive. The diagnosis is based on endo-

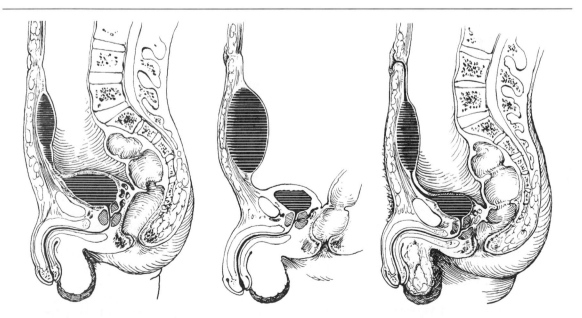

Figure 39–1. Types of persistent urachus. **Left:** Communicating urachus continuous with the bladder. This is a "pseudodiverticulum" and usually causes no symptoms. **Center:** Urachal cyst; usually causes no symptoms or signs unless it becomes larger or infected. **Right:** Patent urachus. There is constant drainage of urine from the umbilicus.

scopic observation, which is an unreliable method. Voiding cystourethrography has been used to depict such narrowing, but interpretation of the films varies from urologist to urologist and radiologist to radiologist.

Nunn (1965) studied the intravesical and urethral pressures during voiding in patients with the signs mentioned previously and found no evidence of bladder neck obstruction. The 2 recorded pressures were essentially equal. It appears that the bladder neck would have to be extremely stenotic to truly obstruct urine flow. It is becoming increasingly clear that in young girls, the obstructive lesion is spasm of the periurethral striated muscle, which develops secondary to distal urethral stenosis (see Chapter 41).

Empirical treatment is often employed; this consists of suprapubic bladder neck revision or transurethral resection. Making the bladder neck incompetent in young boys may cause later retrograde ejaculation and, therefore, infertility. Revision of the bladder neck in females may cause urinary incontinence and is never advised. The diagnosis must therefore be made with caution.

Genuine functional bladder neck obstruction can be detected only in the presence of already high voiding pressures combined with lower resistance in the external sphincteric segment associated with a low flow rate. This condition is highly suggestive of functional bladder neck obstruction, although not 100% diagnostic.

ACQUIRED DISEASES
OF THE BLADDER

INTERSTITIAL CYSTITIS
(Hunner's Ulcer, Submucous Fibrosis)

Interstitial cystitis is primarily a disease of middle-aged women. It is characterized by fibrosis of the vesical wall, with consequent loss of bladder capacity. Frequency, urgency, and pelvic pain with bladder distention are the principal symptoms.

Pathogenesis & Pathology

Infection does not appear to be the cause of fibrosis of the bladder wall, because the urine is usually normal. It has been postulated that the fibrosis is due to obstruction of the vesical lymphatics secondary to pelvic surgery or infection, but many of these patients fail to give such a history. Fibrosis may be secondary to thrombophlebitis complicating acute infections of the bladder or pelvic organs; may be the result of prolonged intrinsic arteriolar spasm secondary to vasculitis or psychogenic impulses; or could be of neuro-

pathic origin. Endocrinologic factors are also suggested. Investigators are currently studying the role of mast cells and bladder surface glycosaminoglycans (GAGs) in the pathogenesis of interstitial cystitis. Currently, it is believed that interstitial cystitis is a neuroimmunoendocrine disorder. It might be primarily a neurogenic inflammation that leads to the release of neuropeptides that activate the differential secretion of potent mast cell mediators. It is thought that mast cells, through their vasoactive and nociceptive secretions, have a major role in the etiology of interstitial cystitis.

The primary change is fibrosis in the deeper layers of the bladder. The capacity of the organ is decreased, sometimes markedly. The mucosa is thinned, especially where mobility is greatest as the bladder fills and empties (ie, over the dome), and small ulcers or cracks in the mucous membrane may be seen in this area. In the most severe cases, the normal mechanism of the ureterovesical junctions is destroyed, leading to vesicoureteral reflux. Hydroureteronephrosis and pyelonephritis may ensue.

Microscopically, the mucosa may be thinned or even denuded. The capillaries of the tunica propria are often engorged, and signs of inflammation are apparent. The muscle is replaced by varying amounts of fibrous tissue, which is often quite avascular. The lymphatics may be engorged. Increased mast cells and lymphocytic infiltration are seen.

There has been a tendency recently to overdiagnose interstitial cystitis, particularly in patients with excessive frequency, urgency, and suprapubic or pelvic pain, even though they lack the pathologic manifestations and usually have normal or large bladder capacity. These patients have voiding dysfunction. Although we may not know the exact cause of their symptoms, these patients should not be labeled as having interstitial cystitis and should not be treated as such.

Clinical Findings

Interstitial cystitis should be considered when a middle-aged woman with clear urine complains of severe frequency and nocturia and suprapubic pain on vesical distention.

A. Symptoms: There is a long history of slowly progressive frequency and nocturia, both of which may be severe. The history does not suggest infection (burning on urination, cloudy urine). Suprapubic pain is usually marked when the bladder is full. Pain may also be experienced in the urethra or perineum; it is relieved on voiding. Gross hematuria is occasionally noted, usually when urination has had to be postponed (ie, following vesical overdistention). The patient is tense and anxious. Whether the anxiety is secondary to the prolonged and severe symptoms or is the primary cause of the vesical changes is not clear. A history of allergy may be obtained.

B. Signs: Physical examination is usually normal. Some tenderness in the suprapubic area may be noted. There may be some tenderness in the region of the bladder when it is palpated through the vagina.

C. Laboratory Findings: If the patient has had no previous treatment (eg, instrumentation), the urine is almost always free of infection. Microscopic hematuria may be noted. Results of renal function tests are normal except in the occasional patient in whom vesical fibrosis has led to vesicoureteral reflux or obstruction.

D. X-Ray Findings: Excretory urograms are usually normal unless reflux has occurred, in which case hydronephrosis is found. The accompanying cystogram reveals a bladder of small capacity; reflux into a dilated upper tract may be noted on cystography.

E. Instrumental Examination: Cystoscopy is usually diagnostic. As the bladder fills, increasing suprapubic pain is experienced. The vesical capacity may be as low as 60 mL. In a patient not previously treated (by fulguration or hydraulic overdistention), the bladder lining may look fairly normal. However, if a second distention is done (Messing and Stamey, 1978), punctate hemorrhagic areas may appear over the most distensible portion of the wall. With further distention, an arcuate split in the mucosa will occur and may bleed profusely. Mucosal changes are usually diffuse. Congestion, edematous reaction, and petechial hemorrhages (glomerulation) are common findings.

Differential Diagnosis

Tuberculosis of the bladder may cause true ulceration but is most apt to involve the region of the ureteral orifice that drains the tuberculous kidney. Typical tubercles may be identified, pyuria is present, and tubercle bacilli usually can be found. Furthermore, urograms often show the typical lesion of renal tuberculosis.

Vesical ulcers due to schistosomiasis cause symptoms similar to those of interstitial cystitis. The diagnosis is suggested if the patient lives in an area in which schistosomiasis is endemic. Most patients are males. The typical ova found in the urine and the pathognomonic appearance of the bladder confirm the diagnosis.

Nonspecific vesical infection seldom causes ulceration. Pus and bacteria are found in the urine. Antimicrobial treatment is effective.

Utz and Zinke (1974) observed that 20% of their male patients who had been diagnosed as having interstitial cystitis actually had carcinoma. They stress the need for cytologic study and transurethral biopsy.

Complications

Gradual ureteral stenosis or reflux and its sequelae (eg, hydronephrosis) may develop.

Treatment

A. Specific Measures: There appears to be no definitive treatment for interstitial cystitis. The therapy usually employed frequently affords partial relief, but it may be completely ineffective.

Hydraulic overdistention, with or without anesthesia, sometimes gradually improves the bladder capacity. Vesical lavage with increasing strengths of silver nitrate (1:5000–1:100) may have the same effect. Superficial (transcystoscopic) electrocoagulation of the split mucosa is commonly performed and may afford temporary relief of pain.

Occasionally, symptomatic relief follows the instillation of 50 mL of 50% dimethyl sulfoxide (DMSO) into the bladder every 2 weeks. It is left in for 15 min.

Messing and Stamey (1978) claim their best results were obtained with vesical irrigations of 0.4% oxychlorosene sodium (Clorpactin WCS-90). At 10 cm of water pressure, the bladder is repeatedly filled to capacity until 1 L has been used. This must be done under anesthesia. Cystography should be done before instituting this therapy. The presence of vesicoureteral reflux has caused ureteral fibrosis (Messing and Freiha, 1979).

Parsons, Schmidt, and Pollen (1983) observed the results obtained in patients who failed to respond to hydraulic distention or the instillation of DMSO. They found that the bladder mucosa needs a layer of sulfonated GAGs on its surface to protect the transitional cells from the effect of urine, and this substance was absent from the mucosa of these patients. They administered sodium pentosanpolysulfate (Elmiron) orally, in doses of either 50 mg 4 times a day or 150 mg twice daily, for 4–8 weeks. Of 24 patients, 20 noted at least 80% relief of urgency, frequency, and nocturia, and 2 noted 50–80% relief. These 22 patients continue to improve. Two patients experienced no apparent relief.

Cortisone acetate, 100 mg, or prednisone (Meticorten), 10–20 mg/d, in divided doses orally for 21 days, followed by decreasing amounts for an additional 21 days, has also been found effective. Transcystoscopic injection of the lesions with prednisone has its proponents.

Antihistamines (eg, tripelennamine [Pyribenzamine], 50 mg 4 times a day) may also afford some relief. Heparin sodium (long-acting), 20,000 units intravenously daily, also blocks the action of histamine, and its use in the treatment of interstitial cystitis is encouraging.

If the bladder becomes fibrotic and the capacity small, ceco- or ileocystoplasty can be done to augment vesical capacity. Most patients are cured or greatly improved; those who are not may require urinary diversion.

Denervation by presacral and sacral neurectomy and perivesical procedures (cystolysis, cystoplasty, transvaginal neurotomy) is to be condemned, as it is rarely of lasting benefit. In severe contracture, augmentation cystoplasty is indicated.

B. General Measures: General or vesical sedatives may be prescribed but seldom afford relief. If urinary infection is found (usually following instrumentation), it should be treated with appropriate antibiotics. If senile urethritis is discovered, diethylstilbestrol vaginal suppositories may prove helpful.

C. Treatment of Complications: If progressive hydronephrosis develops secondary to ureteral stenosis, little will be gained by ureteral dilatations. Diversion of the urinary stream (eg, ureteroileocutaneous anastomosis) may therefore be necessary.

Prognosis

Most patients respond to one of the conservative measures mentioned previously. Those who do not may require surgery.

INTERNAL VESICAL HERNIATION

One side of the bladder may become involved in an inguinal hernia (in men) or a femoral hernia (in women) (Figure 39–2). Such a mass may recede on urination. It is most often found as a previously unsuspected complication during surgical correction of a hernia (Bell and Witherington, 1980). Weitzenfeld et al (1980) reported a case in which the right kidney and ureter as well as the left ureter were in scrotal inguinal hernias.

URINARY INCONTINENCE

Partial or complete urinary incontinence may develop after prostatectomy, particularly radical or transurethral prostatectomy. Intrinsic damage to the smooth muscle urethral sphincter is implied. Although it is common to incriminate damage to or resection of the external voluntary sphincter, this is very rare. Such a patient can stop the voiding stream by contracture of the latter sphincter, but prolonged control is impossible because of fatigue of striated muscle. Only the smooth muscle with its constant tone can afford continence.

Some of the mild cases may respond to ephedrine. Diokno and Taub (1975) prescribed up to 200 mg/d in 4 divided doses, with good response. Children also benefited from the elixir, which contains 11 mg of ephedrine per 5 mL.

Scott, Bradley, and Timm (1974) and Light and Scott (1983) have described an ingenious method for affording urinary control by means of an artificial sphincter. It consists of a reservoir of fluid in a Silastic bag placed deep to the abdominal wall near the bladder and a collar of Silastic material that can encircle either the bladder neck or the bulbar urethra. The former is used in females, the latter in males. One Silastic bulb is implanted in one scrotal (or labial) sac. This bulb has a special pressurized valve that inflates or deflates the cuff around the urethra; compressed fluid passes from the cuff to the reservoir, permitting free voiding. The cuff refills spontaneously after a delay of 2 min. This device has been successful in affording control in most instances. Results are perfect in 75% or more of cases. Most failures follow technical difficulties with the prosthesis, eg, leakage, which requires reoperation.

Tanagho and Smith (1972) have designed a procedure based on sound anatomic principles that has been quite successful in restoring urinary continence. A rectangular flap of the heavy layer of the middle circular layer of the detrusor muscle, anteriorly, is formed into a tube, thus affording sphincteric action. This is anastomosed to the prostatic urethra. With this procedure, 44 of 50 patients suffering from postprostatectomy incontinence were cured. Williams and Snyder (1976) have used this procedure successfully in children.

ENURESIS

Enuresis originally meant incontinence of urine, but usage has caused the term to be restricted to bed-wetting after age 3 years. Most children have achieved normal bladder control by that time, girls earlier than boys. At age 6 years, 10% have enuresis. Even at age 14 years, 5% still wet the bed. It is difficult to be sure, but it seems that more than 50% of cases are caused by delayed maturation of the nervous system or an intrinsic myoneurogenic bladder dysfunction; 30% are of psychological origin; and 20% are secondary to more obvious organic disease. Most children with functional enuresis spontaneously gain nocturnal control by age 10 years. The current thinking is that children with enuresis have high nocturnal urine production; some have normal bladder capacity, others reduced capacity.

Psychodynamics

Training in bladder control should begin after age 1 1/2 years; attempts made before this time are usually fruitless and may be harmful. If the parents fail in this teaching, the child may not develop cerebral inhibitory control over the infantile uninhibited bladder until much later in childhood. If the parents are emotionally unstable, their anxieties may be transmitted to the child, who may express tension through enuresis.

The birth of a sibling may cause loss of the child's paramount position in the family. The child may then regress to an infancy pattern in an attempt to recapture the parents' affection. An acute illness may be accompanied or followed by recurrence of incomplete nocturnal control. Physiologic or psychological stress (fear and anxiety) may reestablish an uninhibited bladder.

Possibly 40% of enuretic children have electroencephalograms that are borderline or compatible with epilepsy or delayed maturation of the central nervous system.

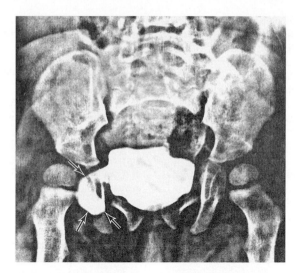

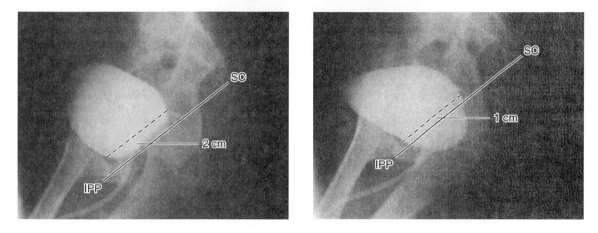

Figure 39–2. Internal vesical hernia; lateral cystograms in stress incontinence. **Top:** Female, 6 months old. Cystogram of excretory urogram showing tongue of bladder in right femoral hernia (see arrows). In the 2 films shown below, the dashed line shows the normal position of the base of the normal bladder. Line SCIPP is a reference line drawn from the sacrococcygeal (SC) joint to the inferior point of the pubic bone (IPP). **Bottom left:** Resting cystogram in a patient with stress incontinence. The bladder base lies 2 cm below the normal position. **Bottom right:** Cystogram taken with straining in a patient with stress incontinence. The base of the bladder descends about 4 cm, revealing poor support of the urethrovesical junction. (Courtesy of John A. Hutch.)

Clinical Findings

A. Symptoms: A child may wet the bed occasionally or regularly. Careful questioning of the parents or observation by the physician reveals that the patient voids a free stream of normal caliber. This tends to rule out obstruction of the lower tract as a cause of the enuresis. Children with daytime incontinence are apt to have more than psychogenic enuresis. Many void frequently and are found to have a diminished vesical capacity, although capacity is normal under anesthesia. This is probably a reflection of delayed maturation. There is no burning, although frequency and urgency are common. The urine is clear.

Observation of the parents often reveals that they are anxious and tense, traits that can only be aggravated by the child's bedwetting.

B. Signs: General physical and urologic examinations are normal.

C. Laboratory Findings: In the emotional and delayed maturation groups, all tests, including urinalysis, are normal. An electroencephalogram may be abnormal, however.

D. X-Ray Findings: Excretory urograms show no abnormality. The accompanying cystogram reveals no trabeculation; a film of the bladder taken immediately after voiding shows no residual urine.

E. Instrumental Examination: A catheter of suitable size passes readily to the bladder, thereby ruling out stricture. If the catheter is passed after urination, no residual urine is found. Urethrocystoscopy is normal. Cystometric studies are usually abnormal, and a curve typical of the "uninhibited" (hyperirritable) neuropathic bladder is often obtained. Unless infection or some more obvious organic disease is discovered, instrumentation, x-ray, and urodynamic studies are not necessary.

Differential Diagnosis

A. Obstruction: Lower tract obstruction (eg, posterior urethral valves, meatal stenosis) causes a urinary stream of decreased caliber. Painful, frequent urination during the day and night, pyuria, and fever (eg, pyelonephritis) are often present, and the bladder may be distended. Urinalysis usually reveals evidence of infection. Anemia and impairment of renal function may be demonstrated.

Excretory urograms may show dilatation of the bladder and the upper urinary tract. Incomplete vesical emptying may be seen on the postvoiding film. Cystography may demonstrate distal urethral stenosis or reflux. Urethrocystoscopy reveals the organic cause.

Severe obstruction from severe spasm of the entire pelvic floor musculature on a psychosomatic basis can cause damage to the bladder and kidneys; infection is the rule.

B. Infection: Chronic urinary tract infection not due to obstruction usually produces frequency both day and night and pain on urination, although such infections may occur without symptoms of vesical irritability. Recurrent fever with exacerbations is common.

General examination may be normal. Anemia may be noted. Urinalysis shows pus cells or bacteria, or both. Renal function may be deficient. Excretory urograms may be essentially normal, although changes compatible with healed pyelonephritis are often seen. Cystoscopy shows the changes caused by infection. Urine specimens obtained by ureteral catheter may reveal renal infection. Cystography may show vesicoureteral reflux.

C. Neurogenic Disease: Children suffering from sacral cord or root abnormality (eg, myelodysplasia) may have incomplete urinary control both day and night. Since they ordinarily have significant amounts of residual urine, infection is usually found on urinalysis. The passage of a catheter or the postvoiding film taken in conjunction with excretory urograms demonstrates the presence of residual urine. A plain film of the abdomen may reveal spina bifida.

The cystometrogram is usually typical of a flaccid neurogenic bladder. Cystoscopy demonstrates an atonic bladder with moderate trabeculation and evidence of infection.

D. Distal Urethral Stenosis: Distal urethral stenosis, a congenital anomaly, is the cause of enuresis in many young girls, even in the absence of cystitis. Urethral calibration establishes this diagnosis.

Complications

The complications of functional enuresis are psychological, not organic. These children are particularly disturbed when they begin to attend school; even more pressure is brought to bear by their parents. These children find it impossible to stay overnight at the homes of their playmates. Unhealthy introversion may be their lot. Enuresis may be prolonged because of undue emphasis on dryness or as a result of punitive or shaming measures.

Late Sequels

Occasionally an adult is seen who, under stress, develops nocturnal frequency without comparable diurnal frequency. Thorough urologic investigation proves to be negative. Many of these people give histories of enuresis of long duration in childhood. It is suggested that their cerebrovesical pathways again break down with excessive emotional tension; nocturnal frequency may be the adult expression of enuresis.

Treatment

Treatment should be considered if enuresis persists after age 3 years.

A. General Measures: Fluids should be limited after supper. The bladder should be completely emptied at bedtime, and the child should be completely awakened a little before the usual time of bedwetting and allowed to void.

Drug therapy has its proponents.

1. Imipramine has been reported to cure 50–70% of patients and is probably the drug of choice. The starting dose is 25 mg before dinner, which is increased as needed to 50 mg. Usually, 25 mg is sufficient.

2. Parasympatholytic drugs such as atropine or belladonna, by decreasing the tone of the detrusor, may at times be of value. Methantheline bromide, 25–75 mg at bedtime, is more potent.

3. Sympathomimetic drugs, eg, dextroamphetamine sulfate, 5–10 mg at bedtime, may cause enough wakefulness so that the child perceives the urge to void.

4. Desmopressin is an antidiuretic that increases renal reabsorption of water, reducing urine output in patients with a decreased nocturnal peak in antidiuretic hormone. Given as a nasal spray by night, it has been successful in 70% of patients with increased nocturnal urine output.

5. Phenytoin has been found to control symptoms in some children whose electroencephalograms are abnormal.

The use of mechanical devices such as metal-covered pads that when wet cause an alarm to ring may be of benefit in cases of delayed maturation by setting up a conditioned reflex.

Urologic treatments (eg, urethral dilation, urethral instillations of silver nitrate), though often recommended, should be condemned in the absence of demonstrable local disease. They are physically and psychologically traumatic and can only cause further apprehension and fear in an already disturbed child.

B. Psychotherapy: Analytic evaluation and treatment may be indicated for some enuretic children and their parents. Responsibility for correction of the patient's feelings of insecurity rests with the parents, who must be cautioned not to punish the child or in any way increase existing feelings of guilt and insecurity. The handling of the parents may prove difficult, in which case psychiatric referral may be necessary.

Prognosis

Retraining the enuretic child and, above all, reeducating the parents are difficult and time-consuming tasks. Psychiatric referral for the parents and, at times, for the child may be necessary. Most patients conquer their enuresis by age 10 years. A few, however, do not, and they may later develop vesical irritability of the psychogenic type in response to acute or chronic tension or anxiety.

FOREIGN BODIES INTRODUCED INTO THE BLADDER & URETHRA

Numerous objects have been found in the urethra and bladder of both men and women. Some of them find their way into the urethra in the course of inquisitive self-exploration. Others are introduced (in the male) as contraceptive devices in the hope that plugging the urethra will block emission of the ejaculate.

The presence of a foreign body causes cystitis. Hematuria is not uncommon. Embarrassment may cause the victim to delay medical consultation. A plain x-ray of the bladder area discloses metal objects. Nonopaque objects sometimes become coated with calcium. Cystoscopy visualizes them all.

Cystoscopic or suprapubic removal of the foreign body is indicated. If not removed, the foreign body will lead to infection of the bladder. If the infecting organisms are urea-splitting, the alkaline urine (which causes increased insolubility of calcium salts) contributes to rapid formation of stone on the foreign object (Figure 17–13).

VESICAL MANIFESTATIONS OF ALLERGY

So many mucous membranes are affected by allergens that the possibility of allergic manifestations involving the bladder must be considered. Hypersensitivity is occasionally suggested in cases of recurrent symptoms of acute "cystitis" in the absence of urinary infection or other demonstrable abnormality. During the attack, general erythema of the vesical mucosa may be seen and some edema of the ureteral orifices noted.

A careful history may reveal that these attacks follow the ingestion of a food not ordinarily eaten (eg, fresh lobster). Sensitivity to spermicidal creams is occasionally observed. If vesical allergy is suspected, it may be aborted by the subcutaneous injection of 0.5–1 mL of 1:1000 epinephrine. Control may also be afforded by the use of one of the antihistamines. Skin testing has not generally proved helpful in determining the source of allergy.

DIVERTICULA

Most vesical diverticula are acquired and are secondary to either obstruction distal to the vesical neck or the upper motor neuron type of neurogenic bladder. Increased intravesical pressure causes vesical mucosa to insinuate itself between hypertrophied muscle bundles, so that a mucosal extravesical sac develops. Often this sac lies just superior to the ureter and causes vesicoureteral reflux (Hutch saccule; Figure 13–6). The diverticulum is devoid of muscle and therefore has no expulsive power; residual urine is the rule, and infection is perpetuated. If the diverticulum has a narrow opening that interferes with its emptying, transurethral resection of its neck will improve drainage. Carcinoma occasionally develops on its wall. Mićić and Ilić (1983) discovered 13 diverticula harboring malignant tumors: 9 transitional cell tumors, 2 squamous cell tumors, and 2 adenocarcinomas. Gerridzen and Futter (1982) saw 48 cases of vesical diverticula. Transitional cell tumors were found in 5 of these patients, but almost all the rest had abnormal histopathology: chronic inflammation and metaplasia. These authors stress the need for visualizing the interior of diverticula during endoscopy. At the time of open prostatectomy, resection of a diverticulum should be considered.

VESICAL FISTULAS

Vesical fistulas are common. The bladder may communicate with the skin, intestinal tract, or female reproductive organs. The primary disease is usually not urologic. The causes are as follows: (1) primary intestinal disease—diverticulitis, 50–60%; cancer of the colon, 20–25%; and Crohn disease, 10% (Badlani et al, 1980); (2) primary gynecologic disease—pressure necrosis during difficult labor; advanced cancer of the cervix; (3) treatment for gynecologic disease following hysterectomy, low cesarean section, or radiotherapy for tumor; and (4) trauma.

Malignant tumors of the small or large bowel, uterus, or cervix may invade and perforate the bladder. Inflammations of adjacent organs may also erode through the vesical wall. Severe injuries involving the bladder may lead to perivesical abscess formation, and these abscesses may rupture through the skin of the perineum or abdomen. The bladder may be inadvertently injured during gynecologic or intestinal surgery; cystotomy for stone or prostatectomy may lead to a persistent cutaneous fistula.

Clinical Findings

A. Vesicointestinal Fistula: Symptoms arising from a vesicointestinal fistula include vesical irritability, the passage of feces and gas through the urethra, and usually a change in bowel habits (eg, constipation, abdominal distention, diarrhea) caused by the primary intestinal disease. Signs of bowel obstruction may be elicited; abdominal tenderness may be found if the cause is inflammatory. The urine is always infected.

A barium enema, upper gastrointestinal series, or sigmoidoscopic examination may demonstrate the communication. Following a barium enema, centrifuged urine should be placed on an x-ray cassette and an exposure made. The presence of radiopaque barium establishes the diagnosis of vesicocolonic fistula. Cystograms may reveal gas in the bladder or reflux of the opaque material into the bowel (Figure 39–3). Cystoscopic examination, the most useful diagnostic procedure, shows a severe localized inflammatory reaction from which bowel contents may exude. Catheterization of the fistulous tract may be feasible; the instillation of radiopaque fluid often establishes the diagnosis.

B. Vesicovaginal Fistula: This relatively common fistula is secondary to obstetric, surgical, or radiation injury or to invasive cancer of the cervix. The constant leakage of urine is most distressing to the patient. Pelvic examination usually reveals the fistulous opening, which also can be visualized with the cystoscope. It may be possible to pass a ureteral catheter through the fistula into the vagina. Vaginography often successfully shows ureterovaginal, vesicovaginal, and rectovaginal fistulas. A 30-mL Foley catheter is inserted into the vagina, and the balloon is distended. A radiopaque solution is then instilled, and appropriate x-rays are taken. Biopsy of the edges of the fistula may show carcinoma. Persky, Forsythe, and Herman (1980) describe vesicovaginal fistulas in 6 children; all occurred as a complication of surgery, 3 following transurethral resection of the bladder neck.

C. Vesicoadnexal Fistula: This rare fistula can be diagnosed by vaginal examination and by seeing the fistulous opening through the cystoscope.

Differential Diagnosis

It is necessary to differentiate ureterovaginal from vesicovaginal fistula. Phenazopyridine (Pyridium) is given by mouth to color the urine orange. One hour later, 3 cotton pledgets are inserted into the vagina, and methylene blue solution is instilled into the bladder. The patient should then walk around, after which the pledgets are examined. If the proximal cotton ball is wet or stained orange, the fistula is ureterovaginal. If the deep cotton pledget contains blue fluid, the diagnosis is vesicovaginal fistula. If only the distal pledget is blue, the patient probably has urinary incontinence (Raghavaiah, 1974).

Treatment

A. Vesicointestinal Fistula: If the lesion is in the rectosigmoid, treatment consists of proximal colostomy. When the inflammatory reaction has subsided, the involved bowel may be resected, with closure of the opening in the bladder. The colostomy can be closed later. Some authors recommend that the entire procedure be performed in one stage, thus avoiding the need for preliminary colostomy. Small bowel or appendiceal vesical fistulas require bowel or appendiceal resection and closure of the vesical defect (Goodwin and Scardino, 1980).

B. Vesicovaginal Fistula: Tiny fistulous openings may become sealed following the introduction of an electrode into the fistula. As the electrode is withdrawn, the fistula is coagulated with the electrosurgical unit to destroy the epithelium of the tract. An indwelling catheter should be left in place for 2 weeks or more. Occasionally, good results are noted in cases of small vesicovaginal fistulas treated by inserting a metal screw through the vaginal end of the fistula. It is moved up and down to act as a curet. The vaginal mucosa is then closed and an indwelling catheter placed for 3 weeks.

Larger fistulas secondary to obstetric or surgical injuries respond readily to surgical repair, which may be done either through the vagina or transvesically (Goodwin and Scardino, 1980). Persky, Herman, and Guerrier (1979) advise repairing such fistulas immediately rather than waiting for 3–6 months as counseled by most surgeons. Fistulas that develop following radiation therapy for cancer of the cervix are much more difficult to close because of the avascularity of the tissues. Surgical closure of fistulas that arise from direct invasion of the bladder by cervical carcinoma is impossible; diversion of the urinary stream above the level of the bladder (eg, ureterosigmoidostomy) is therefore necessary.

C. Vesicoadnexal Fistula: These fistulas are cured by removal of the involved female reproductive organs, with closure of the opening in the bladder (Henricksen, 1981).

Prognosis

The surgical repair of fistulas caused by benign disease or operative trauma is highly successful. Postirradiation necrosis offers a more guarded prognosis. Fistulas secondary to invading cancers present difficult problems.

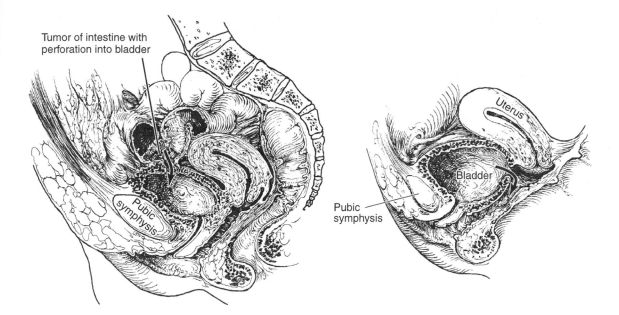

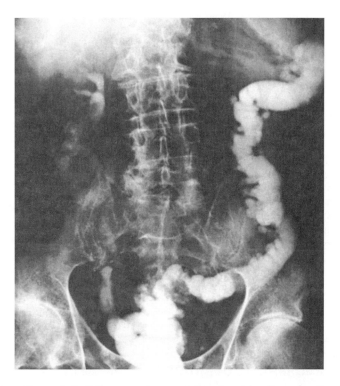

Figure 39–3. Vesical fistulas. **Above left:** Primary carcinoma of the sigmoid, with perforation through bladder wall. **Above right:** Injury to base of bladder following delivery by forceps. **Below:** Cystogram showing radiopaque fluid entering sigmoid containing multiple diverticula; right ureteral reflux, gallbladder calculi.

PERIVESICAL LIPOMATOSIS

The cause of perivesical lipomatosis is not known. The disorder seems to affect principally black men in the 20- to 40-year age group. There are no pathognomonic symptoms. There may be some dysuria or mild urinary obstructive symptoms. Examination may demonstrate a distended or enlarged pear-shaped bladder. Excretory urograms and cystography may show dilatation of both upper tracts and an upward displacement and lateral compression of the bladder. In the perivesical area, x-ray reveals areas of radiolucency compatible with fatty tissue. A barium x-ray may show extrinsic pressure on the rectosigmoid. Angiography shows no evidence of neoplastic vessels.

Computed tomography scan in association with the preceding findings establishes the diagnosis by clearly demonstrating the fatty nature of the perivesical tissue (Levine, Farber, and Lee, 1978; Susmano and Dolin, 1979). Church and Kazam (1979) found sonography equally helpful.

On surgical exploration, lipomatous tissue is found surrounding the bladder and rectosigmoid. Though it is tempting to proceed with its resection, there are no cleavage planes. Such dissections usually fail to relieve the ureteral obstruction.

Ballesteros (1977) believes that surgical excision is feasible and reported excellent results in one such case. Crane and Smith (1977) found, after a 5-year follow-up, that hydronephrosis progressed in most. Many patients finally required urinary diversion.

RADIATION CYSTITIS

Many women receiving radiation treatment for carcinoma of the cervix develop some degree of vesical irritability. These symptoms may develop months after cessation of treatment. The urine may or may not be sterile. Vesical capacity is usually appreciably reduced. Cystoscopy reveals a pale mucous membrane with multiple areas of telangiectatic blood vessels. Vesical ulceration may be noted, and vesicovaginal fistulas may develop. If symptoms are severe and prolonged, diversion of urine from the bladder may be necessary.

NONINFECTIOUS HEMORRHAGIC CYSTITIS

Some patients, following radiotherapy for carcinoma of the cervix or bladder, are prone to intermittent, often serious vesical hemorrhage. The same is true of those given cyclophosphamide.

In the case of the latter, the drug must be stopped. To control bleeding, cystoscopic fulguration can be tried, though it usually fails. The instillation of 3.9% formalin (prepared by diluting the standard 39% solution 10 times) is more efficacious. The catheter is clamped for 30 min and the bladder lavaged with 10% alcohol. A second or third instillation may be necessary on subsequent days. Holstein et al (1973) recommend the transurethral placement of a large balloon in the bladder. The balloon is filled to a pressure level equal to the systolic blood pressure and left in place for 6 h.

Pyeritz et al (1978) were unable to stop the hemorrhage with formalin or silver nitrate, but a continuous intravenous infusion of vasopressin caused it to cease. Giulani et al (1979) report success by selective transcatheter embolization of the internal iliac arteries. Ostroff and Chenault (1982) believe that the best and least harmful method of treatment is continuous irrigation with 1% alum solution (the ammonium or potassium salt) through a 3-way Foley catheter.

Despite these measures, the mortality rate is significant. Droller, Saral, and Santos (1982) have evolved a plan for reducing the incidence of cyclophosphamide-induced hemorrhagic cystitis: they produce diuresis and have the patient void frequently (or use open catheter drainage). This reduces the concentration of cyclophosphamide metabolites and the duration of their contact with bladder mucosa. Before the institution of this regimen, 8 of 97 such patients died; afterward, 1 of 198 patients died.

EMPYEMA OF THE BLADDER

If supravesical diversion of the urine is performed without cystectomy, severe infection of the bladder may develop because of lack of washout. In males, cystostomy or cutaneous vesicostomy may be necessary. In females, the formation of a vesicovaginal fistula permits drainage (Spence and Allen, 1971). Occasionally, cystectomy may be necessary.

CONGENITAL ANOMALIES OF THE PROSTATE & SEMINAL VESICLES

Congenital anomalies of the prostate are rare. Cysts of the prostate and the seminal vesicles have been reported. Enlargements of the prostatic utricle are often found in association with penoscrotal or perineal hypospadias. The cysts are usually small, lying in the midline posterior to the prostate and emptying through the verumontanum. These cysts represent embryologic remnants of the distal end of the müllerian ducts (see Chapter 2). Rarely, they become large enough to be easily palpable rectally or even abdominally. Through local pressure, they may cause symptoms of obstruction of the bladder neck.

BLOODY EJACULATION

Hemospermia is not an uncommon complaint of middle-aged men. It is the wife who usually recognizes the symptom. It is thought by some to be caused by hyperplasia of the mucosa of the seminal vesicles. For this reason, the use of diethylstilbestrol, 5 mg/d for 1 week, has been suggested. In my hands, it has worked well. Thorough urologic investigation of men without other symptoms rarely reveals a pathologic lesion. The cause is therefore not clear. Stein, Prioleau, and Catalona (1980) have observed this symptom to be caused by adenomatous polyps in 3 men and to accompany a prostatic intraductal carcinoma in another. Cattolica (1982) cured 3 patients by electrocoagulation of granulations of the posterior urethra. Van Poppel et al (1983) found the blood to emanate from a utricular cyst. Needle aspiration cured it.

REFERENCES

EXSTROPHY

Ansel JS: Surgical treatment of exstrophy of the bladder with emphasis on neonatal primary closure. Personal experience with 28 consecutive cases treated at the University of Washington hospitals from 1962 to 1977: Techniques and results. J Urol 1979;121:650.

Bellinger MF: Ureterocystoplasty: A unique method for vesical augmentation in children. J Urol 1993;149: 811.

Ben-Chaim J, Gearhart JP: Current management of bladder exstrophy. Tech Urol 1996;2:22.

Ben-Chaim J et al: Bladder exstrophy from childhood into adult life. J R Soc Med 1996;89:39P.

Connor JP et al: Long-term followup of 207 patients with bladder exstrophy: An evolution in treatment. J Urol 1989;142:793, 795.

DeMaria JE et al: Renal function in continent patients after surgical closure of bladder estrophy. J Urol 1980;124:85.

Ganesan GS et al: Lower urinary tract reconstruction using stomach and the artificial sphincter. J Urol 1993; 149:1107.

Gearhart JP: Failed bladder exstrophy repair: Evaluation and management. Urol Clin North Am 1991;18:687.

Gearhart JP, Jeffs RD: Augmentation cystoplasty in the failed exstrophy reconstruction. J Urol 1988;139:790.

Gearhart JP, Jeffs RD: Bladder exstrophy: Increase in capacity following epispadias repair. J Urol 1989; 142:525.

Gearhart JP, Jeffs RD: Management of the failed exstrophy closure. J Urol 1991;146:610.

Gearhart JP et al: Prostate size and configuration in adults with bladder exstrophy. J Urol 1993;149:308.

Gearhart JP et al: Techniques to create continence in the failed bladder exstrophy closure patient. J Urol 1993; 150:441.

Hollowell JG et al: Bladder function and dysfunction in exstrophy and epispadias. Lancet 1991;338:926.

Ikeme AC: Pregnancy in women after repair of bladder exstrophy: Two case reports. Br J Obstet Gynaecol 1981;88:327.

Jeffs RD: Complications of exstrophy surgery. Urol Clin North Am 1983;10:509.

Johnson P et al: Inferior vesical fissure. J Urol 1995; 154:1478.

Lattimer JK et al: Long-term follow-up after exstrophy closure: Late improvement and good quality of life. J Urol 1978;119:664.

Light JK, Scott FB: Treatment of the epispadias-exstrophy complex with the AS792 artificial urinary sphincter. J Urol 1983;129:738.

Lima SVC et al: Bladder exstrophy: Primary reconstruction with human dura mater. Br J Urol 1981;53:119.

Merguerian PA et al: Continence in bladder exstrophy: Determinants of success. J Urol 1991;145:350.

Mitchell ME, Brito CG, Rink RC: Cloacal exstrophy reconstruction for urinary continence. J Urol 1990;144: 554, 562.

Mollard P: Bladder reconstruction in exstrophy. J Urol 1980;124:525.

Oesterling JE, Jeffs RD: The importance of a successful initial bladder closure in the surgical management of classical bladder exstrophy: Analysis of 414 patients at the Johns Hopkins Hospital from 1975 to 1985. J Urol 1987;139:790.

Perlmutter AD, Weinstein MD, Reitelman C: Vesical neck reconstruction in patients with epispadias-exstrophy complex. J Urol 1991;146:613.

Sahoo SP et al: Covered exstrophy: A rare variant of classical bladder exstrophy. Scand J Urol Nephrol 1997;31:103.

Spence HM, Hoffman WW, Pate VA: Exstrophy of the bladder. 1. Long-term results in a series of 37 cases treated by ureterosigmoidostomy. J Urol 1975;114: 133.

Swana HS, Gallagher PG, Weiss RM: Pseudoexstrophy of the bladder: Case report and literature review. J Pediatr Surg 1997;32:1480.

Toguri AG et al: Continence in cases of bladder exstrophy. J Urol 1978;119:538.

Turner WR, Ransley PG, Williams DI: Patterns of renal damage in the management of vesical exstrophy. J Urol 1980;124:412.

Zaontz MR, Packer MG: Abnormalities of the external genitalia. Pediatr Clin North Am 1997;44:1267.

PERSISTENT URACHUS

al-Hindawi MK, Aman S: Benign non-infected urachal cyst in an adult: Review of the literature and a case report. Br J Radiol 1992;65:313.

Bauer SB, Retik AB: Urachal anomalies and related umbilical disorders. Urol Clin North Am 1978;5:195.

Cilento BG Jr et al: Urachal anomalies: Defining the best diagnostic modality. Urology 1998;52:120.

Holten I et al: The ultrasonic diagnosis of urachal anomalies. Australas Radiol 1996;40:2.

Mesrobian HG et al: Ten years of experience with isolated urachal anomalies in children. J Urol 1997;158 (3 Pt 2):1316.

Risher WH, Sardi A, Bolton J: Urachal abnormalities in adults: The Ochsner experience. South Med J 1990;83:1036.

Scheye T et al: Anatomic basis of pathology of the urachus. Surg Radiol Anat 1994;16:135.

Stone NN, Garden RJ, Weber H: Laparoscopic excision of a urachal cyst. Urology 1995;45:161.

Suita S, Nagasaki A: Urachal remnants. Semin Pediatr Surg 1996;5:107.

CONTRACTURE OF THE BLADDER NECK

Elliott JP Jr et al: Post prostatectomy bladder neck contractures. J Miss State Med Assoc 1991;32:41.

Green D, Mitcheson HD, McGuire EJ: Management of the bladder by augmentation ileocecocystoplasty. J Urol 1983;130:133.

Kulb TB et al: Prevention of postprostatectomy vesical neck contracture by prophylactic vesical neck incision. J Urol 1987;137:230.

Nunn IN: Bladder neck obstruction in children. J Urol 1965;93:693.

Salant RL et al: Neodymium: YAG laser treatment of postoperative bladder neck contractures. Urology 1990;35:385.

Smith DR: Critique on the concept of vesical neck obstruction in children. JAMA 1969;207:1686.

INTERSTITIAL CYSTITIS

Andersson KE: Neurotransmitters and neuroreceptors in the lower urinary tract. Curr Opin Obstet Gynecol 1996;8:361.

Awad SA et al: Idiopathic reduced bladder storage versus interstitial cystitis. J Urol 1992;148:409.

Baskin LS, Tanagho EA: Pelvic pain without pelvic organs. J Urol 1992;147:683.

Chaiken DC, Blaivas JG, Blaivas ST: Behavioral therapy for the treatment of refractory interstitial cystitis. J Urol 1993;149:1445.

Duncan JL, Schaeffer AJ: Do infectious agents cause interstitial cystitis? Urology 1997;49(5A Suppl):48.

Elbadawi A: Interstitial cystitis: A critique of current concepts with a new proposal for pathologic diagnosis and pathogenesis. Urology 1997;49(5A Suppl):14.

Fleischmann JD et al: Clinical and immunological response to nifedipine for the treatment of interstitial cystitis. J Urol 1991;146:1235.

Hanno P et al: Diagnosis of interstitial cystitis. J Urol 1990;143:278.

Hohenfellner M et al: Interstitial cystitis: Increased sympathetic innervation and related neuropeptide synthesis. J Urol 1992;147:587.

Holm-Bentzen M et al: Painful bladder disease: Clinical and pathoanatomical differences in 115 patients. J Urol 1987;138:500.

Hurst RE et al: Urinary glycosaminoglycan excretion as a laboratory marker in the diagnosis of interstitial cystitis. J Urol 1993;149:31.

Irwin P, Galloway NT: Impaired bladder perfusion in interstitial cystitis: A study of blood supply using laser Doppler flowmetry. J Urol 1993;149:890.

Johansson SL, Fall M: Clinical features and spectrum of light microscopic changes in interstitial cystitis. J Urol 1990;143:1118.

Jones CA, Nyberg LE: Epidemiology of interstitial cystitis. Urology 1997 (May);49(5A Suppl):2.

Koziol JA et al: The natural history of interstitial cystitis: A survey of 374 patients. J Urol 1993;149:465.

Messing EM, Stamey TA: Interstitial cystitis: Early diagnosis, pathology and treatment. Urology 1978;12: 381.

Nickel JC, Emerson L, Cornish J: The bladder mucus (glycosaminoglycan) layer in interstitial cystitis. J Urol 1993;149:716.

Parsons CL, Mulholland SG: Successful therapy of interstitial cystitis with pentosanpolysulfate. J Urol 1987;138:513.

Parsons CL, Schmidt JD, Pollen JJ: Successful treatment of interstitial cystitis with sodium pentosanpolysulfate. J Urol 1983;130:51.

Parsons CL et al: A quantitatively controlled method to study prospectively interstitial cystitis and demonstrate the efficacy of pentosanpolysulfate. J Urol 1993;150:845.

Pontari MA, Hanno PM, Wein AJ: Logical and systematic approach to the evaluation and management of patients suspected of having interstitial cystitis. Urology 1997;49(5A Suppl):114.

Sant GR, Theoharides TC: The role of the mast cell in interstitial cystitis. Urol Clin North Am 1994;21:41.

Simon LJ et al: The Interstitial Cystitis Data Base Study: Concepts and preliminary baseline descriptive statistics. Urology 1997;49(5A Suppl):64.

Slade D, Ratner V, Chalker R: A collaborative approach to managing interstitial cystitis. Urology 1997;49(5A Suppl):10.

Theoharides TC et al: Interstitial cystitis: A neuroimmunoendocrine disorder. Ann N Y Acad Sci 1998;840: 619.

Utz DC, Zinke H: The masquerade of bladder cancer as interstitial cystitis. J Urol 1974;111:160.

Webster GD, Maggio MI: The management of chronic interstitial cystitis by substitution cystoplasty. J Urol 1989;141:287.

INTERNAL VESICAL HERNIATION

Austin RC, Kaisary A, Winslet MC: Obturator herniation following radical cystoprostatectomy. Br J Urol 1995;76:800.

Bell ED, Witherington R: Bladder hernias. Urology 1980; 15:127.

Catalano O: Incisional herniation of the bladder: CT findings. Rofo Fortschr Geb Rontgenstr Neuen Bildgeb Verfahr 1996;165:508.

Catalano O: US evaluation of inguinoscrotal bladder hernias: Report of three cases. Clin Imaging 1997;21: 126.

Weitzenfeld MB et al: Scrotal kidney and ureter: An unusual hernia. J Urol 1980;123:437.

URINARY INCONTINENCE

Diokno AC, Taub M: Ephedrine in treatment of urinary incontinence. Urology 1975;5:624.

Farghaly SA, Hindmarsh JR: Changes in urethral function following hysterectomy. Proc Int Continence Soc 1985;15:195.

Furlow WL: Postprostatectomy urinary incontinence: Etiology, prevention, and selection of surgical treatment. Urol Clin North Am 1978;5:347.

Gleason DM, Bottaccini MR: The effect of a fine urethral pressure-measuring catheter on urinary flow in females. Neurourol Urodynam 1984;3:163.

Glen ES, Eadie A, Rowan D: Urethral closure pressure profile measurements in female urinary incontinence. Acta Urol Belg 1984;52:174.

Hertogs K, Stanton SL: Mechanism of urinary continence after colposuspension: Barrier studies. Br J Obstet Gynaecol 1985;92:1184.

Hetzenauer A, Bazzanella A, Reider W: Unstable female urethra: Incidence and significance. Proc Int Continence Soc 1985;15:111.

Kramer AEJL, Venema PL: Dynamic urethral pressure measurements in the diagnosis of incontinence in women. World J Urol 1984;2:203.

Langer R et al: Detrusor instability following colposuspension for urinary stress incontinence. Br J Obstet Gynaecol 1988;95:607.

Massey A, Abrams P: Urodynamics of the female lower urinary tract. Urol Clin North Am 1985;12:231.

Ouslander JG: Geriatric urinary incontinence. Dis Mon 1992;38(2):65.

Raezer DM et al: A clinical experience with the Scott genitourinary sphincter in the management of urinary incontinence in the pediatric age group. J Urol 1980;123:546.

Rousseau P, Fuentevilla-Clifton A: Urinary incontinence in the aged. Part 1: Patient evaluation. Geriatrics 1992;47(6):22, 33.

Rousseau P, Fuentevilla-Clifton A: Urinary incontinence in the aged. Part 2: Management strategies. [Published erratum appears in Geriatrics 1992;47(9):87.] Geriatrics 1992;47(6):37, 45, 48.

Scott FB, Bradley WE, Timm GW: Treatment of urinary incontinence by implantable prosthetic urinary sphincter. J Urol 1974;112:75.

Sorensen S et al: Urethral pressure variations in healthy females. Proc Int Continence Soc 1985;15:109.

Stanton SL: Stress urinary incontinence. Ciba Found Symp 1990;151:182, 189.

Tanagho EA: Bladder neck reconstruction for total urinary incontinence: 10 years of experience. J Urol 1981;125:321.

Tanagho EA, Schmidt RA: Bladder pacemaker: Scientific basis and clinical features. Urology 1982;20:614.

Tanagho EA, Smith DR: Clinical evaluation of a surgical technique for the correction of complete urinary incontinence. J Urol 1972;107:402.

Varner RE, Sparks JM: Surgery for stress urinary incontinence. Surg Clin North Am 1991;71:1111.

Westby M, Asmussen M: Anatomical and functional changes in the lower urinary tract after radical hysterectomy with lymph node dissection as studied by dynamic urethrocystography and simultaneous urethrocystometry. Gynecol Oncol 1985;21:261.

Williams DI, Snyder H: Anterior detrusor tube repair for urinary incontinence in children. Br J Urol 1976;48:671.

ENURESIS

Desmopressin for nocturnal enuresis. Med Lett Drugs Ther (April) 1990;32:38.

Djurhuus JC, Rittig S: Current trends, diagnosis, and treatment of enuresis. Eur Urol 1998;33 (Suppl 3):30.

Himsl KK et al: Pediatric urinary incontinence. Urol Clin North Am 1991;18:283.

Hjalmas K: Nocturnal enuresis: Basic facts and new horizons. Eur Urol 1998;33 (Suppl 3):53.

Howe AC, Walker CE: Behavioral management of toilet training, enuresis, and encopresis. Pediatr Clin North Am 1992;39:413.

Klauber GT: Clinical efficacy and safety of desmopressin in the treatment of nocturnal enuresis. J Pediatr 1989;114:719.

Lettgen B: Differential diagnoses for nocturnal enuresis. Scand J Urol Nephrol Suppl 1997;183:47.

Mark SD, Frank JD: Nocturnal enuresis. Br J Urol 1995;75:427.

Meadow SR, Evans JH: Desmopressin for enuresis. Br Med J 1989;298:1596.

Moffatt ME: Nocturnal enuresis: Psychologic implications of treatment and nontreatment. J Pediatr 1989;114:697.

Moffatt ME et al: Desmopressin acetate and nocturnal enuresis: How much do we know? [See comments.] Pediatrics 1993;92:420.

Nørgaard JP, Rittig S, Djurhuus JC: Nocturnal enuresis: An approach to treatment based on pathogenesis. J Pediatr 1989;114:705.

Nørgaard JP et al: Experience and current status of research into the pathophysiology of nocturnal enuresis. Br J Urol 1997;79:825.

Rushton HG: Nocturnal enuresis: Epidemiology, evaluation, and currently available treatment options. J Pediatr 1989;114:691.

Rushton HG: Wetting and functional voiding disorders. Urol Clin North Am 1995;22:75.

Ullom-Minnich MR: Diagnosis and management of nocturnal enuresis. Am Fam Physician 1996;54:2259.

FOREIGN BODIES INTRODUCED INTO THE BLADDER & URETHRA

Bjornerem A, Tollan A: Intrauterine device—primary and secondary perforation of the urinary bladder. Acta Obstet Gynecol Scand 1997;76:383.

Cardozo L: Recurrent intra-vesical foreign bodies. Br J Urol 1997;80:687.

Chitale SV, Burgess NA: Endoscopic removal of a complex foreign body from the bladder. Br J Urol 1998;81:756.

Maskey CP et al: Vesical calculus around an intra-uterine contraceptive device. Br J Urol 1997;79:654.

Najafi E, Maynard JF: Foreign body in lower urinary tract. Urology 1975;5:117.

Prasad S et al: Foreign bodies in urinary bladder. Urology 1973;2:258.

VESICAL MANIFESTATIONS OF ALLERGY

Pastinszky I: The allergic diseases of the male genitourinary tract with special reference to allergic urethritis and cystitis. Urol Int 1960;9:288.

Rubin L, Pincus MD: Eosinophilic cystitis: The relationship of allergy in the urinary tract to eosinophilic cystitis and the pathophysiology of eosinophilia. J Urol 1974;112:457.

DIVERTICULA

Barrett DM, Malek RS, Kelalis PP: Observations on vesical diverticulum in childhood. J Urol 1976;116:234.

Das S, Amar AD: Vesical diverticulum associated with bladder carcinoma: Therapeutic implications. J Urol 1986;136:1013.

Gerridzen R, Futter NG: Ten-year review of vesical diverticula. Urology 1982;10:33.

Keeler LL, Sant GR: Spontaneous rupture of a bladder diverticulum. J Urol 1990;143:349.

Mićić S, Ilić V: Incidence of neoplasm in vesical diverticula. J Urol 1983;129:734.

Shah B et al: Tumour in a giant bladder diverticulum: A case report and review of literature. Int Urol Nephrol 1997;29:173.

Yu CC et al: Intradiverticular tumors of the bladder: Surgical implications—an eleven-year review. Eur Urol 1993;24:190.

VESICAL FISTULAS

Anderson GA, Goldman IL, Mulligan GW: 3-dimensional computerized tomographic reconstruction of colovesical fistulas. J Urol 1997;158(3 Pt 1):795.

Ayhan A et al: Results of treatment in 182 consecutive patients with genital fistulas. Int J Gynaecol Obstet 1995;48:43.

Badlani G et al: Enterovesical fistulas in Crohn disease. Urology 1980;16:599.

Bazeed M et al: Urovaginal fistulae: 20 years' experience. Eur Urol 1995;27:34.

Birkhoff JD, Wechsler M, Romas NA: Urinary fistulas: Vaginal repair using labial fat pad. J Urol 1977;177:595.

Blaivas JG, Heritz DM, Romanzi LJ: Early versus late repair of vesicovaginal fistulas: Vaginal and abdominal approaches. J Urol 1995;153:1110.

Carr LK, Webster GD: Abdominal repair of vesicovaginal fistula. [Editorial]. Urology 1996;48:10.

Cruikshank SH: Early closure of posthysterectomy vesicovaginal fistulas. South Med J 1988;81:1525.

Doherty AP, Whitfield HN: A case of appendico-vesical fistula. J Soc Med 1992;85:757.

Driver CP et al: Vesico-colic fistulae in the Grampian region: Presentation, assessment, management and outcome. J R Coll Surg Edinb 1997;42:182.

Dupont MC, Raz S: Vaginal approach to vesicovaginal fistula repair. (Editorial.) Urology 1996(Jul);48:7.

Elkins TE: Surgery for the obstetric vesicovaginal fistula: A review of 100 operations in 82 patients. Am J Obstet Gynecol 1994;170:1108.

Gokdemir A et al: Superior vesical fistula: A case report. Eur J Pediatr Surg 1991;1:249.

Goodwin WE, Scardino PT: Vesicovaginal and ureterovaginal fistulas: A summary of 25 years of experience. J Urol 1980;123:370.

Henricksen HM: Vesicouterine fistula following cesarean section. J Urol 1981;125:884.

Hsieh JH et al: Enterovesical fistula: 10 years experience. Chung Hua I Hsueh Tsa Chih (Taipei) 1997;59:283.

Iselin CE, Aslan P, Webster GD: Transvaginal repair of vesicovaginal fistulas after hysterectomy by vaginal cuff excision. J Urol 1998;160(3 Pt 1):728.

Kao PF et al: Diuretic renography findings in enterovesical fistula. Br J Radiol 1997;70:421.

Lee RA, Symmonds RE, Williams TJ: Current status of genitourinary fistula. Obstet Gynecol 1988;72:313.

Margolis T, Mercer LJ: Vesicovaginal fistula. Obstet Gynecol Surv 1994;49:840.

Moss RL, Ryan JA Jr: Management of enterovesical fistulas. Am J Surg 1990;159:514.

Persky L, Forsythe WE, Herman G: Vesicovaginal fistulas in childhood. Urology 1980;15:36.

Persky L, Herman G, Guerrier K: Nondelay in vesicovaginal fistula repair. Urology 1979;13:273.

Potter D, Smith D, Shorthouse AJ: Colovesical fistula following ingestion of a foreign body. Br J Urol 1998;81:499.

Raghavaiah NV: Double-dye test to diagnose various types of vaginal fistulas. J Urol 1974;112:811.

Semelka RC et al: Pelvic fistulas: Appearances on MR images. Abdom Imaging 1997;22:91.

Simoneaux SF, Patrick LE: Genitourinary complications of Crohn's disease in pediatric patients. AJR 1997;169:197.

Simsek U, Ozyurt M, Oktay B: Repair of vesical fistulae using lyophilised human dura. Br J Urol 1990;65:550.

Waaldijk K: Surgical classification of obstetric fistulas. Int J Gynaecol Obstet 1995;49:161.

Woo HH, Rosario DJ, Chapple CR: The treatment of vesicovaginal fistulae. Eur Urol 1996;29:1.

PERIVESICAL LIPOMATOSIS

Ambos MA et al: The pear-shaped bladder. Radiology 1977;122:85.

Ballesteros JJ: Surgical treatment of perivesical lipomatosis. J Urol 1977;118:329.

Church PA, Kazam E: Computed tomography and ultrasound in diagnosis of pelvic lipomatosis. Urology 1979;14:631.

Crane DB, Smith MJV: Pelvic lipomatosis: Five-year follow-up. J Urol 1977;118:547.

Halachmi S et al: The use of an ultrasonic assisted lipectomy device for the treatment of obstructive pelvic lipomatosis. Urology 1996;48:128.

Heyns CF et al: Pelvic lipomatosis associated with cystitis glandularis and adenocarcinoma of the bladder. J Urol 1991;145:364.

Joshi KK, Wise HA II: Pelvic lipomatosis: 9-year follow-up in a woman. J Urol 1983;129:1233.

Levine E, Farber B, Lee KR: Computed tomography in diagnosis of pelvic lipomatosis. Urology 1978;12:606.

Mordkin RM et al: The radiographic diagnosis of pelvic lipomatosis. Tech Urol 1997;3:228.

Susmano DE, Dolin EH: Computed tomography in diagnosis of pelvic lipomatosis. Urology 1979;13:215.

Yalla SV et al: Cystitis glandularis with perivesical lipomatosis: Frequent association of two unusual proliferative conditions. Urology 1975;5:383.

RADIATION CYSTITIS

Del Pizzo JJ et al: Treatment of radiation induced hemorrhagic cystitis with hyperbaric oxygen: Long-term followup. J Urol 1998;160(3 Pt 1):731.

Levenback C et al: Hemorrhagic cystitis following radiotherapy for stage Ib cancer of the cervix. Gynecol Oncol 1994;55:206.

Lowe BA, Stamey TA: Endoscopic topical placement of formalin soaked pledgets to control localized hemorrhage due to radiation cystitis. J Urol 1997;158:528.

Maatman TJ et al: Radiation-induced cystitis following intracavitary irradiation for superficial bladder cancer. J Urol 1983;130:338.

Neustein P, Heins PS, Goergen TG: Chronic hemospermia due to müllerian duct cyst: Diagnosis by magnetic resonance imaging. J Urol 1989;142:828.

Norkool DM et al: Hyperbaric oxygen therapy for radiation-induced hemorrhagic cystitis. J Urol 1993;150:332.

Sanchiz F et al: Prevention of radioinduced cystitis by orgotein: A randomized study. Anticancer Res 1996;16:2025.

Suzuki K et al: Successful treatment of radiation cystitis with hyperbaric oxygen therapy: Resolution of bleeding event and changes of histopathological findings of the bladder mucosa. Int Urol Nephrol 1998;30:267.

Weiss JP, Neville EC: Hyperbaric oxygen: Primary treatment of radiation-induced hemorrhagic cystitis. J Urol 1989;142:43.

NONINFECTIOUS HEMORRHAGIC CYSTITIS

Bennett AH: Cyclophosphamide and hemorrhagic cystitis. J Urol 1974;111:603.

deVries CR, Freiha FS: Hemorrhagic cystitis: A review. J Urol 1990;143:1.

Donahue LA, Frank IN: Intravesical formalin for hemorrhagic cystitis: Analysis of therapy. J Urol 1989;141:809.

Droller MJ, Saral K, Santos G: Prevention of cyclophosphamide-induced hemorrhagic cystitis. Urology 1982;20:256.

Giulani L et al: Gelatin foam and isobutyl-2-cyanoacrylate in the treatment of life-threatening bladder haemorrhage by selective transcatheter embolisation of the internal iliac arteries. Br J Urol 1979;51:125.

Hampson SJ, Woodhouse CR: Sodium pentosanpolysulphate in the management of haemorrhagic cystitis: Experience with 14 patients. Eur Urol 1994;25:40.

Holstein P et al: Intravesical hydrostatic pressure treatment: New method for control of bleeding from bladder mucosa. J Urol 1973;109:234.

Ilhan O et al: Hemorrhagic cystitis as a complication of bone marrow transplantation. J Chemother 1997;9:56.

Marshall FF, Klinefelter HF: Late hemorrhagic cystitis following low-dose cyclophosphamide therapy. Urology 1979;14:573.

Miller J, Burfield GD, Moretti KL: Oral conjugated estrogen therapy for treatment of hemorrhagic cystitis. J Urol 1994;151:1348.

Moinuddin SM, Upton DW: Urothelial carcinoma after cyclophosphamide therapy. J Urol 1983;129:143.

Ostroff EB, Chenault OW Jr: Alum irrigation for the control of massive bladder hemorrhage. J Urol 1982;128:929.

Pyeritz RE et al: An approach to the control of massive hemorrhage in cyclophosphamide-induced cystitis by intravenous vasopressin: A case report. J Urol 1978;120:253.

Ratliff TR, Williams RD: Hemorrhagic cystitis, chemotherapy, and bladder toxicity. (Editorial.) J Urol 1998;159:1044.

Stillwell TJ, Benson RC Jr: Cyclophosphamide-induced hemorrhagic cystitis. A review of 100 patients. Cancer 1988;61:451.

West NJ: Prevention and treatment of hemorrhagic cystitis. Pharmacotherapy 1997;17:696.

EMPYEMA OF THE BLADDER

Adeyoju AB, Lynch TH, Thornhill JA: The defunctionalized bladder. Int Urogynecol J Pelvic Floor Dysfunct 1998;9:48.

Dretler SP: The occurrence of empyema cystitis: Management of the bladder to be defunctionalized. J Urol 1972;108:82.

Spence HM, Allen TD: Vaginal vesicostomy for empyema of the defunctionalized bladder. J Urol 1971;106:862.

CONGENITAL ANOMALIES OF THE PROSTATE & SEMINAL VESICLES

Barzilai M, Ginesin Y: A müllerian prostatic cyst protruding into the base of the urinary bladder. Urol Int 1998;60:194.

Donohue RE, Greenslade NF: Seminal vesical cyst and ipsilateral renal agenesis. Urology 1973;2:66.

Feldman RA, Weiss RM: Urinary retention secondary to Müllerian duct cyst in a child. J Urol 1972;108:647.

McDermott VG et al: Prostatic and periprostatic cysts: Findings on MR imaging. AJR 1995;164:123.

Ng KJ, Milroy EJ, Rickards D: Intraprostatic cyst—a cause of bladder outflow obstruction. J R Soc Med 1996;89:708.

Sanchez-Chapado M, Angulo JC: Giant Müllerian duct cyst mimicking prostatic malignancy. Scand J Urol Nephrol 1995;29:229.

Terris MK: Transrectal ultrasound guided drainage of prostatic cysts. J Urol 1997;158:179.

Yasumoto R et al: Is a cystic lesion located at the midline of the prostate a müllerian duct cyst? Analysis of aspirated fluid and histopathological study of the cyst wall. Eur Urol 1997;31:187.

BLOODY EJACULATION

Cattolica EV: Massive hemospermia: A new etiology and simplified treatment. J Urol 1982;128:151.

Munkel witz R et al: Current perspectives on hematospermia: A review. J Androl 1997;18:6.

Neustein P, Hein PS, Goergen TG: Chronic hemospermia due to Müllerian duct cyst: Diagnosis by magnetic resonance imaging. J Urol 1989;142:828.

Stein AJ, Prioleau PG, Catalona WJ: Adenomatous polyps of the prostatic urethra: A cause of hematospermia. J Urol 1980;124:298.

Van Poppel R et al: Hemospermia owing to utricular cyst: Embryological summary and surgical review. J Urol 1983;129:608.

Disorders of the Penis & Male Urethra

40

Jack W. McAninch, MD

CONGENITAL ANOMALIES OF THE PENIS

APENIA

Congenital absence of the penis (apenia) is extremely rare. In this condition, the urethra generally opens on the perineum or inside the rectum.

Patients with apenia must be assigned the female gender. Castration should be done and vaginoplasty performed in combination with estrogen treatment as the child develops.

MEGALOPENIS

The penis enlarges rapidly in childhood (megalopenis) in boys with abnormalities that have increased the production of testosterone, eg, interstitial cell tumors of the testicle, hyperplasia, or tumors of the adrenal cortex. Management is by correction of the underlying endocrine problem.

MICROPENIS

Micropenis is a more common anomaly and has been attributed to a testosterone deficiency that results in poor growth of organs that are targets of this hormone. A penis smaller than 2 standard deviations from the norm is considered a micropenis (see Table 40–1). The testicles are small and frequently undescended. Other organs, including the scrotum, may be involved. Early evidence suggests that the ability of the hypothalamus to secrete luteinizing hormone-releasing hormone (LHRH) is decreased. The pituitary-gonadal axis appears to be intact, since the organs respond to testosterone, although this response may be sluggish at times. Studies have shown that topical application of 5% testosterone cream causes

increased penile growth, but its effect is due to absorption of the hormone, which systemically stimulates genital growth. Patients with micropenis must be carefully evaluated for other endocrine and central nervous system anomalies. Retarded bone growth, anosmia, learning disabilities, and deficiencies of adrenocorticotropic hormone and thyrotropin have been associated with micropenis. In addition, the possibility of intersex problems must be carefully investigated before therapy is begun.

The approach to management of micropenis has undergone gradual change in recent years, but androgen replacement is the basic requirement. The objective is to provide sufficient testosterone to stimulate penile growth without altering growth and closure of the epiphyses. Allen (1980) recommends giving testosterone in doses of 25 mg orally every 3 weeks for no more than 4 doses. Penile growth is assessed by measuring the length of the stretched penis (pubis to glans) before and after treatment. Therapy should be started by age 1 year and aimed at maintaining genital growth commensurate with general body growth. Repeat courses of therapy may be required if the size of the penis falls behind as the child grows. For undescended testicles, orchiopexy should be done before the child is 2 years old. In the future, treatment with LHRH may correct micropenis as well as cause descent of the testicles, but at present, LHRH is not approved for such use.

ADULT PENILE SIZE

In recent years, penile augmentation and enhancement procedures have been done with increasing frequency, although no validation of success has been documented. Suspensory ligament release with pubic fat pad advancement, fat injections, and dermal fat grafts have been used in attempts to enhance penile size. Many consider that these procedures have not been proved safe or efficacious in normal men. Recently, Wessells, Lue, and McAninch (1996) evaluated penile size in the flaccid and erect state in other-

Table 40–1. Size of unstretched penis and testis from infancy to adulthood.

Age (Years)	Length of Penis (cm ± SD)	Diameter of Testis (cm ± SD)
0.2–2	2.7 ± 0.5	1.4 ± 0.4
2.1–4	3.3 ± 0.4	1.2 ± 0.4
4.1–6	3.9 ± 0.9	1.5 ± 0.6
6.1–8	4.2 ± 0.8	1.8 ± 0.3
8.1–10	4.9 ± 1	2 ± 0.5
10.1–12	5.2 ± 1.3	2.7 ± 0.7
12.1–14	6.2 ± 2	3.4 ± 0.8
14.1–16	8.6 ± 2.4	4.1 ± 1
16.1–18	9.9 ± 1.7	5 ± 0.5
18.1–20	11 ± 1.1	5 ± 0.3
20.1–25	12.4 ± 1.6	5.2 ± 0.6

Source: Reproduced, with permission, from Winter JSD, Faiman C: Pituitary-gonadal relations in male children and adolescents. Pediatr Res 1972;6:126.

Table 40–2. Adult penile size: Relationships among flaccid, stretched, and erect measurements.[1]

Penile State	Length (cm)	Circumference (cm)
Flaccid	8.8	9.7
Stretched	12.4	—
Erect	12.9	12.3

[1] Data represent the mean of measurements in 80 men and are drawn from Wessells H, Lue TF, McAninch JW: Penile length in the flaccid and erect states: Guidelines for penile augmentation. J Urol 1996;156:995.

wise normal adult men and found very good correlation between stretched and erect length ($R^2 = 0.793$; Table 40–2). This information can provide a guideline for physicians whose patients are concerned with their penile dimensions.

CONGENITAL ANOMALIES OF THE URETHRA

DUPLICATION OF THE URETHRA

Duplication of the urethra is rare. The structures may be complete or incomplete (Wirtshafter et al, 1980). Resection of all but one complete urethra is recommended.

URETHRAL STRICTURE

Congenital urethral stricture is uncommon in infant boys. The fossa navicularis and membranous urethra are the 2 most common sites. Severe strictures may cause bladder damage and hydronephrosis (see Chapter 12), with symptoms of obstruction (urinary frequency and urgency) or urinary infection. A careful history and physical examination are indicated in patients with these complaints. Excretory urography and excretory voiding urethrography often define the lesion and the extent of obstruction. Retrograde urethrography (Figure 40–1) may also be helpful. Cystoscopy and urethroscopy should be performed in all patients in whom urethral stricture is suspected.

Strictures can be treated at the time of endoscopy. Diaphragmatic strictures may respond to dilation or visual urethrotomy. Other strictures should be treated under direct vision by internal urethrotomy with the currently available pediatric urethrotome. It may be necessary to repeat these procedures in order to stabilize the stricture. Single-stage open surgical repair by anastomotic urethroplasty, buccal mucosa graft, or penile flap is desirable if the obstruction recurs.

POSTERIOR URETHRAL VALVES

Posterior urethral valves, the most common obstructive urethral lesions in infants and newborns, occur only in males and are found at the distal prostatic urethra. The valves are mucosal folds that look like thin membranes; they may cause varying degrees of obstruction when the child attempts to void (Figure 40–2).

Clinical Findings

A. Symptoms and Signs: Children with posterior urethral valves may present with mild, moderate, or severe symptoms of obstruction. They often have a poor, intermittent, dribbling urinary stream. Urinary infection and sepsis occur frequently. Severe obstruction may cause hydronephrosis (see Chapter 12), which is apparent as a palpable abdominal mass. A palpable midline mass in the lower abdomen is typical of a distended bladder. Occasionally, palpable flank masses indicate hydronephrotic kidneys. In many patients, failure to thrive may be the only significant symptom, and examination may reveal nothing more than evidence of chronic illness.

B. Laboratory Findings: Azotemia and poor concentrating ability of the kidney are common findings. The urine is often infected, and anemia may be found if infection is chronic. Serum creatinine and blood urea nitrogen levels and creatinine clearance are the best indicators of the extent of renal failure.

C. X-Ray Findings: Voiding cystourethrography is the best radiographic study available to establish the diagnosis of posterior urethral valves. The presence of large amounts of residual urine is apparent on initial catheterization done in conjunction with radiographic studies, and an uncontaminated urine spec-

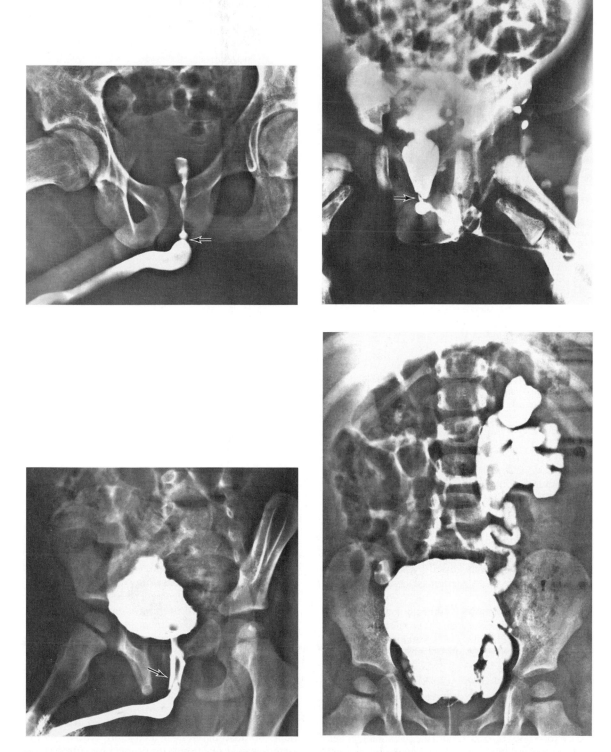

Figure 40–1. Upper left: Retrograde urethrogram showing congenital diaphragmatic stricture. **Upper right:** Posterior urethral valves revealed on voiding cystourethrography. Arrow points to area of severe stenosis at distal end of prostatic urethra. **Lower left:** Posterior urethral valves. Patient would not void with cystography. Retrograde urethrogram showing valves (arrow). **Lower right:** Cystogram, same patient. Free vesicoureteral reflux and vesical trabeculation with diverticula.

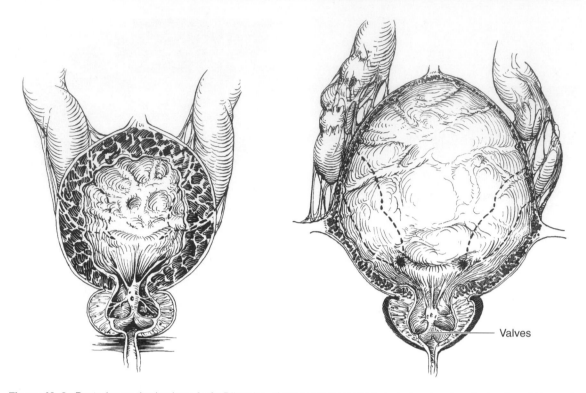

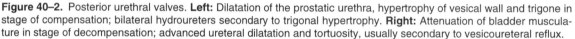

Figure 40–2. Posterior urethral valves. **Left:** Dilatation of the prostatic urethra, hypertrophy of vesical wall and trigone in stage of compensation; bilateral hydroureters secondary to trigonal hypertrophy. **Right:** Attenuation of bladder musculature in stage of decompensation; advanced ureteral dilatation and tortuosity, usually secondary to vesicoureteral reflux.

imen should be obtained via the catheter and sent for culture. The cystogram may show vesicoureteral reflux and the severe trabeculations of long-standing obstruction, and the voiding cystourethrogram often demonstrates elongation and dilatation of the posterior urethra, with a prominent bladder neck (Figure 40–1). Excretory urograms may reveal hydroureter and hydronephrosis when obstruction is severe and long-standing.

D. Ultrasonography: Ultrasonography can be used to detect hydronephrosis, hydroureter, and bladder distention in children with severe azotemia. It can also detect fetal hydronephrosis, which is typical of urethral valves, as early as 28 weeks of gestation; when the obstruction is from valves, an enlarged bladder with bilateral hydroureteronephrosis is usually present (Figure 40–3).

E. Instrumental Examination: Urethroscopy and cystoscopy, performed with the patient under general anesthesia, show vesical trabeculation and cellules and, occasionally, vesical diverticula. The bladder neck and trigone may be hypertrophied. The diagnosis is confirmed by visual identification of the valves at the distal prostatic urethra. Supravesical compression shows that the valves cause obstruction.

Treatment

Treatment consists of destruction of the valves, but the approach depends on the degree of obstruction and the general health of the child. In children with mild to moderate obstruction and minimal azotemia, transurethral fulguration of the valves is usually successful. Occasionally, catheterization, cystoscopy, or urethral dilation by perineal urethrostomy destroys the valves.

The more severe degrees of obstruction create varying grades of hydronephrosis requiring individualized management. Treatment of children with urosepsis and azotemia associated with hydronephrosis includes use of antibiotics, catheter drainage of the bladder, and correction of the fluid and electrolyte imbalance. Vesicostomy may be of benefit in patients with reflux and renal dysplasia.

In the most severe cases of hydronephrosis, vesicostomy or removal of the valves may not be sufficient, because of ureteral atony, obstruction of the ureterovesical junction from trigonal hypertrophy, or both. In such cases, percutaneous loop ureterostomies may be done to preserve renal function and allow resolution of the hydronephrosis. After renal function is stabilized, valve ablation and reconstruction of the urinary tract can be done.

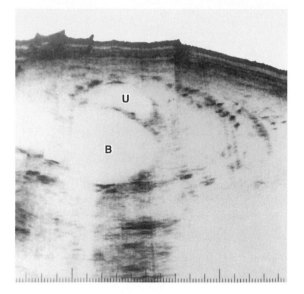

Figure 40–3. Intrauterine ultrasonogram demonstrating fetal hydronephrosis at 32 weeks of gestation. Massive enlarged bladder (B) and ureter (U) are typical of posterior urethral valves.

The period of proximal diversion should be as short as possible, since vesical contracture can be permanent after prolonged supravesical diversion.

Johnston (1979) found that approximately 50% of children with urethral valves had vesicoureteral reflux and that the prognosis is worse if the reflux is bilateral. After removal of the obstruction, reflux ceases spontaneously in about one-third of patients. In the remaining two-thirds of patients, the reflux should be corrected surgically.

Long-term use of antimicrobial drugs is often required to prevent recurrent urosepsis and urinary tract infection even though the obstruction has been relieved.

Prognosis

Early detection is the best way to preserve kidney and bladder function. This can be accomplished by ultrasonography in utero, by careful physical examination and observation of voiding in the newborn, and by thorough evaluation of children who have urinary tract infections. Children in whom azotemia and infection persist after relief of obstruction have a poor prognosis.

ANTERIOR URETHRAL VALVES

Signs of anterior urethral valves, a rare congenital anomaly, are urethral dilatation or diverticula proximal to the valve, bladder outlet obstruction, postvoiding incontinence, and infection. Enuresis may be present. Urethroscopy and voiding cystourethrography will demonstrate the lesion, and endoscopic electrofulguration will effectively correct the obstruction.

URETHRORECTAL & VESICORECTAL FISTULAS

Urethrorectal and vesicorectal fistulas are rare and are almost always associated with imperforate anus. Failure of the urorectal septum to develop completely and separate the rectum from the urogenital tract permits communication between the 2 systems (see Chapter 2). The child with such a fistula passes fecal material and gas through the urethra. If the anus has developed normally (ie, if it opens externally), urine may pass through the rectum.

Cystoscopy and panendoscopy usually show the fistulous opening. Radiographic contrast material given by mouth will reach the blind rectal pouch, and the distance between the end of the rectum and the perineum can be seen on appropriate radiograms.

Imperforate anus must be opened immediately and the fistula closed, or if the rectum lies quite high, temporary sigmoid colostomy should be performed. Definitive surgery, with repair of the urethral fistula, can be done later.

HYPOSPADIAS

In hypospadias, the urethral meatus opens on the ventral side of the penis proximal to the tip of the glans penis (Figure 40–4).

Sexual differentiation and urethral development begin in utero at approximately 8 weeks and are complete by 15 weeks. The urethra is formed by the fusion of the urethral folds along the ventral surface of the penis, which extends to the corona on the distal shaft. The glandular urethra is formed by canalization of an ectodermal cord that has grown through the glans to communicate with the fused urethral folds (see Chapter 2). Hypospadias results when fusion of the urethral folds is incomplete.

Hypospadias occurs in one in every 300 male children. Estrogens and progestins given during pregnancy are known to increase the incidence. Although a familial pattern of hypospadias has been recognized, no specific genetic traits have been established.

Classification

There are several forms of hypospadias, classified according to location: (1) glandular, ie, opening on the proximal glans penis; (2) coronal, ie, opening at the coronal sulcus; (3) penile shaft; (4) penoscrotal; and (5) perineal. About 70% of all cases of hypospadias are distal penile or coronal.

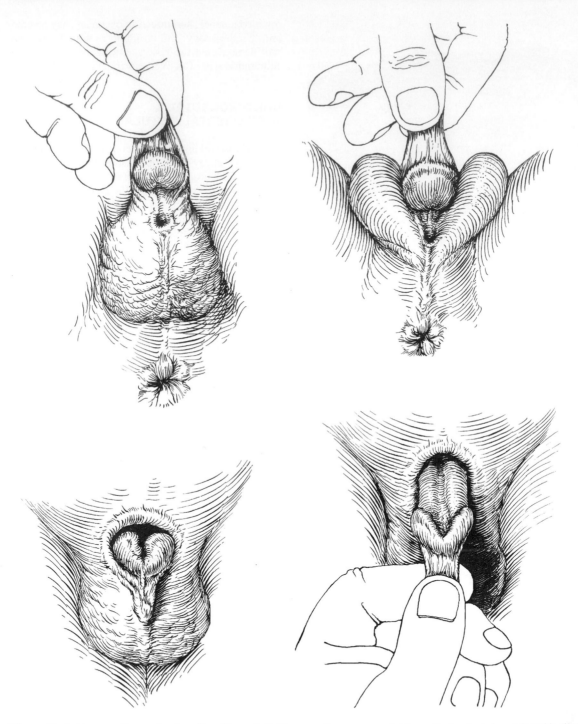

Figure 40–4. Hypospadias and epispadias. **Upper left:** Hypospadias, penoscrotal type. Redundant dorsal foreskin that is deficient ventrally; ventral chordee. **Upper right:** Hypospadias, midscrotal type. Chordee more marked. Penis often small. **Lower left:** Epispadias. Redundant ventral foreskin that is absent dorsally; severe dorsal chordee. **Lower right:** Traction on foreskin reveals dorsal defect.

Hypospadias in the male is evidence of feminization. Patients with penoscrotal and perineal openings should be considered to have potential intersex problems requiring appropriate evaluation. Hypospadiac newborns should not be circumcised, because the preputial skin may be useful for future reconstruction.

Clinical Findings

A. Symptoms and Signs: Although newborns and young children seldom have symptoms related to hypospadias, older children and adults may complain of difficulty directing the urinary stream and stream spraying. Chordee (curvature of the penis) causes ventral bending and bowing of the penile shaft, which can prevent sexual intercourse. Perineal or penoscrotal hypospadias necessitates voiding in the sitting position, and these proximal forms of hypospadias in adults can be the cause of infertility. An additional complaint of almost all patients is the abnormal (hooded) appearance of the penis, caused by deficient or absent ventral foreskin. The hypospadiac meatus may be stenotic and should be carefully examined and calibrated. (A meatotomy should be done when stenosis exists.) There is an increased incidence of undescended testicles in children with hypospadias; scrotal examination is necessary to establish the position of the testicles.

B. Laboratory, X-Ray, and Endoscopic Findings: Since children with penoscrotal and perineal hypospadias often have a bifid scrotum and ambiguous genitalia, a buccal smear and karyotyping are indicated to help establish the genetic sex. Urethroscopy and cystoscopy are of value to determine whether internal male sexual organs are normally developed. Excretory urography is also indicated in these patients to detect additional congenital anomalies of the kidneys and ureters.

Some authors recommend routine use of excretory urography for all patients with hypospadias; however, this seems to be of little value in the more distal types of the disorder, because there appears to be no increased incidence of upper urinary tract anomalies.

Differential Diagnosis

Any degree of hypospadias is an expression of feminization. Perineal and scrotal urethral openings should be carefully evaluated to ascertain that the patient is not a female with androgenized adrenogenital syndrome. Urethroscopy and cystoscopy will aid in evaluating the development of internal reproductive organs.

Treatment

For psychological reasons, hypospadias should be repaired before the patient reaches school age; in most cases, this can be done before age 2.

More than 150 methods of corrective surgery for hypospadias have been described. Currently, one-stage repairs using island flap grafts are performed by more and more urologists. Bladder epithelium has also been used successfully (Keating, Cartwright, and Duckett, 1990; Mollard et al, 1989). It now appears that buccal mucosa grafts are more advantageous than others and should be considered the primary grafting technique (Baskin and Duckett, 1995). Fistulas occur in 15–30% of patients, but the fistula repair is considered a small, second-stage reconstruction.

All types of repair involve straightening the penis by removal of the chordee. The chordee removal can be confirmed by producing an artificial erection in the operating room following urethral reconstruction and advancement. Most successful techniques for repair of hypospadias use local skin and foreskin in developing the neourethra. In recent years, advancement of the urethra to the glans penis has become technically feasible and cosmetically acceptable.

Prognosis

After corrective surgery, most patients are able to void in the standing position as well as to deposit semen into the vagina. The overall cosmetic appearance and the prevention of fistula formation remain the greatest challenges in these repairs.

CHORDEE WITHOUT HYPOSPADIAS

Congenital ventral chordee without hypospadias is seen occasionally and is caused by a short urethra, fibrous tissues surrounding the corpus spongiosum, or both. The urethral opening is in the normal position on the glans penis; only with erection does the penis bow, thus preventing satisfactory vaginal penetration. During examination, if the patient cannot achieve an erection naturally, erection can be induced by injecting saline solution into the corpus cavernosum after placing a tourniquet at the base of the penis. This technique should also be used during corrective surgery to be certain that the penis will be straight after the operation.

If the penis is adequate in length, the dorsal surface can be shortened (1) by excising elliptic portions of the tunica albuginea on the dorsum of the penis on either side of the midline (Redman, 1978) or (2) by making transverse cuts in a similar position and then closing them longitudinally, thus shortening the dorsum (Udall, 1980). Fibrous tissue found in association with the urethra and corpus spongiosum should be totally excised.

EPISPADIAS

The incidence of complete epispadias is approximately 1 in 120,000 males and 1 in 450,000 females. The urethra is displaced dorsally, and classification is based on its position in males. In glandular epispadias, the urethra opens on the dorsal aspect of the glans, which is broad and flattened. In the penile type, the urethral meatus, which is often broad and gaping, is located between the pubic symphysis and the coronal sulcus. A distal groove usually extends from the meatus through the splayed glans. The penopubic type has the urethral opening at the penopubic junction, and the entire penis has a distal dorsal groove extending through the glans.

Patients with glandular epispadias seldom have urinary incontinence. However, with penopubic and penile epispadias, incontinence is present in 95% and 75% of cases, respectively (Kramer and Kelalis, 1982).

Females with epispadias have a bifid clitoris and separation of the labia. Most are incontinent.

Urinary incontinence is a common problem because of maldevelopment of the urinary sphincters. Dorsal curvature of the penis (dorsal chordee) is also present (Figure 40–4). The pubic bones are separated as in exstrophy of the bladder. Epispadias is a mild form of bladder exstrophy, and in severe cases, exstrophy and epispadias coexist.

Surgery is required to correct the incontinence, remove the chordee to straighten the penis, and extend the urethra out onto the glans penis. Repair of the urinary sphincter has not been very successful, but Tanagho and Smith (1972) obtained complete continence by interposing a tube graft of anterior bladder wall between the bladder and prostatic urethra. Chordee excision and urethroplasty with advancement of the meatus have been successful in achieving acceptable cosmetic and functional results (Kramer and Kelalis, 1982). Bladder augmentation combined with the artificial sphincter may be required in patients in whom incontinence cannot be corrected.

ACQUIRED DISEASES & DISORDERS OF THE PENIS & MALE URETHRA

PRIAPISM

Priapism is an uncommon condition of prolonged erection. It is usually painful for the patient, and no sexual excitement or desire is present. The disorder is idiopathic in 60% of cases, while the remaining 40% of cases are associated with diseases (eg, leukemia, sickle cell disease, pelvic tumors, pelvic infections), penile trauma, spinal cord trauma, or use of medications. Currently, intracavernous injection therapy for impotence may be the most common cause. Although the idiopathic type often is initially associated with prolonged sexual stimulation, cases of priapism due to the other causes are unrelated to psychic sexual excitement.

Priapism may be classified into high- and low-flow types. High-flow priapism usually occurs secondary to perineal trauma, which injures the central penile arteries and results in loss of penile blood-flow regulation. Aneurysms of one or both central arteries have been observed. Aspiration of penile blood for blood-gas determination demonstrates high oxygen and normal carbon dioxide levels. Arteriography is useful to demonstrate aneurysms that will respond to embolization; erectile function is usually preserved.

The patient with low-flow priapism usually presents with a history of several hours of painful erection. The glans penis and corpus spongiosum are soft and uninvolved in the process. The corpora cavernosa are tense with congested blood and tender to palpation. The current theories regarding the mechanism of priapism remain in debate, but most authorities believe the major abnormality to be physiologic obstruction of the venous drainage. This obstruction causes buildup of highly viscous, poorly oxygenated blood (low O_2, high CO_2) within the corpora cavernosa. If the process continues for several days, interstitial edema and fibrosis of the corpora cavernosa will develop, causing impotence.

Priapism must be considered a urologic emergency. Sedation followed by enemas of ice-cold saline solution may induce subsidence of the erection. Epidural or spinal anesthesia can also be used. The sludged blood can then be evacuated from the corpora cavernosa through a large needle placed through the glans. The addition of adrenergic agents administered via intracavernous irrigation has proved helpful. Monitoring intracavernous pressure ensures that recurrence is not imminent (Lue et al, 1986). Multiple wedges of tissue can be removed via a Travenol biopsy needle to create a shunting fistula between the glans penis and corpora cavernosa (Winter and McDowell, 1988). This technique, which has been very successful, provides an internal fistula to keep the corpora cavernosa decompressed. To maintain continuous fistula drainage, pressure should be exerted intermittently (every 15 min) on the body of the penis. The patient can do this manually after he has recovered from anesthesia.

If the shunt described fails, another shunting technique may be used. Barry (1976) described an easy method of accomplishing shunting by anastomosing the superficial dorsal vein to the corpora cavernosa. Other effective shunting methods are corpora cavernosa to corpus spongiosum shunt by perineal anastomosis; saphenous vein to corpora cavernosa shunt; and pump decompression.

Patients with sickle cell disease have benefited from massive blood transfusions, exchange transfusions, or both. Hyperbaric oxygen also has been suggested for these patients. Patients with leukemia should receive prompt chemotherapy. Appropriate management of any underlying cause should be instituted without delay. Such treatment should not prevent aggressive management of the priapism if the erection persists for several hours.

Impotence is the worst sequel of priapism. It is more common after prolonged priapism (several days). Early recognition (within hours) and prompt treatment of priapism offer the best opportunity to avoid this major problem.

PEYRONIE DISEASE

Peyronie disease (plastic induration of the penis) was first described in 1742 and is a well-recognized clinical problem affecting middle-aged and older men. Patients present with complaints of painful erection, curvature of the penis, and poor erection distal to the involved area. The penile deformity may be so severe that it prevents satisfactory vaginal penetration. The patient has no pain when the penis is in the nonerect state.

Examination of the penile shaft reveals a palpable dense, fibrous plaque of varying size involving the tunica albuginea. The plaque is usually near the dorsal midline of the shaft. Multiple plaques are sometimes seen. In severe cases, calcification and ossification are noted and confirmed by radiography. Although the cause of Peyronie disease remains obscure, the dense fibrous plaque is microscopically consistent with findings in severe vasculitis. The condition has been noted in association with Dupuytren's contracture of the tendons of the hand, in which the fibrosis resembles that of Peyronie disease when examined microscopically.

There is no satisfactory treatment for this disease. However, spontaneous remission occurs in about 50% of cases. Initially, observation and emotional support are advised. If remission does not occur, *p*-aminobenzoic acid powder or tablets or vitamin E tablets may be tried for several months. However, these medications have limited success. In recent years, a number of operative procedures have been used in refractory cases. Excision of the plaque with replacement with a dermal graft has been successful, as has the use of tunica vaginalis grafts after plaque incision. Other authors have incised the plaque and inserted penile prostheses in the corpora cavernosa. Additional methods include radiation therapy and injection of steroids, dimethyl sulfoxide, or parathyroid hormone into the plaque. The success of such treatments is poorly documented.

PHIMOSIS

Phimosis is a condition in which the contracted foreskin cannot be retracted over the glans. Chronic infection from poor local hygiene is its most common cause. Most cases occur in uncircumcised males, although excessive skin left after circumcision can become stenotic and cause phimosis. Calculi and squamous cell carcinoma may develop under the foreskin. Phimosis can occur at any age. In diabetic older men, chronic balanoposthitis may lead to phimosis and may be the initial presenting complaint. Children under 2 years of age seldom have true phimosis; their relatively narrow preputial opening gradually widens and allows for normal retraction of foreskin over the glans. Circumcision for phimosis should be avoided in children requiring general anesthesia; except in cases with recurrent infections, the procedure should be postponed until the child reaches an age when local anesthesia can be used.

Edema, erythema, and tenderness of the prepuce and the presence of purulent discharge usually cause the patient to seek medical attention. Inability to retract the foreskin is a less common complaint.

The initial infection should be treated with broad-spectrum antimicrobial drugs. The dorsal foreskin can be slit if improved drainage is necessary. Circumcision, if indicated, should be done after the infection is controlled.

PARAPHIMOSIS

Paraphimosis is the condition in which the foreskin, once retracted over the glans, cannot be replaced in its normal position. This is due to chronic inflammation under the redundant foreskin, which leads to contracture of the preputial opening (phimosis) and formation of a tight ring of skin when the foreskin is retracted behind the glans. The skin ring causes venous congestion leading to edema and enlargement of the glans, which make the condition worse. As the condition progresses, arterial occlusion and necrosis of the glans may occur.

Paraphimosis usually can be treated by firmly squeezing the glans for 5 min to reduce the tissue edema and decrease the size of the glans. The skin can then be drawn forward over the glans. Occasionally, the constricting ring requires incision under local anesthesia. Antibiotics should be administered and circumcision should be done after inflammation has subsided.

CIRCUMCISION

Although circumcision is routinely performed in some countries for religious or cultural reasons, it is usually not necessary if adequate penile cleanliness and good hygiene can be maintained. There is a higher incidence of penile carcinoma in uncircumcised males, but chronic infection and poor hygiene are usually underlying factors in such instances. Circumcision is indicated in patients with infection, phimosis, or paraphimosis (see preceding sections).

URETHRAL STRICTURE

Acquired urethral stricture is common in men but rare in women. (Congenital urethral stricture is discussed earlier in the chapter.) Most acquired strictures are due to infection or trauma. Although gonococcal urethritis is seldom a cause of stricture today, infection remains a major cause—particularly infection from long-term use of indwelling urethral catheters. Large catheters and instruments are more likely than small ones to cause ischemia and internal trauma. External trauma, eg, pelvic fractures (see Chapter 19) can partially or completely sever the membranous urethra and cause severe and complex strictures. Straddle injuries can produce bulbar strictures.

Urethral strictures are fibrotic narrowings composed of dense collagen and fibroblasts. Fibrosis usually extends into the surrounding corpus spongiosum, causing spongiofibrosis. These narrowings restrict urine flow and cause dilation of the proximal urethra and prostatic ducts. Prostatitis is a common complication of urethral stricture. The bladder muscle may become hypertrophic, and increased residual urine may be noted. Severe, prolonged obstruction can result in decompensation of the ureterovesical junction, reflux, hydronephrosis, and renal failure. Chronic urinary stasis makes infection likely. Urethral fistulas and periurethral abscesses commonly develop in association with chronic, severe strictures.

Clinical Findings

A. Symptoms and Signs: A decrease in urinary stream is the most common complaint. Spraying or double stream is often noted, as is postvoiding dribbling. Chronic urethral discharge, occasionally a major complaint, is likely to be associated with chronic prostatitis. Acute cystitis or symptoms of infection are seen at times. Acute urinary retention seldom occurs unless infection or prostatic obstruction develops. Urinary frequency and mild dysuria may also be initial complaints.

Induration in the area of the stricture may be palpable. Tender enlarged masses along the urethra usually represent periurethral abscesses. Urethrocutaneous fistulas may be present. The bladder may be palpable if there is chronic retention of urine.

B. Laboratory Findings: If urethral stricture is suspected, urinary flow rates should be determined. The patient is instructed to accumulate urine until the bladder is full and then begin voiding; a 5-s collection of urine should be obtained during midstream maximal flow and its volume recorded. After the patient repeats this procedure 8–10 times over several days in a relaxed atmosphere, the mean peak flow can be calculated. With strictures creating significant problems, the flow rate will be less than 10 mL/s (normal, 20 mL/s).

Urine culture may be indicated. The midstream specimen is usually bacteria-free, with some pyuria [8–10 white blood cells (leukocytes) per high-power field] in a carefully obtained first aliquot of urine. If the prostate is infected, bacteria will be present in a specimen obtained after prostatic massage. In the presence of cystitis, the urine will be grossly infected.

C. X-Ray Findings: A urethrogram or voiding cystourethrogram (or both) will demonstrate the location and extent of the stricture. Sonography has also been a useful method of evaluating the urethral stricture (McAninch, Laing, and Jeffrey, 1988). Urethral fistulas and diverticula are sometimes noted. Vesical stones, trabeculations, or diverticula may also be seen.

D. Instrumental Examination: Urethroscopy allows visualization of the stricture. Small-caliber strictures prevent passage of the instrument through the area. Direct visualization and sonourethrography aid in determining the extent, location, and degree of scarring. Additional areas of scar formation adjacent to the stricture may be detected by urethroscopy.

The stricture can be calibrated by passage of bougies à boule (see Chapter 10).

Differential Diagnosis

Benign or malignant prostatic obstruction can cause symptoms similar to those of stricture. After prostatic surgery, bladder neck contracture can develop and induce stricturelike symptoms. Rectal examination and panendoscopy adequately define such abnormalities of the prostate. Urethral carcinoma is often associated with stricture; urethroscopy demonstrates a definite irregular lesion, and biopsy establishes the diagnosis of carcinoma.

Complications

Complications include chronic prostatitis, cystitis, chronic urinary infection, diverticula, urethrocutaneous fistulas, periurethral abscesses, and urethral carcinoma. Vesical calculi may develop from chronic urinary stasis and infection.

Treatment

A. Specific Measures:

1. Dilation–Dilation of urethral strictures is not usually curative, but it fractures the scar tissue of the stricture and temporarily enlarges the lumen. As healing occurs, the scar tissue re-forms.

Dilation may initially be required because of severe symptoms of chronic retention of urine. The urethra should be liberally lubricated with a water-soluble medium before instrumentation. A filiform is passed down the urethra and gently manipulated through the narrow area into the bladder. A follower can then be attached (see Chapter 11) and the area gradually dilated (with successively larger sizes) to approximately 22F. A 16F silicone catheter can then be inserted. If difficulty arises in passing the filiform through the stricture, urethroscopy should be used to guide the filiform under direct vision.

An alternative method of urethral dilation employs Van Buren sounds. These instruments are best used by an experienced urologist familiar with the size and extent of the stricture involved. First, a 22F sound should be passed down to the stricture site and gentle pressure applied. If this fails, a 20F sound should be used. Smaller sounds should not be used, because they can easily perforate the urethral wall and produce false passages. Bleeding and pain are major problems caused by dilation.

2. Urethrotomy under endoscopic direct vision–Lysis of urethral strictures can be accomplished using a sharp knife attached to an endoscope. The endoscope provides direct vision of the stricture during cutting. A filiform should be passed through the stricture and used as a guide during lysis. The stricture is usually incised dorsally, but multiple incisions in other areas may be required to open a narrow segment. A 22F instrument should pass with ease. A catheter is left in place for a short time to prevent bleeding and pain. Results of this procedure have been satisfactory in short-term follow-up in 70–80% of patients (Walther, Parsons, and Schmidt, 1980), but long-term success rates are much lower. The procedure has several advantages: (1) Minimal anesthesia is required—in some cases, only topical anesthesia combined with sedation; (2) it is easily repeated if the stricture recurs; and (3) it is very safe, with few complications.

3. Surgical reconstruction–If urethrotomy under direct vision fails, open surgical repair should be performed. Short strictures (≤ 2.0 cm) of the anterior urethra should be completely excised and primary anastomosis done. If possible, the segment to be excised should extend 1 cm beyond each end of the stricture to allow for removal of any existing spongiofibrosis and improve postoperative healing.

Strictures more than 2 cm in length can be managed by patch graft urethroplasty. The urethra is incised in the midline for the full length of the stricture plus an additional 1.5 cm proximal and distal to its ends. A full-thickness skin graft is obtained—preferably from the penile skin or buccal mucosa—and all subcutaneous tissue is carefully removed. The graft is then tailored to cover the defect and meticulously sutured into place (Figure 40–5).

In very long, densely fibrotic strictures, the distal penile fasciocutaneous flap technique has been successful in more than 80% (McAninch and Morey, 1998). This single-stage procedure can be combined with buccal mucosa grafting in panurethral strictures (Wessells, Morey and McAninch, 1997). In adults, grafts from buccal mucosa or penile skin should be applied with an onlay technique in the bulbar region of the urethra to maximize graft vascularization from the corpus spongiosum (Morey and McAninch, 1996b).

Strictures involving the membranous urethra ordinarily result from external trauma (see Chapter 19) and present problems in reconstruction. Most can be corrected by a perineal approach with excision of the urethral rupture defect and direct anastomosis of the bulbar urethra to the prostatic urethra (Figure 40–6). At times, partial pubectomy from the perineal approach can be done to improve urethral approximation without tension on the anastomosis. Rarely, total pubectomy combined with the perineal approach is required to accomplish the direct end-to-end anastomosis.

These single-stage procedures have a high success

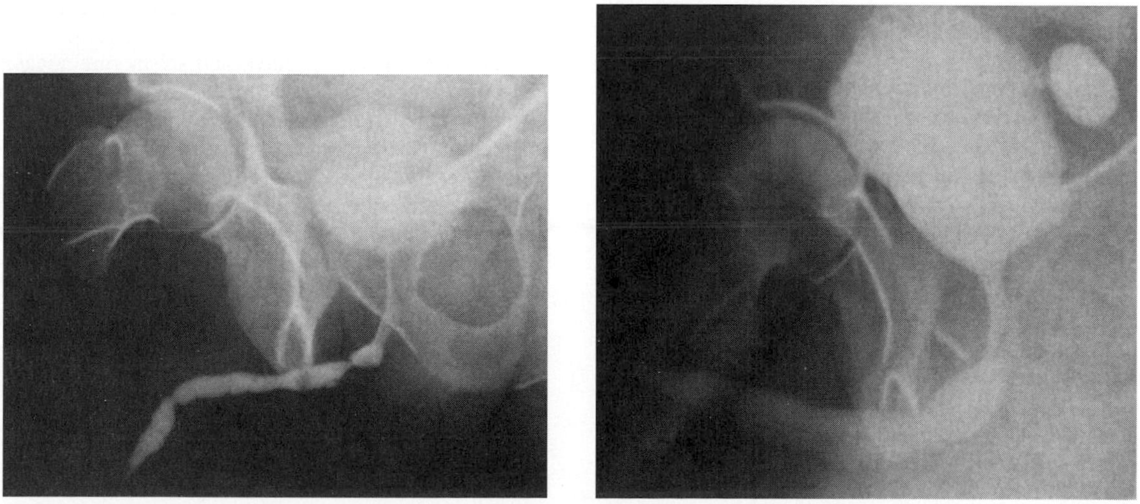

Figure 40–5. Left: Urethrogram demonstrating multiple anterior urethral strictures. **Right:** Voiding cystourethrogram following a patch skin graft of 14 cm in the same patient. There are no residual strictures.

rate and create a urethra free of hair—a major problem seen with 2-stage procedures. Although seldom required, 2-stage procedures are important reconstructive techniques to be considered in complex urethral strictures.

B. Treatment of Complications: Urinary tract infection in patients with strictures requires specific antimicrobial therapy, followed by long-term prophylactic therapy until the stricture has been corrected. Periurethral abscesses require drainage and use of antimicrobial drugs. Urethral fistulas usually require surgical repair.

Prognosis

A stricture should not be considered "cured" until it has been observed for at least 1 year after therapy, since it may recur at any time during that period. Urinary flow rate measurements and urethrograms are helpful to determine the extent of residual obstruction.

URETHRAL CONDYLOMATA ACUMINATA (Urethral Warts)

Condylomata acuminata are uncommon in the urethra and are almost always preceded by lesions on the skin (see **p 697**). They are wartlike papillomas caused by a papilloma virus and are usually transmitted by direct sexual contact but may be transmitted nonsexually.

Patients commonly complain of bloody spotting from the urethra and occasionally have dysuria and

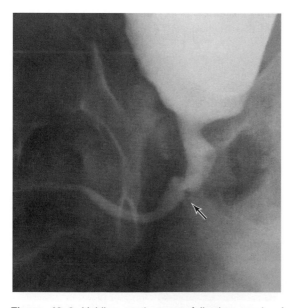

Figure 40–6. Voiding urethrogram following repair of traumatic posterior urethral stricture. Arrow indicates that area of repair is stricture-free.

urethral discharge. Examination of the urethral meatus often reveals a small, protruding papilloma. If a lesion is not found in this location, the meatus should be separated with the examining fingers so that the distal urethra can be inspected. About 90% of such lesions are situated in the distal urethra. Complete urethroscopy must be done to be certain other lesions do not exist.

Lesions of the meatus can be treated by local excision. A local anesthetic is applied to the area at the base of the lesions, and the pedunculated lesions are sharply incised with small scissors. The area is then fulgurated by electrocautery. Meatotomy may be indicated for excision of lesions in the fossa navicularis and glandular urethra.

Deeper lesions may be fulgurated transurethrally with a resectoscope or Bugby electrode. Recently, lesions have been successfully destroyed using a carbon dioxide laser. Laser therapy does minimal damage to the urethral mucosa, and stricture formation seems less likely with its use.

Multiple lesions have also been treated with fluorouracil, 5% solution or cream. The drug is instilled in the urethra for 20 min twice a week for 5 weeks. Care must be taken to protect the penile skin and scrotum from coming in contact with the medication, since it may produce severe irritation.

Lesions may become infected and ulcerated. This suggests carcinoma, and histopathologic confirmation of the diagnosis should be obtained. Rarely, giant condylomata (Buschke-Löwenstein tumors) involving the glans penis and often the urethra may be seen. Such lesions suggest carcinoma and must be biopsied. Surgical excision is the treatment of choice.

To prevent recurrence of condylomata acuminata, the sexual partner must also be examined and treated if necessary.

STENOSIS OF THE URETHRAL MEATUS

Newborns are often suspected of having meatal stenosis of some degree. This condition is thought to be secondary to ammonia dermatitis following circumcision and resulting in prolonged irritative meatitis.

Calibration is important, since the visual appearance of the meatus does not correlate well with its actual size. The urethra should easily accept the tip of an 8F pediatric feeding tube. The significance of meatal stenosis is debated, but a meatal caliber less than 5F in children under 10 years of age is an indication for meatotomy.

PENILE PHLEBOTHROMBOSIS & LYMPHATIC OCCLUSION

Superficial veins and lymphatic vessels of the dorsal penile shaft just proximal to the corona may become irritated and inflamed. A careful history usually indicates that minor trauma to the area (eg, from prolonged sexual intercourse) has occurred. Examination reveals a tender, indurated, cordlike structure on the distal penile shaft. Slight erythema may be present.

For clinical purposes, there is no need to distinguish lymphatic and venous causes, since both penile phlebothrombosis and lymphatic occlusion will resolve spontaneously. The patient must be reassured.

REFERENCES

CONGENITAL ANOMALIES

Penis & Urethra
Allen TD: Congenital microphallus. In: Kaufman JJ (editor): *Current Urologic Therapy.* Saunders, 1980.

Churchill BM et al: The dartos flap as an adjunct in preventing urethrocutaneous fistulas in repeat hypospadias surgery. J Urol 1996;156:2047.

Gad YZ et al: 5 alpha-reductase deficiency in patients with micropenis. J Inherit Metab Dis 1997;20:95.

Hinman F Jr: Microphallus: Distinction between anomalous and endocrine types. J Urol 1980;123:412.

Karnak I et al: Rare congenital abnormalities of the anterior urethra. Pediatr Surg Int 1997;12:407.

Kennedy HA et al: Collateral urethral duplication in the frontal plane: A spectrum of cases. J Urol 1988;139:332.

Klugo RC, Cerny JC: Response of micropenis to topical testosterone and gonadotropin. J Urol 1978;119:667.

Kogan SJ, Williams DI: The micropenis syndrome: Clinical observations and expectations for growth. J Urol 1977;118:311.

Wessells H, Lue TF, McAninch JW: Penile length in the flaccid and erect states: Guidelines for penile augmentation. J Urol 1996;156:995.

Wilson SA, Walker RD: Megalourethra and hypospadias. J Urol 1983;129:556.

Wirtshafter A et al: Complete trifurcation of the urethra. J Urol 1980;123:431.

Urethral Stricture
Aragona F et al: Familial occurrence of congenital stricture of bulbar urethra. Urol Int 1991;46:112.

Hoebeke PB et al: Membrano-bulbo-urethral junction stenosis. Posterior urethra obstruction due to extreme caliber disproportion in the male urethra. Eur Urol 1997;32:480.

Narborough GC, Elliott S, Minford JE: Congenital stricture of the urethra. Clin Radiol 1990;42:402.

Scherz HC, Kaplan GW: Etiology, diagnosis, and management of urethral strictures in children. Urol Clin North Am 1990;17:389.

Posterior Urethral Valves
Ewalt DH, Bauer SB: Pediatric neurourology. Urol Clin North Am 1996;23:501.

Hulbert WC et al: The predictive value of ultrasonography in evaluation of infants with posterior urethral valves. J Urol 1992;148:122.

Johnston JH: Vesicoureteric reflux with urethral valves. Br J Urol 1979;51:100.

Parkhouse HF, Woodhouse CR: Long-term status of patients with posterior urethral valves. Urol Clin North Am 1990;17:373.

Peters CA et al: The urodynamic consequences of posterior urethral valves. J Urol 1990;144:122.

Reinberg Y, de Castano I, Gonzalez R: Influence of initial therapy on progression of renal failure and body growth in children with posterior urethral valves. J Urol 1992;148:532.

Reinberg Y, de Castano I, Gonzalez R: Prognosis for patients with prenatally diagnosed posterior urethral valves. J Urol 1992;148:125.

Scott JE, Renwick M: Urological anomalies in the Northern Region Fetal Abnormality Survey. Arch Dis Child 1993;68(1 Spec No):22.

Anterior Urethral Valves
Churchill BM et al: The dartos flap as an adjunct in preventing urethrocutaneous fistulas in repeat hypospadias surgery. J Urol 1996;156:2047.

Firlit RS, Firlit CF, King LR: Obstructing anterior urethral valves in children. J Urol 1978;119:819.

Golimbu M et al: Anterior urethral valves. Urology 1978;12:343.

Takeda M et al: Application of flexible renoureteroscope for antegrade urethroscopy in the treatment of congenital anterior urethral valve. Eur Urol 1992;22:190.

Urethrorectal, Vesicorectal, & Urethroperineal Fistulas
Bates DG, Lebowitz RL: Congenital urethroperineal fistula. Radiology 1995;194:501.

Brown WC, Dillon PW, Hensle TW: Congenital urethral-perineal fistula: Diagnosis and new surgical management. Urology 1990;36:157.

Glenn JF: Eccentric flap repair of urethral fistulas. J Urol 1983;129:510.

Hong AR et al: Congenital urethral fistula with normal anus: A report of two cases. J Pediatr Surg 1992;27:1278.

Hypospadias
Asopa HS: Newer concepts in the management of hypospadias and its complications. Ann R Coll Surg Engl 1998;80:161.

Baskin LS, Duckett JW: Buccal mucosa grafts in hypospadias surgery. Br J Urol 1995;76(Suppl 3):23.

Baskin LS, Duckett JW, Lue TF: Penile curvature. Urology 1996;48:347.

Belman BA, Kass EJ: Hypospadias repair in children less than 1 year old. J Urol 1982;128:1273.

Duckett JW: Island flap technique for hypospadias repair. Urol Clin North Am 1981;8:503.

Duckett JW, Snyder HM III: Meatal advancement and glanuloplasty hypospadias repair after 1,000 cases: Avoidance of meatal stenosis and regression. J Urol 1992;147:665.

Gearhart JP et al: Androgen receptor levels and 5 alpha-re-ductase activities in preputial skin and chordee tissue of boys with isolated hypospadias. J Urol 1988;140:1243.

Gearhart JP et al: Endocrine evaluation of adults with mild hypospadias. J Urol 1990;144:274.

Hendren WH, Horton CE Jr: Experience with 1-stage re-pair of hypospadias and chordee using free graft of prepuce. J Urol 1988;140:1259.

Hinman F JR: The blood supply to preputial island flaps. J Urol 1991;145:1232.

Kass EJ, Bolong D: Single stage hypospadias recon-struction without fistula. J Urol 1990;144:520, 530.

Keating MA, Cartwright PC, Duckett JW: Bladder mu-cosa in urethral reconstructions. J Urol 1990;144:827.

Mollard P et al: Repair of hypospadias using a bladder mucosal graft in 76 cases. J Urol 1989;142:1548.

Rober PE, Perlmutter AD, Reitelman C: Experience with 81, 1-stage hypospadias/chordee repairs with free graft urethroplasties. J Urol 1990;144:526.

Smith EP, Wacksman J: Evaluation of severe hypospa-dias. J Pediatr 1997;131:344.

Chordee without Hypospadias

Devine CJ Jr et al: The surgical treatment of chordee without hypospadias in men. J Urol 1991;146:325.

Kaplan GW, Lamm DL: Embryogenesis of chordee. J Urol 1975;114:769.

Redman JF: Extended application of Nesbit ellipses in the correction of childhood penile curvature. J Urol 1978;119:122.

Udall DA: Correction of 3 types of congenital curvature of the penis, including the first reported case of dorsal curvature. J Urol 1980;124:50.

Epispadias

Arap S et al: Incontinent epispadias: Surgical treatment of 38 cases. J Urol 1988;140:577.

Ben-Chaim J, Gearhart JP: Current management of blad-der exstrophy. Scand J Urol Nephrol 1997;31:103.

Diamond DA, Ransley PG: Male epispadias. J Urol 1995;154:2150.

Kaefer M et al: Continent urinary diversion: The Chil-dren's Hospital experience. J Urol 1997;157:1394.

Kramer SA, Kelalis PP: Assessment of urinary conti-nence in epispadias: Review of 94 patients. J Urol 1982;128:290.

Perlmutter AD, Weinstein MD, Reitelman C: Vesical neck reconstruction in patients with epispadias-exstrophy complex. J Urol 1991;146:613.

Peters CA, Gearhart JP, Jeffs RD: Epispadias and incon-tinence: The challenge of the small bladder. J Urol 1988;140:1199.

Silver RI et al: Urolithiasis in the exstrophy-epispadias complex. J Urol 1997;158(3 Pt 2):1322.

Tanagho EA, Smith DR: Clinical evaluation of a surgi-cal technique for the correction of complete urinary incontinence. J Urol 1972;107:402.

ACQUIRED DISEASES & DISORDERS

Priapism

Barry JM: Priapism: Treatment with corpus cavernosum to dorsal vein of penis shunts. J Urol 1976;116:754.

Brock G et al: High flow priapism: A spectrum of dis-ease. J Urol 1993;150:968.

Hamre MR et al: Priapism as a complication of sickle-cell disease. J Urol 1991;145:1.

Ilkay AK, Levine LA: Conservative management of high-flow priapism. Urology 1995;46:419.

Lakin MM et al: Intracavernous injection therapy: Analy-sis of results and complications. J Urol 1990;143:1138.

Levine JF et al: Recurrent prolonged erections and pri-apism as a sequela of priapism: Pathophysiology and management. J Urol 1991;145:764.

Lue TF et al: Priapism: Refined approach to diagnosis and treatment. J Urol 1986;136:104.

Meriob P, Livne PM: Incidence, possible causes and fol-lowup of idiopathic prolonged penile erection in the newborn. J Urol 1989;141:1410.

Mulhall JP, Honig SC: Priapism: Etiology and manage-ment. Acad Emerg Med 1996;3:810.

Patel AG, Mukherji K, Lee A: Priapism associated with psychotropic drugs. Br J Hosp Med 1996;55:315.

Ricciardi R Jr et al: Delayed high flow priapism: Patho-physiology and management. J Urol 1993;149:119.

Sayer J, Parsons CL: Successful treatment of priapism with intracorporeal epinephrine. J Urol 1988;140:827.

Shapiro RH, Berger RE: Post-traumatic priapism treated with selective cavernosal artery ligation. Urology 1997;49:638.

Winter CC, McDowell G: Experience with 105 patients with priapism: Update review of all aspects. J Urol 1988;140:980.

Peyronie Disease

Carson CC: Penile prosthesis implantation in the treat-ment of Peyronie's disease. Int J Impotence Res 1998;10:125.

Ganem JP et al: Unusual complications of the vacuum erection device. Urology 1998;51:627.

Gelbard MK, Dorey F, James K: The natural history of Peyronie's disease. J Urol 1990;144:1376.

Jordan GH, Angermeier KW: Preoperative evaluation of erectile function with dynamic infusion cavernosome-try/cavernosography in patients undergoing surgery for Peyronie's disease: Correlation with postoperative results. J Urol 1993;150:1138.

Lopez JA, Jarow JP: Penile vascular evaluation of men with Peyronie's disease. J Urol 1993;149:53.

Lue TF, El-Sakka AI: Venous patch graft for Peyronie's disease. Part I: technique. J Urol 1998;160:2047.

Mufti GR et al: Corporeal plication for surgical correc-tion of Peyronie's disease. J Urol 1990;144:281.

O'Donnell PD: Results of surgical management of Pey-ronie's disease. J Urol 1992;148:1184.

Pryor JP: Correction of penile curvature and Peyronie's disease: Why I prefer the Nesbit technique. Int J Im-potence Res 1998;10:129.

Somers KD et al: Isolation and characterization of colla-gen in Peyronie's disease. J Urol 1989;141:629.

Phimosis

Fakjian N et al: An argument for circumcision. Preven-tion of balanitis in the adult. Arch Dermatol 1990;126:1046.

Langer JC, Coplen DE: Circumcision and pediatric disor-ders of the penis. Pediatr Clin North Am 1998;45:801.

Simpson ET, Barraclough P: The management of the paediatric foreskin. Aust Fam Physician 1998;27:381.

Paraphimosis

Hamdy FC, Hastie KJ: Treatment for paraphimosis: The "puncture" technique. (See comments.) Br J Surg 1990;77:1186.

Olson C: Emergency treatment of paraphimosis. Can Fam Physician 1998;44:1253.

Raveenthiran V: Reduction of paraphimosis: A technique based on pathophysiology. Br J Surg 1996;83:1247.

Circumcision

American Academy of Pediatrics: Report of the Task Force on Circumcision [published erratum appears in Pediatrics 1989;84:761]. Pediatrics 1989;84:388.

Baskin LS et al: Treating complications of circumcision. Pediatr Emerg Care 1996;12:62.

Fergusson DM, Lawton JM, Shannon FT: Neonatal circumcision and penile problems: An 8-year longitudinal study. Pediatrics 1988;81:537.

Langer JC, Coplen DE: Circumcision and pediatric disorders of the penis. Pediatr Clin North Am 1998;45:801.

Niku SD, Stock JA, Kaplan GW: Neonatal circumcision. Urol Clin North Am 1995;22:57.

Stull TL, LiPuma JJ: Epidemiology and natural history of urinary tract infections in children. Med Clin North Am 1991;75:287.

Urethral Stricture

Angermeier KW, Jordan GH, Schlossberg SM: Complex urethral reconstruction. Urol Clin North Am 1994;21:567.

Barry JM: Visual urethrotomy in the management of the obliterated membranous urethra. Urol Clin North Am 1989;16:319.

Benet AE et al: Surgical management of long urethral strictures. J Urol 1990;143:917.

el-Kasaby AW et al: The use of buccal mucosa patch graft in the management of anterior urethral strictures. J Urol 1993;149:276.

Gary R, Cass AS, Koos G: Vascular complications of transurethral incision of post-traumatic urethral strictures. J Urol 1988;140:1539.

McAninch JW: Pubectomy in repair of membranous urethral stricture. Urol Clin North Am 1989;16:297.

McAninch JW, Laing FC, Jeffrey RB Jr: Sonourethrography in the evaluation of urethral strictures: A preliminary report. J Urol 1988;139:294.

McAninch JW, Morey AF: Penile circular fasciocutaneous skin flap in one-stage reconstruction of complex anterior urethral strictures. J Urol 1998;159:1209.

Morey AF, McAninch JW: Reconstruction of posterior urethral disruption injuries: Outcome analysis in 82 patients. J Urol 1997a;157:506.

Morey AF, McAninch JW: Reconstruction of traumatic posterior urethral strictures. Tech Urol 1997b;3:103.

Morey AF, McAninch JW: Ultrasound evaluation of the male urethra for assessment of urethral stricture. J Clin Ultrasound 1996a;24:473.

Morey AF, McAninch, JW: When and how to use buccal mucosal grafts in adult bulbar urethroplasty. Urology 1996b;48:194.

Schreiter F: Mesh-graft urethroplasty: Our experience with a new procedure. Eur Urol 1984;10:338.

Stormont TJ, Suman VJ, Oesterling JE: Newly diagnosed bulbar urethral strictures: Etiology and outcome of various treatments. J Urol 1993;150:1725.

Walther PC, Parsons CL, Schmidt JD: Direct vision internal urethrotomy in the management of urethral strictures. J Urol 1980;123:497.

Webster GD: Perineal repair of membranous urethral stricture. Urol Clin North Am 1989;16:303.

Webster GD, Ramon J: Repair of pelvic fracture posterior urethral defects using an elaborated perineal approach: Experience with 74 cases. J Urol 1991;145:744.

Wessells H, Morey AF, McAninch JW: Single-stage reconstruction of complex anterior urethral strictures: Combined tissue-transfer techniques. J Urol 1997;157:1271.

Urethral Condylomata Acuminata

Chacho MS et al: Influence of human papillomavirus on DNA ploidy determination in genital condylomas. Cancer 1990;65:2291.

Fralick RA et al: Urethroscopy and urethral cytology in men with external genital condyloma. Urology 1994;43:361.

Rock B, Shah KV, Farmer ER: A morphologic, pathologic, and virologic study of anogenital warts in men. Arch Dermatol 1992;128:495.

Volz LR, Carpiniello VL, Malloy TR: Laser treatment of urethral condyloma: A five-year experience. Urology 1994;43:81.

Penile Thrombophlebitis & Lymphatic Occlusion

Bird V et al: Traumatic thrombophlebitis of the superficial dorsal vein of the penis: An occupational hazard. Am J Emerg Med 1997;15:67.

Shapiro RS: Superficial dorsal penile vein thrombosis (penile Mondor's phlebitis): Ultrasound diagnosis. J Clin Ultrasound 1996;24:272.

41

Disorders of the Female Urethra

Emil A. Tanagho, MD

CONGENITAL ANOMALIES OF THE FEMALE URETHRA

DISTAL URETHRAL STENOSIS IN INFANCY & CHILDHOOD
(Spasm of the External Urinary Sphincter)

There has been considerable confusion about the site of lower tract obstruction in young girls who suffer from enuresis, a slow and interrupted urinary stream, recurrent cystitis, and pyelonephritis, and who, on thorough examination, often exhibit vesicoureteral reflux. Treatment has been directed largely to the bladder neck on rather empiric grounds. Most of these children, however, have congenital distal urethral stenosis with secondary spasm of the striated external sphincter rather than bladder neck obstruction due to functional or organic causes.

At birth, calibration of the urethra with bougies à boule reveals no evidence of a distal ring of urethral stenosis (Fisher et al, 1969). Within a few months, however, such a ring develops as a normal anatomic structure. After puberty, the ring disappears. The inference is that the absence of estrogens leads to the development of this lesion. Lyon and Tanagho (1965) found that the ring calibrates at 14F at age 2 and at 16F between the ages of 4 and 10. Even though from the hydrodynamic standpoint such a stenotic area should not be obstructive, almost all observers agree that dilatation of the ring does relieve symptoms in these children and that it results in cure or amelioration of persistent infection or vesical dysfunction in 80% of cases. Lyon and Tanagho thought it possible that the basic cause of these urinary difficulties might be reflex spasm of periurethral striated sphincter and noted that voiding cystourethrograms supported that view (Figure 41–1).

Tanagho et al (1971) measured pressures in the bladder and in the proximal and mid urethra simultaneously in symptomatic girls and found high resting pressures, some as high as 200 cm of water (normal, 100 cm of water) in the midurethral segment. Attempts at voiding caused intravesical pressures as high as 225 cm of water (normal, 30–40 cm of water) to develop. Under curare, the urethral closing pressures dropped to normal (40–50 cm of water), proving that these obstructing pressures were caused by spasm of the striated sphincter muscle. If the distal urethral ring was treated and symptoms abated, repeat pressure studies showed normal midurethral and intravesical voiding pressures. If, on the other hand, symptoms persisted, pressures were found to remain at extremely high levels. It seems clear, therefore, that the major cause of urinary problems in young girls is spasm of the external sphincter and not vesical neck stenosis (Smith, 1969).

In addition to recurrent urinary tract infections, these patients have hesitancy in initiating micturition and a slow, hesitant, or interrupted urinary stream. Enuresis and involuntary loss of urine during the day are common complaints. Abdominal straining may be required in order to void. Small amounts of residual urine are found, which impair the vesical defense mechanism (Hinman, 1966). A voiding cystourethrogram may reveal an open bladder neck and ballooning of the proximal urethra secondary to spasm of the external sphincter (Figure 41–1).

The voiding cystourethrogram may reveal evidence of the distal ring, but typical findings are not always seen, particularly if the flow rate is slow. Definitive diagnosis is made by bougienage.

The simplest and least harmful treatment is overdilatation with sounds up to 32–36F or with the Kollmann dilator (Lyon and Tanagho, 1965; Lyon and Marshall, 1971; Hendry, Stanton, and Williams, 1973). With either method, the ring "cracks" anteriorly, with some bleeding. Recurrence of the ring is rare. Internal urethrotomy has its proponents (Immergut and Gilbert, 1973; Hradec et al, 1973), but Kaplan, Sammons, and King (1973) found that results with urethrotomy were poor, since incising the urethra along its entire length does not cut the external sphincter, whose abnormal tone is the cause of the obstruction, whereas "cracking" the ring by overdilatation accomplishes this purpose.

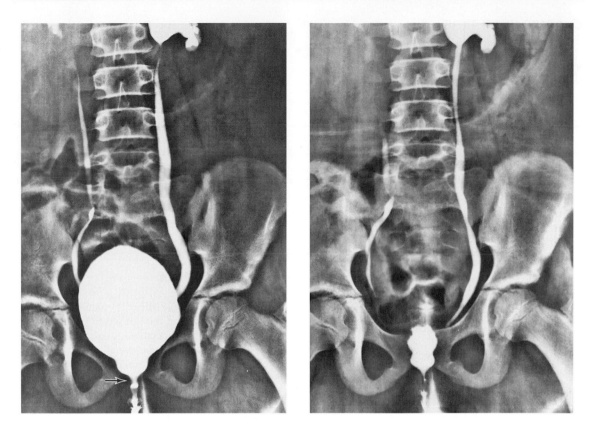

Figure 41–1. Distal urethral stenosis with reflux spasm of voluntary urethral sphincter. **Left:** Voiding cystourethrogram showing bilateral vesicoureteral reflux, a wide-open vesical neck, and severe spasm of the striated urethral sphincter in the mid portion of the urethra (arrow) secondary to distal urethral stenosis. **Right:** Postvoiding film. The bladder is empty and the vesical neck open, but the dilated urethra contains radiopaque fluid proximal to the stenotic zone. Bacteria in the urethra thus can flow back into the bladder. (Courtesy of AD Amar.)

In 80% of affected children, destruction of the ring of distal urethral stenosis helps to overcome enuresis and achieve a normal free voiding pattern and to cure recurrent cystitis or persistent bacteriuria (Lyon and Marshall, 1971). Spontaneous resolution of reflux is possible only in the case of "borderline" values that tend to give way in the presence of increased voiding pressure and infection.

Since the ring normally disappears at puberty, it is possible to await spontaneous cure; however, the ring should be broken if symptoms have been severe enough to bring the child to the attention of a urologist.

LABIAL FUSION
(Synechia Vulvae)

Some children with recurring urinary infection are found to have fused labia minora, which are apt to obstruct the flow of urine, causing it to pool in the vagina. Local application of estrogen cream twice daily for 2–4 weeks usually causes spontaneous sepa-

ration. Forceful separation or dissection has its advocates (Christensen and Oster, 1971).

ACQUIRED DISEASES
OF THE FEMALE URETHRA

ACUTE URETHRITIS

Acute urethritis frequently occurs with gonorrheal infection in women. Urinary symptoms are often present at the onset of the disease. Cultures and smears establish the diagnosis. Prompt cure can be achieved with antimicrobial drugs.

The detergents in bubble bath and some spermicidal jellies may cause vaginitis and urethritis. Symptoms of vesical irritability may occur.

CHRONIC URETHRITIS

Chronic urethritis is one of the most common urologic problems of females. The distal urethra normally harbors pathogens, and the risk of infection may be increased by wearing contaminated diapers, by insertion of an indwelling catheter, by spread from cervical or vaginal infections, or by intercourse with an infected partner. Urethral inflammation may also occur from the trauma of intercourse or childbirth, particularly if urethral stenosis, either congenital or following childbirth, is present.

Clinical Findings

The urethral mucosa is reddened, quite sensitive, and often stenotic. Granular areas are often seen, and polypoid masses may be noted just distal to the bladder neck.

A. Symptoms: The symptoms resemble those of cystitis, although the urine may be clear. Complaints include burning on urination, frequency, and nocturia. Discomfort in the urethra may be felt, particularly when walking.

B. Signs: Examination may disclose redness of the meatus, hypersensitivity of the meatus and of the urethra on vaginal palpation, and evidence of cervicitis or vaginitis. There is no urethral discharge.

C. Laboratory Findings: When the initial and midstream urine are collected in separate containers, the first glass contains pus and the second does not (Marshall, Lyon, and Schieble, 1970). *Ureaplasma urealyticum* (formerly called T strains of mycoplasmas) is often identifiable in the first glass. These findings are similar to those of nongonococcal (chlamydial) urethritis in males. Clinically, the presence of white blood cells (leukocytes) in the absence of bacteria on a routine stain or culture suggests nongonococcal urethritis. In other cases, various bacteria (eg, *Streptococcus faecalis, Escherichia coli*) may be cultured from both the urethral washings and a specimen taken from the introitus.

D. Instrumental Examination: A catheter, bougie à boule, or sound may meet resistance because of urethral stenosis. Panendoscopy reveals redness and a granular appearance of the mucosa. Inflammatory polyps may be seen in the proximal portion of the urethra. Cystoscopy may show increased injection of the trigone (trigonitis), which often accompanies urethritis.

Differential Diagnosis

Differentiation of urethritis from cystitis depends on bacteriologic study of the urine; panendoscopy demonstrates the urethral lesion. Both urethritis and cystitis may be present.

Psychological disorders may cause symptoms identical to those of chronic urethritis. A history of short bouts of frequency without nocturia is suggestive of functional illness. The neurotic makeup of the patient is usually obvious.

Treatment & Prognosis

Gradual urethral dilatations (up to 36F in adults) are indicated for urethral stenosis; this allows for some inevitable contracture. Immergut and Gilbert (1973) prefer internal urethrotomy. *U urealyticum* is fairly sensitive to tetracycline or erythromycin. Chlamydial urethritis usually responds to sulfonamides or tetracyclines. For ascending bacterial infections, Bruce et al (1973) recommend the regular, local application of an antiseptic (eg, hexachlorophene, chlorhexidine cream) to the introitus in order to prevent bacteria from the area of the perineum, vagina, and vulva from reinfecting the urethra.

SENILE URETHRITIS

After physiologic (or surgical) menopause, hypoestrogenism occurs and retrogressive (senile) changes take place in the vaginal epithelium, so that it becomes rather dry and pale. Similar changes develop in the lower urinary tract, which arises from the same embryologic tissues as the female reproductive organs. Some eversion of the mucosa about the urethral orifice, from foreshortening of the vaginal canal, is usually seen. This is commonly misdiagnosed as caruncle.

Clinical Findings

A. Symptoms: Many postmenopausal women have symptoms of vesical irritability (burning, frequency, urgency) and stress incontinence. They may complain of vaginal and vulval itching and some discharge.

B. Signs: The vaginal epithelium is dry and pale. The mucosa at the urethral orifice is often reddened and hypersensitive; eversion of its posterior lip from foreshortening of the urethrovaginal wall is common.

C. Laboratory Findings: The urine is usually free of microorganisms. The diagnosis can be made by the following procedure: A dry smear of vaginal epithelial cells is stained with Lugol's solution. The slide is then washed with water and immediately examined microscopically while wet. In hypoestrogenism, the cells take up the iodine poorly and are therefore yellow. When the mucosa is normal, these cells stain a deep brown because of their glycogen content. The diagnosis may also be confirmed by a Papanicolaou smear.

D. Instrumental Examination: Panendoscopy usually demonstrates a reddened and granular urethral mucosa. Some urethral stenosis may be noted.

Differential Diagnosis

Senile urethritis is often mistaken for urethral caruncle. Eversion of the posterior lip of the urinary meatus is evident in both conditions; however, a hypersensitive vascular tumor is not present in senile urethritis.

Before operations to relieve stress incontinence are performed, estrogen (or androgen) therapy should be tried.

Treatment

Senile urethritis responds well to diethylstilbestrol vaginal suppositories, 0.1 mg nightly for 3 weeks. Estrogen creams applied locally are also effective. Estrogen urethral suppositories have been recommended, but they offer no advantages and are difficult to insert. After 3 weeks of treatment, the drug is withheld for 1 week and the course is repeated. Three or more courses are occasionally indicated, depending on the symptoms and the appearance of the vaginal smear stained as outlined previously.

If vaginal irritation or bleeding on discontinuation of estrogen suppositories is a problem, methyltestosterone buccal tablets can be used as vaginal suppositories. One 5-mg tablet is inserted vaginally daily for 5–8 weeks. Diethylstilbestrol, 0.1 mg/d orally, is also effective.

Prognosis

Senile urethritis usually responds promptly to estrogen or androgen therapy.

URETHRAL CARUNCLE

Urethral caruncle is a benign, red, raspberrylike, friable vascular tumor involving the posterior lip of the external urinary meatus. It is rare before the menopause. Microscopically, it consists of connective tissue containing many inflammatory cells and blood vessels and is covered by an epithelial layer.

Clinical Findings

Symptoms include pain on urination, pain with intercourse, and bloody spotting from even mild trauma. A sessile or pedunculated red, friable, tender mass is seen at the posterior lip of the meatus.

Differential Diagnosis

Carcinoma of the urethra may involve the urethral meatus. Palpation reveals definite induration. Biopsy establishes the true diagnosis.

Senile urethritis is often associated with a polypoid reaction of the urinary meatus and in fact is the most common cause of masses in this region. The diagnosis can be made by verifying the patient's hypoestrogenic status and by demonstrating a favorable response to estrogen replacement therapy. Biopsy should be done if doubt exists.

Thrombosis of the urethral vein presents as a bluish, swollen, tender lesion involving the posterior lip of the urinary meatus. It has the appearance of the thrombosed hemorrhoid. It subsides without treatment.

Treatment

Local excision is indicated only if symptoms are troublesome.

Prognosis

True caruncle is usually cured by excision, but in a few instances it does recur.

PROLAPSE OF THE URETHRA

Prolapse of the female urethra is not common. It usually occurs only in children or in paraplegics suffering from a lower motor neuron lesion. The protruding urethral mucosa presents as an angry red mass that may become gangrenous if it is not reduced promptly. When a young girl has a protruding mass, urethral prolapse must be differentiated from prolapse of a ureterocele.

After reduction, cystoscopy should be done to rule out ureterocele. Recurrences are rare following reduction; the accompanying inflammation probably "fixes" the tissue in place as healing progresses. If the prolapsed urethra cannot be reduced or if it recurs, an indwelling catheter should be inserted, traction placed on it, and a heavy piece of suture material tightly tied over the tissue and catheter just proximal to the mass. The tissue later sloughs off. Using this same technique, the tissue can be resected, preferably with an electrosurgical cautery.

URETHROVAGINAL FISTULA

Urethrovaginal fistulas may follow local injury secondary to fracture of the pelvis or obstetric or surgical injury (see Chapter 17). A common cause is accidental trauma to the urethra or its blood supply in the course of surgical repair of a cystocele or excision of urethral diverticula. Vaginal urethroplasty is indicated.

URETHRAL DIVERTICULUM

Diverticulation of the urethral wall is not common. Diverticula are at times multiple. Most cases are probably secondary to obstetric urethral trauma or severe urethral infection. A few cases of carcinoma in such diverticula have been reported. Urethral diverticula are usually associated with recurrent attacks of cystitis. Purulent urethral discharge is sometimes noted as the infected diverticulum empties. Dyspareunia sometimes results. On occasion, the diverticulum may be large enough to be discovered by the patient.

The diagnosis is usually made on feeling a rounded cystic mass in the anterior wall of the vagina that leaks pus from the urethral orifice when pressure is applied. Endoscopy may reveal the urethral opening. The postvoiding film of an excretory urographic series may demonstrate the lesion. It may be possible to introduce a small catheter through which radiopaque fluid can be instilled. Appropriate x-ray films are then exposed (Figure 41–2). The plain film may show a stone in the diverticulum. If these methods fail, the following procedures can be used:

(1) Empty the diverticulum manually. Via a catheter, instill 5 mL of indigo carmine and 60 mL of contrast medium into the bladder. Remove the catheter and have the patient begin to void. Occlude the meatus with a finger. This maneuver usually causes the diverticulum to fill with the test solution. Take appropriate x-rays, and perform panendoscopy to look for leakage of blue dye from the mouth of the diverticulum.

(2) Insert a Davis-TeLinde catheter. This looks like a Foley catheter but is surrounded by a second movable balloon. Pass the catheter to the bladder and inflate the proximal balloon. While exerting tension on the catheter, slide the second balloon against the urinary meatus and inflate it. Then inject contrast medium into the catheter. The radiopaque fluid will escape from the catheter through a hole between the balloons and will fill the urethra and diverticulum, after which x-rays can be exposed. Occasionally, urethral diverticulum is elusive and difficult to visualize. Transvaginal ultrasonography or pelvic magnetic resonance imaging can be helpful in diagnosis.

Treatment consists of removal of the sac through an incision in the anterior vaginal wall, care being taken not to injure the urethral sphincteric musculature. Incision is carried down to the diverticular mucosa, and the plane of cleavage is followed all around to the neck of the diverticulum. The diverticular sac is completely excised and the defect in the urethra repaired. Elik (1957) recommends that the diverticulum be opened, stuffed with absorbable cellulose (Oxycel), and then closed; the resulting inflammatory reaction destroys the cyst. A suprapubic cystostomy should be left in place for 15 days following surgical excision of the diverticulum.

The outcome is usually good unless the diverticulum is so situated that its excision injures the external urinary sphincter mechanism. In a few cases, urethrovaginal fistula may develop. If the fistula does not close with adequate suprapubic drainage, surgical repair will be necessary 2–3 months later.

URETHRAL STRICTURE

True organic stricture of the adult female urethra is not common. (Functional urethral obstruction is more common.) It may be congenital or acquired. The trauma of intercourse and especially of childbirth may lead to periurethral fibrosis with contracture, or the stricture may be caused by the surgeon during vaginal repair. It may develop secondary to acute or chronic urethritis.

Persistent hesitancy in initiating urination and a slow urinary stream are the principal symptoms of stricture. Burning, frequency, nocturia, and urethral pain may occur from secondary urethritis or cystitis. If secondary infection of the bladder is present, pus and bacteria will be found in the urine. A fairly large catheter (22F) may pass to the bladder only with dif-

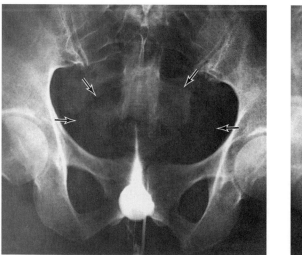 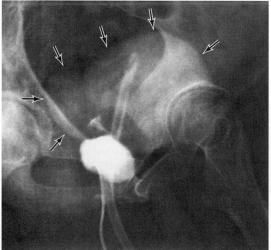

Figure 41–2. Urethral diverticulum containing stone. **Left:** Plain film showing stone. Arrows outline bladder. **Right:** Diverticulum filled with radiopaque fluid instilled through ureteral catheter. Bladder outlined by arrows.

ficulty. Panendoscopy may demonstrate the point of narrowness and disclose evidence of urethritis. Cystoscopy often reveals trabeculation (hypertrophy) of the bladder wall.

Chronic cystitis may cause similar symptoms, but urinalysis reveals evidence of infection. Cancer of the urethra causes progressive narrowing of the urethra, but induration and infiltration of the urethra are found on vaginal examination. Panendoscopy with biopsy establishes the diagnosis. Vesical tumor involving the bladder neck causes hesitancy and impairment of the urinary stream. Cystoscopy is definitive. Chronic ure-

thritis commonly accompanies urethral stenosis; either may be primary. Recurrent or chronic cystitis is often secondary to stenosis.

Treatment consists of gradual urethral dilatation (up to 36F) at weekly intervals. Slight overstretching is necessary, since some contracture will occur after therapy is discontinued. Measures to combat urethritis and cystitis also must be employed. Internal urethrotomy has its proponents.

With proper overdilatation of the urethra and specific therapy of the urethritis that is usually present, the prognosis is good.

REFERENCES

DISTAL URETHRAL STENOSIS

Archimbaud JP, Leriche A, Mottet N: Urethral stenosis and urinary incontinence in the female: 149 cases. Ann Urol 1989;23:340.

Farrar DJ, Green NA, Ashken MH: An evaluation of the Otis urethrotomy in female patients with recurrent urinary tract infections: A review after 6 years. Br J Urol 1980;52:68.

Firlit CF: Urethral anomalies. Urol Clin North Am 1978; 5:31.

Fisher RE et al: Urethral calibration in newborn girls. J Urol 1969;102:67.

Hendry WF, Stanton SL, Williams DI: Recurrent urinary infections in girls: Effects of urethral dilatation. Br J Urol 1973;45:72.

Hinman F Jr: Mechanisms for the entry of bacteria and the establishment of urinary infection in female children. J Urol 1966;96:546.

Hojsgaard A: The urethral pressure profile in female patients with meatal stenosis. Scand J Urol Nephrol 1976;10:97.

Hradec E et al: Significance of urethral obstruction in girls. Urol Int 1973;28:440.

Immergut MA, Gilbert EC: Internal urethrotomy in recurring urinary infections in girls. J Urol 1973;109: 126.

Kaplan GW, Sammons TA, King LR: A blind comparison of dilatation, urethrotomy and medication alone in the treatment of urinary tract infection in girls. J Urol 1973;109:917.

Leadbetter GW: Re: Internal urethrotomy in girls and its impact on the urethral intrinsic and extrinsic continence mechanisms. (Letter.) J Urol 1988;139:142.

Lyon RP, Marshall S: Urinary tract infections and difficult urination in girls: Long-term follow-up. J Urol 1971;105:314.

Lyon RP, Tanagho EA: Distal urethral stenosis in little girls. J Urol 1965;93:379.

Obrink A, Bunne G, Hedlund PO: Cultures from different parts of the urethra in female urethral syndrome. Urol Int 1979;34:70.

Smith DR: Critique on the concept of vesical neck obstruction in children. JAMA 1969;207:1686.

Tanagho EA, Lyon RP: Urethral dilatation versus internal urethrotomy. J Urol 1971;105:242.

Tanagho EA et al: Spastic external sphincter and urinary tract infection in girls. Br J Urol 1971;43:69.

Uehling DT: The normal caliber of the adult female urethra. J Urol 1978;120:176.

Van Gool J, Tanagho EA: External sphincter activity and recurrent urinary tract infection in girls. Urology 1977;10:348.

Vermillion CD, Halverstadt DB, Leadbetter GW Jr: Internal urethrotomy and recurrent urinary tract infection in female children. 2. Long-term results in the management of infection. J Urol 1971;106:154.

Walker D, Richard GA: A critical evaluation of urethral obstruction in female children. Pediatrics 1973;51: 272.

LABIAL FUSION

Aribarg A: Topical oestrogen therapy for labial adhesions in children. Br J Obstet Gynaecol 1975;82:424.

Christensen EH, Oster J: Adhesions of labia minora (synechia vulvae) in childhood: A review and report of fourteen cases. Acta Paediatr Scand 1971;60:709.

Evruke C et al: Labial fusion in a pubertal girl: A case report. J Pediatr Adolesc Gynecol 1996;9:81.

Johnson N, Lilford RJ, Sharpe D: A new surgical technique to treat refractory labial fusion in the elderly. Am J Obstet Gynecol 1989;161:289.

Leung AK, Robson WL, Tay-Uyboco J: The incidence of labial fusion in children. J Paediatr Child Health 1993;29:235.

McCann J, Voris J, Simon M: Labial adhesions and posterior fourchette injuries in childhood sexual abuse. Am J Dis Child 1988;142:659.

Norbeck JC, Ritchey MR, Bloom DA: Labial fusion causing upper urinary tract obstruction. Urology 1993;42:209.

Runsza ME: Gonorrheal vulvovaginitis, labial fusion and imperforate hymen. Am J Dis Child 1989;143:381.

Wheeler RA, Burge DM: Urinary obstruction due to labial fusion. Br J Urol 1991;67:102.

ACUTE URETHRITIS

Bass HN: "Bubble bath" as an irritant to the urinary tract of children. Clin Pediatr 1968;7:174.

Fihn SD, Johnson C, Stamm WE: *Escherichia coli* urethritis in women with symptoms of acute urinary tract infection. J Infect Dis 1988;157:196.

Horner PJ et al: Association of *Mycoplasma genitalium* with acute non-gonococcal urethritis. Lancet 1993; 342:582.

Marshall S: The effect of bubble bath on the urinary tract. J Urol 1965;93:112.

Taylor-Robinson D, Furr PM: Genital mycoplasma infections. Wien Klin Wochenschr 1997;109(14–15): 5785.

Taylor-Robinson D, Gilroy CB, Hay PE: Occurrence of *Mycoplasma genitalium* in different populations and its clinical significance. Clin Infect Dis 1993;17 (Suppl 1):S66.

Waugh MA: Azithromycin in gonorrhoea. Int J STD AIDS 1996;7(Suppl 1):2.

CHRONIC URETHRITIS

Batra SC, Iosif CS: Female urethra: Target for estrogen action. J Urol 1983;129:418.

Bodner DR: The urethral syndrome. Urol Clin North Am 1988;15:699.

Bruce AW et al: Recurrent urethritis in women. Can Med Assoc J 1973;108:973.

Farrar DJ, Green NA, Ashken MH: An evaluation of Otis urethrotomy in female patients with recurrent urinary tract infections: A review after 6 years. Br J Urol 1980;52:68.

Gittes RF, Nakamura RM: Female urethral syndrome. A female prostatitis? West J Med 1996;164:435.

Immergut MA, Gilbert EC: The clinical response of women to intestinal urethrotomy. J Urol 1973;109:90.

Karafin LJ, Coll ME: Lower urinary tract disorders in the postmenopausal woman. Med Clin North Am 1987;71:111.

Krieger JN et al: Evaluation of chronic urethritis: Defining the role for endoscopic procedures. Arch Intern Med 1988;148:703.

Marshall S, Lyon RP, Schieble J: Nonspecific urethritis in females. Calif Med (June) 1970;112:9.

O'Neil AGB: The bacterial content of the female urethra: A new method of study. Br J Urol 1981;53:368.

SENILE URETHRITIS

Murphy JT: Urological problems in aged patients. Aust Fam Physician 1977;6:17, 21, 25.

Quinlivan LG: The treatment of senile vaginitis with low doses of synthetic estrogens. Am J Obstet Gynecol 1965;92:172.

Smith P: Age changes in the female urethra. Br J Urol 1972;44:667.

Zweig S: Urinary tract infections in the elderly. Am Fam Physician 1987;35:123.

URETHRAL CARUNCLE

Lee WH, Tan KH, Lee YW: The aetiology of postmenopausal bleeding—a study of 163 consecutive cases in Singapore. Singapore Med J 1995;36:164.

Neilson D, Grant JB, Smith CE: Squamous intra-epithelial neoplasia presenting as a urethral caruncle. Br J Urol 1989;64:200.

Young RH et al: Urethral caruncle with atypical stromal cells simulating lymphoma or sarcoma—a distinctive pseudoneoplastic lesion of females. A report of six cases. Am J Surg Pathol 1996;20:1190.

PROLAPSE OF THE URETHRA

Anveden-Hertzberg L, Gauderer MW, Elder JS: Urethral prolapse: An often misdiagnosed cause of urogenital bleeding in girls. Pediatr Emerg Care 1995;11:212.

Devine PC, Kessel HC: Surgical correction of urethral prolapse. J Urol 1980;123:856.

Fernandes ET et al: Urethral prolapse in children. Urology 1993;41:240.

Gilpin SA et al: The pathogenesis of genitourinary prolapse and stress incontinence of urine: A histological and histochemical study. Br J Obstet Gynaecol 1989; 96:15.

Johnson CF: Prolapse of the urethra: Confusion of clinical and anatomic characteristics with sexual abuse. Pediatrics 1991;87:722.

Klaus H, Stein RT: Urethral prolapse in young girls. Pediatrics 1973;52:645.

Kleinjan JH, Vos P: Strangulated urethral prolapse. Urology 1996;47:599.

Low JA, Armstrong JB, Mauger GM: The unstable urethra in the female. Obstet Gynecol 1989;74:69.

Mitre A et al: Urethral prolapse in girls: Familial case. J Urol 1987;137:115.

Okada A et al: A case of urethral prolapse in a young girl. Acta Paediatr Jpn 1993;35:267.

Rudin JE, Geldt VG, Alecseev EB: Prolapse of urethral mucosa in white female children: Experience with 58 cases. J Pediatr Surg 1997;32:423.

URETHROVAGINAL FISTULA

Creatsas G et al: Reconstruction of urethrovaginal fistula and vaginal atresia in an adolescent girl after an abdominoperineal-vaginal pull-through procedure. Fertil Steril 1997;68:556.

Fall M: Vaginal wall bipedicled flap and other techniques in complicated urethral diverticulum and urethrovaginal fistula. J Am Coll Surg 1995;180:150.

Gil-Vernet JM, Gil-Vernet A, Campos JA: New surgical approach for treatment of complex vesicovaginal fistula. J Urol 1989;141:513.

Gray L: Urethrovaginal fistulas. Am J Obstet Gynecol 1968;101:28.

Hedlund H, Lindstedt E: Urovaginal fistulas: 20 years of experience with 45 cases. J Urol 1987;137:926.

Hendren WH: Construction of female urethra from vaginal wall and perineal flap. J Urol 1980;123:657.

Hilton P: Urodynamic findings in patients with urogenital fistulae. Br J Urol 1998;81:539.

Kliment J, Berats T: Urovaginal fistulas: Experience with the management of 41 cases. Int Urol Nephrol 1992;24:119.

Krogh J, Kay L, Hjortrup A: Treatment of urethrovaginal fistula. Br J Urol 1989;63:555.

Leach GE: Urethrovaginal fistula repair with Martius labial fat pad graft. Urol Clin North Am 1991;18:409.

Tancer ML: A report of thirty-four instances of urethrovaginal and bladder neck fistulas. Surg Gynecol Obstet 1993;177:77.

Tehan TJ, Nardi JA, Baker R: Complications associated

with surgical repair of urethrovaginal fistula. Urology 1980;15:31.

URETHRAL DIVERTICULUM

Baert L, Willemen P, Oyen R: Endovaginal sonography: New diagnostic approach for urethral diverticula. J Urol 1992;147:464.

Bracken RB et al: Primary carcinoma of the female urethra. J Urol 1976;116:188.

Debaere C et al: MR imaging of a diverticulum in a female urethra. J Belge Radiol 1995;78:345.

Dretler SP, Vermillion CD, McCullough DL: The roentgenographic diagnosis of female urethral diverticula. J Urol 1972;107:72.

Elik M: Diverticulum of the female urethra: A new method of ablation. J Urol 1957;77:243.

Fall M: Vaginal wall bipedicled flap and other techniques in complicated urethral diverticulum and urethrovaginal fistula. J Am Coll Surg 1995;180:150.

Fortunato P, Schettini M, Gallucci M: Diverticula of the female urethra. Br J Urol 1997;80:628.

Ganabathi K et al: Experience with the management of urethral diverticulum in 63 women. J Urol 1994;152 (5 Pt 1):1445.

Glassman TA, Weinerth JL, Glenn JF: Neonatal female urethral diverticulum. Urology 1975;5:249.

Golimbu M, al-Askari S: High pressure voiding urethrography. Urology 1974;3:717.

Jensen LM et al: Female urethral diverticulum. Clinical aspects and a presentation of 15 cases. Act Obstet Gynecol Scand 1996;75:748.

Kato H et al: Carcinoembryonic antigen positive adenocarcinoma of a female urethral diverticulum: Case report and review of the literature. Int J Urol 1998;5:291.

Keefe B et al: Diverticula of the female urethra: Diagnosis by endovaginal and transperineal sonography. AJR 1991;156:1195.

Kim B, Hricak H, Tanagho EA: Diagnosis of urethral diverticula in women: Value of MR imaging. AJR 1993;161:809.

Marshall S, Hirsch K: Carcinoma within urethral diverticula. Urology 1977;10:161.

Moran PA, Carey MP, Dwyer PL: Urethral diverticula in pregnancy. Aust N Z J Obstet Gynaecol 1998;38:102.

Mouritsen L, Bernstein I: Vaginal ultrasonography: A diagnostic tool for urethral diverticulum. Acta Obstet Gynecol Scand 1996;75:188.

Mueller EJ, Drake GL: A new surgical procedure for the removal of the wide-mouthed urethral diverticulum in females. Surg Gynecol Obstet 1989;168:269.

Nakamura Y et al: A case of adenocarcinoma arising within a urethral diverticulum diagnosed only by the surgical specimen. Gynecol Obstet Invest 1995;40:69.

Neitlich JD et al: Detection of urethral diverticula in women: Comparison of a high resolution fast spin echo technique with double balloon urethrography. J Urol 1998;159:408.

Niemiec TR et al: Unusual urethral diverticulum lined by colonic epithelium with Paneth cell metaplasia. Am J Obstet Gynecol 1989;160:186.

Pauwels M, Wyndaele JJ: Female urethral diverticula: A report of 5 cases. Acta Urol Belg 1996;64:27.

Presman D, Rolnick D, Zumerchek J: Calculus formation within a diverticulum of the female urethra. J Urol 1964;91:376.

Siegel CL et al: Sonography of the female urethra. AJR 1998;170:1269.

Spence HM, Duckett JW Jr: Diverticulum of the female urethra: Clinical aspects and presentation of a simple operative technique for cure. J Urol 1970;104:432.

Spencer WF, Streem SB: Diverticulum of the female urethral roof managed endoscopically. J Urol 1987;138:147.

Summit RL Jr, Stovall TG: Urethral diverticula: Evaluation by urethral pressure profilometry, cystourethroscopy, and the voiding cystourethrogram. Obstet Gynecol 1992;80:695.

Vargas-Serrano B et al: Transrectal ultrasonography in the diagnosis of urethral diverticula in women. J Clin Ultrasound 1997;25:21.

URETHRAL STRICTURE

Essenhigh DM, Ardran GM, Cope V: A study of the bladder outlet in lower urinary tract infections in women. Br J Urol 1968;40:268.

Immergut MA, Gilbert EC: The clinical response of women to internal urethrotomy. J Urol 1973;109:90.

Palou J, Caparros J, Vicente J: Use of proximal-based vaginal flap in stricture of the female urethra. Urology 1996;47:747.

Spirnak JP: Pelvic fracture and injury to the lower urinary tract. Surg Clin North Am 1988;68:1057.

SURGICAL REPAIR

Bass JS, Leach GE: Surgical treatment of concomitant urethral diverticulum and stress incontinence. Urol Clin North Am 1991;18:365.

Hricak H et al: Female urethra: MR imaging. Radiology 1991;178:527.

Steward M, Bretland PM, Stidolph NE: Urethral diverticula in the adult female. Br J Urol 1981;53:353.

Symmonds RE, Hill LM: Loss of the urethra: A report on 50 patients. Am J Obstet Gynecol 1978;53:130.

van Geelen JM et al: The clinical and urodynamic effects of anterior vaginal repair and Burch colposuspension. Am J Obstet Gynecol 1988;159:137.

Woodhouse CRJ et al: Urethral diverticulum in females. Br J Urol 1980;52:305.

42

Disorders of the Testis, Scrotum, & Spermatic Cord

Jack W. McAninch, MD

DISORDERS OF THE SCROTUM

Hypoplasia of the scrotum accompanies cryptorchidism. Bifid scrotum is present with midscrotal or perineal hypospadias and in certain cases of intersexuality. In both instances, the 2 scrotal sacs simulate labia majora.

Idiopathic edema of the scrotum is occasionally seen in children. It may involve one or both sacs and also the penis, the perineum, or the inguinal region. The exact cause is not known; the condition may represent an allergic response or angioneurotic edema. Antihistamines may be of value, although the condition resolves spontaneously.

Scrotal edema has been observed consequent to development of a fistula between the peritoneum and the subcutaneous tissue following paracentesis for cirrhosis of the liver. A patent processus vaginalis may fill with fluid during peritoneal dialysis (Deshmukh, Kjellberg, and Shaw, 1995). In women, the edema involves the labia. Three instances of scrotal emphysema have been observed: (1) following treatment of rectal polyp, (2) following an open renal biopsy, and (3) in traumatic pneumothorax. It must be remembered, however, that torsion of the spermatic cord may affect the scrotal skin in a similar manner. Acute scrotal swelling in an infant may be a sign of acute peritonitis. Such a reaction requires a patent processus vaginalis.

In association with healed meconium peritonitis, masses may develop in the scrotum (or in the inguinal area). Examination at birth may lead to the diagnosis of hydrocele, but a month later, the scrotal masses become firm. A plain film of the abdomen reveals calcification in both the masses and the abdomen; this differentiates the masses from teratoma.

CONGENITAL ANOMALIES OF THE TESTIS

ANOMALIES OF NUMBER

Absence of one or both testes is very rare. Brothers, Weber, and Ball (1978) stress the need for a careful search for the absent organ. They cite 13 cases of testicular tumor in intra-abdominal cryptorchidism, most of which were seminomas. Selective gonadal venography, sonography, computed tomography scanning, and laparoscopy are useful in locating nonpalpable testes. Magnetic resonance imaging is particularly useful as a noninvasive method of detecting the nonpalpable testicle (Kogan, Hricak, and Tanagho, 1987).

A review of the literature shows fewer than 100 instances of polyorchidism. A spermatocele or tumor of the spermatic cord is often mistaken for a third gonad.

Jarow et al (1986) noted an elevation of serum gonadotropins in prepubertal boys with bilateral anorchism.

HYPOGONADISM

Males suffering from either congenital or prepubertal primary testicular eunuchoidism or pituitary hypogonadism (congenital or secondary to a brain lesion) are tall and have disproportionately long extremities because of delay in fusion of the epiphyses. The testes are small, and there is lack of development of secondary sexual characteristics associated with some deficiency in libido and potency. These men are sterile. A somewhat feminine fat distribution may be noted, and there are wrinkles about the eyes. The primary gonadal defect is often associated with color blindness and mental retardation.

X-ray studies of the bones reveal delay in closure of the epiphyses. The differential diagnosis of these 2 disorders often depends on determination of follicle-stimulating hormone (FSH) and 17-ketosteroid (or serum testosterone) excretion in the urine. In the pituitary type, the patient excretes no FSH; the androgen level is very low. The gonadal eunuch excretes high levels of FSH but only moderately decreased amounts of urinary 17-ketosteroids and has a low serum testosterone level. The pituitary eunuchoid male may have an enlarged sella turcica or visual field defects secondary to tumor.

Both conditions in the adult are treated with long-acting esters of testosterone, 200 mg/month intramuscularly, or transdermal testosterone (McClellan and Goa, 1998).

For a discussion of Klinefelter syndrome, see Chapter 44.

ECTOPY & CRYPTORCHIDISM

In ectopy, the testis has strayed from the path of normal descent; in cryptorchidism, it is arrested in the normal path of descent. Ectopy may be due to an abnormal connection of the distal end of the gubernaculum testis that leads the gonad to an abnormal position. The ectopic sites are as follows (Figure 42–1):
- Superficial inguinal (most common site): After passing through the external inguinal ring, the testis proceeds superolaterally to a position superficial to the aponeurosis of the external oblique muscle.
- Perineal (rare): The testis is found just in front of the anus and to one side of the midline.
- Femoral or crural (rare): The testis is found in Scarpa's triangle superficial to the femoral vessels. The cord passes under the inguinal ligament.
- Penile (rare): The testis is placed under the skin at the root of the dorsum of the penis.

- Transverse or paradoxic descent (rare): Both testes descend the same inguinal canal. Some 85 examples have been collected from the literature.
- Pelvic (rare): The testis is found in the true pelvis (discovered only by surgical exploration).

Cryptorchidism is a condition in which a testicle is arrested at some point in its normal descent anywhere between the renal and scrotal areas. Unilateral arrest is more common than bilateral arrest. At the time of birth (9-month gestation), the incidence of maldescent is 3.4%; half of such testicles descend in the first month of life. The incidence of cryptorchidism in adults is 0.7–0.8%. In premature infants, it is 30%. A few cryptorchid testes may descend at puberty.

Chromosomal studies in cases of cryptorchidism have revealed no abnormalities. Bartone and Schmidt (1982) found normal chromosomes in 48 of 50 consecutive cases of cryptorchidism. One of the two patients with abnormal chromosomes was found to have Klinefelter syndrome.

Etiology
The cause of maldescent is not clear. The following possibilities must be considered.

A. Abnormality of the Gubernaculum Testis: Differential growth of the embryo appears to cause descent of the gonad from its lumbar origin. Descent is guided by the gubernaculum, a cordlike structure that extends from the lower pole of the testis to the scrotum. In the embryo, of course, it is very short. Absence or abnormality of this structure may be a cause of maldescent.

B. Intrinsic Testicular Defect: Maldescent may be caused by a congenital gonadal (dysgenetic) defect that makes the testicle insensitive to go-

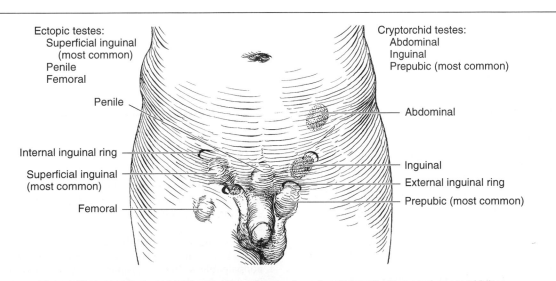

Figure 42–1. Undescended testes. Position of testes in various types of ectopy and cryptorchidism.

nadotropins. This theory is the best explanation for unilateral cryptorchidism. It would also explain why many patients with bilateral cryptorchidism are sterile, even when given definitive therapy at the optimum age.

C. Deficient Gonadotropic Hormonal Stimulation: Lack of adequate maternal gonadotropins may be a cause of incomplete descent. This seems to be the obvious explanation for bilateral cryptorchidism in premature infants, since the elaboration of maternal gonadotropins remains at a low level until the last 2 weeks of gestation. It is difficult, however, to apply this theory to unilateral cryptorchidism.

Rajfer et al (1986) have shown that testicular descent is an androgen-mediated event regulated by pituitary gonadotropin. This process leads to high levels of dihydrotestosterone. They point out that the testis also must have free access to the scrotum for normal descent.

Pathogenesis & Pathology

The scrotum is an effective temperature regulator for the testes, which are kept about 1 °C (1.8 °F) cooler than body temperature. The spermatogenic cells are sensitive to body temperature. Mininberg, Rodger, and Bedford (1982) studied the ultrastructure of the cryptorchid testis and found deleterious changes in the first year of life. By age 4 years, massive collagen deposition was evident. They concluded that the testes had to be in the scrotum by age 1 year.

After age 6 years, changes become more obvious. The diameter of the tubules is smaller than normal. The number of spermatogonia decreases, and fibrosis between the tubules becomes marked. The cryptorchid testis after puberty may be fairly normal in size, but it is markedly deficient in spermatogenic components; infertility is the rule.

It must be remembered that about 10% of these testes are congenitally defective (primary hypogonadism, hypogonadism secondary to hypopituitarism). These gonads show subnormal spermatogenic activity despite treatment.

Fortunately, the Leydig cells are not affected by body temperature and are therefore usually found in normal numbers in the cryptorchid organ. An endocrinologic cause of impotence is rare in this group.

In a study employing the latest analytic methods, no chromosomal abnormalities could be found in biopsies of undescended testes. Maldescent and carcinomatous degeneration cannot be attributed to defects in chromosomes in the undescended organ.

DePalma, Carter, and Weiss (1988) and Koff and Scaletscky (1990) point out that epididymal abnormalities are commonly found in these testes. The anomalies include agenesis, atresia, and elongated epididymides poorly connected to the gonad.

Clinical Findings

A. Symptoms: The cardinal symptom of ectopy or cryptorchidism is the absence of one or both testes from the scrotum. The patient may complain of pain from trauma to the testis, which may be situated in a vulnerable position (eg, over the pubic bone). The adult patient with bilateral cryptorchidism may present with a complaint of infertility.

B. Signs: In true maldescent, the scrotum on the affected side is atrophic. The testis either is not palpable (lying within or even proximal to the inguinal canal) or can be felt external to the inguinal ring. It cannot be manipulated into the scrotum. A common position for such a testis is in the region of the inguinal canal. A testis felt in this area would have to be a superficial inguinal ectopic testis (lying subcutaneously), for it is unlikely that a small testis could be palpated through the heavy external oblique aponeurosis. Inguinal hernia is often present on the affected side.

C. Laboratory Findings: Studies of the urinary 17-ketosteroids, gonadotropins, and serum testosterone may help in tracing the cause of cryptorchidism. In primary hypogonadism, the urinary gonadotropins (FSH) are markedly elevated, whereas the androgens are moderately reduced. In primary hypopituitarism, the androgens and pituitary gonadotropins are definitely depressed. In "primary" bilateral cryptorchidism, the androgens and pituitary gonadotropins are often moderately diminished.

If neither testis can be demonstrated, success has been achieved by herniography, venography, and arteriography. If these are unrevealing, one may use the human chorionic gonadotropin (hCG) test. This is done by establishing a baseline serum testosterone level and then giving hCG, 2000 units daily for 4 days. On the fifth day, the serum testosterone estimation should be repeated. If testes are present, this hormone will be elevated as much as 10-fold.

D. X-Ray Findings: Selective gonadal venography appears to be one of the most consistently useful tests for proving the presence and position of a testis. Demonstration of a pampiniform plexus makes it almost certain that a testis is attached. However, Greenberg et al (1981) described 2 cases in which no testes were found although pampiniform plexuses were present.

E. Computed Tomography: Computed tomography scanning is more useful in postpubertal patients when the intra-abdominal testicle is sufficiently enlarged to be detected.

F. Ultrasonography: Using ultrasonography, numerous authors have had no difficulty in identifying testes in the groin but were less successful if the organ was in the pelvis. Testes within the inguinal canal or positioned just inside the internal ring can easily be detected.

G. Magnetic Resonance Imaging: Recent studies indicate a high success rate in detecting the nonpalpable testicle with magnetic resonance imaging. One limiting factor of this technique in children is the requirement of remaining in a fixed position for a prolonged period of time.

H. Laparoscopy: Laparoscopy has been particularly useful as an aid in identifying the impalpable testis. Cortes et al (1995) examined 100 patients laparoscopically and found either blind-ending cord structures above the inguinal ring or an intra-abdominal testis in 50%. The remaining 50% had cord structures passing through the internal ring, indicating an inguinal location of the impalpable gonad. Laparoscopy was also useful in patients with bilateral nonpalpable testes.

Differential Diagnosis

Physiologic cryptorchidism (retractile or migratory testis) is a common phenomenon requiring no treatment. Because of the small mass of the prepubertal testis and the strength of the cremaster muscle, which inserts on the spermatic cord, the testes are apt to be involuntarily retracted out of the scrotum in cold weather or with excitement or physical activity. The diagnosis is made by noting that the scrotum on the suspected side is normally developed and that the "inguinal" testis can be pushed into and to the bottom of the scrotum. It may be necessary to place the child in a warm tub to afford maximum muscular relaxation, in which case the testis is found in the normal position. Such a testis descends at puberty and has been found to be normal.

Complications

Associated inguinal hernia is found in 25% of patients with maldescent. At surgery, 95% of such patients are found to have a patent processus vaginalis.

Torsion of the spermatic cord is occasionally seen as a complication of cryptorchidism. Some authors believe it is most commonly seen in spastic neurologic disease. Torsion of the cord must be differentiated from strangulated hernia, appendicitis, and diverticulitis.

Most authorities agree that cancer is 35–48 times more common in a misplaced testis than in the normally descended organ. This fact further substantiates the theory that many of these testes are dysgenetic. Martin (1979) collected 220 instances of cancer in undescended testes. Seminoma is the most common tumor; it is rare before age 10. Because of this evidence, Martin suggests that the undescended testis in a patient 10 years of age or older should be removed rather than treated by orchiopexy. Hinman (1979) recommends orchidectomy for the unilateral abdominal testis because it is less likely to be fertile, more prone to cancer, and more difficult to place in the scrotum.

Treatment

Since definite histologic change can be demonstrated in the cryptorchid testis by age 1 year, placement of the testis in the scrotum should be accomplished by that age. Most authors recommend surgical correction at about 1 year of age. A successful operation does not ensure fertility if the testis is congenitally defective.

A. Hormone Therapy: Job et al (1982) suggest the use of hormone therapy before surgery is attempted. They find that although the optimal age for hormone therapy is 5 years of age, it can be effective at age 3 years. One may give hCG, 1500 units/wk intramuscularly every other day or 3 times a week, for a total of 9 injections. The inguinal testis responds best. In addition, luteinizing hormone releasing hormone analog has been effective in treating the undescended testis (Hadžiselimovic et al, 1987; Rajfer et al, 1986).

If physiologic cryptorchidism has been ruled out, hormone therapy will cause descent in about a month in 10–20% of cases, with more success in bilateral than unilateral cryptorchidism. Some of these cases may have been physiologic retractile testes that were misdiagnosed despite frequent examination. Descent with hormone therapy will save the child an operation and the surgeon embarrassment, although if this treatment is successful, the testis probably would have descended spontaneously at puberty.

B. Surgical Treatment: If hormone therapy fails, or if inguinal hernia can be demonstrated, orchiopexy (and hernioplasty) should be done immediately. The testis must be placed at the bottom of the scrotum, without tension; the blood supply to the organ must be meticulously preserved. Dissection of the inguinal area sometimes reveals that the vascular pedicle is too short to allow placement of the testis in the bottom of the scrotum. If so, the organ should be placed as low as possible, and 2 years later, the testicle should be advanced to the scrotum. This form of management results in testicular atrophy in approximately 17% of cases, and orchiectomy is required. In the past, a few authors have recommended division of the spermatic artery if the vascular pedicle was too short, claiming that viability of the testis was preserved. Some have divided this artery at the internal ring (taking care to preserve collateral arteries to the vas deferens, cremaster muscle, and scrotum) and have observed radionuclide evidence of normal vascular perfusion of the testicle. This is probably the procedure of choice for the short cord. Microsurgery has been used to place the abdominal testis in the scrotum by anastomosing the artery and vein of the testis to the inferior epigastric artery and vein. If the testis is not discovered or is very atrophic and is therefore removed, a prosthesis can be placed in the scrotum. Orchiopexy can be done as an outpatient procedure.

Prognosis

The testicle that is properly placed in the scrotum provides adequate hormonal function and gives the scrotum a normal appearance. Approximately 20% of males with unilateral undescended testis remain infertile even though orchiopexy is performed at an appropriate age. A man with one untreated cryptorchid testis produces sperm of a lower concentration and poorer quality than a man with normally descended testes. In bilateral undescended testes, treated or untreated, fertility rates are uniformly poor.

CONGENITAL ANOMALIES OF THE EPIDIDYMIS

Congenital absence of the epididymis is rare. At times the epididymis may be anterior rather than posterior to the testis. Fusion of the epididymis and testis may not occur.

DISORDERS OF THE SPERMATIC CORD*

SPERMATOCELE

A spermatocele is a painless cystic mass containing sperms. It lies just above and posterior to the testis but is separate from it (Figure 42–2). Most spermatoceles are less than 1 cm in diameter, although they are occasionally quite large and may be mistaken for hydroceles. They may be firm, simulating solid tumor. The cause is not entirely clear, although they probably arise from the tubules that connect the rete testis to the head of the epididymides (vasa efferentia) or from cystic structures on the upper pole of the testis or epididymis.

Since they are relatively small, spermatoceles are usually discovered by the physician during routine examination of the genitalia; at times they may be large enough to come to the attention of the patient. Examination reveals a freely movable transilluminating cystic mass lying above the testicle. Microscopic examination of aspirated contents reveals sperms, usually dead. Grossly, the fluid is thin, white, and cloudy.

Spermatocele is differentiated from hydrocele of the tunica vaginalis in that the latter covers the entire anterior surface of the testicle. Aspiration of hydrocele recovers yellow but clear fluid. A tumor of the cover-

ings of the spermatic cord (eg, mesothelioma, fibroma) may feel like a tense spermatocele. It does not contain fluid, however, and will not transilluminate.

Spermatocele requires no therapy unless it is large enough to annoy the patient, in which case it should be excised.

VARICOCELE
(See also Male Infertility, Chapter 46)

Varicocele is found in approximately 10% of young men and consists of dilatation of the pampiniform plexus above the testis, with the left side most commonly affected. These veins drain into the internal spermatic vein in the region of the internal inguinal ring. The internal spermatic vein passes lateral to the vas deferens at the internal inguinal ring and, on the left side, drains into the renal vein. On the right it empties into the vena cava.

Incompetent valves are more common in the left internal spermatic vein. This condition, combined with the effect of gravity, may lead to poor drainage of the pampiniform plexus, the veins of which gradually undergo dilation and elongation. The area may be painful, particularly in sexually continent men.

The sudden development of a varicocele in an older man is sometimes a late sign of renal tumor when tumor cells have invaded the renal vein, thereby occluding the spermatic vein.

Examination of a man with varicocele when he is upright reveals a mass of dilated, tortuous veins lying posterior to and above the testis. It may extend up to the external inguinal ring and is often tender. The degree of dilatation can be increased by the Valsalva maneuver. In the recumbent position, venous distention abates. Testicular atrophy from impaired circulation may be present.

Sperm concentration and motility are significantly decreased in 65–75% of subjects. Infertility is often observed and can be reversed in a high percentage of patients by correction of the varicocele. The most useful surgical procedure is ligation of the internal spermatic veins at or above the internal inguinal ring. This can be done as an outpatient procedure (Thomas and Geisinger, 1990). Recently, percutaneous methods, eg, balloon catheter, sclerosing fluids, have been used to occlude the veins. These procedures are particularly useful when the infertile patient is undergoing percutaneous internal spermatic venography. One or both veins can be occluded as indicated (Hunter, Bildsoe, and Amplatz, 1989). A trial of scrotal support can be helpful in patients with chronic pain.

HYDROCELE

A hydrocele consists of a collection of fluid within the tunica or processus vaginalis. Although it may oc-

---

*The primary congenital anomaly that affects the spermatic cord is absence of the vas deferens. If the vas is absent on both sides, infertility results.

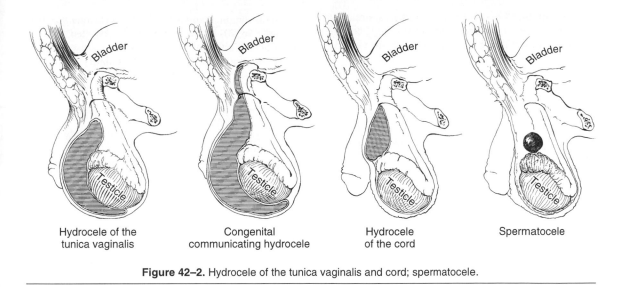

| Hydrocele of the tunica vaginalis | Congenital communicating hydrocele | Hydrocele of the cord | Spermatocele |

Figure 42–2. Hydrocele of the tunica vaginalis and cord; spermatocele.

cur within the spermatic cord, it is most often seen surrounding the testis. A number of cases of hydrocele of the canal of Nuck have been reported. A hydrocele may develop rapidly secondary to local injury, radiotherapy, acute nonspecific or tuberculous epididymitis, or orchitis. It may complicate testicular neoplasm. Chronic hydrocele is more common. Its cause is usually unknown, and it usually occurs in men past the age of 40 years. Fluid collects about the testis, and the mass grows gradually (Figure 42–2). It may be soft and cystic or quite tense. The fluid is clear and yellow.

Communicating hydrocele of infancy and childhood is caused by a patent processus vaginalis, which is continuous with the peritoneal cavity. It is also a form of indirect inguinal hernia. If the hydrocele is large, bowel may be found within the contents. Most communicating hydroceles of infancy close spontaneously before 1 year of age. If the presence of bowel in the sac is suspected, surgical correction should be done.

Clinical Findings

Young boys with hydrocele commonly have a history of a cystic mass that is small and soft in the morning but larger and more tense at night. This indicates that a small communication exists in the processus vaginalis (Figure 42–2). Hernia or communicating hydrocele is therefore the proper diagnosis. Hydrocele is usually painless unless it is accompanied by acute epididymal infection. The patient may, however, complain of its bulk or weight.

The diagnosis is made by finding a rounded cystic intrascrotal mass that is not tender unless underlying inflammatory disease is present. The mass transilluminates. If the hydrocele is enclosed within the spermatic cord, a cystic fusiform swelling is noted in the

groin or in the upper scrotum. Sonography should be done if the diagnosis is in question.

A tense hydrocele must be differentiated from tumor of the testis, which does not transilluminate. However, if hydrocele develops in a young man without apparent cause, careful evaluation of the testicle and epididymis should be done in order to rule out cancer or infection. This is best done by sonography.

Complications include compression of the blood supply of the testicle, which leads to atrophy, and hemorrhage into the hydrocele sac following trauma.

Treatment

Unless complications are present, active therapy is not required. The indications for treatment are a very tense hydrocele that might embarrass circulation to the testicle or a large, bulky mass that is cosmetically unsightly and perhaps uncomfortable for the patient.

Spontaneous closure and resolution of the hydrocele may occur in infancy. If it persists beyond 1 year of age, closure is unlikely. When treatment is necessary, surgical therapy is definitive. In children, high ligation of the patent processus vaginalis at the internal inguinal ring followed by excision of the distal sac corrects the problem. Inguinal incisions should be made in all children undergoing hydrocele repair in order to correct the patent processus. In adults, Lord (1970) has described a simple operation wherein the hydrocele sac, after being opened, is merely stitched together to collapse the wall. The results of both procedures are good, though occasionally the hydrocele recurs.

TORSION OF THE SPERMATIC CORD

Torsion of the spermatic cord (torsion of the testicle) is an uncommon affliction that is most commonly seen in adolescent males. It causes strangulation of the blood supply to the testis. Unless treatment is given within 5 or 6 h, testicular atrophy may occur.

The cryptorchid testis is prone to undergo torsion. Many cases of torsion occur in the neonatal period (Ryken, Turner, and Haynes, 1990; Das and Singer, 1990). Witherington and Jarrell (1990) have found a significant number of patients with torsion who were over age 21. Trauma may be an initiating factor. A few intra-abdominal cancerous testes have undergone torsion. In about half of patients, this disorder occurs during sleep. In most instances, congenital abnormality of the tunica vaginalis or spermatic cord is present. Torsion seems to be due most often to a voluminous tunica vaginalis that inserts well up on the cord. This allows the testis to rotate within the tunica. The initiating factor seems to be spasm of the cremaster muscle, which inserts obliquely on the cord. The contraction of this muscle causes the patient's left testis to rotate counterclockwise and his right testis clockwise (as the physician observes the patient from the foot of the bed). With vascular occlusion, there is edema of the testis and the cord up to the point of occlusion. This leads to ischemic death of the testis and epididymis.

Clinical Findings

The diagnosis is suggested when a young boy suddenly develops severe pain in one testicle, followed by swelling of the organ, reddening of the scrotal skin, lower abdominal pain, and nausea and vomiting. However, torsion of the cord may be accompanied only by moderate scrotal swelling and little or no pain.

Examination usually reveals a swollen, tender organ that is retracted upward as a result of shortening of the cord by volvulus. Testes that are apt to undergo torsion lie horizontally with the patient standing. This abnormality has been recognized in a number of boys who had, in the past, suffered from transient testicular pain representing torsion with spontaneous detorsion. Acute testicular torsion results in a very painful testicle and absence of the cremasteric reflex (Kadish and Bolte, 1998). Pain may be increased by lifting the testicle up over the symphysis. (The pain from epididymitis is usually alleviated by this maneuver.) Within a few hours after onset, leukocytosis may develop.

The diagnosis may be made in the early stages if the epididymis can be felt in an abnormal position (eg, anterior). After a few hours, however, the entire gonad becomes so swollen that the epididymis cannot be distinguished from the testis by palpation. Torsion can be differentiated from epididymitis with reasonable success by color Doppler sonography (Burks et al, 1990). Absence of arterial flow is typical of torsion. Hypervascularity suggests inflammatory lesions. The most definitive test appears to be the scintillation scan using ^{99m}Tc-pertechnetate. It is accurate in 90–100% of cases. The twisted testis is avascular. Testicular tumors show increased vascularity; trauma shows decreased vascularity.

Differential Diagnosis

The differential diagnosis includes acute epididymitis, acute orchitis, and trauma. Epididymitis is rare before puberty and is often accompanied by pyuria. Mumps orchitis, also rare before puberty, is usually accompanied by parotitis. Without a history or findings of injury, traumatic orchitis may be misdiagnosed as torsion of the cord.

Epididymitis is unusual before age 16. Differential diagnosis from tension may be difficult if epididymitis is not complicated by pyuria. In case of doubt, scintillation scanning is indicated.

Treatment

If the patient is seen within a few hours of onset, manual detorsion may be attempted. Torsion causes the left testis to rotate counterclockwise and the right one clockwise; therefore, one may twist a testis in the opposite direction. The right testis should be "unscrewed" and the left one "screwed up." This maneuver is facilitated by infiltration of the spermatic cord, near the external inguinal ring, with 10–20 mL of 1% lidocaine hydrochloride. Even if this is successful, surgical fixation of both testes should be done within the next few days. If manual detorsion fails, immediate surgical detorsion must be performed, although after 5–6 h infarction usually occurs in testes subjected to a 720-degree twist of the cord. Using early surgery, Cattolica et al (1982) obtained viable testes in 79% of their cases of torsion. Discounting the cases that they saw late, the salvage rate was 93%. Whether the testis appears to be viable or not, it probably should be sutured down to preclude subsequent torsion. Even though the seminiferous tubules may become necrotic, the more hardy interstitial cells may remain viable. Excision of the parietal tunica vaginalis causes agglutination of the testicle to the scrotal wall. Because the opposite testicle usually is affected by the same abnormal attachments, prophylactic fixation of that organ is imperative.

Prognosis

Unfortunately, the diagnosis is usually made and treatment instituted too late, and atrophy is to be expected in these instances. It has been observed that detorsion within 6 h of onset affords a good result; that recovery is possible if treatment is given 8–10 h later; and that preservation is doubtful after 12 h. If detorsion is delayed beyond 24 h, orchiectomy is advised.

TORSION OF THE APPENDICES OF THE TESTIS & EPIDIDYMIS

On the upper poles of both the testis and epididymis, there are small vestigial appendages that may be sessile or pedunculated (Figure 1–8). The latter type may spontaneously undergo torsion, which leads to an inflammatory reaction followed by ischemic necrosis and absorption.

This phenomenon usually affects boys up to age 16 years, though Altaffer and Steele (1980) were able to find reports of 350 instances of appendiceal torsion in adults. Sudden onset of testicular pain is noted. Shortly after onset, a small tender lump may be felt at the upper pole of the testis or epididymis; this sign is pathognomonic, particularly if the lump appears to be blue when the skin is held tight over the mass (Dresner, 1973).

At later examination, the entire testicle is swollen and tender. The differential diagnosis is then between torsion of these appendages and torsion of the spermatic cord. Immediate surgical exploration is indicated unless the diagnosis is clearly established, for time is a critical factor in the treatment of torsion of the cord. If an appendix is twisted, it should be excised. Holland, Graham, and Ignatoff (1981) advise that if the examination shows the problem to be torsion of an appendix of the testis or epididymis, no surgical intervention is necessary. The pain will slowly subside over 5–7 days and the scrotal swelling resolve.

REFERENCES

SCROTUM

Brandes SB, Chelsky MJ, Hanno PM: Adult acute idiopathic scrotal edema. Urology 1994;44:602.

Deshmukh N, Kjellberg SI, Shaw PM: Occult inguinal hernia, a cause of rapid onset of penile and scrotal edema in patients on chronic peritoneal dialysis. Milit Med 1995;160:597.

Krieger JN, Wang K, Mack L: Preliminary evaluation of color Doppler imaging for investigation of intrascrotal pathology. J Urol 1990;144:904.

Lerner RM et al: Color Doppler US in the evaluation of acute scrotal disease. Radiology 1990;176:355.

Melekos MD, Asbach HW, Markou SA: Etiology of acute scrotum in 100 boys with regard to age distribution. J Urol 1988;139:1023.

Najmaldin A, Burge DM: Acute idiopathic scrotal oedema: Incidence, manifestations and aetiology. Br J Surg 1987;74:634.

Serra AD et al: Inconclusive clinical and ultrasound evaluation of the scrotum: Impact of magnetic resonance imaging on patient management and cost. Urology 1998;51:1018.

Wilbert DM et al: Evaluation of the acute scrotum by color-coded Doppler ultrasonography. J Urol 1993; 149:1475.

Ziegelbaum M, Kovach C, Siegel S: The use of technetium-99m in the diagnosis of patent processus vaginalis. J Urol 1988;139:599.

TESTIS

Anomalies of Number

Brothers LR III, Weber CH Jr, Ball TP Jr: Anorchism versus cryptorchidism: The importance of a diligent search for intra-abdominal testes. J Urol 1978;119: 707.

Cadigan P: Polyorchidism diagnosed by ultrasound. Br J Radiol 1989;62:82.

Hazebroek FW, Molenaar JC: The management of the impalpable testis by surgery alone. J Urol 1992;148:629.

Huff DS et al: Evidence in favor of the mechanical (intrauterine torsion) theory over the endocrinopathy (cryptorchidism) theory in the pathogenesis of testicular agenesis. J Urol 1991;146:630.

Jarow JP et al: Elevation of serum gonadotropins establishes the diagnosis of anorchism in prepubertal boys with bilateral cryptorchidism. J Urol 1986;136:277.

Kogan BA, Hricak H, Tanagho EA: Magnetic resonance imaging in genital anomalies. J Urol 1987; 138:1028.

Kuyumcuoglu U et al: Bilateral perineal ectopic testes. Int Urol Nephrol 1990;22:271.

Thum G: Polyorchidism: Case report and review of literature. J Urol 1991;145:370.

Hypogonadism

Korenman SG et al: Secondary hypogonadism in older men: Its relation to impotence. J Clin Endocrinol Metab 1990;712:963.

Levy JB, Husmann DA: The hormonal control of testicular descent. J Androl 1995;16:459.

McClellan KJ, Goa KL: Transdermal testosterone. Drugs 1998;55:253.

Tzvetkova P et al: hCG stimulation test for diagnosis of androgen deficiency. Arch Androl 1997;39:163.

Whitcomb RW, Crowley WF Jr: Diagnosis and treatment of isolated gonadotropin-releasing hormone deficiency in men. J Clin Endocrinol Metab 1990;70:3.

Ectopy & Cryptorchidism

Bartone FF, Schmidt MA: Cryptorchidism: Incidence of chromosomal anomalies in 50 cases. J Urol 1982; 127:1105.

Benson RC Jr et al: Malignant potential of the cryptorchid testis. Mayo Clin Proc 1991;66:372.

Berkowitz GS et al: Prevalence and natural history of cryptorchidism. Pediatrics 1993;92:44.

Bhasin S: Clinical review 34: Androgen treatment of hypogonadal men. J Clin Endocrinol Metab 1992;74: 1221.

Cortes D et al: Laparoscopy in 100 consecutive patients with 128 impalpable testes. Br J Urol 1995;75:281.

Cryptorchidism: A prospective study of 7500 consecutive

male births, 1984–8. John Radcliffe Hospital Crypt-orchidism Study Group. Arch Dis Child 1992;67:892.

DePalma L, Carter D, Weiss RM: Epididymal and vas deferens immaturity in cryptorchidism. J Urol 1988; 140:1194.

Elder JS: The undescended testis: Hormonal and surgical management. Surg Clin North Am 1988;68:983.

Giuliani L, Carmignani G: Microsurgical testis auto-transplantation: A critical review. Eur Urol 1983;9: 129.

Greenberg SH et al: The falsely positive gonadal venogram: Presence of a pampiniform plexus without a gonad. J Urol 1981;125:887.

Hadžiselimovic F et al: Long-term effect of luteinizing hormone-releasing hormone analogue (buserelin) on cryptorchid testes. J Urol 1987;138:1043.

Hinman F Jr: Unilateral abdominal cryptorchidism. J Urol 1979;122:71.

Job JC et al: Hormonal therapy of cryptorchidism with human chorionic gonadotropin (HCG). Urol Clin North Am 1982;9:405.

John Radcliffe Hospital Cryptorchidism Study Group. Clinical diagnosis of cryptorchidism. Arch Dis Child 1988;63:587.

Koff WJ, Scaletscky R: Malformations of the epididymis in undescended testis. J Urol 1990;143:340.

Martin DC: Germinal cell tumors of the testis after orchiopexy. J Urol 1979;121:422.

Martinetti M et al: Immunogenetic and hormonal study of cryptorchidism. J Clin Endocrinol Metab 1992;74:39.

Mininberg DT, Rodger JC, Bedford JM: Ultrastructural evidence of the onset of testicular pathological conditions in the cryptorchid human testis within the first year of life. J Urol 1982;128:782.

Puri P, O'Donnell B: Semen analysis of patients who had orchidopexy at or after seven years of age. Lancet 1988;2:1051.

Rajfer J et al: Hormonal therapy of cryptorchidism. A randomized, double-blind study comparing human chorionic gonadotropin and gonadotropin-releasing hormone. N Engl J Med 1986;314:466.

Saggese G et al: Hormonal therapy for cryptorchidism with a combination of human chorionic gonadotropin and follicle-stimulating hormone: Success and relapse rate. Am J Dis Child 1989;143:980.

SPERMATIC CORD

Spermatocele

Clarke BG, Bamford SB, Gherardi GJ: Spermatocele: Pathologic and surgical anatomy. Arch Surg 1963;86: 351.

Lord PH: A bloodless operation for spermatocele or cyst of the epididymis. Br J Surg 1970;57:641.

Rockey KE, Cusack TJ: Ultrasound imaging of the scrotum. A pictorial guide to its varied capabilities. Postgrad Med 1987;82:219.

Varicocele

Beck EM, Schlegel PN, Goldstein M: Intraoperative varicocele anatomy: A macroscopic and microscopic study. J Urol 1992;148:1190.

Dubinsky TJ, Chen P, Maklad N: Color-flow and power Doppler imaging of the testes. World J Urol 1998; 16:35.

Gill IS, Kerbl K, Clayman RV: Laparoscopic surgery in urology: Current applications. AJR 1993;160:1167.

Hunter DW, Bildsoe MC, Amplatz K: Aid for safer sclerotherapy of the internal spermatic vein. Radiology 1989;173:282.

Kass EJ, Marcol B et al: Results of varicocele surgery in adolescents: A comparison of techniques. J Urol 1992;148:694.

Lemack GE et al: Microsurgical repair of the adolescent varicocele. J Urol 1998;160:179.

McClure RD et al: Subclinical varicocele: The effectiveness of varicocelectomy. J Urol 1991;145:789.

Palmer LS et al: The influence of surgical approach and intraoperative venography on successful varicocelectomy in adolescents. J Urol 1997;158:1201.

Ross LS, Ruppman N: Varicocele vein ligation in 565 patients under local anesthesia: A long-term review of technique, results and complications in light of proposed management by laparoscopy. J Urol 1993; 149:1361.

Sayfan J, Soffer Y, Orda R: Varicocele treatment: Prospective randomized trial of 3 methods. J Urol 1992;148:1447.

Thomas AJ Jr, Geisinger MA: Current management of varicoceles. Urol Clin North Am 1990;17:893.

Wishahi MM et al: Anatomy of the spermatic venous plexus (pampiniform plexus) in men with and without varicocele: Intraoperative venographic study. J Urol 1992;147:1285.

Hydrocele

Dandapat MC, Padhi NC, Patra AP: Effect of hydrocele on testis and spermatogenesis. Br J Surg 1990;77: 1293.

Kapur P, Caty MG, Glick PL: Pediatric hernias and hydroceles. Pediatr Clin North Am 1998;45:773.

Lord PH: A bloodless operation for spermatocele or cyst of the epididymis. Br J Surg 1970;57:641.

Rodriguez WC, Rodriguez DD, Fortuo RF: The operative treatment of hydrocele: A comparison of 4 basic techniques. J Urol 1981;125:804.

Ross LS, Flom LS: Azoospermia: A complication of hydrocele repair in a fertile population. J Urol 1991; 146:852.

Torsion of the Spermatic Cord

Anderson MJ et al: Semen quality and endocrine parameters after acute testicular torsion. J Urol 1992;147: 1545.

Anderson PA, Giacomantonio JM: The acutely painful scrotum in children: Review of 113 consecutive cases. Can Med Assoc J 1985;132:1153.

Barada JH, Weingarten JL, Cromie WJ: Testicular salvage and age-related delay in the presentation of testicular torsion. J Urol 1989;142:746.

Burks DD et al: Suspected testicular torsion and ischemia: Evaluation with color Doppler sonography. Radiology 1990;175:815.

Cattolica EV et al: High testicular salvage rate in torsion of the spermatic cord. J Urol 1982;128:66.

Das S, Singer A: Controversies of perinatal torsion of the spermatic cord: A review, survey and recommendations. J Urol 1990;143:231.

Hadžiselimovic F, Geneto R, Emmons LR: Increased apoptosis in the contralateral testes of patients with testicular torsion as a factor for infertility. J Urol 1998;160:1158.

Jones DJ: Recurrent subacute torsion: Prospective study of effects on testicular morphology and function. J Urol 1991;145:297.

Kadish HA, Bolte RG: A retrospective review of pediatric patients with epididymitis, testicular torsion, and torsion of testicular appendages. Pediatrics 1998;102:73.

Middleton WD et al: Sonographic prediction of viability in testicular torsion: Preliminary observations. J Ultrasound Med 1997;16:23.

Ryken TC, Turner JW, Haynes T: Bilateral testicular torsion in a pre-term neonate. J Urol 1990;143:102.

Schulsinger D, Glassberg K, Strashun A: Intermittent torsion: Association with horizontal lie of the testicle. J Urol 1991;145:1053.

Sellu DP, Lynn JA: Intermittent torsion of the testis. J R Coll Surg Edinb 1984;29:107.

Witherington R, Jarrell TS: Torsion of the spermatic cord in adults. J Urol 1990;143:62.

Torsion of Appendices of the Testis & Epididymis

Altaffer LF III, Steele SM Jr: Torsion of testicular appendages in men. J Urol 1980;124:56.

Dresner ML: Torsed appendage diagnosis and management: Blue dot sign. Urology 1973;1:63.

Holland JM, Graham JB, Ignatoff JM: Conservative management of twisted testicular appendages. J Urol 1981;125:213.

Skin Diseases of the External Genitalia*

Timothy G. Berger, MD

INFLAMMATORY DERMATOSES

Almost any skin condition can affect the external genitalia and perineum. The patient with lesions of the external genitalia should be questioned about and examined for other possible areas of involvement. In any case of itching or infected dermatitis in this area, it is important to rule out diabetes and pediculosis or scabies.

Associated vaginal and other urologic conditions should be corrected. Self-treatment and overtreatment may alter and complicate genital lesions. Emotional factors associated with repeated scratching and rubbing tend to prolong and complicate genital conditions.

Many people with involvement in this area have a fear of sexually transmitted disease; if there is any question of this, appropriate evaluation should be performed, and the fear should be dispelled, if it is unfounded.

CONTACT DERMATITIS

Contact dermatitis includes changes produced by both primary irritants and true allergic sensitizers. Possible causes are cosmetics, feminine deodorant sprays, douches, contraceptives, soaps, local medications (overtreatment dermatitis), wearing apparel, and plants (poison oak and ivy).

Treatment must include removal of the suspected agent, if possible. Cool wet dressings constitute excellent initial treatment, and corticosteroid creams may be used topically if infection is not present. The fluori-

---

*Sexually transmitted disease is discussed in Chapter 16; tumors in Chapter 24.

nated corticosteroid creams are more likely to produce atrophic striae in the groin than is hydrocortisone.

CIRCUMSCRIBED NEURODERMATITIS (Lichen Simplex Chronicus)

The thickened lesions of circumscribed neurodermatitis are of great importance in the persistence of any vulval or scrotal skin condition regardless of the original cause. Rubbing and scratching can prolong any eruption indefinitely, and it is usually this problem that causes the patient to seek medical care. The rubbing or scratching may be done almost subconsciously. A continuing itch-scratch cycle is established that must be broken before healing can occur.

The treatment is the same as that for contact dermatitis (described previously) plus stopping the rubbing or scratching. The addition of pramoxine hydrochloride 1% lotion to topical steroid treatment may be of great benefit.

ATOPIC DERMATITIS

Atopic dermatitis presents as dry lichenified dermatitis on the penis and scrotum, in the groin, or on the vulva. Similar changes are usually present on the face and neck and in the antecubital and popliteal spaces. Generalized dryness is present. There is usually a personal or family history of asthma or hay fever.

The treatment of this condition is the same as that for contact dermatitis (see preceding section) plus an oral antihistamine (hydroxyzine or diphenhydramine).

INTERTRIGO

Intertrigo (sodden, macerated dermatitis) is due to chafing and friction of contiguous surfaces. It occurs in the groin, inframammary areas, skin folds, and other such areas, usually in obese individuals, and is more common in hot, humid weather. Superficial bacterial or candidal infection is often present. Treatment consists of applying cool soaks to dry the lesions, followed by a combination of a nonfluorinated topical steroid and an anticandidal cream (see Candidiasis, following).

DRUG ERUPTIONS

Most drug eruptions are widespread, but they may first appear in the genital area. A fixed drug eruption, due usually to laxatives (phenolphthalein), sulfonamides, nonsteroidal anti-inflammatory drugs (NSAIDs), or barbiturates, may present as a perfectly round, bright red to violaceous macule that quickly vesiculates and produces a superficial erosion. It occurs in the same site with reexposure to the drug. Lesions of erythema multiforme in the genital area have a similar clinical appearance. Treatment is to stop the offending medication.

PSORIASIS

Psoriasis may involve flexural surfaces (inverse psoriasis), such as the groin and the perianal cleft, and inframammary areas. It tends to be bright red and moist and is usually free of scales. Itching may be intense. Occasionally, the only involvement may be in the anogenital area. A solitary plaque may present on the penis, leading to confusion with Bowen disease or some other more serious disorder. The diagnosis usually can be made by inspection and by noting other areas of involvement such as on the scalp, elbows, and knees. Pitting of the nails, when present, is almost pathognomonic of psoriasis. Hydrocortisone cream, 1%, mixed with an imidazole cream (clotrimazole, 1%; miconazole, 2%; or ketoconazole, 2%) is usually efficacious.

SEBORRHEIC DERMATITIS

Seborrheic dermatitis may appear as scaly erythematous patches and is easily confused with candidiasis, intertrigo, and psoriasis. Involvement is usually present elsewhere, typically on the scalp or brows, in creases of the cheeks and chin, in and around the ears, on the presternum, and in the axillae. Corticosteroid creams are very useful, especially in combination with an imidazole cream. Highly potent corticosteroid creams should not be used because temporary atrophy and atrophic striae may appear.

LICHEN PLANUS

Lichen planus may appear on the glans penis or on the labia and introitus. The lesions are small, polygonal, violet-hued papules about 0.5–1 cm in diameter,

with milky striations over their shiny surfaces. They may become clustered together to form plaques. Itching is usually a problem. There may be generalized involvement or typical lesions in the buccal mucosa that are lacelike in appearance. Erosions may occur on the vulva and in the vagina causing severe pain. The condition may mimic lichen sclerosus, and biopsy may be required for diagnosis.

Corticosteroid creams may be helpful in relieving the pruritus. The disease may disappear after a course of several months to years.

LICHEN SCLEROSUS ET ATROPHICUS

Lichen sclerosus et atrophicus is a distinct entity characterized by flat-topped white papules that coalesce to form white patches without infiltration. The surface may show comedolike plugs or dells. The end stages may resemble very thin parchment or tissue paper. The condition occurs most frequently in patches on the upper back, chest, and breasts, mostly in women. It almost inevitably involves the anogenital regions, where painful erosions may develop and severe itching may be a distressing symptom. On the penis, this condition occurs as balanitis xerotica obliterans, which may lead to urethral stenosis and atrophy with telangiectasia about the meatus and on the glans and may cause phimosis. There is a direct relationship between these conditions and carcinoma; the occurrence of carcinoma is rare, however, and prophylactic surgery of these genital lesions is not called for. Anogenital lichen sclerosus et atrophicus may be misdiagnosed as leukoplakia.

Lichen sclerosus et atrophicus may involute spontaneously, especially in young girls. Circumcision for balanitis xerotica obliterans is not particularly helpful.

Super potent topical steroids are the treatment of choice for all forms of genital lichen sclerosus, in children and adults. Initially treatment is twice daily, with gradual tapering to once daily, then several times weekly. An initial trial should be 6 weeks of treatment. Atrophy reverses despite the use of potent steroids on thin genital skin. Once the patient is in remission, milder steroids or bland emollients may be used for maintenance. Topical testosterone has limited benefit when compared with potent topical steroids.

COMMON SUPERFICIAL INFECTIONS

ARTHROPODS

Pediculosis Pubis
(Pubic Lice, Crabs)

Pediculosis is a parasitic infestation of the skin of the scalp, trunk, or pubic area. Pediculosis pubis may be sexually or nonsexually transmitted.

Itching may be intense, leading to scratching, which may lead to pyoderma. The nits are found on the hair shafts. Treatment consists of application of lindane (gamma benzene hexachloride), 1% lotion or cream, which should remain in place for 8 h and then be washed out. All hairy areas contiguous with the genital area, which may be a significant portion of the male body (chest, abdomen, legs, and axilla), should be treated. Pyrethrins in lotion form (RID, NIX) are equally effective. The sexual partner(s) should also be examined and treated. All clothing, bedding, and towels should be washed in very hot water or dry-cleaned. If lice are found 1 week later, the treatment should be repeated.

Scabies

A severely pruritic, widespread dermatitis frequently involving the genital area is caused by the mite *Sarcoptes scabiei*. In males, very itchy papules or nodules with a central crust are common on the glans or shaft of the penis or on the scrotum and are virtually pathognomonic of scabies. These nodules often persist for weeks to months after effective treatment. In adults, scabies is often a sexually transmitted disease. Treatment consists of overnight (8–12 h) application of 5% permethrin cream (Elimite). The treatment may be repeated in 1 week. All members of the household and all sexual partners of the index case should be treated simultaneously. Lindane, 1% lotion, may be used similarly. All clothing, bedding, and towels should be washed or dry-cleaned. Topical steroids or tar gels may be used to treat persistent genital nodules.

FUNGAL INFECTIONS
(Tinea Cruris)

Tinea cruris is characterized by marginated, slightly elevated, scaling patches on the inner thighs and in the groin with an active border. Tinea cruris does not affect the scrotum and is less intense deep in the inguinal folds (clears centrally). This is in contrast to candidiasis, which characteristically affects the scrotum and is accentuated deep in the inguinal folds (the moistest area). Pruritus may be intense.

Heat, moisture, and darkness favor these infections. Direct microscopic examination of skin scrapings in potassium hydroxide solution reveals hyphae.

Miconazole, 2% cream; clotrimazole, 1% cream; ketoconazole, 2% cream; econazole, 1% cream; ciclopirox olamine, 1% cream; and terbinafine and butenafine 1% creams are all effective. All are applied twice daily except the last two, which are applied once daily. If the medications are irritating, 1% hydrocortisone cream may be used concomitantly. In severe or refractory cases, oral antifungal treatment may be required. Griseofulvin ultramicronized (Grispeg), 250 mg twice daily for 4–6 weeks; itraconazole, 200 mg twice daily with food and an acid beverage for 7 days; or terbinafine, 250 mg once daily for 2–4 weeks, is usually adequate, even in the most severe cases. The infections are frequently aggravated by overtreatment.

CANDIDIASIS

Infection with *Candida albicans* is characterized by erythematous, weeping, circumscribed lesions with peripheral satellite vesiculopustules. Lesions occur most commonly on the inner thighs, with a predilection for the creases. Scrotal involvement is common in candidiasis and rare in tinea cruris. "Ping-pong" infections between sexual partners may occur. Pregnancy, diabetes, obesity, and immunosuppression are predisposing factors. Broad-spectrum antibiotic therapy or estrogen therapy may be followed by an overgrowth of *Candida*. The skin involvement may be secondary to vaginal infection. Lesions occur under the prepuce. High-power microscopic examination of skin scrapings in potassium hydroxide solution shows clusters of tiny spores and fine mycelial filaments. Nystatin appears to be effective in most instances. It is available as dusting powder, cream, vaginal inserts, and oral tablets. Miconazole, 2% cream or lotion; clotrimazole, 1% cream or lotion; ketoconazole, 2% cream; and econazole, 1% cream, applied twice daily, are good alternatives to nystatin but may cause burning on application. The nystatin comes as a heavier ointment that can be applied to eroded areas. In severe cases in women, fluconazole tablets (100–200 mg) once daily for 1 week, followed by 150 mg once weekly, is often dramatically effective.

BACTERIAL INFECTIONS
(Pyoderma)

Staphylococcus aureus is the most common cause of primary bacterial infections in the genital area. In addition, many inflammatory dermatoses may be secondarily infected by *S aureus* or other bacteria. A Gram's-stained smear shows clumps of cocci and many polymorphonuclear leukocytes. Culture may confirm the diagnosis. *S aureus* produces 2 types of primary lesions, a follicular pustule (folliculitis) and a superficial blister (impetigo).

Staphylococcal folliculitis begins as a superficial infection of the follicle but may extend deeply (furunculosis). It is usually acute but may be chronic or recurrent. Chronic folliculitis is usually due to nasal carriage of *Staphylococcus*. Deep, draining abscesses are rarely due to bacteria alone and suggest the presence of a chronic suppurative disorder, eg, histiocytosis X, regional enteritis, lymphogranuloma venereum, hidradenitis suppurativa, schistosomiasis, or amebiasis. Recurrent folliculitis in the groin is common in acquired immunodeficiency syndrome (AIDS).

Topical treatment alone is often inadequate for bacterial folliculitis. A penicillinase-resistant penicillin (dicloxacillin) is the treatment of choice. Penicillin-allergic individuals may be treated with a first-generation cephalosporin or erythromycin. Treatment is continued until all lesions are healed. Adding rifampin to the described treatment is recommended for frequent recurrences. Washing the affected area with an antibacterial soap or a benzoyl peroxide wash may be useful adjunctively and may help to suppress recurrences.

Staphylococcal impetigo starts as a very superficial blister that quickly breaks, leaving a crusted, weeping erosion. Treatment is the same as for staphylococcal folliculitis but usually of shorter duration.

VIRAL INFECTIONS

Genital Warts

Genital warts, caused by certain types of human papilloma viruses (HPV), are the most common sexually transmitted disease, with an up to 80% lifetime risk. One percent of all sexually active adults have genital warts, and up to 10% can be documented to have active HPV infection by sensitive techniques such as polymerase chain reaction. Genital warts, also called condyloma acuminata, are most common on the vulva, under the prepuce (in uncircumcised men) and on the penile shaft. Although they tend to involve the external genitalia, anal or oral intercourse may lead to involvement of the anal canal or the mouth. They must be differentiated from condylomata lata, the lesions of syphilis.

Since HPV infection is so prevalent, and current treatments can eradicate only the clinical lesions (the warts) and not the infectious agent (the virus), recurrence is very common (> 25%). In addition, it appears that treating the sexual partners of infected persons has no effect on the outcome of the treatment in the index case. Warts may spontaneously resolve. For these reasons the treatment should be no worse than the disease. It is no longer recommended to search for and treat "subclinical warts"—those seen with acetic acid soaking or identified by special immunologic techniques. The goal of treatment is to provide wart-free intervals with the least discomfort and long-term sequelae to the patient. In monogamous couples the option of no treatment should be discussed. Since certain HPV types (high-risk types) are associated with genital dysplasia (especially cervical dysplasia), regular gynecologic examination with Pap smears is recommended.

After careful discussion with the patient, a choice of the form of treatment is made. There are two basic forms of therapy: patient applied and health care worker applied. Patient-applied treatment is either podophyllotoxin or imiquimod. Podophyllotoxin is applied twice daily for 3 days per week. A treatment course is 6–10 weeks, and about half of patients clear their warts with such treatment. It is less irritating and more effective than health care worker–applied podophyllum resin. It is contraindicated in pregnancy. Imiquimod is an immune modulator that results in the local production of antiviral substances, including interferon. It is applied once daily for 3 days a week (usually Monday, Wednesday, Friday). The response rate is about 40% for men and over 75% for women. Treatment duration is prolonged, with average time to final response being over 2 months. Physician-applied treatments include liquid nitrogen cryotherapy (75% response, 50% durable remission), electrocautery (100% response, 75% durable remission), and snip excision with light electrocautery of the base. Laser therapy and intralesional or systemic interferon are second-line treatments and are rarely indicated.

Molluscum Contagiosum

Molluscum contagiosum is a common cutaneous infection that is sexually transmitted in adults. It is caused by a poxvirus. The characteristic lesion is a smooth-surfaced, firm, pearly papule 2–5 mm in diameter with a central umbilication. Most infected persons have 5–15 lesions located on the lower abdomen, upper thighs, or skin of the genitalia. Extensive molluscum contagiosum outside the genital area in adults is rare except in immunosuppressed patients, especially those infected with human immunodeficiency virus (HIV). Treatment involves local destruction of the lesions by curettage, cryotherapy, or light electrodesiccation.

Herpes Simplex

Genital eruptions due to herpes simplex virus (HSV) are usually caused by HSV 2, but, increasingly, HSV 1 genital herpes due to orogenital sex has been reported. Infection often occurs initially as a more severe, bilateral blistering eruption that lasts several weeks if untreated. Viral culture or Tzanck smear will confirm the diagnosis. Initial genital HSV is treated with acyclovir (200 mg) 5 times daily, valacyclovir (500 mg) twice daily, or famciclovir (250 mg) twice daily, for 7–10 days.

Recurrent disease following the initial episode is frequent, often preceded by itching or tingling at the soon-to-be-affected site (the prodrome). It is virtually always caused by HSV 2. It presents as grouped blisters localized to 1 site and lasting about 1 week. Most patients do not require treatment if the outbreaks are mild. For individual outbreaks, acyclovir (200 mg) 5 times daily, valacyclovir (500 mg) twice daily, or famciclovir (125 mg) twice daily may be used to shorten the duration and severity of the eruption. For frequent recurrences (> 6–12/year), suppression may be better than intermittent treatment. Acyclovir (400

mg) twice daily (or 800 mg once daily), valacyclovir (500 mg–1 g) once daily, or famciclovir (250 mg) twice daily may be used. This treatment will reduce outbreaks by 85% and reduce the amount of virus shed by 95%.

Herpes simplex is the most common cause of persistent genital ulceration in immunosuppressed patients. A viral culture is indicated in all cases, and treatment with acyclovir (400 mg) 5 times daily, valacyclovir (500 mg) twice daily, or famciclovir (250 mg) twice daily is begun. In severe cases, intravenous acyclovir may be required. Acyclovir resistance can occur in the setting of immunosuppression and is treated with foscarnet intravenously.

REFERENCES

GENERAL

Fitzpatrick TB et al: *Dermatology in General Medicine,* 4th ed. McGraw-Hill, 1993.

Holmes KK et al (editors): *Sexually Transmitted Diseases,* 2nd ed. McGraw-Hill, 1990.

INFLAMMATORY DERMATOSES

Bonnez W et al: Efficacy and safety of 0.5% podofilox solution in the treatment and suppression of anogenital warts. Am J Med 1994;96:420.

Drake LA et al: Guidelines for the care of superficial mycotic infections of the skin. J Am Acad Dermatol 1996;34:282.

Meffert JJ et al: Lichen sclerosus. J Am Acad Dermatol 1995;32:393.

Pereira FA: Herpes simplex: Evolving concepts. J Am Acad Dermatol 1996;35:503.

COMMON SUPERFICIAL INFECTIONS

Bertner KR et al: Genital warts and their treatment. Clin Inf Dis 1999;28:537–56.

Feingold DS, Wagner RF Jr: Antibacterial therapy. J Am Acad Dermatol 1986;14:535.

Lesher JL, Jr: Oral therapy of common superficial fungal infections. J Am Acad Dermatol 1999;40:531–4.

Sacks SL. Improving the management of genital herpes. Hospital Practice 1999;34:41–9.

Abnormalities of Sexual Determination & Differentiation

44

Felix A. Conte, MD, & Melvin M. Grumbach, MD, DM (hon)

Advances in molecular genetics, experimental embryology, steroid biochemistry, and methods of evaluation of the interaction between the hypothalamus, pituitary, and gonads have helped to clarify problems of sexual determination and differentiation. Anomalies may occur at any stage of intrauterine maturation and lead to gross ambisexual development or to subtle abnormalities that do not become manifest until sexual maturity is achieved.

NORMAL SEX DIFFERENTIATION

Chromosomal Sex

The normal human diploid cell contains 22 autosomal pairs of chromosomes and 2 sex chromosomes (2 X or 1 X and 1 Y). When arranged serially and numbered according to size and centromeric position, they are known as a karyotype. Advances in the techniques of staining chromosomes (Figure 44–1) permit positive identification of each chromosome by its unique "banding" pattern. Bands can be produced in the region of the centromere (C bands), with the fluorescent dye quinacrine (Q bands), and with Giemsa stain (G bands). Fluorescent banding (Figure 44–2) is particularly useful because the Y chromosome stains so brightly that it can be identified easily in both interphase and metaphase cells. A new technique called fluorescence in situ hybridization has been developed. This technique has been found to be particularly useful in identifying "marker" chromosomes, especially deleted sex chromosomes that are not readily identifiable by standard banding techniques. The standard nomenclature for describing the human karyotype is shown in Table 44–1. Recently, a complete clone map of the euchromatic region of the Y chromosome was described. This is the first map of this type for a human chromosome, and it spans about 35 million base pairs.

Studies in animals as well as humans with abnormalities of sexual differentiation indicate that the sex chromosomes (the X and Y chromosomes) and the autosomes carry genes that influence sexual differentiation by causing the bipotential gonad to develop either as a testis or as an ovary. Two intact and normally functioning X chromosomes, in the absence of a Y chromosome (and the genes for testicular organogenesis), lead to the formation of an ovary, whereas a Y chromosome or the presence of the male-determining region on the short arm of the Y chromosome—the **testis-determining factor**—will lead to testicular organogenesis.

In humans, there is a marked discrepancy in size between the X and Y chromosomes. Gene dosage compensation is achieved in all persons with 2 or more X chromosomes in their genetic constitution by partial inactivation of all X chromosomes except one. This phenomenon is thought to be a random process that occurs in each cell in the late blastocyst stage of embryonic development in which either the maternally or the paternally derived X chromosome undergoes heterochromatinization. The result of this process is formation of an X chromatin body (Barr body) in the interphase cells of persons having 2 or more X chromosomes (Figure 44–3). A gene termed *XIST* (X inactive-specific transcripts) is located in the region of the putative X inactivation center at Xq13.2 on the paracentromeric region of the long arm of the X chromosome. *XIST* is expressed only by the inactive X chromosome. The *XIST* gene encodes a large RNA that appears to "coat" the X chromosome and facilitate inactivation of genes on the X chromosome.

The distal portion of the short arm of the X chromosome escapes inactivation and has a short (2.5-megabase) segment homologous to a segment on the distal portion of the short arm of the Y chromosome. This segment is called the **pseudoautosomal** region; it is these 2 limited regions of the X and Y that pair during meiosis, undergo obligatory chiasm formation, and allow for exchange of DNA between these specific regions of the X and Y chromosomes. At least 7 genes have been localized to the pseudoautosomal region on the short arm of the X and Y chromosomes. Among these are *MIC2,* a gene coding for a cell surface antigen recognized by the monoclonal antibody, 12E7; the gene for the granulocyte-macrophage colony-stimulating factor receptor (GM-

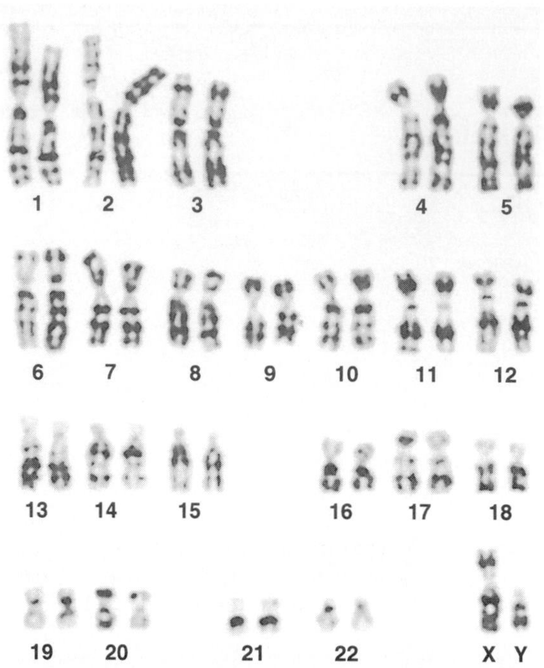

CSF); the human interleukin-3 receptor; and a gene for short stature, *PHOG/SHOX*. This gene is expressed in bone and is associated with idiopathic short stature as well as dyschondrosteosis in heterozygotes. Homozygous mutations of this gene are associated with a more severe form of short stature, Langer mesomelic dwarfism. A pseudoautosomal region has also been described for the distal ends of the long arms of the X and Y chromosomes. Only one gene has been localized to this region (Figures 44–4 and 44–5).

In buccal mucosal smears of 46,XX females, a sex chromatin body is evident in 20–30% of the interphase nuclei examined, whereas in normal 46,XY males, a comparable sex chromatin body is absent. In patients with more than 2 X chromosomes, the maximum number of sex chromatin bodies in any diploid nucleus is one less than the total number of X chromosomes. Using sex chromatin and Y fluorescent staining, one can determine indirectly the sex chromosome complement of an individual (Table 44–2).

Sex Determination (SRY = Testis-Determining Factor)

Over the past 20 years, interest has focused on several proteins as candidates for the testis-determining factor produced by a gene on the Y chromosome. Experimental and clinical data do not support the candidacy of H-Y antigen or zinc finger Y as the testis-determining factor. In studies of 46,XX males with very small Y-to-X translocations, a gene was localized to the region just proximal to the pseudoautosomal boundary of the Y chromosome (Figure 44–5). This gene has been cloned, expressed, and named sex-determining region Y (*SRY*). *Sry* (the mouse analog of the human *SRY* gene) is expressed in the embryonic genital ridge of the mouse between days 10.5

Figure 44–1. A normal 46,XY karyotype stained with Giemsa stain to produce G bands. Note that each chromosome has a specific banding pattern. (Reproduced, with permission, from Grumbach MM, Conte FA: Disorders of sex differentiation. In: Wilson JD et al [editors]: *Williams Textbook of Endocrinology,* 9th ed. Saunders, 1998.

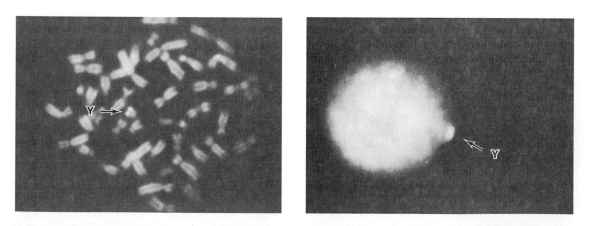

Figure 44–2. Metaphase chromosomes stained with quinacrine and examined through a fluorescence microscope. Note the bright fluorescence of the distal arms of the Y chromosome, which can also be seen in interphase cells ("Y body" at right). (Reproduced, with permission, from Grumbach MM, Conte FA: Disorders of sex differentiation. In: Wilson JD et al [editors]: *Williams Textbook of Endocrinology,* 9th ed. Saunders, 1998.

Table 44–1. Nomenclature for describing the human karyotype pertinent to designating sex chromosome abnormalities.

ISCN 1995	Description	Former Nomenclature
46,XX	Normal female karyotype	XX
46,XY	Normal male karyotype	XY
47,XXY	Karyotype with 47 chromosomes including an extra Y chromosome	XXY
45,X	Monosomy X	XO
45,X/46,XY	Mosaic karyotype composed of 45,X and 46,XY cell lines	XO/XY
p	Short arm	p
q	Long arm	q
46,X,del (X) (p21)	Deletion of the short arm of the X distal to band Xp21	XXp–
46,X,del (X) (q21)	Deletion of the long arm of the X distal to band Xq21	XXq–
46,X,i(Xq10)	Isochromosome of the long arm of X. q10 = centromeric band	XXqi
46,Xr(X)(p22q25)	Ring X chromosome with breaks at p22 and q25	XXr
46,XY,der(7)t(Y;7)(q11;q13)	Translocation of the distal fluorescent portion of the Y chromosome to the long arm of chromosome 7	46,XYt (Yq–7q+)

(Reproduced, with permission, from Grumbach MM, Conte FA: Disorders of sex differentiation. In: Wilson JD et al [editors]: *Williams Textbook of Endocrinology,* 9th ed. Saunders, 1998.)

and 12.5, just before and during the time at which testis differentiation first occurs. Furthermore, deletions or mutations of the human *SRY* gene occur in about 15–20% of 46,XY females with complete XY gonadal dysgenesis. However, the most compelling evidence to indicate that *SRY* is the testis-determining factor is that transfection of the *SRY* gene into 46,XX mouse embryos results in transgenic 46,XX mice with testes and male sex differentiation.

The *SRY* gene encodes a DNA-binding protein that has an 80–amino acid domain similar to that found in high mobility group (HMG) proteins. This domain binds to DNA in a sequence-specific manner (A/TAA-CAAT). It bends the DNA and is thus thought to facilitate interaction between DNA-bound proteins to affect the transcription of "downstream genes." Almost all the mutations thus far described in 46,XY females

with gonadal dysgenesis have occurred in the nucleotides of the *SRY* gene encoding the DNA binding region (the HMG box) of the SRY protein.

An unknown number of genes are involved in the testis-determining cascade (Figure 44–6A). Heterozygous mutations and deletions of the Wilms tumor repressor gene (*WT-1*) located on 11p13 result in urogenital malformations as well as Wilms tumors. Knockout of the *WT-1* gene in mice results in apoptosis of the metanephric blastema with the resultant absence of the kidneys and gonads. Thus, *WT-1,* a transcriptional regulator, appears to act on metanephric blastema early in urogenital development.

SF-1 (steroidogenic factor-1) is an orphan nuclear receptor involved in transcriptional regulation. It is expressed in both the female and male urogenital ridges as well as in steroidogenic tissues, where it is required for the synthesis of testosterone, and in Sertoli cells, where it regulates the antimüllerian hormone gene. SF-1 is encoded by the mammalian homolog of the *Drosophila* gene *FTZ-F1.* Knockout of the *SF-1* gene in mice results in apoptosis of the cells of the genital ridge that give rise to the adrenals and gonads and thus lack of gonadal and adrenal gland morphogenesis in both males and females. This gene thus appears to play a critical role in the formation of all steroid-secreting glands, ie, the adrenals, testes, and ovaries.

XY gonadal dysgenesis with resulting female differentiation in 46,XY patients with intact *SRY* function has been reported in individuals with duplications of Xp21. A locus at this site has been called DSS (dosage-sensitive sex reversal). A mutation or deletion of a gene in this locus called *AHCH,* which encodes a transcriptional factor termed DAX-1, results in X-linked congenital adrenal hypoplasia and hypogonadotropic hypogonadism. Deletion or mutation of the *AHCH* gene (DAX-1) in 46,XY individuals has not resulted in an abnormality of testicular differentiation. Similarly, duplication of the *AHCH*

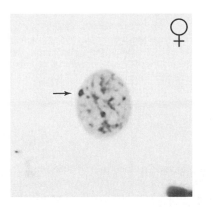

Figure 44–3. X chromatin (Barr) body in the nucleus of a buccal mucosal cell from a normal 46,XX female. (Reproduced, with permission, from Grumbach MM, Conte FA: Disorders of sex differentiation. In: Wilson JD et al [editors]: *Williams Textbook of Endocrinology,* 9th ed. Saunders, 1998.

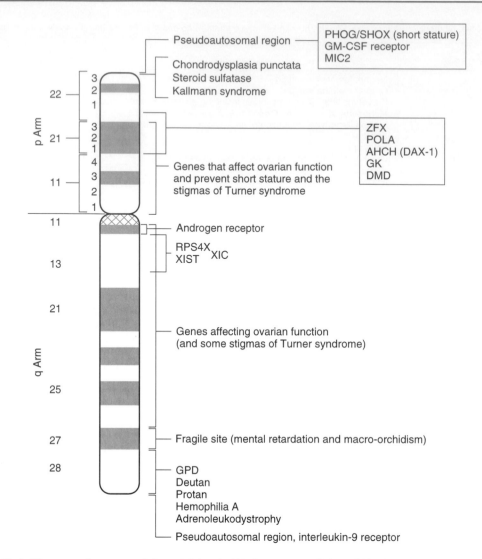

Figure 44–4. Diagrammatic representation of G-banded X chromosome. Selected X-linked genes are shown. (PHOG, pseudoautosomal homeobox osteogenic gene; SHOX, short-stature homeobox gene; GM-CSF, granulocyte-macrophage colony-stimulating factor; MIC2, a cell surface antigen recognized by monoclonal antibody 12E7; ZFX, zinc finger X; POLA, RNA polymerase; AHCH, adrenal hypoplasia congenita, hypogonadotropic hypogonadism; DAX-1, DSS-AHC-critical region on the X chromosome gene 1; GPD, glucose-6-phosphate dehydrogenase; deutan and protan, color blindness genes; GK, glycerol kinase; DMD, Duchenne muscular dystrophy; RPS4X, ribosomal protein S4; XIST, Xi-specific transcripts; XIC, X-inactivation center.) (Reproduced, with permission, from Grumbach MM, Conte FA: Disorders of sex differentiation. In: Wilson JD et al [editors]: *Williams Textbook of Endocrinology,* 9th ed. Saunders, 1998.)

gene (DAX-1) appears not to affect ovarian morphogenesis and function in 46,XX females. Duplication of the *Ahch* (Dax-1) (mouse homolog) gene in 46,XY mice has caused sex reversal when tested against weak alleles of *Sry.* Hence, it appears that duplication of *AHCH* (DAX-1) is responsible for dosage-sensitive sex reversal in humans. It has been suggested that *Ahch* (Dax-1) is an "antitestes" factor rather than an ovary-determining gene. This hypothe-

sis is supported by the finding that mutations of the *Ahch* (Dax-1) locus in the female mouse with loss of function do not affect ovarian differentiation or fertility (Figure 44–6B).

Campomelic dysplasia is a skeletal dysplasia associated with sex reversal due to gonadal dysgenesis in 46,XY individuals. The gene for campomelic dysplasia (*CMPD1*) has been localized to 17q24.3–q25.1. Mutations in one allele of the *SOX 9* gene, a gene re-

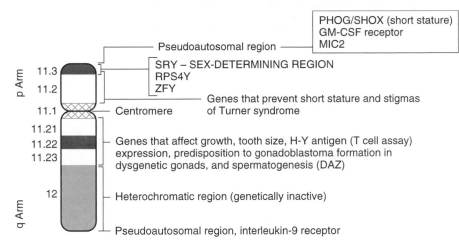

Figure 44–5. Diagrammatic representation of a G-banded Y chromosome. Y-linked genes are shown. (ZFY, zinc finger Y; SRY, sex-determining region Y; *PHOG,* pseudoautosomal homeobox osteogenic gene; *SHOX,* short-stature homeobox gene; GM-CSF, granulocyte-macrophage colony-stimulating factor; MIC2, gene for a cell surface antigen recognized by monoclonal antibody 12E7; RPS4Y, ribosomal protein S4; DAZ, deleted in azoospermia.) (Reproduced, with permission, from Grumbach MM, Conte FA: Disorders of sex differentiation. In: Wilson JD et al [editors]: *Williams Textbook of Endocrinology,* 9th ed. Saunders, 1998.)

lated to *SRY* (called a *SOX* gene because it has an SRY HMG box that is more than 60% homologous to that of SRY), can result in both *CMPD1* and XY gonadal dysgenesis with sex reversal. XY individuals with 9p– or 10q– deletions exhibit gonadal dysgenesis and male pseudohermaphroditism, which suggests that autosomal genes at these loci are important in the gonadal differentiation cascade (Figure 44–6B).

TESTICULAR & OVARIAN DIFFERENTIATION

Until the 12-mm stage (approximately 42 days of gestation), the embryonic gonads of males and females are indistinguishable. By 42 days, 300–1300 primordial germ cells have seeded the undifferentiated gonad from their extragonadal origin in the yolk sac dorsal endoderm. These large cells are the progenitors of oogonia and spermatogonia; lack of these cells is incompatible with further ovarian differentiation but not testicular differentiation. Under the influence of SRY and other genes that encode male sex determination (Figure 44–6B), the gonad will begin to differentiate as a testis at 43–50 days of gestation. Leydig cells are apparent by about 60 days, and differentiation of male external genitalia occurs by 65–77 days of gestation.

In the gonad destined to be an ovary, the lack of differentiation persists. At 77–84 days—long after differentiation of the testis in the male fetus—a significant number of germ cells enter meiotic prophase to characterize the transition of oogonia into oocytes, which marks the onset of ovarian differentiation from the undifferentiated gonads. Primordial follicles (small oocytes surrounded by a single layer of flat granulosa cells and a basement membrane) are evident after 90 days. Preantral follicles are seen after 6 months, and fully developed oocytes with fluid-filled

Table 44–2. Sex chromosome complement correlated with X chromatin and Y bodies in somatic interphase nuclei.[1]

Sex Chromosomes	Maximum Number in Diploid Somatic Nuclei	
	X Bodies	Y Bodies
45,X	0	0
46,XX	1	0
46,XY	0	1
47,XXX	2	0
47,XXY	1	1
47,XYY	0	2
48,XXXX	3	0
48,XXXY	2	1
48,XXYY	1	2
49,XXXXX	4	0
49,XXXXY	3	1
49,XXXYY	2	2

[1]The maximum number of X chromatin bodies in diploid somatic nuclei is one less than the number of Xs, whereas the maximum number of Y fluorescent bodies is equivalent to the number of Ys in the chromosome constitution. (Reproduced, with permission, from Grumbach MM, Conte FA: Disorders of sex differentiation. In: Wilson JD et al [editors]: *Williams Textbook of Endocrinology,* 9th ed. Saunders, 1998.)

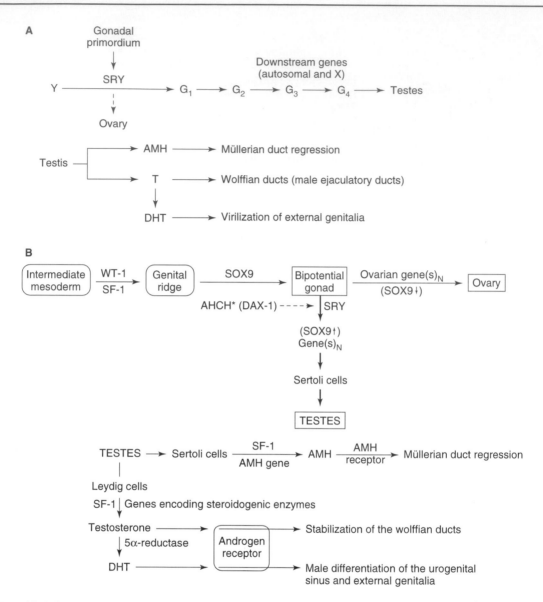

Figure 44–6. Hypothetical diagrammatic representation of the cascade of genes involved in testes determination and hormones involved in male sex differentiation. WT-1, Wilms tumor suppressor; SF-1, steroidogenic factor-1; AHCH, adrenal hypoplasia congenita, hypogonadotropic hypogonadism; Asterisk, a double dose of AHCH inhibits SRY and results in inhibition of testes determination; DAX-1, DSS-AHC critical region on the X chromosome; SRY, sex-determining region Y; SOX 9, SRY-like HMG box gene 9; AMH, antimüllerian hormone; DHT, dihydrotestosterone. (Reproduced, with permission, from Grumbach MM, Conte FA: Disorders of sex differentiation. In: Wilson JD et al [editors]: *Williams Textbook of Endocrinology,* 9th ed. Saunders, 1998.)

cavities and multiple layers of granulosa cells are present at birth. As opposed to the testes, there is little evidence of hormone production by the fetal ovaries (Figure 44–7).

Differentiation of Genital Ducts (Figure 44–8)

By the seventh week of intrauterine life, the fetus is equipped with the primordia of both male and female genital ducts. The müllerian ducts, if allowed to persist, form the uterine (fallopian) tubes, the corpus and cervix of the uterus, and the upper third of the vagina. The wolffian ducts, on the other hand, have the potential for differentiating into the epididymis, vas deferens, seminal vesicles, and ejaculatory ducts of the male. In the presence of a functional testis, the müllerian ducts involute under the influence of antimüllerian hormone (AMH), a dimeric glycoprotein secreted by

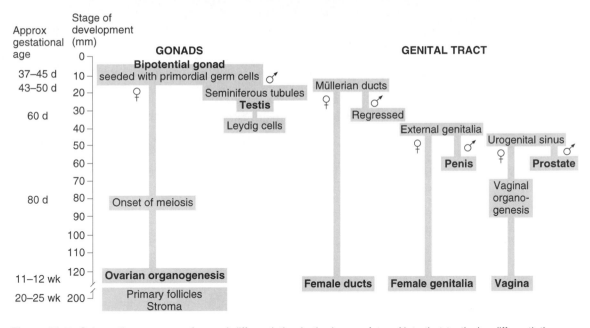

Figure 44–7. Schematic sequence of sexual differentiation in the human fetus. Note that testicular differentiation precedes all other forms of differentiation. (Reproduced, with permission, from Grumbach MM, Conte FA: Disorders of sex differentiation. In: Wilson JD et al [editors]: *Williams Textbook of Endocrinology,* 9th ed. Saunders, 1998.)

fetal Sertoli cells. This hormone acts "locally" to cause müllerian duct repression ipsilaterally. The differentiation of the wolffian duct is stimulated by testosterone secretion from the testis. In the presence of an ovary or in the absence of a functional fetal testis, müllerian duct differentiation occurs, and the wolffian ducts involute. Data indicate that *SF-1* regulates steroidogenesis by the Leydig cell by binding to the promoter of the genes encoding P450scc and P450c17.

The gene for AMH encodes a 560–amino acid protein whose carboxyl terminal domain shows marked homology with transforming growth factor (TGF)-β and the B chain of inhibin and activin. The gene has been localized on the short arm of chromosome 19. AMH is secreted by human fetal and postnatal Sertoli cells until 8–10 years of age and can be used as a marker for the presence of these cells. *SF-1,* an orphan nuclear receptor, has been shown to regulate AMH gene expression. The human AMH receptor gene has been cloned and mapped to the q13 band of chromosome 12. The receptor has been identified as being similar to other type II receptors of the TGF-β family.

Differentiation of External Genitalia (Figure 44–9)

Up to the eighth week of fetal life, the external genitalia of both sexes are identical and have the capacity to differentiate into the genitalia of either sex. Female sex differentiation will occur in the presence

of an ovary or streak gonads or if no gonad is present (Figure 44–10). Differentiation of the external genitalia along male lines depends on the action of testosterone and particularly dihydrotestosterone, the 5α-reduced metabolite of testosterone. In the male fetus, testosterone is secreted by the Leydig cells, perhaps autonomously at first and thereafter under the influence of human chorionic gonadotropin (hCG), and then by stimulation from fetal pituitary luteinizing hormone (LH). Masculinization of the external genitalia and urogenital sinus of the fetus results from the action of dihydrotestosterone, which is converted from testosterone in the target cells by the enzyme 5α-reductase. Dihydrotestosterone (as well as testosterone) is bound to a specific protein receptor in the nucleus of the target cell. The transformed steroid-receptor complex dimerizes and binds with high affinity to specific DNA domains, initiating DNA-directed, RNA-mediated transcription. This results in androgen-induced proteins that lead to differentiation and growth of the cell. The gene that encodes the intracellular androgen-binding protein has been localized to the paracentromeric portion of the long arm of the X chromosome (Figure 44–4). Thus, an X-linked gene controls the androgen response of all somatic cell types by specifying the androgen receptor protein.

As in the case of the genital ducts, there is an inherent tendency for the external genitalia and urogenital sinus to develop along female lines. Differentiation of the external genitalia along male lines requires andro-

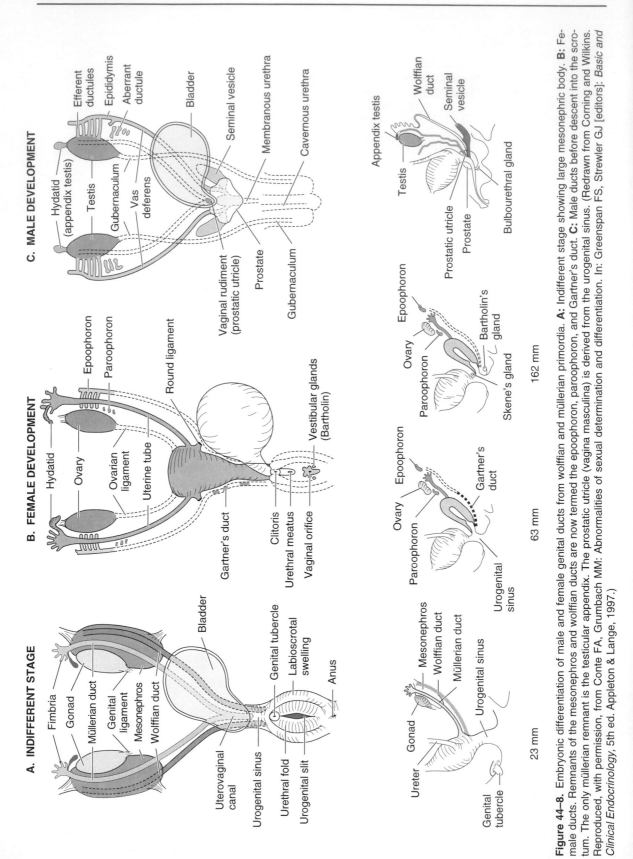

Figure 44–8. Embryonic differentiation of male and female genital ducts from wolffian and müllerian primordia. **A:** Indifferent stage showing large mesonephric body. **B:** Female ducts. Remnants of the mesonephros and wolffian ducts are now termed the epoophoron, paroophoron, and Gartner's duct. **C:** Male ducts before descent into the scrotum. The only müllerian remnant is the testicular appendix. The prostatic utricle (vagina masculina) is derived from the urogenital sinus. (Redrawn from Corning and Wilkins. Reproduced, with permission, from Conte FA, Grumbach MM: Abnormalities of sexual determination and differentiation. In: Greenspan FS, Strewler GJ [editors]: *Basic and Clinical Endocrinology*, 5th ed. Appleton & Lange, 1997.)

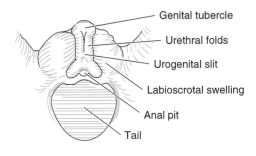

16.8 mm

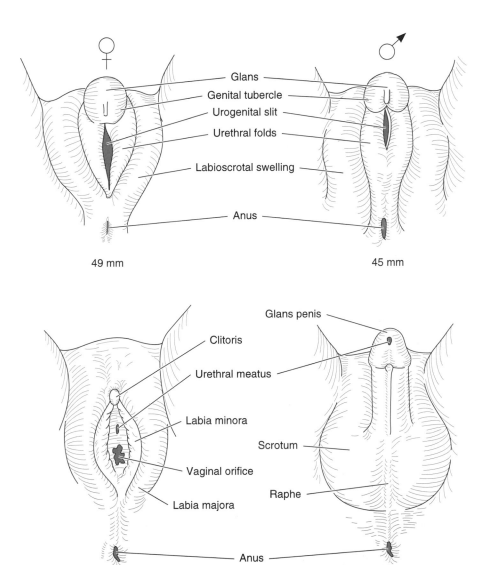

49 mm

45 mm

Figure 44–9. Differentiation of male and female external genitalia from bipotential primordia. (Reproduced, with permission, from Grumbach MM, Conte FA: Disorders of sex differentiation. In: Wilson JD et al [editors]: *Williams Textbook of Endocrinology,* 9th ed. Saunders, 1998.)

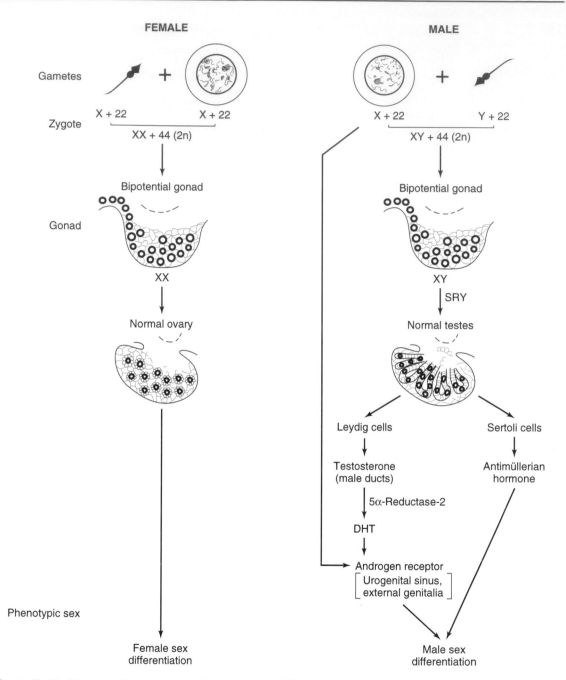

Figure 44–10. Diagrammatic summation of human sexual differentiation. (DHT, dihydrotestosterone; SRY, sex-determining region Y.) (Reproduced, with permission, from Grumbach MM, Conte FA: Disorders of sex differentiation. In: Wilson JD et al [editors]: *Williams Textbook of Endocrinology,* 9th ed. Saunders, 1998.)

genic stimulation early in fetal life. The testosterone metabolite dihydrotestosterone and its specific nuclear receptor must be present to effect masculinization of the external genitalia of the fetus. Dihydrotestosterone stimulates growth of the genital tubercle, fusion of the urethral folds, and descent of the labioscrotal swellings to form the penis and scrotum. Androgens also inhibit descent and growth of the vesicovaginal septum and differentiation of the vagina. There is a critical period for action of the androgen. After about the 12th week of gestation, fusion of the labioscrotal folds will not occur even under intense androgen stimulation, although phallic growth can be induced. Incomplete masculinization of the male fetus results from

(1) impairment in the synthesis or secretion of fetal testosterone or in its conversion to dihydrotestosterone, (2) deficient or defective androgen receptor activity, or (3) defective production and local action of antimüllerian hormone. Exposure of the female fetus to abnormal amounts of androgens from either endogenous or exogenous sources, especially before the 12th week of gestation, can result in virilization of the external genitalia.

PSYCHOSEXUAL DIFFERENTIATION

Psychosexual differentiation may be classified into 4 broad categories: (1) gender identity, defined as the identification of self as either male or female; (2) gender role, ie, those aspects of behavior in which males and females differ from one another in our culture at this time; (3) gender orientation, the choice of sexual partner; and (4) cognitive differences.

Over the past 30 years, the prevailing dogma has been that newborns are born psychosexually neutral and that gender identity is imprinted postnatally by words, attitudes, and comparisons of one's body with that of others. Recently, this hypothesis has been rigorously challenged by Diamond and Sigmundson as well as Reiner. Their studies, and others, suggest that prenatal exposure to androgen and the presence of genes on the Y chromosome can influence gender identity in the patient with ambiguous genitalia. Gender identity has been hypothesized to be established by 18–30 months of age; however, it appears to be more plastic than previously thought. If, at puberty, discordant secondary sexual characteristics are allowed to mature, some individuals, especially those with 5α-reductase deficiency, 45,X/46,XY mosaicism, or 17-hydroxysteroid dehydrogenase-3, have had doubts about their gender identity and have chosen to change their assigned sex from female to male. Further studies on patients with ambiguous genitalia and, in particular, long-term outcomes of gender identity, gender role, and sexual activity in intersex patients are necessary before this nature versus nurture controversy can be resolved and more comprehensive, enlightened, less doctrinaire guidelines developed. Until further data are available, experience obtained from a pragmatic approach to the assignment of sex in individuals with ambiguous genitalia suggests that the most critical elements in the development of gender identity are the assigned sex of rearing, its psychological and social reinforcement during infancy and childhood, and its reinforcement by appropriate gonadal steroid secretion or replacement therapy at the normal age of puberty. Also of critical importance is the long-term psychological and clinical support of the patients and their families.

ABNORMAL SEX DIFFERENTIATION

Classification of Errors in Sex Differentiation (Table 44–3)

Disorders of sexual differentiation are the result of abnormalities in complex processes that originate in genetic information on the X and Y chromosomes as well as on the autosomes. A true hermaphrodite is defined as a person who possesses both ovarian and testicular tissue. A male pseudohermaphrodite is one whose gonads are exclusively testes but whose genital ducts or external genitalia (or both) exhibit incomplete masculinization. A female pseudohermaphrodite is a person whose gonadal tissue is exclusively ovarian but whose genital development exhibits ambiguous or male appearance.

SEMINIFEROUS TUBULE DYSGENESIS: CHROMATIN-POSITIVE KLINEFELTER SYNDROME & ITS VARIANTS

Klinefelter syndrome is one of the most common forms of primary hypogonadism and infertility in males. The invariable clinical features in adults are a male phenotype, firm testes less than 3 cm in length, and azoospermia. Gynecomastia is common. Affected patients usually have a 47,XXY sex chromosome constitution and an X chromatin-positive buccal smear, although subjects with a variety of sex chromosome constitutions, including mosaicism, have been described. Virtually all of these variants have in common the presence of at least 2 X chromosomes and a Y chromosome, except for the rare group in which only an XX sex chromosome complement is found.

Surveys of the prevalence of 47,XXY fetuses by karyotype analysis of unselected newborn infants indicate an incidence of about 1:1000 newborn males. Prepubertally, the disorder is characterized by small testes, disproportionately long legs, personality and behavioral disorders, and a lower mean verbal IQ score when compared with that of control subjects but no significant difference in full-scale IQ. Severe mental retardation requiring special schooling is uncommon. Gynecomastia and other signs of androgen deficiency such as diminished facial and body hair, a small phallus, poor muscular development, and a eunuchoid body habitus occur postpubertally in affected patients. Adult males with a 47,XXY karyotype tend to be taller than average, with adult height close to the 75th percentile, mainly because of the disproportionate length of their legs. Untreated adult males, especially those with subnormal sex steroid levels, are at increased risk for the development of osteoporosis. They also have an increased incidence of mild diabetes mellitus, varicose veins, stasis dermatitis, cerebrovascular disease, chronic pulmonary disease, and carcinoma of the

Table 44–3. Classification of anomalous sexual development.

I. Disorders of gonadal differentiation
  A. Seminiferous tubule dysgenesis (Klinefelter syndrome)
  B. Syndrome of gonadal dysgenesis and its variants (Turner syndrome)
  C. Complete and incomplete forms of XX and XY gonadal dysgenesis
  D. True hermaphroditism
II. Female pseudohermaphroditism
  A. Congenital virilizing adrenal hyperplasia
  B. P450 aromatase (placental) deficiency
  C. Androgens and synthetic progestins transferred from maternal circulation
  D. Associated with malformations of intestine and urinary tract (non-androgen-induced female pseudohermaphroditism)
  E. Other teratologic factors
III. Male pseudohermaphroditism
  A. Testicular unresponsiveness to hCG and LH (Leydig cell agenesis or hypoplasia due to hcG/LH receptor defect)
  B. Inborn errors of testosterone biosynthesis
    1. Enzyme defects affecting synthesis of both corticosteroids and testosterone (variants of congenital adrenal hyperplasia)
      a. StAR deficiency (congenital lipoid adrenal hyperplasia)
      b. 3β-Hydrosysteroid dehydrogenase deficiency
      c. P450c17 (17α-hydroxylase) deficiency
    2. Enzyme defects primarily affecting testosterone biosynthesis by the testes
      a. P450c17 (17,20-lyase) deficiency
      b. 17β-Hydroxysteroid oxidoreductase deficiency
  C. Defects in androgen-dependent target tissues
    1 End-organ resistance to androgenic hormones (androgen receptor and postreceptor defects)
      a. Syndrome of complete androgen resistance and its variants (testicular feminization and its variant forms)
      b. Syndrome of partial androgen resistance and its variants (Reifenstein syndrome)
      c. Androgen resistance in infertile men
      d. Androgen resistance in fertile men
    2. Defects in testosterone metabolism by peripheral tissues
      a. 5α-Reductase deficiency (pseudovaginal perineoscrotal hypospadias)
  D. Dysgenetic male pseudohermaphroditism
    1. XY gonadal dysgenesis (incomplete)
    2. 45,X/46,XY mosaicism, structurally abnormal Y chromosome, Xp+, 9p–, 10q–
    3. Denys-Drash (*WT-1* mutation)
    4. WAGR (*WT-1* deletion)
    5. Campomelic dysplasia (SOX 9 mutation)
    6. SF-1 mutation
    7. Testicular regression syndrome
  E. Defects in synthesis, secretion, or response to AMH
    1. Female genital ducts in otherwise normal men—"herniae uteri inguinale"; persistant müllerian duct syndrome
  F. ?Environmental chemicals
IV. Unclassified forms of abnormal sexual development
  A. In males
    1. Hypospadias
    2. Ambiguous external genitalia in 46,XY males with multiple congenital anomalies
  B. In females
    1. Absence or anomalous development of the vagina, uterus, and uterine tubes (Rokitansky-Küster syndrome)

(Reproduced, with permission, from Grumbach MM, Conte FA: Disorders of sex differentiation. In: Wilson JD et al [editors]: *Williams Textbook of Endocrinology,* 9th ed. Saunders, 1998.)

breast; the incidence of breast carcinoma in patients with Klinefelter syndrome is 20 times higher than that in normal men. Patients with Klinefelter syndrome often have a delay in the onset of adolescence. There is an increased risk for developing malignant extragonadal germ cell tumors, including central nervous system germinomas and mediastinal tumors, which may be hCG-secreting and cause sexual precocity in the prepubertal patient.

The testicular lesion is progressive and gonadotropin-dependent. It is characterized in the adult by extensive seminiferous tubular hyalinization and fibrosis, absent or severely deficient spermatogenesis, and pseudoadenomatous clumping of the Leydig cells.

Although hyalinization of the tubules is usually extensive, it varies considerably from patient to patient and even between testes in the same patient. Azoospermia is the rule, and patients who have been reported to be fertile invariably have been 46,XY/47,XXY mosaics.

Nondisjunction during the first or second meiotic division of gametogenesis plays an important role in the genesis of a 47,XXY karyotype. Fifty-three percent of cases appear to result from paternal nondisjunction at the first meiotic division, 34% from meiotic nondisjunction during the first maternal meiotic division, and 9% from nondisjunction at the second meiotic division. Only 3% of patients appear to have arisen from postzygotic meiotic nondisjunction.

The diagnosis of Klinefelter syndrome is suggested by the classic phenotype and hormonal changes. It is confirmed by the finding of an X chromatin-positive buccal smear and demonstration of a 47,XXY karyotype in blood, skin, or gonads. After puberty, levels of serum and urinary gonadotropins (especially follicle-stimulating hormone [FSH]) are raised. The testosterone production rate, the total and free levels of testosterone, and the metabolic clearance rates of testosterone and estradiol tend to be low, while plasma estradiol levels are normal or high. Testicular biopsy reveals the classic findings of hyalinization of the seminiferous tubules, severe deficiency of spermatogonia, and pseudoadenomatous clumping of Leydig cells.

Treatment of patients with Klinefelter syndrome is directed toward androgen replacement, especially in patients in whom puberty is delayed or fails to progress or in those who have subnormal testosterone levels for age and developmental stage. Testosterone therapy may help to enhance secondary sexual characteristics and sexual performance, prevent osteoporosis, prevent or cause regression of gynecomastia, and improve general well-being in most patients. If testosterone deficiency is present, testosterone therapy early in adolescence should commence with 50 mg of testosterone enanthate in oil intramuscularly every 4 weeks, gradually increasing to the adult replacement dose of 200 mg every 2 weeks. Thereafter, transdermal testosterone therapy (testosterone patch) may be used for adult replacement. A marked decrease in gynecomastia may result from testosterone therapy; however, once advanced, gynecomastia may not be amenable to hormone therapy but can be surgically corrected if it is severe or psychologically disturbing to the patient. Early diagnosis, support, and appropriate counseling may improve the overall prognosis.

Variants of Chromatin-Positive Seminiferous Tubule Dysgenesis

A. Variants of Klinefelter Syndrome: Variants of Klinefelter syndrome include 46,XY/47,XXY mosaics as well as patients with multiple X and Y chromosomes. With increasing numbers of X chromosomes in the genome, both mental retardation and other developmental anomalies such as radioulnar synostosis become prevalent.

B. 46,XX Males: Phenotypic males with a 46,XX karyotype have been described since 1964; the incidence of 46,XX males is approximately 1:20,000 births. In general, these individuals have a male phenotype, male psychosocial gender identity, and testes with histologic features similar to those observed in patients with a 47,XXY karyotype. At least 10% of patients have hypospadias or ambiguous external genitalia. XX males have normal body proportions and a mean final height that is shorter than that of patients with an XXY sex chromosome constitution or normal males but taller than that of normal females. As in XXY patients, testosterone levels are low or low normal, gonadotropins are elevated, and spermatogenesis is impaired postpubertally. Gynecomastia is present in approximately one-third of cases.

The presence of testes and male sexual differentiation in 46,XX individuals has been a perplexing problem. However, the paradox has been clarified by the use of recombinant DNA studies. Males with a 46,XX karyotype have been shown by genetic linkage studies and X chromosome restriction fragment length polymorphisms (RFLPs) to possess one X chromosome from each of their parents. Approximately 80% of XX males have a Y chromosome–specific DNA segment from the distal portion of the Y short arm translocated to the distal portion of the short arm of the paternal X chromosome. This translocated segment is heterologous in length but always includes the *SRY* gene, which encodes testis-determining factor as well as the pseudoautosomal region of the Y chromosome. Thus, in 80% of XX males, an abnormal X-Y terminal exchange during paternal meiosis has resulted in 2 products: an X chromosome with an *SRY* gene and a Y chromosome deficient in this gene (the latter would result in a female with XY gonadal dysgenesis). Fewer than 20% of XX males tested have been shown to lack Y chromosome–specific DNA sequences, including the *SRY* gene and the pseudoautosomal region of the Y chromosome. These XX, Y DNA–negative males tend to have hypospadias and may have relatives with true hermaphroditism.

The finding of XX males who lack any evidence of Y chromosome–specific genes suggests that testicular determination—and, thus, male differentiation—can occur in the absence of a gene or genes from the Y chromosome. This could be a result of (1) mutation of a "downstream" autosomal gene involved in male sex determination; or (2) mutation, deletion, or aberrant inactivation of a gene sequence on the X chromosome, critical to testis determination and differentiation; or (3) circumscribed Y chromosome mosaicism (eg, occurring only in the gonads). Further studies will be necessary to elucidate the pathogenesis of male sex determination and differentiation in those 46,XX males who lack ascertainable Y-to-X chromosome translocations.

SYNDROME OF GONADAL DYSGENESIS: TURNER SYNDROME & ITS VARIANTS

Turner Syndrome: 45,X Gonadal Dysgenesis

One in 5000 newborn females has a 45,X sex chromosome constitution. It has been estimated that 99% of 45,X fetuses do not survive beyond 28 weeks of gestation, and 15% of all first-trimester abortuses have a 45,X karyotype. In about 70–80% of instances, the origin of the normal X chromosome is maternal. Patients with a 45,X karyotype represent approximately

50% of all patients with X chromosome abnormalities. The cardinal features of 45,X gonadal dysgenesis are a variety of somatic anomalies, sexual infantilism at puberty secondary to gonadal dysgenesis, and short stature. Patients with a 45,X karyotype can be recognized in infancy, usually because of lymphedema of the extremities and loose skin folds over the nape of the neck. In later life, the typical patient is often recognizable by her distinctive facies in which micrognathia, epicanthal folds, prominent low-set ears, a fishlike mouth, and ptosis are present to varying degrees. The chest is shieldlike and the neck short, broad, and webbed (40% of patients). Additional anomalies associated with Turner syndrome include coarctation of the aorta (10%), hypertension, renal abnormalities (50%), pigmented nevi, cubitus valgus, a tendency to keloid formation, puffiness of the dorsum of the hands and feet, short fourth metacarpals and metatarsals, Madelung deformity of the wrist, scoliosis, and recurrent otitis media, which may lead to conductive hearing loss. Routine intravenous urography or renal sonography is indicated for all patients to rule out a surgically correctable renal abnormality. The internal ducts as well as the external genitalia of these patients are invariably female except in rare patients with a 45,X karyotype, in whom a Y-to-autosome or Y-to-X chromosome translocation has been found.

Short stature is an invariable feature of the syndrome of gonadal dysgenesis. Mean final height in 45,X patients is 143 cm, with a range of 133–153 cm. Current data suggest that the short stature found in patients with the syndrome of gonadal dysgenesis is not due to a deficiency of growth hormone, somatomedin, sex steroids, or thyroid hormone. It appears to be related at least in part to haploinsufficiency of the *PHOG/SHOX* gene in the pseudoautosomal region of the X and Y chromosome (see earlier section). However, administration of high-dose biosynthetic human growth hormone results in an increase in final height.

Gonadal dysgenesis is another feature of patients with a 45,X chromosome constitution. The gonads are typically streaklike and usually contain only fibrous stroma arranged in whorls. Longitudinal studies of both basal and gonadotropin-releasing hormone (GnRH)-evoked gonadotropin secretion in patients with gonadal dysgenesis indicate a lack of feedback inhibition of the hypothalamic-pituitary axis by the dysgenetic gonads in affected infants and children (Figure 44–11). Thus, plasma and urinary gonadotropin levels, particularly FSH levels, are high during early infancy and after 9–10 years of age. Since ovarian function is impaired, puberty does not usually ensue spontaneously; hence, sexual infantilism is a hallmark of this syndrome. Rarely, patients with a 45,X karyotype may undergo spontaneous pubertal maturation, menarche, and pregnancy.

A variety of disorders are associated with this syndrome, including obesity, osteoporosis, diabetes mellitus, Hashimoto thyroiditis, rheumatoid arthritis, inflammatory bowel disease, intestinal telangiectasia with bleeding, and anorexia nervosa. Because an increased prevalence of bicuspid aortic valve, coarctation of the aorta, and aortic dilation with aneurysm formation and rupture has been reported in patients

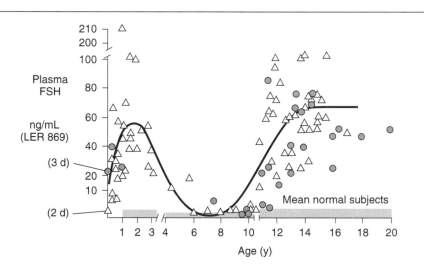

Figure 44–11. Diphasic variation in basal levels of plasma follicle-stimulating hormone (FSH) (ng/mL-LER 869) in patients with a 45,X karyotype (triangles) and patients with structural abnormalities of the X chromosome and mosaics (circles). Note that mean basal levels of plasma FSH in patients with gonadal dysgenesis are in the castrate range before 4 years and after 10 years of age. (Reproduced, with permission, from Conte FA, Grumbach MM, Kaplan SL: A diphasic pattern of gonadotropin secretion in patients with the syndrome of gonadal dysgenesis. J Clin Endocrinol Metab 1975;40:670.)

with Turner syndrome, screening and periodic echo-cardiography are indicated in all patients with a 45,X cell line.

Phenotypic females with the following features should have a karyotype analysis: (1) short stature (> 2.5 SD below the mean value for age); (2) somatic anomalies associated with the syndrome of gonadal dysgenesis; and (3) delayed adolescence with an increased level of plasma FSH.

Therapy should be directed toward maximizing final height and inducing secondary sexual characteristics and menarche at an age commensurate with that of normal peers. The results of recent clinical trials suggest that patients treated with recombinant growth hormone (0.375 mg/kg/wk divided into 7 once-daily doses), with or without oxandrolone (0.0625 mg/kg/d by mouth), had an increase in growth rate that was sustained and resulted in a mean 8–10 cm increase in height after 3–7 years of therapy. Before initiation of growth hormone therapy, a thorough analysis of the costs, benefits, and possible side effects must be discussed with the parents and the child. Long-term studies with low-dose estrogen therapy have not demonstrated a positive effect on final height in girls with Turner syndrome. No synergistic effect of combined estrogen and growth hormone therapy on final height has been found. In patients who have been treated with growth hormone and have achieved an acceptable height and in those who have refused growth hormone therapy, estrogen replacement therapy is usually initiated after 12–13 years of age. Conjugated estrogens (0.3 mg or less) or ethinyl estradiol (5 μg) are given orally for the first 21 days of the calendar month. Thereafter, the dose of estrogen is gradually increased over the next several years to 0.6–1.25 mg of conjugated estrogens or 10 μg of ethinyl estradiol daily for the first 21 days of the month. The minimum dose of estrogen necessary to maintain secondary sexual characteristics and menses and prevent osteoporosis should be administered. After the first year of estrogen therapy, medroxyprogesterone acetate, 5 mg daily, or a comparable progestin is given on the 10th–21st days of the menstrual cycle to ensure physiologic menses and to reduce the risk of endometrial carcinoma, which is associated with unopposed estrogen stimulation.

X Chromatin-Positive Variants of the Syndrome of Gonadal Dysgenesis

Patients with structural abnormalities of the X chromosome (deletions and additions) and sex chromosome mosaicism with a 45,X cell line may manifest the somatic as well as the gonadal features of the syndrome of gonadal dysgenesis (Table 44–4). Evidence suggests that genes on both the long and short arms of the X chromosome control gonadal differentiation, whereas genes primarily on the short arms of the X prevent the short stature and somatic anomalies that are seen in 45,X patients (Figure 44–4). In general, 45,X/46,XX mosaicism will modify the 45,X phenotype toward normal and can even result in normal gonadal function. Some patients with mosaicism and a 45,X/46,Xr(X) karyotype may manifest mental retardation and congenital anomalies not usually associated with Turner syndrome. Recent data indicate that these abnormalities are related to lack of inactivation of small ring X chromosomes and, hence, functional disomy for genes on the ring X chromosome and the normal X chromosome.

X Chromatin-Negative Variants of the Syndrome of Gonadal Dysgenesis

These patients usually have mosaicism with a 45,X and a Y-bearing cell line—45,X/46,XY; 45,X/47, XXY; 45,X/46,XY/47,XYY—or perhaps a structurally abnormal Y chromosome. They range from phenotypic females with the features of Turner syndrome through patients with ambiguous genitalia to completely virilized males with few stigmas of Turner syndrome. The variations in gonadal differentiation range from bilateral streaks to bilateral dysgenetic testes to apparently "normal" testes, and there may be asymmetric development, ie, a streak on one side and a dysgenetic testicle or, rarely, a normal testis on the other side—sometimes called **mixed gonadal dysgenesis.** The development of the external genitalia and of the internal ducts correlates with the degree of testicular differentiation and, presumably, the capacity of the fetal testes to secrete antimüllerian hormone and testosterone.

The risk of development of gonadal tumors is greatly increased in patients with 45,X/46,XY mosaicism and streak or dysgenetic gonads; hence, prophylactic removal of streak gonads or dysgenetic undescended testes in this syndrome is indicated. Breast development at or after the age of puberty in these patients is commonly associated with a gonadal neoplasm, usually a gonadoblastoma. Pelvic sonography, computed tomography scanning, or magnetic resonance imaging may be useful in screening for neoplasms in these patients. Gonadoblastomas are calcified and so may be visible even on a plain film of the abdomen.

The diagnosis of 45,X/46,XY mosaicism can be established by the demonstration of both 45,X and 46,XY cells in blood, skin, or gonadal tissue. In some mosaics, a marker chromosome is found that is cytogenetically indistinguishable as X or Y. In these cases, either fluorescence in situ hybridization or molecular analyses with X- and Y-specific probes is indicated to definitively determine the origin of the marker chromosome, since gonadoblastomas have been reported in patients with deleted Y chromosomes—even those with deletions of the *SRY* gene. The decision regarding the sex of rearing should be based on the age at diagnosis and the potential for normal function of the external genitalia. Most patients with 45,X/46,XY mo-

Table 44–4. Relationship of structural abnormalities of the X and Y to clinical manifestations of the syndrome of gonadal dysgenesis.

Type of Sex Chromosome Abnormality	Karyotype	Phenotype	Sexual Infantilism	Short Stature	Somatic Anomalies of Turner Syndrome
Loss of an X or Y	45,X	Female	+	+	+
Deletion of short arm of an X[1]	46,XXqi	Female	+ (occ. ±)	+	+
	46,XXp–	Female	+, ±, or –	+	+ (–)
Deletion of long arm of an X[1]	46,XXq–	Female	+	– (+)	– or (±)
Deletion of ends of both arms of an X[2]	46,XXr	Female	– or +	+	+ or (±)
Deletion of short arm of Y	46,XYp–	Female	+	+	+

[1]In Xp and Xq–, the extent and site of the deleted segment are variable.
Xqi = Isochromosome for long arm of an X; Xp– = deletion of short arm of an X; Xq– = deletion of long arm of an X; Xr = ring chromosome derived from an X.
[2]Patients with small ring X chromosomes can have mental retardation and somatic abnormalities not usually associated with the Turner phenotype owing to noninactivation of genes on the small ring X chromosome.
(Reproduced, with permission, from Grumbach MM, Conte FA: Disorders of sex differentiation. In: Wilson JD et al [editors]: *Williams Textbook of Endocrinology,* 9th ed. Saunders, 1998.)

saicism ascertained by amniocentesis have normal male genitalia and normal testicular histology. Thus, the ambiguity of the genitalia invariably described in patients with 45,X/46,XY mosaicism is due to ascertainment bias. We have observed a short, 30-year-old male with documented 45,X/46,XY mosaicism who has normal male genitalia and is fertile.

In patients assigned a female gender role, the gonads should be removed and the external genitalia repaired as soon as feasible. Estrogen therapy should be initiated at the age of puberty, as in patients with a 45,X karyotype (see above). In affected infants who are assigned a male gender role, all gonadal tissue except that which appears functionally and histologically normal and is in the scrotum should be removed. Removal of the müllerian structures and repair of hypospadias are also indicated. At puberty, depending on the functional integrity of the retained gonads, androgen replacement therapy may be indicated in doses similar to those for patients with the incomplete form of XY gonadal dysgenesis. In patients with retained scrotal testes, a repeat gonadal biopsy is indicated postpubertally to rule out the possibility of carcinoma in situ, a premalignant lesion (see below).

In infants and children with 45,X/46,XY mosaicism who have normal genitalia, and normal testicular integrity as assessed by gonadotropin levels and pelvic magnetic resonance imaging, gonadal biopsy may be deferred until adolescence. The risk of gonadal malignancies in males with 45,X/46,XY mosaicism who have normal male genitalia and histologically and functionally normal testes in the scrotum is still to be ascertained.

46,XX & 46,XY GONADAL DYSGENESIS

The terms XX and XY gonadal dysgenesis have been applied to 46,XX or 46,XY patients who have bilateral streak gonads, a female phenotype, and no somatic stigmas of Turner syndrome. After the age of puberty, these patients exhibit sexual infantilism, castrate levels of plasma and urinary gonadotropins, normal or tall stature, and eunuchoid proportions.

46,XX Gonadal Dysgenesis

Familial and sporadic cases of XX gonadal dysgenesis have been reported with an incidence as high as 1:8300 females in Finland. Pedigree analysis of familial cases is consistent with autosomal recessive inheritance.

Analysis of familial cases in Finland revealed that a locus on chromosome 2p was linked to XX gonadal dysgenesis in females. The gene for the FSH receptor has been localized to chromosome 2p. Analysis of this gene revealed a mutation in exon 7 of the FSH receptor that segregated with XX gonadal dysgenesis. This mutation affected the extracellular ligand-binding domain of the FSH receptor and reduced the binding capacity of the receptor and consequently signal transduction, resulting in variable ovarian function, including "streak ovaries" and hypergonadotropic hypogonadism in some XX females at puberty. Further studies in Western Europe and the United States of females with 46,XX gonadal dysgenesis have been negative for FSH receptor gene mutations, suggesting that a mutation in this gene is rare and that other causes for this phenotype are more common. Preliminary data suggest that males homozygous for this mutation are phenotypically normal, with spermatogenesis varying from normal to absent.

Studies of familial cohorts have revealed apparent marked heterogeneity in pathogenesis. Siblings, one with a 46,XX karyotype and the other with a 46,XY karyotype, both with gonadal "agenesis," have been reported, supporting the involvement of an autosomal gene in this family. However, in view of the normal phenotype in XY males observed with a mutation in the FSH receptor, it seems unlikely that these patients have an FSH receptor defect. Rather, they may have a mutation in an autosomal recessive gene involved in gonadal determination. In one family, 4 affected women had an inherited interstitial deletion of the long arm of the X chromosome involving the q21–q27 region. This region seems to contain a gene or genes critical to ovarian development and function. In 3 families, XX gonadal dysgenesis was associated with deafness of the sensorineural type. In several affected groups of siblings, a spectrum of clinical findings occurred, eg, varying degrees of ovarian function, including breast development and menses followed by secondary amenorrhea. In contrast to Turner syndrome, stature is normal. The diagnosis of 46,XX gonadal dysgenesis should be suspected in phenotypic females with sexual infantilism and normal müllerian structures who lack the somatic stigmas of the syndrome of gonadal dysgenesis (Turner syndrome). Karyotype analysis reveals only 46,XX cells. As in Turner syndrome, gonadotropin levels are high, estrogen levels are low, and treatment consists of cyclic estrogen and progesterone replacement.

Sporadic cases of XX gonadal dysgenesis, similar to familial cases, may represent a heterogeneous group of patients from a pathogenetic point of view. XX gonadal dysgenesis should be distinguished from ovarian failure due to infections such as mumps, antibodies to gonadotropin receptors, biologically inactive FSH, gonadotropin-insensitive ovaries, and galactosemia as well as errors in steroid (estrogen) biosynthesis. In the latter group, ultrasound or magnetic resonance imaging should reveal polycystic ovaries.

46,XY Gonadal Dysgenesis

46,XY gonadal dysgenesis occurs both sporadically and in familial aggregates. Patients with the complete form of this syndrome have female external genitalia, normal or tall stature, bilateral streak gonads, müllerian duct development, sexual infantilism, eunuchoid habitus, and a 46,XY karyotype. Clitorimegaly is quite common, and, in familial cases, a continuum of involvement ranging from the complete syndrome to ambiguity of the external genitalia has been described. The phenotypic difference between the complete and incomplete forms of XY gonadal dysgenesis is due to the degree of differentiation of testicular tissue and the functional capacity of the fetal testis to produce testosterone and antimüllerian hormone. Early in infancy and after the age of puberty, plasma and urinary gonadotropin levels are markedly elevated.

Analysis of familial and sporadic cases of 46,XY gonadal dysgenesis indicates that about 15–20% of patients have a mutation in the HMG box of the *SRY* gene that affects DNA binding and/or bending by the SRY protein. So far, all patients in whom mutations have been detected have had "complete" gonadal dysgenesis. Patients with large deletions of the short arm of the

Y chromosome may have, in addition to gonadal dysgenesis, stigmas of Turner syndrome. Mutations outside the HMG box region of the *SRY* gene as well as in X-linked or autosomal genes may be responsible for those patients in whom no molecular abnormality has as yet been found. A mutation in the HMG box of the *SRY* gene has been described in 3 normal 46,XY fathers and their "daughters" with 46,XY gonadal dysgenesis. These 3 familial cohorts suggest that these mutations may affect either the level or the timing of *SRY* expression and in this manner result in either normal or abnormal testicular differentiation.

More than 20 patients with 46,XY gonadal dysgenesis have been reported with a duplication of the Xp21.2 → p22.11 region of the X chromosome. This region contains a gene, *AHCH,* that encodes DAX-1. Deletion or mutation of *AHCH* in males causes adrenal hypoplasia congenita and hypogonadotropic hypogonadism. The finding that 46,XY males with adrenal hypoplasia and hypogonadotropic hypogonadism have normal sex differentiation suggests that *AHCH* is not required for testicular differentiation; duplicating *AHCH,* however, impairs testes differentiation. Thus, *AHCH* (DAX-1) appears to be an antitestes gene. (See earlier section.)

XY gonadal dysgenesis associated with campomelic dysplasia is due to a mutation of one allelle of an *SRY*-related gene, *SOX 9* on chromosome 17. In addition, XY gonadal dysgenesis has been associated with 9p– and 10q– deletions, which suggests the presence of other autosomal genes that affect testicular morphogenesis.

Therapy for patients with 46,XY gonadal dysgenesis who have female external genitalia involves prophylactic gonadectomy at diagnosis and estrogen substitution at puberty. In the incomplete form of XY gonadal dysgenesis, assignment of a male gender role should be carefully weighed. It depends upon the degree of ambiguity of the genitalia and the potential for normal sexual function. Prophylactic gonadectomy must be considered, since fertility is unlikely and there is an increased risk of malignant transformation of the dysgenetic gonads in these patients. Biopsy of all retained gonads should be done pre- and postpubertally in order to detect early malignant changes (carcinoma in situ). In affected individuals raised as males, prosthetic testes should be implanted at the time of gonadectomy, and androgen substitution therapy is instituted at the age of puberty. Testosterone enanthate in oil (or another long-acting testosterone ester) is used, beginning with 50 mg intramuscularly every 4 weeks and gradually increasing over 3–4 years to a full replacement dose of 200 mg intramuscularly every 2 weeks.

TRUE HERMAPHRODITISM

In true hermaphroditism, both ovarian and testicular tissue are present in one or both gonads. Differentiation of the internal and external genitalia is highly variable. The external genitalia may simulate those of a male or female, but most often they are ambiguous. Cryptorchidism and hypospadias are common. A testis or ovotestis, if present, is located in the labioscrotal folds in one-third of patients, in the inguinal canal in one-third, and in the abdomen in the remainder. A uterus is usually present, though it may be hypoplastic or unicornuate. The differentiation of the genital ducts usually follows that of the ipsilateral gonad. The ovotestis is the most common gonad found in true hermaphrodites (60%), followed by the ovary and, least commonly, by the testis. At puberty, breast development is usual in untreated patients, and menses occur in over 50% of cases. Whereas the ovary or the ovarian portion of an ovotestis may function normally, the testis or testicular portion of an ovotestis is almost always dysgenetic.

Sixty percent of true hermaphrodites have been reported to have a 46,XX karyotype, 20% 46,XY, and about 20% mosaicism or 46,XX/46,XY chimerism. 46,XX true hermaphroditism appears to be a genetically heterogeneous entity. A small proportion of 46,XX true hermaphrodites, including some in family cohorts with 46,XX males, have been reported to be *SRY*-positive. Hence, Y-to-X and Y-to-autosome translocations, hidden sex chromosome mosaicism, or chimerism can explain the pathogenesis in these patients. The majority of 46,XX true hermaphrodites, however, are *SRY*-negative. A number of families have been reported that had both *SRY*-negative 46,XX males and 46,XX true hermaphrodites. This latter observation suggests a common genetic pathogenesis in these patients. Possible genetic mechanisms to explain *SRY*-negative true hermaphroditism include (1) mutation of a downstream autosomal gene or genes involved in testicular determination; (2) mutation, deletion, duplication, or anomalous inactivation of an X-linked locus involved in testes determination; or (3) circumscribed chimerism or mosaicism that occurred only in the gonads.

The diagnosis of true hermaphroditism should be considered in all patients with ambiguous genitalia. The finding of a 46,XX/46,XY karyotype or a bilobate gonad compatible with an ovotestis in the inguinal region or labioscrotal folds suggests the diagnosis. Basal plasma testosterone levels are elevated above 40 ng/dL in affected patients under 6 months of age, and testosterone levels increase after hCG stimulation. The estradiol response to human menopausal gonadotropins has been shown to be a reliable test for differentiating infants with true hermaphroditism from those with other disorders of sexual differentiation. If all other forms of male and female pseudohermaphroditism have been excluded, laparotomy and histologic confirmation of both ovarian and testicular tissue establish the diagnosis. The management of true hermaphroditism is contingent upon the age at diagnosis and a careful assessment of the functional capacity of the gonads, genital ducts, and external genitalia.

Gonadal Neoplasms in Dysgenetic Gonads

While gonadal tumors are rare in patients with 47,XXY Klinefelter syndrome and 45,X gonadal dysgenesis, the prevalence of gonadal neoplasms is greatly increased in patients with certain types of dysgenetic gonads. The frequency is increased in 45,X/46,XY mosaicism, especially in those with female or ambiguous genitalia; in patients with a structurally abnormal Y chromosome; and in those with XY gonadal dysgenesis, either with a female phenotype or with ambiguous genitalia. Gonadoblastomas, germinomas, seminomas, and teratomas are found most frequently. Prophylactic gonadectomy is advised in these patients as well as in those with gonadal dysgenesis who manifest signs of virilization, regardless of karyotype. Gonadoblastomas have been reported in patients with marker chromosomes of Y origin lacking the *SRY* gene. The testis should be preserved in patients who are to be raised as males only if it is histologically normal and is or can be situated in the scrotum. The fact that a testis is palpable in the scrotum does not preclude malignant degeneration and tumor dissemination, as seminomas tend to metastasize at an early stage before a mass is obvious. If a testis is preserved in the scrotum in a patient with 45,X/46,XY mosaicism or in rare cases of true hermaphroditism, it is prudent to follow the patient closely with sonography or pelvic magnetic resonance imaging and a biopsy postpubertally in order to monitor for the development of a premalignant or malignant lesion.

FEMALE PSEUDOHERMAPHRODITISM

Affected individuals have normal ovaries and müllerian derivatives associated with ambiguous external genitalia. In the absence of testes, a female fetus will be masculinized if subjected to increased circulating levels of androgens derived from a fetal or maternal source. The degree of masculinization depends upon the stage of differentiation at the time of exposure (Figure 44–12). After 12 weeks of gestation, androgens will produce only clitoral hypertrophy. Rarely, ambiguous genitalia that superficially resemble those produced by androgens are the result of other teratogenic factors.

Congenital Adrenal Hyperplasia (Figure 44–13)

There are 6 major types of congenital adrenal hyperplasia (CAH), all transmitted as autosomal recessive disorders. The common denominator of all 6 types is a defect in the synthesis of cortisol that results in an increase in ACTH and consequently in adrenal

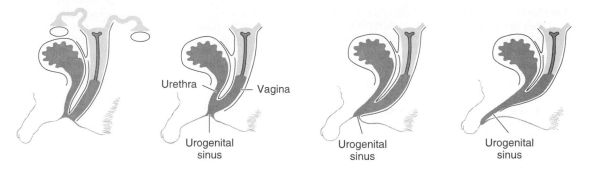

Figure 44–12. Female pseudohermaphroditism induced by prenatal exposure to androgens. Exposure after the 12th fetal week leads only to clitoral hypertrophy (diagram at left). Exposure at progressively earlier stages of differentiation (depicted from left to right in drawings) leads to retention of the urogenital sinus and labioscrotal fusion. If exposure occurs sufficiently early, the labia will fuse to form a penile urethra. (Reproduced, with permission, from Grumbach MM, Ducharme J: The effects of androgens on fetal sexual development: Androgen-induced female pseudohermaphroditism. Fertil Steril 1960;11:757.)

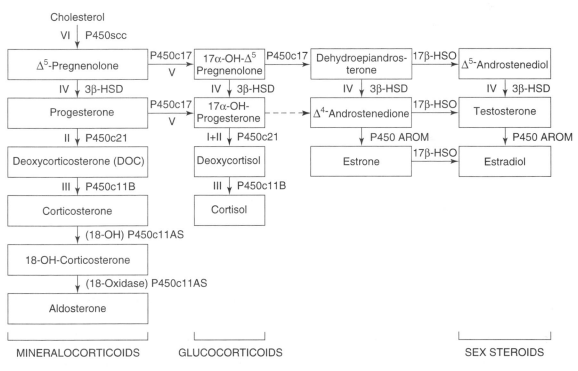

Figure 44–13. A diagrammatic representation of the steroid biosynthetic pathways in the adrenal and gonads. I–VI correspond to enzymes whose deficiency results in congenital adrenal hyperplasia. (OH, hydroxy or hydroxylase; 3β-HSD, 3β-hydroxysteroid dehydrogenase and Δ⁵-isomerase; 17β-HSO, 17β-hydroxysteroid oxidoreductase (dehydrogenase); P450scc, cholesterol side-chain cleavage, previously termed 20,22 desmolase; P450c21, 21-hydroxylase; P450c17, 17-hydroxylase; P450arom, aromatase. P450c17 also mediates 17,20-lyase activity; P450c11AS (aldosterone synthetase) mediates 18-hydroxylase and 18-oxidase reactions; P450c11B mediates 11-hydroxylation of deoxycortisol to cortisol and DOC to corticosterone. The dashed arrow indicates that conversion of 17a-OH progesterone to Δ⁴ androstenedione occurs at a low rate in humans. (Modified and reproduced, with permission, from Conte FA, Grumbach MM. Pathogenesis, classification, diagnosis, and treatment of anomalies of sex. In: DeGroot L [editor]: *Endocrinology.* Grune & Stratton, 1989.)

hyperplasia. Both males and females can be affected, but males are rarely diagnosed at birth unless they have ambiguous genitalia, are salt losers and manifest adrenal crises, are identified during newborn screening, or are at known risk because they have an affected sibling. Defects of types I–III are confined to the adrenal gland and produce virilization. Defects of types IV–VI have in common blocks in cortisol and sex steroid synthesis in both the adrenals and the gonads. The latter 3 types produce chiefly incomplete masculinization in the male and little or no virilization in the female (Table 44–5). Consequently, these will be discussed primarily as forms of male pseudohermaphroditism.

P450c21 Hydroxylase Deficiency

21-Hydroxylase activity in mediated by P450c21, a microsomal cytochrome P450 enzyme. A deficiency of this enzyme results in the most common type of adrenal hyperplasia, with an overall prevalence of 1:14,000 live births in whites. Over 95% of patients with CAH have 21-hydroxylase deficiency. The locus for the gene that encodes 21-hydroxylation is on the short arm of chromosome 6, close to the locus for C4 (complement) between HLA-B and HLA-D. DNA analysis has detected 2 genes, designated *P450c21A* and *P450c21B*, in this region in tandem with the 2 genes for complement, *C4A* and *C4B*. *P450c21A* is a nonfunctional "pseudogene," ie, it is missing critical sequences and does not encode a functional 21-hydroxylase. Patients with P450c21B (21α-hydroxylase) deficiency have either a point mutation, a deletion, or a "gene conversion" (the transfer of nonfunctioning sequences from the *21-OHA* gene to the *21-OHB* gene)

in the *P450c21B* gene. Seventy-five percent of patients with "classic" P450c21 deficiency have point mutations that change a small portion of the *P450c21B* to a sequence similar to that in the nonfunctional *P450c21A* gene—hence a "microgene conversion." The remainder have gene deletions and macrogene conversions. Recent work has demonstrated that classic salt-wasting 21-hydroxylase deficiency is associated with a mutation, deletion, or gene conversion that abolishes or severely reduces 21-hydroxylase activity. Most patients with 21-hydroxylase deficiency are compound heterozygotes, ie, they have a different genetic lesion in each of their *P450c21B* allelic genes. The phenotypic spectrum observed—salt loss, simple virilization, or late onset of virilization—is a consequence of the degree of enzymatic deficiency. The latter is determined by the functionally less severely mutated *P450c21B* allele. The gene for P450c21 (21-hydroxylase) deficiency is not only closely linked to the HLA supergene complex, but certain specific HLA subtypes are found to be statistically increased in patients with 21-hydroxylase deficiency. These include Bw51 in the simple virilizing form, Bw47 in the salt-losing form, and B14 in the nonclassic form.

A. Type I—P450c21 Hydroxylase Deficiency With Virilization: This defect in P450c21 (21-hydroxylase) activity results in impaired cortisol synthesis, increased ACTH levels, and increased adrenal androgen precursor and androgen secretion. Before 12 weeks of gestation, high fetal androgen levels lead to a varying degree of labioscrotal fusion and clitoral enlargement in the female fetus; exposure to androgen after 12 weeks induces clitoromegaly alone. In the male fetus, no abnormalities in the external genitalia are evident at birth, but the phallus may be enlarged.

Table 44–5. Clinical manifestations of the various types of congenital adrenal hyperplasia.

Enzymatic Defect Type	StAR[1] VI		3β-Hydroxysteroid Dehydrogenase IV		P-450c17 (17 α-Hydroxylase) V		P-450c11 (11β-Hydroxylase) III		P-450c21 (21α-Hydroxylase) II and I	
Chromosomal	XX	XY	XX	XY	XX	XY	XX	XY	XX	XY
External genitalia	Female	Female	Female (clitorimegaly)[2]	Ambiguous	Female	Female or ambiguous	Ambiguous[2]	Male	Ambiguous[2]	Male
Postnatal virilization	Puberty 2° amenorrhea	Sexual infantilism at puberty	±	Mild to moderate	(Sexual infantilism at puberty)		+		+	
Addisonian crises	+		±		–		–		+ in 80% (type II)	
Hypertension	–		–		+		+		–	

[1]StAR: Steroidogenic acute regulatory protein. StAR deficiency leads secondarily to P450scc deficiency.
[2]Normal female in late-onset and "cryptic" forms.
(Reproduced, with permission, from Grumbach MM, Conte FA: Disorders of sex differentiation. In: Wilson JD et al [editors]: *Williams Textbook of Endocrinology*, 9th ed. Saunders, 1998.)

These patients produce sufficient amounts of aldosterone to prevent the signs and symptoms of mineralocorticoid deficiency, although they may have a defect in mineralocorticoid synthesis as evidenced by an elevated plasma renin level. Virilization continues after birth in untreated patients. This results in rapid growth and bone maturation as well as the physical signs of excess androgen secretion (eg, acne, seborrhea, increased muscular development, premature development of pubic or axillary hair, and phallic enlargement). True (central) precocious puberty can occur following initiation of glucocorticoid therapy in affected children with peripubertal bone ages.

Mild defects in P450c21 (21-hydroxylase) activity have been reported. Patients can be symptomatic (late-onset or nonclassic) or asymptomatic ("cryptic" form). These mild forms of P450c21 hydroxylase deficiency are HLA-linked, as is "classic" P450c21 hydroxylase deficiency; however, they occur much more frequently than the classic form of the disease. It has been postulated that "nonclassic" P450c21 hydroxylase deficiency is the most common autosomal recessive disorder, affecting about 1 in 100 persons of all ethnic groups but having an incidence 2–3 times higher in Hispanics and Ashkenazi Jews. Females with late-onset P450c21 hydroxylase deficiency have normal female genitalia at birth and do not have an electrolyte abnormality. Mild virilization occurs later in childhood and adolescence, resulting in the premature development of pubic or axillary hair, slight clitoral enlargement, menstrual irregularities, acne, hirsutism, polycystic ovary syndrome, and an advanced bone age. Affected males have normal male genitalia at birth, rapid growth, and advanced skeletal maturation. Later in childhood, they exhibit premature growth of pubic or axillary hair, sexual precocity with inappropriately small testes, and increased muscular development. While tall as children, they end up as short adults due to advanced bone maturation and premature epiphysial fusion. Asymptomatic individuals who have the same biochemical abnormalities as patients with mild forms of P450c21 hydroxylase deficiency have been detected by hormonal testing of families in which there is at least one member with symptoms.

B. P450c21 Hydroxylase Deficiency With Virilization and Salt Loss: The salt-losing variant of P450c21 hydroxylase deficiency accounts for about 80% of patients with classic 21-hydroxylase deficiency and involves a more severe deficit of P450c21 hydroxylase, which leads to impaired secretion of both cortisol and aldosterone. This results in electrolyte and fluid losses after the fifth day of life and, as a consequence, hyponatremia, hyperkalemia, acidosis, dehydration, and vascular collapse. Masculinization of the external genitalia of affected females tends to be more severe than that found in patients with simple P450c21 hydroxylase deficiency. Affected males may have macrogenitosomia.

The diagnosis of P450c21 hydroxylase deficiency should always be considered (1) in patients with ambiguous genitalia who have a 46,XX karyotype (and are thus female pseudohermaphrodites); (2) in apparent cryptorchid males; (3) in any infant who presents with shock, hypoglycemia, and chemical findings compatible with adrenal insufficiency; and (4) in males and females with signs of virilization before puberty, including premature adrenarche. In the past, the diagnosis of P450c21 hydroxylase deficiency was based on the finding of elevated levels of 17-ketosteroids and pregnanetriol in the urine. Although still valid and useful, urinary steroid determinations have been replaced by the simpler and more cost-effective measurement of plasma 17-hydroxyprogesterone, androstenedione, and testosterone levels.

The concentration of plasma 17-hydroxyprogesterone is elevated in umbilical cord blood but rapidly decreases into the range of 1–2 µg/L (3–6 nmol/L) by 24 h after delivery. In premature infants and in stressed full-term newborns, the levels of 17-hydroxyprogesterone are higher than those observed in nonstressed full-term infants. In patients with P450c21 hydroxylase deficiency, the 17-hydroxyprogesterone values usually range from 50 to 400 µg/L (150–1200 nmol/L), depending on the age of the patient and the severity of P450c21 hydroxylase deficiency. Patients with mild P450c21 hydroxylase deficiency, ie, late-onset and cryptic forms, may have borderline basal 17-hydroxyprogesterone values, but they can be distinguished from heterozygotes by the magnitude of the 17-hydroxyprogesterone response to the parenteral administration of ACTH.

Salt losers may be ascertained clinically or by chemical evidence of hyponatremia and hyperkalemia on a regular infant diet. In these patients, aldosterone levels in both plasma and urine are low in relation to the serum sodium concentration, while plasma renin activity is elevated. Breast milk and many infant formulas have a low concentration of sodium.

HLA typing, measurement of amniotic fluid 17-hydroxyprogesterone levels, and chorionic villus biopsy with HLA typing and gene analysis have been used in the prenatal diagnosis of affected fetuses. Data indicate that prenatal therapy with dexamethasone given to the mother early in pregnancy can lessen the genital ambiguity seen in affected newborn females; however, the use of this therapy is controversial. While the immediate effects of maternal dexamethasone therapy on reducing masculinization of the female external genitalia may be striking, long-term studies are needed to exclude late untoward effects.

Heterozygosity has been ascertained by HLA typing in informative families, by the use of ACTH-induced rises in plasma 17-hydroxyprogesterone levels, and by genetic analysis. Measurement of plasma 17-hydroxyprogesterone levels using heel-stick capillary blood specimens blotted onto paper has been shown to be a useful and valid screening tool for the diagnosis of 21-hydroxylase deficiency in newborn infants.

C. P450c11 Hydroxylase Deficiency: (Virilization with hypertension.) Classic P450c11 hydroxylase deficiency is rare; however, it is the second most common form of CAH, representing 5–8% of all cases. It occurs in 1:100,000 births in persons of European ancestry. However, in Middle Eastern people, it is much more common. In the classic patient, a defect in 11-hydroxylation leads to decreased cortisol levels with a consequent increase in ACTH and the hypersecretion of 11-deoxycorticosterone and 11-deoxycortisol in addition to adrenal androgens. Marked heterogeneity in the clinical and hormonal manifestations of this defect has been described, including mild, late-onset, and even "cryptic" forms. Patients with this form of adrenal hyperplasia classically exhibit virilization secondary to increased androgen production and hypertension related to increased 11-deoxycorticosterone secretion. Plasma renin activity is either normal or suppressed. The hypertension is not invariable; it occurs in approximately two-thirds of patients and may be associated with hypokalemic alkalosis.

Two P450c11 hydroxlyase genes have been localized to the long arm of chromosome 8: *P450c11β* and *P450c11AS*. Similar to 21-hydroxylase, these 2 genes are 95% homologous. *P450c11β* encodes the enzyme for 11-hydroxylation and is expressed in the zona fasciculata and reticularis and is ACTH-dependent. It primarily mediates 11-hydroxylation of 11-deoxycortisol to cortisol and deoxycorticosterone (DOC) to corticosterone. It has about one-twelfth the capacity of P450c11AS for 18-hydroxylation and does not oxidize 18-hydroxycorticosterone to aldosterone. *P450c11AS* encodes the angiotensin-dependent isozyme aldosterone synthetase and is only expressed in the zona glomerulosa, where it mediates 11-hydroxylation, 18-hydroxylation, and 18 oxidation. Mutations, deletions, and gene duplications can produce a wide variety of clinical manifestations from virilization and hypertension (*P450c11β* deficiency) to isolated salt wasting (P450c11AS-aldosterone synthetase deficiency) to glucocorticoid remedial hypertension (due to fusion of the ACTH-dependent regulatory region of the 11-hydroxylase gene with the coding region of aldosterone synthetase). Both the gene encoding *P450c11β* and *P450c11AS* are located on chromosome 8, and as such are not linked to HLA. ACTH stimulation tests have thus far failed to demonstrate a consistent biochemical abnormality in obligate heterozygotes.

The diagnosis of P450c11β-hydroxylase deficiency can be confirmed by demonstration of elevated plasma levels of 11-deoxycortisol and 11-deoxycorticosterone and increased excretion of their metabolites in urine (mainly tetrahydro-11-deoxycortisol) either in the basal state or after the administration of ACTH. Prenatal diagnosis can be made by genetic analysis of chorionic tissue or amniotic fluid cells.

D. Type IV—3β-Hydroxysteroid Dehydrogenase Deficiency: (Male or female pseudohermaphroditism and adrenal insufficiency.) See below.

E. Type V—P450c17 Deficiency: (Male pseudohermaphroditism, sexual infantilism, hypertension and hypokalemic alkalosis.) See below.

F. Type VI—StAR Deficiency: (Congenital lipoid adrenal hyperplasia, male pseudohermaphroditism, sexual infantilism, and adrenal insufficiency.) See below.

Treatment

Treatment of patients with adrenal hyperplasia may be divided into acute and chronic phases. In acute adrenal crises, a deficiency of both cortisol and aldosterone results in hypoglycemia, hyponatremia, hyperkalemia, hypovolemia, acidosis, and shock. If the patient is hypoglycemic, an intravenous bolus of glucose, 0.25–0.5 g/kg (maximum 25 g) should be administered. If the patient is in shock, an infusion of normal saline (20 mL/kg) may be given over the first hour; thereafter, replacement of glucose, fluid, and electrolytes is calculated on the basis of deficits and standard maintenance requirements. Hydrocortisone sodium succinate, 50 mg/m^2, should be given as a bolus and another 50–100 mg/m^2 added to the infusion fluid over the first 24 h of therapy. If hyponatremia and hyperkalemia are present, 0.05–0.1 mg of fludrocortisone by mouth may be given along with the intravenous saline and hydrocortisone. Since hydrocortisone has mineralocorticoid activity, it may suffice to correct the electrolyte abnormality along with the saline. In extreme cases of hyponatremia, hyperkalemia, and acidosis, sodium bicarbonate and a cation exchange resin (eg, sodium polystyrene sulfonate) may be needed.

Once the patient is stabilized and a definitive diagnosis has been arrived at by means of appropriate steroid studies, the patient should receive maintenance doses of glucocorticoids to permit normal growth, development, and bone maturation (hydrocortisone, approximately 12–18 mg/m^2/d by mouth in 3 divided doses). The dose of hydrocortisone must be titrated in each patient, depending on steroid hormone levels in plasma and urine, linear growth, bone maturation, and clinical signs of steroid overdose or of virilization. Salt losers need treatment with mineralocorticoid (fludrocortisone, 0.05–0.2 mg/d by mouth) and added dietary salt (1–3 g/d). The dose of mineralocorticoid should be adjusted so that the electrolytes and blood pressure, as well as the plasma renin activity, are in the normal range.

Patients with ambiguous external genitalia should have plastic repair before age 1 year. Clitoral recession or clitoroplasty—*not clitoridectomy!*—is indicated. Of major importance to the family with an affected child is the assurance that the child will grow and develop into a normal adult. In patients with the most common form of adrenal hyperplasia—21-hydroxylase deficiency—fertility in males and feminization, menstruation, and fertility in females can be expected with adequate treatment. Long-term psychological guidance and support by the physician for the patient and family is essential.

Adrenal rests in the testes of males with P450c21 hydroxylase deficiency (especially salt losers) may enlarge under the stimulus of ACTH and be mistaken for testicular neoplasms. These adrenal rests are often bilateral and are made up of cells that appear indistinguishable from Leydig cells histologically except that they lack Reinke crystalloids. The rests are usually seen in noncompliant or undertreated patients. To prevent this complication as well as the risk of adrenal crisis, pituitary basophil hyperplasia, and adrenal carcinoma, continuous treatment with a glucocorticoid (and, if indicated, a mineralocorticoid) is recommended even in adult males.

P450 AROMATASE DEFICIENCY

Recently, a new form of androgen-induced female pseudohermaphroditism has been defined that is due to aromatase deficiency. Mutations in the gene encoding P450arom result in defective placental conversion of C_{19} steroids to estrogens leading to exposure of the fetus to excessive amounts of testosterone and masculinization of the external genitalia of the female fetus. Virilization of the mother during gestation can also occur. At puberty, defective aromatase activity in the gonads leads to pubertal failure, hypergonadotropic hypogonadism, polycystic ovaries, mild virilization, tall stature, and osteoporosis. A striking delay in bone age occurs despite increased concentrations of plasma testosterone, supporting the concept that estrogens rather than androgens are the major sex steroids affecting bone maturation and bone turnover in females as well as males. The diagnosis of aromatase deficiency is suggested by the finding of the above clinical picture and elevated plasma androstenedione and testosterone levels in the face of low estrogen levels.

MATERNAL ANDROGENS & PROGESTOGENS

Masculinization of the external genitalia of a female infant can occur if the mother is given testosterone, other androgenic steroids, or certain synthetic progestational agents during pregnancy. After the 12th week of gestation, exposure results in clitorimegaly alone. Norethindrone, ethisterone, norethynodrel, and medroxyprogesterone acetate have all been implicated in masculinization of the female fetus. Nonadrenal female pseudohermaphroditism can occur as a consequence of maternal ingestion of danazol, the 2,3-*d*-isoxazole derivative of 17α-ethinyl testosterone. In rare instances, masculinization of a female fetus is due to a virilizing maternal ovarian or adrenal tumor, congenital virilizing adrenal hyperplasia in the mother, or a luteoma of pregnancy. The fetus is protected from excess androgen exposure by the ability of the fetal-placental unit to aromatize androgens to estrogens, especially after the first trimester.

The diagnosis of female pseudohermaphroditism arising from transplacental passage of androgenic steroids is based on exclusion of other forms of female pseudohermaphroditism and a history of drug exposure. Surgical correction of the genitalia, if needed, is the only therapy necessary.

Nonadrenal female pseudohermaphroditism can be associated with imperforate anus, renal anomalies, and other malformations of the lower intestine and urinary tract. Sporadic as well as familial cases have been reported.

MALE PSEUDOHERMAPHRODITISM

Male pseudohermaphrodites have gonads that are testes, but the genital ducts or external genitalia, or both, are not completely masculinized. Male pseudohermaphroditism can result from deficient testosterone secretion as a consequence of (1) defective testicular differentiation (testicular dysgenesis), (2) impaired secretion of testosterone or antimüllerian hormone, (3) failure of target tissue response to testosterone and dihydrotestosterone or antimüllerian hormone, and (4) failure of conversion of testosterone to dihydrotestosterone.

Testicular Unresponsiveness to hCG & LH

Male sexual differentiation is dependent upon the production of testosterone by fetal Leydig cells. Leydig cell testosterone secretion is under the influence of placental hCG during the critical period of male sexual differentiation and, thereafter, fetal pituitary LH during gestation.

The finding of normal male sexual differentiation in XY males with anencephaly, apituitarism, or congenital hypothalamic hypopituitarism suggests that male sex differentiation in the human occurs independently of the secretion of fetal pituitary gonadotropins.

Absence, hypoplasia, or unresponsiveness of Leydig cells to hCG-LH results in deficient testosterone production and, consequently, male pseudohermaphroditism. The extent of the genital ambiguity is a function of the degree of testosterone deficiency, and the phenotype has ranged from extreme forms with female external genitalia to milder forms with micropenis and to males with normal male genitalia and hypergonadotropic hypogonadism at puberty. A small number of patients with absent, hypoplastic, or unresponsive Leydig cells due to a mutation in the gene encoding the LH-hCG receptor have been reported as well as an animal model, the "vet" rat. In most of the patients thus far reported, the defect resulted in female-appearing genitalia and a short blind-ending vagina. Müllerian duct regression was complete. Basal gonadotropin levels as well as GnRH-evoked responses were elevated in postpubertal patients. Plasma 17α-hydroxyprogesterone, androstenedione, and testosterone levels were low, and hCG elicited little or no response in testosterone or its precursors. In 2 siblings with the extreme phenotype of this syndrome, a homozygous missense mutation in exon 11 of the LH receptor gene was found. This mutation resulted in an alanine-to-proline change in the sixth transmembrane domain of the LH receptor and a nonfunctional receptor. At least 7 other inactivating mutations of the LH receptor gene have been described in unrelated families with LH resistance. These mutations have resulted in a variable degree of hCG-LH resistance and a variable phenotype in the affected XY individual. The phenotype extends from that of a female, to that of am-biguous external genitalia, to that of a male with micropenis. Treatment depends on the age at diagnosis and the extent of masculinization. A female sex assignment has usually been chosen in patients with female-appearing genitalia.

Inborn Errors of Testosterone Biosynthesis

Figure 44–14 demonstrates the major pathways in testosterone biosynthesis in the gonads; each step is associated with an inherited defect that results in testosterone deficiency and, consequently, male pseudohermaphroditism. Steps 1, 2, and 3 are enzymatic deficiencies that occur in both the adrenals and gonads and result in defective synthesis of both corticosteroids and testosterone. Thus, they represent forms of congenital adrenal hyperplasia.

A. StAR Deficiency and Congenital Lipoid Adrenal Hyperplasia: (Male pseudohermaphroditism, sexual infantilism, and adrenal insufficiency.) This is a very early defect in the synthesis of all

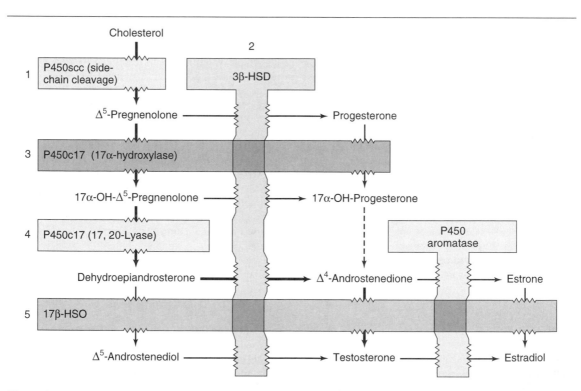

Figure 44–14. Enzymatic defects in the biosynthetic pathway for testosterone. All 5 of the enzymatic defects cause male pseudohermaphroditism in affected males. Although all of the blocks affect gonadal steroidogenesis, those at steps 1, 2, and 3 are associated with major abnormalities in the biosynthesis of glucocorticoids and mineralocorticoids in the adrenal. Patients with apparent P450scc deficiency have a mutation in StAR (steroidogenic acute regulatory protein), a protein necessary for the transport of cholesterol from outer to inner mitochondrial membrane where P450scc resides. (OH, hydroxy; 3β-HSD, 3β-hydroxysteroid dehydrogenase; 17β-HSO, 17β-hydroxysteroid oxidoreductase (dehydrogenase). Chemical names for enzymes are shown with traditional names in parentheses. (Modified and reproduced, with permission, from Conte FA, Grumbach MM. Pathogenesis, classification, diagnosis, and treatment of anomalies of sex. In: DeGroot L [editor]: *Endocrinology.* Grune & Stratton, 1989.)

steroids affecting the conversion of cholesterol to Δ^5-pregnenolone and results in severe adrenal and gonadal deficiency. The *P450scc* gene has been isolated, cloned, and localized to chromosome 15. However, thus far, molecular analysis of this gene has not revealed a defect in affected patients with this syndrome. Mutations in a steroidogenic acute regulatory protein (StAR) that is necessary for the transport of cholesterol from the outer to the inner mitochondrial membrane, the site of P450scc, have been identified in patients with the clinical syndrome of congenital lipoid adrenal hyperplasia. StAR is expressed in the adrenals and gonads but not in the placenta; hence, placental synthesis of progesterone, which is required to maintain pregnancy in humans, is apparently not affected. A mutation in the *P450scc* gene resulting in a deficit of side-chain cleavage enzymatic activity most likely would be lethal, as it is essential for progesterone synthesis by the human fetoplacental unit.

Affected males usually have female external genitalia with a blind vaginal pouch and hypoplastic male genital ducts but no müllerian derivatives; the genitalia of affected females are normal. Large lipid-laden adrenals that displace the kidneys downward may be demonstrated by intravenous urography, abdominal ultrasonography, or computed tomography scan. Death in early infancy from adrenal insufficiency is not uncommon. The diagnosis is confirmed by the lack of or low levels of all C_{21}, C_{19}, and C_{18} steroids in plasma and urine and an absent response to ACTH and hCG stimulation. Treatment involves replacement with appropriate doses of glucocorticoids and mineralocorticoids.

B. 3β-Hydroxysteroid Dehydrogenase and D⁵-Isomerase Deficiency: (Male or female pseudohermaphroditism and adrenal insufficiency.) 3β-Hydroxysteroid dehydrogenase and Δ^5-isomerase deficiency is an early defect in steroid synthesis that results in inability of the adrenals and gonads to convert 3β-hydroxy-Δ^5 steroids to 3-keto-Δ^4 steroids. This enzyme is encoded for by a gene on the short arm of chromosome number 1. Recent data indicate that there are 2 highly homologous genes encoding 3β-hydroxysteroid dehydrogenase on chromosome 1. The type I 3β-hydroxysteroid dehydrogenase gene is expressed in the placenta and peripheral tissues, while type II is expressed in the adrenals and gonads. 3β-Hydroxysteroid dehydrogenase is not a cytochrome P450 enzyme, and it requires NAD^+ as a cofactor. Mutations causing frame shifts, stops, and missense have been reported in the type II gene in affected patients. This defect in its complete form results in a severe deficiency of aldosterone, cortisol, testosterone, and estradiol secretion. Males with this defect are incompletely masculinized, and females have mild clitorimegaly. Salt loss and adrenal crises usually occur in early infancy in affected patients. Affected males may experience normal male puberty but often have prominent gynecomastia. Patients with a mild non-salt-losing form of 3β-hydroxysteroid dehydrogenase deficiency have been described as well as late-onset patients presenting with only premature pubarche. These patients were shown to have elevated Δ^5 steroids as well as mutations in the 3β-hydroxysteroid type II gene.

The diagnosis of 3β-hydroxysteroid dehydrogenase deficiency is based on finding elevated concentrations of Δ^5-pregnenolone, Δ^5-17α-hydroxypregnenolone, dehydroepiandrosterone (DHEA) and its sulfate, and other 3β-hydroxy-Δ^5 steroids in the plasma and urine of patients with a consistent clinical picture. 3-keto-Δ^4 steroids, ie, 17-hydroxyprogesterone and androstenedione, may be elevated owing to peripheral conversion of 3β-hydroxy-Δ^5 to 3-keto-Δ^4 steroids by the enzyme encoded by the type 1 gene. The diagnosis of 3β-hydroxysteroid dehydrogenase deficiency may be facilitated by detecting abnormal levels of serum Δ^5-17α-hydroxypregnenolone and DHEA and its sulfates as well as abnormal ratios of Δ^5 to Δ^4 steroids after intravenous administration of 0.25 mg of synthetic ACTH. It can be confirmed by detecting a mutation in the type II β-hydroxysteroid dehydrogenase Δ^5 isomerase gene. Suppression of the increased plasma and urinary 3β-hydroxy-Δ^5 steroids by the administration of dexamethasone distinguishes 3β-hydroxysteroid dehydrogenase deficiency from a virilizing adrenal tumor. Treatment of this condition is similar to that of other forms of adrenal hyperplasia (see above).

C. P450c17 Deficiency, 17α-Hydroxylase Deficiency: (Male pseudohermaphroditism, sexual infantilism, hypertension, and hypokalemic alkalosis.) A defect in 17α-hydroxylation in the zona fasciculata of the adrenal and in the gonads results in impaired synthesis of 17-hydroxyprogesterone and 17-hydroxypregnenolone and, consequently, cortisol and sex steroids. The secretion of large amounts of corticosterone and DOC leads to hypertension, hypokalemia, and alkalosis. Increased DOC secretion with resultant hypertension produces suppression of renin and, consequently, decreased aldosterone secretion.

A single gene on chromosome 10 encodes both adrenal and testicular P450c17 hydroxylase as well as 17,20-lyase activity. This enzyme catalyzes the 17-hydroxylation of pregnenolone and progesterone to 17-hydroxypregnenolone and 17-hydroxyprogesterone as well as the scission (lyase) of 17-hydroxypregnenolone to the c19 steroid—dehydroepiandrosterone—in the adrenal cortex and gonads. Mutations affecting 17-hydroxylase activity have included stop codons, frame shifts, deletions, and missense substitutions.

The clinical manifestations result from the adrenal and gonadal defect. Affected XX females have normal development of the internal ducts and external genitalia but manifest sexual infantilism with elevated gonadotropin concentrations at puberty. Affected males have impaired testosterone synthesis by the fetal testes, which results in female or ambiguous genitalia. At adolescence, sexual infantilism, low renin hypertension, and often hypokalemia are the hallmarks of this defect.

The diagnosis of 17-hydroxylase deficiency should be suspected in XY males with female or ambiguous genitalia or XX females with sexual infantilism who also manifest hypertension associated with hypokalemic alkalosis. High levels of progesterone, Δ^5-pregnenolone, DOC, corticosterone, and 18-hydroxycorticosterone in plasma and increased excretion of their urinary metabolites establish the diagnosis. Plasma renin activity and aldosterone secretion are diminished in these patients.

Note: The following errors affect testosterone and estrogen biosynthesis in the gonads primarily.

D. P450c17 Deficiency (17,20-Lyase Deficiency): The enzyme P450c17 mediates the 17-hydroxylation of pregnenolone and progesterone to 17-hydroxypregnenolone and 17-hydroxyprogesterone as well as the scission of the $C_{17,20}$ bond of 17-hydroxypregnenolone to yield DHEA. In the human, the scission of 17-hydroxyprogesterone to androstenedione has not yet been demonstrated. Rare patients are reported to have a putative defect primarily in the scission of the C_{21} steroids to C_{19} steroids, which results in a defect in testosterone synthesis and subsequently pseudohermaphroditism in the male and impaired sex steroid synthesis and secretion in the affected 46,XX female. Two male pseudohermaphrodites from consanguineous marriages who had micropenis, perineal hypospadias, bifid scrotum, a blind vaginal pouch, and cryptorchidism have recently been studied. The administration of hCG resulted in a marked rise in plasma 17-hydroxyprogesterone with a paucity of response in plasma DHEA, androstenedione, and testosterone consistent with a diagnosis of isolated 17,20-lyase deficiency. Analyses of the 17-hydroxylase gene in these patients demonstrated one to be homozygous for an Arg347 → His mutation and the other to have an Arg358 → Gln mutation. Both of these mutations result in a specific decrease in 17,20-lyase activity of the *P450c17* gene. The finding of wolffian ducts associated with female external genitalia in these patients is as yet unexplained. Müllerian derivatives were absent as a result of the secretion of antimüllerian hormone by the fetal testes.

Patients with 17,20-lyase deficiency have low circulating levels of testosterone, androstenedione, DHEA, and estradiol. The diagnosis can be confirmed by demonstration of an increased ratio of 17-hydroxy C_{21} steroids to C_{19} steroids (testosterone, DHEA, Δ^5-androstenediol, and androstenedione) after stimulation with ACTH or hCG and by DNA analysis of the *P450c17* gene.

E. 17β-Hydroxysteroid Oxidoreductase (Dehydrogenase) Deficiency: The last step in testosterone and estradiol biosynthesis by the gonads involves the reduction of androstenedione to testosterone and estrone to estradiol. 17-Hydroxysteroid oxidoreductase is an NADPH-dependent microsomal enzyme. Two genes are found in tandem on the long arm of chromosome 17. They are 89% homologous. One gene appears to be a pseudogene because of the presence of a stop codon. A third gene has been found on chromosome 9q22. This gene is expressed primarily in the testes, and its product is 23% homologous to the other 17β-hydroxysteroid oxidoreductase enzyme. This enzyme utilizes NADPH as a cofactor and catalyzes the reduction of androstenedione to testosterone. Mutations in this gene have been described in male pseudohermaphrodites. At birth, males with a deficiency of the enzyme 17-hydroxysteroid oxidoreductase have predominantly female or mildly ambiguous external genitalia resulting from testosterone deficiency during male differentiation. They have male duct development, absent müllerian structures with a blind vaginal pouch, and inguinal or intra-abdominal testes. At puberty, progressive virilization with clitoral hypertrophy occurs, often associated with the concurrent development of gynecomastia. Plasma gonadotropin, androstenedione, and estrone levels are elevated, whereas testosterone and estradiol concentration are relatively low. A putative late-onset form of 17-hydroxysteroid oxidoreductase deficiency has been reported in a small number of postadolescent males with gynecomastia and normal male genitalia.

Analysis of 17 patients with classic 17β-hydroxysteroid dehydrogenase deficiency, including 4 from San Francisco, has revealed 14 mutations in the 17β-hydroxysteroid oxidoreductase-3 gene. Twelve patients had homozygous mutations, 4 were compound heterozygotes, and one was a presumed heterozygote. In a large cohort from the Gaza Strip, an Arg80 → Gln mutation was found with partial (15–20%) enzymatic activity.

17-Hydroxysteroid oxidoreductase deficiency should be included in the differential diagnosis of (1) male pseudohermaphrodites with absent müllerian derivatives who have no abnormality in glucocorticoid or mineralocorticoid synthesis; and (2) male pseudohermaphrodites who virilize at puberty, especially if they also exhibit gynecomastia. The diagnosis of 17-hydroxysteroid oxidoreductase deficiency is confirmed by the demonstration of inappropriately high plasma levels of estrone and androstenedione and increased ratios of plasma androstenedione to testosterone and estrone to estradiol before and after stimulation with hCG.

Management of the patients, as of those with other forms of male pseudohermaphroditism, depends on the age at diagnosis and the degree of ambiguity of the external genitalia. In the patient assigned a male gender identity, plastic repair of the genitalia and testosterone augmentation of phallic growth prepubertally as well as testosterone replacement therapy at puberty is indicated. In patients reared as females (the usual case), the appropriate treatment is castration, followed by estrogen replacement therapy at puberty.

Defects in Androgen-Dependent Target Tissues

The complex mechanism of action of steroid hormones at the cellular level has recently been clarified (Figure 44–15).

Free testosterone enters the target cells and undergoes 5α reduction to dihydrotestosterone. Dihydrotestosterone binds to the intracellular androgen receptor, inducing a conformational change that facilitates the release of heat shock protein, nuclear transport, dimerization, and binding to the specific hormone response elements of DNA. It initiates transcription, translation, and protein synthesis that leads to androgenic actions. A lack of androgen effect at the end organ and, consequently, male pseudohermaphroditism may result from abnormalities in 5α-reductase activity, transformation of the steroid-receptor complex, receptor binding of dihydrotestosterone, receptor-ligand complex binding to DNA, transcription, exportation, or translation.

End-Organ Resistance to Androgenic Hormones (Androgen Receptor Defects)

A. Syndrome of Complete Androgen Resistance and Its Variants (Testicular Feminization): The syndrome of complete androgen resistance (testicular feminization) is characterized by a 46,XY karyotype, bilateral testes, absent or hypoplastic wolffian ducts, female-appearing external genitalia with a hypoplastic clitoris and labia minora, a blind vaginal pouch, and absent or rudimentary müllerian derivatives (33%). At puberty, female secondary sexual characteristics develop, but menarche does not ensue. Pubic and axillary hair is usually sparse and in one-third of patients is totally absent. Affected patients are taller than average females. Some patients have a variant form of this syndrome and exhibit slight clitoral enlargement. These patients may exhibit mild virilization in addition to the development of breasts and a female habitus.

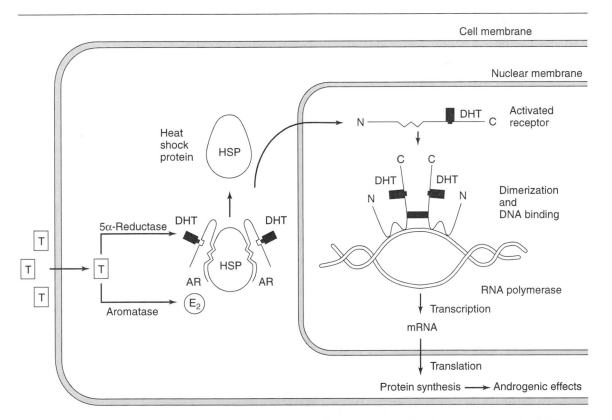

Figure 44–15. Diagrammatic representation of the putative mechanism of action of testosterone on target cells. Testosterone (T) enters the cells, where it is either 5α-reduced to dihydrotestosterone (DHT) or aromatized to estradiol (E₂). Dihydrotestosterone binds to the androgen receptor (AR) in the nucleus and "activates" it with the release of heat shock proteins (HSP). The activated AR complex then binds as a dimer (not shown) to specific hormone response elements of the DNA and initiates transcription, translation, and protein synthesis, with consequent androgenic effects. N, amino terminus; C, COOH terminus. (Reproduced, with permission, from Conte FA, Grumbach MM: Abnormalities of sexual determination and differentiation. In: Greenspan FS, Strewler GJ [editors]: *Basic and Clinical Endocrinology,* 5th ed. Appleton & Lange, 1997.)

Androgen resistance during embryogenesis prevents masculinization of the external genitalia and differentiation of the wolffian ducts. Secretion of antimüllerian hormone by the fetal Sertoli cells leads to regression of the müllerian ducts. Thus, affected patients are born with female external genitalia and a blind vaginal pouch. At puberty, androgen resistance results in augmented LH secretion with subsequent increases in testosterone and estradiol. Estradiol arises from peripheral conversion of testosterone and androstenedione as well as from direct secretion by the testes. Androgen resistance coupled with increased testicular estradiol secretion and conversion of androgens to estrogens result in the development of female secondary sexual characteristics at puberty.

The androgen receptor gene is located on the X chromosome between Xq11 and Xq13. The gene is composed of 8 exons, numbered 1 through 8. Exon 1 encodes the amino-terminal end of the androgen receptor protein and is thought to play a role in transcription. Exons 2 and 3 encode the DNA-binding zinc finger of the androgen receptor protein. The 5′ portion of exon 4 is called the hinge region and plays a role in nuclear targeting. Exons 5–8 specify the carboxyl terminal portion of the androgen receptor, which is the androgen binding domain (Figure 44–16).

Patients with complete androgen resistance have been found to be heterogeneous with respect to dihydrotestosterone binding to the androgen receptor. Receptor-negative and receptor-positive individuals with qualitative defects such as thermolability, instability, and impaired binding affinity as well as individuals with presumed normal binding have been described. Analysis of the androgen receptor gene has shed light on the pathogenesis of the heterogeneity in receptor studies found in patients with complete androgen resistance. Patients with the receptor-negative form of complete androgen resistance have been found to have primarily point mutations or substitutions in exons 5–8, which encode the androgen-binding domain of the receptor. Most of the mutations are familial in nature. Other defects such as deletions, mutations in a splice donor site, and point mutations causing premature termination codons are less common in this group of patients. Mutations in exon 3 (which encodes the DNA-binding segment of the androgen receptor) are associated with normal binding of androgen to the receptor but inability of the ligand-receptor complex to bind to DNA and thus to initiate mRNA transcription. These mutations result in receptor-positive complete androgen resistance. The phenotype of the affected patient does not correlate as well with the receptor studies but does correlate with the transcriptional activity of the ligand-androgen receptor complex.

The diagnosis of complete androgen resistance can be suspected from the clinical features. Before puberty, the presence of testislike masses in the inguinal canal or labia in a phenotypic female suggests the

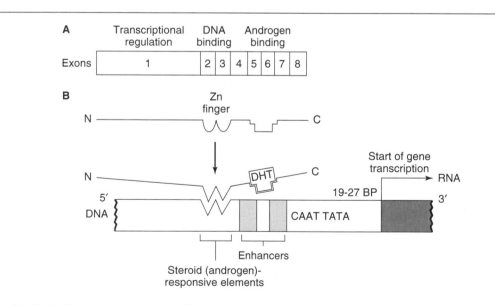

Figure 44–16. A: Diagrammatic representation of the androgen receptor gene divided into its 8 exons. Exon 1 encodes the NH$_2$-terminal domain and regulates transcription. Exons 2 and 3 encode 2 zinc fingers. Exons 4–8 encode the androgen-binding domain of the receptor. **B:** The organization of a steroid-responsive gene. Ligand binding activates the receptor, and it binds to the steroid response elements of the gene (as a dimer; not shown). Enhancers as well as a CAAT and a TATA box are present. Gene transcription begins 19–27 base pairs downstream of the TATA box. (Reproduced, with permission, from Grumbach MM, Conte FA: Disorders of sex differentiation. In: Wilson JD et al [editors]: *Williams Textbook of Endocrinology,* 9th ed. Saunders, 1998.)

diagnosis. Postpubertally, the patients present with primary amenorrhea, normal breast development, and absent or sparse pubic or axillary hair. Pelvic examination or ultrasound confirms the absence of a cervix and uterus.

The complete and incomplete forms (Reifenstein syndrome) of androgen resistance must be distinguished from other forms of male pseudohermaphroditism due to androgen deficiency or to 5α-reductase deficiency. Unfortunately, there is no readily available, rapid in vivo or in vitro assay for androgen sensitivity. The diagnosis is suggested by the clinical picture, the family history, and the presence of elevated basal and hCG-induced testosterone levels with normal levels of dihydrotestosterone. A lack of decrease in sex hormone-binding globulin levels after a short course of the anabolic steroid stanozolol has been suggested as a biologic test for androgen resistance. However, few or no confirmatory data on this assay have yet been reported. Also, one would expect that some patients with incomplete androgen resistance might respond to this test in somewhat the same way as normal individuals. It has been suggested that an elevated antimüllerian hormone level is a marker of androgen resistance and androgen deficiency. Abnormalities in androgen binding and mutational analysis as well as studies of transactivation are all diagnostic, but they are time-consuming, labor-intensive, and not universally available. In the infant with ambiguous genitalia in whom the sex of rearing is in question, we have used a trial of testosterone enanthate in oil, 25 mg intramuscularly monthly for 3 months, as a predictive test of androgen responsiveness and future phallic growth before deciding on a sex of rearing.

Therapy of patients with complete androgen resistance involves affirmation and reinforcement of their female gender identity. Castration, either before or after puberty, is indicated because of the increased risk of gonadal neoplasms with age. Estrogen replacement therapy is required at the age of puberty in orchidectomized patients. In most cases, vaginal reconstructive surgery is not required.

B. Syndrome of Incomplete Androgen Resistance and Its Variants (Reifenstein Syndrome): Patients with incomplete androgen resistance manifest a wide spectrum of phenotypes as far as the degree of masculinization is concerned. The external genitalia at birth can range from ambiguous, with a blind vaginal pouch, to hypoplastic male genitalia. Müllerian duct derivatives are absent and wolffian duct derivatives present, but they are usually hypoplastic. At puberty, virilization recapitulates that seen in utero and is generally poor; pubic and axillary hair as well as gynecomastia are usually present. The most common phenotype postpubertally is the male with perineoscrotal hypospadias and gynecomastia. Axillary and pubic hair are normal. The testes remain small and exhibit azoospermia as a consequence of germinal cell arrest. As in the case of patients with

complete androgen resistance, there are elevated levels of plasma LH, testosterone, and estradiol. However, the degree of feminization in these patients despite high estradiol levels is less than that found in the syndrome of complete androgen resistance.

Androgen receptor studies in these patients have usually shown quantitative or qualitative abnormalities in androgen binding. It would be expected that mutations that lead to partial reduction of androgen action would result in incomplete virilization. As previously noted, the best correlation to phenotype is the degree of impairment of transcriptional activity of the ligand-androgen receptor complex. A wide variety of androgen receptor gene mutations can result in the same phenotype, and a specific mutation may not always be associated with the same phenotype in all affected patients. In general, point mutations that result in more conservative amino acid substitutions are more likely to result in partial rather than complete androgen resistance.

Androgen Resistance in Men With Normal Male Genitalia

Partial androgen resistance has been described in a group of infertile men who have a normal male phenotype but may exhibit gynecomastia. Unlike other patients with androgen resistance, some of these patients have normal plasma LH and testosterone levels. Infertility in otherwise normal men may be the only clinical manifestation of androgen resistance. However, infertility may not always be associated with androgen resistance. A family has been described in which there were 5 males with gynecomastia, all of them with a small phallus. Plasma testosterone levels were elevated, and a subtle qualitative abnormality in ligand binding was noted. Fertility was documented in 4 of the 5 males. These patients represent the mildest form of androgen resistance presently documented.

Defects in Testosterone Metabolism by Peripheral Tissues; 5α-Reductase Deficiency (Pseudovaginal Perineoscrotal Hypospadias)

The defective conversion of testosterone to dihydrotestosterone produces a unique form of male pseudohermaphroditism (Figure 44–17). Phenotypically, these patients may vary from those with a microphallus to patients with pseudovaginal perineoscrotal hypospadias. At birth, in the most severely affected patients, ambiguous external genitalia are manifested by a small hypospadiac phallus bound down in chordee, a bifid scrotum, and a urogenital sinus that opens onto the perineum. A blind vaginal pouch is present, opening either into the urogenital sinus or onto the urethra, immediately behind the urethral orifice. The testes are either inguinal or labial. Müllerian structures are absent, and the wolffian structures are well-differentiated. At puberty, affected males virilize; the voice deepens, muscle mass increases, and the phallus enlarges. The bifid scrotum becomes rugose and pigmented. The testes enlarge and descend into the labioscrotal folds, and spermatogenesis may ensue. Gynecomastia is notably absent in these patients. Of note is the absence of acne and the presence of temporal hair recession and hirsutism. A remarkable feature of this form of male pseudohermaphroditism in some cultural isolates has been the reported change in gender identity from female to male at puberty.

After the onset of puberty, patients with 5α-reductase deficiency have normal to elevated testosterone levels and slightly elevated plasma concentrations of LH. As expected, plasma dihydrotestosterone is low, and the testosterone-dihydrotestosterone ratio is abnormally high. Apparently, lack of 5α reduction of testosterone to dihydrotestosterone in utero during the critical phases of male sex differentiation results in incomplete masculinization of the urogenital sinus and external genitalia, while testosterone-dependent wolffian structures are normally developed. Partial and mild forms of 5α-reductase deficiency have been described. These patients can present with hypospadias or microphallus (or both).

5α-Reductase deficiency is transmitted as an autosomal recessive trait, and the enzymatic defect exhibits genetic heterogeneity. There are 2 classes of affected individuals: those with absent enzyme activity and those with a measurable but unstable enzyme. Two genes catalyze the conversion of testosterone to dihydrotestosterone, and they are termed type I and type II. The type I enzyme is not expressed in the fetus but is expressed in skin, especially from puberty onward. The type II isoenzyme is the enzyme found in fetal genital skin, male accessory glands, and the prostate. In patients with 5α-reductase deficiency, the isozyme with a pH 5.5 optimum is deficient (type II). The gene encoding this enzyme contains 5 exons and is localized to chromosome 2, band p23. A variety of mutations are reported including deletions, nonsense,

splicing defects, and the more common missense mutations. Two-thirds of patients are homozygous for a single mutation, while the remainder are compound heterozygotes. It has been suggested that the marked virilization noted at puberty as opposed to its absence in utero may be the result of the expression and function of the type I gene at puberty and, consequently, the generation of sufficient amounts of dihydrotestosterone by peripheral conversion to induce phallic growth and other signs of masculinization.

5α-Reductase deficiency should be suspected in male pseudohermaphrodites with a blind vaginal pouch and in males with hypospadias or microphallus. The diagnosis can be confirmed by demonstration of an abnormally high plasma testosterone-dihydrotestosterone ratio, either under basal conditions or after hCG stimulation. Other confirmatory findings, especially in newborns, include an increased 5β:5α ratio of urinary C_{19} and C_{21} steroid metabolites. One can also examine the level of 5α-reductase activity in cultures of genital skin and the degree of conversion of infused labeled testosterone to dihydrotestosterone in vivo.

The early diagnosis of this condition is particularly critical. In view of the natural history of this disorder, a male gender assignment may be considered, and dihydrotestosterone (if available) or high-dose testosterone therapy should be initiated in order to augment phallic size. Repair of hypospadias should be performed as soon as possible in infancy. In patients who are diagnosed after infancy in whom gender identity is unequivocally female, prophylactic orchiectomy and estrogen substitution therapy may still be considered the treatment of choice until further experience with this biochemical entity and sex reversal in our culture is available.

Dysgenetic Male Pseudohermaphroditism (Ambiguous Genitalia Due to Dysgenetic Gonads)

Defective gonadogenesis of the testes results in ambiguous development of the genital ducts, urogenital

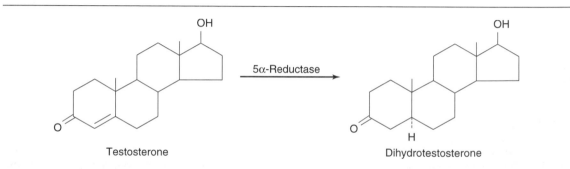

Figure 44–17. Metabolism of testosterone. (Reproduced, with permission, from Conte FA, Grumbach MM: Abnormalities of sexual determination and differentiation. In: Greenspan FS, Strewler GJ [editors]: *Basic and Clinical Endocrinology,* 5th ed. Appleton & Lange, 1997.)

sinus, and external genitalia. Patients with 45,X/46,XY mosaicism, structural abnormalities of the Y chromosome, and forms of XY gonadal dysgenesis manifest defective gonadogenesis and thus defective virilization. These disorders are classified under disorders of gonadal differentiation but are included also as a subgroup of male pseudohermaphroditism. 46,XY gonadal dysgenesis has been associated with deletion and mutation of the *SRY* gene on the Y chromosome, duplication of the *AHCH* (DAX-1) gene of the X chromosome, and chromosome 9p– or 10q– deletions.

Male pseudohermaphroditism can occur in association with degenerative renal disease and hypertension as well as with Wilms tumor (Denys-Drash syndrome). In this syndrome, both the kidneys and the testes are dysgenetic, and a predisposition for renal neoplasms exists. Patients with the Wilms tumor–aniridia–genital anomalies–mental retardation (WAGR) syndrome have been described. These patients exhibit various forms of ambiguous or hypoplastic male genitalia, including bifid scrotum, hypospadias, and cryptorchidism. Recent data indicate that the Denys-Drash and WAGR syndromes are due to heterozygous mutations (Denys-Drash) or deletions (WAGR) involving the Wilms tumor repressor gene *WT-1* on chromosome 11.

A mutation in SF-1 has recently been reported in a 46,XY patient. Similar to the mouse knockout experiment, the patient had female sex differentiation including müllerian derivatives and severe, neonatal onset adrenal insufficiency. However, in the human the mutation was heterozygous (present in only one allele of the SF-1 gene) and gonadotropin secretion was preserved as opposed to the deficiency of gonadotropins observed in the homozygous SF-1 knockout mouse. This illuminating patient demonstrates that SF-1 plays a critical role in adrenal and gonadal development and function in the human being.

Testicular Regression Syndrome (Vanishing Testes Syndrome; XY Agonadism; Rudimentary Testes Syndrome; Congenital Anorchia)

Cessation of testicular function during the critical phases of male sex differentiation can lead to various clinical syndromes depending on when testicular function ceases. At one end of the clinical spectrum of these heterogeneous conditions are the XY patients in whom testicular deficiency occurred before 8 weeks of gestation, which results in female differentiation of the internal and external genitalia—so-called XY gonadal dysgenesis.

At the other end of the spectrum are the patients with "anorchia" or "vanishing testes" in which the testes are lost later in gestation. These patients have perfectly normal male differentiation of their internal and external structures, but gonadal tissue is absent. The diagnosis of anorchia should be considered in all cryptorchid males. Administration of chorionic go-

nadotropin, 1000–2000 units per m^2 injected intramuscularly every other day for 2 weeks (total of 7 injections), is a useful test of Leydig cell function. In the presence of normal Leydig cell function, there is a rise in serum testosterone from concentrations of less than 20 ng/dL (0.69 nmol/L) to over 200 ng/dL (6.9 nmol/L) in prepubertal males. In infants under 4 years of age and children over 10 years of age, plasma FSH levels are a sensitive index of gonadal integrity. The gonadotropin response to a 100 μg intravenous injection of GnRH can also be used to diagnose the absence of gonadal feedback on the hypothalamus and pituitary. In agonadal children, GnRH elicits a rise in LH and FSH levels that is greater than that achieved in prepubertal children with normal gonadal function. Patients with high gonadotropin levels and no testosterone response to chorionic gonadotropin usually lack recognizable testicular tissue at surgery. Recent data indicate that both antimüllerian hormone and inhibin levels may be useful in ascertaining the absence of functioning Sertoli cells and, hence, presumed anorchia.

Persistent Müllerian Duct Syndrome (Defects in the Synthesis, Secretion, or Response to Antimüllerian Hormone)

Patients have been described in whom normal male development of the external genitalia has occurred but in whom the müllerian ducts persist. The retention of müllerian structures can be ascribed to failure of the Sertoli cells to synthesize antimüllerian hormone and to an end-organ defect in the response of the duct to antimüllerian hormone. This condition is transmitted as an autosomal recessive trait. The gene for antimüllerian hormone has been cloned and mapped to chromosome 19, and mutations in the antimüllerian gene have been reported. More recently, the gene encoding the antimüllerian receptor has been isolated, and patients with mutations in the AMH receptor have been described. In these patients müllerian ducts are present despite the presence of normal to high levels of AMH in plasma. Therapy involves removal of the müllerian structures.

Environmental Chemicals

An increase in disorders of development and function of the urogenital tract in males has been noted over the past 50 years. It has been hypothesized that this increased incidence of reproductive abnormalities observed in human males is related to increasing exposure in utero to "estrogens" found in the diet both naturally and as a result of chemical contamination. Recently, it has been demonstrated that *p,p'*-DDE (dichlorodiphenyldichloroethylene)—the major and persistent DDT metabolite—binds to the androgen receptor and inhibits androgen action in developing rodents.

Further studies on the levels as well as the risks to humans of environmental chemicals are necessary before abnormalities of the reproductive tract can be ascribed to these agents (Figure 44–19).

UNCLASSIFIED FORMS OF ABNORMAL SEXUAL DEVELOPMENT IN MALES

Hypospadias

Hypospadias occurs as an isolated finding in 1:300 newborn males. It is often associated with ventral contraction and bowing of the penis, called chordee. Deficient virilization of the external genitalia of the male fetus implies subnormal Leydig cell function in utero, end-organ resistance, or an inappropriate temporal correlation of the rise in fetal plasma testosterone and the critical period for tissue response. Although in most patients there is little reason to suspect these mechanisms, recent reports in a small number of patients have suggested that simple hypospadias can be associated with an abnormality (or competitive inhibition) of the androgen receptor, the nuclear localization of the ligand-receptor complex, an aberration in the maturation of the hypothalamic-pituitary-gonadal axis, and 5α-reductase deficiency. Further studies are necessary to determine the prevalence and role of these abnormalities in the pathogenesis of simple hypospadias. Nonendocrine factors that affect differentiation of the primordia may be found in a variety of genetic syndromes. A study of 100 patients with hypospadias reported one patient to be an XX female with congenital adrenal hyperplasia; 5 had sex chromosome abnormalities; and one had the incomplete form of XY gonadal dysgenesis. Nine affected males were the product of pregnancies in which the mother had taken progestational compounds during the first trimester. Thus, a presumed pathogenetic mechanism was found in 15% of patients.

Micropenis

Microphallus without hypospadias—micropenis—can result from a heterogeneous group of disorders, but by far the most common cause is fetal testosterone deficiency; more rarely, 5α-reductase deficiency or mild defects in the androgen receptor are implicated (Table 44–6). In the human male fetus, testosterone synthesis by the fetal Leydig cell during the critical period of male differentiation (8–12 weeks) is under the influence of placental hCG. After midgestation, fetal pituitary LH modulates fetal testosterone synthesis by the Leydig cell and, consequently, affects the growth of the differentiated penis. Thus, males with congenital hypopituitarism as well as isolated gonadotropin deficiency and "late" fetal testicular failure can present with normal male differentiation and micropenis at birth (penis < 2.5

Table 44–6. Etiology of micropenis.

I. Deficient testosterone secretion
  A. Hypogonadotropic hypogonadism
    1. Isolated, including Kallmann syndrome
    2. Associated with other pituitary hormone deficiencies
    3. Prader-Willi syndrome
    4. Laurence-Moon syndrome
    5. Bardet-Biedel syndrome
    6. Rudd syndrome
  B. Primary hypogonadism
    1. Anorchia
    2. Klinefelter and poly X syndromes
    3. Gonadal dysgenesis (incomplete form)
    4. LH receptor defects (incomplete forms)
    5. Genetic defects in testosterone steroidogenesis (incomplete forms)
    6. Noonan syndrome
    7. Trisomy 21
    8. Robinow syndrome
    9. Bardet-Biedel syndrome
    10. Laurence-Moon syndrome
II. Defects in testosterone action
  A. GH/IGF-1 deficiency
  B. Androgen receptor defects (incomplete forms)
  C. 5-α-reductase deficiency (incomplete forms)
  D. Fetal hydantoin syndrome
III. Developmental anomalies
  A. Aphallia
  B. Cloacal exstrophy
IV. Idiopathic
V. Associated with other congenital malformations

LH, luteinizing hormone; GH, growth hormone; IGF, insulin-like growth factor.
Source: Bin Abbas B et al: Congenital hypogonadotrophic hypogonadism and micropenis. Effect of testosterone treatment on adult penile size. Why sex reversal is not indicated. J Pediatr, 1999;134:579.

cm in length) (Table 44–7). Patients with hypothalamic hypopituitarism or pituitary aplasia may also have midline craniofacial defects, hypoglycemia, and giant cell hepatitis. After appropriate evaluation of anterior pituitary function (ie, determination of the plasma concentration of growth hormone, ACTH, cortisol, thryoid-stimulating hormone, thyroxine, and gonadotropins), stabilization of the patient with hormone replacement should be achieved. Thereafter, all patients with micropenis should receive a trial of testosterone therapy before definitive gender assignment is made. Patients with fetal testosterone deficiency as a cause of micropenis—whether due to gonadotropin deficiency or to a primary testicular disorder—respond to 25–50 mg of testosterone enanthate intramuscularly monthly for 3 months with a mean increase of 2 cm in penile length (Figure 44–18). A long-term study of 8 males with micropenis due to congenital hypogonadotropic hypogonadism who were followed up in our clinic revealed that fetal deficiency of gonadotropins and testosterone did not prevent the penis from responding to testosterone in infancy and at the age of puberty. Final penile length for all patients who were treated with one or more short courses of repository testos-

Table 44–7. Normal values for stretched penile length

Age	Length (cm) (mean ± SD)
Newborn: 30 wk[1]	2.5 ± 0.4
Newborn: full term[1]	3.5 ± 0.4
0–5 mo[2]	3.9 ± 0.8
6–12 mo[2]	4.3 ± 0.8
1–2 y[2]	4.7 ± 0.8
2–3 y[2]	5.1 ± 0.9
3–4 y[2]	5.5 ± 0.9
5–6 y[2]	6.0 ± 0.9
10–11 y[2]	6.4 ± 1.1
Adult[3]	12.4 ± 2.7

[1]Data from Feldman and Smith (1975); see Tuladhar et al (1998) for the normal range of penile length in preterm infants between 24 and 36 weeks of gestational age.
[2]Data from Schonfeld and Beebe (1942).
[3]Data from Wessels et al (1996).
Source: Bin Abbas B et al: Congenital hypogonadotrophic hypogonadism and micropenis. Effect of testosterone treatment on adult penile size. Why sex reversal is not indicated. J Pediatr, 1999;134:579.

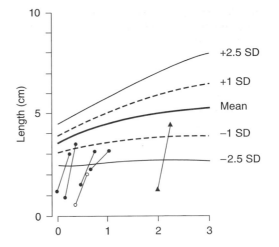

Figure 44–18. The response in phallic length to a 3-month course of testosterone in 6 patients with microphallus. Patients were under 2 years of age. Each patient was given 25 mg of testosterone enanthate in oil intramuscularly monthly for 3 months. Lines set off with solid triangles and open circles indicate 2 patients who subsequently underwent a second course of testosterone therapy. (Reproduced, with permission, from Burstein S, Grumbach MM, Kaplan SL: Early determination of androgen-responsiveness is important in the management of microphallus. Lancet 1979;2:983.)

terone in infancy or childhood and with replacement doses of testosterone in adolescence was in the normal adult range. Furthermore, these patients had a male gender identity, erections, ejaculation, and orgasm (Table 44–8). We found no clinical, psychological, or physiologic indications to support conversion of males with micropenis secondary to diminished testosterone secretion during gestation to females. In the rare patient in whom a trial of testosterone therapy does not result in an increase in phallic size due to an intrinsic penis defect, castration and assignment of a female gender has been the course followed in the past. However, there is a scarcity of long term data on these patients and their outcome, and thus this approach remains controversial.

Complete absence of the phallus is a rare anomaly. The urethra may open on the perineum or into the rectum. Assignment of a female gender, castration, and plastic repair of the genitalia and urethra have been the treatment of choice in the past, but questions about this approach have been raised recently.

Table 44–8. Treatment of 8 males with micropenis secondary to congenital hypogonadotropic hypogonadism, followed from infancy or childhood to maturity (ages 18–27 years).[1]

Characteristics of Patients	Group I	Group II
Age at start of testosterone	4 mo–2 y	6–13 y
Mean penile length and range	1.1 cm (–4 SD) (range 0.5–1.5 cm)	2.7 cm (–3.4 SD) (range 1.5–3.5 cm)
Mean penile length and range after 3 mo testosterone	3.3 cm (–1.6 SD) (range 2.5–4 cm)	4.8 cm (–1.4 SD) (range 2.5–7.5 cm)
Age of replacement testosterone	13–15 y	13–15 y
Mean final adult penile length	10.3 cm (–0.8 SD) (range 8–12 cm)	10.3 cm (–0.8 SD) (range 8.5–14 cm)

[1]Four patients were treated with testosterone before 2 years of age (group I), and 4 were treated between 6 and 13 years of age (group II). All patients received one or more courses of 3 intramuscular injections of testosterone enanthate (25 or 50 mg) at 4-week intervals in infancy or childhood to induce penile growth. At the age of puberty, the dose was gradually increased to adult replacement doses. Final adult penile length in both groups was 10.3 cm ± 2.7 cm with a range of 8–14 cm, which was within the normal range for mean adult stretched penile length in white men.
Source: Bin Abbas B et al: Congenital hypogonadotrophic hypogonadism and micropenis. Effect of testosterone treatment on adult penile size. Why sex reversal is not indicated. J Pediatr, 1999;134:579.

UNCLASSIFIED FORMS OF ABNORMAL SEXUAL DEVELOPMENT IN FEMALES

Congenital absence of the vagina occurs in 1:5000 female births. It can be associated with müllerian derivatives that vary from normal to absent. Ovarian function is usually normal. Therapy may involve plastic repair of the vagina.

Müllerian agenesis may be associated with renal aplasia (an absent kidney) and cervicothoracic somite dysplasia ("MURCS").

MANAGEMENT OF PATIENTS WITH INTERSEX PROBLEMS

Choice of Sex

The goal of the physician in management of patients with ambiguous genitalia is to establish a diagnosis and to assign a sex for rearing that is most compatible with a well-adjusted life and sexual adequacy. Once the sex for rearing is assigned, the gender role is reinforced by the use of appropriate surgical, hormonal, or psychological measures. Except in female pseudohermaphrodites, ambiguities of the genitalia are caused by lesions that almost always make the patient infertile. In recommending male sex assignment, the adequacy of the size of the phallus has been the most important consideration. However, recent recommendations for sex assignment have focused on the effect of prenatal androgen exposure on central nervous system organization and gender identity. As noted previously, there is a paucity of hard data on long-term follow-up in patients with intersex problems. Until further data are available, many years of experience from a pragmatic approach to the assignment of sex in individuals with ambiguous genitalia still suggest that the most critical elements in the development of gender identity are the assigned sex of rearing, its surgical and psychosocial reinforcement during infancy and childhood, and its further reinforcement by appropriate gonadal steroid secretion replacement therapy at the normal age of puberty.

A comprehensive discussion with the parents about the cause of their child's atypical genitalia, the natural history of other patients with similar parthophysiology, and the possible hormonal and therapeutic options is critical to their coming to an informed decision on the sex rearing of their child. This discussion must take into account the parental anxieties, religious views, social mores, cultural factors and, most important, the level of understanding of the parents. The evaluation, management and continuing follow-up of the child with ambiguous genitalia and his/her family is best facilitated by a coordinated team approach involving the pediatric endocrinologist, psychiatrist, and surgeon.

The steps in the diagnosis of intersexuality are set forth in Figures 44–19 and 44–20.

Reassignment of sex in infancy and childhood is always a difficult psychosocial problem for the patient, the parents, and the physicians involved. While easier in infancy than after 2 years of age, it should only be undertaken after deliberation and with provision for long-term medical and psychiatric supervision and counseling.

It is desirable to initiate plastic repair of the external genitalia before 6–12 months of age. In children raised as females, the clitoris should be salvaged. Surgical procedures, if necessary, should be designed to maintain the functional capacity of the clitoris. Reconstruction of a vagina, if necessary, can be deferred until adolescence.

Removal of the gonads in children with Y chromosome material and gonadal dysgenesis should be performed at the time of initial repair of the external genitalia, because gonadoblastomas, seminomas, and germinomas can occur during the first decade.

In a patient with complete androgen resistance, the gonads may be left in situ (provided they are not situated in the labia majora) to provide estrogen until late adolescence. The patient may then undergo prophylactic castration, having had her female identity reinforced by normal feminization at puberty. However, it is reasonable to remove the gonads prepubertally, especially if herniorrhaphy is necessary. In this circumstance, sex steroid replacement therapy at the time of puberty is indicated.

In patients with incomplete androgen resistance reared as females or in patients with errors of testosterone biosynthesis in whom some degree of masculinization occurs at puberty, gonadectomy should be performed before puberty.

Cyclic estrogen and progestin are used in individuals reared as females in whom a uterus is present. In males, virilization is achieved by the administration of a repository preparation of testosterone.

Sex is not a single biologic feature but the sum of many morphogenetic, functional, and psychological potentialities. The physician should not express to the parent or child any doubts about the sex of rearing. Chromosomal and gonadal sex are secondary considerations; the sex of rearing is paramount. With proper surgical reconstruction, hormone substitution, and continuing psychological support and reinforcement of the sex of rearing, the individual whose psychosexual gender is discordant with chromosomal sex need not have any psychological catastrophes as long as the sex of rearing is accepted with conviction by the family and others during the critical early years. These individuals can reach adulthood as well-adjusted men or women capable of normal sexual interaction, though usually not of procreation.

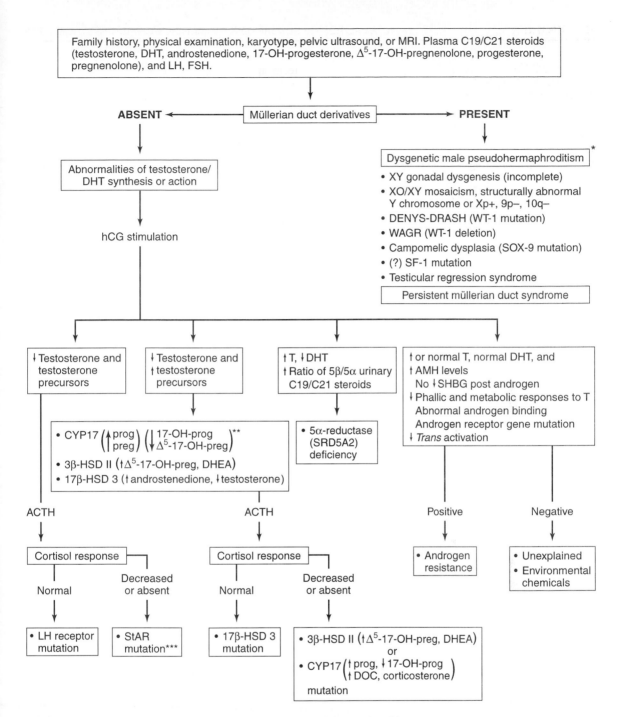

Figure 44–19. Steps in the differential diagnosis of male pseudohermaphroditism.
*Patients with dysgenetic male pseudohermaphroditism may manifest varying degrees of testicular dysgenesis with consequent testosterone/DHT and/or AMH deficiency. Therefore, not all patients may manifest either ambiguous genitalia or the presence of müllerian ducts.
**CYP17 (P450c17) catalyzes the 17-hydroxylation of progesterone and pregnenolone to 17-hydroxyprogesterone and Δ^5-17-hydroxypregnenolone as well as the scission (lyase) of 17-hydroxypregnenolone to DHEA. Patients with 17,20-lyase deficiency have elevated levels of 17-hydroxyprogesterone and Δ^5-17-hydroxypregnenolone in relation to androstenedione and DHEA either before or after hCG stimulation.
***The StAR (steroidogenic acute regulatory) protein is involved in the transport of cholesterol from the outer to the inner mitochondrial membrane where the enzyme CYP11A1 (P450scc) resides. Patients with a mutation in the gene for this protein have a markedly diminished ability to convert cholesterol to Δ^5-17-hydroxypregnenolone, although their CYP11A1 enzymatic activity is intact, and they manifest congenital lipoid adrenal hyperplasia. WAGR, Wilms tumor, aniridia, genital anomalies, and mental retardation; SF-1, steroidogenic factor-1; CYP17, 17α-hydroxylase/17,20-lyase; 3β-HSD II, 3β-hydroxysteroid dehydrogenase/Δ^5-isomerase; 17β-HSD 3, 17β-hydroxysteroid dehydrogenase (oxidoreductase); T, testosterone; DHT, dihydrotestosterone; AMH, antimüllerian hormone; SHBG, sex hormone binding globulin; DHEA, dehydroepiandrosterone. (Reproduced, with permission, from Grumbach MM, Conte FA: Disorders of sex differentiation. In: Wilson JD et al [editors]: *Williams Textbook of Endocrinology,* 9th ed. Saunders, 1998.)

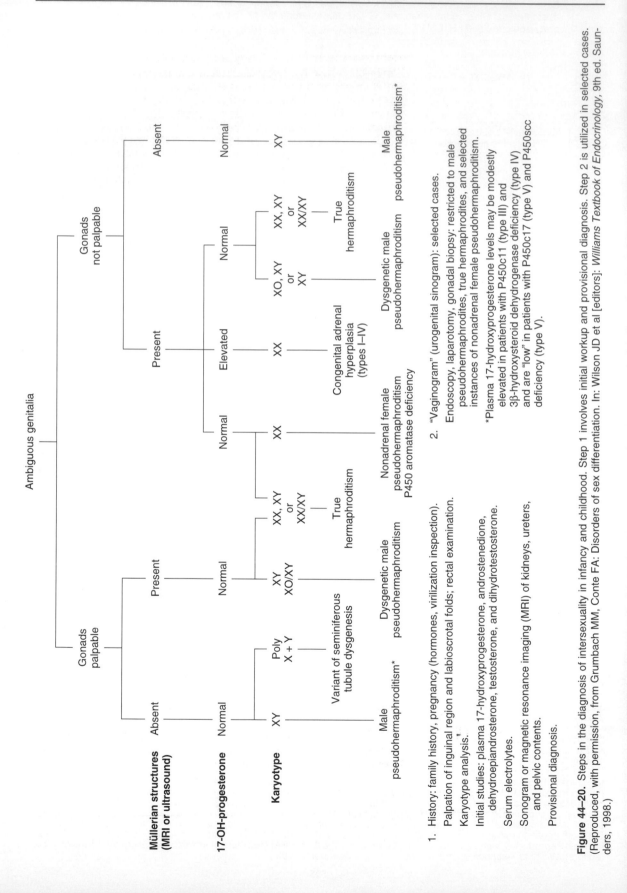

Figure 44–20. Steps in the diagnosis of intersexuality in infancy and childhood. Step 1 involves initial workup and provisional diagnosis. Step 2 is utilized in selected cases. (Reproduced, with permission, from Grumbach MM, Conte FA: Disorders of sex differentiation. In: Wilson JD et al [editors]: *Williams Textbook of Endocrinology,* 9th ed. Saunders, 1998.)

1. History: family history, pregnancy (hormones, virilization inspection).
   Palpation of inguinal region and labioscrotal folds; rectal examination.
   Karyotype analysis.
   Initial studies: plasma 17-hydroxyprogesterone, androstenedione, dehydroepiandrosterone, testosterone, and dihydrotestosterone.
   Serum electrolytes.
   Sonogram or magnetic resonance imaging (MRI) of kidneys, ureters, and pelvic contents.
   Provisional diagnosis.

2. "Vaginogram" (urogenital sinogram): selected cases.
   Endoscopy, laparotomy, gonadal biopsy: restricted to male pseudohermaphrodites, true hermaphrodites, and selected instances of nonadrenal female pseudohermaphroditism.

   *Plasma 17-hydroxyprogesterone levels may be modestly elevated in patients with P450c11 (type III) and 3β-hydroxysteroid dehydrogenase deficiency (type IV) and are "low" in patients with P450c17 (type V) and P450scc deficiency (type V).

REFERENCES

Achermann JC et al: A mutation in the gene encoding steroidogenic factor-1 causes XY sex reversal and adrenal failure in humans. Nat Genet 1999;22:125.

Aittomaki K et al: Mutation in the follicle-stimulating hormone receptor gene causes hereditary hypergonadotrophic ovarian failure. Cell 1995;82:954.

Andersson S et al: Molecular genetics and pathophysiology of 17β-hydroxysteroid dehydrogenase 3 deficiency. J Clin Endocrinol Metab 1996;81:130.

Bardoni B et al: A dosage sensitive locus at chromosome Xp21 is involved in male to female sex reversal. Nat Genet 1994;7:497.

Beau I et al: A novel phenotype related to partial loss of function: Mutations of the follicle stimulating hormone receptor. J Clin Invest 1998;102:1352.

Behringer RR: The in vivo role of müllerian-inhibiting substance. Curr Top Dev Biol 1994;29:171.

Berkovitz GD et al: Clinical and pathologic spectrum of 46,XY gonadal dysgenesis: Its relevance to the understanding of sex differentiation. Medicine 1991;70:375.

Berkovitz GD et al: The role of the sex-determining region of the Y chromosome (SRY) in the etiology of 46,XX true hermaphroditism. Hum Genet 1992;88:411.

Bin Abbas B et al: Congenital hypogonadotrophic hypogonadism and micropenis: Effect of testosterone treatment on adult penile size. Why sex reversal is not indicated. J Pediatr 1999;134:579.

Bose HS et al: The physiology and genetics of congenital lipoid adrenal hyperplasia. N Engl J Med 1996;335:1870.

Capel B: Sex in the 90s: SRY and the switch to the male pathway. Annu Rev Physiol 1998;60:497.

Cerame, BI et al: Prenatal diagnosis and treatment of beta-hydroxylase deficiency congenital adrenal hyperplasia resulting in normal female genitalia. J Clin Endo Metab 1999;84:3129.

Conte FA et al: A syndrome of female pseudohermaphroditism, hypergonadotrophic hypogonadism, and multicystic ovaries associated with missense mutations in the gene encoding aromatase (P450arom). J Clin Endocrinol Metab 1994;78:1287.

da Silva SM et al: Sox9 expression during gonadal development implies a conserved role for the gene in testis differentiation in mammals and birds. Nat Genet 1996;14:62.

Diamond M, Sigmundson HK: Sex reassignment at birth. Long-term review and clinical implications. Arch Pediatr Adolesc Med 1997;151:298.

Donahoue PA et al: Congenital adrenal hyperplasia. In: Scriver CR et al (editors): *The Metabolic and Molecular Bases of Inherited Disease,* 7th ed. McGraw-Hill, 1995.

Ellison JW et al: PHOG, a candidate gene for the involvement in the short stature of Turner syndrome. Hum Mol Genet 1997;6:1341.

Evans JA et al: Agenesis of the penis: patterns of associated malformations. Amer J Med Genet 1999;84:47.

Fechner PY et al: Report of a kindred with X-linked (or autosome dominant sex linked) 46,XY partial gonadal dysgenesis. J Clin Endocrinol Metab 1993;76:1248.

Feldman KW, Smith DW: Fetal phallic growth and penile standards for newborn male infants. J Pediatr 1975;86:395.

Ferguson-Smith MA, Goodfellow PN: SRY and primary sex reversal syndromes. In: Scriver CR et al (editors): *The Metabolic and Molecular Bases of Inherited Disease,* 7th ed. McGraw-Hill, 1995.

Forest MG et al: Prenatal treatment of congenital adrenal hyperplasia. Trends Endocrinol Metab 1998;9:284.

Geissler WM et al: Male pseudohermaphroditism caused by mutations of testicular 17β-hydroxysteroid dehydrogenase 3. Nat Genet 1994;7:34.

Geller DH et al: The genetic and functional basis of isolated 17,20-lyase deficiency. Nat Genet 1997;17:201.

Goodfellow P, Lovell-Badge R: SRY and sex determination in mammals. Ann Rev Genet 1993;27:71.

Griffen JE, Wilson JD: The androgen resistance syndromes: Steroid 5α reductase 2 deficiency, testicular feminization and related syndromes. In: Scriver CR et al (editors): *The Metabolic and Molecular Bases of Inherited Disease,* 7th ed. McGraw-Hill, 1995.

Grumbach MM, Conte FA: Disorders of sex differentiation. In: Wilson JD et al (editors): *Williams Textbook of Endocrinology,* 9th ed. Saunders, 1998.

Hadjiathanasiou CG et al: True hermaphroditism: Genetic variants and clinical management. J Pediatr 1994;125:738.

Harada N et al: Biochemical and molecular genetic analyses on placental aromatase (P450arom) deficiency. J Biol Chem 1992;267:4781.

Harly VR et al: DNA binding activity of recombinant SRY from normal males and XY females. Science 1992;255:453.

Hawkins JR. Sex determination. Hum Mol Genet 1994;3:1463.

Hawkins JR et al: Mutational analysis of SRY: Nonsense and missense mutations in XY sex reversal. Hum Genet 1992;88:471.

Hibi I, Takano K (editors): *Basic and Clinical Approach to Turner Syndrome.* International Congress Series 1014, Amsterdam, Excerpta Medica, 1993.

Imbeaud S et al: Insensitivity to anti-müllerian hormone due to a mutation in the human anti-müllerian hormone receptor. Nat Genet 1995;11:382.

Imbeaud S et al: A 27 base-pair deletion of the anti-müllerian Type II receptor gene is the most common cause of the persistent müllerian duct syndrome. Hum Mol Genet 1996;5:1269.

Jimenez R, Burgos M: Mammalian sex determination: Joining pieces of the genetic puzzle. Bioessays 1998;20:696.

Kay GF: Xist and X chromosome inactivation. Mol Cell Endocrinol 1998;140:71.

Knebelmann B et al: Anti-Müllerian hormone Bruxelles: A nonsense mutation associated with the persistent Müllerian duct syndrome. Proc Natl Acad Sci USA 1991;88:3767.

Koopman P et al: Male development of chromosomally female mice transgenic for SRY. Nature 1991;351:117.

Kreidberg JA et al: WT-1 is required in early kidney development. Cell 1993;74:679.

Kremer H et al: Male pseudohermaphroditism due to a homozygous missense mutation of the luteinizing hormone receptor gene. Nat Genet 1994;9:160.

Labrie F et al: Structure, regulation and role of 3β-hydroxysteroid dehydrogenase, 17β-hydroxysteroid dehydrogenase and aromatase enzymes in the formation of sex steroids in classical and peripheral intracrine tissues. Bailliere's Clin Endocrinol Metab 1994;8:451.

Latronico AC et al: A homozygous microdeletion in helix 7 of the luteinizing hormone receptor associated with familial testicular and ovarian resistance is due to both decreased cell surface expression and impaired effector activation by the cell surface receptor. Mol Endocrinol 1998;123:442.

Lin D et al: Role of steroidogenic acute regulatory protein in adrenal and gonadal steroidogenesis. Science 1995;267:1828.

Lo, JC et al: Normal female infants born of mothers with classic congenital adrenal hyperplasia due to 21-hydroxylase deficiency. J Clin Endocrinol Metab 1999;84:930.

Luo X et al: A cell specific receptor is essential for adrenal and gonadal development and sexual differentiation. Cell 1994;77:481.

Mendez JP et al: A reliable endocrine test with human menopausal gonadotrophin for diagnosis of true hermaphrodism in early infancy. J Clin Endocrinol Metab 1998;83:3523.

Mendonca BB et al: Mutation in 3β-hydroxysteroid dehydrogenase type II associated with pseudohermaphroditism in males and premature pubarche or cryptic expression in females. J Mol Endocrinol 1994;12:119.

Meyer-Bahlburg HFL: Gender assignment in intersexuality. J of Hum Psychol & Hum Sexuality 1999;10:1.

Miller WL: Genetics, diagnosis and management of 21-hydroxylase deficiency. J Clin Endocrinol Metab 1994;78:241.

Miller WL: Prenatal treatment of congenital adrenal hyperplasia: A promising experimental therapy of unproven safety. Trends Endocrinol Metab 1998;9:290.

Moghrabi N, Andersson S: 17β-Hydroxysteroid dehydrogenases: Physiologic roles in health and disease. Trends Endocrinol Metab 1998;9:265.

Morel Y, Miller W: Clinical and molecular genetics of congenital adrenal hyperplasia due to 21-hydroxylase deficiency. Adv Genet 1991;20:1.

Morishima A et al: Aromatase deficiency in male and female siblings caused by a novel mutation and the physiological role of estrogens. J Clin Endocrinol Metab 1995;80:3689.

Nachtigall MW et al: Wilms tumor 1 and Dax-1 modulate the orphan nuclear receptor SF-1 in sex-specific gene expression. Cell 1998;93:445.

Pelletier J et al: Germline mutations in the Wilms tumor suppressor gene are associated with abnormal urogenital development in Denys-Drash syndrome. Cell 1991;67:437.

Petit C et al: An abnormal terminal X-Y interchange accounts for most but not all cases of human XX maleness. Cell 1987;49:595.

Pontiggia A et al: Sex-reversing mutations affect the architecture of SRY-DNA complexes. EMBO J 1994;13:6115.

Quigley CA et al: Androgen receptor defects: Historical, clinical and molecular properties. Endocr Rev 1995;6:271.

Rao et al: Pseudoautosomal deletions encompassing a novel homeobox gene cause growth failure in idiopathic short stature and Turner syndrome. Nat Genet 1997;16:54.

Raymond CS et al: A region of human chromosome 9 required for testis development contains two genes related to known sexual regulators. Hum Mol Genet 1999;8:989.

Reiner WG: Sex assignment in the neonate with intersex or inadequate genitalia. Arch Pediatr Adolesc Med 1997;151:1044.

Rey R: Endocrine, paracrine and cellular regulation of postnatal anti-müllerian hormone secretion by Sertoli cells. Trends Endocrinol Metab 1998;9:271.

Russell DW, Wilson JD: Steroid 5α-reductase: Two genes/two enzymes. Annu Rev Biochem 1994;63:25.

Schafer AJ: Sex determination and its pathology in man. Adv Genet 1995;33:275.

Schonfeld WA, Beebe GW: Normal growth and variation in male genitalia from birth to maturity. J Urol 1942;64:759.

Simard J et al: Molecular basis of human 3 beta-hydroxysteroid dehydrogenase deficiency. J Steroid Biochem Mol Biol 1995;53:127.

Sliiper FME et al: Long term psychological evaluation of future sex. Children Archiv Sex Behavior 1998;27:125.

Speiser PW, White PC: Congenital adrenal hyperplasia due to 21-hydroxylase deficiency. Clin Endocrinol 1998;49:411.

Speiser PW et al: Disease expression and molecular genotype in congenital adrenal hyperplasia due to 21-hydroxylase deficiency. J Clin Invest 1992;90:584.

Sutherland RS et al: The effect of prepubertal androgen exposure on adult penile length. J Urol 1996;156:783.

Swain A et al: Dax-1 antagonizes Sry action in mammalian sex determination. Nature 1998;391:761.

Thigpen AE et al: Molecular genetics of steroid 5α-reductase deficiency. J Clin Invest 1992;90:799.

Tuladhar R et al: Establishment of a normal range of penile length in preterm infants. J Paediatr Child Health 1998;34:471.

Van Niekerk WA: *True Hermaphroditism.* Harper & Row, 1974.

Wagner T et al: Autosomal sex reversal and campomelic dysplasia. Cell 1994;79:1111.

Wessels H et al: Penile length in the flaccid and erect status: Guidelines for penile augmentation. J Urol 1996;156:995.

Wilson JD et al: Steroid 5α-reductase deficiency. Endocr Rev 1993;14:577.

Yanese T: 17α-Hydroxylase/17,20-lyase defects. J Steroid Biochem Mol Biol 1995;53:153.

Yanese T et al: 17α-Hydroxylase/17,20-lyase deficiency: From clinical investigation to molecular definitions. Endocr Rev 1991;12:91.

Yanese T et al: Molecular basis of apparent isolated 17,20-lyase deficiency: Compound heterozygous mutations in the C-terminal region [Arg(496) → Cys, Gln(461) → Stop] actually cause combined 17α-hydroxylase/17,20-lyase deficiency. Biochim Biophys Acta 1992;1139:275.

Yu RN et al: Role of AHCH in gonadal development and gametogenesis. Nat Genet 1998;20:353.

Zanaria E et al: An unusual member of the hormone receptor superfamily responsible for X-linked adrenal hypoplasia congenita. Nature 1994;372:635.

Renovascular Hypertension

45

R. Ernest Sosa, MD, & E. Darracott Vaughan, Jr., MD

Renovascular disease is one of the most common causes of secondary hypertension. Renovascular hypertension is underdiagnosed in clinical practice. Although emphasis has been placed on developing accurate tests to identify the 5% of hypertensive patients who suffer from renovascular hypertension, there are no perfect screening tests for its detection. Improved detection is possible because of a better understanding of clinical clues and pathophysiology of renovascular hypertension (Table 45–1). The diagnosing of renovascular hypertension is important for several reasons. (1) Renovascular hypertension can be difficult to manage medically. (2) Many renal artery lesions are progressive and may result in complete renal artery occlusion despite adequate medical management. Renovascular disease is a major cause of end-stage renal disease, especially in elderly patients. (3) High-renin hypertension is associated with an increased rate of cerebrovascular and cardiovascular complications. (4) Renal revascularization can potentially cure or better control the hypertension and reverse renal insufficiency.

Renal parenchymal diseases can also cause hypertension (Table 45–2). In many cases the hypertension is correctable if properly diagnosed and treated.

Etiology

Renal disease in association with hypertension has been recognized since the early nineteenth century. In 1898, Tigerstadt and Bergman demonstrated that a water-soluble substance—extracted from the renal cortex of a healthy rabbit and termed **renin**—produced marked and sustained hypertension when injected intravenously into a second healthy rabbit.

In 1934 Goldblatt described 2 models of experimental hypertension. In a 2-kidney animal, clipping of one renal artery results in sustained hypertension. Removal of the clip or of the ischemic kidney returns the blood pressure to normal. This model is analogous to unilateral renal artery stenosis in humans: The hypertension is renin-dependent. In humans, as in the Goldblatt 2-kidney, 1-clip model of hypertension, unilateral renal ischemia has been shown to produce high-renin, angiotensin-dependent hypertension that can be cured by reconstruction of the renal artery, percutaneous balloon catheter dilation of the stenosed artery, or nephrectomy (Figure 45–1). In the second model—1 clip, 1 kidney—the hypertension is sodium volume–dependent. Blockade of the renin-angiotensin system has little effect on blood pressure, unless the animal is sodium-depleted. This model is analogous to renal artery stenosis in a solitary kidney. It may also resemble bilateral renal artery stenosis.

Natural History

Atheromatous renal arterial disease predominantly occurs in the proximal third of the renal artery and is often part of diffuse atherosclerosis, affecting many other vascular beds (eg, coronary, carotid, and pudendal arteries). In many cases, a plaque in the wall of the aorta may encroach on the ostium of the renal artery. Atheromatous disease of the renal artery most commonly afflicts older men. The disease is often bilateral (40%) and progressive (44%), resulting in total occlusion (16%) despite medical treatment of the hypertension.

Fibromuscular dysplasia of the renal arteries is the most common cause of renovascular hypertension in younger patients. It is diagnosed in one-third of patients with renovascular hypertension. These lesions can be progressive in up to 33% of cases but rarely result in total arterial occlusion. There are 4 different pathologic types of fibromuscular dysplasia. Medial fibroplasia is the most common and accounts for 70% of cases. The angiographic appearance is that of a string of beads owing to thickening of the media interspersed with areas of aneurysmal dilation. These lesions are rare in children.

In a study of potential renal donors, 27% of the normotensive patients with incidentally found fibromuscular dysplasia subsequently became hypertensive over the ensuing 7.5 years.

Thus, renal arterial lesions are often progressive. This fact provides strong support for angioplasty or

Table 45–1. Causes of renovascular hypertension.

Common causes
  Atherosclerosis (66%)
  Fibromuscular dysplasia (33%)
    Intimal fibroplasia (about 5%)
    Fibromuscular hyperplasia (about 2%)
    Medial fibroplasia (about 80%)
    Perimedial fibroplasia (about 15%)
Rare causes
  Polyarteritis nodosa
  Takayasu's arteritis
  Arteriovenous fistula
  Aortic aneurysm
  Coarctation of the aorta
  Middle aortic syndrome
  Radiation arteritis
  Cholesterol emboli

Table 45–2. Nonvascular causes of renal hypertension in unilateral renal parenchymal disease.

Surgery indicated
  Renal cell carcinoma
  Wilms tumor
  Reninoma
  Obstructive uropathy
  Nonfunctioning atrophic kidney
Surgery only upon proved indications
  Chronic pyelonephritis associated with
    vesicoureteral reflux
  Polycystic kidney
  Radiation nephritis
  Perinephric scarring (Page kidney)
  Segmental hypoplasia (Ask-Upmark kidney)
  Renal tuberculosis

surgical revascularization to maintain renal function and correct hypertension.

Pathogenesis

The renin-angiotensin-aldosterone system (Figure 45–2) is an integrated hormonal cascade that simultaneously controls blood pressure and sodium and potassium balance, and influences regional blood flow. Renin is a proteolytic enzyme produced in the juxtaglomerular cells of the afferent arterioles. It acts on renin substrate (angiotensinogen), an alpha-2 globulin produced in the liver, to form the decapep-

tide angiotensin I. Converting enzyme cleaves 2 amino acids from angiotensin I to form the octapeptide angiotensin II, a potent arterial vasoconstrictor. Angiotensin II also stimulates the zona glomerulosa of the adrenal gland to secrete aldosterone. Elevation of blood pressure and restoration of sodium balance inhibit further renin secretion.

The mechanisms responsible for renin secretion include an afferent arteriolar baroreceptor responding to decreased renal perfusion pressure, a sensor at the macula densa responding to decreased delivery of sodium and chloride to the distal tubule, and increased

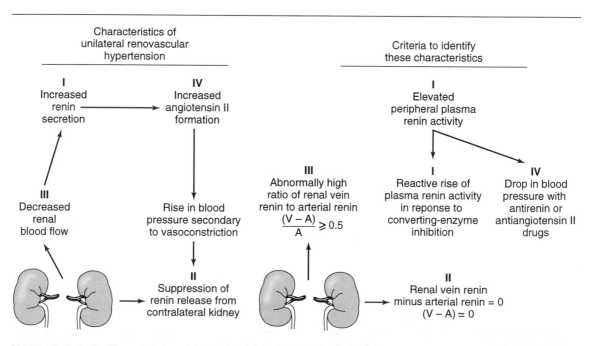

Figure 45–1. Left: Characteristics of the early phase of 2-kidney, 1-clip Goldblatt hypertension in the rat. **Right:** The criteria derived from the animal model that serve to identify patients with correctable renal hypertension. Roman numerals relate left and right parts of figure. (Modified and reproduced, with permission, from Vaughan ED Jr et al: Clinical evaluation of renovascular hypertension and therapeutic decisions. Urol Clin North Am 1984;11:393.)

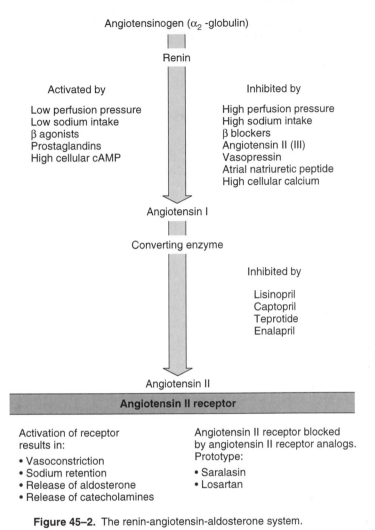

Angiotensinogen (α_2 -globulin)

Renin

Activated by	Inhibited by
Low perfusion pressure	High perfusion pressure
Low sodium intake	High sodium intake
β agonists	β blockers
Prostaglandins	Angiotensin II (III)
High cellular cAMP	Vasopressin
	Atrial natriuretic peptide
	High cellular calcium

Angiotensin I

Converting enzyme

Inhibited by

Lisinopril
Captopril
Teprotide
Enalapril

Angiotensin II

Angiotensin II receptor

Activation of receptor
results in:

• Vasoconstriction
• Sodium retention
• Release of aldosterone
• Release of catecholamines

Angiotensin II receptor blocked
by angiotensin II receptor analogs.
Prototype:

• Saralasin
• Losartan

Figure 45–2. The renin-angiotensin-aldosterone system.

activity of the sympathetic nervous system, mediated by beta-1-adrenergic receptors. Frequent causes of hypersecretion of renin include sodium depletion, hemorrhage, shock, congestive heart failure, and renal artery stenosis.

Plasma renin activity is closely related to the patient's sodium intake and urinary sodium excretion, ie, sodium balance. The renin-angiotensin-aldosterone system is activated in response to sodium restriction and suppressed by sodium loading. Plasma renin activity must therefore be correlated with the sodium balance in order to be meaningful. Figure 45–3 illustrates how the plasma renin activity varies with the sodium balance, which is determined by measuring the urinary excretion of sodium in a 24-h specimen.

The renin angiotensin system is undoubtedly the main mechanism responsible for renovascular hypertension. However, other mechanisms appear to play a causative role. There is evidence that activity of the

sympathetic nervous system may be increased. Two-kidney, 1-clip rats have a high rate of norepinephrine release. Sympathetic blockade with chlorisondamine reduces both norepinephrine levels and blood pressure. Nitrous oxide appears to play a role as well. Feeding a nitric oxide inhibitor to dogs exacerbated the hypertension produced by clipping one of 2 healthy kidneys. It is believed that nitric oxide may counter the vasoconstrictor effects of angiotensin.

Pathology

Stenosis of the renal artery (and, therefore, renovascular hypertension) is most commonly caused by arteriosclerotic plaques or fibromuscular dysplasia (Table 45–1). Not all renal artery stenoses are physiologically significant and cause hypertension, however. A lesion must produce a reduction in luminal diameter of at least 70% before renal plasma flow is reduced to the point that clinically significant is-

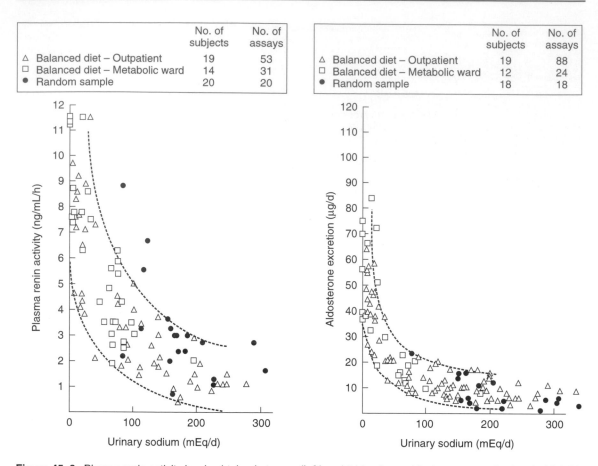

	No. of subjects	No. of assays
△ Balanced diet – Outpatient	19	53
□ Balanced diet – Metabolic ward	14	31
● Random sample	20	20

	No. of subjects	No. of assays
△ Balanced diet – Outpatient	19	88
□ Balanced diet – Metabolic ward	12	24
● Random sample	18	18

Figure 45–3. Plasma renin activity levels obtained at noon (**left**) and 24-h urinary aldosterone excretion levels (**right**) in relation to daily urinary sodium excretion levels in normal subjects. In such subjects, plasma renin activity and excretion of aldosterone describe similar hyperbolic curves in relation to sodium excretion. The fact that a random sampling of nonhospitalized subjects consuming uncontrolled diets yielded similar results enhances the validity of this nomogram for use in studies of outpatients or subjects not consuming a constant diet. (Reproduced, with permission, from Laragh JH: *Hypertension Manual.* York Medical Books, 1973.)

chemia results. The clinical significance of an anatomic stenosis noted on angiography (Figure 45–4) is assessed by renin assays, as discussed subsequently.

Other urologic lesions that may cause renin-dependent hypertension include obstructive uropathy, benign and malignant renal masses, and chronic pyelonephritis, the latter most commonly associated with vesicoureteral reflux (Table 45–2). In some patients, elevated levels of plasma renin activity return to normal, and hypertension is alleviated after appropriate surgical treatment of the underlying urologic disorder. However, hypertension due to renal parenchymal disease usually is not curable by surgical means. Most patients require medical management to control blood pressure.

History & Physical Examination

A. History: A complete and thorough medical history and physical examination provide important information about the patient's current general health, past medical history, and family medical history. Clinical clues and other factors suggestive of renovascular hypertension are set forth in Table 45–3. The patient's age and circumstances at onset of hypertension, recorded blood pressure ranges, previous treatment, results of therapy, and history of end-organ damage are noted. The past history is investigated for evidence of diseases (eg, glomerulonephritis, chronic pyelonephritis with or without vesicoureteral reflux, hydronephrosis, urolithiasis) or other factors (eg, renal trauma, radiation therapy to the abdomen) that could contribute to the development of hypertension.

Hypertension may have an abrupt onset and progress rapidly in children with Wilms tumor, in young adults with fibromuscular dysplasia, and in older patients with arteriosclerotic occlusion of the

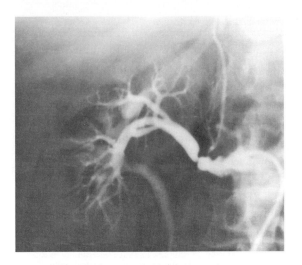

Figure 45–4. Selective renal arteriogram showing severe renal artery stenosis in a 65-year-old patient with normal blood pressure. (Reproduced, with permission, from Vaughan ED Jr: Laboratory tests in the evaluation of renal hypertension. Urol Clin North Am 1979;6:485.)

renal artery. Anorexia, weight loss, and malaise may be signs of malignant disease leading to elevated blood pressure. However, the absence of symptoms is not sufficient to rule out a diagnosis of curable hypertension.

Pulmonary edema is relatively frequent in patients with advanced renovascular hypertension with bilateral disease and azotemia.

B. Physical Examination: Physical examination should include serial measurements of the patient's blood pressure to establish the degree of hypertension. Measurements are taken in each arm with an appropriate-sized cuff while the patient is standing, sitting, and lying down. If 3 measurements are higher than 140/90 mm Hg in an adult, further evaluation is warranted. A funduscopic examination should be performed to look for hemorrhage, exudates and papilledema. The physician should palpate all peripheral pulses. Diminution of pulses and decreased blood pressure in the lower extremities in a young patient may signify coarctation of the aorta; an intrascapular murmur is another characteristic sign. In patients with renal artery stenosis, a continuous abdominal bruit may be heard on either side of the midline immediately above the umbilicus.

Laboratory Evaluation

A. Renovascular Hypertension: The low prevalence of renovascular hypertension among hypertensive patients, together with the cost and less than perfect accuracy of screening tests for renovascular hypertension, makes screening for this disease impractical. Pickering and colleagues have suggested

that for patients with a low index of suspected disease, only basic evaluation is needed (see below). These include patients with borderline, mild, or moderate hypertension in the absence of clinical clues (Table 45–3), and patients with low renin hypertension. For patients with a moderate index of suspected disease, noninvasive tests should be performed as described below. For this group the prevalence of renovascular hypertension is between 5% and 15%. For these patients, the predictive value of a negative result of a diagnostic test with a sensitivity and specificity of 90% would exceed 98%. The predictive value of a positive test would be 32%, which would justify arteriography.

For patients with a high index of suspected disease, eg, those with severe hypertension (diastolic > 120 mm Hg) refractory to aggressive medical treatment or with an increase in creatinine, or patients with malignant hypertension (type III or IV retinopathy), arteriography is justified even if the noninvasive diagnostic tests are negative or inconclusive. These patients are likely to suffer deterioration in renal function when treated with converting-enzyme inhibitors and are at high risk for ischemic nephropathy.

1. Basic tests–Laboratory examination of patients with suspected renovascular hypertension (Figure 45–5) should begin with basic tests that assess the patient's general health: complete blood count, serum electrolytes and fasting blood glucose determinations, blood urea nitrogen and serum creatinine measurements, urinalysis and urine culture, and an electrocardiogram.

2. Plasma renin activity profile–In patients in whom the diagnosis of hypertension has been definitively established, evaluation with a plasma renin activity profile (plasma renin activity must be plotted against 24-h urinary sodium excretion) is performed. These measurements should be obtained while the patient is on a diet containing normal amounts of sodium; antihypertensive medication must be withheld for 2 weeks before sampling. The blood sample for the renin determination is drawn at the end of the 24-h period in which the urine is collected and after 4 h of ambulatory activity. This test will reveal elevated plasma renin activity levels in about 80% of patients with renovascular hypertension (Figure 45–6, left). However, 15% of patients with essential hypertension also have high renin, which lowers the predictive value of the test (Table 45–4).

3. Captopril challenge test–Peripheral plasma renin activity is measured before and 1 h after administration of captopril (a converting-enzyme inhibitor), 25 mg orally. In renin-dependent hypertension, inhibition of the converting enzyme occurs. If the 3 criteria found by Muller (Table 45–5) are present in a patient with normal renal function who is not taking diuretics, renovascular hypertension can be distinguished from essential hypertension. Other investiga-

Table 45–3. Clinical clues suggestive of renovascular hypertension.

	Comment
Clues from history	
Hypertension in the absence of any family history of hypertensive disease	Suspect renovascular hypertension if the family history is negative; however, about one-third of patients with renovascular hypertension have a positive family history.
Age of onset of hypertension is under 25 years or over 45 years	Average age of onset of essential hypertension is 31 ± 10 (SD) years. Children and young adults usually have fibromuscular disease, whereas adults over age 45 years are more likely to have atherosclerotic narrowing of the arteries.
Abrupt onset of moderate to severe hypertension	Essential hypertension usually begins with a labile phase before mild hypertension becomes established, whereas the natural history in renovascular hypertension is usually more compressed, with the disease often appearing initially as moderate hypertension of recent onset.
Development of severe or malignant hypertension	Renovascular hypertension often becomes moderately severe and may cause accelerated or malignant hypertension; both forms of hypertension involve markedly increased secretion of renin.
Headaches	Essential hypertension is usually asymptomatic; headaches occur more commonly with renovascular hypertension and may be related to its greater severity or the high levels of angiotensin II (a potent cerebrovascular vasoconstrictor) associated with this disease.
Cigarette smoking	A recent survey showed that 74% of patients with fibromuscular renal artery stenosis are smokers; 88% of those with atherosclerotic disease smoke.
White race	Renovascular hypertension is uncommon in blacks.
Resistance to or escape from adequate control of blood pressure with standard diuretic or antiadrenergic therapy	Renovascular hypertension typically responds poorly to diuretics and ofen responds only transiently to antiadrenergic drugs.
Excellent antihypertensive response to converting enzyme inhibitors, eg, captopril	Converting-enzyme inhibitors block the renin-angiotensin-aldosterone system most effectively and are highly specific agents.
Clues from physical examination and routine laboratory studies	
Retinopathy	Hemorrhage, exudates, or papilledema indicates accelerated or malignant hypertension.
Abdominal or flank bruit	Bruits are not pathognomonic of renovascular hypertension, since they are common in elderly persons and occasionally occur in younger patients who have no apparent vascular stenosis.
Carotid bruits or other evidence of large-vessel disease	Vascular pathologic processes are not limited to the renal bed.
Hypokalemia exists in the untreated state or persists even after administration of a thiazide diuretic	Increased aldosterone secretion by the renin-angiotensin-aldosterone system reduces serum potassium level. This does not occur in untreated *essential* hypertension. Thiazide diuretics accentuate this phenomenon in *renovascular* hypertension.

tors confirmed the value of the captopril test, although they found it less reliable than first reported. The overall sensitivity is approximately 61%, and specificity is 86%. Differences in the reported accuracy of the test may be attributed to a number of factors. The assay used, the patient selection, and position during testing can all alter outcomes. Previous sodium depletion due to use of diuretics, dietary restrictions, and chronic treatment with captopril increases plasma renin activity and causes the captopril challenge test to be nonspecific. Patients taking beta blockers remain responsive to the test as described previously, unless the baseline plasma renin activity is less than 2.5 ng/mL/h, in which case the test may be unreliable.

Most studies have found the test to be less reliable in azotemic patients, and it does not discriminate be-

tween unilateral and bilateral disease. Moreover, the test may be less reliable in black patients than in white patients.

4. Captopril renography–A recently introduced addition to the captopril test is the comparison of both ^{131}I-hippurate and ^{99m}Tc-diethylenetriaminepentaacetic acid (^{99m}Tc-DTPA) renography before and after single-dose captopril. Patients with renal artery stenosis show a fall in glomerular filtration confined to the affected kidney and thus a selective fall in ^{99m}Tc-DTPA uptake with preservation or even an increase in ^{131}I-hippurate and ^{99m}Tc-DTPA uptake to the normal side. Captopril renography has been found to have 90–92% sensitivity and 86–93% sensitivity in various studies. It has become one of the most popular noninvasive tests for renovascular hypertension. Captopril renography may be less reli-

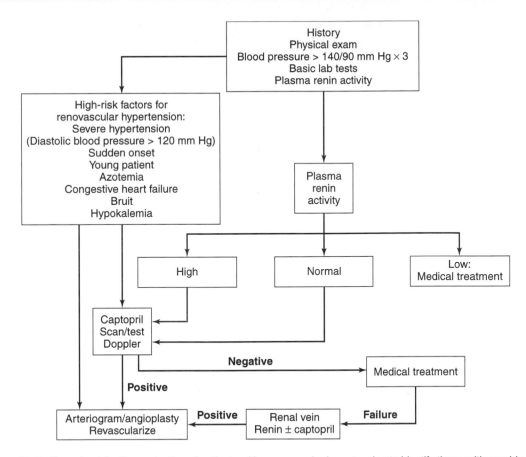

Figure 45–5. Flow sheet for the evaluation of patients with renovascular hypertension to identify those with curable renovascular disease. (Modified and reproduced, with permission, from Sosa RE, Vaughan ED Jr: World J Urol 1989;7:64.)

able in patients with impaired renal function or in patients with severe renal artery stenosis.

5. Renal vein renin sampling–Patients with high peripheral plasma renin activity levels or those in whom the captopril challenge test is positive may undergo further evaluation with renal vein sampling for renin. Samples are collected from each renal vein (V1 and V2) and from the distal inferior vena cava before and after administration of captopril, 25 mg orally (Table 45–6).

According to criteria established by Vaughan et al (1973), potentially reversible hypertension is characterized by ipsilateral hypersecretion of renin ([V1 – A] divided by A ≤ 0.50), contralateral suppression of renin secretion ([V2 – A] divided by A = 0), and an increase in the peripheral plasma renin activity level (Table 45–6). In patients with stenoses of both renal arteries, the pattern of renal vein renins often shows the same degree of asymmetry as in unilateral stenosis, lateralizing to the kidney with the greater degree of stenosis. The most marked asymmetry is seen in patients who have complete occlusion of one renal artery.

Renal vein renins are performed less widely today, in part because of high cost, but also owing to the high false-negative rate that tends to exclude patients from the benefit of renal revascularization.

6. Ultrasound scans–Renal Doppler ultrasound scanning is gaining widespread use for the evaluation of renovascular disease. Doppler ultrasound scanning can record velocity profiles of blood flow from the renal arteries and parenchyma. A number of criteria have been used to identify a stenosis. One is to take the ratio of the peak systolic velocity between the aorta and the renal artery. A renal-aortic ratio of 3.5 or more and peak systolic velocity of more than 200 cm/s are considered indicative of a significant stenosis. Another is the "tardus-parvus" pattern, which occurs distal to a stenosis and is characterized by a smaller and more rounded waveform.

Doppler exam of the main renal arteries may fail technically in up to 40% of patients. An alternative strategy is to use the flow profile from the interlobar arteries. This can be quantified as the renal resistive index, which is defined as the peak systolic flow veloc-

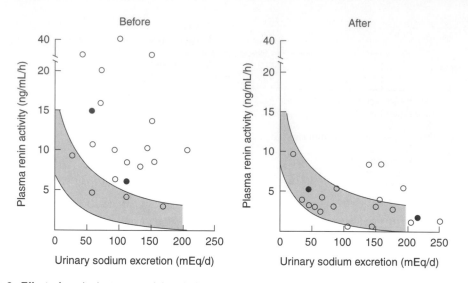

Figure 45–6. Effect of angioplasty on peripheral plasma renin activity level plotted against 24-h urinary sodium excretion. **Left:** Before angioplasty. **Right:** Six months after angioplasty. Hatched area shows normal range. o = Cured or improved, • = Failed to improve. (Reproduced, with permission, from Pickering TG et al: Predictive value and changes of renin secretion in hypertensive patients with unilateral renovascular disease undergoing successful renal angioplasty. Am J Med 1984;76:398.)

Table 45–4. Predictive value of screening tests for renovascular hypertension.

		IVP[1]	DIVA[2]	PRA[3]	Single-Dose[4] Captopril
Sensitivity	(%)	75	88	80	100
Specificity	(%)	86	89	84	95
False positive	(%)	14	11	16	5
False negative	(%)	25	12	20	0
Predictive value (%)					
Prevalence	2%	9.9	14.6	9.3	29
	5%	22.1	30.5	20.8	51.3
	10%	37.5	48.1	35.7	69
Exclusion value (%)					
Prevalence	2%	99.4	99.7	99.5	100
	5%	98.5	99.3	98.8	100
	10%	96.7	98.5	97.4	100

Predictive value =

$$\frac{Sensitivity \times Prevalence}{(Sensitivity \times Prevalence) + False\text{-}positive\ rate \times (100 - Prevalence)} \times 100$$

Exclusion value =

$$\frac{Specificity \times (100 - Prevalence)}{Specificity \times (100 - Prevalence) + (False\text{-}negative\ rate) \times Prevalence} \times 100$$

[1]Harvey RJ et al: Screening for renovascular hypertension. JAMA 1985;254:388.
[2]Pickering TG et al: Predictive value and changes of renin secretion in hypertensive patients with unilateral renovascular disease undergoing successful renal angioplasty. Am J Med 1985;76:398.
[3]Brunner HR et al: Angiotensin II blockade in man by SAR[1]-ALA[1]—Angiotensin for understanding and treatment of high blood pressure. Lancet 1973;2:1045.
[4]Muller FB et al: The captopril test for identifying renovascular disease in hypertensive patients. Am J Med 1986;80:633.

Table 45–5. Single-dose captopril test. Criteria distinguishing patients with renovascular hypertension from those with essential hypertension.

Stimulated plasma renin activity of 12 ng/mL/h or more **and**
Absolute increase in plasma renin activity of 10 ng/mL/h **or more and**
Percent increase in plasma renin activity of 150% or more **or** of 400% if the baseline plasma renin activity is less than 3 ng/mL/h.

Source: Reproduced, with permission, from Muller FB et al: The captopril test for identifying renovascular disease in hypertensive patients. Am J Med 1986;80:633.

ity – peak end-diastolic flow velocity/peak systolic flow velocity × 100. A difference of resistive index between the 2 kidneys of more than 5% has been used as an indication of renal artery stenosis. Also, the absence of flow in the artery and a low-amplitude parenchymal signal is diagnostic of occlusion of the renal artery. In a meta-analysis of the cost-effectiveness of different methods for diagnosing renovascular hypertension, Blaufox et al (1996) concluded that the sensitivity of

Table 45–6. Renin values for reversibility of renovascular hypertension.

Collection of samples (Patient should have moderate sodium intake, ie, 40–100 mEq/d).
1. With patient ambulatory, measure peripheral plasma renin level and 24-h urinary excretion of sodium under steady-state conditions (ie, not on the day of arteriography).
2. Before and after blockade with converting-enzyme inhibitor, collect blood for measurement of plasma renin levels.
3. With patient supine, collect blood samples for measurement of renin levels[1]: sample from renal vein of kidney thought to be affected (V1), matching sample from aorta (A1) or inferior vena cava (IVC1), sample from renal vein of contralateral kidney (V2), and second matching sample from aorta (A2) or inferior vena cava (IVC2).
4. If results of initial renin determinations are inconclusive, enhance renin secretion by using converting-enzyme inhibitor blockade.
Criteria for predicting reversibility
  High plasma renin level in relation to urinary sodium level. Indicates hypersecretion of renin.
  Marked reactive rise in plasma renin level and fall in blood pressure in response to converting-enzyme inhibitor.
  In contralateral kidney, $V2 - A2 \approx 0$. Indicates suppression of renin secretion in this kidney.
  In affected kidney, $(V1 - A1) \div A1 > 0.5$. Indicates unilateral renin secretion and reduced renal blood flow.
  In patients with high plasma renin levels, low ratios of renal vein renin to aorta renin ($[V1 - A1] \div A1 + [V2 - A2] \div A2 \leq 0.5$) indicate incorrect sampling or segmental sampling. Repeat measurements with segmental samplings.

[1]Renin levels in inferior vena cava (IVC) can be substituted for those in aorta (A); values are identical (Sealey et al, 1973).
Source: Modified and reproduced, with permission, from Vaughan ED Jr: Renal artery stenosis. In: Brenner BM, Stein JH (editors): *Hypertension,* vol. 8 of *Contemporary Issues in Nephrology.* Churchill Livingstone, 1981.

Doppler testing was no better than captopril renography and that, although the specificity was higher, this was offset by the high technical failure rate of 17%.

The advantages of duplex scanning are that it is noninvasive and free of adverse effects. For the patient with an elevated serum creatinine in whom the physician wants to determine, with a high degree of likelihood, whether significant renal artery disease is contributing to the azotemia, duplex scanning is useful. It can also be used for following up patients after percutaneous transluminal renal angioplasty, renal artery stents, or bypass surgery.

An interesting new development has been to use the hemodynamic effects of captopril to improve the diagnostic accuracy of Doppler scanning. Rene et al (1995) found that the pulsus tardus pattern was more likely to be seen after captopril in stenotic renal arteries; 68% of stenoses could be diagnosed before captopril, and 100% could be diagnosed after captopril. Another technique is to compare the resistive index of the ischemic and nonischemic kidneys before and after captopril.

7. Magnetic resonance angiography (MRA)– Magnetic resonance angiography is a new technique that has the ability to visualize arteries noninvasively without contrast. Using phase contrast imaging, the gadolinium-enhanced MRA with 3-dimensional reconstruction of the images, sensitivities and specificities have been reported to be > 90% when compared with conventional angiography. Magnetic resonance angiography is much better at detecting proximal than peripheral lesions. The low false-negative rate for detecting major atherosclerotic lesions means that a normal MRA obviates the need for traditional angiography in high-risk patients. Its expense and the high degree of expertise required to obtain and correctly interpret good images precludes its use as a general screening test.

8. Helical (spiral) computed tomography– Computed tomography (CT) can be used to visualize arteries as well as solid tissues. Spiral CT differs from conventional CT in that it incorporates a rapidly rotating gantry, which enables acquisition of images with sufficient rapidity to visualize arteries as the contrast passes through. The resolution compares very favorably with that of MRA, although both techniques have limited ability to detect accessory renal arteries. The main appeal of spiral CT is that it enables construction of 3-dimensional images of the aorta, renal arteries, and kidneys all at the same time, using one of 2 procedures (maximal intensity projection or surface shaded display). Both are time-consuming to construct and require a highly skilled radiologist or technician. The sensitivity and specificity of spiral CT for detecting renal artery stenoses have been reported to be in the region of 95%. Unlike MRA, it can be used to examine the patency of renal arteries with intravascular stents. The chief disadvantages are the cost and the much greater volume of contrast agents needed to obtain adequate images (about 150 mL, compared with 15 mL for conventional digital subtraction angiography). This greatly limits its use in patients with impaired renal function.

9. Other tests–Excretory urography is not generally recommended as an initial screening test for renovascular hypertension because it has a sensitivity of only 75% and a specificity of 86% (Harvey et al, 1985). It is nonetheless useful in patients with a history of verified or suspected urologic disease and in the localization of anatomic defects before surgery.

Arteriography or digital intravenous subtraction angiography (see Chapter 6) has not greatly increased the predictive value of screening tests for identifying renovascular hypertension (Table 45–4). These methods involve intravenous injection of contrast material to delineate the anatomy of the renal arteries and urinary tract. However, arteriographic or angiographic demonstration of an arterial lesion must be supplemented by evidence of abnormal levels of renin secretion to prove that unilateral ischemia is the cause of renovascular hypertension.

B. Renal Parenchymal Disease: In patients with suspected renal parenchymal disease, preoperative evaluation of plasma renin activity is similar to that described for patients with renovascular hypertension. The captopril challenge test is recommended in these patients to elicit evidence of a reactive rise in plasma renin activity and a fall in blood pressure. Hypertension due to renal parenchymal disease is less frequently curable by surgical treatment than is renovascular hypertension. Nephrectomy should be avoided if the blood pressure can be controlled with antihypertensive medication and if the glomerular filtration rate in the involved kidney is sufficient to ensure the patient's survival if removal of the contralateral kidney ever becomes necessary.

Treatment

Patients with known or suspected hypertension must be methodically evaluated to identify those with renin-dependent hypertension and to plan individualized treatment.

There are 3 principal modes of treatment for renovascular hypertension: medical, surgical, and angioplasty with and without stents. Because renal artery stenoses impair renal function and cause hypertension, renal revascularization is preferred over medical management.

A. Medical Measures: Medical management of patients was difficult before the advent of modern antihypertensive therapy, and survival has improved with surgical treatment. Currently, blood pressure can be controlled effectively but renal function may deteriorate, especially in patients with atherosclerotic disease. Converting-enzyme inhibitors are the most powerful drugs for patients with renovascular hypertension. However, the inhibition of angiotensin II constriction of the efferent glomerular arteriole may lead to decreased glomerular filtration rate and even renal failure in patients with bilateral renal arterial disease. In patients with bilateral renal artery stenosis or stenosis of a renal artery in a solitary kidney, use of converting-enzyme inhibitors may increase creatinine and blood urea nitrogen. Moreover, renal artery stenosis is progressive, with 15% of patients suffering complete occlusion despite adequate blood pressure control. Angiotensin receptor blockers are being used to treat renovascular hypertension. As yet the clinical data as to the effectiveness of these medications are limited. Calcium channel blockers vasodilate the afferent arteriole and have been shown to lower blood pressure with less impairment of function than converting-enzyme inhibitors. In summary, medical management is limited to patients who are not candidates for intervention or in whom revascularization has failed. In these patients both blood pressure and renal function must be monitored carefully.

B. Transluminal Angioplasty: Patients who meet the criteria for reversible renovascular hypertension can now be treated with percutaneous transluminal balloon dilation of the stenotic renal artery (transluminal angioplasty; see Chapter 8). In successful cases, angiograms obtained after transluminal angioplasty show enlargement of the diameter of the renal artery (Figure 45–7), and measurements show that the renin activity returns to normal levels and the blood pressure likewise returns to normal or near-normal levels (Figures 45–6 and 45–8). Angioplasty is now the initial treatment of choice in all patients with fibromuscular hyperplasia and in patients with atherosclerotic disease, excluding those with osteal lesions and total occlusion. Successful dilation in more than 80% of these patients precludes the need for major surgery and can lower blood pressure while preserving or improving renal function. The results in patients with fibromuscular dysplasia are good. There is an overall benefit of 93% (58% cured, 35% improved, and 7% failed). Restenosis is uncommon in these patients. In patients with renal artery stenosis due to atheroma, the benefit is about 80% (22% cured, 58% improved, and 20% failed). The restenosis in patients with atheromatous disease is 19% after 9 months. It has been shown that failed angioplasty does not reduce the success rate of subsequent surgical renal revascularization.

C. Renal Artery Stents: Renal artery stents can be placed to maintain patency of the renal artery following angioplasty. The indications for stent placement include renal ostial stenoses that have a high restenosis rate following angioplasty. Other atheromatous lesions that were dilated unsuccessfully or have restenosed can be stented as well. The restenosis rate for these high-risk patients is less than that for angioplasty alone.

D. Surgical Measures: Surgery is indicated for patients with total renal artery occlusion and preservation of function, osteal lesions, and complex lesions,

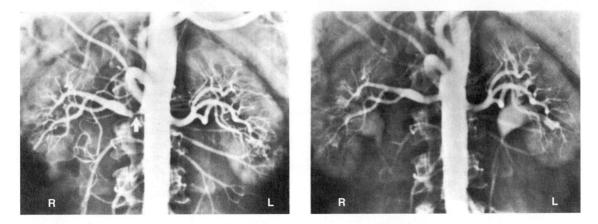

Figure 45–7. Aortograms showing unilateral right renal artery stenosis before (**left**) and after (**right**) successful percutaneous transluminal angioplasty. (Reproduced, with permission, from Vaughan ED Jr: Renal artery stenosis. In: Brenner BM, Stein JH [editors]: *Hypertension,* vol. 8 of *Contemporary Issues in Nephrology.* Churchill Livingstone, 1981.)

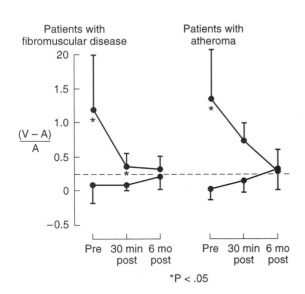

Figure 45–8. Effect of angioplasty on renal vein renin levels. Blood samples were drawn immediately before, 30 min after, and 6 months after angioplasty. The higher values are for the ischemic kidney; the lower ones, for the contralateral kidney. The asterisks indicate a significant difference between the 2 kidneys, and the dashed line represents the normal level of (V − A) divided by A (0.24). (Reproduced, with permission, from Pickering TG et al: Predictive value and changes of renin secretion in hypertensive patients with unilateral renovascular disease undergoing successful renal angioplasty. Am J Med 1984;76:398.)

and those in whom percutaneous transluminal dilation is not successful. The first surgical cure of hypertension was achieved by unilateral nephrectomy. However, unilateral nephrectomy has benefited only 26–37% of the large group of unselected patients with hypertension who have been so treated. Unilateral nephrectomy is now reserved for treatment of 2 groups of patients with hypertension: (1) those who have poor or absent renal function in the involved kidney but normal function in the contralateral kidney and in whom attempts at revascularization have failed, and (2) those at such high risk that the loss of functioning nephrons is offset by the elimination of the cause of significant excess renin secretion. Partial nephrectomy may be performed if the kidney has multiple renal arteries and only one is stenotic.

Today, surgical treatment emphasizes preservation of renal function. Accordingly, various methods may be used to attempt to revascularize an ischemic kidney; these include endarterectomy, aortorenal bypass graft using the saphenous vein or hypogastric artery, and hepatorenal and splenorenal bypass procedures for patients with severely diseased aortas. Hypertension has been cured or improved in more than 90% of the carefully selected patients treated surgically by experienced operating teams; the mortality rate has been about 2%. More favorable results have been achieved in patients with fibromuscular disease, who tend to be younger and healthier than the patients presenting with atheromatous disease. Renal revascularization for preservation of renal function in azotemic patients with renal arterial disease is gaining wider acceptance irrespective of blood pressure or renin values. All azotemic patients without a clear cause of renal failure should be evaluated for renal arterial disease.

REFERENCES

Abdi A, Johns EJ: The effect of angiotensin II receptor antagonists on kidney function in two-kidney, two-clip Goldblatt hypertensive rats. Eur J Pharmacol 1997;331:185.

Abdi A, Johns EJ: Importance of the renin-angiotensin system in the generation of kidney failure in renovascular hypertension. J Hypertens 1996;14:1131.

Bedoya L et al: The effect of baseline renal function on the outcome following renal revascularization. Cleve Clin J Med 1989;56:415.

Beregi JP et al: Helical CT angiography compared with arteriography in the detection of renal artery stenosis [see comments]. AJR 1996;167:495.

Blaufox MD et al: Cost efficacy of the diagnosis and therapy of renovascular hypertension. J Nucl Med 1996;37:171.

Brunner HR et al: Essential hypertension: Renin and aldosterone, heart attack, and stroke. N Engl J Med 1972;286:441.

Brunner HR et al: Hypertension of renal origin: Evidence for two different mechanisms. Science 1971;174:1344.

Cragg AH et al: Incidental fibromuscular dysplasia in potential renal donors: Long-term clinical follow-up. Radiology 1989;172:145.

Davidson RA, Wilcox CS: New tests for the diagnosis of renovascular disease. JAMA 1992;268:3353.

Elliott WJ, Martin WB, Murphy MB: Comparison of two noninvasive screening tests for renovascular hypertension. Arch Intern Med 1993;153:755.

Eyler WR et al: Angiography of the renal areas, including a comparative study of renal arterial stenosis in patients with and without hypertension. Radiology 1962;78:879.

Frederickson ED et al: A prospective evaluation of a simplified captopril test for the detection of renovascular hypertension [see comments]. Arch Intern Med 1990;150:569.

Gaul MK, Linn WD, Mulrow CD: Captopril-stimulated renin secretion in the diagnosis of renovascular hypertension. Am J Hypertens 1989;2:335.

Gavras H et al: Reciprocation of renin dependency in renal hypertension. Science 1979;188:1316.

Goldblatt H, Lynch J, Hangel R: Studies on experimental hypertension. J Exp Med 1934;59:347.

Gosse P et al: Captopril test in the detection of renovascular hypertension in a population with low prevalence of the disease. A prospective study. Am J Hypertens 1989;2:191.

Harvey RJ et al: Screening for renovascular hypertension. JAMA 1985;254:388.

Holley KE et al: Renal artery stenosis: A clinical-pathologic study in normotensive patients. Am J Med 1964;37:14.

Holm EA, Randlov A, Strandgaard S: Brief report: Acute renal failure after losartan treatment in a patient with bilateral renal artery stenosis. Blood Press 1996;5:360.

Howard JE et al: Hypertension resulting from unilateral renovascular disease and its relief by nephrectomy. Bull Johns Hopkins Hosp 1954;94:51.

Hunt JC, Strong CS: Renovascular hypertension: Mechanisms, natural history and treatment. Am J Cardiol 1973;32:562.

Idrissi A et al: The captopril challenge test as a screening test for renovascular hypertension. Kidney Int Suppl 1988;25:S138.

Jacobson HR: Ischemic renal disease: An overlooked clinical entity. Kidney Int 1988;34:729.

Jenni R et al: Combined two-dimensional ultrasound Doppler technique. New possibilities for the screening of renovascular and parenchymatous hypertension? Nephron 1986;44(Suppl 1):2.

Kohler TR et al: Noninvasive diagnosis of renal artery stenosis by ultrasonic duplex scanning. J Vasc Surg 1986;4:450.

Kooner JS, Peart WS, Mathias CJ: The sympathetic nervous system in hypertension due to unilateral renal artery stenosis in man. Clin Auton Res 1991;1:195.

Kutkuhn B et al: Validity of the captopril test for identifying correctable unilateral renovascular hypertension. Clin Exp Hypertens (A) 1991;13:143.

Laragh JH, Brenner BM: *Hypertension: Pathophysiology, Diagnosis and Management.* Raven Press, 1990.

Laragh JH, Sealy JE: The renin-angiotensin-aldosterone system and the renal regulation of sodium, potassium, and blood pressure homeostasis. In: Windhager EE (editor): *Handbook of Physiology,* section 8, vol. 2. Oxford Univ Press, 1992.

MacLeod M et al: Renal artery stenosis managed by Palmaz stent insertion: Technical and clinical outcome. J Hypertens 1995;13:1791.

Mann SJ, Pickering TG: Detection of renovascular hypertension. State of the art: 1992 [see comments]. Ann Intern Med 1992;117:845.

Maxwell MH, Lupu AN: Excretory urogram in renal arterial hypertension. J Urol 1968;100:395.

Maxwell MH, Lupu AN, Kaufman JJ: Individual kidney function tests in renal arterial hypertension. J Urol 1968;100:384.

Maxwell MH, Lupu AN, Taplin GV: Radioisotope renogram in renal arterial hypertension. J Urol 1968;100:376.

Miller ED Jr, Samuels AI, Haber E: Inhibition of angiotensin conversion in experimental renovascular hypertension. Science 1972;177:1108.

Miyajima E et al: Muscle sympathetic nerve activity in renovascular hypertension and primary hyperaldosteronism. Hypertension 1991;17:1057.

Muller FB et al: The captopril test for identifying renovascular disease in hypertensive patients. Am J Med 1986;80:633.

Nakamoto H et al: Angiotensin-(1-7) and nitric oxide interaction in renovascular hypertension. Hypertension 1995;25:796.

Novick AC: Selection of patients with atherosclerosis for renal reconstruction to preserve renal function. World J Urol 1989;7:98.

Novick AC et al: Diminished operative morbidity and mortality following revascularization for atherosclerotic renovascular disease. JAMA 1981;246:749.

Olbricht CJ et al: Minimally invasive diagnosis of renal artery stenosis by spiral computed tomography angiography. Kidney Int 1995;48:1332.

Pickering TG: Medical management of renovascular hypertension. World J Urol 1989;7:77.

Pickering TG, Mann SJ: Is there a role for non-invasive screening tests in diagnosing renal artery stenosis? (Editorial.) J Hypertens 1996;14:1265.

Pickering TG et al: Predictive value and changes of renin secretion in hypertensive patients with unilateral renovascular disease undergoing successful renal angioplasty. Am J Med 1984;76:398.

Plouin PF et al: Restenosis after a first percutaneous transluminal renal angioplasty. Hypertension 1993;21:89.

Postma CT et al: The captopril test in the detection of renovascular disease in hypertensive patients [see comments]. Arch Intern Med 1990;150:625.

Prince MR et al: Hemodynamically significant atherosclerotic renal artery stenosis: MR angiographic features. Radiology 1997;205:128.

Ratliff NB: Renal vascular disease: pathology of large blood vessel disease. In: Porush JG (editor): *Hypertension and the Kidney.* Grune and Stratton, 1985.

Rees CR et al: Palmaz stent in atherosclerotic stenoses involving the ostia of the renal arteries: Preliminary report of a multicenter study. Radiology 1991;181:507.

Rene PC et al: Renal artery stenosis: Evaluation of Doppler US after inhibition of angiotensin-converting enzyme with captopril [see comments]. Radiology 1995;196:675.

Ribstein J, Mourad G, Mimran A: Contrasting acute effects of captopril and nifedipine on renal function in renovascular hypertension. Am J Hypertens 1988;1:239.

Schreiber MJ, Novick AC, Pohl MA: The natural history of atherosclerotic and fibrous renal artery disease. World J Urol 1989;7:59.

Sealey JE et al: On the renal basis for essential hypertension: Nephron heterogeneity with discordant renin secretion and sodium excretion causing a hypertensive vasoconstriction-volume relationship. J Hypertens 1988;6:763.

Sealey JE et al: The physiology of renin secretion in essential hypertension: Estimation of renin secretion rate and renal plasma flow from peripheral and renal vein renin levels. Am J Med 1973;55:391.

Sinaiko AR, Wells TG: Childhood hypertension. In: Laragh JH, Brenner BM (editors): *Hypertension: Pathophysiology, Diagnosis, and Management.* Raven Press, 1990.

Sos TA et al: Percutaneous transluminal renal angioplasty in renovascular hypertension due to atheroma or fibromuscular dysplasia. N Engl J Med 1983;309:274.

Svetkey LP et al: Prospective analysis of strategies for diagnosing renovascular hypertension. Hypertension 1989;14:247.

Textor SC, Novick AC, Tarazi RC: Critical perfusion pressure for renal function in patients with bilateral atherosclerotic renal vascular disease. Ann Intern Med 1985;120:308.

Update of the working group reports on chronic renal failure and renovascular hypertension. National High Blood Pressure Education Program Working Group. Arch Intern Med 1996;156:1938.

Vaughan ED Jr, Sosa RE: Renovascular hypertension. In: Walsh PC et al (editors): *Campbell's Urology,* 6th ed. Saunders, 1992.

Vaughan ED Jr et al: Hypertension and unilateral parenchymal renal disease: Evidence for abnormal vasoconstriction-volume interaction. JAMA 1975;233:1177.

Vaughan ED Jr et al: Renovascular hypertension: Renin measurements to indicate hypersecretion and contralateral suppression, estimate renal plasma flow, and score for surgical curability. Am J Med 1973;55:402.

Veglio F et al: Assessment of renal resistance index after captopril test by Doppler in essential and renovascular hypertension. Kidney Int 1995;48:1611.

Wilcox GF, Smith TP, Fredrickson ED: Captopril glomerular filtration rate renogram in renovascular hypertension. Clin Nucl Med 1989;14:1.

46

Male Infertility

Paul J. Turek, MD

Infertility is defined as the inability to conceive after 1 year of unprotected sexual intercourse. Infertility affects approximately 15% of couples. Roughly 40% of cases involve a male contribution or factor, 40% involve a female factor, and the remainder involve both sexes. The evaluation of male infertility is undertaken methodically to acquire several kinds of information. Before discussing the diagnosis and treatment of male infertility, a review of basic reproductive tract physiology is in order.

MALE REPRODUCTIVE PHYSIOLOGY

THE HYPOTHALAMIC-PITUITARY-GONADAL AXIS

The physiology of the hypothalamic-pituitary-gonadal (HPG) axis was dramatically advanced from experiments in which hormones were purified from the brains of slaughterhouse animals in the 1950s and, more recently, from the development of radioimmunoassay techniques for accurate hormone measurement. The physiology of reproduction is centered on the HPG axis. It plays a critical role in each of the following processes, the last 2 of which will be discussed in this chapter:

1. Phenotypic gender development during embryogenesis
2. Sexual maturation during puberty
3. Endocrine function of the testis: testosterone production
4. Exocrine function of the testis: sperm production

Because of its importance in normal and pathologic states of reproductive health, an understanding of the HPG axis is vital for the evaluation and management of the infertile male.

Basic Endocrine Concepts

A. Hormone Classes (Figure 46–1): Two kinds of hormones classically mediate intercellular communication in the reproductive hormone axis: peptide and steroid. Peptide hormones are small secretory proteins that act via receptors located in the cell surface membrane. Hormone signals are transduced by one of 3 second-messenger pathways, as outlined in Figure 46–1. Ultimately, most peptide hormones induce the phosphorylation of various proteins that alter cell function. Examples of peptide hormones are luteinizing hormone (LH) and follicle-stimulating hormone (FSH).

In contrast, steroid hormones are derived from cholesterol and are not stored in secretory granules; consequently, steroid secretion rates directly reflect production rates. In plasma, these hormones are usually bound to carrier proteins. Since they are lipophilic substances, steroid hormones are generally cell membrane–permeable. After binding to an intracellular receptor, steroids are translocated to DNA recognition sites within the nucleus and regulate the transcription of target genes. Examples of reproductive steroid hormones are testosterone and estradiol.

B. Hormone Assays: Hormones can be quantified by biologic activity (bioassay) or by measuring hormone binding to specific, high-affinity antibodies (immunoassay). In vivo and in vitro bioassays are very useful for determining hormone potency but are tedious to perform and greatly influenced by the serum stability of the hormone. Immunoassays are usually more sensitive and much faster to perform. However, they do not monitor the biologic activities of hormones. In fact, the bioreactivity-immunoreactivity (B-I) ratio of hormones can change with variations in hormone concentration, binding proteins, and subunit composition of the hormone. Most commonly, a monoclonal-based "sandwich" assay (ELISA) is used for the evaluation of pituitary and gonadal hormone concentrations.

C. Feedback Loops: Normal reproduction depends on the cooperation of numerous hormones, and thus the signals that hormones generate must be well controlled. Feedback control is the principal mecha-

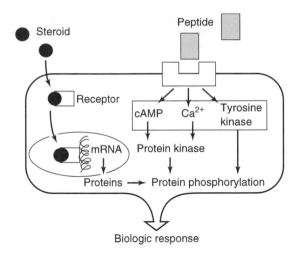

Figure 46–1. Two kinds of hormone classes mediate intercellular communication in the reproductive hormone axis: peptide and steroid.

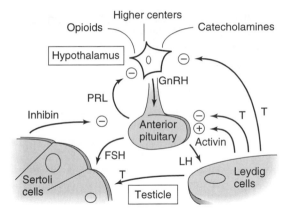

Figure 46–2. Major components of the HPG axis and recognized hormone feedback pathways. GnRH = gonadotropin-releasing hormone; PRL = prolactin; T = testosterone; FSH = follicle-stimulating hormone; LH = luteinizing hormone; + = positive feedback; − = negative feedback.

nism through which this occurs. With feedback, a hormone can regulate the synthesis and action of itself or of another hormone. Further coordination is provided by hormone action at multiple sites and eliciting multiple responses. In the HPG axis, negative feedback activity is responsible for the reduced pituitary LH secretion in the presence of elevated testosterone or estradiol. Thus, feedback control provides an exquisitely sensitive system for minimizing hormonal perturbations and returning to a homeostatic set point.

Components of the HPG Axis (Figure 46–2)

A. Hypothalamus: The hypothalamus weighs 4 g and is located caudal to the ventricles of the brain. As the integrative center of the HPG axis, the hypothalamus receives neuronal input from many brain centers, including the amygdala, thalamus, pons, retina, and cortex, and is the pulse generator for the cyclical secretion of pituitary and gonadal hormones. It is anatomically linked to the pituitary gland by both a portal vascular system and neuronal pathways. By avoiding the systemic circulation, the portal vascular system provides a direct mechanism for the delivery of hypothalamic hormones to the anterior pituitary. In addition, reverse flow through this vascular tree may allow pituitary hormones direct access to the hypothalamus.

Of the several hypothalamic hormones that act on the pituitary gland, the most important one for reproduction is gonadotropin-releasing or LH-releasing hormone (GnRH or LHRH), a 10–amino acid peptide secreted from the neuronal cell bodies in the preoptic and arcuate nuclei. At present, the only known func-

tion of GnRH is to stimulate the secretion of LH and FSH from the anterior pituitary. Although present in various brain regions and in other organs, the physiologic function of GnRH in extrapituitary locations is unknown. Once secreted into the pituitary portal circulation, GnRH has a half-life of approximately 5–7 min, almost entirely removed on the first pass through the pituitary either by receptor internalization or enzymatic degradation.

GnRH secretion by the hypothalamus is the result of integrated input from a variety of influences, including the effects of stress, exercise, and diet from the higher brain centers, gonadotropins secreted from the pituitary, and circulating gonadal hormones. It is important that the GnRH nerve terminals within the hypothalamus are outside the impermeable blood-brain barrier. This exposes the HPG axis to the effects of hormones present within the peripheral circulation. Known substances that regulate GnRH secretion are listed in Table 46–1. By far the most important of these are the gonadal steroid hormones.

GnRH secretion is pulsatile in nature. This secretory pattern governs the concomitant cyclic release of

Table 46–1. Substances that modulate GnRH secretion.

GnRH Modulator	Type of Feedback	Examples
Opioids	Negative/inhibitory	β-Endorphin
Catecholamines	Variable	Dopamine
Peptide hormones	Negative/inhibitory	FSH, LH
Sex steroids	Negative/inhibitory	Testosterone
Prostaglandins	Positive/stimulatory	PGE$_2$

FSH, follicle-stimulating hormone; LH, luteinizing hormone; PGE$_2$, prostaglandin E-2.

the gonadotropins LH and FSH (to a lesser extent) from the pituitary. The pulse frequency appears to vary from once hourly to as seldom as once or twice in 24 h. The demonstration of pulsatile activity in immortalized GnRH neurons in culture has led to the belief that a free-running, GnRH pulse-generator exists within the hypothalamus that is held in check primarily by the negative feedback of testicular hormones. The importance of the pulsatile GnRH secretory pattern in normal reproductive function is aptly demonstrated by the ability of the exogenously given GnRH agonists Lupron or Zoladex (leuprolide acetate) to halt testosterone production within the testicle by changing the pituitary exposure to GnRH from a cyclic to a constant pattern. As a consequence, pituitary receptors become downregulated through changes in the receptivity of Ca^{2+} ion channels.

B. Anterior Pituitary: The anterior pituitary gland, located within the bony sella turcica of the cranium, is the site of action of GnRH. The anterior pituitary has the highest blood flow of any organ in the body (0.8 mL/g/min) and receives > 80% of its nutrient blood supply as effluent from the hypothalamus through the portal vessels. GnRH stimulates the production and release of FSH and LH by a calcium flux-dependent mechanism. These peptide hormones were named after their elucidation in the female, but it is recognized that they are equally important in the male. The sensitivity of the pituitary gonadotrophs for GnRH varies with patient age and hormonal status.

LH and FSH are the primary pituitary hormones that regulate testis function. They are both glycoproteins composed of 2 polypeptide chain subunits, termed α and β, each coded by a separate gene. The α subunit of each hormone is identical and is similar to that of all other pituitary hormones; biologic and immunologic activity are conferred by the unique β subunit. Both subunits are required for endocrine activity. Sugars linked to these peptide subunits, consisting of oligosaccharides with sialic acid residues, differ in content between FSH and LH and may account for differences in signal transduction and plasma clearance of these hormones. Because of the increased carbohydrate content of FSH, it is cleared more slowly from the serum than is LH (Table 46–2).

Secretory pulses of LH vary in frequency from 8 to 16 pulses in 24 h and vary in amplitude by 1- to 3-fold. These pulse patterns generally reflect GnRH release. Both androgens and estrogens regulate LH secretion through negative feedback. The effect of GnRH on the pulsatile secretion of FSH is less well described. On average, FSH pulses occur approximately every 1.5 h and vary in amplitude by 25%. The FSH response to GnRH is more difficult to measure than that of LH because of a smaller amplitude response and a longer serum half-life. The recently discovered gonadal proteins inhibin and activin may exert significant effects on FSH secretion and are thought to account for the relative secretory independence of FSH from GnRH secretion. They will be discussed in the Testis section.

The only known effects of FSH and LH are in the gonads. They activate adenylate cyclase which leads to increases in intracellular cAMP. In the testis, LH stimulates steroidogenesis within Leydig cells by inducing the mitochondrial conversion of cholesterol to pregnenolone and eventually to testosterone. FSH binds to Sertoli cells and spermatogonial membranes within the testis and is the major stimulator of seminiferous tubule growth during development. FSH is essential for the initiation of spermatogenesis at puberty. In the adult, the major physiologic role of FSH is to stimulate quantitatively normal levels of spermatogenesis.

A third anterior pituitary hormone, prolactin, can also have effects on the HPG axis and fertility. Prolactin is a large, globular protein of 199 amino acids (23 kDa) that is known to affect milk synthesis during pregnancy and lactation in women. The normal role of prolactin in men is less clear, but it appears to be primarily involved with reproductive function. In rodents, prolactin receptors are present in Leydig cells of the testes and also in the prostate and seminal vesicles. Prolactin increases the concentration of LH receptors on the Leydig cell and therefore may help sustain normal, high intratesticular testosterone levels. It may also potentiate the effects of androgens on the growth and secretions of the male accessory sex glands. Normal prolactin levels may be important in the maintenance of libido. Although low prolactin levels are not necessarily pathologic, evidence suggests that hyperprolactinemia abolishes gonadotropin pulsatility by interfering with episodic GnRH release.

C. The Testis: Normal male virility and fertility requires the collaboration of both exocrine and endocrine compartments of the testis. Both of these units are under the direct control of the HPG axis. The interstitial compartment, composed mainly of Leydig cells, has an endocrine function and is responsible for steroidogenesis. The seminiferous tubules have an exocrine function with spermatozoa as the product.

1. Endocrine testis–Normal testosterone production in men is approximately 5 g/d, and secretion occurs in a damped, irregular, pulsatile manner. In normal men, approximately 2% of testosterone is "free" or unbound and considered the biologically active fraction. The remainder is almost equally bound to al-

Table 46–2. Structural and clearance characteristics of the gonadotropins.

	Molecular Mass (kDa)	No. Sialic Acid Residues	Serum Half-Life (h)
LH	28	1 or 2	0.5
FSH	33	5	4.0

bumin or sex hormone-binding globulin (SHBG) within the blood. SHBG can also bind estradiol in the peripheral blood, but the binding affinity is lower than that of testosterone. Several pathologic conditions can alter SHBG levels within the blood and, as a consequence, change the amount of free or bioactive testosterone available for tissues. Elevated estrogens and thyroid hormone decrease plasma SHBG and therefore increase the free testosterone fraction, whereas androgens, growth hormone, and obesity depress SHBG levels and decrease the active androgen fraction. Testosterone is a profound regulator of its own production through negative feedback on the HPG axis.

Testosterone is metabolized into 2 major active metabolites in the target tissue: (1) the major androgen dihydrotestosterone (DHT) from the action of 5α-reductase and (2) the estrogen estradiol through the action of aromatases. DHT is a much more potent androgen than is testosterone. In most peripheral tissues, testosterone reduction to DHT is required for androgen action, but in the testis and probably skeletal muscle, conversion to DHT is not essential for hormonal activity.

2. Exocrine testis–The primary site of FSH action is on Sertoli cells within the seminiferous tubules of the testis. In response to FSH binding, Sertoli cells are stimulated to make a host of secretory products important for germ cell growth, including androgen-binding protein (an effect augmented by testosterone), transferrin, lactate, ceruloplasmin, clusterin, plasminogen activator, prostaglandins, and several growth factors. Through these FSH-mediated actions on the testis, seminiferous tubule growth is stimulated during development and sperm production is initiated during puberty. In adults the FSH requirement for spermatogenesis is less clear, since spermatogenesis can occur in the absence of FSH. It is thought, however, that FSH is required to achieve normal levels of spermatogenesis.

3. Inhibin and activin–Since the early 1930s, it has been postulated that a gonadal substance exists that can decrease FSH release from the anterior pituitary. This was confirmed by the purification and cloning of a hormone called inhibin, a 32-kDa protein derived from Sertoli cells that specifically inhibits FSH release from the pituitary. Within the testis, inhibin production is stimulated by FSH and acts by negative feedback at the pituitary or hypothalamus to decrease FSH secretion. Recently, activin, a protein hormone with close structural homology to transforming growth factor-β has also been purified and cloned and appears to exert a specific stimulatory effect on FSH secretion. Activin consists of a combination of 2 of the same β subunits found in inhibin and is also derived from the testis. Activin receptors are found in a host of extragonadal tissues, suggesting that this hormone may have a variety of growth factor or regulatory roles throughout the body.

SPERMATOGENESIS

Spermatogenesis is a complex process by which primitive, totipotent stem cells divide to either renew themselves or produce daughter cells that become spermatozoa. These processes occur within the seminiferous tubule, a highly specialized environment of the testis. In fact, 90% of testis volume is determined by the seminiferous tubules and constituent germ cells at various developmental stages.

Sertoli Cells

The seminiferous tubules are lined with Sertoli cells that rest on the tubular basement membrane and extend into its lumen with a complex ramification of cytoplasm. Sertoli cells are linked by tight junctions, the strongest intercellular barriers in the body. These junctional complexes divide the seminiferous tubule space into basal (basement membrane) and adluminal (lumen) compartments. This anatomic arrangement, complemented by closely aligned myoid cells that surround the seminiferous tubule, form the basis for the blood-testis barrier. This barrier supports a microenvironment that is like no other in the body, in that spermatogenesis occurs in an immunologically privileged site. The importance of this sanctuary effect becomes clear when we remember that spermatozoa are produced at puberty and are considered foreign to an immune system that develops an ability for self-recognition long before this, during the first year of life.

Sertoli cells serve as "nurse" cells for spermatogenesis, nourishing germ cells as they develop. These highly specialized support cells also participate in germ cell phagocytosis. It is understood, but still unproved, that multiple sites of communication exist between Sertoli cells and developing germ cells for the maintenance of spermatogenesis within an appropriate hormonal milieu. It is clear that high-affinity FSH receptors exist on Sertoli cells and that FSH binding to its receptors induces the production of androgen-binding protein, which is then secreted into the tubular luminal fluid. By binding testosterone, androgen-binding protein ensures that high levels of androgen (20–50× that of serum) are present within the seminiferous tubule. Evidence also suggests that inhibin is Sertoli cell–derived and may be a key macromolecule in pituitary FSH regulation. Most recently, ligand-receptor complexes, such as c-*kit* and kit ligand, that may mediate communication between germinal and Sertoli cells have been described.

Germ Cells

Within the tubule, germ cells are arranged in a highly ordered sequence from the basement membrane to the lumen. Spermatogonia lie directly on the basement membrane, followed by primary spermatocytes, secondary spermatocytes, and spermatids as one progresses toward the tubule lumen. Thirteen different germ cell stages have been identified in the human spermatogenetic process. The tight junction barrier supports spermatogonia and early spermatocytes within the basal compartment and all subsequent germ cells within the adluminal compartment. Germ cells are staged by their morphologic appearance; there are dark type A (Ad) and pale type A (Ap) and type B spermatogonia and preloptotene, leptotene, zygotene, and pachytene primary spermatocytes, secondary spermatocytes, and Sa, Sb, Sc, Sd_1, and Sd_2 spermatids.

Cycles and Waves

A cycle of spermatogenesis involves the division of primitive spermatogonial stem cells into subsequent germ cell types through the process of meiosis. Since type A spermatogonial divisions occur at a shorter time interval than the entire process of spermatogenesis, several cycles of spermatogenesis coexist within the germinal epithelium at any one time. The duration of an entire spermatogenic cycle within the human testis is 74 days. During spermatogenesis, cohorts of germ cells at the same point in development are linked by cytoplasmic bridges and pass through the process together. Groups of such cells at different stages can be observed histologically on cross section; remarkably, many germ cell cohorts are seen only in association with certain other germ cells. This has led to the description of 6 stages of the seminiferous tubule epithelium in men. To add another level of complexity, there is a specific organization of the steps of the spermatogenic cycle within the space of seminiferous tubules, termed spermatogenic waves. In humans, this appears to be a spiral cellular arrangement as one progresses down the tubule. This spatial arrangement probably exists to ensure that sperm production is a continuous and not a pulsatile process.

MEIOSIS AND MITOSIS

Basic Processes

Somatic cells replicate by mitosis, in which genetically identical daughter cells are formed. Germ cells replicate by meiosis, in which the genetic material is halved to allow for reproduction. The processes of meiosis and sexual reproduction generate genetic diversity, providing a richer source of material on which natural selection can act. The life of a cell can

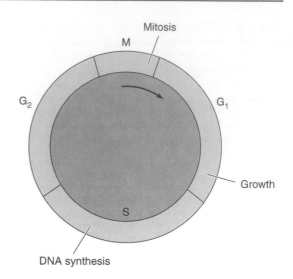

Figure 46–3. Recognized periods of the cell cycle. G = growth phase; S = DNA synthesis phase; M = mitotic phase.

be divided into several cycles, each of which is associated with different activities, as shown in Figure 46–3. There are growth phases, such as G_1, and a DNA synthesis (S) phase. About 5–10% of the cell cycle is spent in the mitotic phase (M), in which DNA and cellular division occurs. The process of cell replication by mitosis is a precise, well-orchestrated sequence of events involving duplication of the genetic material (chromosomes), breakdown of the nuclear envelope, and equal division of the chromosomes and cytoplasm into 2 daughter cells. Table 46–3 describes the phases of this process.

The essential difference between mitotic and meiotic replication is that a single DNA duplication step is followed by only 1 cell division in mitosis, but 2 cell divisions in meiosis (4 daughter cells). As a consequence, the daughter cells contain only half of the chromosome content of the parent cell. Thus, a diploid ($2n$) parent cell becomes a haploid (n) gamete. Meiosis is characterized by prophase, metaphase, anaphase, and telophase. Because of the 2 cell divisions, however, each of these phases occurs twice before the entire process is complete (divisions I and II). The 2 nuclei that result from meiosis I are haploid with respect to the parent cell. Thus, meiosis I is called a reduction division. The second meiotic cell

Table 46–3. Phases of the cell cycle and mitosis.

Mitotic Phase	Cell Cycle	Description of Events
Interphase	G_1, S, G_2	DNA doubling occurs.
Prophase	M	Nuclear envelope dissolves; spindle forms.
Metaphase	M	Chromosomes align at cell equator.
Anaphase	M	Duplicated chromosomes separate.
Telophase	M	Chromosomes to poles, cytoplasm divides.

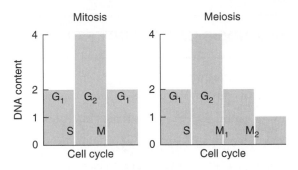

Figure 46–4. Changes in nuclear DNA content with mitosis and meiosis. G = growth phase; S = DNA synthesis phase; M = mitotic phase.

division, meiosis II, is called equational division. Figure 46–4 illustrates how the DNA content of the dividing cell changes with mitosis and meiosis. Other major differences between mitosis and meiosis are outlined in Table 46–4.

Making Sperm

The mature spermatozoan is an elaborate, highly specialized cell produced in massive quantity, up to 300 per g of testis per second. As a consequence, spermatogenesis is quite a complex and dramatic process that involves both mitotic and meiotic proliferation as well as extensive cell remodeling. Type B spermatogonia divide mitotically to produce diploid resting primary spermatocytes ($2n$), the germ cells that initiate the meiotic cycle. The clones of resting spermatocytes duplicate their DNA during interphase and then push their way into the adluminal compartment of the Sertoli cell cytoplasm. After the first meiotic division, each daughter cell contains one partner of the homologous chromosome pair, and they are called secondary spermatocytes ($2n$). These cells rapidly enter the second meiotic division in which the chromatids then separate at the centromere to yield haploid early round spermatids (n). Thus, each primary spermatocyte can theoretically yield 4

spermatids, although fewer actually result, as the complexity of meiosis is associated with a loss of some germ cells.

The process by which spermatids become mature spermatozoa can take several weeks and is one of the most elaborate differentiation events of any mammalian cell. This process requires the synthesis of hundreds of new proteins and the assembly of unique organelles. Within the purview of the Sertoli cell, several events occur during this differentiation of spermatid to sperm:

1. The acrosome is formed from the Golgi apparatus.
2. A flagellum is constructed from the centriole.
3. Mitochondria reorganize around the midpiece.
4. The nucleus is compacted to about 10% of its former size.
5. Residual cell cytoplasm is eliminated.

Early on, the nucleus of the round spermatid is spherical and is located in the center of the cell. Subsequently, the shape changes from spherical to asymmetric, as chromatin condenses. It is theorized that many cellular elements contribute to the reshaping process, including chromosome structure, associated chromosomal proteins, the perinuclear cytoskeletal theca layer, the manchette of microtubules in the nucleus, subacrosomal actin, and Sertoli cell interactions.

As spermiogenesis proceeds, the spermatid is moved toward the seminiferous tubule lumen. With completion of spermatid elongation, the Sertoli cell cytoplasm retracts around the developing sperm, stripping it of all unnecessary cytoplasm and extruding it into the tubule lumen. The mature sperm has remarkably little cytoplasm left after extrusion.

Sperm Maturation: The Epididymis

Spermatozoa within the testis have very poor or no motility and are incapable of fertilizing an egg. They become functional only after traversing the epididymis and the additional maturation process that it entails. Anatomically, the epididymis is classically divided into 3 regions: caput or head, corpus or body,

Table 46–4. Essential differences between mitosis and meiosis.

Mitosis	Meiosis
Occurs in somatic cells	Occurs in sexual cycle cells
1 cell division, 2 daughter cells	2 cell divisions, 4 daughter cells
Chromosome number maintained	Chromosome number halved
No pairing, chromosome homologs	Synapse of homologs, prophase I
No crossovers	> 1 crossover per homolog pair
Centromeres divide, anaphase	Centromeres divide, anaphase II
Identical daughter genotype	Genetic variation in daughter cells

and cauda or tail. Passage through these regions of the epididymis induces many changes to the newly formed sperm, including alterations in net surface charge, membrane protein composition, immunoreactivity, phospholipid and fatty acid content, and adenylate cyclase activity. Many of these changes are thought to improve the structural integrity of the sperm membrane and increase fertilization ability. The capacities for protein secretion and storage within the epididymis are known to be extremely sensitive to temperature and reproductive hormone levels, including estrogens. The transit time of sperm through the fine tubules of the epididymis is thought to be 10–15 days in humans.

FERTILIZATION

Fertilization normally occurs within the ampullary portion of the fallopian tubes. During the middle of the female menstrual cycle the cervical mucus changes, becoming more abundant and watery. These changes facilitate the entry of sperm into the uterus and protect the sperm from the highly acidic vaginal secretions. During this period of transit within the female reproductive tract, sperm undergo several physiologic changes, generally referred to as capacitation. During sperm contact with the egg, a new type of flagellar motion is initiated, termed hyperactive motility, that is characterized by large, lashing motions of the sperm tail. Sperm release lytic enzymes from the acrosome region to help penetrate the egg investments, a process known as the acrosome reaction. Direct contact between the sperm and egg appears to be mediated by specific receptors on the surface of each gamete. In the mouse, several glycoproteins, including ZP1, ZP2, and ZP3, have been demonstrated on the egg zona pellucida that are thought to mediate sperm-egg binding in this species. As a result of the interactions and changes, the sperm is incorporated into the cytoplasm of the egg.

After penetration of the egg, a "zona reaction" occurs in which the inner zona pellucida becomes impenetrable to more sperm, providing a block to polyspermy. In addition, the egg resumes its meiosis and begins to form a metaphase II spindle of sister chromatids. Recent evidence suggests that the sperm centriole within the midpiece is crucial for early spindle formation within the fertilized egg. The microtubule aster assembly that governs chromatid alignment in the metaphase spindle appears to be completely derived from the sperm and not the egg. This stage of fertilization is generally observed in vitro 14–19 h after penetration of the egg.

DIAGNOSIS OF MALE INFERTILITY

Given that a male problem or factor can be identified as the cause of infertility in 30–40% of couples and a contributing factor in 50% of cases, it is important to evaluate the male and female partners in parallel. Although the definition of infertility is a failure to conceive after 1 year of unprotected sexual intercourse, couples may be anxious to proceed with an evaluation sooner and this may be appropriate. Indeed, it is often more cost-effective to evaluate the male partner first, especially if there are significant infertility risk factors involved. A well-performed male evaluation should be rapid, cost-effective, and noninvasive. A complete urologic evaluation is important because male infertility may be the presenting symptom of otherwise occult but significant systemic disease. The evaluation involves an assessment of 4 types of information, as outlined in Figure 46–5.

HISTORY

The cornerstone of the male partner evaluation is the history. It should note the duration of infertility, earlier pregnancies with present or past partners, and whether there was previous difficulty with conception. A comprehensive list of information relevant to the fertility history is given in Table 46–5.

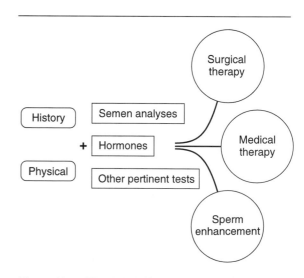

Figure 46–5. The male infertility evaluation consists of 4 kinds of information: the history, physical examination, semen analysis, and hormone assessment. Several therapeutic directions are possible once this information is collected.

Table 46–5. Components of the infertility history.

Medical history
  Fevers
  Systemic illness—diabetes, cancer, infection
  Genetic diseases—cystic fibrosis, Kleinfelter syndrome
Surgical history
  Orchidopexy, cryptorchidism
  Herniorrhaphy
  Trauma, torsion
  Pelvic, bladder, or retroperitoneal surgery
  Transurethral resection for prostatism
  Pubertal onset
Fertility history
  Previous pregnancies (present and with other partners)
  Duration of infertility
  Previous infertility treatments
  Female evaluation
Sexual history
  Erections
  Timing and frequency
  Lubricants
Family history
  Cryptorchidism
  Midline defects (Kartagener syndrome)
  Hypospadias
  Exposure to diethylstilbestrol
  Other rare syndromes—prune belly, etc.
Medication history
  Nitrofurantoin
  Cimetidine
  Sulfasalazine
  Spironolactone
  Alpha blockers
Social history
  Ethanol
  Smoking/tobacco
  Cocaine
  Anabolic steroids
Occupational history
  Exposure to ionizing radiation
  Chronic heat exposure (saunas)
  Aniline dyes
  Pesticides
  Heavy metals (lead)

A sexual history should be addressed. Most men (80%) do not know how to precisely time intercourse to achieve a pregnancy. Simple problems of timing and frequency can be corrected by a review of the couple's sexual habits. Normally, sperm reside within the cervical mucus and crypts for 1–2 days; thus, an appropriate frequency of intercourse is every 2 days for most men. Lubricants can influence sperm motility and are important to review. Commonly used products such as K-Y Jelly, Surgilube, Lubifax, most skin lotions, and saliva significantly reduce sperm motility in vitro. Couples should be counseled to avoid lubricants if at all possible; if needed, a lubricant that does not inhibit sperm motility should be used. Acceptable lubricants include vegetable, safflower, and peanut oils.

A general medical and surgical history is also important. Any generalized insult such as a fever, viremia, or other acute infection can decrease testis function and semen quality. The effects of such insults are not noted in the semen until 2–3 months after the event, because spermatogenesis and sperm transport require a full 75 days to complete. In essence, at ejaculation, sperm are already 3 months old. In general, uncontrolled diseases in any organ system of the body can reduce sperm quality; medical conditions should therefore be diagnosed and treated to maximize reproductive potential. Surgical procedures on the bladder, retroperitoneum, or pelvis can also lead to infertility, by causing either retrograde ejaculation of sperm into the bladder or anejaculation (aspermia), in which the muscular function within the entire reproductive tract is inhibited. A classic example of this is in patients with testicular cancer who have been treated with a retroperitoneal lymph node dissection. This procedure can interrupt the sympathetic chain either at the level of postganglionic nerves in the pelvis or by disruption of the sacral or inferior hypogastric plexi and cause either retrograde or anejaculation. Fortunately, newer "nerve-sparing" surgical techniques have significantly reduced this risk. Hernia surgery can also result in vas deferens obstruction in 1% of cases; this incidence may be rising because of the recent increased use of mesh patches that tend to be inflammatory to tissues.

Childhood diseases may also affect fertility. A history of mumps can be significant if the infection occurs postpubertally. After age 11, unilateral orchitis is found in 30% of mumps infections and bilateral orchitis in 10%. Mumps orchitis is thought to cause pressure necrosis of testis tissue as a sequelae of viral edema within the fixed and confined space of the testis. Marked testis atrophy is usually obvious later in life. Cryptorchidism is also associated with decreased sperm production. This is true for both unilateral and bilateral cases. Longitudinal studies of affected boys have shown that abnormally low sperm counts can be found in 30% of men with unilateral cryptorchidism and 50% of men with bilateral undescended testes. Differences in fertility have not been as easy to demonstrate, but it appears that boys with unilateral cryptorchidism have a slightly higher risk of infertility. However, only 50% of men with a history of bilateral undescended testes are fertile. It is important to remember that orchidopexy performed for this problem does not improve sperm production and semen quality later in life.

Exposure and medication histories are very relevant to fertility. Decreased sperm counts have been demonstrated in workers exposed to specific pesticides, an effect that is thought to result from a shift in the normal testosterone/estrogen hormonal balance. Ionizing radiation is also a well-described exposure risk, with temporary reductions in sperm production seen at doses as low as 10 cGy. Medications such as sulfasalazine, cimetidine, and Ca^{2+} channel-blocking agents, and ingestants such as tobacco, cocaine, and marijuana have all been implicated as gonadotoxins. The effects of these agents are usually reversible on withdrawal. Androgenic steroids, often taken by bodybuilders to increase muscle mass and development, act as contraceptives with respect to fertility. Excess testosterone inhibits the pituitary-gonadal hormone axis and virtually shuts down sperm production within the testis. Again, the effect of anabolic steroids is usually, but not necessarily, reversible on withdrawal of the medication. The routine use of hot tubs or saunas should be discouraged, as these activities can elevate intratesticular temperature and impair sperm production. In general, it is safe to say that an overall healthy body is best for a reproductively healthy body.

The family and developmental histories may also provide clues about infertility. A family history of cystic fibrosis (CF), a condition associated with congenital absence of the vas deferens (CAVD), or intersex conditions is important. The existence of siblings with fertility problems may suggest that a Y chromosome microdeletion or a cytogenetic (karyotype) abnormality is present in the family. A history of delayed onset of puberty could suggest Kallmann or Klinefelter syndrome. A history of recurrent respiratory tract infections may suggest a ciliary defect characteristic of the immotile cilia syndromes. This kind of information is more important than ever to uncover since reproductive technologies enable most men afflicted with such conditions to become fathers and therefore allow for the perpetuation of genetic abnormalities that may not be normally sustained.

PHYSICAL EXAMINATION

A complete examination of the infertile male is important, as factors that affect health in general can be associated with infertility. The patient should be adequately virilized; signs of decreased body hair, gynecomastia, and eunuchoid proportions (arm span greater than height) may suggest states of androgen deficiency.

The scrotal contents should be carefully palpated with the patient standing. As it is often psychologically uncomfortable for young men to be examined, one helpful hint for the clinician is to make the examination as efficient and as matter of fact as possible. Two features should be noted about the testis: size and consistency. Size can be assessed by measuring the long axis and width; as an alternative, an orchidometer can be placed next to the testis for volume determination (Figure 46–6). Standard values of testis size have been reported for normal men and include a mean testis length of 4.6 cm (range 3.6–5.5 cm), a mean width of 2.6 cm (range 2.1–3.2 cm), and a mean volume of 18.6 mL (+/- 4.6 mL) (Figure 46–7). Consistency is more difficult to assess but can be described as firm (normal) or soft (abnormal). Testis size and consistency are relevant because 90% of testis volume is contributed by germ cells and seminiferous tubules. Therefore, a smaller or softer than normal testis usually indicates impaired spermatogenesis.

The peritesticular area is an important component

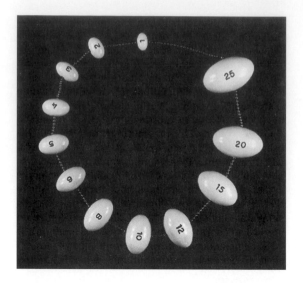

Figure 46–6. Prader orchidometer for measuring testicular volume. (Reproduced, with permission, from McClure RD: Endocrine investigation and therapy. Urol Clin North Am 1987;14:471.)

of the examination. Irregularities of the epididymis, located posterior-lateral to the testis, include induration, tenderness, or cysts. The presence or absence of the scrotal vas deferens is critical to observe, as 2% of infertile men may present with CAVD. Engorgement of the pampiniform plexus of veins in the scrotum is an important finding indicative of a varicocele. The exam should be performed while the patient is standing in a

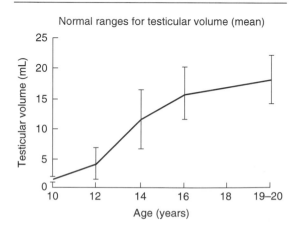

Figure 46–7. Normal values for testicular volume in relation to age. (Redrawn and reproduced, with permission, from Zachman M et al: Testicular volume during adolescence: Cross-sectional and longitudinal studies. Helv Paediatr Acta 1974;29:61, and McClure RD: Endocrine investigation and therapy. Urol Clin North Am 1987;14:471.)

warm room. Asymmetry of the spermatic cords is the usual initial observation, followed by the feeling of an "impulse" with the increased intra-abdominal pressure associated with a Valsalva maneuver. Varicoceles are usually found on the left side and are commonly associated with atrophy of the left testis. A discrepancy in testis size between the right and left sides should alert the clinician to the possibility of a varicocele.

Prostate or penile abnormalities should also be noted during the examination for infertility. Penile abnormalities such as hypospadias, abnormal curvature, or phimosis could result in inadequate delivery of semen to the upper vaginal vault during intercourse. Prostatic infection may be detected by the finding of a boggy, tender prostate on rectal examination. Prostate cancer, often suspected with the finding of unusual firmness or a nodule within the prostate, can occasionally be diagnosed among men who present with infertility. Enlarged seminal vesicles, indicative of ejaculatory duct obstruction, may also be palpable on digital rectal examination.

LABORATORY

Laboratory testing is an important component of the male infertility evaluation.

Urinalysis

A urinalysis is a simple and informative test that can be performed as part of the initial office visit. It may indicate the presence of infection, hematuria, glucosuria, or renal disease, and as such may suggest anatomic or medical problems within the urinary tract or elsewhere.

Semen Analysis

A carefully performed semen analysis is the primary source of information on sperm production, hormone integrity and reproductive tract patency. However, it must be stated that it is not a measure of fertility. An abnormal semen analysis simply suggests the likelihood of decreased fertility. Studies of infertile men have established that there are certain limits of adequacy below which it may be difficult to initiate a pregnancy. These semen analysis values were identified by the World Health Organization (1992) and are considered the minimum criteria for "normal" semen quality (Table 46–6). It is statistically more difficult to achieve a pregnancy if a semen parameter falls below any of those listed in the table. Of these routine semen variables, the count and motility appear to correlate best with fertility.

A. Semen Collection: It is important to remember that semen quality can vary widely in a normal individual from day to day and that semen analysis results are very dependent on collection technique. For example, the period of sexual abstinence before sample collection is a large source of variability. With

Table 46–6. Semen analysis—minimal standards of adequacy.

Ejaculate volume	1.5–5.5 mL
Sperm concentration	$> 20 \times 10^6$ sperm/mL
Motility	> 50%
Forward progression	2 (scale 1–4)
Morphology	> 30% WHO normal forms (> 4% Kruger normal forms)

No agglutination (clumping), white cells, or increased viscosity

each day of abstinence (up to 1 week) semen volume can rise by up to 0.4 mL, and sperm concentration can increase by 10–15 million/mL. Sperm motility tends to fall when the abstinence period is longer than 7 days. For this reason, it is recommended that semen collection be undertaken at a consistent time: after 48–72 h of sexual abstinence.

To establish a baseline of semen quality, several semen samples may be needed. Classic teaching has been to obtain 3 semen analyses to establish this baseline. However, in the era of cost-effective medicine, if 2 semen analyses show a discrepancy of < 20%, then a third sample may not be needed. Semen should be collected by self-stimulation, by coitus interruptus (less ideal), or with a special, nonspermicidal condom into a wide-mouthed, clean (not necessarily sterile) clear glass or plastic container. Because sperm motility decreases after ejaculation, it is important to have the specimen analyzed within 1 h of procurement. During transit, the specimen should be kept at body temperature.

B. Physical Characteristics and Measured Variables: Fresh semen is a coagulum that liquefies 5–30 min after ejaculation. The seminal vesicles contribute the coagulation factors, and the proteolytic factors (such as prostate-specific antigen) are derived from the prostate. After liquefaction, semen viscosity is measured and should not show evidence of stranding. Ejaculate volume should be at least 1.5 mL, as smaller volumes may not sufficiently buffer against vaginal acidity. Low ejaculate volume may indicate retrograde ejaculation, ejaculatory duct obstruction, incomplete collection or androgen deficiency. Sperm concentration should be > 20 million sperm/mL, as lower concentrations may make pregnancy less probable. Sperm motility is the single most important measure of semen quality. It should be evaluated within 1–2 h of collection and is usually rated in 2 ways: the fraction or percentage of all sperm that are moving and the quality of sperm movement (how fast, how straight they swim). A normal value for sperm motility is 50–60% motile and quality or progression score of at least 2 (on a scale of 0 [no movement] to 4 [excellent forward progression]).

Sperm cytology or morphology is another measure of semen quality. By assessing the exact dimensions and shape characteristics of the sperm head, midpiece, and tail, sperm can be classified as "normal" or not. In the strictest classification system (Kruger morphology), only 14% of sperm in the entire ejaculate are truly normal looking. In fact, this number correlates with the success of egg fertilization in in vitro treatments for infertility and thus is ascribed real clinical significance. Thus, sperm morphology may correlate with a man's fertility potential. It is accepted that sperm morphology is a sensitive indicator of overall testicular health, because the sperm morphologic characteristics are determined during spermatogenesis. The main role of sperm morphology assessment in the male infertility evaluation is to complement other information and to better estimate the chances of fertility.

C. Computer-assisted Semen Analysis (CASA): In an effort to remove the subjective variables inherent in the manual semen analysis, there have been attempts to quantify the reading of sperm motility, concentration, and morphology with the use of computers. Computer-aided semen analyses couple video technology with digitalization and microchip information processing to categorize sperm features by set algorithms. Most commonly, CASA systems report sperm concentration, motilities, and velocities (curvilinear, straight-line) and can be used to analyze sperm shape by examination of nuclear features. Although the technology is very promising, when manual semen analysis findings have been compared with those from CASA on identical specimens, CASA can overestimate sperm counts by 30% in the presence of high levels of contaminating cells such as immature sperm or leukocytes. In addition, at high sperm concentrations, motility can be underestimated with CASA. Last, despite the use of technology, CASA is still a user-dependent technique since the machine's variables are set by the operator. At this point, CASA has accepted value in the research setting and is beginning to gain further clinical acceptance as machines become more standardized.

D. Seminal Fructose and Postejaculate Urinalysis: Fructose is a carbohydrate derived from the seminal vesicles and is normally present in the ejaculate. If absent, the condition of seminal vesicle agenesis or obstruction may exist. Seminal fructose testing is indicated in men with low ejaculate volumes and no sperm present. It is measured by a chemical reaction using resorcinol, which turns color in the presence of fructose. A postejaculate urinalysis is a microscopic inspection of the first voided urine after

Table 46–7. Frequency of semen analysis findings in infertile men.

	Percent
All normal	55
Isolated abnormal	37
Low motility	26
Low count	8
Volume	2
Morphology	1
No sperm	8

ejaculation for the presence of sperm. If sperm are found in the voided urine, then retrograde ejaculation is diagnosed and treated. Such an analysis is indicated in diabetic patients with low semen volume and sperm counts, patients with a history of pelvic, bladder, or retroperitoneal surgery, and patients receiving medical therapy for prostatic enlargement. In general, the semen analyses of infertile men have identifiable patterns that may suggest a diagnosis. Frequently identified patterns are listed in Table 46–7.

Hormone Assessment

An evaluation of the pituitary-gonadal axis can provide valuable information on the state of sperm production. In turn, this evaluation can reveal problems with the pituitary axis that can cause infertility (hyperprolactinemia, gonadotropin deficiency, congenital adrenal hyperplasia). It is recommended that FSH and testosterone levels be measured in infertile men with sperm densities of $< 10 \times 10^6$ sperm/mL. Testosterone, as a final product of the pituitary axis, is a measure of the overall integrity of the axis and endocrine balance in general. FSH reflects more on the state of sperm production (the exocrine testis) than on overall endocrine balance. This combination of tests will detect virtually all (99%) endocrine abnormalities (Sigman and Jarow, 1997). Serum LH and prolactin levels may be obtained if testosterone and FSH are abnormal, to help pinpoint the endocrine defect in the axis. Thyroid hormone, liver function, and other organ-specific tests should be obtained if there is clinical evidence of active disease, as uncontrolled systemic illnesses can affect sperm production. The common patterns of hormonal disorders observed in infertility are given in Table 46–8.

In men with hypogonadotropic hypogonadism,

Table 46–8. Characteristic endocrine profiles in infertile men.

Condition	T	FSH	LH	PRL
Normal	NL	NL	NL	NL
Primary testis failure	Low	High	NL/High	NL
Hypogonadotropic hypogonadism	Low	Low	Low	NL
Hyperprolactinemia	Low	Low/NL	Low	High
Androgen resistance	High	High	High	NL

T, testosterone; FSH, follicle-stimulating hormone; LH, luteinizing hormone; PRL, prolactin; NL, normal.

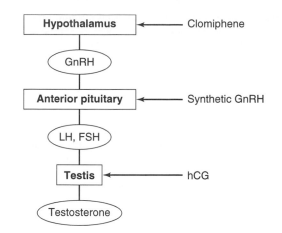

Figure 46–8. Dynamic hormone testing can be undertaken at all levels of the HPG axis. GnRH = gonadotropin-releasing hormone; FSH = follicle-stimulating hormone; LH = luteinizing hormone; hCG = human chorionic gonadotropin.

other pituitary hormones besides FSH and LH should be assessed, including adrenal cortical-stimulating hormone, thyrotropin-stimulating hormone, and growth hormone. With relatively normal spermatogenesis, low levels of plasma LH and FSH have no clinical meaning; likewise, an isolated low LH with normal testosterone is not significant. The measurement of plasma estradiol should be reserved for those men who appear underandrogenized or have gynecomastia in association with low, normal, or elevated testosterone levels.

Dynamic hormone testing can also be performed at all levels of the pituitary-gonadal axis, as shown in Figure 46–8, but is only rarely indicated clinically. The concept behind dynamic stimulation of the axis is that subtle abnormalities may be elucidated by perturbing the system. Dynamic testing may reveal dysfunction in feedback inhibition or demonstrate a lack of endocrine "reserve" within an endocrine gland that would not be picked up on simpler tests. These tests are limited in clinical application, as the response ranges in normal and infertile men are very broad, making reliable interpretation difficult.

A large retrospective study on 1035 infertility patients has been conducted and the prevalence of endocrine disorders examined (Sigman and Jarow, 1997). In general, 20% of infertile men had an abnormal hormone level on initial testing, but only 9.6% of men harbored a true endocrinopathy on repeat testing. If FSH elevations are excluded, the incidence of clinically significant endocrinopathies in infertile men is 1.7%.

In summary, the indications for hormonal evaluation of the infertile male are:

1. Sperm density of $< 10 \times 10^6$ sperm/mL on semen analysis
2. Evidence of impaired sexual function (impotence, low libido)
3. Findings suggestive of a specific endocrinopathy (eg, thyroid)

ADJUNCTIVE TESTS

Many adjunctive tests are available to help evaluate male-factor infertility if the initial evaluation fails to lead to a diagnosis. One guiding principle in this era of cost-containment is to order these tests only if they will change the way the patient is managed.

Semen Leukocyte Analysis

White blood cells (leukocytes) are present in all ejaculates and may play important roles in immune surveillance and clearance of abnormal sperm. Leukocytospermia or pyospermia, an increase in leukocytes in the ejaculate, is defined as $> 1 \times 10^6$ leukocytes/mL semen and may be a significant cause of male subfertility. The prevalence of pyospermia ranges from 2.8 to 23% of infertile men. In general, neutrophils predominate among inflammatory cells (Table 46–9). This condition is detected by a variety of diagnostic assays. With routine microscopy, leukocytes look similar to immature sperm forms (ie, spermatocytes) and cannot be distinguished. They are identified simply as "round cells." In over 70% of cases in which elevated numbers of round cells are observed in the ejaculate, they are usually immature sperm forms, the significance of which is unclear. Differential stains (eg, Papanicolaou) can distinguish leukocytes from immature sperm, as can a simple peroxidase stain that detects the peroxidase enzyme in neutrophils. Immunocytology is the present "gold-standard" technique to distinguish these cell types; it uses a monoclonal antibody specific to leukocyte surface antigens.

The reason for, and origin of, the immune cell infiltrate in pyospermia is poorly understood, although some proposed causes include an inflammatory response associated with infection, sensitization of the immune system to sperm antigens, or a reaction to

Table 46–9. Cells involved in leukocytospermia.

Cell Type	Relative Abundance
Neutrophils	++++
Monocyte/macrophage	+
T-helper lymphocytes	+
T-suppressor lymphocytes	++
B lymphocytes	+

low-grade toxins like cigarette smoke or alcohol. Regardless of the mechanism, it is believed that the inflammatory cells recruited to the ejaculate are in an activated state. The treatment of pyospermia is discussed later in this chapter.

Antisperm Antibody Test

The testis is a curious organ in that it is an immunologically privileged site, probably owing to the blood-testis barrier. Autoimmune infertility may occur when the blood-testis barrier is broken and the body is exposed to sperm antigens. Trauma to the testis and vasectomy are 2 common ways in which there is exposure to abnormal amounts of sperm antigen, and by which antisperm antibodies (ASA) are generated. The presence of ASA may be associated with impaired sperm transport through the reproductive tract or impairment in egg fertilization. An assay for ASA should be obtained when:

1. The semen analysis shows sperm agglutination or clumping.
2. Low sperm motility exists with history of testis injury or surgery.
3. There is confirmation that increased round cells are leukocytes.
4. There is unexplained infertility.

Antisperm antibodies can be found in 3 locations: serum, seminal plasma, and sperm-bound. Serum ASA are clinically less important than sperm-bound antibodies. The antibody classes that appear to be clinically relevant for sperm binding include IgG and IgA. IgG antibody is derived from local production and from transudation from the bloodstream (1%). IgA is thought to be purely locally derived. Many assays are available to detect ASA. The most widely used assay system is the immunobead test (Bioscreen Inc, New York). Polyacrylamide beads are coated with antihuman antibody and exposed to washed, motile sperm. Attachment of beads to sperm indicates the presence of antibody.

Hypoosmotic Swelling Test

The most clinically useful measure of sperm viability is cell motility. It is important to note, however, that the lack of sperm motility does not necessarily signify an absence of viability. Indeed, there are clinical conditions, such as immotile-cilia syndrome and extracted testicular sperm, in which there may be an immotile population of otherwise presumably healthy sperm. Such sperm can now be used clinically for micromanipulation and in vitro fertilization (IVF). Cell viability can be evaluated noninvasively by using the physiologic principle of hypoosmotic swelling. Conceptually, viable cells with functional membranes should swell when placed in a hypoosmotic environment (25 mM citrate and 75 mM fructose). Since sperm have tails, the swelling

response is very obvious in that tail coiling often accompanies head swelling. The fraction of total sperm that exhibit swelling can be calculated; in addition, the individual swollen sperm can be chosen for use with assisted reproductive technology. This sperm test is indicated in cases of complete absence of sperm motility.

Sperm Penetration Assay (SPA)

It is possible to measure the ability of human sperm to penetrate a specially prepared hamster egg in the laboratory setting. The hamster egg allows interspecies fertilization but no further development. This form of bioassay can give important information about the ability of sperm to undergo the capacitation process as well as penetrate and fertilize the egg. Infertile sperm would be expected to penetrate and fertilize a lower fraction of eggs than normal sperm. The SPA has undergone several generations of revisions, and its role in the prediction of human fertility potential is controversial. Most studies show that SPA results correlate with routine semen variables, and there is evidence to suggest that poor SPA results may correlate with lower pregnancy rates with intercourse or with IVF. The indications for the diagnostic SPA are limited to situations in which functional information about sperm are needed, ie, to further evaluate couples with unexplained infertility and to help couples decide whether intrauterine insemination (IUI) (good SPA result) or IVF and micromanipulation (poor SPA result) is an appropriate next therapeutic step.

An additional assessment of sperm fertilizing ability can be obtained with the hemizona assay. Unlike the SPA, which uses oocytes that are stripped of the zona pellucida, this bioassay specifically assesses sperm binding to the zona pellucida from nonfertilized, nonliving human oocytes. Each whole zona pellucida is divided in half under a microscope, and each half is incubated with either fertile sperm from a donor or with the patient's sperm. The number of sperm bound to each zona half is determined, and a binding ratio or index is calculated. It is not a widely used assay because of the expertise required to manipulate the zona for assay preparation. It is indicated in the setting of failed IVF to help determine whether poor sperm penetration was a factor.

Sperm–Cervical Mucus Interaction

Infertility can be caused by impaired sperm transport in the female reproductive tract. An evaluation of interaction between sperm and cervical mucus is one way to assess the quality of the transport process. The postcoital test involves the microscopic examination of the cervical mucus 2–8 h after intercourse near the time of ovulation. A positive result implies that cervical mucus has an appropriately thin consistency and that moving sperm are found within it. A poor or negative test implies that one or the other of these is abnormal and may indicate the presence of ASA or another sperm transport problem. This assay has not been standardized and has a considerable number of variables associated with it, including the timing of ovulation, specimen collection, and the interpretation of results.

A more sophisticated way to examine sperm-mucus interaction is by measuring the rate of sperm movement through a pool of cervical mucus on a microscope slide or within a capillary tube. This assay involves controls, in which sperm are placed in seminal fluid instead of cervical mucus, that add an important level of standardization to the assay when compared with the postcoital test. An abnormal cervical mucus–sperm interaction may suggest infertility treatment in which sperm are placed beyond the cervix into the uterus (IUI).

Chromosomal Studies

Subtle genetic abnormalities can present as male infertility. It is estimated that between 2% and 15% of infertile men with azoospermia or severe oligospermia (low sperm counts) will harbor a chromosomal abnormality, which can be found on either the sex chromosomes or on autosomes. A blood test for cytogenetic analysis (karyotype) can determine if such a genetic anomaly is present. Patients at risk for abnormal cytogenetic findings include men with small, atrophic testes, elevated FSH values, and azoospermia. Klinefelter syndrome (XXY) is the most frequently detected sex chromosomal abnormality among infertile men.

Cystic Fibrosis Mutation Testing

A blood test is indicated for infertile men who present with CF or the much more subtle condition, CAVD. Similar genetic mutations are found in patients with CAVD and those with CF, although the former group are generally considered to have only a form fruste of CF, in which the scrotal vas deferens is nonpalpable. Approximately 80% of men without palpable vasa will harbor a CF gene mutation. There are also recent data to indicate that azoospermic men with idiopathic obstruction and men with a clinical triad of chronic sinusitis, bronchiectasis, and obstructive azoospermia (Young syndrome) may be at higher risk for CF gene mutations.

Y Chromosome Microdeletion Analysis

As many as 7% of men with oligospermia and 15% of azoospermic men with testis failure have small, underlying deletions in one or more gene regions on the long arm of the Y chromosome (Yq). Several regions of the Y chromosome have been implicated in spermatogenic failure, identified as *AZFa, b,* and *c* (Figure 46–9). Deletion of the *DAZ* (deleted in azoospermia) gene in the *AZFc* region is the most commonly observed microdeletion in infertile men. No case of deletion of this gene family has been reported in fertile

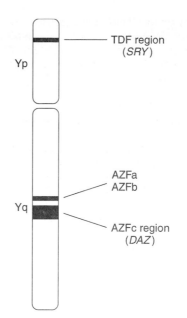

Figure 46–9. Regions of the Y chromosome that have been associated with male infertility include azoospermia factor (AZF) regions *a, b,* and *c*. The *AZFc* region contains the *DAZ* gene, one of the few true infertility genes isolated to date. TDF = testis-determining factor.

men. Fertility has been reported in men with these deletions with the use of IVF and micromanipulation of sperm that are present. A polymerase chain reaction–based blood test can examine the Y chromosome from peripheral leukocytes for these gene deletions and is recommended for men with low or no sperm counts and small, atrophic testes.

Radiologic Testing

A. Scrotal Ultrasound: High-frequency (7.5–10 mHz) ultrasound of the scrotum has become a mainstay in the evaluation of testicular and scrotal lesions. In men who have a hydrocele within the tunica vaginalis space, the testis may be nonpalpable and should undergo ultrasound to confirm that it is normal. Any abnormality of the peritesticular region should also undergo a scrotal ultrasound to determine its characteristics or origin.

Recently, scrotal color Doppler ultrasonography has been used to investigate varicoceles (Figure 46–10). By combining measurements of blood-flow patterns and vein size, both physiologic and anatomic information can be derived for the accurate assessment of this lesion. The diagnostic criteria that define a varicocele vary from study to study, but in general, a pampiniform venous diameter of > 2–3 mm is considered abnormal. Retrograde blood flow through the veins with a Valsalva maneuver may also be an im-

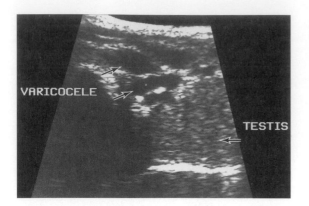

Figure 46–10. Scrotal ultrasound. Varicoceles are imaged as tubular echo-free structures. (Reproduced, with permission, from McClure RD, Hricak H: Scrotal ultrasound in the infertile male. Detection of subclinical unilateral and bilateral varicoceles. J Urol 1986;135:711.)

portant feature of a varicocele and has become a criterion in its definition.

B. Venography: Venography is generally accepted as the most accurate diagnostic method and can be considered a gold standard of varicocele detection. Although found by palpation in approximately 30–40% of subfertile men, varicoceles can be detected by venography in 70% of patients. Renal and spermatic venography is fairly invasive and is usually performed through percutaneous cannulization of the internal jugular vein or common femoral vein. Venographically, a varicocele is defined by a Valsalva-induced, retrograde flow of contrast material from the renal vein into the scrotal pampiniform plexus. This test is quite expensive and technician-dependent; at present its main indications are to assist in concurrent percutaneous treatment of varicoceles or for the diagnosis of varicocele recurrence after previous surgical treatment.

C. Transrectal Ultrasound (TRUS): High-frequency (5–7 mHz) TRUS offers superb imaging of the prostate, seminal vesicles, and ejaculatory ducts. Transrectal ultrasound has virtually replaced surgical vasography in the diagnosis of obstructive lesions that can cause infertility. Demonstration by TRUS of dilated seminal vesicles (> 1.5 cm in width) or dilated ejaculatory ducts (> 2.3 mm) in association with a cyst, calcification, or stones along the duct is highly suggestive of ejaculatory duct obstruction (Figure 46–11). This technique can also be used as a real-time guide during transurethral surgery for blockages in the ejaculatory duct. In addition, prostatic abnormalities such as tumors and congenital - anomalies of the vas, seminal vesicle, or ejaculatory ducts are easily defined with this technique. The indications for TRUS in infertility include low ejaculate volumes in association with azoospermia or severe oligospermia and decreased motility.

D. Computed Tomography Scan or Magnetic Resonance Imaging of the Pelvis: The general imaging techniques CT and MRI can help define reproductive tract anatomy. However, since the advent of TRUS, these studies have relatively few indications. They include evaluation of a patient with a solitary right varicocele, a condition that can be associated with retroperitoneal pathology, and evaluation of the nonpalpable testis.

Testis Biopsy and Vasography

The testis biopsy is a useful adjunct in the male infertility evaluation because it can provide a more precise clinical diagnosis in, and assist in treatment selection for, several infertility disorders. Most commonly, the technique involves a small, open incision in the scrotal wall and testis tunica albuginea under local anesthesia. A small wedge of testis tissue is removed and examined histologically. Abnormalities of seminiferous tubule architecture and cellular composition can be assessed and categorized into several patterns that aid in therapeutic decision-making.

A testis biopsy is most useful in the azoospermic patient. It is often difficult to distinguish between a failure of sperm production and obstruction within the reproductive tract ducts in men with azoospermia. In this situation, a testis biopsy provides critically important information about spermatogenesis that allows delineation between these 2 conditions. In cases of obstruction, formal investigation of the reproductive tract is warranted, beginning with a vasogram. A vasogram involves the injection of dye or contrast media into the vas deferens toward the bladder from the region of the scrotum (Figure 46–12). In plain film radiographs of the pelvis, contrast can then delineate the proximal vas

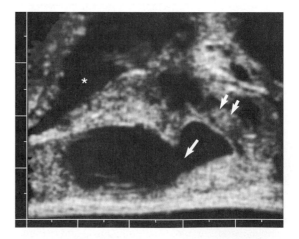

Figure 46–11. Transrectal ultrasonography (sagittal view) in a man with low ejaculate volume and low sperm counts and motility. Ejaculatory duct cyst (white arrow); urethra (double white arrows); bladder (asterisk).

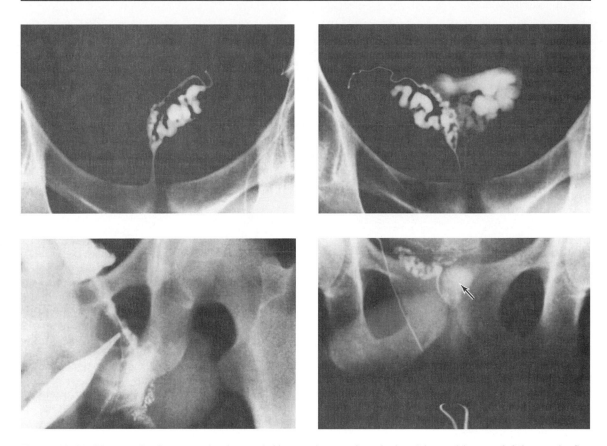

Figure 46–12. Vasography demonstrating (**upper left**) normal vas and seminal vesicles and (**upper right**) normal reflux into the bladder, confirming duct patency. Epididymal imaging showing extravasation (**lower left**) that demonstrates the difficulty of vasal dye injection toward the testis. **Lower right:** Azoospermia from a midline ejaculatory duct cyst is shown with contrast filling the cyst (arrow). (Reproduced, with permission, from McClure RD: Evaluation of the infertile male. In: deVere White R [editor]: *Problems in Urology*. Lippincott, 1987.)

deferens, seminal vesicle, and ejaculatory duct anatomy and determine whether or not obstruction is present. Sampling of vasal fluid during the same procedure can also determine whether sperm are present within the scrotal vas deferens. The presence of sperm there implies that there is no obstruction in the testis or epididymis. With such information, the site of obstruction can be accurately determined.

Whether a biopsy is indicated in cases of oligospermia is controversial. There may be rare cases of partial reproductive tract obstruction that can be diagnosed if a biopsy is performed, but the incidence of these disorders is low. While unilateral testis biopsies suffice in most cases, the finding of 2 asymmetric testes may warrant bilateral testis biopsies. A low sperm count may result when a unilateral unobstructed failing testis is paired with a normal obstructed testis. In this scenario, bilateral biopsies are indicated and will add valuable information for treatment decisions. Testis biopsies may also be indicated to identify patients at high risk for intratubular germ cell neoplasia. This pre-

malignant condition exists in 5.5% of men with a contralateral germ cell tumor of the testis and may be more prevalent in infertile men than in normal men.

Last, a relatively new indication for the testis biopsy is to determine whether men with atrophic, failing testes and elevated FSH levels actually have mature sperm present within the seminiferous tubules that may be used for high technology pregnancies with IVF and intracytoplasmic sperm injection (ICSI). It has been reported that a single testis biopsy can detect the presence of sperm in 30% of men with azoospermia, elevated FSH levels, and atrophic testes. Testicular sperm that are harvested in vitro after tissue procurement by biopsy are now routinely used to help men with severe male-factor infertility to achieve fatherhood.

Fine-Needle Aspiration "Mapping" of Testes
(Figure 46–13)

Although it is possible to use testicular sperm with

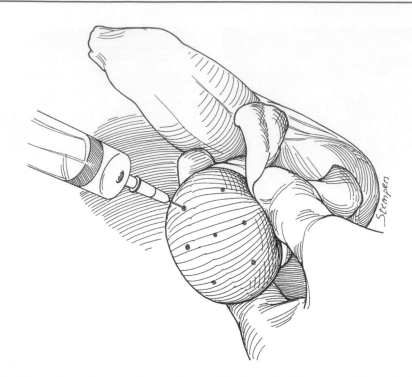

Figure 46–13. Technique of percutaneous fine-needle aspiration "mapping" for sperm in the testis. Cytologic samples are taken from various systematically sampled areas of the testis, guided by marks on the scrotum. (Reproduced, with permission, from Turek PJ, Cha I, Ljung B-M: Systematic fine needle aspiration of the testis: Correlation to biopsy and the results of organ "mapping" for mature sperm in azoospermic men. Urology 1997;49:743.)

IVF and ICSI to achieve pregnancies, there is a failure to obtain sperm in 25–50% of men with severe testis failure who are not obstructed. When testis biopsies fail to retrieve sperm, IVF cycles are canceled at great emotional and financial cost to couples. To minimize the chance of failed sperm retrieval, a diagnostic technique of systematically mapping the testis for sperm with percutaneous fine-needle aspiration has been described. This technique can detect sperm in 60% of men with nonobstructed azoospermia and has also confirmed that spermatogenesis can vary geographically in the failing testis such that pockets of sperm can exist.

The fine-needle aspiration procedure is performed under local anesthesia in the office. Systematically placed sites of aspiration are marked on the skin overlying the testis, and a needle is placed percutaneously into the testis to generate a core of tissue. The aspirated seminiferous tubules (5–10 mg) are smeared on a slide, fixed, stained, and read by a cytologist for the presence or absence of sperm. This technique eliminates the need for a diagnostic testis biopsy and is more of a "testis-sparing" procedure than a biopsy. The information gained from this technique can fully inform patients of their chances of subsequent sperm retrieval for IVF and ICSI.

Semen Culture

Seminal fluid that passes through the urethra is routinely contaminated with bacteria that colonize this area. This can make the interpretation of semen culture difficult. Thus, semen cultures should not be obtained at random, but only in selected situations. The unselected use of semen cultures is wasteful, given that 83% of all infertile men will have positive semen cultures and that the relationship between bacterial cultures and infertility is at best inconclusive. Semen cultures should be obtained when there is suspicion that a clinical or subclinical genital tract infection exists. Features suggestive of infection may include: (1) a history of genital tract infection, (2) abnormal expressed prostatic secretion, (3) the presence of more than 1000 pathogenic bacteria per milliliter of semen, and (4) the presence of $> 1 \times 10^6$ leukocytes per milliliter of semen (pyospermia).

The agents most commonly responsible for male genital tract infections are listed in Table 46–10. Gonorrhea is the most common infection. Ten percent to 25% of chlamydial infections may be asymptomatic. *Trichomonas vaginalis* is a protozoan parasite responsible for 1–5% of nongonococcal infections; it is usually symptomatic. *Ureaplasma urealyticum* is a common inhabitant of the urethra in sexually active men (30–50% of normal men) and is

Table 46–10. Most common organisms in male genital infection.

Neisseria gonorrhoeae	Cytomegalovirus
Chlamydia trachomatis	Herpes simplex II
Trichomonas vaginalis	Human papilloma virus
Ureaplasma urealyticum	Epstein-Barr virus
Escherichia coli (other	Hepatits B virus
gram-negative bacilli)	Human immunodeficiency
Mycoplasma hominis	virus

responsible for one-fourth of all cases of nongono-coccal infections. *Escherichia coli* infections are relatively uncommon in young men and are usually symptomatic. The relationship of *E coli* to infertility is unknown. Mycoplasmas are aerobic bacteria that are known to colonize the male reproductive tract. The true relationship of this organism to abnormal semen parameters or infertility has not been established. Rarer but possible causes of infection include anaerobic bacteria and tuberculosis.

CAUSES OF MALE INFERTILITY

The causes underlying male infertility are myriad in number but can be conveniently grouped by their effects at one or more of the following levels: pretesticular, testicular, and posttesticular.

PRETESTICULAR

Conditions that cause infertility that act at the pretesticular level tend to be hormonal in nature (Table 46–11).

Hypothalamic Disease
A.   Gonadotropin Deficiency (Kallmann Syndrome): Kallmann syndrome is a rare (1:50,000 per-

Table 46–11. Pretesticular causes of infertility.

Hypothalamic disease
  Gonadotropin deficiency (Kallmann syndrome)
  Isolated LH deficiency ("fertile eunuch")
  Isolated FSH deficiency
  Congenital hypogonadotropic syndromes
Pituitary disease
  Pituitary insufficiency (tumors, infiltrative processes, operation, radiation, deposits)
  Hyperprolactinemia
  Exogenous hormones (estrogen-androgen excess, glucocorticoid excess, hyper- and hypothyroidism)
  Growth hormone deficiency

sons), genetically heterogeneous disorder that occurs in familial and sporadic forms. The X-linked form of the disease is a consequence of a single gene deletion (Xp22.3 region, termed KALIG-1). It may also be autosomally transmitted with sex limitation to males. In either case, a disturbance of fetal neuron migration from the olfactory placode occurs during development. This neural region contains not only precursors for the olfactory nerves but also the LH-releasing cells of the hypothalamus, which explains the 2 most common clinical deficits in the disorder: anosmia and absence of GnRH. Pituitary function is normal. The clinical features include anosmia, facial asymmetry, color blindness, renal anomalies, microphallus, and cryptorchidism. The hallmark of the syndrome is a delay in pubertal development. The differential diagnosis includes constitutionally delayed puberty. Patients have severely atrophic testes (< 2 cm) with biopsies showing germ cell arrest and Leydig cell hypoplasia. Hormone evaluation reveals low testosterone, low LH, and low FSH levels. These men can be fertile when given FSH and LH to stimulate sperm production. Virilization can be obtained with testosterone or human chorionic gonadotropin (hCG).

B.   Isolated LH Deficiency ("Fertile Eunuch"): The cause of this very rare condition appears to be a partial gonadotropin deficiency in which there is enough LH produced to stimulate intratesticular testosterone production so that spermatogenesis is present but insufficient testosterone to promote adequate virilization. Affected individuals have eunuchoid body proportions, variable degrees of virilization, and often gynecomastia. These men characteristically have normal testis size, but the ejaculate contains reduced numbers of sperm. Plasma FSH levels are normal, but serum LH and testosterone levels are low-normal.

C.   Isolated FSH Deficiency: In this extremely rare condition, there is a lack of sufficient FSH production by the pituitary gland. Patients are normally virilized, as LH production is present. Testicular size is normal, and LH and testosterone levels are normal. FSH levels are uniformly low and do not respond to stimulation with GnRH. Sperm counts range from azoospermia to severely low numbers (oligospermia).

D.   Congenital Hypogonadotropic Syndromes: Several syndromes are associated with secondary hypogonadism in addition to other somatic findings. Prader-Willi syndrome (1:20,000 persons) is characterized by genetic obesity, retardation, small hands and feet, and hypogonadism. A deficiency of hypothalamic GnRH is present. The single gene deletion associated with this condition is found on chromosome 15. Similar to Kallmann syndrome, spermatogenesis can be induced with exogenous FSH and LH. Bardet-Biedl syndrome is another rare, autosomal recessive form of hypogonadotropic hypogonadism that results from GnRH deficiency. It is characterized by retardation, retinitis pigmentosa, polydactyly, and hypogonadism. The presentation is similar to Kallmann syndrome except that the patient has genetic obesity. The hypogonadism can also be treated with FSH and LH. Cerebellar ataxia can be associated with hypogonadotropic hypogonadism. This is a rare condition that can result from consanguineous unions. Cerebellar involvement includes abnormalities of speech and gait. These patients can be eunuchoid-looking with atrophic testes. Hypothalamic-pituitary dysfunction is thought to be the cause of infertility in this disease, and the basis for the dysfunction may be pathologic changes in cerebral white matter.

Pituitary Disease

A. Pituitary Insufficiency: Pituitary insufficiency may result from tumors, infarcts, surgery, radiation, or one of several infiltrative and granulomatous processes. In sickle cell anemia, pituitary and testicular microinfarcts are theorized to occur and result in infertility. Sickling of red blood cells (erythrocytes) occurs at low oxygen tension and, as a result, the viscosity of the blood increases and stasis of flow occurs in small vessels. Men with sickle cell anemia have decreased testosterone and variable LH and FSH levels. β-Thalassemia patients have mutations in the β-globin gene that lead to an imbalance in the α and β globin composition of hemoglobin; these patients are mainly of Mediterranean or African origin. Infertility is also believed to result from the deposition of iron in the pituitary gland and testes. Similarly, hemochromatosis results in iron deposition within the liver, testis, and pituitary and is associated with testicular dysfunction in 80% of cases.

B. Hyperprolactinemia: Another form of hypogonadotropic hypogonadism is due to elevated circulating prolactin. If hyperprolactinemia is present, secondary causes such as stress during the blood draw, systemic diseases, and medications should be ruled out. With these causes excluded, the most common and important cause of hyperprolactinemia is a prolactin-secreting pituitary adenoma. The use of high-resolution CT scanning or MRI of the sella turcica has classically been used to distinguish between microadenoma (< 10 mm) and macroadenoma (> 10 mm) forms of tumor. Functional or idiopathic hyperprolactinemia refers to elevations in prolactin without radiologic evidence of tumor. Unfortunately, stratification of disease into these groups based on radiologic diagnosis alone is misleading, as surgery for hyperprolactinemia almost always reveals a pituitary tumor. Since basal prolactin levels generally reflect tumor size, the degree of prolactin elevation has been added to radiologic assessment to categorize hyperprolactinemia (Table 46–12). Elevated prolactin usually results in decreased FSH, LH, and testosterone levels and causes infertility. Associated symptoms include loss of libido, impotence, galactorrhea, and gynecomastia. Signs and symptoms of other pituitary hormone derangements (adrenocorticotropic hormone,

Table 46–12. Correlation of serum prolactin levels and pathologic findings.

Prolactin Level (ng/mL)	Diagnosis
0–25	Normal
25–150	Pituitary stalk compression[1]
25–250	Microadenoma
> 250	Macroadenoma

[1]From a non-prolactin-secreting adenoma of the pituitary.

thyroid-stimulating hormone) should also be investigated.

C. Exogenous or Endogenous Hormones

1. Estrogens–An excess of sex steroids, either estrogens or androgens, can result in male infertility because of an imbalance in the testosterone-estrogen ratio. Hepatic cirrhosis is associated with an increase in endogenous estrogens because of augmented aromatase activity within the diseased liver. Likewise, excessive obesity may be associated with testosterone-estrogen imbalance owing to increased peripheral aromatase activity. Less commonly, adrenocortical tumors, Sertoli cell tumors, and interstitial testis tumors may also produce estrogens. Excess estrogens mediate infertility by decreasing pituitary gonadotropin secretion and inducing a secondary testis failure. Exposure to exogenous estrogens has been implicated as a reason for the controversial finding of decreased sperm concentrations in men over the last 50 years. Supporters of this claim suggest that men are overexposed to estrogenic compounds during fetal life, which results in compromised semen quality later in life (Carlsen et al, 1992). Postulated sources of exposure include anabolic estrogen use in livestock, consumed plant estrogens, and environmental estrogenic chemicals like pesticides. This xenoestrogen exposure theory, however, remains unproved as a cause of impaired sperm quality.

2. Androgens–An excess of androgens can also suppress pituitary gonadotropin secretion and lead to secondary testis failure. The use of exogenous androgenic steroids (anabolic steroids) by as many as 15% of high school athletes, 30% of college athletes, and 70% of professional athletes may actually result in temporary sterility because of this effect. Initial treatment for such exposures is to discontinue the steroids and reevaluate semen quality every 3–6 months until spermatogenesis returns. The most common reason for excess endogenous androgens is congenital adrenal hyperplasia, in which the enzyme 21-hydroxylase is most commonly deficient. As a result, there is defective cortisol synthesis and excessive adrenocorticotropic hormone production, which leads to abnormally high production of androgenic steroids by the adrenal cortex. High levels of androgens in prepubertal boys results in precocious puberty, in which there is premature development of secondary sex characteristics and abnormal enlargement of the phallus. The testes are characteristically small because of central gonadotropin inhibition by androgens. In young girls, virilization and clitoral enlargement may be obvious. In cases of the classic 21-hydroxylase-deficient congenital adrenal hyperplasia that present in childhood, normal sperm counts and fertility have been reported, even without treatment with glucocorticoids. This disorder is one of the few intersex conditions that are associated with fertility later in life. Other sources of endogenous androgens include hormonally active adrenocortical tumors or Leydig cell tumors of the testis.

3. Glucocorticoids–Exposure to excess glucocorticoids either endogenously or exogenously can result in decreased spermatogenesis. Elevated plasma cortisone levels depress LH secretion from the pituitary and induce secondary testis failure. Sources of exogenous glucocorticoids include chronic therapy for ulcerative colitis, asthma, or rheumatoid arthritis. Cushing syndrome is a common reason for excess endogenous glucocorticoids. Correction of the problem usually results in improved spermatogenesis.

4. Hyper- and hypothyroidism–Abnormally high or low levels of serum thyroid hormone affect spermatogenesis at the level of both the pituitary and testis. Thyroid balance is important for normal hypothalamic hormone secretion and for a normal balance of sex hormone-binding proteins that determine the testosterone-estrogen ratio. Thyroid abnormalities are a rare cause (0.5%) of male infertility.

5. Growth hormone–There is emerging evidence that growth hormone balance may play a role in male infertility. Some infertile men have deficient responses to growth hormone challenge tests and may respond to growth hormone treatment with improvements in semen quality. Growth hormone is an anterior pituitary hormone that has receptors in the testis. It induces insulin-like growth factor-1, a growth factor that may be important for spermatogenesis. The routine measurement of serum growth hormone is presently not indicated for the male infertility evaluation.

TESTICULAR

Conditions that cause infertility that act at the testicular level are listed in Table 46–13. Unlike most pretesticular conditions, which are treatable with hormone manipulation, most testicular effects are, at present, largely irreversible. If sperm are observed, however, assisted reproductive technology can provide biological children for affected men.

Chromosomal Causes

Abnormalities in chromosomal constitution are well-recognized causes of male infertility. In a study of 1263 infertile couples, one study found a 6.2% over-

Table 46–13. Testicular causes of infertility.

Chromosomal (Klinefelter syndrome [XXY], XX sex reversal, XYY syndrome)
Noonan syndrome (male Turner syndrome)
Myotonic dystrophy
Vanishing testis syndrome (bilateral anorchia)
Sertoli-cell-only syndrome (germ cell aplasia)
Y chromosome microdeletions (*DAZ*)
Gonadotoxins (radiation, drugs)
Systemic disease (renal failure, liver failure, sickle cell anemia)
Defective androgen activity
Testis injury (orchitis, torsion, trauma)
Cryptorchidism
Varicocele
Idiopathic

all incidence of chromosomal abnormalities. Among men whose sperm count was < 10 million/mL, the incidence rose to 11%. In azoospermic men, 21% had significant chromosomal abnormalities. For this reason, cytogenetic analysis (karyotype) of autosomal and sex chromosomal anomalies should be considered in men with severe oligospermia and azoospermia.

A. Klinefelter syndrome (Figure 46–14): Klinefelter syndrome is the most common genetic reason for azoospermia. accounting for 14% of cases (overall incidence 1:500 males). It has a classic associated triad: small, firm testes; gynecomastia; and azoospermia. This syndrome may present with delayed sexual maturation, increased height, decreased intelligence, varicosities, obesity, diabetes, leukemia, increased likelihood of extragonadal germ cell tumors, and breast cancer (20-fold higher than in normal males). In this abnormality of chromosomal number, 90% of men carry an extra X chromosome (47,XXY) and 10% of men are mosaic, with a combination of XXY/XY chromosomes. Paternity with this syndrome is rare but is more likely in the mosaic or milder form of the disease. The testes are usually < 2.0 cm in length and always < 3.5 cm; biopsies show sclerosis and hyalinization of the seminiferous tubules with normal numbers of Leydig cells. Hormones usually demonstrate decreased testosterone and frankly elevated LH and FSH levels. Serum estradiol levels are commonly elevated. Since testosterone tends to decrease with age, these men will require androgen replacement therapy both for virilization and for normal sexual function.

B. XX Male Syndrome: XX male syndrome is a structural and numerical chromosomal condition, a variant of Klinefelter syndrome, that presents in boys with gynecomastia at puberty or in men with azoospermia. The average height of these men is below normal, and hypospadias is common. Male external and internal genitalia are otherwise normal. The incidence of mental deficiency is not increased. Hormone evaluation shows elevated FSH and LH and low or normal testosterone levels. Testis biopsy

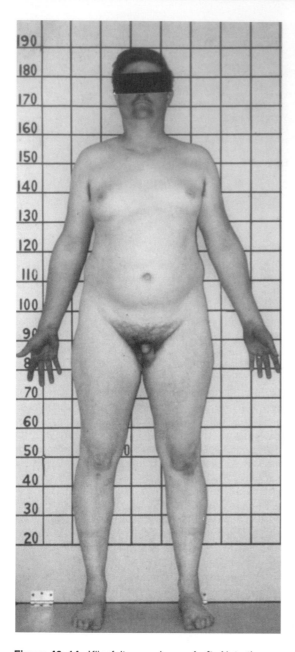

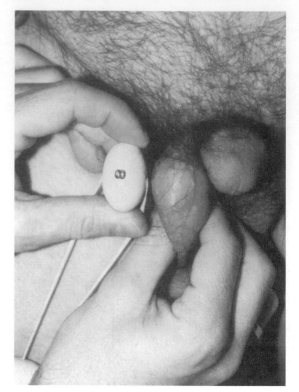

Figure 46–14. Klinefelter syndrome. **Left:** Note the eunuchoid habitus, female escutcheon, gynecomastia, and lack of temporal blading. **Right:** Characteristic firm, small testes. (Reproduced, with permission, from McClure RD: Endocrine investigation and therapy. Urol Clin North Am 1987;14:471.)

reveals an absence of spermatogenesis with hyalinization, fibrosis, and Leydig cell clumping. The most obvious explanation for the disease is that the SRY, or testis-determining region, is translocated from the Y to the X chromosome so that testis differentiation is present. However, the genes that may control spermatogenesis on the Y chromosome are not similarly translocated, resulting in azoospermia.

C. XYY Syndrome: The incidence of XYY syndrome is similar to that of Klinefelter, but the clinical presentation is more variable. Typically, men with 47,XYY are tall, and 2% exhibit aggressive, antisocial, and often criminal behavior. Hormone evaluation reveals elevated FSH and normal testosterone and LH levels. Semen analyses show either oligospermia or azoospermia. Testis biopsies vary widely but usually demonstrate arrest of maturation or Sertoli-cell-only syndrome.

Other Syndromes

A. Noonan Syndrome: Also called male Turner syndrome, Noonan syndrome is associated with clinical features of Turner syndrome (45,X). However, the karyotype in these men is either normal (46,XY) or mosaic (X/XY). Typically, these men have dysmorphic features like webbed neck, short stature, low-set ears, wide-set eyes, and cardiovascular abnormalities. At birth, 75% will have cryptorchidism that limits fertility in adulthood. If testes are fully descended, then fertility is possible and likely. Associated FSH and LH levels depend on the degree of testicular function.

B. Myotonic Dystrophy: Myotonic dystrophy is the most common reason for adult-onset muscular dystrophy. In addition to having the defining feature of mytotonia, or delayed relaxation after muscle contraction, patients usually present with cataracts, muscle atrophy, and various endocrinopathies. Most men with this condition are noted to have testis atrophy, but fertility has been reported. Infertile men may have elevated FSH and LH with low or normal testosterone, and testis biopsies show seminiferous tubule damage in 75% of cases. Pubertal development is normal; the testis damage seems to occur later in life.

C. Vanishing Testis Syndrome: Also called bilateral anorchia, vanishing testis syndrome is extremely rare, occurring in 1:20,000 males. Patients present with bilateral nonpalpable testes and sexual immaturity because of the lack of testicular androgens. The testes may have been lost owing to fetal torsion, trauma, vascular injury, or infection. In general, functioning testis tissue must have been present during weeks 14–16 of fetal life, since wolffian duct growth and müllerian duct inhibition occur along with appropriate growth of male external genitalia. These patients have eunuchoid body proportions but do not have gynecomastia. The karyotype is normal. Serum LH and FSH levels are elevated, and serum testosterone levels are extremely low. There is no treatment for this form of infertility; patients receive lifelong testosterone for normal virilization and sexual function.

D. Sertoli-Cell-Only Syndrome: Also referred to as germ cell aplasia, the hallmarks of Sertoli-cell-only syndrome are an azoospermic male with testes biopsies that show the presence of all testis cell types except for the germinal epithelium. Several causes have been proposed, including genetic defects, congenital absence of germ cells, and androgen resistance. Clinically, these men have normal virilization and testes of normal consistency but of slightly smaller size. There is no gynecomastia. Testosterone and LH levels are normal, but FSH levels are usually (90%) elevated. The use of the word syndrome implies that no recognized insult has occurred to the patient, since it is known that gonadotoxins like ionizing radiation, chemotherapy, and mumps orchitis can also render the testes aplastic of germ cells. There is no known treatment for this condition. In some patients, extensive testis sampling with fine-needle aspiration mapping or multiple biopsies can reveal the focal presence of sperm that can be used for pregnancy with assisted reproductive technologies.

E. Y Chromosome Microdeletions: Approximately 7% of men with low sperm counts and 13% with azoospermia have a structural alteration in the long arm of the Y chromosome (Yq). The testis-determining region genes that control testis differentiation are intact, but there may be gross deletions in other regions that may lead to defective spermatogenesis. This idea, originally postulated in 1976, was based on small structural changes in the Y chromosome seen on karyotyping. This led to the concept that an azoospermic factor (AZF) exists and that its absence (or mutation) accounts for the azoospermia. Since then, an explosion in molecular genetics technology has allowed for more sophisticated analysis of the Y chromosome. At present, 3 gene sites are being investigated as putative AZF candidates: *AZFa, b,* and *c.* The most promising site to date is *AZFc,* which contains the *DAZ* gene region. No fertile man has been observed to be missing the *DAZ* gene. The gene, of which there are at least 7 copies in this region, appears to encode an RNA-binding protein that may be involved in the genetics of the meiotic pathway of germ cell production. Homologs of the *DAZ* gene are found in many other animals, including mouse and *Drosophila.* A quantitative polymerase chain reaction–based assay is used to test the patient's blood for these deletions. In the future, sperm DNA may also be testable as part of a semen analysis. Since men with these microdeletions can have sperm in the ejaculate, they are certainly likely to pass them on to offspring if assisted reproductive technology is used to achieve biologic pregnancies.

Gonadotoxins

A. Radiation: The effects of radiotherapy on sperm production within the testis are well described. They are derived mainly from a series of remarkable experiments performed during the "atomic age" but only recently published. In a study of healthy prisoners in Oregon and Washington in the 1960s, Clifton and Bremner (1983) examined the effects of ionizing irradiation on semen quality and spermatogenesis. Before a vasectomy, each of 111 volunteers was exposed to a different level of radiation, from 7.5 to 600 cGy. Sperm counts were analyzed weekly both before and during the experiment; each prisoner served as his own control. There was a distinct dose-dependent, inverse relationship between irradiation and sperm count. A significant reduction in sperm count was manifested at 15 cGy, and sperm count was temporarily abolished at 50 cGy. Azoospermia was induced at 400 cGy in 4 of 5 patients; this persisted for at least 40 weeks. Despite these profound effects, sperm counts rebounded to preirradiation levels in most patients in follow-up.

From examination of the testis tissue after irradiation, it was concluded that spermatogonia are the germ cells most sensitive to irradiation at all doses. Given the dramatic sensitivity of testis tissue to irradiation, there is justifiable concern about radiation doses received through "scatter" to testes of men undergoing radiation therapy for cancer. In a study of patients with testis cancer who were subjected to abdominal radiation with gonadal shielding, the estimated mean unintended gonadal exposure was approximately 75 cGy. During treatment for Hodgkin disease, the testes receive approximately 200 cGy of scatter exposure. There does not appear to be an increase in congenital birth defects in the offspring of irradiated men.

B. Drugs: Medications are usually tested extensively for their potential as reproductive hazards before marketing. Despite this, it is wise to discontinue any unnecessary medications that can be safely stopped during attempts to conceive. A list of gonadotoxic medications can be found in Table 46–14. Medications may result in infertility by various mechanisms. Ketoconazole, spironolactone, and alcohol inhibit testosterone synthesis, whereas cimetidine is an androgen antagonist. Recreational drugs such as marijuana, heroin, and methadone are associated with lower testosterone levels unaccompanied by elevated LH levels, suggesting a centrally acting mechanism of action. Certain pesticides, like dibromochloropropane, have been found to have estrogen-like activity.

Cancer chemotherapy is designed to kill rapidly dividing cells; an undesired outcome is the cytotoxic effect on normally proliferating tissues such as the testes. The differentiating spermatogonia appear to be the germinal cells most sensitive to cytotoxic chemotherapy; alkylating agents such as cyclophosphamide, chlorambucil, and nitrogen mustard are considered the most toxic agents. The toxic effects of chemotherapeutic drugs vary according to dose and duration of treatment, type and stage of disease, age and health of the patient, and baseline testis function before therapy. Despite the toxicity of chemotherapeutic agents to the testis, the mutagenic effects do not appear to be significant enough to increase the chance of congenital defects or genetically linked diseases among offspring of treated men. However, patients should wait at least 6 months after chemotherapy is finished before attempting to conceive.

Systemic Disease

A. Renal Failure: Uremia is associated with infertility in addition to decreased libido, erectile dysfunction, and gynecomastia. The cause of hypogonadism is controversial and probably multifactorial. Testosterone levels are decreased, and FSH and LH levels can be elevated. Serum prolactin levels are elevated in 25% of patients. It is likely that estrogen excess plays a role in hormone axis derangement and contributes to hypogonadism. Medications and uremic neuropathy may play a role in uremic-related impotence and changes in libido. After successful renal transplantation, the hypogonadism usually improves.

B. Liver Cirrhosis: The hypogonadism related to liver failure may have various contributing factors. The reason for organ failure is important. Hepatitis may be associated with viremia and fevers, both of which can affect spermatogenesis. Excessive alcohol intake directly inhibits testicular testosterone synthesis, an action independent of its effect on the liver. Liver failure and cirrhosis are associated with testicular atrophy, impotence, and gynecomastia. Levels of testosterone and its metabolic clearance are decreased; estrogen levels are increased owing to augmented conversion of androgens to estrogens by aromatases. Decreased testosterone levels are not accompanied by proportionate elevations in LH and FSH levels, suggesting that a central inhibition of the HPG axis may also exist in liver failure.

C. Sickle Cell Disease: As mentioned earlier, sickle cell disease can cause pituitary dysfunction, most likely to the sludging of erythrocytes and associated microinfarcts within the organ. This same disease mechanism may also be active within testis tissue and may contribute to a primary hypogonadism in addition to the pituitary effect. As a result, spermatogenesis is decreased, accompanied by lower serum testosterone levels.

Defective Androgen Activity

Peripheral resistance to androgens occurs as a result of 2 basic defects: (1) a deficiency of androgen production through the absence of 5α-reductase or (2) a deficiency in the androgen receptor. In general, these diseases are a consequence of single gene deletions. Figure 46–15 shows the algorithm of normal male development. Androgen insensitivity syndromes are due to aberrations in this pathway.

A. 5α-Reductase Deficiency: 5α-Reductase deficiency causes normal development of the testes and wolffian duct structures (internal genitalia) but ambiguous external genitalia. The ambiguity results from an inborn deficiency of the 5α-reductase enzyme responsible for conversion of testosterone to

Table 46–14. Medications associated with infertility.

Calcium channel blockers	Allopurinol
Cimetidine	Alpha blockers
Sulfasalazine	Nitrofurantoin
Valproic acid	Lithium
Spironolactone	Tricyclic antidepressants
Colchicine	Antipsychotics

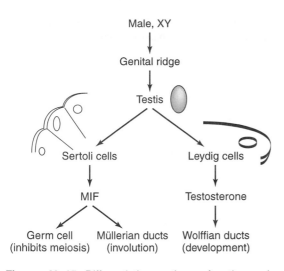

Figure 46–15. Differentiation pathway for the male. Aberrations in the pathway result in androgen insensitivity syndromes. MIF = müllerian inhibiting factor.

DHT in androgen-sensitive tissues like the prostate, seminal vesicle, and external genitalia. Thus far, 29 mutations have been described for the culprit enzyme in this syndrome. The diagnosis is made by measuring the ratio of testosterone metabolites in the urine and is confirmed by the finding of decreased 5α-reductase in genital skin fibroblasts. Spermatogenesis has been described in descended testes; however, fertility has not been reported in these patients. The lack of fertility may be due largely to functional abnormalities of the external genitalia.

B. Androgen Receptor Deficiency: Androgen receptor deficiency is an X-linked genetic condition marked by a resistance to androgens. The androgen receptor, a nuclear protein, is absent or functionally altered such that testosterone or DHT cannot bind to it and activate target cell genes. Since androgens have no effect on tissues, both internal and external genitalia are affected. Fertility effects depend on the receptor abnormality. Some patients are 46,XY males with complete end-organ resistance to androgens. They have female external genitalia with intra-abdominal testes. Testes show immature tubules and Sertoli cells, and the risk of testis cancer is elevated: Tumors will develop in 10–30% of patients without orchiectomy. Fertility is absent. Patients with mild receptor defects may present as normal-appearing infertile men. Spermatogenesis may be present, although impaired. It is unclear exactly how common this presentation is among infertile men.

Testis Injury

A. Orchitis: Inflammation of testis tissue occurs most commonly as a result of bacterial infection, termed epididymo-orchitis. Viral infections also occur in the testis in the form of mumps orchitis. Orchitis is observed in approximately 30% of postpubertal males who contract parotitis. Testis atrophy is a significant and frequent result of viral orchitis but is less commonly noted with bacterial infections.

B. Torsion: Ischemic injury to the testis secondary to twisting of the testis on the spermatic cord pedicle is not uncommon in prepubertal and early postpubertal boys. When diagnosed and corrected surgically within 6 h of the occurrence, the testis can usually be saved. Torsion may result in inoculation of the immune system with testis antigens that may predispose to later immunologically based infertility. It is well recognized that the "normal" contralateral mate of a torsed testis can exhibit histologic abnormalities as well. It has not been clearly demonstrated whether this is related to the torsion event or to an underlying abnormality in testes predisposed to torsion.

C. Trauma: Because of the peculiar immunologic status of the testis in the body (ie, it is an immunologically privileged site), trauma to the testis can invoke an abnormal immune response in addition to atrophy resulting directly from injury. Both may contribute to infertility. Trauma to the testis that results in fracture of the testis tunica albugineal layer should be surgically explored and repaired to minimize exposure of testis tissue to the body.

Cryptorchidism

The undescended testis is a very common urologic problem, observed in 0.8% of boys at 1 year of age. It is considered a developmental defect and places the affected testis at higher risk of developing testicular cancer. Although the newborn undescended testis is morphologically fairly normal, deterioration in early germ cell numbers is often seen by 2 years of age. The contralateral, normally descended testis is also at increased risk of harboring morphologic abnormalities in germ cell number. Thus, males with either unilaterally or bilaterally undescended testes are at risk for infertility later in life. Prophylactic orchidopexy is generally performed by 2 years of age to allow the testis to be palpated for cancer detection. It is unclear whether orchidopexy alters fertility potential in cryptorchidism.

Varicocele

A varicocele is defined as dilated and tortuous veins within the pampiniform plexus of scrotal veins. It constitutes the most surgically correctable cause of male subfertility. The varicocele is a disease of puberty and is only rarely detected in boys under 10 years of age. A left-sided varicocele is found in 15% of healthy young men. In contrast, the incidence of a left varicocele in subfertile men approaches 40%. Bilateral varicoceles are uncommon in healthy men (< 10%) but are palpated in up to 20% of subfertile men. In general, varicoceles do not spontaneously regress. The cornerstone of varicocele diagnosis rests on an accurate physical examination.

Several anatomic features contribute to the predominance of left-sided varicoceles. The left internal spermatic vein is 10 cm longer than the right; in addition, it usually joins the left renal vein at right angles. The right internal spermatic vein has a more oblique insertion into the inferior vena cava. This side-to-side difference in anatomy in the standing man may cause higher venous pressures to be transmitted to the left scrotal veins and result in retrograde reflux of blood within the pampiniform plexus.

It is well established that varicoceles are associated with testicular atrophy. It has also been reliably demonstrated that varicocele correction can reverse this atrophy in adolescent patients. There is also indisputable evidence that the varicocele affects semen quality. In fact, based on the work of MacLeod, a classic semen analysis pattern has been attributed to varicoceles. In a study of 200 men with varicoceles, MacLeod and Gold (1951) noted a mean sperm density of $< 20 \times 10^6$ sperm/mL and low motility in 90% of patients, a shift in sperm shape from oval to tapered and amorphous forms, and an increase in immature sperm forms. The finding of semen abnormalities constitutes the main indication for varicocele surgery in infertile men.

Precisely how a varicocele exerts an effect on the testicle remains unclear. Several theories have been postulated; it is likely that a combination of effects results in decreased spermatogenesis. Because pituitary-gonadal hormonal dysfunction has been found in varicocele patients, it has been suggested that a hormonal imbalance within the axis may be caused by a varicocele-induced decrease in testosterone production by Leydig cells. A second theory stems from early anatomic work that demonstrated internal spermatic vein reflux in varicocele patients. Presumably, if renal vein blood refluxes retrograde down the internal spermatic vein, then potentially toxic renal or adrenal metabolites can bathe and damage the testis. A third theory implicates an increase in hydrostatic pressure that is associated with venous reflux within the scrotal veins of varicocele patients. Increased hydrostatic pressures may reduce the efficiency of blood return and result in venous stasis, intratesticular venous congestion, and possibly testis hypoxia. The most intriguing theory of how varicoceles affect testis function invokes an inhibition of spermatogenesis through the reflux of warm corporeal blood into the pampiniform plexus, with consequent disruption of the normal countercurrent heat exchange balance. This theory ascribes a decrease in sperm production to the stasis of warm, refluxing venous blood within the scrotum, with the secondary effect of elevated intratesticular temperature.

Idiopathic

It has been estimated that at least 25% of male in-

fertility has no identifiable cause. As our knowledge expands, it is likely that causes will be assigned in these cases, especially with respect to genetic and environmental factors.

POSTTESTICULAR
(Table 46–15)

Reproductive Tract Obstruction

The posttesticular portion of the reproductive tract includes the epididymis, vas deferens, seminal vesicles, and associated ejaculatory apparatus. Abnormalities of these organs can result in infertility.

A. Congenital Blockages:

1. Cystic fibrosis–Cystic fibrosis is the most common autosomal recessive genetic disorder in the United States and is fatal. It is associated with fluid and electrolyte abnormalities (abnormal chloride-sweat test) and presents with chronic lung obstruction and infections, pancreatic insufficiency, and infertility. Interestingly, 98% of men with CF are missing parts of the epididymis; the vas deferens, seminal vesicles, and ejaculatory ducts are usually atrophic, fibrotic, or completely absent, causing reproductive tract obstruction. Spermatogenesis is usually normal. Congenital absence of the vas deferens accounts for 1–2% of all cases of infertility. On physical examination, no palpable vas deferens is observed on one or both sides. As in CF, the rest of the reproductive tract ducts may also be abnormal and unreconstructable. This disease has been demonstrated to be related to CF. Despite the fact that the vast majority of these men fail to demonstrate symptoms of CF, up to 65% of patients will harbor a de-

---

Table 46–15. Posttesticular causes of infertility.

Reproductive tract obstruction
  Congenital blockages
    Congenital absence of the vas deferens (CAVD)
    Young syndrome
    Idiopathic epididymal obstruction
    Polycystic kidney disease
    Ejaculatory duct obstruction
  Acquired blockages
    Vasectomy
    Groin surgery
    Infection
  Functional blockages
    Sympathetic nerve injury
    Pharmacologic
Disorders of sperm function or motility
  Immotile cilia syndromes
  Maturation defects
  Immunologic infertility
  Infection
Disorders of coitus
  Impotence
  Hypospadias
  Timing and frequency

tectable CF mutation. In addition, 15% of these men will have renal malformations, most commonly unilateral renal agenesis.

2. Young syndrome–Young syndrome presents with the clinical triad of chronic sinusitis, bronchiectasis, and obstructive azoospermia. The obstruction is located in the epididymis. The pathophysiology of the condition is unclear but may involve abnormal ciliary function or abnormal mucus quality. Although spermatogenesis is usually normal, reconstructive surgery is associated with lower success rates than are observed with other obstructed conditions.

3. Idiopathic epididymal obstruction–Idiopathic epididymal obstruction is a relatively uncommon condition found in otherwise healthy men. There is recent evidence linking this condition to CF in that one-third of men so obstructed may harbor CF gene mutations.

4. Adult polycystic kidney disease–Adult polycystic kidney disease is an autosomal dominant disorder associated with numerous cysts of the kidney, liver, spleen, pancreas, epididymis, seminal vesicle, and testis. Disease onset usually occurs in the twenties or thirties with symptoms of abdominal pain, hypertension, and renal failure. Infertility with this disease is usually secondary to obstructing cysts in the epididymis or seminal vesicle.

5. Blockage of the ejaculatory ducts–Blockage of the ejaculatory ducts, the delicate, paired, collagenous tubes that begin at the vas deferens–seminal vesicle junction, course through the prostate, and empty into the urethra at the verumontanum, is termed ejaculatory duct obstruction. It is the cause of infertility in 5% of azoospermic men. Such obstruction can be congenital and result from müllerian duct (utricular) cysts, wolffian duct (diverticular) cysts, or congenital atresia or can be acquired from seminal vesicle calculi or postsurgical or inflammatory scar tissue. It presents as hematospermia, painful ejaculation, or infertility. The diagnosis is confirmed by the finding of a low-volume ejaculate and TRUS showing dilated seminal vesicles or dilated ejaculatory ducts.

B. Acquired Blockages:

1. Vasectomy–Vasectomy is performed on 750,000 men per year in the United States for the purpose of contraception. Subsequently, approximately 5% of these men have the vasectomy reversed, most commonly because of remarriage.

2. Groin and hernia surgery–Groin and hernia surgery can result in inguinal vas deferens obstruction in 1% of cases. There has been concern that marlex mesh used for hernia repairs may add to perivasal inflammation and increase the likelihood of vasal obstruction.

3. Bacterial infections–Bacterial infections (*E coli* in men age > 35) or *Chlamydia trachomatis* in young men may involve the epididymis, with scarring and obstruction.

C. Functional Blockages: Besides physical obstruction, functional obstruction of the seminal vesicles may exist. Functional blockages may be the result of nerve injury or medications that impair the contractility of seminal vesicle or vasal musculature. A classic example of nerve injury affecting ejaculation can occur with a retroperitoneal lymph node dissection performed for testis cancer. This surgery can result in either retrograde ejaculation or true anejaculation, depending on the degree of injury to the postganglionic sympathetic fibers arising from the thoracolumbar region of the spinal cord. These autonomic nerves overlie the inferior aorta and coalesce as the hypogastric plexus within the pelvis. These nerves supply the ampullary vas deferens, seminal vesicle, periurethral glands, and the internal sphincter closure mechanism and thus control seminal emission. Multiple sclerosis and diabetes are other conditions that result in disordered ejaculation.

Evidence from animal models indicates that the seminal vesicles, as hollow smooth-muscle organs, possess contractile properties similar to those of the urinary bladder, making it conceivable that seminal vesicle organ dysfunction may actually underlie some cases of ejaculatory duct "obstruction." Many medications that are implicated in this functional problem are those classically associated with ejaculatory impairment. Table 46–16 presents a list of these medications.

Disorders of Sperm Function or Motility

A. Immotile Cilia Syndromes: Immotile cilia syndromes are a heterogeneous group of disorders (1:20,000 males) in which sperm motility is reduced or absent. The sperm defects are based on the presence of abnormalities in the motor apparatus or axoneme of sperm and other ciliated cells. Normally, 9 pairs of microtubules are organized around a central pair within the sperm tail and are connected by dynein arms (ATPase) that regulate microtubule and therefore sperm tail motion. Various defects in the dynein arms cause deficits in ciliary and sperm activity. Kartagener syn-

Table 46–16. Medications associated with impaired ejaculation.

Antihypertensive agents
Alpha-adrenergic blockers (Prazosin, Phentolamine)
Thiazides
Antipsychotic agents
Mellaril (thioridazine)
Haldol (haloperidol)
Librium
Antidepressants
Imipramine
Amitriptyline

drome is a subset of this disorder (1:40,000 males) that presents with the triad of chronic sinusitis, bronchiectasis, and situs inversus. Most immotile cilia cases are diagnosed in childhood and are due to respiratory and sinus difficulties. Cilia present in the retina and ear may also be defective and lead to retinitis pigmentosa and deafness in Usher syndrome. Men with immotile cilia characteristically have completely nonmotile but viable sperm in normal numbers. Sperm nuclear material is thought to be unaffected. The diagnosis is made with electron microscopy of sperm.

B. Maturation Defects: After vasectomy reversal, normal sperm counts but low motility can be observed in some cases. This is thought to be due to elevated epididymal intratubular pressure and epididymal dysfunction, a consequence of time after vasectomy-induced blockage. As a result, sperm may not gain the usual maturation and motility capacities during their transit through the epididymis.

C. Immunologic Infertility: Autoimmune infertility has been implicated as a cause of infertility in up to 10% of infertile couples. The testis is a curious organ in that sperm are highly antigenic, yet normally coexist within the host; it is an immunologically privileged site, probably owing to the blood-testis barrier. The blood-testis barrier theory is not conclusive, because anatomic gaps have been observed. In these unprotected areas, there may be a downregulation of cellular immunity that protects the sperm. This theory is termed active immunosuppression and explains how autoimmune infertility can occur: A larger than normal exposure to sperm antigens after, for example, vasectomy, testis torsion, or biopsy, incites a pathologic immune response.

Clinically, ASA are found in 3–12% of men who undergo evaluation for infertility. Antibodies may result in infertility by disturbances of sperm transport or disruptions in sperm-egg interaction. Sperm antibodies may cause clumping or agglutination of sperm, which inhibits passage, or may be destroyed within the uterus. Closer to the egg, ASA may block normal sperm binding to the oocyte. Many assays are available to detect ASA. The most widely used assay system is the immunobead test. Polyacrylamide beads are coated with antihuman antibody and then exposed to motile sperm. Attachment of beads to sperm indicates the presence of antibodies.

D. Infection: The agents most commonly responsible for male genital tract infections are listed in Table 46–10. Various products of activated leukocytes have been shown to exist in infected semen. A significant correlation has been demonstrated between leukocytes in semen and the generation of superoxide anions, hydrogen peroxide, and hydroxyl radicals, all of which are reactive oxygen species that can damage sperm membranes. Sperm are highly susceptible to the effects of oxidative stress because they possess little cytoplasm and therefore little antioxidant activity. Damage to sperm from oxidative

stress has been correlated to loss of function as assessed by motility and fertilization. Although genital tract infection has been linked to infertility in epidemiologic studies, the correlation between specific organisms and infertility is unclear. Uncontrolled studies suggest that pregnancy rates may improve after treatment, but in general, controlled studies do not confirm these findings. It is important to remember that seminal fluid that passes through the urethra is routinely contaminated with bacteria that colonize this area. This makes interpretation of semen cultures difficult. Thus, semen cultures should be obtained selectively.

Disorders of Coitus

A. Impotence: Sexual dysfunction stemming from low libido or impotence is a not infrequent cause of infertility. The male hormonal evaluation can detect organic causes for such problems. Most cases of situational impotence, in which the stress of attempting to conceive results in poor erections, are simply treated with sexual counseling.

B. Hypospadias: Anatomic problems like hypospadias can cause inappropriate placement of the seminal coagulum too far away from the cervix and result in infertility.

C. Timing and Frequency: Simple problems of coital timing and frequency can be corrected by a review of the couple's sexual habits. An appropriate frequency of intercourse is every 2 days for most men, performed within the periovulatory period, the window of time surrounding ovulation when egg fertilization is possible. Charting of basal body temperature by the female partner allows for the calculation of that period for the next ovulatory cycle. Home kits that detect the LH surge in the urine before ovulation are equally helpful or more so, because of their simplicity. Couples should be counseled to avoid lubricants if at all possible. It is also wise to discontinue any unnecessary medications that can be safely stopped during attempts to conceive. Other coital toxins include heat exposure from regular saunas, hot tubs, or jacuzzis and the use of cigarettes, cocaine, marijuana, and excessive alcohol.

TREATMENT OF MALE INFERTILITY

SURGICAL TREATMENTS

The role of surgical therapy in the treatment of male infertility is well established and cost-effective when compared with high-technology approaches. Surgical therapy also attempts to reverse specific pathophysiologic effects and may allow for conception at home rather than in the laboratory.

Microsurgery in Urology

The rise of microsurgery as a surgical discipline followed 3 advances. The first was refinements in optical magnification; the second, the development of more precise microsuture and microneedles; and the third, the ability to manufacture smaller and more refined surgical instruments. In urology, microsurgical techniques were first applied to the vasculature in renal transplantation and for vasectomy reversal. The evolution of these procedures progressed quickly from humble beginnings with the use of small, borrowed forceps from the local jewelry store (the still aptly named "jeweler's forcep") and the application of human hair for fine suture material.

Because of the small dimensions of reproductive tract organs, urologic procedures are some of the most difficult cases in all of microsurgery. The fine motor control of the human hand is so well developed that controlled movements of as little as 1 μm at a time are possible. To achieve this level of control, however, it is necessary for the surgeon to be completely relaxed during microsurgical procedures. Microsurgery is an acquired skill that demands practice and coordination and can be quite physically and mentally demanding. Under the surgical microscope at 30× magnification, even the smallest of movements becomes significant; precise control is required for operative success. Microsurgery in urology is one of the most challenging disciplines in the field.

Varicocele

Although most men with varicoceles are fertile, the association of varicoceles with infertility is well established by observational, retrospective, and prospective studies. Several treatment modalities, both surgical and nonsurgical, are available for varicoceles. These include incisional ligation of the veins through the retroperitoneal, inguinal, or subinguinal approaches; percutaneous embolization; and laparoscopy. The common goal of all treatments is to eliminate the retrograde reflux of venous blood through the internal spermatic veins. Treatments can be compared in terms of expected success rates (semen improvement and pregnancy), cost, and outcomes (pain pills, return to work or other activity), and their relative merits can be analyzed. A basic comparison of the 3 treatment options is outlined in Table 46–17. Remember that if watchful waiting is chosen as a treatment, a pregnancy rate of 16% can be expected. If IVF is chosen, a pregnancy rate of 35% can be expected. An overall complication rate of 1% is expected for the incisional approach, compared with a 4% complication rate for laparoscopy and 10–15% for radiologic occlusion. A significant complication with the radiologic approach is the technical failure rate, meaning the inability to access and occlude the internal spermatic vein.

Vasovasostomy

About 35,000 men per year undergo vasectomy reversal in the United States. The most common reason is remarriage and the desire for more children. Others in long-standing relationships have merely "changed their minds." Occasionally, an unfortunate individual will have lost a child and desire another. Infection, deformities, trauma, and previous surgery in the reproductive tract are less frequent indications for vasovasostomy or epididymovasostomy. A problem with duct obstruction is suspected in men with normal hormones and normal testis size and no sperm in the ejaculate.

There are several methods for performing a vasovasostomy. None has been proved superior to any other. It is well established that magnification with an operating microscope allows for a more precise surgical reconnection. Generally, either a single-layer anastomosis or a strict, two-layer anastomosis is performed (Figure 46–16). Although these procedures are technically different, the experience of the surgeon is the most important factor for success. Evidence of epididymal inflammation or infection after the vasectomy, or a period from vasectomy to reversal of > 14 years are both associated with a decrease in success. A long (> 2.7 cm) vas deferens between the testis and the vasectomy site and the presence of clear fluid with sperm from the reopened vas on the testicular side are both good signs for success. Depending on these factors, 95% or more of patients may have a return of sperm after a vasovasostomy. If

Table 46–17. Varicocele treatments: Comparison of outcomes.

Outcome Parameter	Treatment		
	Incisional	Laparoscopic	Radiologic
Semen improvement	66%	50–70%	60%
Pregnancy rate	35%	12–32%	10–50%
Recurrence	0–15%	5–25%	0–10%
Technical failure	Negligible	Small	10–15%
Pain pills	9.4	11	Minimal
Days to work	5.0	5.3	1

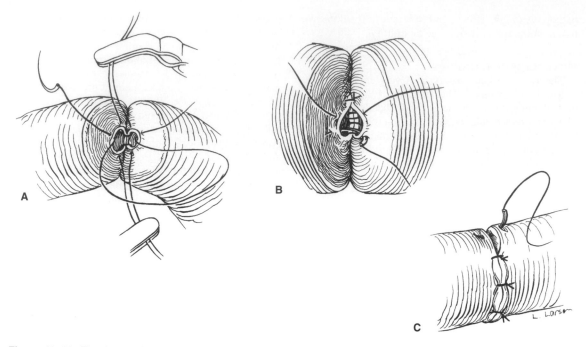

Figure 46–16. Two-layer microsurgical vasovasostomy. **A:** Mucosal stitches of 10-0 nylon are placed in the "back wall" of the vas lumen, incorporating mucosa and a small amount of submucosal tissue. **B:** The "front wall" mucosal sutures are then placed. **C:** Finally, serosal sutures of 9-0 nylon are placed in the outside wall of the vas deferens to complete the anastomosis. (Reproduced, with permission, from McClure RD: Microsurgery of the male reproductive system. World J Urol 1986;4:105.)

the vas fluid contains no sperm, a second problem may exist in the delicate tubules of the epididymis. The longer the time since vasectomy, the greater the "back-pressure" behind the blocked vas deferens. This may cause a blowout at some point in the single, 18-foot-long epididymal tubule, the weakest point in the system. A blowout results in blockage of the tubule as it heals. In this case, the vas must be connected to the epididymis above the blowout to allow sperm to travel through the reproductive tract. This is called an epididymovasostomy. After epididymovasostomy, approximately 60–65% of men will have sperm in the ejaculate. These rates, however, have improved remarkably during the last several years, with the development of newer surgical techniques and equipment.

The achievement of sperm in the ejaculate after vasovasostomy depends on 2 individuals, the surgeon and the patient, but pregnancy after surgery obviously involves a third party. It is rare that more than 67% of men who have normal sperm counts after vasectomy reversal surgery will impregnate a woman. Therefore, it is critical to delve into the reproductive health of the female partner before embarking on the procedure. Other reasons that reproductive tract microsurgery fails: (1) the quality of preblockage semen may not have been normal; (2) roughly 30% of men who have

had vasectomies develop ASA (high antibody levels may impair fertility); (3) postsurgical scar tissue can develop at the anastomotic site, causing another blockage; (4) when the vas deferens has been blocked for a long time, the epididymis is adversely affected and sperm maturation may be compromised.

Ejaculatory Duct Obstruction

For more than 20 years, transurethral resection of the ejaculatory ducts (TURED) has been used to relieve pain due to ejaculatory duct obstruction. More recently, it has become obvious that ejaculatory duct obstruction is the cause of infertility in 5% of azoospermic men. Ejaculatory duct obstruction is suspected when the ejaculate volume is < 2.0 mL and no sperm or fructose is present. Clinical suspicion can be confirmed by TRUS demonstration of dilated seminal vesicles or dilated ejaculatory ducts. Patients with ejaculatory duct obstruction sufficient to cause coital discomfort, recurrent hematospermia, or infertility should be considered candidates for treatment.

Transurethral resection of the ejaculatory ducts is performed cystoscopically (Figure 46–17). A small resectoscope and electrocautery loop are inserted, and the verumontanum is resected in the midline. Since the area of resection is at the prostatic apex, near both the external urethral sphincter and the rectum, careful po-

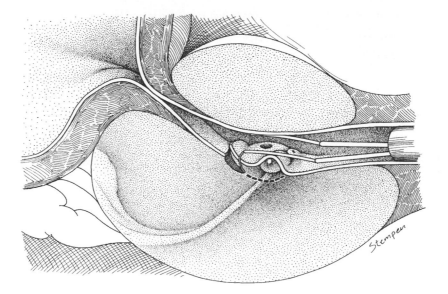

Figure 46–17. Transurethral resection of the ejaculatory ducts. A cystoscope with a resecting loop is used to remove the verumontanum and unroof an associated obstructing cyst that has compressed and obstructed the ejaculatory ducts. (Reproduced, with permission, from Turek PJ: Seminal vesicle and ejaculatory duct surgery. In: Graham SD [editor]: *Glenn's Urologic Surgery*, 5th ed. Lippincott, 1998.)

sitioning of the resectoscope is essential. A small Foley catheter is placed for 24–48 h and removed on an outpatient basis. Long-term relief of postcoital pain after TURED can be expected in 60% of patients. Hematospermia has also been effectively treated with TURED, but this literature is anecdotal. There is convincing evidence from several large studies of patients treated for infertility that 65–70% of men show significant improvements in semen quality after TURED and that a 20–30% pregnancy rate can be expected. The complication rate from TURED is approximately 20%. The most common complications are self-limited and include hematospermia, hematuria, urinary tract infection, epididymitis, and a watery ejaculate. Watery ejaculate is presumed to be secondary to the reflux of urine through the ejaculatory ducts and into the seminal vesicles. Rarely reported complications include retrograde ejaculation, rectal perforation, and urinary incontinence.

Electroejaculation

A complete failure of emission and ejaculation occurs most commonly from spinal cord injury (10,000 cases per year in the United States) and as a result of deep pelvic or retroperitoneal surgery that injures the pelvic sympathetic nerves. With rectal probe electroejaculation, the pelvic sympathetic nerves undergo controlled stimulation, with contraction of the vas deferens, seminal vesicle, and prostate, such that a reflex ejaculation is induced. The semen is collected from the penis and the bladder, as retrograde ejacula-

tion is often an associated finding with electroejaculation. Semen acquired in this way generally requires some form of assisted reproductive technology for success.

In men with anejaculation after retroperitoneal surgery for testis cancer, successful recovery of sperm with electroejaculation is possible in the vast majority of patients. Sperm motility tends to be lower than normal when obtained in this manner, an effect that appears independent of electrical or heat effects inherent to the procedure. In men with spinal cord injuries above the T5 level, it is often possible to induce a reflex ejaculation with high-frequency penile vibration, termed vibratory stimulation. With the use of handheld vibrators set to a frequency of 100 cycles/s at an amplitude of 2–3 mm, patients may be taught to perform the procedure and attempt to conceive at home with the use of cervical cap insemination.

Sperm Aspiration

Sperm aspiration techniques are indicated for men in whom the transport of sperm is not possible because the ductal system is absent or not surgically reconstructable. An example of this is vasal agenesis, a condition in which the vas deferens fails to develop normally. Acquired forms of obstruction may also exist; one common condition is failed vasectomy reversal. Aspiration procedures can involve microsurgery to collect sperm from the sperm reservoirs within the genital tract. At present, sperm are routinely aspirated from the vas deferens, epididymis, or testicle. It is im-

Table 46–18. Sources of aspirated sperm and associated reproductive technologies.

Procedure	Source	IVF	Micromanipulation
Vasal aspiration	Vas deferens	Usually	No
Epididymal aspiration	Epididymis	Yes	Yes
Testis biopsy	Testicle	Yes	Yes

IVF, in vitro fertilization.

portant to realize that IVF is required to achieve a pregnancy with these procedures. Thus, success rates are intimately tied to a complex program of assisted reproduction for both partners (Table 46–18). In cases of sperm aspiration from the testicle and epididymis, IVF along with micromanipulation is required to achieve pregnancy. An obvious prerequisite for these procedures is ongoing sperm production. Although evaluated indirectly by means of hormone levels and testis volume, the most direct way to verify sperm production is with a testis biopsy, performed as part of the evaluation or just before an aspiration attempt.

A. Vasal Aspiration: Vasal aspiration is performed with local anesthesia through a scrotal incision. With the use of an operating microscope, a vasotomy is made, and leaking sperm are aspirated into culture medium. Once enough sperm are obtained (> 10–20 million), the vasotomy is closed with microscopic sutures. Of the 3 procurement procedures, vasal aspiration provides the most mature or fertilizable sperm, as they have already passed through the epididymis, where maturation processes take place during normal sperm development.

B. Epididymal Sperm Aspiration: Epididymal sperm aspiration is performed when the vas either is not present or is scarred from previous surgery, trauma, or infection to the point that it is not usable. It is performed through an incision similar to that in vasal aspiration (or often percutaneously). Sperm are directly collected from a single, isolated epididymal tubule (Figure 46–18). When 10–20 million sperm are obtained, the epididymal tubule is closed with microscopic suture, and the sperm are processed for insemination of the partner's eggs. Epididymal sperm are not as mature as sperm that have traversed the entire length of the epididymis and reside in the vas deferens; as a consequence, epididymal sperm require micromanipulation to fertilize the egg. Egg fertilization rates of 65% and pregnancy rates of 50% are possible with epididymal sperm, but results vary among individuals because of differences in sperm and egg quality.

C. Testis Sperm Retrieval: The most recently developed aspiration technique is testicular sperm retrieval, begun in 1995. It is a breakthrough in the sense that it demonstrates that sperm do not have to pass through the epididymis to fertilize the egg. Testicular sperm extraction is indicated for patients in whom there is a blockage in the epididymis very

close to where it connects to the testis, or a blockage in the testis efferent ductules. It is also a valuable technique in cases of severe testis failure, in which so few sperm are produced that they cannot reach the ejaculate. In this procedure, a small piece of testis tissue is taken in a manner similar to that of a regular testis biopsy under local anesthesia. The testis tissue is specially treated in the laboratory to separate sperm from other cells. High egg fertilization rates (50–65%) and pregnancy rates (40–50%) are possible with testis sperm.

Orchidopexy

An undescended testis occurs in 0.8% of male infants at 1 year of age. Spontaneous descent into the scrotum is unlikely after 1 year. Although the most important reason for orchidopexy is to make testicles with a higher risk of future cancer palpable and assessable, preservation of fertility is a second and more debatable reason. Histologic studies of undescended testis show that significant decreases in spermatogo-

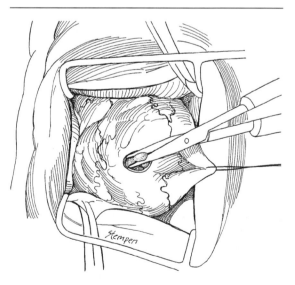

Figure 46–18. Microscopic epididymal sperm aspiration. A small "window" incision is made in the scrotum and held open with a small retractor. Under 20× magnification, the epididymis is dissected, and a single epididymal tubule is incised with microscissors. Fluid containing sperm is aspirated for use with in vitro fertilization.

nial numbers occur between birth and 2 years of age. Orchidopexy has been recommended within 2 years of age with the idea that some of this germ cell degeneration might be prevented, although proof of this is poor. Given that sperm can be retrieved from even the smallest failing testis and used for biologic pregnancies, orchidopexy and not orchiectomy should be the primary goal in these cases.

Torsion of the testis is a urologic emergency. There are significant data from animal studies but little literature in humans to suggest that the unaffected, contralateral testis can become infertile after torsion of its mate. This has been termed sympathetic orchidopathia and is assumed to be immunologic in nature. It is the basis for the recommendation that the nonviable torsed testicle be removed at diagnosis. However, given the advances in assisted reproductive technologies, such as fine-needle aspiration mapping procedures that can detect sperm in small, failing testis, such recommendations should be reconsidered.

Pituitary Ablation

Elevated serum prolactin levels stemming from a pituitary adenoma can be treated both medically and surgically. If the adenoma is radiologically visible (macroadenoma), then transphenoidal surgical ablation of the lesion is possible. If the adenoma is not visible (microadenoma), then medical therapy with the dopamine agonist bromocriptine is indicated.

NONSURGICAL TREATMENTS

Specific Therapy

Specific therapy seeks to reverse known pathophysiologic effects to improve fertility. For the most part, they are cost-effective treatments for infertility.

A. Pyospermia: The presence of elevated numbers of leukocytes in semen is termed pyospermia and has been associated with (1) subclinical genital tract infection, (2) elevated reactive oxygen species, and (3) poor sperm function and infertility. Sperm are highly susceptible to the effects of oxidative stress induced by leukocytes or infection because they possess little cytoplasm and therefore little antioxidant activity. The treatment of pyospermia is controversial in the absence of overt bacteriologic infection. It is important to evaluate the patient for sexually transmitted diseases, penile discharge, prostatitis, or epididymitis. An expressed prostatic secretion is examined for leukocytes, and urethral cultures are obtained for chlamydia and mycoplasma. The use of broad-spectrum antibiotics like doxycyline and trimethoprim-sulfamethoxazole has been shown to reduce seminal leukocyte concentrations, improve sperm function, and increase conception. Generally, the female partner is also treated.

In pyospermia with a documented prostatic source (> 20 leukocytes per high-power field in expressed prostatic secretion), frequent ejaculation (more than every 3 days) and doxycycline may result in a more durable resolution of pyospermia (55% of treated men) than either treatment alone (5–17% resolution) (Branigan and Muller, 1994). There is increasing evidence that the antioxidant vitamins (A, C, and E) as well as glutathione and other antioxidants may help to scavenge reactive oxygen species within the semen and improve sperm motility in pyospermic men (Baker et al, 1996).

B. Coital Therapy: Simple counseling on issues of coital timing, frequency, and gonadotoxin avoidance can help couples achieve fertility. It is important to review the essentials of basal body temperature charting or home kits that detect the LH surge in the urine immediately (< 24 h) before ovulation. Since sperm reside in the cervical mucus for 48 h and are released continuously, it is not necessary that coitus and ovulation occur at exactly the same time, a fact that can reduce the stress associated with infertility. Coitus every other day around ovulation is the usual recommendation. Coital lubricants should be avoided if possible. If necessary, vegetable oils, olive oil, and petroleum jelly are the safest.

Retrograde ejaculation results from a failure of the bladder neck to appropriately close during ejaculation. This condition is diagnosed by the finding of sperm within the postejaculate bladder urine. Initial treatment is a trial of sympathomimetic medications, to which approximately 30% of men will respond with some degree of antegrade ejaculation. Begun several days before ejaculation, imipramine (25–50 mg twice a day), Nasal-D (twice a day), Ornade (twice a day), or Sudafed Plus (60 mg 4 times a day) have all been used with varying success. The side effects associated with these medications usually limit the efficacy of this therapy. For medication failure, sperm harvesting techniques can often be used with IUI to achieve a pregnancy. Premature ejaculation occurs when men ejaculate before the partner is ready. Sexual counseling combined with tricyclic antidepressants, Prozac, or other serotoninergic uptake inhibitors can be very effective.

C. Immunologic Infertility: Antisperm antibodies are a complex problem underlying male infertility. Available treatment options include corticosteroid suppression (Table 46–19), sperm washing, IUI, IVF, and ICSI. Steroid suppression is based on the concept that an overactive immune system can be weakened or altered to reduce the number of antibodies on sperm. Intrauterine insemination places more sperm nearer the ovulated egg to optimize the sperm-egg environment. Pregnancy rates with this technique generally fall in the 10–20% range. Assisted reproductive technology with IVF and ICSI offers high pregnancy rates, equivalent to those achieved with otherwise normal sperm. In general, if > 50% of sperm are bound with antibodies, then treatment should be offered. In addition, head-directed or mid-

Table 46–19. Corticosteroid therapy for immunologic infertility.

Year	Investigator	Control	Daily Dose	No. of Patients	% Pregnant
1983	Alexander	Yes	60 mg pred.	19	45
1986	Hendry	No	40/80 mg predl.	76	33
1987	Hass	Yes	96 mg methylpred.	20	15
1988	Smarr	No	15 mg pred.	60	43
1990	Hendry	Yes	20/5 mg predl.	29	31
1990	Hendry		Placebo	21	9

pred., prednisone; methylpred., methylprednisolone; predl., prednisolone.

piece-directed sperm antibodies appear more relevant than tail-directed antibodies. Since the presence of ASA is associated with obstruction in the genital tract, these lesions should be sought and corrected. There is renewed interest in the causes and possible treatments of this interesting problem, as several animal models exist that mimic the condition in humans.

D. Medical Therapy: Effective hormonal therapy can be offered to patients with certain diseases that also predispose to infertility. Hormone therapy is effective when it is used as specific and not empiric treatment. Specific replacement therapy seeks to reverse well-established, pathophysiologic states. Empiric treatments attempt to overcome pathologic conditions that are ill-defined or have no proven treatment.

1. Hyperprolactinemia–Normal levels of prolactin in men appear to help sustain high intratesticular testosterone levels and affect the growth and secretions of the accessory sex glands. Hyperprolactinemia abolishes gonadotropin pulsatility by interfering with episodic GnRH release. Visible lesions are generally treated with transphenoidal surgery, and nonvisible lesions are treated with bromocriptine, 5–10 mg daily, to restore the normal pituitary balance of LH and FSH.

2. Hypothyroidism–Both elevated and depressed levels of thyroid hormone alter spermatogenesis. States of thyroid dysfunction account for about 0.5% of infertility cases but are very treatable. Replacement or removal of low or excessive thyroid hormone is cost-effective treatment for infertility. As these diseases are clinically very evident, routine thyroid screening is not recommended for infertility patients.

3. Congenital adrenal hyperplasia–Most commonly, the 21-hydroxylase enzyme is deficient, and defective cortisol production results. The testes fail to mature because of gonadotropin inhibition due to excessive androgens. The diagnosis is rare and classically presents as precocious puberty; careful laboratory evaluation is essential. In both sexes, the condition and the infertility associated with it are both treated with corticosteroids.

4. Testosterone excess/deficiency–Patients with Kallmann syndrome lack GnRH that stimulates normal pituitary function. Infertility associated with this condition can be very effectively treated with hCG, 1000–2000 U 3 times weekly, and human menopausal gonadotropin (hMG), 75 U twice weekly, to replace LH and FSH. It is also possible to give GnRH replacement in a pulsatile manner, 25–50 ng/kg every 2 h, by a portable infusion pump. Pituitary diseases associated with testis failure are not amenable to GnRH treatment but respond well to hCG and hMG therapy. Individuals with fertile eunuch syndrome or isolated LH deficiency respond well to hCG therapy alone. Since injectable drug regimens in these conditions are involved and costly, it is good practice for men to cryopreserve motile sperm once achieved in the ejaculate. One can expect to find sperm in the ejaculate beginning 6–9 months after therapy is started. Anabolic steroids are a common and probably underdiagnosed reason for testicular failure in which excess exogenous testosterone and metabolites depress the pituitary-gonadal axis and spermatogenesis. Initially, the patient should discontinue the offending hormones to allow for the return of the normal homeostatic balance. Second-line therapy generally consists of "jump-starting" the testis with hCG and hMG as with Kallmann syndrome.

Empiric Medical Therapy

In 25% of infertile men who present with infertility, no identifiable cause can be attributed to the problem. Because the pathophysiology is ill-defined, this is termed idiopathic infertility. There is a second group of men in whom a cause of infertility may be identified but no specific therapy is available to treat the problem. Both groups of men are candidates for empiric medical therapy. This form of therapy seeks to overcome pathologic conditions that are ill-defined or have no proven treatment. Some of the pitfalls and variables that plague studies on this form of therapy are that (1) men diagnosed as "idiopathic" are a very heterogeneous group; (2) the definition of male infertility varies between studies; (3) the definition of semen analysis "improvement" also varies; (4) most studies lack placebo controls; and (5) treatment regimens (doses, intervals) are not standardized. As a rule, it is important to establish a timeline of therapy and decide with the patient when empiric treatment is to be discontinued and when other avenues are to be pursued.

A. Clomiphene Citrate: Clomiphene citrate is a synthetic nonsteroidal drug that acts as an antiestrogen and competitively binds to estrogen receptors in the hypothalamus and pituitary. This effectively blocks the action of the normally low levels of estrogen on the male hormone axis and results in increased secretion of GnRH, FSH, and LH. The enhanced output of these hormones increases testosterone production and sperm production within the testis. Clomiphene therapy is given for the treatment of idiopathic low sperm counts. It is less effective as a treatment for low motility. The dose is 12.5–50 mg/d either continuously or with a 5-day rest period each month. Serum gonadotropins and testosterone should be monitored at 2–4 weeks and the dose adjusted to keep the testosterone level within the normal range. Higher than normal testosterone levels may result in a decrease in semen quality. Therapy should be discontinued if no semen quality response is observed in 6 months. Although there have been over 30 published trials on clomiphene since 1964, only a few included control arms. In general, there are as many trials showing that clomiphene is equivalent to placebo as there are showing that it improves sperm density and pregnancy rates. Decreased sperm densities have also been observed on this therapy.

B. Tamoxifen: Tamoxifen is commonly used for the treatment of metastatic breast cancer in women. It is another antiestrogen that works in a manner similar to that of clomiphene citrate. It may have less estrogenic activity than clomiphene, however. Also indicated for idiopathic oligospermia, the dose of tamoxifen is 10–15 mg twice daily for 3–6 months. Serum testosterone, LH, and FSH should be measured 2–4 weeks after initiating therapy. Semen analyses are taken at 3 months and regularly thereafter.

C. Kallikreins: The kallikrein-kinin system is involved with tissue proliferation, the coagulation cascade, and the complement system. Components of this system are also present in reproductive tract secretions from men. They are postulated to be involved in sperm transport through the female genital tract, induction of sperm motility, and stimulation of spermatogenesis. Kallikrein is a pancreatic enzyme that acts on kininogens to release kinins. It has been used in cases of idiopathic oligospermia with the idea that it may enhance sperm metabolism, increase testis blood flow, stimulate Sertoli cells, and stimulate accessory sex gland secretions. For the treatment of low sperm motility, oral porcine pancreatic kallikrein is used in Europe at a dose of 600 IU/d. A recent placebo-controlled clinical trial with 90 subjects showed significant improvements in sperm density, motility, and forward progression in the treated men. Pregnancy rates were 38% in the treatment arm and 16% in the placebo arm.

D. Antioxidant Therapy: There is evidence that up to 40% of infertile men have increased levels of reactive oxygen species in the reproductive tract. These species (OH, O_2 radicals, and hydrogen peroxide) are thought to cause lipid peroxidation damage to sperm membranes. Treatment with scavengers of these radicals may protect sperm from oxidative damage: glutathione, 600 mg daily for 3–6 months, or vitamin E, 400–1200 U/d. These agents may be useful in a subgroup of infertile men with elevated levels of seminal reactive oxygen species.

E. Growth Hormone: There is emerging evidence that growth hormone–induced insulin-like growth factor-1 may be important for spermatogenesis in the testicle. Growth hormone is an established anabolic hormone used by bodybuilders worldwide. In recent European trials of growth hormone in infertile men, individuals with maturation arrest and azoospermia developed sperm counts. The use of growth hormone or its releasing factor may become a new and effective treatment for oligospermia.

ASSISTED REPRODUCTIVE TECHNOLOGIES

If neither surgery nor medical therapy is appropriate for male infertility treatment, assisted reproductive techniques can be used to achieve a pregnancy.

Intrauterine Insemination

Intrauterine insemination (IUI) involves the placement of a washed pellet of ejaculated sperm within the female uterus, beyond the cervical barrier. The principal indication for IUI is for a cervical factor; if the cervix is bypassed, then pregnancies may ensue. IUI is also used for low sperm quality, for immunologic infertility, and for men with mechanical problems of sperm delivery (eg, hypospadias). There should be at least 5–40 million motile sperm in the ejaculate (volume × concentration × motility) to make this procedure worthwhile. The success rates vary widely and are directly related to female reproductive potential; given this, pregnancy rates of 8–16% per cycle have been reported with the use of IUI as a treatment for male infertility. Success rates are improved if ultrasound is used to document that follicles are enlarging and if urine testing is used to predict ovulation precisely.

In Vitro Fertilization and ICSI (Figure 46–19)

In vitro fertilization is a more complex technique than IUI and removes even more of the formidable obstacles to sperm in the female reproductive tract. It involves controlled ovarian stimulation and ultrasound-guided transvaginal egg retrieval from the ovaries before normal ovulation. Eggs are then fertilized in petri dishes with anywhere from 500,000 to 5 million

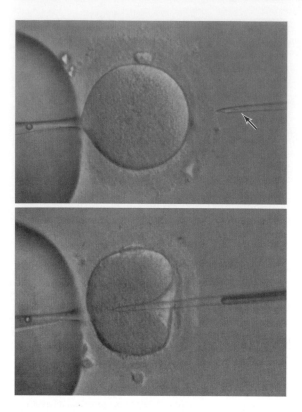

Figure 46–19. The intracytoplasmic sperm injection procedure. (**Top**) A mature oocyte (left) is readied for injection with a sperm (arrow) in a micropipet under the microscope. (**Bottom**) The micropipet is placed directly into the oocyte, and the sperm is deposited into the cytoplasm.

motile sperm. This is an excellent technology with which to bypass moderate to severe forms of male infertility in which low numbers of motile sperm are present. Most recently, a revolutionary addition to IVF has been described that is referred to as sperm micromanipulation or ICSI. The sperm requirement for egg fertilization has dropped from hundreds of thousands for IVF to 1 viable sperm for ICSI. This has led to the development of aggressive new surgical techniques to provide viable sperm for egg fertilization from men with apparent azoospermia (no ejaculated sperm). The availability of these techniques has pushed urologists to look beyond the ejaculate and into the male reproductive tract to find sperm for biologic pregnancies. At present, sources of sperm in otherwise azoospermic patients include the vas deferens, epididymis, and testicle. Two notes of concern are that, since IVF and ICSI eliminate many of the natural selection barriers

that exist during natural fertilization, genetic defects that caused the infertility are expected to be passed on to offspring unabated. This has large ethical implications, especially with respect to X-linked diseases like Klinefelter syndrome that might be expected to resurface again in grandchildren of the affected but treatable infertile male. Second, there are recent data that offspring born to infertile couples with this technique have a 4-fold higher incidence of sex chromosomal anomalies than do children who are naturally conceived.

Gamete Intrafallopian Transfer (GIFT)

As in IVF, oocytes are retrieved from the female partner with GIFT. Unlike IVF, sperm and oocytes are mixed together and then injected into the fallopian tubes with laparoscopy before fertilization. This technique has the theoretical advantage of allowing fertilization to occur in the fallopian tube but is associated with the increased expense of laparoscopy. Several variations of GIFT and IVF seek to take advantage of fertilization in vitro followed by early-stage embryo transfer into the fallopian tube, where embryo development naturally begins. These techniques are known by various names, including ZIFT (zygote intrafallopian transfer), TET (tubal embryo transfer), and PROUST (pronuclear stage tubal embryo transfer).

Preimplantation Genetic Diagnosis

Preimplantation genetic diagnosis is a highly specialized technique that enables the laboratory to precisely define the genetic normality of embryos. In patients with inheritable, possibly life-threatening diseases, it is possible that offspring conceived with IVF and ICSI may have these diseases transmitted to them. This complex technique involves the removal of single cells from the embryo while the embryo is grown in petri dishes before transfer to the uterus. The genetic material from these "biopsied" cells can then be examined to determine whether that embryo carries an abnormal chromosome or gene. Through preimplantation genetic diagnosis, early human embryos that result from IVF and ICSI can be individually examined as they develop for the presence or absence of these suspected genetic traits. Because of the real-time nature of the technique, decisions as to which embryos should be transferred to the female partner for pregnancy can be made within 24 h and will help to ensure that lethal diseases are not transmitted to offspring. Remarkably, the removal of a few cells from the embryo is not detrimental to the survival and normal development of the embryo.

REFERENCES

MALE REPRODUCTIVE PHYSIOLOGY

Aitken RJ, West K, Buckingham D: Leukocytic infiltration into the human ejaculate and its association with semen quality, oxidative stress, and sperm function. J Androl 1994;15:343.

Amann RP, Howards SS: Daily spermatozoal production and epididymal spermatozoal reserves of the human male. J Urol 1980;124:211.

DeGroot LJ: *Endocrinology,* 3rd ed. Saunders, 1995.

Griffin JE, Wilson JD: Disorders of the testes and male reproductive tract. In: Wilson JD, Foster DW (editors): *Williams Textbook of Endocrinology,* 8th ed. Saunders, 1991.

Hess RA et al: A role for estrogens in the male reproductive system. Nature 1997;390:509.

Mather JP, Woodruff TK, Krummen LA: Paracrine regulation of reproductive function by inhibin and activin. Proc Soc Exp Biol Med 1992;20:1.

Turek PJ: Immunopathology and infertility. In: Lipshultz LI, Howards SS (editors): *Infertility in the Male,* 3rd ed. Mosby Year Book, 1997.

Turek PJ et al: Observations on seminal vesicle dynamics in an in vivo rat model. J Urol 1998;159:1731.

Turek PJ et al: The role of the sertoli cell in active immunosuppression in the human testis. Br J Urol 1996; 77:891.

Veldhuis JD: Male hypothalamic-pituitary-gonadal axis. In: Lipshultz LI, Howards SS (editors): *Infertility in the Male,* 3rd ed. Mosby Year Book, 1997.

Whitmore WF, Kars L, Gittes, RF: The role of germinal epithelium and spermatogenesis in the privileged survival of intratesticular grafts. J Urol 1985;134:782.

Wolff H, Anderson DJ: Immunohistologic characterization and quantification of leukocyte subpopulations in human semen. Fertil Steril 1988;49:497.

EVALUATION OF MALE INFERTILITY

Aitken R et al: Analysis of the relationship between defective sperm function and the generation of reactive oxygen species in cases of oligozoospermia. J Androl 1989;10:214.

Carlsen E. et al: Evidence for decreasing quality of semen during the past 50 years. Br Med J 1992;105:609.

Carter SS, Shinohara K, Lipshultz LI: Transrectal ultrasonography in disorders of the seminal vesicles and ejaculatory ducts. Urol Clin North Am 1989;16:773.

Clarke GN, Elliot PJ, Smaila C: Detection of sperm antibodies in semen using the immunobead test. A survey of 813 consecutive patients. Am J Reprod Immunol Microbiol 1985;7:118.

Clifton DK, Bremner WJ: The effect of testicular X-irradiation on spermatogenesis in man. J Androl 1983;4: 387.

Davis RO, Katz DF: Computer-aided sperm analysis: Technology at a crossroads. Fertil Steril 1993;59:953.

Dubin L, Amelar RD: Varicocele size and results of varicocelectomy in selected subfertile men with varicocele. Fertil Steril 1970;21:606.

Jeyendran RS et al: Development of an assay to assess the functional integrity of the human sperm membrane and its relationship to other serum characteristics. J Reprod Fertil 1984;70:219.

Kruger TF et al: Predictive value of abnormal sperm morphology in in vitro fertilization. Fertil Steril 1988; 49:112.

Liu DY, Baker WHG: Tests of human sperm function and fertilization in vitro. Fertil Steril 1992;58:465.

MacLeod J, Gold RZ: The male factor in fertility and infertility: Spermatozoan counts in 1000 men of known fertility and in 1000 cases of infertile marriage. J Urol 1951;66:436.

MacLeod J, Hitchkiss RS: The effects of hyperpyrexia on spermatozoa counts in men. Endocrinology 1941; 28:780.

McClure RD: Endocrine investigation and therapy. Urol Clin North Am 1987;14:471.

McClure RD: Evaluation of the infertile male. In: deVere White R (editor): *Problems in Urology.* Lippincott, 1987.

McClure RD, Hricak H: Scrotal ultrasound in the infertile man: Detection of subclinical unilateral and bilateral varicoceles. J Urol 1986;135:711.

Meacham RB, Hellerstein DK, Lipshultz LI: Evaluation and treatment of ejaculatory duct obstruction in the infertile male. Fertil Steril 1993;59:393.

Meinertz H et al: Antisperm antibodies and fertility after vasovasostomy: A follow-up study of 216 men. Fertil Steril 1990;54:315.

Petros JA et al: Correlation of testicular color Doppler ultrasonography, physical examination and venography in the detection of left varicoceles in men with infertility. J Urol 1991;145:785.

Rodriguez-Rigau LJ, Smith KD, Steinberger E: Varicocele and the morphology of spermatozoa. Fertil Steril 1981;35:54.

Schlegel PN, Chang TSK, Marshall FF: Antibiotics: Potential hazards to male fertility. Fertil Steril 1991;55: 235.

Sigman M, Jarow JP: Medical evaluation of infertile men. Urology 1997;50:659.

Sigman M, Lipshultz LI, Howards SS: Evaluation of the subfertile male. In: Lipshultz LI, Howards SS (editors): *Infertility in the Male,* 3rd ed. Mosby Year Book, 1997.

Smikle CB, Turek PJ: Hypoosmotic swelling can accurately determine the viability of nonmotile sperm. Mol Reprod Dev 1997;47:200.

Turek PJ, Cha I, Ljung B-M: Systematic fine-needle aspiration of the testis: Correlation to biopsy and results of organ "mapping" for mature sperm in azoospermic men. Urology 1997;49:743.

Turek PJ, Gilbaugh JH, Lipshultz LI: Imaging in the diagnosis and treatment of male infertility. Curr Opin Urol 1994;4:156.

Urban MD, Lee PA, Migeon CJ: Adult height and fertility in men with congenital virilizing adrenal hyperplasia. N Engl J Med 1978;299:1392.

Weintraub MP, De Mouy E, Hellstrom WJG: Newer modalities in the diagnosis and treatment of ejaculatory duct obstruction. J Urol 1993;150:1150.

World Health Organization: *WHO Laboratory Manual for the Examination of Human Semen and Sperm-*

Cervical Mucus Interaction, 3rd ed. Cambridge Univ Press, 1992.

Zamboni L: The ultrastructural pathology of the spermatozoa as a cause of infertility: The role of electron microscopy in the evaluation of semen quality. Fertil Steril 1987;48:711.

CAUSES OF MALE INFERTILITY—PRETESTICULAR

Carter JN et al: Prolactin-secreting tumors and hypogonadism in 22 men. N Engl J Med 1978;299:847.

Fairman C et al: The "fertile eunuch" syndrome: Demonstration of isolated luteinizing hormone deficiency by radioimmunoassay technique. Mayo Clin Proc 1968;43:661.

Griffin JE: Androgen resistance: The clinical and molecular spectrum. N Engl J Med 1992;326:611.

Lieblich JM et al: Syndrome of anosmia with hypogonadotropic hypogonadism (Kallmann syndrome): Clinical and laboratory studies in 23 cases. Am J Med 1982;73:506.

Mozaffarian GA, Higley M, Paulsen CA: Clinical studies in an adult male patient with "isolated follicle stimulating hormone (FSH) deficiency." J Androl 1983;4:393.

CAUSES OF MALE INFERTILITY—TESTICULAR

Aiman J, Griffin JE: The frequency of androgen receptor deficiency in infertile men. J Clin Endocrinol Metab 1982;54:725.

Aynsley-Green A et al: Congenital bilateral anorchia in childhood: A clinical, endocrine and therapeutic evaluation of twenty-one cases. Clin Endocrinol 1976;5: 381.

Coburn M, Wheeler TM, Lipshultz LI: Testicular biopsy: Its uses and limitations. Urol Clin North Am 1987;14:551.

Gorelick J, Goldstein M: Loss of fertility in men with varicocele. Fertil Steril 1993;59:613.

Kass EJ, Belman B: Reversal of testicular growth failure by varicocele ligation. J Urol 1987;137:475.

Kjessler B: Chromosomal constitution and male reproductive failure. In: Mancini RE, Martini L (editors): *Male Fertility and Sterility.* Academic Press, 1974.

Lipshultz LI et al: Testicular function after orchiopexy for unilaterally undescended testis. N Engl J Med 1976;295:15.

Okuyama M et al: Surgical repair of varicocele at puberty: Preventive treatment for fertility improvement. J Urol 1988;139:562.

Turek PJ, Lowther DN, Carroll PA: Fertility issues and their management in men with testis cancer. Urol Clin North Am 1998;25:517.

Turek PJ et al: The clinical characteristics of 82 patients with sertoli-cell only syndrome. Fertil Steril 1995;64: 1197.

Turek PJ et al: The reversibility of anabolic-induced azoospermia. J Urol 1995;153:1628.

Whorton MD: Male occupational reproductive hazards. West J Med 1982;137:521.

World Health Organization: The influence of varicocele on parameters of fertility in a large group of men presenting to infertility clinics. Fertil Steril 1992;57: 1289.

Yarborough MA, Burns JR, Keller FS: Incidence and clinical significance of subclinical scrotal varicoceles. J Urol 1989;141:1372.

CAUSES OF MALE INFERTILITY—POSTTESTICULAR

Afzelius BA, Mossberg B: The immotile-cilia syndrome including Kartagener's syndrome. In: Stanbury JB et al (editor): *The Metabolic Basis of Inherited Disease,* 5th ed. McGraw-Hill, 1983.

Chillon M et al: Mutations in the cystic fibrosis gene in patients with congenital absence of the vas deferens. N Engl J Med 1995;332:1475.

Handelsman DJ et al: Young's syndrome: Obstructive azoospermia and chronic sinopulmonary infections. N Engl J Med 1984;310:3.

Jaffe T, Oates RD: Genetic abnormalities and reproductive failure. Urol Clin North Am 1994;21:389.

Matsuda T, Horii Y, Yoshida O: Obstructive azoospermia of unknown origin: Sites of obstruction and surgical outcomes. J Urol 1994;151:1543.

Matsumiya K et al: Clinical study of azoospermia. Int J Androl 1994;17:140.

Nagler HM, Deitch AD, deVere White R: Testicular torsion: Temporal considerations. Fertil Steril 1984;42: 257.

Turek PJ: Immunopathology and infertility. In: Lipshultz LI, Howards SS (editors): *Infertility in the Male,* 3rd ed. Mosby Year Book, 1997.

GENETIC CAUSES OF MALE INFERTILITY

Kent-First MG et al: Infertility in intracytoplasmic-sperm-injection-derived sons. Lancet 1996;348:332.

Mak V, Jarvi K: The genetics of male infertility. J Urol 1996;156:1245.

Mulhall JP et al: Azoospermic men with deletion of the DAZ gene cluster are capable of completing spermatogenesis: Fertilization, normal embryonic development and pregnancy occur when retrieved testicular spermatozoa are used for intracytoplasmic sperm injection. Hum Reprod 1997;12:503.

Pryor JL et al: Microdeletions in the Y chromosome of infertile men. N Engl J Med 1997;336:534.

Reijo R et al: Diverse spermatogenic defects in humans caused by Y chromosome deletions encompassing a novel RNA-binding protein gene. Nat Genet 1995;10: 383.

Reijo R et al: Severe oligospermia resulting from deletions of the Azoospermia Factor gene on the Y chromosome. Lancet 1996;347:1290.

Tiepolo L, Zuffardi O: Localization of factors controlling spermatogenesis in the nonfluorescent portion of the human Y chromosome long arm. Hum Genet 1976;34:119.

TREATMENT

Anguiano A et al: Congenital bilateral absence of the vas deferens: A primarily genital form of cystic fibrosis. JAMA 1992;267:1794.

Baker WHG et al: Protective effect of antioxidants on the impairment of semen motility by activated polymorphonuclear leukocytes. Fertil Steril 1996;65:411.

Belker AM et al: Results of 1,469 microsurgical vasectomy reversals by the vasovasostomy study group. J Urol 1991;145:505.

Bennett CJ et al: Sexual dysfunction and electroejaculation in men with spinal cord injury: Review. J Urol 1988;139:453.

Branigan EF, Muller CH: Efficacy of treatment and recurrence rate of leukocytospermia in infertile men with prostatitis. Fertil Steril 1994;62:580.

Burris AS et al: A low sperm concentration does not preclude fertility in men with isolated hypogonadotropic hypogonadism after gonadotropin therapy. Fertil Steril 1988;50:343.

Cohen J et al: In vitro fertilization: A treatment for male infertility. Fertil Steril 1985;43:422.

Devroey P et al: Pregnancies after testicular sperm extraction and intracytoplasmic sperm injection in nonobstructive azoospermia. Hum Reprod 1995;10:1457.

Enquist E, Stein BS, Sigman M: Laparoscopic versus subinguinal varicocelectomy: A comparative study. Fertil Steril 1994;61:1092.

Goldstein M. *The Surgery of Male Infertility.* Saunders, 1995.

Goldstein M et al: Microsurgical inguinal varicocelectomy with delivery of the testis: An artery and lymphatic sparing technique. J Urol 1992;148:1808.

Haas GG Jr, Manganiello P: A double-blind, placebo-controlled study of the use of methylprednisolone in infertile men with sperm-associated immunoglobulins. Fertil Steril 1987;47:295.

Hendry WF et al: Comparison of prednisolone and placebo in subfertile men with antibodies to spermatozoa. Lancet 1990;335:85.

Kerin JFP et al: Improved conception rate after poor intrauterine insemination of washed spermatozoa from men with poor quality semen. Lancet 1984;1:533.

Madgar I et al: Controlled trial of high spermatic vein ligation for varicocele in infertile men. Fertil Steril 1995;63:120.

Matthews GJ, Schlegel PN, Goldstein M: Patency following microsurgical vasoepididymostomy and vasovasostomy: Temporal considerations. J Urol 1993; 154:2070.

McClure RD: Microsurgery of the male reproductive system. World J Urol 1986;4:105.

Nudell DM et al: The mini-MESA for sperm retrieval: A study of urological outcomes. Hum Reprod 1998;13: 1260.

Ovesen P et al: Growth hormone treatment of subfertile males. Fertil Steril 1996;66:292.

Royle MG, Hendry WF: Why does vasectomy reversal fail? Br J Urol 1988;57:780.

Schoysman R et al: Pregnancy after fertilisation with human testicular spermatozoa. (Letter.) Lancet 1993; 342:1237.

Sharlip ID: What is the best pregnancy rate that may be expected from vasectomy reversal? J Urol 1993;149: 1469.

Steckel J, Dicker AP, Goldstein M: Relationship between varicocele size and response to varicocelectomy. J Urol 1993;149:769.

Tournaye H et al: Are there predictive factors for successful testicular sperm recovery in azoospermic patients? Hum Reprod 1997;12:80.

Turek PJ, Magana JO, Lipshultz LI: Semen parameters before and after transurethral surgery for ejaculatory duct obstruction. J Urol 1996;155:1291.

Van Steirteghem AC et al: High fertilization and implantation rates after intracytoplasmic sperm injection. Hum Reprod 1993;8:1061.

47

Male Sexual Dysfunction

Tom F. Lue, MD

A better understanding of male sexual dysfunction has been made possible by innovative laboratory and clinical research in the hemodynamics, neurophysiology, and pharmacology of penile erection. Erectile function can now be evaluated in the office setting by intracavernous injection of vasoactive agents or the response to oral phosphodiesterase inhibitor at home. Improved diagnostic tests can differentiate among types of impotence. More treatment options, such as oral and transurethral drugs, are being added, and the latest generation of penile prostheses is more sophisticated and durable than earlier ones. Continuing research offers the possibility of a more physiologic solution to erectile dysfunction.

PHYSIOLOGY OF PENILE ERECTION

Innervation of the Penis

The autonomic erection center is located in the intermediolateral nucleus of the spinal cord at levels S_2–S_4 and T_{12}–L_2. Branches of the thoracolumbar segments join the inferior hypogastric plexus, which sends branches to the pelvic plexus, which is formed by contributions from sacral nerves. Bundles from these plexuses radiate to the pelvic organs. The fibers innervating the penis (the cavernous nerves) travel along the posterolateral aspect of the seminal vesicles and prostate and then accompany the membranous urethra through the genitourinary diaphragm (Walsh and Donker, 1982). At the prostatic urethra, these fibers are located at the 5 and 7 o'clock positions, and at the membranous urethra, they are at the 3 and 9 o'clock positions; they ascend gradually to the 1 and 11 o'clock positions (at the level of the midurethral bulb) and finally enter the hilum of the penis at the level of the distal urethral bulb (Figure 47–1). Some fibers enter the corpora cavernosa and corpus spongiosum with the cavernous and urethral arteries. Others travel further distally with the dorsal nerve and enter the corpus cavernosum and corpus spongiosum in various locations to supply the mid and distal portions of the penis. The terminal branches of the cavernous nerves innervate the helicine arteries and the trabecular smooth muscle and are responsible for the vascular events during tumescence and detumescence.

The center for somatic motor nerves is located at the Onuf nucleus of the ventral horn of the S_2–S_4 segment (de Araujo, Schmidt, and Tanagho, 1982). The motor fibers join the pudendal nerve to innervate the bulbocavernosus and ischiocavernosus muscles. The somatic sensory nerves originate at the receptors in the penile skin and glans. Sensations of pain and temperature ascend via the spinothalamic tract; vibratory stimuli are carried in the dorsal column; touch and pressure sensations are transmitted via both pathways to the thalamus. The perception of pleasant or unpleasant emotions probably involves past experiences and cortical interpretation.

The brain has a modulatory effect on the spinal pathways of erection. Various supraspinal areas that have a role in erectile function include the hypothalamus and limbic system (Perachio, Marr, and Alexander, 1979), ventral thalamus, tegmentum of mid brain and lateral substantia nigra (MacLean, 1975), and ventrolateral pons and medulla. Specifically, the medial preoptic area (MPOA) and the paraventricular nucleus of the hypothalamus, the periaqueductal gray of the mid brain and the nucleus paragigantocellularis of the medulla are the centers intimately involved in the control of penile erection (McKenna, 1998).

Three types of erections are noted in humans: genital-stimulated (contact or reflexogenic), central-stimulated (noncontact or psychogenic), and central-originated (nocturnal). Genital-stimulated erection is induced by tactile stimulation of the genital area. Afferent fibers ascend from the pudendal nerves to the sacral dorsal horn and dorsal gray commissure. The messages are then processed by the interneurons and carried to the parasympathetic and motor neurons in the sacral spinal centers. The efferent impulses are carried in the cavernous and dorsal nerves to the genitalia. This kind of erection can be preserved in upper spinal cord lesions, although erections are usually short in duration and poorly controlled by the individual. Central-stimulated erection is more complex, resulting from memory, fantasy, or visual or auditory stimuli. After the stimuli are processed in various

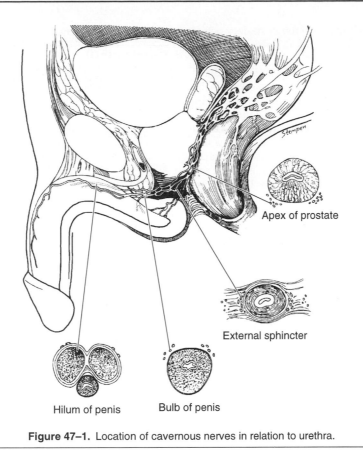

Figure 47–1. Location of cavernous nerves in relation to urethra.

brain centers, the messages are then conveyed through the thoracolumbar and sacral centers to the external genitalia. The fact that only a small percentage of patients with complete sacral cord lesion can retain erection suggests that the sacral center exerts major control of the erectile process. The central-originated erection can occur spontaneously without stimulation or during sleep. The exact neural mechanism of nocturnal erection is unknown. Most of the sleep erections occur during rapid eye movement sleep, and the number and duration of erections are markedly reduced in hypogonadism and in men receiving antiandrogen therapy.

Anatomy & Hemodynamics of Penile Erection

The tunica of the corpora cavernosa is a bilayered structure with multiple sublayers. (1) The inner circular bundles support and contain the cavernous tissue. From this inner layer radiate intracavernosal pillars that act as struts to augment the septum, which provides essential support to the erectile tissue. (2) The outer-layer bundles are oriented longitudinally and extend from the glans penis to the proximal crura. These insert into the inferior pubic ramus but

are absent between the 5 and 7 o'clock positions. In contrast, the corpus spongiosum lacks an outer layer or intracorporeal struts, ensuring a low-pressure structure during erection.

The tunica is composed of elastic fibers forming a network resembling an irregular lattice on which the collagen fibers rest. The detailed histologic composition of the tunica varies with anatomic location and function. Emissary veins run between the inner and outer layers for a short distance, often piercing the outer bundles obliquely. Branches of the dorsal artery take a more direct perpendicular route, however, and are surrounded by a periarterial fibrous sheath. The outer layer appears to play an additional role in compression of the veins during erection (Hsu et al, 1992).

The paired internal pudendal artery is the major carrier of the blood supply to the penis. The terminal portion of this artery divides into 3 branches: the bulbourethral artery, the dorsal artery, and the cavernous artery (deep artery). The cavernous artery supplies the corpora cavernosa; the dorsal artery, the glans penis; and the bulbourethral artery, the corpus spongiosum. Accessory pudendal arteries from external iliac or obturator arteries may supply a major portion of the penis in some cases. Collaterals among the 3 branches are often observed (Breza et al, 1989). The venous drainage of the glans is mainly through the deep dorsal vein. The corpus spongiosum is drained via the circumflex, urethral, and bulbar veins, but the drainage of the corpora cavernosa is more complex: The mid and distal shafts are drained by the deep dorsal vein to the preprostatic plexus; the proximal portion is drained by the cavernous and the crural veins to the preprostatic plexus and internal pudendal vein. The drainage of all 3 corpora originates in the subtunical venules, which unite to form emissary veins that pierce the tunica albuginea. The emissary veins may drain into the deep dorsal vein (dorsal group), circumflex or lateral veins (lateral group), and periurethral veins or corpus spongiosum (ventral group) (Tudoriu, 1989). The emissary veins may empty directly or through the circumflex veins into the deep dorsal vein. The glans penis possesses numerous large and small veins that communicate freely with the dorsal veins. The penile skin and subcutaneous tissue are drained by superficial dorsal veins, which then empty into the saphenous veins.

Investigations of human penile blood flow have included Newman's infusion study in cadavers (Newman, Northrup, and Devlin, 1964) and the radioactive xenon washout studies of Wagner and Uhrenholdt (1980) and Shirai et al (1978) in volunteers during visual erotic stimulation. Although the contribution of increased arterial flow has been well established, the role of the venous system has remained controversial. However, studies in dogs and monkeys after electrical stimulation of the cavernous and pudendal nerves and in humans during papaverine-induced erection have finally clarified the role of the arterial, venous, and sinusoidal systems.

The erection process can be divided into phases as shown in Table 47–1 and Figure 47–2.

Studies of erection during visual sexual stimulation (Wagner, 1986 [personal communication]) and rapid eye movement sleep (Karacan, Aslan, and Hirshkowitz, 1983) have shown synergistic activity of the bulbocavernosus and ischiocavernosus muscles during the erectile process. Separate electrode implantation on the cavernous and pudendal nerves in the animal model as well as papaverine injection in humans and animals have made it possible to study the relative contribution of the autonomic and somatic nerves in the erectile process. Autonomic neural stimulation is responsible for the **vascular stage of erection,** ie, filling and trapping of blood in the cavernous bodies. After full erection is achieved, contraction of the ischiocavernosus muscle compresses the proximal corpora and raises the pressure in the entire corpora well above the systolic blood pressure, resulting in rigid erection (Table 47–1) (**skeletal muscle stage of erection**). This rigid phase occurs naturally during masturbation or sexual intercourse but can also occur from slight bending of the penis, without muscular action. Studies in animal models (Lue, 1986) have shown markedly decreased flow in the internal pudendal artery during the rigid erection phase; because this phase usually lasts

Table 47–1. Phases of the erection process.[1]

Flaccid phase (1)
Minimal arterial and venous flow; blood gas values equal those of venous blood. Flow rate: 2.5–8 mL/100 g/min (Wagner and Uhrenholdt, 1980); 0.5–6.5 mL/100 g/min (Shirai et al, 1978).

Latent (filling) phase (2)
Increased flow in the internal pudendal artery during both systolic and diastolic phases. Decreased pressure in the internal pudendal artery; unchanged intracavernous pressure. Some elongation of the penis.

Tumescent phase (3)
Rising intracavernous pressure until full erection is achieved. Penis shows more expansion and elongation with pulsation. The arterial flow rate decreases as the pressure rises. When intracavernous pressure rises above diastolic pressure, flow occurs only in the systolic phases.

Full erection phase (4)
Intracavernous pressure can rise to as much as 80–90% of the systolic pressure. Pressure in the internal pudendal artery increases but remains slightly below systemic pressure. Arterial flow is much less than in the initial filling phase but is still higher than in the flaccid phase. Although the venous channels are mostly compressed, the venous flow rate is slightly higher than during the flaccid phase. Blood gas values approach those of arterial blood.

Skeletal or rigid erection phase (5)
As a result of contraction of the ischiocavernous muscle, the intracavernous pressure rises well above the systolic pressure, resulting in rigid erection. During this phase, almost no blood flows through the cavernous artery; however, the short duration prevents the development of ischemia or tissue damage.

Detumescent phase (6)
After ejaculation or cessation of erotic stimuli, sympathetic tonic discharge resumes, resulting in contraction of the smooth muscles around the sinusoids and arterioles. This effectively diminishes the arterial flow to flaccid levels, expels a large portion of blood from the sinusoidal spaces, and reopens the venous channels. The penis returns to its flaccid length and girth.

[1]Numbers 1–6 correspond to phases shown in Fig 47–2.

only a short period of time, however, ischemia or tissue damage does not occur.

The hemodynamics of the glans penis are somewhat different. Arterial flow increases in the glans in a manner similar to that in the shaft. Because it lacks the tunica albuginea, however, the glans functions as an arteriovenous fistula during the full erection phase. Partial compression of the deep dorsal vein (1) within Buck's fascia by the expanded corpora and (2) between the corpora cavernosa and the pubic bone does contribute to the pressure increase in the glans and deep dorsal vein. Nevertheless, during rigid erection, most of the venous channels are temporarily compressed, and further engorgement of the glans can be observed.

Mechanism of Penile Erection

Based on human cadaveric dissections, Conti (1952) proposed the theory that penile erection is

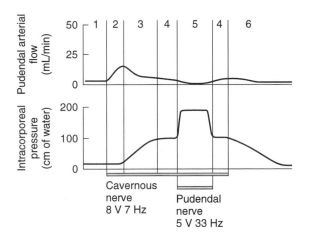

Figure 47–2. Phases of penile erection (induced in monkeys via neurostimulation). Numbers correspond to phases outlined in Table 47–1. (Lower tracing = intracavernous pressure; upper tracing = flow within the internal pudendal artery.)

ial and arteriolar vasodilatation and easy expansion of the sinusoids to receive a large increase of flow. Trapping of blood owing to increased compliance of the entire sinusoidal system causes the penis to lengthen and widen rapidly until the capacity of the tunica albuginea is reached. Meanwhile, expansion of the sinusoidal walls against one another and against the tunica albuginea results in compression of the subtunical venular plexus. Further expansion stretches the tunica albuginea, strangulates the emissary veins, and effectively reduces the venous flow to a minimum (Figure 47–3A and B). Because flow to the penis is not constant (as evidenced by the tremendous flow increase in the internal pudendal artery during erection), there is no need to have an arteriovenous shunt to divert excess blood from the penis. Thus, polsters, if they do exist, serve no necessary function. Furthermore, it becomes obvious that contraction and relaxation of the smooth muscles of the trabeculae and the arteriolar tree are the mechanisms that control erection.

regulated by polsters in the penile arteries and veins. Synergistic contraction or relaxation of these polsters would control the arteriovenous shunting of blood and result in erection or detumescence. This theory was challenged by Newman and Tchertkoff (1980), who could not find polsters in newborns, and by Benson et al (1980), who believe that what Conti described were not polsters but atherosclerotic lesions.

The controversy about the anatomic changes of penile erection was finally settled in the 1980s by electron microscopy of corrosion penile casts made in the flaccid state and during erection (Fournier et al, 1987; Banya et al, 1989). In these models, the flaccid corpus cavernosum shows contracted sinusoids and constricted arteries and arterioles, and the draining venules form a plexus under the tunica albuginea. During erection, dilation of the arterial tree, expansion of the sinusoids, and compression of the subtunical and emissary veins are clearly seen. From these studies and observation of vasodilator-induced erections, it appears that the smooth muscles in the arterial tree and the trabeculae are the key to the erectile process.

The intrinsic smooth-muscle tone and, possibly, the adrenergic tonic discharge maintain contraction of the smooth muscles in the flaccid state. This high peripheral resistance distributed throughout the contracted sinusoids and tortuous and constricted arteriolar and arterial tree allows only a minimal amount of flow to enter the sinusoidal spaces. When the smooth muscles relax owing to release of neurotransmitters or injection of alpha blockers or a smooth-muscle relaxant, the compliance of the sinusoidal spaces and the arterial tree increases, and the resistance to incoming flow drops to a minimum. This allows arter-

Hormones & Sexual Function

Androgens are essential for male sexual maturity. Testosterone regulates gonadotropin secretion and muscle development; dihydrotestosterone mediates all other aspects of male sexual maturation, including hair growth, acne, male pattern baldness, and spermatogenesis. Androgens are known to act on the hypothalamus, which is an important site for modulation of erectile function. The hormones can also modulate synaptic transmission, including storage, synthesis, uptake, and release of neurotransmitters as well as receptor sensitivity (Crowley and Selman, 1981; Johnston and Davison, 1972; McEwen, 1981). In adults, androgen deficiency results in loss of sexual interest and impaired seminal emission. The frequency, magnitude, and latency of nocturnal penile erections are reduced. However, studies have shown that erection in response to visual sexual stimulation is not affected by androgen withdrawal in hypogonadal men, suggesting that androgen enhances but is not essential for erection (Bancroft and Wu, 1983; Kwan et al, 1983).

A progressive decline in testosterone occurs after the seventh decade. Studies suggest that this decline may be partly of testicular origin and partly due to hypothalamic-pituitary dysfunction (Deslypere and Vermeulen, 1984). It is not known whether there is a threshold level of androgen above which a further increase would have no effect on sexual interest. However, it has been shown that exogenous testosterone does increase sexual interest in some men with levels in the "laboratory normal" range. Further studies are needed to determine if there is such a threshold and whether it changes with age (O'Carroll and Bancroft, 1984).

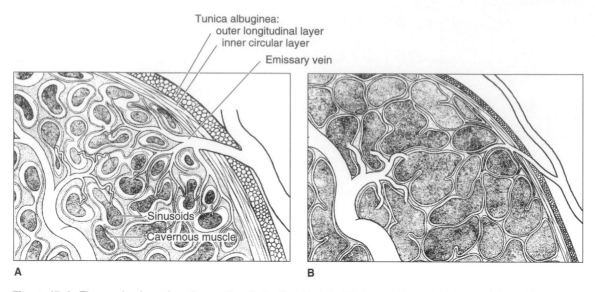

Figure 47–3. The mechanism of penile erection. In the flaccid state (**A**), the arteries, arterioles, and sinusoids are contracted. The intersinusoidal and subtunical venular plexuses are wide open, with free flow to the emissary veins. In the erect state (**B**), the muscles of the sinusoidal wall and the arterioles relax, allowing maximal flow to the compliant sinusoidal spaces. Most of the venules are compressed between the expanding sinusoids. Even the larger intermediary venules are sandwiched and flattened by distended sinusoids and the noncompliant tunica albuginea. This effectively reduces the venous capacity to a minimum.

Neurotransmitters & the Pharmacology of Erection

Neural control of penile erection involves the adrenergic, cholinergic, and nonadrenergic-noncholinergic (NANC) neuroeffector systems. Adrenergic nerves mediate intracavernous smooth-muscle contraction, which causes detumescence of an erect penis. Cholinergic nerves may contribute to smooth-muscle relaxation and penile erection through (1) inhibition of adrenergic nerves via inhibitory interneurons and (2) release of nitric oxide from the endothelium by acetylcholine (Saenz de Tejada et al, 1988a; Kim et al, 1991).

Ignarro et al (1990) reported the release of nitric oxide (NO), accumulation of cyclic GMP (cGMP), and relaxation of rabbit corpus cavernosum muscles in in vitro stimulation of NANC neurotransmission. Saenz de Tejada et al (1988a) also demonstrated NANC neurogenic relaxation of human corpus cavernosum muscle and attenuation of the relaxation by substances that interfere with the synthesis or the effects of NO in in vitro experiments. Trigo-Rocha et al (1993a, b) showed that the NO-cGMP pathway is the principal mechanism in canine penile erection. Other studies have proposed that NO is a NANC inhibitory neurotransmitter in various organs (Bult et al, 1990). Furthermore, NO synthase has been localized in the peripheral autonomic nerves innervating vascular and nonvascular smooth muscles (Bredt, Hwang, and Snyder, 1990). In biopsy specimens of human penile tissue, NO synthase staining within the cavernous nerves was found to be reduced significantly after non-nerve-sparing radical prostatectomy (Brock et al, 1993).

In addition, substances secreted by endothelium lining the sinusoidal spaces may also be involved in penile erection. These include prostaglandins (Saenz de Tejada et al, 1988b), EDRF, and endothelium-derived contracting factor. Because both nitrovasodilators and EDRF increase intracellular cGMP and activate soluble guanylate cyclase in vascular smooth muscle, NO released from L-arginine has been suggested to be the EDRF (Moncada, 1990). On the other hand, endothelin-1, -2, and -3 have been suggested as the endothelium-derived contracting factor (Holmquist, Andersson, and Hedlund, 1990).

Direct injection of vasoactive agents, on the other hand, has helped in the understanding of the pharmacology of the penis and changed diagnosis and treatment strategies. The agents capable of inducing erection and causing detumescence are summarized in Table 47–2. Although the actions of different agents vary, when given in large doses, all erection-inducing agents cause the smooth muscles to relax, and all detumescence-inducing agents cause them to contract.

Molecular Mechanism of Smooth-Muscle Contraction & Relaxation

Smooth muscles have molecular structures similar to those in striated muscles, but the actin and myosin

Table 47–2. Agents that induce or inhibit penile erection in human males.

Inducers	Inhibitors
Vasoactive intestinal polypeptide (VIP)[1]	Metaraminol
Phentolamine[1]	Epinephrine
Papaverine[1]	Norepinephrine
Nitroglycerin	Ephedrine
Thymoxamine	Dopamine
Imipramine	Phenylephrine
Verapamil	Guanethidine
Phenoxybenzamine	
Prostaglandin E_1	
Nitric oxide donors	
Calcitonin-gene-related peptide	
Sildenafil	

[1]Alone and in combination.

filaments are not arrayed regularly to generate the striated appearance. Smooth-muscle myosin contains light chains that control the binding of the myosin head to actin.

Smooth-muscle contraction is regulated by Ca^{2+}. When the cytosolic free Ca^{2+} increases from a resting level of 120–270 to 500–700 nM, calmodulin-4 Ca^{2+} complex binds to the myosin light-chain kinase (Murray, 1996). The activated kinase then phosphorylates the light chain, which ceases to inhibit the myosin-actin interaction and initiates a contraction cycle.

When cytosolic free Ca^{2+} falls to the resting level, the Ca^{2+} dissociates from calmodulin, which in turn dissociates from the myosin light-chain kinase, thus inactivating it. Dephosphorylated myosin light chain resumes its action of inhibiting the binding of the myosin head to actin and relaxes the smooth muscle (Murray, 1996).

Signal Transduction in Penile Erection

Peptide hormones and many local regulators derived from amino acids are unable to pass through the plasma membrane of the target cells. However, they are able to bind to specific sites on receptor proteins embedded within the cell's plasma membrane. The receptors are components of signal transduction pathways that convert the hormone's extracellular signal to intracellular signals, which alter the behavior of the target cells.

Binding of a receptor with the regulatory factor (ligand) induces a conformational change in the receptor protein, which either directly or indirectly activates or inhibits a cascade of molecular events that lead to the biologic response. Direct activation occurs when the receptor protein is an enzyme or an ion channel. Indirect activation requires a coupling factor, eg, a GTP-binding regulatory protein (G protein) to activate separate effector molecules, including enzymes and ion channels. The enzymes then produce

intracellular mediator molecules (messengers), which relay the signal to the cytoplasm. The major second messengers are cyclic AMP (cAMP), cGMP, inositol triphosphate, and diacylglycerol. Calcium ion is considered a third messenger because its rise in cytoplasm is mediated through inositol triphosphate (Campbell, 1996).

All of the above signal pathways may be involved in penile erection and detumescence. For example, soluble cGMP is a second messenger between NO-guanylyl cyclase and smooth-muscle relaxation. cAMP is a second messenger for prostaglandin E_1, vasoactive intestinal polypeptide, and calcitonin gene-related peptide. Norepinephrine, phenylephrine, and endothelin appear to activate phospholipase C, which leads to the formation of inositol triphosphate and diacylglycerol, which in turn increases cytoplasmic calcium and induces smooth-muscle relaxation.

In smooth muscle, both cGMP and cAMP induce relaxation by decreasing intracellular Ca^{2+} concentration via activation of specific protein kinases and by modifying the activity of ion channels. Degradation of cGMP and cAMP to GMP and AMP, respectively, is achieved by specific phosphodiesterases. Ten classes of phosphodiesterases have been identified. The penis is rich in phosphodiesterase type V (GMP specific), and therefore a specific type V phosphodiesterase inhibitor (sildenafil) has been shown to improve penile erections in patients with erectile dysfunction.

Ion Channels

The presence of voltage-dependent L-type calcium channels (long-duration current, slow calcium channel) on isolated cavernous smooth muscle and cultured muscle cells has been documented. Christ et al (1993) have reported that both calcium influx via calcium channels and mobilization of intracellular calcium stores are involved during phenylephrine and endothelin-induced contraction, but only calcium channel influx is apparent for KCl-induced contraction.

Studies have shown at least 4 types of potassium channel subtypes in the cavernous smooth muscle: (1) the calcium-sensitive K channels (eg, maxi-K); (2) the metabolically regulated K channels (K_{ATP}); (3) the delayed rectifier, and (4) the fast transient A current (I_A) (Christ et al, 1993). The calcium-sensitive K channels may be involved in cAMP-mediated smooth-muscle relaxation.

Intercellular Communication

Gap junctions are aqueous intercellular channels that have been demonstrated to interconnect the cytoplasm of adjacent cells in many tissues. In the penis, the millions of individual smooth-muscle cells are sparsely innervated by the terminal branches of the cavernous nerves. Therefore, gap junctions play a vital role in the intercellular communication within the corpus cavernosum, which enables the penis to function as a unit. In human cavernous smooth muscle, intercellular communication through gap junctions appears to modulate alpha-1-adrenergic- and endothelin-induced contractility. The gap junctions may also be involved in muscle contraction and relaxation involving the second messenger systems. It is also postulated that alteration of the gap junction protein connexin 43 may be involved in erectile dysfunction in some patients (Moreno et al, 1993).

MALE SEXUAL DYSFUNCTION

Male sexual dysfunction, denoting the inability to achieve a satisfactory sexual relationship, may involve inadequacy of erection or problems with emission, ejaculation, or orgasm.

Erectile dysfunction (impotence) is the consistent inability to obtain or maintain an erection for satisfactory sexual relations (NIH Consensus Conference, 1993).

Premature ejaculation refers to uncontrolled ejaculation before or shortly after the vagina is entered.

Retarded ejaculation is unusually delayed ejaculation.

Retrograde ejaculation denotes backflow of semen into the bladder during ejaculation owing to an incompetent bladder neck mechanism.

EPIDEMIOLOGY

In the Massachusetts Male Aging Study, a community-based survey of men between 40 and 70 years of age, 52% of respondents reported some degree of erectile dysfunction: 17% mild, 25% moderate, and 10% complete. Although the prevalence of mild erectile dysfunction remained constant (17%) between the age of 40 and 70, there was a doubling in the number of men reporting moderate erectile dysfunction (from 17% to 34%) and a tripling in the number of men reporting complete erectile dysfunction (from 5% to 15%). Among the major predictors of erectile dysfunction are diabetes mellitus, heart disease, hypertension, and decreased high-density lipoprotein level. There is a higher prevalence of erectile dysfunction in men who have undergone radiation or surgery for prostate cancer. The psychological correlates of erectile dysfunction include depression and anger (Feldman et al, 1994). In the National Health and Social Life Survey in men aged 18–59, other male sexual dysfunctions were also found to be highly prevalent: premature ejaculation (28.5%), lack of sexual interest (15.8%), anxiety about sexual performance (17%), and lack of pleasure in sex (8.1%) (Laumann et al, 1994).

PATHOGENESIS

Erection involves psychological, neurologic, hormonal, arterial, and cavernosal factors (Figure 47–4). Impotence of clearly defined origin is discussed under the appropriate heading. Cases resulting from more than one factor or from causes that cannot be precisely determined are discussed under Other Causes.

Psychological Disorders
Early theories attributed erectile failure to anxiety (Wolpe, 1958; Ellis, 1962). Masters and Johnson (1976) introduced the concept of performance anxiety and the spectator role. LoPiccolo (1986) refined the differentiation of various psychological causes as religious orthodoxy, obsessive-compulsive or anhedonic personality, sexual phobias or deviation, widower's syndrome, depression, lack of physical attraction or poor body image, the "madonna-prostitute" syndrome, concern over aging, and lack of knowledge of physiologic changes with age. In the 1950s, 90% of cases of impotence were believed to be psychogenic. Most authors now believe that more than 50% have an organic cause, and in the older population the percentage is probably higher (Montague et al, 1979; Spark, White, and Connolly, 1980). The pathogenesis of psychogenic impotence is unknown. Sympathetic overactivity and inhibition of neurotransmitter release are some of the proposed causes.

Neurogenic Disorders
Erectile impotence can be caused by disease or dysfunction of the brain, spinal cord, cavernous and pudendal nerves, and terminal nerve endings and receptors. Among these, spinal cord injury is particularly intriguing. Bors and Comarr (1971) found that about 95% of patients with complete upper motor neuron lesions are capable of erection (reflexogenic), while only about 25% of those with complete lower motor neuron lesions can have erections (psychogenic). With incomplete lesions, however, more than 90% of patients in both groups retain erectile ability. It is suggested that diseases at the level of the brain (eg, tumors, epilepsy, cerebrovascular accidents, and Parkinson or Alzheimer disease) probably cause erectile failure through decreased sexual interest or overinhibition of the spinal erection centers. Diseases at the spinal level (eg, spina bifida, disk herniation, syringomyelia, cord tumor, tabes dorsalis, and multiple sclerosis) may affect either the afferent or efferent nerve pathway to the penis. Peripheral neuropathy as seen in diabetes mellitus, chronic alcohol consumption, or vitamin deficiency may affect the nerve endings and result in a deficiency of neuro-

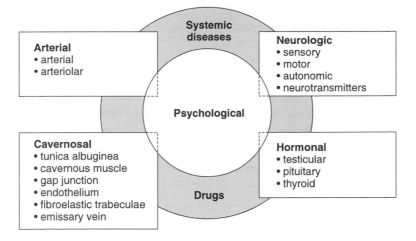

Figure 47–4. Erection involves psychological, neurologic, hormonal, arterial, and cavernosal factors.

transmitters. Direct injury to the cavernous or pudendal nerves from trauma or radical prostatic or rectal surgery also can cause disruption of the neural pathway and result in impotence.

Hormonal Disorders

Diabetes mellitus is the most common hormonal disease associated with erectile failure. However, impotence in diabetics is due mostly to vascular, neurogenic, or psychological factors (or a combination of these) rather than to the hormonal aberration per se. Hypogonadism due to hypothalamic or pituitary tumors, estrogen or antiandrogen therapy, or orchiectomy for prostatic cancer can suppress sexual interest and nocturnal erections. However, these patients can achieve normal erection during visual sexual stimulation (Bancroft and Wu, 1983), and thus, the erectile ability is intact. Similarly, impotence resulting from hyperprolactinemia is probably caused by suppressed sexual interest. Hyperthyroidism, hypothyroidism, Cushing syndrome, and Addison disease are all reported to cause decreased libido and impotence. Whether the hormonal disturbance or other factors are responsible for the impotence needs further investigation.

Arterial Disorders

When the penis is in the flaccid state, a minimal amount of blood enters the corpora cavernosa to meet the metabolic needs, and the corporeal blood gas levels are the same as in venous blood. After sexual stimulation, a large amount of arterial flow instantaneously passes through the dilated arterioles to expand the entire sinusoidal system (tumescence), until a new equilibrium is established at approximately 100 mm Hg (full erection), when only a small amount of flow enters and leaves the corpora to maintain the erection.

In animal experiments, the time required to achieve full erection gradually increases with increasing arterial insufficiency. Narrowing of the arterial lumen (or hardening of the arterial wall in humans) results in low pressure in the cavernous arteries and poor arterial flow that can only partially fill the sinusoidal system and is not adequate to expand the sinusoidal wall fully to compress most of the venules. This insufficiency results in partial erection, difficulty in maintaining erection, or early detumescence—the most frequent complaints.

Michal, Kovac, and Belan (1984) found that the incidence and age at onset of coronary disease and impotence are parallel. Although arteriogenic impotence may be due to trauma or may be congenital, most often it is probably a component of generalized systemic arterial disease. The distribution and severity of the disease, however, differ from person to person. Some patients with severe arterial disease may still be potent as long as the arterial flow exceeds the venous flow; conversely, some patients with minimal arterial disease may be partially or completely impotent because of relatively large venous outflow, cavernous smooth-muscle dysfunction, or inadequate neurotransmitter release. In evaluating the arterial system, therefore, additional contributing factors must be taken into consideration.

Arterial disease can be classified as extra- or intrapenile arterial insufficiency. Extrapenile arterial disease is amenable to surgical repair and comprises diseases of the internal pudendal artery, internal and common iliac arteries, and aorta (Leriche syndrome [Leriche and Morel, 1968]); the pelvic steal syndrome (Michal and Pospichal, 1978); and pelvic trauma. Intrapenile arterial disease such as that resulting from aging, arteriosclerosis, or diabetes mellitus does not respond well to currently available surgical techniques.

Cavernosal Disorders

The relationship between aberrant venous flow and erectile dysfunction was confirmed by Ebbehoj and Wagner (1979), who used cavernosography during visual erotic stimulation. Animal experiments have shown that venous compression by the expanding sinusoidal wall and tunica albuginea depends on trabecular smooth-muscle relaxation and a compliant sinusoidal system. Cavernous (venous) impotence can be divided into 5 types according to cause: In type 1, large veins exit the corpus cavernosum (this type is probably congenital); in type 2, venous channels are enlarged as a result of distortion of the tunica albuginea (as in Peyronie disease or the weakening associated with aging); in type 3, the cavernous smooth muscle is unable to relax because of fibrosis, degeneration, or dysfunction of gap junctions; in type 4, there is inadequate neurotransmitter release (in neurologic or psychological impotence or endothelial dysfunction); and in type 5, there is abnormal communication between the corpus cavernosum and the spongiosum or glans (either congenital, traumatic, or consequent to shunt procedure for priapism) (Lue, 1988).

With an insufficient venous occlusion mechanism, erection is only partial or short-lived. Patients may have primary impotence or may become impotent at a young age, in their early thirties or forties. Local disease such as Peyronie disease, penile tumor, scleroderma, penile contusion, or penile fracture may involve the sinusoids and prevent erection. Impotence occurs in more than 50% of patients after priapism due to fibrosis of the corpora (Winter, 1979).

Electron microscope studies of cavernous erectile tissue obtained during implantation of penile prostheses reveals a high incidence of smooth-muscle atrophy, fibrous replacement, and endothelial disruption in patients with diabetes mellitus and atherosclerosis. In addition, changes of the terminal erectile nerves are common in chronic alcoholics and diabetics (Mersdorf et al, 1991; Persson et al, 1989).

Studies of penile tissue obtained by needle biopsy have also revealed changes in the smooth muscle–collagen ratio, decreased endothelium, and diminished elastic fibers in impotent patients (Sattar, Schulman, and Wespes, 1995). Additional studies also suggest that a decrease of intracavernous smooth-muscle fibers may contribute to decreased oxygen tension during erection (Sattar et al, 1995b) and venous leakage (Nehra et al, 1996).

Other Causes

Other causes may affect one or more of the factors controlling the erectile mechanism. Because of the lack of scientific studies, however, their precise pathogenetic relationship remains speculative.

A. Drugs: In older patients taking several medications for different diseases, it is often difficult to determine whether sexual dysfunction results from a specific drug, from interactions among several drugs, from underlying diseases, or from associated psychological factors (Van Arsdalen, Malloy, and Wein, 1983).

Almost all antihypertensive drugs have been implicated in impotence, especially the central-acting sympatholytics such as methyldopa, clonidine, and reserpine. Their major effect is probably through central nervous system depression, elevated prolactin levels, and decreased libido (Reichgott, 1979). The peripheral alpha-adrenergic blockers such as phenoxybenzamine or prazosin rarely affect erection, although retrograde ejaculation is a known side effect. The beta blockers such as propranolol reportedly decrease libido, as does spironolactone, which causes gynecomastia in some patients. Theoretically, diuretics and vasodilators should not cause erectile dysfunction; however, patients with severe atherosclerosis may require higher blood pressure to deliver sufficient flow to the penis, and the lowering of blood pressure by these agents may result in partial erection.

Antidepressants such as tricyclics and monoamineoxidase inhibitors depress the libido, probably through their sedative and anticholinergic effects. The major and minor tranquilizers and hypnotics have also been reported to cause decreased libido. Suggested mechanisms are sedation, an anticholinergic effect, and prolactin release through the inhibition of dopamine receptors. These 2 groups of medications include phenothiazines, benzodiazepines, meprobamate, and barbiturates.

Other drugs or chemicals known to cause impotence include estrogen and antiandrogens (cimetidine, ketoconazole, cyproterone acetate). Marijuana depresses the testosterone level; alcohol may induce alcoholic neuropathy or increase estrogen owing to hepatic dysfunction; narcotics decrease the libido; and cigarette smoking contributes to vasoconstriction and venous leakage. Digoxin has also been reported to cause erectile dysfunction in some men. A recent study suggests that it may be related to inhibition of sodium/potassium adenosine triphosphatase activity in the corpus cavernosum (Gupta et al, 1998).

B. Systemic Disease and Other Disorders:

1. Diabetes mellitus–Impotence reportedly occurs in 25% of young diabetics and in almost 75% of older patients (Rubin and Babbott, 1958). However, insulin dosage and duration and adequacy of control appear unrelated to sexual dysfunction. Although diabetes is an endocrine disorder, most studies reveal no other hormonal dysfunction or androgen deficiency that might contribute to impotence (Jensen et al, 1979). Psychogenic impotence is probably rare; however, secondary psychological factors compounding organic impotence are common.

The major impact of diabetes is on the nervous and vascular systems. After 10–15 years, a functional abnormality of the somatic and autonomic nervous system can often be found on neurologic testing.

Faerman et al (1974) showed a good correlation between sexual dysfunction and the presence of peripheral neuropathy but not retinopathy or arrhythmia. The pathogenesis of neurogenic impotence in diabetes is still under investigation. Recently, decreased levels of vasoactive intestinal polypeptide (Crowe et al, 1983) and norepinephrine (Melman and Henry, 1979) have been reported. Diabetes is also known to affect both large and small vessels. Rubarsk and Michal (1977) reported fibrotic lesions of the cavernous arteries with intimal proliferation, calcification, and stenosis of the lumen in 15 men with diabetes of an average of 13 years' duration. Jevtich et al (1980) reported a high incidence of abnormal results on Doppler examination of the penile arteries. Although a neurologic deficit or arterial disease alone may not cause impotence if adequate compensation can be recruited, the presence of both simultaneously will certainly aggravate the disability.

2. Renal disease–Impotence occurs in about 50% of patients undergoing dialysis (Sherman, 1975). Multiple factors are involved, including decreased testosterone levels; autonomic neuropathy; accelerated vascular disease; multiple medications; worsening of the primary disease; and psychological stress. In a study of patients who underwent successful renal transplantation, potency was restored in 75% (Salvatierra, Fortmann, and Belzer, 1975). Bilateral renal transplantation with end-to-end anastomosis to internal iliac arteries can result in postoperative impotence owing to compromised internal pudendal arterial flow.

3. Other diseases–Patients who have recently recovered from myocardial infarction and those with angina or heart failure can develop impotence owing to anxiety, arterial insufficiency, or the effects of drugs. Patients with severe pulmonary emphysema with dyspnea often develop impotence because of anxiety, which may exacerbate the dyspnea and cause interpersonal conflicts with the sexual partner. In patients who have colostomies, ileostomies, or ileal conduits, problems may occur owing to depression and loss of self-esteem. Cirrhosis of the liver, scleroderma, chronic debilitation, and cachexia are also known to cause impotence.

Although hypertension is common among impotent patients, Newman and Marcus (1985) found that the frequency of erectile failure was little different from that in a control group of men of similar age. They also found that aging has a negative impact in all groups, with or without hypertension or diabetes.

DIAGNOSIS & TREATMENT

A detailed medical and sexual history and a thorough physical examination are the most important steps in the differential diagnosis of sexual dysfunction. Interviewing the partner, if available, is indispensable in eliciting a reliable history, planning treatment, and obtaining a successful outcome. Because multiple contributing factors may exist, a routine noninvasive workup aimed at determining the major cause should be performed in all patients. This should include basic laboratory tests such as a complete blood count, urinalysis, fasting blood glucose, serum creatinine, morning serum testosterone, and prolactin levels. In patients with symptoms of prostatic disease, expressed prostatic secretions should be examined.

At our institution, my colleagues and I have adopted a method called the patient's goal-directed approach for the diagnosis and treatment of all impotent patients (Lue, 1989). After the history, physical examination, and laboratory testing are completed, the patient is given a pamphlet explaining the treatment options currently available. Further tests are conducted according to the patient's general health, motivation, and desired treatment (Table 47–3).

Psychological Impotence

In the past, impotence was arbitrarily classified as either organic or psychogenic. When it was associated with a disease known to cause erectile failure, impotence was classified as organic; all other cases were labeled psychogenic. In fact, the pattern of sexual dysfunction, rather than the presence or absence of an organic factor, is probably the most important factor in making a diagnosis. Because psychogenic impotence is the result of changes in affect and mood, it usually occurs in a specific pattern. A suggestive history includes sudden onset, selective dysfunction (eg, rigid erection with one partner and poor

---

Table 47–3. Tests suggested for various treatment options (Lue, 1989).[1]

1. **Oral medication, transurethral therapy, or vacuum constriction device**
   No further testing
2. **Intracavernous injection therapy**
   CIS test
3. **Penile prosthesis**
   CIS test or NPT test or duplex scanning
4. **Venous surgery**
   CIS test
   Duplex scanning or cavernous arterial occlusion pressure test
   Cavernosometry and cavernosography
5. **Arterial surgery (or combined arterial and venous surgery)**
   CIS test
   Duplex scanning or cavernous arterial occlusion pressure
   Cavernosometry and cavernosography
   Pharmacologic arteriography

CIS, combined injection and stimulation; NPT, noctunal penile tumescence.
[1]Regardless of desired treatment, all patients must undergo history, physical examination, and basic laboratory testing.

erection with others, or normal erection during masturbation or fantasy but not during intercourse), and normal pattern of nocturnal erections but abnormal pattern during waking hours. This is often associated with anxiety, guilt, fear, emotional stress, and religious or parental inhibition.

Complementary psychometric testing (eg, Minnesota Multiphasic Personality Inventory, Walker Sex Form, and Derogatis Sexual Function Inventory) is reported to be helpful in assessing psychological status. However, some researchers find that these tests do not provide much information. Because patients with psychogenic impotence usually have normal nocturnal erections (3–5 per night, each lasting 25–35 min), whereas those with physiologic impotence have impaired nocturnal erections, monitoring of the nocturnal erectile activity has been used to differentiate psychogenic from physiologic impotence (Karacan et al, 1978). A formal sleep laboratory study usually records electroencephalogram, electrooculogram, electromyogram, and penile erectile activity simultaneously. Several modifications with the advantage of home monitoring and addition of penile rigidity measurement have been proposed. These include the stamp test (Barry, Blank, and Boileau, 1980), snap gauge band (Ek, Bradley, and Krane, 1983), and the Rigiscan device (Bradley et al, 1985). The major criticism is the lack of sleep quality documentation in these tests (Karacan, 1988).

The intracavernous injection test (with or without sexual stimulation [Lue, 1989]) can be used to help establish the diagnosis. When a neurologic deficit and hormonal disease are absent, the positive result (sustained full erection after injection) strongly suggests a psychogenic cause.

Theoretically, the preferred treatment of psychogenic impotence should be psychotherapy. Several techniques have been developed. Individual therapy using the psychoanalytic method is based on Freud's theory that erectile failure is the result of unconscious fears centering on the Oedipus complex. Subsequently, Masters and Johnson (1976) developed individual and couple counseling based on the concept of performance anxiety. This was followed by psychodynamically oriented couple therapy developed by Kaplan (1979). Other techniques include behaviorist therapy, feedback training, and hypnotherapy. Because of the urologist's limited knowledge of psychotherapy, referral to a sex therapist or psychotherapist is recommended. If the patient refuses to undergo psychotherapy or fails to improve after a reasonable number of sessions, an alternative treatment can be recommended. Options include a vacuum constriction device, transurethral or intracavernous injection of vasodilators, and a penile prosthesis. The recently approved oral phosphodiesterase inhibitor sildenafil has been shown to be very effective in patients with psychogenic impotence (84% improved erection and 70% successful in intercourse versus 26% and 29%, respectively, with placebo). Because of its efficacy, some even suggest that sildenafil might be used as a screening tool to rule out psychogenic impotence.

Neurologic Impotence

Ideally, neurologic examination should assess the integrity of the entire nervous system, including the afferent and efferent components of the central and peripheral nervous system and the autonomic and somatic functions. However, such a thorough examination is time-consuming and unrewarding in most cases. Furthermore, since erectile capability can be retained in the presence of neuropathy (eg, in some diabetics), an abnormal neurologic finding may not be the cause of impotence. Correlation with the history and other test results is essential before neurogenic impotence can be diagnosed.

A practical approach should begin with a detailed medical history. Particular attention should be directed to the autonomic and somatic functions of the sacral nerves (urinary, bowel, and sphincter control; sensation of the external genitalia, including the experience of pleasure or pain with penile stimulation; and direction and force of ejaculation). A history of diabetes, alcoholism, trauma or lesion of the head and spinal cord, or multiple sclerosis should be sought. If the medical history reveals no neurologic disease or deficit, a simple neurologic examination, including pinprick, touch, and vibratory stimulation of the external genitalia, perineum, and lower extremities and evaluation of the bulbocavernous reflex, is probably sufficient. When responses are normal, the chance of finding a neurologic lesion is rare.

In patients with a history of neurologic disease or deficit or abnormal findings on testing, more sophisticated testing is warranted. The patient should be referred to a neurologist if the urologist does not have the equipment for the following tests.

A. Somatosensory and Motor Function: Biothesiometry (Newman, 1970; Padma-Nathan, Goldstein, and Krane, 1986a) can be used to quantify dorsal nerve dysfunction, because loss of vibratory sense is one of the early signs of diabetic peripheral neuropathy. Evoked potential techniques are useful to determine dorsal nerve conduction velocity (Gerstenberg and Bradley, 1983), sacral evoked potential (Ertekin and Reel, 1976; Krane and Siroky, 1980), and genitocerebral responses (Haldeman et al, 1982).

B. Autonomic Afferent and Efferent Components: There are several procedures for assessing autonomic neuropathy: (1) heart rate variations during deep breathing (Watkins and Mackay, 1980), which indicate abnormal cardiac reflex—an early sign of autonomic neuropathy; (2) pupillary response to light; (3) cystometry with bethanechol testing and urethral pressure profile; and (4) bulbocavernous reflex to stimulation of the prostatic urethra. However, all these tests are indirect; direct testing of erectile function is not yet available.

Several researchers have suggested that recording electromyographic activity from the tissue of the corpus cavernosum may detect penile neuropathy. Further studies are required to validate this work (Jünemann, Buhrle, and Stief, 1993; Truss et al, 1993; Wagner, Gerstenberg, and Levin, 1989).

C. Central Nervous System: Nocturnal penile tumescence testing represents the standard evaluation of nocturnal erections. Karacan and Moore (1982) have perfected this technique by adding electroencephalography, electromyography, and electrocardiography. Irregularities revealed by these tests combined with abnormal nocturnal penile tumescence results may suggest a central nervous system abnormality.

Because dissociation between penile tumescence and rigidity has been noted in some patients during nocturnal testing, several techniques have been introduced to measure rigidity, such as the stamp test (Barry, Blank, and Boileau, 1980), the snap gauge band (Ek, Bradley, and Krane, 1983), and the Rigiscan continuous testing technique (Kaneko and Bradley, 1986).

Spark, Wills, and Royal (1984) identified a group of men with sexual dysfunction and temporal lobe epilepsy. They suggested that sleep-deprived electroencephalography or single photon emission computed tomography (SPECT) be used to locate lesions causing the sexual dysfunction.

Treatment of neurogenic impotence depends on the severity of the disease and associated factors. Patients with purely neurogenic disease may be treated with a vacuum constriction device, intracavernous injection of vasodilators, or a penile prosthesis. The newly approved oral agent sildenafil has also been shown to be quite effective in patients with spinal cord injury (83% improved erection and 59% successful intercourse versus 12% and 13%, respectively, with placebo). Clinical trials in postradical prostatectomy patients to test whether sildenafil can speed up nerve recovery are currently ongoing. Because patients with neurogenic impotence usually have an exaggerated erectile response to vasodilator injection and a higher rate of priapism, careful titration of the amount of vasodilator is mandatory before injection therapy is instituted. Starting with 0.1 mL (3 mg) of papaverine followed by 0.1-mL increments or starting with 1 μg of prostaglandin E_1 followed by 1-μg increments until adequate erection lasting for less than 1 h can be achieved is recommended. In patients with diminished genital sensation, warning about the harmful effect of the penile constricting ring must be given, and patients should be instructed to remove the ring within 30 min. A higher rate of prosthetic complications such as protrusion or infection also occurs in patients with neurogenic impotence. Therefore, careful pre- and postoperative instruction is essential in this group of patients. Implantation of electrodes on the erectile nerves is currently under investigation. In patients whose neuropathy is due to alcoholism or nutritional deficiency, vitamin supplements and a decrease in alcohol consumption may be helpful.

Hormonal Impotence

Evaluation of endocrine function should begin with a thorough medical history and systemic review. The hypothalamic-pituitary-gonadal axis should be assessed, as should thyroid and adrenal function. Diabetes mellitus is the most common endocrine disorder, although its effect is mainly on vascular and neurologic functions. A history of chemotherapy; irradiation; exposure to toxins, alcohol, or drugs; or chronic renal failure should be elicited. Most patients with endocrine abnormalities report decreased sexual interest rather than erectile failure, so a detailed sexual history is helpful in differential diagnosis.

During physical examination, particular attention should be directed toward signs of hypogonadism (small atrophic testes, loss of beard and body hair, and gynecomastia). If Leydig cell failure occurs before puberty, signs of eunuchoidism are apparent (sparse facial, pubic, and axillary hair; infantile genitalia; and a high-pitched voice). Laboratory tests should include testosterone and prolactin levels. Because 97% of the testosterone in plasma is bound to protein, a free testosterone determination may be necessary if a protein-building problem is suspected.

Patients with an elevated prolactin level should undergo repeat testing; if the result is still abnormal, they should be referred to an endocrinologist for investigation of a pituitary tumor. Patients with low morning testosterone levels also should have repeat studies and determination of luteinizing hormone (LH) and follicle-stimulating hormone (FSH) levels. When testosterone levels are low but LH and FSH levels are not elevated, endocrine consultation should be requested for investigation of pituitary or hypothalamic dysfunction. When LH and FSH levels are appropriately elevated in the presence of low testosterone levels, primary testicular failure is the cause of impotence.

Patients with diseases of the thyroid, adrenal, or pituitary gland should be referred to an endocrinologist for treatment. Diseases of the testicle such as primary testicular failure can be treated with sublingual, oral, or intramuscular testosterone. Because of the possibility of hepatotoxicity associated with oral or sublingual forms, intramuscular injection of testosterone (cypionate or enanthate, 200 mg every 2–3 weeks) is recommended (McClure, 1988). Luteinizing hormone-releasing hormone has also been reported to be useful in patients with hypothalamic-pituitary-gonadal axis abnormalities. In patients with hypopituitarism, human chorionic gonadotropin can be used to stimulate the production of testosterone in the testicle. In patients with hyperprolactinemia, treatment with a dopaminergic drug, bromocriptine, has been reported to improve sexual function. In patients with a pituitary tumor secreting excessive prolactin, treatment with bromocriptine or surgery also restores potency.

Arterial Impotence

Except in traumatic cases, arterial disease is a generalized systemic disorder and usually involves multiple organ systems. A history of peripheral vascular disease, intermittent claudication, and atrophic change of the extremities provides clues to the possible involvement of the penile arteries. Patients with coronary or peripheral vascular bypass have a high incidence of impotence due to arterial disease. The physical examination should include palpation of the carotid, brachial, femoral, and dorsal penile arteries.

Measurement of the penile blood pressure has been advocated as a screening test for penile arterial disease. The ratio of penile systolic blood pressure to brachial systolic pressure, expressed as the penile brachial pressure index (PBI), is reportedly a good indicator of arterial disease. A ratio below 0.6 is strongly indicative of arteriogenic impotence. Continuous-wave Doppler analysis is used for the PBI. This technique measures a mixture of signals from all the penile arteries rather than signals from a single artery; thus, a low value (eg, 0.6) correlates well with arteriography showing severe arterial disease. However, a normal PBI does not indicate normal penile blood flow. Pressure is measured in the flaccid penis and is not predictive of erectile function. Nevertheless, if this test is combined with pelvic exercise, the pelvic steal syndrome may be unmasked (Goldstein et al, 1982). Some authors report a better correlation between penile arteriography and other techniques (eg, determining the difference between mean arterial pressure and penile blood pressure [Montague et al, 1979]; pulse wave form analysis [Velcek et al, 1980]; and pulse volume recording [Merchant and DePalma, 1981]).

A. Functional Evaluation of Penile Arteries: The xenon washout technique performed during visual erotic stimulation provides an excellent functional test of psychogenic erection (Wagner, 1981). Different washout curves can be demonstrated in patients with abnormal venous leakage or arterial disease. However, this technique requires a radioisotope; also, the individual response to erotic videotapes varies greatly.

The introduction of intracavernous injection of vasoactive agents opened a new era in the functional study of penile vasculature. Although in rare situations psychological apprehension can affect the patient's response (Buvat et al, 1986), in most situations intracavernous injection can reliably assess penile vascular status (Abber et al, 1986). A negative response (no erection or partial erection) is not diagnostic; however, if the patient develops a fully rigid erection within 12 min of injection of 60 mg of papaverine or 10 μg of prostaglandin E_1 and the rigid erection is sustained for more than 30 min, adequate arterial flow and an intact venous mechanism can be assumed. Patients with less than full erection after papaverine injection can be further evaluated with high-resolution ultrasonography combined with pulsed Doppler analysis of the penile arteries during papaverine-induced erection (Lue et al, 1986a). This technique can scan the architecture of the penis, define the thickness of Peyronie plaque, measure changes in the diameter of the cavernous arteries before and after vasodilator injection, and visually assess the pulsation of the penile arteries. Pulsed color Doppler wave analysis can also measure the velocity of the flow through individual vessels in the penis. Sonography combined with Doppler analysis is a noninvasive way of assessing the individual penile arteries and is much more accurate than the PBI (Figure 47–5). Recording of Doppler signals from cavernous arteries after intracavernous injection of a vasodilator and infusion of saline (cavernous artery occlusion pressure) has also been reported to be a reliable functional assessment of the cavernous artery (Padma-Nathan, 1992).

Internal iliac or pudendal arteriography is indicated in selected cases of pelvic injury or in young healthy patients suspected of having isolated arterial disease. In most instances, the cavernous arteries are poorly visualized if arteriography is performed under local anesthesia owing to high resistance and minimal flow in the flaccid state. Intracavernous and intra-arterial injection of a vasodilator before imaging aids in assessment of the functional capacity of the penile arteries (Figure 47–6) (Virag et al, 1984; Zorgniotti and Lefleur, 1985; Bookstein et al, 1987).

B. Treatment of Arterial Impotence: Most patients with mild to moderate arterial impotence respond well to nonsurgical therapies, such as oral phosphodiesterase inhibitor, vacuum constriction device, and transurethral or intracavernous therapy. In those with severe arterial disease, surgical treatments such as arterial revascularization or penile prosthesis may be required to restore erectile function.

Sildenafil citrate (Viagra) is an oral phosphodiesterase type 5 inhibitor that prolongs the relaxant effect of NO in penile smooth muscle. During sexual stimulation, NO is released into the penile smooth muscle from NANC neurons (Gruetter et al, 1979). NO activates guanylyl cyclase, leading to increased levels of cGMP, which then relaxes cavernous smooth muscle and increases the penile blood flow necessary for erection. When the breakdown of cGMP is blocked by sildenafil, cGMP's concentration increases and its relaxant effects on penile smooth muscle are prolonged. It is important to note that sildenafil has no effect in the absence of sexual stimulation when NO and cGMP are at basal levels.

Clinical response to sildenafil is dose-dependent; 63% of patients taking a 25-mg dose reported im-

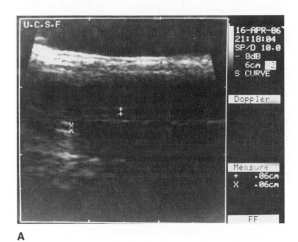

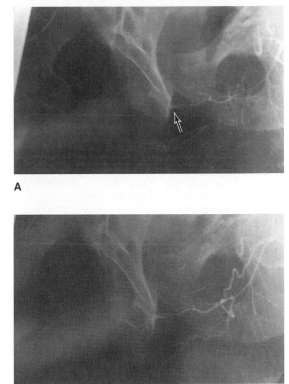

A

B

Figure 47–6. Internal iliac arteriogram in the flaccid penis (**A**) shows poor visualization of penile arteries, simulating occlusion (arrow). After intracavernous injection of 60 mg of papaverine (**B**), all the branches of the penile artery are well visualized.

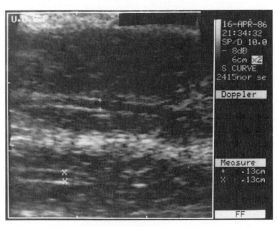

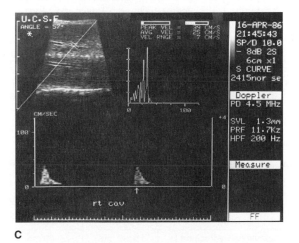

C

Figure 47–5. Duplex ultrasonography and Doppler analysis of the arterial response to intracavernous papaverine injection. In the flaccid state (**A**), the luminal diameter of the cavernous artery is 0.06 cm; after papaverine injection (**B**), this increases to 0.13 cm. Wave analysis (**C**) shows normal flow in the cavernous artery (peak velocity, 39 cm/s).

proved erection, and 82% reported improvement with 100 mg (Goldstein et al, 1998). Successful intercourse rates averaged 1.3 per week with 50–100 mg of sildenafil as compared with 0.4 with placebo. However, there was no effect on sexual drive.

Most adverse events were mild to moderate. Common complaints include headache (16%), flushing (10%), dyspepsia (7%), nasal congestion (4%), and abnormal vision (3%), described as a mild and transient color tinge or increased sensitivity to light. The incidence of adverse effects increased with larger doses. At 100 mg, dyspepsia occurred in 17% and abnormal vision in 11%. Adverse cardiovascular events were mild and transient in most cases, with a similar percentage between placebo and sildenafil groups. The rate of serious cardiovascular events, such as myocardial infarctions, was similar, at 1.7 and 1.4 events (per 1000 man-years of treatment) for the sildenafil and placebo groups, respectively (Morales et al, 1998). A word of caution is warranted, however; because most of the 128 US men who died after taking sildenafil had severe underlying cardiovascular disease, the patient's cardiovascular status must be carefully assessed before treatment.

The recommended starting dose is 50 mg taken 1 h before sexual activity. Depending on effectiveness and side effects, the dose may be increased to 100 mg or decreased to 25 mg. The maximal recommended frequency is once per day. Sildenafil is mainly metabolized by the liver. In patients over 65, those with hepatic or renal impairment, and those concomitantly receiving p450 3A4 inhibitors (eg, erythromycin, ketoconazole, itraconazole), a lower starting dose of 25 mg should be used. Patients taking nitrates should not take sildenafil, as severe hypotension and cardiac compromise may result.

Transurethral pharmacotherapy is also an effective treatment for erectile dysfunction. Delivered into the urethra, alprostadil can be absorbed directly through the urethral mucosa and act locally. Transurethral alprostadil (MUSE) has been shown to be effective in patients with erectile dysfunction from various organic causes. In clinical trials, during initial dose titration, 64–66% of patients achieved an adequate erection sufficient for intercourse. Responders were then given either alprostadil or placebo for home treatment. Sixty-five to sixty-nine percent of those treated with alprostadil reported successful intercourse at least once, thus gives an overall success rate of 43% compared with only 11–18% in the placebo arms (Padma-Nathan et al, 1997; Williams et al, 1998). The most common side effects were penile pain (11%) and urethral pain/burning (7%). Most patients (83%) reported minimal to no discomfort. The incidence of fibrosis (including curvature, nodules, and Peyronie plaque) and priapism was 1.4% and < 1%, respectively. To maximize response of the transurethral approach, researchers have reported the use of an adjustable constriction device (Actis) that is placed at the base of the penis to facilitate drug transport from the corpus spongiosum to the cavernosum. The rate of adequate erection for sexual intercourse with the added use of Actis was reported to be about 71% (Lewis, 1998).

To minimize systemic absorption, the patient is advised to sit down or stand up for 10 min after application to decrease penile venous return. MUSE has been shown to be embryotoxic when administered subcutaneously to pregnant rats. Thus, a condom barrier is strongly recommended if the female partner is pregnant. Other contraindications include abnormal or inflammatory penile and urethral diseases and diseases that are prone to priapism such as sickle cell anemia, thrombocythemia, polycythemia, and multiple myeloma.

Intracavernous injection of vasoactive agents provides an attractive alternative to surgery. The reported agents are papaverine alone (Virag, 1982b) or with phentolamine (Zorgniotti and Lefleur, 1985; Sidi et al, 1986), and prostaglandin E_1 (Ishii et al, 1986). In the United States, 2 prostaglandin E_1 (alprostadil) preparations have been approved by the

Food and Drug Administration: Caverject and Edex. Both are available in different dosages with an injection kit. When single-agent injection is not effective or produces undesirable side effects (eg, painful erection with alprostadil), injection of a combination of papaverine, phentolamine, and alprostadil have been shown to be quite useful. These substances cause prolonged arterial dilatation and venous compression, and a large number of patients have been able to achieve and maintain erections better than previously. The recommended dosages of vasodilators for patients with arterial or combined arterial and venous insufficiency are listed in Table 47–4. Repeated injection can improve penile hemodynamics; after short-term treatment, some patients have achieved good erections without injection. Several complications have been reported: ecchymosis at the injection site, transient dizziness or a drop in blood pressure, fibrosis, Peyronie disease, failure of ejaculation, painful erection, infection, and priapism.

Prolonged erection or priapism can be treated by aspiration or intracavernous injection of alpha-adrenergic agents. The alpha-adrenergic agents for priapism therapy are listed in Table 47–5. In priapism lasting more than 24 h, a shunting procedure may be required; several patients reportedly have become completely impotent owing to fibrosis of the corpora after prolonged priapism (Halsted et al, 1986).

Other reported complications of intracavernous injections include elevated liver enzymes and fibrosis. In a summary of about 4000 patients treated worldwide with papaverine with or without phentolamine, fibrotic nodule was reported in 1.5–60% of patients and prolonged erection in 2.3–15% of patients in the titration period and less than 1% after therapy had begun. Prostaglandin E_1 seems to have a lower incidence of prolonged erection and fibrosis (Stackl, Hasun, and Marberger, 1988). However, penile pain of various degrees in up to 50% of patients treated is a significant drawback (Schramek and Waldhauser, 1989).

Another alternative is the use of a vacuum constriction device with a constrictive band placed at the base of the penis. With proper use, a number of patients have been able to achieve and maintain erec-

Table 47–4. Intracavernous vasodilator injection therapy.[1]

Drug	Test Dose	Dose Range
Papaverine hydrochloride Papaverine 30 mg/mL;	15–30 mg	15–60 mg
phentolamine 1 mg/mL	0.5 mL	0.2–1 mL
Prostaglandin E_1	10 µg	5–15 µg
Papaverine (12 mg);		
phentolamine (1 mg);		
prostaglandin E_1 (9 µg)	0.1–0.5 mL	0.1–0.5 mL

[1]Lower doses for management of neurogenic and psychogenic impotence.

Table 47–5. Intravenous vasoconstrictor therapy for priapism.[1]

Drug	Usual Dose
Epinephrine	10–20 µg
Phenylephrine	250–500 µg
Ephedrine	50–100 µg

[1]Intracavernous injection every 5 min until detumescence after aspiration of 10–20 mL of blood.

tions adequate for sexual intercourse. Complications include ejaculatory difficulty (12%), initial penile pain (41%) (Witherington, 1988), ecchymosis (10%), and petechiae (27%) (Nadig, Ware, and Blumoff, 1986). This therapy is not recommended in patients with sickle cell disease or trait and in patients with bleeding diathesis.

Isolated stenosis or occlusion of the extrapenile arteries is amenable to surgical repair. Restoration of potency has been reported after surgery of the internal iliac, internal pudendal, and dorsal arteries. Michal et al (1977) pioneered the use of extrapenile vessels to revascularize the corpora cavernosa (epigastric-corporeal anastomosis). Subsequent modifications include epigastric-dorsal artery anastomosis, a venous graft for femorocorporeal anastomosis, and direct anastomosis of the epigastric artery to the cavernous artery (Crespo et al, 1982). Although short-term results for all 4 techniques are good, long-term results are less than satisfactory. Anastomosis of the epigastric artery to the deep dorsal vein (Virag, 1982b; Furlow et al, 1990) or to both the deep dorsal vein and artery (Hauri, 1986) has been reported to achieve a better result because of the higher flow and better anastomotic patency rate. However, the exact mechanism of vascular improvement is still controversial.

Penile prostheses continue to be refined (Table 47–6). In addition to the improved durability of the semirigid prostheses (AMS and Mentor malleable), there has been upgrading of the mechanics and strength of the 2-piece and 3-piece inflatable prostheses (eg, AMS inflatable, Mentor inflatable). Other

Table 47–6. Types of penile prostheses.

Semirigid
AMS 600 and 650 (malleable)
Mentor malleable
Acu-Form
Hinged
DuraPhase
One-piece inflatable
DynaFlex
Two-piece inflatable
Mark II (Mentor)
Ambicor (AMS)
Three-piece inflatable
Alpha-1, Alpha-1 narrow base (Mentor)
CX, CXM, Ultrex (AMS)

prostheses are also available. One is the single-component inflatable prosthesis (DynaFlex) with inflating and deflating mechanisms contained within a single cylinder for easier implantation. Another (DuraPhase) consists of a segmented hinge and a cable that runs through the center of each segment with or without a mechanical activator on one end. Gratifying results have been achieved in more than 95% of cases after penile prosthesis insertion, especially if preoperative counseling is given to both the patient and the partner (Kaufman, Lindner, and Raz, 1982; Montague, 1983). The major complications are infection, prolonged pain, tenderness, and problems resulting from inadequate length (SST syndrome).

In general, patients should try an oral agent, transurethral therapy, or vacuum constriction device first, followed by intracavernous injection. A penile prosthesis is recommended for patients in whom these treatments have failed or who are unwilling to accept them. Vascular surgery is an acceptable alternative in young patients with localized arterial disease.

Cavernosal Impotence

A. Diagnosis: Detection of penile venous incompetence was pioneered by Wagner's group, who used cavernosography during visual erotic stimulation (Wagner, 1981). Virag (1982a) and Wespes et al (1984) modified this approach and introduced the technique of cavernosometry (ie, measuring the rate of saline perfusion required to achieve and maintain erection) before cavernosography. A further refinement with the addition of intracavernous vasodilator injection is probably a better way to study the functional status of the penile venous occlusion mechanism. Wespes' group (1986) has determined that in potent volunteers, the maintenance rate after papaverine is less than 5 mL/min.

Padma-Nathan (1989) observed that after injection of papaverine and phentolamine, and saline infusion to raise the intracavernous pressure, patients with a normal veno-occlusive mechanism have a minimal drop of intracavernous pressure (< 40 mm Hg in the first 30 s from 150 mm Hg). Freidenberg et al (1987) reported that intracavernous pressure remains higher than 60 mm Hg after 5 min in patients with a normal veno-occlusive mechanism after papaverine and saline infusion. Because of the wide variation of penile size, monitoring the pressure drop seems to be a better assessment of venous function. Pharmacologic cavernosography involves intracavernous injection of contrast after injection of vasodilators (Lue et al, 1986a). Patients with a normal veno-occlusive mechanism should show minimal or no visualization of the penile veins (Figure 47–7). Because of its relative invasiveness, use of cavernosography is limited to visualization of abnormal outflow channels prior to surgery. Visualization of the penile veins depends on the amount of contrast medium present in the venous system. Therefore, a high maintenance rate results in

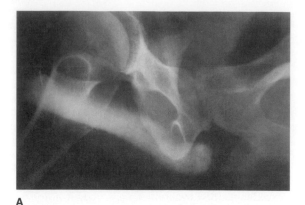

A

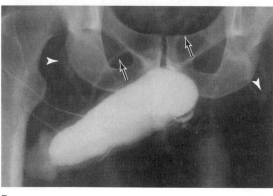

B

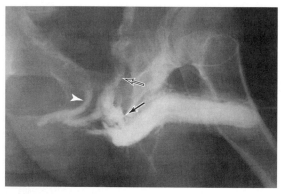

C

Figure 47–7. Cavernosography after intracavernous injection of papaverine. In a normal man (**A**), the cavernosogram shows opacification of the erect corpora cavernosa and nonvisualization of penile veins. In (**B**), the patient has a large leak through both superficial dorsal veins (arrows) to the saphenous veins (arrowheads). Film (**C**) shows abnormal venous drainage via the cavernous veins (solid arrow) into the preprostatic plexus (open arrow) and the internal pudendal veins (arrowhead). (Reproduced, with permission, from Lue TF, Tanagho EA: Physiology of erection and pharmacological management of impotence. J Urol 1987;137:829. © by Williams & Wilkins, 1987.)

visualization of abnormal venous systems, and a low rate shows minimal or no venous drainage outside the corpora cavernosa (Figure 47–7). An abnormal communication between the corpora cavernosa and the corpus spongiosum or the glans penis can sometimes be demonstrated.

A history of rapid detumescence or partial erection, especially in young men, is strongly suggestive of venous incompetence, although arterial insufficiency can produce the same symptoms. Dizziness, facial flushing, or even a drop in systemic blood pressure after vasodilator injection can be due to vasovagal reflex or a large venous leak. Confirmation with cavernosometry is necessary. For practical purposes, reliance on the speed of detumescence during the combined injection and stimulation test for the diagnosis of venogenic impotence is recommended. After intracavernous injection of 30 mg of papaverine or 10 µg of prostaglandin E_1 and manual genital stimulation, rapid detumescence within 5 min is diagnostic of an incompetent veno-occlusive mechanism (Donatucci and Lue, 1992a; Lue, 1989). Because of its minimal invasiveness and the addition of sexual stimulation, we believe this is a more physiologic test for venogenic impotence.

The most widely recognized disease of the cavernous muscle is fibrosis after priapism and local replacement with fibrotic plaque in Peyronie disease. A recent electron microscope study of the cavernous erectile tissue revealed a high incidence of smooth-muscle atrophy, endothelial defects, and replacement of smooth muscles by collagen fibers in patients with diabetes and atherosclerosis (Persson et al, 1989). Nerve degeneration is common in diabetics and alcoholics. Although duplex ultrasonography can detect vascular insufficiency, which is a major cause of the ultrastructural changes, biopsy of the cavernous erectile tissue may be necessary in selected cases (Wespes et al, 1991).

B. Treatment: In some patients with mild venous leakage, sildenafil, transurethral alprostadil, vacuum constriction device or intracavernous injection may be sufficient to produce adequate erection. Surgical therapy is recommended only for those who do not accept or are not satisfied with the less invasive treatments.

Although improvement of potency after ligation of the penile veins was described in the early twentieth century, urologists were skeptical until cavernosography and cavernosometry provided a scientific demonstration of venous leakage. Ligation and excision of the superficial and deep dorsal veins and repair of a fistula between the glans and the cavernous bodies are the procedures reported. Virag's technique of anastomosis of the epigastric artery to the deep dorsal vein probably also decreases venous outflow because of higher venous resistance. Although this technique appears promising, only a few series have been reported, and long-term results are not very satisfactory (Wespes and Schulman, 1985; Lewis and Puyau, 1986).

For practical purposes my colleagues and I believe that venous surgery can be recommended as an acceptable alternative to a penile prosthesis in young patients with veno-occlusive dysfunction and adequate arterial function.

Because cavernous erectile tissue changes vary from the microscopic foci of pathology to diffuse involvement of most of the corpus cavernosum, less invasive therapy such as a vacuum constriction device or intracavernous injection should always be tried before surgical treatment is contemplated. Correction of a localized disorder such as Peyronie disease by collagenase (Gelbard, Lindner, and Kaufman, 1985) or surgery such as plaque excision and grafting (Horton, Sadove, and Devine, 1987), incision and grafting (Gelbard and Hayden, 1991; Lue and El-Sakka, 1998), or plication (Donatucci and Lue, 1992b) may improve the erectile function. When diffuse fibrosis such as that after cavernosal infection, priapism, or scleroderma is present, a penile prosthesis is usually the only option.

Impotence Due to Other Causes

The medical history, systemic review, laboratory examination, and drug history cannot always reveal the precise cause of erectile dysfunction. Evaluation of potency after systemic disease has been adequately treated or a medication discontinued or changed sometimes is the only way of diagnosing the cause of impotence. Conservative management should always be tried first, with surgery considered as a last resort.

MALE SEXUAL DYSFUNCTION INVOLVING EMISSION, EJACULATION, & ORGASM

Physiology of Emission, Ejaculation, & Orgasm

Different mechanisms are involved in erection, emission, ejaculation, and orgasm, and these events can be dissociated from one another (eg, a frequent complaint of impotent patients is ejaculating through a "limp penis"). Except for nocturnal emissions, or "wet dreams," emission and ejaculation require stimulation of the external genitalia. Impulses traveling from the pudendal nerves reach the upper lumbar spinal sympathetic nuclei. Efferent signals traveling in the hypogastric nerve activate secretions and transport sperm from the distal epididymis, vasa deferentia, seminal vesicles, and prostate to the prostatic urethra. Coordinated closing of the internal urethral sphincter and relaxation of the external sphincter direct the semen into the bulbous urethra (emission). Subsequent rhythmic contractions of the bulbocavernous muscles force the semen through a pressur-

ized conduit—the much narrowed urethral lumen compressed by the engorged corpora cavernosa—to produce the 2- to 5-mL ejaculate. The external ejaculation process involves the somatomotor efferent of the pudendal nerve to contract the bulbocavernous muscle. Since this action is involuntary, however, integrated autonomic and somatic action is required.

The mechanism of orgasm is the least understood of the sexual processes. It probably involves cerebral interpretation and response to sexual stimulation. Along with emission and ejaculation, several nongenital responses also occur. These include involuntary rhythmic contractions of the anal sphincter, hyperventilation, tachycardia, and elevation of blood pressure.

Disorders Affecting Emission, Ejaculation, & Orgasm

Bilateral sympathectomy at the L2 level has resulted in ejaculatory dysfunction in about 40% of patients. High bilateral retroperitoneal lymphadenectomy causes an even higher percentage of emission failures.

Retrograde ejaculation is usually the result of dysfunction of the internal sphincter or the bladder neck, as seen after prostatectomy, with alpha-blocker therapy, and in autonomic neuropathy due to diabetes.

Successful emission and ejaculation without orgasm occur in some patients with spinal cord injury. Phantom orgasm in a paraplegic man also has been described. A history of disease or surgery is helpful in differentiating emission failure from retrograde ejaculation. If microscopic examination confirms the presence of sperm in bladder urine after a dry ejaculation, retrograde ejaculation can be diagnosed. If no sperm is found, emission failure is the cause.

Treatment

Elimination of alpha blockers results in cure for some patients with emission failure or retrograde ejaculation. Alpha sympathomimetics such as ephedrine or a combination of chlorpheniramine maleate and phenylpropanolamine hydrochloride (Ornade) have been used successfully in patients with retrograde ejaculation. Electroejaculation via a rectal probe has been applied in patients suffering from spinal cord injury with some success (Brindley, 1981; Perkash et al, 1985; Ohl et al, 1991). Patients who have normal wet dreams but cannot achieve orgasm and ejaculation may benefit from psychosexual counseling. Premature ejaculation can be treated by desensitization, the squeezing technique (Masters and Johnson, 1976), or application of a local anesthetic (Berkovitch, Keresteci, and Koren, 1995; Xin et al, 1997) or a condom to reduce the sensitivity of the glans and frenulum. Recently, selective serotonin reuptake inhibitors (fluoxetine, sertraline, and clomipramine) are also reported to be useful in prolonging the intravaginal ejaculation latency time in patients with premature ejaculation (Kim and Seo, 1998).

REFERENCES

PHYSIOLOGY OF PENILE ERECTION

Adaikan PG, Kottegoda SR, Ratnam SS: Is vasoactive intestinal polypeptide the principal transmitter involved in human penile erection? J Urol 1986;135: 638.

Adaikan PG et al: Cholinoreceptors in the corpus cavernosum muscle of the human penis. J Auton Pharmacol 1983;3:107.

Bancroft J, Wu FCW: Changes in erectile responsiveness during androgen replacement therapy. Arch Sex Behav 1983;12:59.

Banya Y et al: Two circulatory routes within the human corpus cavernosum penis: A scanning electron microscopic study of corrosion casts. J Urol 1989;142:879.

Benson GS et al: Neuromorphology and neuropharmacology of the human penis: An in vitro study. J Clin Invest 1980;65:506.

Bredt DS, Hwang PM, Snyder SH: Localization of nitric oxide synthase indicating a neural role for nitric oxide. Nature 1990;347:68.

Breza J et al: Detailed anatomy of penile neurovascular structures: Surgical significance. J Urol 1989;141: 437.

Brock G et al: Nitric oxide synthase: A new diagnostic tool for neurogenic impotence. Urology 1993;42:412.

Bult H et al: Nitric oxide as an inhibitory non-adrenergic non-cholinergic neurotransmitter. Nature 1990;345: 346.

Campbell NA: *Biology,* 4th ed. Benjamin/Cummings, 1996.

Carati CJ et al: Pharmacology of the erectile tissue of the canine penis. Pharmacol Res Commun 1985;3:951.

Christ GJ et al: The role of gap junctions and ion channels in the modulation of electrical and chemical signals in human corpus cavernosum smooth muscle. Int J Impotence Res 1993;5:77.

Conti G: L'erection du penis humain et ses bases morphologico-vasculaires. Acta Anat 1952;14:217.

Crowley WR, Selman FP: The neurochemical control of mating behavior. In: Adler, NT (editor): *Neuroendocrinology of Reproduction, Physiology and Behavior.* Plenum, 1981.

de Araujo CG, Schmidt RA, Tanagho EA: Neural pathways to lower urinary tract identified by retrograde axonal transport of horseradish peroxidase. Urology 1982;19:290.

Deslypere JP, Vermeulen A: Leydig cell function in normal men: Effect of age, life-style, residence, diet, and activity. J Clin Endocrinol Metab 1984;59:955.

Fournier GR Jr et al: Mechanism of venous occlusion during canine penile erection: Anatomic demonstration. J Urol 1987;137:163.

Hedlund H, Andersson KE: Contraction and relaxation induced by some prostanoids in isolated human penile erectile tissue and cavernous artery. J Urol 1985; 134:1245.

Holmquist F, Andersson K-E, Hedlund H: Actions of endothelin on isolated corpus cavernosum from rabbit and man. Acta Physiol Scand 1990;139:113.

Hsu G-L et al: The three dimensional structure of the human tunica albuginea: Anatomical and ultrastructure levels. Int J Impotence Res 1992;4:117.

Ignarro LJ et al: Nitric oxide and cyclic GMP formation upon electrical stimulation cause relaxation of corpus cavernosum smooth muscle. Biochem Biophys Res Commun 1990;170:843.

Johnston P, Davidson JM: Intracerebral androgens and sexual behavior in the male rat. Horm Behav 1972; 3:345.

Jünemann KP et al: Hemodynamics of papaverine- and phentolamine-induced penile erection. J Urol 1986; 136:158.

Karacan I, Aslan C, Hirshkowitz M: Erectile mechanisms in man. Science 1983;220:1080.

Kawatani M, Nagel J, de Groat WC: Identification of neuropeptides in pelvic and pudendal nerve afferent pathways to the sacral spinal cord of the cat. J Comp Neurol 1986;249:117.

Kim N et al: A nitric oxide-like factor mediates non-adrenergic-noncholinergic neurogenic relaxation of penile corpus cavernosum smooth muscle. J Clin Invest 1991;88:12.

Kwan M et al: The nature of androgen action on male sexuality: A combined laboratory/self-report study on hypogonadal men. J Clin Endocrinol Metab 1983;57: 557.

Lue TF: The mechanism of penile erection in the monkey. Semin Urol 1986;4:217.

Lue TF, Tanagho EA: Functional anatomy and mechanism of penile erection. In: Tanagho EA, Lue TF, McClure RD (editors): *Contemporary Management of Impotence and Infertility.* Williams & Wilkins, 1988.

Lue TF et al: Hemodynamics of erection in the monkey. J Urol 1983;130:1237.

MacLean PD: Brain mechanisms of primal sexual functions and related behavior. In: Sandler M, Gessa GL (editors): *Sexual Behavior: Pharmacology and Biochemistry.* Raven Press, 1975.

Marberger H: The mechanisms of ejaculation. In: Coutinho E, Fuchs F (editors): *Physiology and Genetics of Reproduction.* Plenum Press, 1974.

McEwen BX: Neural gonadal steroid actions. Science 1981;211:1303.

McKenna KE: Central control of penile erection. Int J Impotence Res 1998;(Suppl 1):S25.

Moncada S: The first Robert Furchgott lecture: From endothelium-dependent relaxation to the L-arginine: NO pathway. Blood Vessels 1990;27:208.

Moreno AP et al: Gap junctions between human corpus cavernosum smooth muscle cells: Gating properties and unitary conductance. Am J Physiol 1993;264:C80.

Murray RK: Muscle. In: Murray RK et al (editors): *Harper's Biochemistry,* 24th ed. Appleton & Lange, 1996.

Newman HF, Northup JP, Devlin J: Mechanism of human penile erection. Invest Urol 1964;1:350.

Newman HF, Tchertkoff V: Penile vascular cushions and erection. Invest Urol 1980;18:43.

O'Carroll R, Bancroft J: Testosterone therapy for low sexual interest and erectile dysfunction in men: A controlled study. Br J Psychiatry 1984;145:146.

Padma-Nathan H et al: In vivo and in vitro studies on the physiology of penile erection. Semin Urol 1986;4: 209.

Perachio AA, Marr LD, Alexander M: Sexual behavior in male rhesus monkeys elicited by electrical stimulation of preoptic and hypothalamic areas. Brain Res 1979;177:127.

Saenz de Tejada I et al: Cholinergic neurotransmission in human corpus cavernosum. I. Response of isolated tissue. Am J Physiol 1988a;254:H459.

Saenz de Tejada I et al: Impaired neurogenic and endothelium-mediated relaxation of penile smooth muscle from diabetic men with impotence. N Engl J Med 1989;320:1025.

Saenz de Tejada I et al: Prostaglandin production by human corpus cavernosum endothelial cells (HCC EC) in culture. J Urol 1988b;139:252A.

Shirai M et al: Hemodynamic mechanism of erection in the human penis. Arch Androl 1978;1:345.

Trigo-Rocha F et al: Nitric oxide and cyclic guanosine monophosphate: Mediators of pelvic nerve-stimulated erection in dogs. Am J Physiol 1993a;264(Heart Circ Physiol 33):H419.

Trigo-Rocha F et al: The role of cyclic AMP, cyclic GMP, endothelium and non-adrenergic non-cholinergic neurotransmission in canine penile erection. J Urol 1993b;149:872.

Tudoriu T: My views about the applied anatomy of the penis and the physiopathology of erection. Arch Ital Urol 1989;61:249.

Virag R: Intracavernous injection of papaverine for erectile failure. Lancet 1982;2:938.

Wagner G, Uhrenholdt A: Blood flow measurement by the clearance method in the human corpus cavernosum in the flaccid and erect states. In: Zorgniotti AW, Rossi G (editors): *Vasculogenic Impotence.* (Proceedings of the First International Conference on Corpus Cavernosum Revascularization.) Thomas, 1980.

Wagner G et al: New theory on the mechanism of erection involving hitherto undescribed vessels. Lancet 1982;1:416.

Walsh PC, Donker PJ: Impotence following radical prostatectomy: Insight into etiology and prevention. J Urol 1982;128:492.

Willis E et al: Vasoactive intestinal polypeptide (VIP) as a possible neurotransmitter involved in penile erection. Acta Physiol Scand 1981;113:545.

MALE SEXUAL DYSFUNCTION

Abber JC et al: Diagnostic tests for impotence: Comparison of papaverine injection with penile-brachial index and nocturnal penile tumescence monitoring. J Urol 1986;135:923.

Abelson D: Diagnostic value of the penile pulse and blood pressure: A Doppler study of impotence in diabetics. J Urol 1975;113:636.

Aboseif SR et al: Local and systemic effects of chronic intracavernous injection of papaverine, prostaglandin E1 and saline in primates. J Urol 1989;142:403.

Bancroft J, Wu FCW: Changes in erectile responsiveness during androgen therapy. Arch Sex Behav 1983;12:59.

Barry JM, Blank B, Boileau M: Nocturnal penile tumescence monitoring with stamps. Urology 1980;15:171.

Bennett AH: Revascularization using the dorsal vein of the penis in vasculogenic impotence. Semin Urol 1986;4:259.

Berkovitch M, Keresteci AG, Koren G: Efficacy of prilocaine-lidocaine cream in the treatment of premature ejaculation. J Urol 1995;154:1360.

Bookstein JJ et al: Pharmacoarteriography in the evaluation of impotence. J Urol 1987;137:333.

Bors E, Comarr AE: *Neurological Urology.* University Park Press, 1971.

Bradley WE et al: New method for continuous measurement of nocturnal penile tumescence and rigidity. Urology 1985;26:4.

Brindley GS: Electroejaculation: Its technique, neurological implication and uses. J Neurol Neurosurg Psychiatry 1981;44:9.

Britt DB, Kemmerer WT, Robison JR: Penile blood flow determination by mercury strain gauge plethysmography. Invest Urol 1971;8:673.

Buvat J et al: Is intracavernous injection of papaverine a reliable screening test for vascular impotence? J Urol 1986;135:476.

Crespo E et al: Treatment of vasculogenic sexual impotence by revascularizing of cavernous and/or dorsal arteries using microvascular techniques. Urology 1982;20:271.

Crowe R et al: Vasoactive intestinal polypeptide-like immunoreactive nerves in diabetic penis: A comparison between streptozotocin-treated rats and man. Diabetes 1983;32:1075.

DePalma RG, Levine SB, Feldman S: Preservation of erectile function after aortoiliac reconstruction. Arch Surg 1978;113:958.

Donatucci CF, Lue TF: The combined intracavernous injection and stimulation test: Diagnostic accuracy. J Urol 1992a;148:61.

Donatucci CF, Lue TF: Correction of penile deformity assisted by intracavernous injection of papaverine. J Urol 1992b;147:1108.

Ebbehoj J, Wagner G: Insufficient penile erection due to abnormal drainage of cavernous bodies. Urology 1979;13:507.

Ek A, Bradley WE, Krane RJ: Nocturnal penile rigidity measured by the snap gauge band. J Urol 1983;129:964.

Ellis A: *Reason and Emotion in Psychotherapy.* Lyle Stuart, 1962.

Ertekin C, Reel F: Bulbocavernosus reflex in normal men and in patients with neurogenic bladder and/or impotence. J Neurol Sci 1976;28:1.

Faerman J et al: Impotence and diabetes: Histological studies of the autonomic nervous fibers of the corpora cavernosa in impotent diabetic males. Diabetes 1974;23:971.

Feldman HA et al: Impotence and its medical and psychosocial correlates: Results of the Massachusetts Male Aging Study. J Urol 1994;151:54.

Finney RP: Finney flexirod prosthesis. Urology 1984;23(5 Spec No):79.

Finney RP: Flexi-flate penile prosthesis. Semin Urol 1986;4:244.

Fishman IJ: Experience with the Hydroflex penile prosthesis. Semin Urol 1986;4:239.

Fishman IJ, Shabsign R, Scott FB: A comparison of the hydroflex and inflatable penile prosthesis. J Urol 1986;135:358.

Flanigan DP et al: Internal iliac artery revascularization in the treatment of vasculogenic impotence. Arch Surg 1985;120:271.

Freidenberg DH et al: Quantitation of corporeal venous outflow resistance in man by corporeal pressure flow evaluation. J Urol 1987;138:533.

Furlow WL et al: Penile revascularization: Experience with the Furlow-Fisher technique of deep dorsal vein arterialization. J Urol 1990;143:318A.

Gelbard MK, Hayden B: Expanding contractures of the tunica albuginea due to Peyronie's disease with temporalis fascia free grafts. J Urol 1991;145:772.

Gelbard MK, Lindner A, Kaufman JJ: The use of collagenase in the treatment of Peyronie's disease. J Urol 1985;134:280.

Gerstenberg TC, Bradley WE: Nerve conduction velocity measurement of dorsal nerve of the penis in normal and impotent males. Urology 1983;21:90.

Ginestie J, Romieu A: *Radiologic Exploration of Impotence.* Martinus Nijhoff, 1978.

Goldstein I: Arterial revascularization procedures. Semin Urol 1986;4:252.

Goldstein I: Neurologic impotence. In: Krane RJ, Siroky MG, Goldstein I (editors): *Male Sexual Dysfunction.* Little, Brown, 1983.

Goldstein I et al: Oral sildenafil in the treatment of erectile dysfunction. Sildenafil Study Group. N Engl J Med 1998;338:1397.

Goldstein I et al: Vasculogenic impotence: Role of the pelvic steal test. J Urol 1982;128:300.

Gordon GG et al: Effect of alcohol (ethanol) administration on sex-hormone metabolism in normal men. N Engl J Med 1976;295:793.

Gruetter CA et al: Relaxation of bovine coronary artery and activation of coronary arterial guanylate cyclase by nitric oxide, nitroprusside and a carcinogenic nitrosoamine. J Cyclic Nucl Res 1979;5:211.

Gupta S et al: A possible mechanism for alteration of human erectile function by digoxin: Inhibition of corpus cavernosum sodium/potassium adenosine triphosphatase activity. J Urol 1998;159:1529.

Haldeman S, Bradley WE, Bhatia N: Evoked responses from the pudendal nerve. J Urol 1982;128:974.

Haldeman S et al: Pudendal evoked responses. Arch Neurol 1982;39:280.

Halsted DS et al: Papaverine-induced priapism. J Urol 1986;136:109.

Hauri D: A new operative technique in vasculogenic erectile impotence. World J Urol 1986;4:237.

Horton CE, Sadove RC, Devine CJ Jr: Peyronie's disease. Ann Plast Surg 1987;18:122.

Ishii N et al: Therapeutic trial with prostaglandin E for organic impotence. Jpn J Urol 1986;77:954.

Jensen SB et al: Sexual function and pituitary axis in insulin treated diabetic men. Acta Med Scand 1979;624 (Suppl):65.

Jevtich MJ: Importance of penile arterial pulse sound examination in impotence. J Urol 1980;124:820.

Jünemann KP, Buhrle CP, Stief CG: Current trends in corpus cavernosum EMG. Int J Impotence Res 1993; 5:105.

Kaneko S, Bradley WE: Evaluation of erectile dysfunction with continuous monitoring of penile rigidity. J Urol 1986;136:1026.

Kaplan HS: *Disorders of Sexual Desire.* Brunner/Mazel, 1979.

Karacan I: Sleep environment important in assessing NPT. Urology 1988;32:180.

Karacan I, Moore CA: Nocturnal penile tumescence: An objective diagnostic aid for erectile dysfunction. In: Bennett AH (editor): *Management of Male Impotence.* Williams & Wilkins, 1982.

Karacan I et al: Nocturnal penile tumescence and diagnosis in diabetic impotence. Am J Psychiatry 1978; 135:191.

Kaufman JJ, Lindner A, Raz S: Complications of penile prosthesis surgery for impotence. J Urol 1982;128: 1192.

Kedia KR, Markland C: The effect of pharmacologic agents on ejaculation. J Urol 1975;114:237.

Kedia KR, Markland C, Fraley EE: Sexual function following high retroperitoneal lymphadenectomy. J Urol 1975;114:237.

Kim SC, Seo KK: Efficacy and safety of fluoxetine, sertraline and clomipramine in patients with premature ejaculation: a double-blind, placebo controlled study. J Urology 1998;159:425.

Kolodny RC et al: Depression of plasma testosterone levels after chronic intensive marihuana use. N Engl J Med 1974;290:872.

Krane RJ: Omniphase penile prosthesis. Semin Urol 1986;4:247.

Krane RJ, Goldstein I, Saenz de Tejada I: Impotence. N Engl J Med 1989;321:1648.

Krane RJ, Siroky MB: Studies on sacral-evoked potentials. J Urol 1980;124:872.

Laumann EO et al: *The Social Organization of Sexuality: Sexual Practice in the United States.* University of Chicago Press, 1994.

Leriche A, Morel A: The syndrome of thrombotic obliteration of aortic bifurcation. Ann Surg 1968;127:193.

Lewis R: Combined use of transurethral alprostadil and an adjustable penile constriction band in men with erectile dysfunction: Results from a multicenter trial. Int J Impotence Res 1998;10:S49.

Lewis RW, Puyau FA: Procedures for decreasing venous drainage. Semin Urol 1986;4:263.

LoPiccolo J: Diagnosis and treatment of male sexual dysfunction. J Sex Marital Ther 1986;11:215.

Lowsley OS, Bray JL: The surgical relief of impotence: Further experiences with a new operative procedure. JAMA 1936;107:2029.

Lue TF: Patient's goal-directed impotence management. Urol Grand Rounds 1989;29:1.

Lue TF: Treatment of venogenic impotence. In: Tanagho EA, Lue TF, McClure RD (editors): *Contemporary Management of Impotence and Infertility.* Williams & Wilkins, 1988.

Lue TF, El-Sakka AI: Venous patch graft for Peyronie's disease. Part I: technique. J Urol 1998;2047.

Lue TF et al: Functional evaluation of penile veins by cavernosography in papaverine-induced erection. J Urol 1986a;135:479.

Lue TF et al: Priapism: A refined approach to diagnosis and treatment. J Urol 1986b;136:104.

Lue TF et al: Vasculogenic impotence evaluated by high-resolution ultrasonography and pulsed Doppler spectrum analysis. Radiology 1985;155:777.

MacKay JD et al: Diabetic autonomic neuropathy: The diagnostic value of heart rate monitoring. Diabetologia 1980;18:471.

Masters WH, Johnson VE: Principles of the new sex therapy. Am J Psychol 1976;133:548.

McClure RD: Endocrine evaluation and therapy. In: Tanagho EA, Lue TF, McClure RD (editors): *Contemporary Management of Impotence and Fertility.* Williams & Wilkins, 1988.

Melman A, Henry D: The possible role of the catecholamines of the corpora in penile erection. J Urol 1979;121:419.

Merchant RF Jr, DePalma RG: Effects of femorofemoral grafts on postoperative sexual function: Correlation with penile pulse volume recordings. Surgery 1981; 90:962.

Merrill DC: Clinical experience with Mentor inflatable penile prosthesis in 206 patients. Urology 1986;28:185.

Mersdorf A et al: Ultrastructural changes in impotent penile tissue: Comparison of 65 patients. J Urol 1991; 145:749.

Michal V, Kovac J, Belan A: Arterial lesions in impotence: Phalloarteriography. Int Angiol 1984;3:247.

Michal V, Kramar R, Pospichal J: External iliac "steal syndrome." J Cardiovasc Surg 1978;19:355.

Michal V, Pospichal J: Phalloarteriography in the diagnosis of erectile impotence. World J Surg 1978;2:239.

Michal V et al: Arterial epigastricocavernous anastomosis for the treatment of sexual impotence. World J Surg 1977;1:515.

Money J: Phantom orgasm in the dreams of paraplegic men and women. Arch Gen Psychiatry 1960;3:373.

Montague DK: Experience with semirigid rod and inflatable penile prostheses. J Urol 1983;129:967.

Montague DK et al: Diagnostic evaluation, classification, and treatment of men with sexual dysfunction. Urology 1979;14:545.

Morales A et al: Clinical safety of oral sildenafil citrate (VIAGRA) in the treatment of erectile dysfunction. Int J Impotence Res 1998;10:69.

Morales A et al: Nonhormonal pharmacological treatment of organic impotence. J Urol 1982;128:45.

Morley JE, Melmed S: Gonadal dysfunction in systemic disorders. Metabolism 1979;28:1051.

Moul JW, McLeod DG: Experience with the AMS 600 malleable penile prosthesis. J Urol 1986;135:929.

Nadig PW, Ware JC, Blumoff R: A noninvasive device to produce and maintain an erection-like state. Urology 1986;27:126.

Nehra A et al: Mechanisms of venous leakage: A prospective clinicopathological correlation of corporeal function and structure. J Urol 1996;156:1320.

Newman HF: Vibratory sensitivity of the penis. Fertil Steril 1970;21:791.

Newman HF, Marcus H: Erectile dysfunction in diabetes and hypertension. Urology 1985;26:135.

NIH Consensus Panel on Impotence: Impotence. JAMA 1993;270:83.

Ohl DA et al: Electroejaculation following retroperitoneal lymphadenectomy. J Urol 1991;145:980.

Padma-Nathan H: Dynamic infusion cavernosometry and cavernosography (DICC) and the cavernosal artery systolic occlusion pressure gradient: A complete evaluation of the hemodynamic events of penile erection. In: Lue TF (editor): *World Book of Impotence.* Smith-Gordon, 1992.

Padma-Nathan H: Evaluation of the corporal veno-occlusive mechanism: Dynamic infusion cavernosometry and cavernosography. Semin Interventional Radiol 1989;6:205.

Padma-Nathan H, Goldstein I, Krane RJ: Evaluation of the impotent patient. Semin Urol 1986a;4:225.

Padma-Nathan H, Goldstein I, Krane RJ: Treatment of prolonged or priapistic erections following intracavernosal papaverine therapy. Semin Urol 1986b;4:236.

Padma-Nathan H et al: Treatment of men with erectile dysfunction with transurethral alprostadil. Medicated Urethral System for Erection (MUSE) Study Group. N Engl J Med 1997;336:1.

Papadopoulos C: Cardiovascular drugs and sexuality: A cardiologist's review. Arch Intern Med 1980;140: 1341.

Perkash I et al: Reproductive biology of paraplegics: Results of semen collection, testicular biopsy and serum hormone evaluation. J Urol 1985;134:284.

Persson C et al: Correlation of altered penile ultrastructure with clinical arterial evaluation. J Urol 1989;149: 1462.

Reichgott MJ: Problems of sexual function in patients with hypertension. Cardiovasc Med 1979;4:149.

Rubarsk V, Michal V: Morphologic changes in the arterial bed of the penis with aging: Relationship to the pathogenesis of impotence. Invest Urol 1977;15:194.

Rubin A, Babbott D: Impotence and diabetes mellitus. JAMA 1958;168:498.

Salvatierra O, Fortmann JL, Belzer FO: Sexual function of males before and after renal transplantation. Urology 1975;5:64.

Sattar AA, Schulman CC, Wespes E: Objective quantification of cavernous endothelium in potent and impotent men. J Urol 1995;153:1136.

Sattar AA et al: Cavernous oxygen tension and smooth muscle fibers: Relation and function. J Urol 1995; 154:1736.

Schramek P, Waldhauser M: Dose-dependent and side-effect of prostaglandin E1 in erectile dysfunction. Br J Clin Pharmacol 1989;28:567.

Sharlip ID: Penile arteriography in impotence after pelvic trauma. J Urol 1981a;126:477.

Sharlip ID: Penile revascularization in the treatment of impotence. West J Med 1981b;134:206.

Sherman FP: Impotence in patients with chronic renal failure on dialysis: Its frequency and etiology. Fertil Steril 1975;26:221.

Sidi AA et al: Intracavernous drug-induced erections in the management of male erectile dysfunction: Experience with 100 patients. J Urol 1986;135:704.

Siroky MB, Krane RJ: Physiology of sexual function. In: Krane RJ, Siroky MB (editors): *Clinical Neuro-Urology.* Little, Brown, 1979.

Small MP: Surgical treatment of impotence with Small-Carrion prosthesis: Preoperative, intraoperative, and postoperative considerations. J Urol 1984;23(5 Spec No):93.

Spark RF, White RA, Connolly PB: Impotence is not always psychogenic: Newer insights into hypothalamic-pituitary-gonadal dysfunction. JAMA 1980;243: 750.

Spark RF, Wills CA, Royal H: Hypogonadism, hyperprolactinaemia, and temporal lobe epilepsy in hyposexual men. Lancet 1984;1:413.

Stackl W, Hasun R, Marberger M: Intracavernous injection of prostaglandin E1 in impotent men. J Urol 1988;140:66.

Truss MC et al: Single potential analysis of cavernous

electrical activity: Four years' experience in more than 500 patients with erectile dysfunction. Eur Urol 1993;24:358.

Tudoriu T, Bourmer H: The hemodynamics of erection at the level of the penis and its local deterioration. J Urol 1983;129:741.

Van Arsdalen KN, Malloy TR, Wein AJ: Erectile physiology, dysfunction and evaluation. 2. Etiology and evaluation of erectile dysfunction. Monogr Urol 1983;4:165.

Van Thiel DH et al: Hypothalamic-pituitary-gonadal dysfunction in men using cimetidine. N Engl J Med 1979;300:1012.

Velcek D et al: Penile flow index utilizing a Doppler pulse wave analysis to identify penile vascular insufficiency. J Urol 1980;123:669.

Virag R: Arterial and venous hemodynamics in male impotence. In: Bennett AH (editor): *Management of Male Impotence*. Williams & Wilkins, 1982a.

Virag R: Revascularization of the penis. In: Bennett AH (editor): *Management of Male Impotence*. Williams & Wilkins, 1982b.

Virag R et al: Intracavernous injection of papaverine as a diagnostic and therapeutic method in erectile failure. Angiology 1984;35:79.

Wagner G: Methods for differential diagnosis of psychogenic and organic erectile failure. In: Wagner G, Green R (editors): *Impotence: Physiological, Psychological, Surgical Diagnosis and Treatment*. Plenum Press, 1981.

Wagner G, Gerstenberg T, Levin RJ: Electrical activity of corpus cavernosum during flaccidity and erection of the human penis: A new diagnostic method? J Urol 1989;142:723.

Wagner G, Uhrenholdt A: Blood flow measurement by the clearance method in the human corpus cavernosum in the flaccid and erect status. In: Zorgniotti AW, Rossi G (editors): *Vasculogenic Impotence*. Thomas, 1980.

Walsh PC, Donker PJ: Impotence following radical prostatectomy: Insight into etiology and preservation. J Urol 1982;128:492.

Waltzer WC: Sexual and reproductive function in men treated with hemodialysis and renal transplantation. J Urol 1981;126:713.

Watkins PJ, Mackay JD: Assessment of diabetic autonomic neuropathy using heart rate monitoring. Horm Metab Res 1980(Suppl);9:69.

Weinstein MH, Roberts M: Sexual potency following surgery for rectal carcinoma: A follow-up of 44 patients. Ann Surg 1977;185:295.

Wespes E, Schulman CC: Parameters of erection. Br J Urol 1984;56:416.

Wespes E, Schulman CC: Venous leakage: Surgical treatment of a curable cause of impotence. J Urol 1985;133:796.

Wespes E et al: Cavernometry-cavernography: Its role in organic impotence. Eur Urol 1984;10:229.

Wespes E et al: Computerized analysis of smooth muscle fibers in potent and impotent patients. J Urol 1991;146:1015.

Wespes E et al: Pharmacocavernometry-cavernography in impotence. Br J Urol 1986;58:429.

Whitelaw GP, Smithwick RA: Some secondary effects of sympathectomy with particular reference to sexual function. N Engl J Med 1951;245:121.

Winter CC: Priapism treated by modification of creation of fistulas between glans penis and corpora cavernosa. J Urol 1979;121:743.

Williams G et al: Efficacy and safety of transurethral alprostadil therapy in men with erectile dysfunction. MUSE Study Group. Br J Urol 1998;81:889.

Witherington R: Suction device therapy in the management of erectile impotence. Urol Clin North Am 1988;15:123.

Wolpe J: *Psychotherapy by Reciprocal Inhibition*. Stanford Univ Press, 1958.

Wooten JS: Ligation of the dorsal vein of the penis as a cure for atonic impotence. Tex Med J 1902–1903;18:325.

Xin ZC et al: Efficacy of a topical agent SS-cream in the treatment of premature ejaculation: Preliminary clinical studies. Yonsei Med J 1997;38:91.

Zorgniotti AW: Corpus cavernosum blockade for impotence: Practical aspects and results in 250 cases. J Urol 1985;135:306.

Zorgniotti AW, Lefleur RS: Auto-injection of the corpus cavernosum with a vasoactive drug combination for vasculogenic impotence. J Urol 1985;133:39.

Appendix: Normal Laboratory Values*

Marcus A. Krupp, AB, MD

Values may vary with method of measurement and population.

HEMATOLOGY

Antithrombin III: [P] 86–120%.

Bleeding time: Template method, 3–9 min (180–540 s).

Cellular measurements of red blood cells (erythrocytes): Average diameter = 7.3 μm (5.5–8.8 μm).
Mean corpuscular volume (MCV): Men, 80–94 fL; women, 81–99 fL (by Coulter counter).
Mean corpuscular hemoglobin (MCH): 27–32 pg.
Mean corpuscular hemoglobin concentration (MCHC): 32–36 g/dL erythrocytes (32–36%).
Color, saturation, and volume indices: 1 (0.9–1.1).

Clot retraction: Begins in 1–3 h; complete in 6–24 h. No clot lysis in 24 h.

Fibrin D-dimer: [P] 0–250 ng/mL.

Fibrinogen split products: < 10 μg.

Fragility of erythrocytes: Begins at 0.45–0.38% NaCl; complete at 0.36–0.3% NaCl.

Glucose-6-phosphate dehydrogenase (G6-PD): [B] 4–8 μg/g Hb.

Hematocrit (PCV): Men, 40–52%; women, 37–47%.

Hemoglobin: [B] Men, 14–18 g/dL (2.09–2.79 mmol/L as Hb tetramer); women, 12–16 g/dL (1.86–2.48 mmol/L). [S] 2–3 mg/dL.

Partial thromboplastin time: Activated, 25–37 s.

Platelets: 150,000–400,000/mL (0.15–0.4 × 10^{12}/L).

Prothrombin: INR, 1–1.4.

Erythrocyte count: Men, 4.5–6.2 million/μL (4.5–6.2 × 10^{12}/L); women, 4–5.5 million/μL (4–5.5 × 10^{12}/L).

Reticulocytes: 0.6–1.8% of erythrocytes.

Sedimentation rate: Less than 20 mm/h (Westergren).

White blood count (leukocytes) and differential: 5000–10,000/μL (5–10 × 10^9/L).

Segmented neutrophils	40–70%
Myelocytes	0%
Juvenile neutrophils	0%
Band neutrophils	0–15%
Lymphocytes	15–45%
Eosinophils	1–3 %
Basophils	0–5 %
Monocytes	0–7 %

Lymphocytes: Total, 1500–4000/μL	
B cell	5–25%
T cell	60–88%
Suppressor	10–43%
Helper	32–66%
H:S	> 1

BLOOD, PLASMA, OR SERUM CHEMICAL CONSTITUENTS
(Values vary with method used.)

Acetone and acetoacetate: [S] 0.3–2 mg/dL (3–20 mg/L).

Aldolase: [S] Values vary with method used.

α-Amino acid nitrogen: [S, fasting] 3–5.5 mg/dL (2.2–3.9 mmol/L).

Aminotransferases:
Aspartate aminotransferase (AST; SGOT): [S] 15–55 IU/L.
Alanine aminotransferase (ALT; SGPT): [S] 10–70 IU/L. Values vary with method used.

Ammonia: [B] 9–33 μmol/L.

Amylase: [S] 80–180 units/dL (Somogyi). Values vary with method used.

---

*Blood [B], Plasma [P], Serum [S], Urine [U].

α_1-**Antitrypsin:** [S] > 180 mg/dL.

Ascorbic acid: [P] 0.4–1.5 mg/dL (23–85 μmol/L).

Base, total serum: [S] 145–160 mEq/L (145–160 mmol/L).

Bicarbonate: [S] 24–28 mEq/L (24–28 mmol/L).

Bilirubin: [S] Total, 0.2–1.2 mg/dL (3.5–20.5 μmol/L). Direct conjugated, 0.1–0.4 mg/dL (< 7 μmol/L). Indirect, 0.2–0.7 mg/dL (< 12 μmol/L).

Calcium: [S] 8.5–10.3 mg/dL (2.1–2.6 mmol/L). Values vary with albumin concentration.

Calcium, ionized: [S] 4.25–5.25 mg/dL; 2.1–2.6 mEq/L (1.05–1.3 mmol/L).

β-**Carotene:** [S, fasting] 50–300 μg/dL (0.9–5.58 μmol/L).

Ceruloplasmin: [S] 25–43 mg/dL (1.7–2.9 μmol/L).

Chloride: [S or P] 96–106 mEq/L (96–106 mmol/L).

Cholesterol: [S or P] 150–240 mg/dL (3.9–6.2 mmol/L). (See Lipid fractions.) Values vary with age.

Cholesteryl esters: [S] 65–75% of total cholesterol.

CO_2 content: [S or P] 24–29 mEq/L (24–29 mmol/L).

Complement: [S] C3 (b1C), 90–250 mg/dL. C4 (β_{1E}), 10–60 mg/dL. Total (CH_{50}), 75–160 mg/dL.

Copper: [S or P] 100–200 μg/dL (16–31 μmol/L).

Cortisol: [P] 8:00 AM, 5–25 μg/dL (138–690 nmol/L); 8:00 PM, < 14 μg/dL (385 nmol/L).

Creatine kinase (CK): [S] 10–50 IU/L at 30 °C. Values vary with method used.

Creatine kinase MB fraction: [S] < 4% total CK.

Creatinine: [S or P] 0.7–1.5 mg/dL (62–132 μmol/L).

Cyanocobalamin: [S] 200 pg/mL (148 pmol/L).

Epinephrine: [P] Supine, < 0.1 μg/L (< 0.55 nmol/L).

Erythropoietin: [S] 5–20% IU/L.

Ferritin: [S] Adult women, 20–120 ng/mL; men, 30–300 ng/mL. Child to 15 years, 7–140 ng/mL.

α-**Fetoprotein:** [S] 0–8.5 ng/mL.

Folic acid: [S] 2–20 ng/mL (4.5–45 nmol/L). [Erythrocytes] > 100 ng/mL (> 318 nmol/L).

Glucose: [S or P] 65–110 mg/dL (3.6–6.1 mmol/L).

α-**Glutamyl transpeptidase:** [S] 8–78 IU/L.

Glycosylated hemoglobin (HbA_{10}): [B] 4–7%.

Haptoglobin: [S] 40–200 mg of hemoglobin-binding capacity.

Iron: [S] 40–175 μg/dL (9–31.3 μmol/dL).

Iron-binding capacity: [S] Total, 250–410 μg/dL (44.7–73.4 μmol/L). Percent saturation, 20–55%.

Lactate: [B, special handling] Venous, 4–16 mg/dL (0.44–1.8 mmol/L).

Lactate dehydrogenase (LDH): [S] 55–140 IU/L. Values vary with method used.

Lipase: [S] 0.2–1.5 units.

Lipid fractions: [S or P] Desirable levels: HDL cholesterol, > 40 mg/dL; LDL cholesterol, < 150 mg/dL; VLDL cholesterol, < 40 mg/dL. (To convert to mmol/L, multiply by 0.026.)

Lipids, total: [S] 450–1000 mg/dL (4.5–10 g/L).

Magnesium: [S or P] 1.8–3 mg/dL (0.75–1.25 mmol/L).

Myoglobin: [P] 15–100 ng/mL.

Norepinephrine: [P] Supine, < 0.5 μg/L (< 3 nmol/L).

Osmolality: [S] 280–296 mOsm/kg water.

Oxygen:
Capacity: [B] 16–24 vol%. Values vary with hemoglobin concentration.
Arterial content: [B] 15–23 vol%. Values vary with hemoglobin concentration.
Arterial % saturation: 94–100% of capacity.
Arterial PO_2 (PaO_2): 80–100 mm Hg (10.67–13.33 kPa) (sea level). Values vary with age.

$PaCO_2$: [B, arterial] 35–45 mm Hg (4.7–6 kPa).

pH (reaction): [B, arterial] 7.35–7.45 (H^+ 44.7–45.5 nmol/L).

Phosphatase, acid: [S] 1–5 units (King-Armstrong), 0.1–0.63 units (Bessey-Lowry).

Phosphatase, alkaline: [S] 38–126 IU/L.

Phospholipid: [S] 145–200 mg/dL (1.45–2 g/L).

Phosphorus, inorganic: [S, fasting] 3–4.5 mg/dL (1–1.5 mmol/L).

Potassium: [S or P] 3.5–5 mEq/L (3.5–5 mmol/L).

Prostate-specific antigen (PSA): [S] 0–4 ng/mL.

Protein:
Total: [S] 6–8 g/dL (60–80 g/L).
Albumin: [S] 3.5–5.5 g/dL (35–55 g/L).
Globulin: [S] 2–3.6 g/dL (20–36 g/L).
Immunoglobulin: [S] IgA 78–400 mg/dL. IgG 690–1400 mg/dL. IgM 35–240 mg/dL.
Fibrinogen: [P] 0.2–0.6 g/dL (2–6 g/L).

Prothrombin clotting time: [P] By control. INR, 1–1.4.

Pyruvate: [B] 0.6–1 mg/dL (70–114 mmol/L).

Serotonin: [B] 0.05–0.2 µg/mL (0.28–1.14 µmol/L).

Sodium: [S or P] 136–145 mEq/L (136–145 mmol/L).

Specific gravity: [B] 1.056 (varies with hemoglobin and protein concentration). [S] 1.0254–1.0288 (varies with protein concentration).

Sulfate: [S or P] As sulfur, 0.5–1.5 mg/dL (156–468 µmol/L).

Transferrin: [S] 200–400 mg/dL (23–45 µmol/L).

Triglycerides: [S] < 165 mg/dL (1.9 mmol/L). (See Lipid fractions.)

Troponin: [S] < 0.5 ng/mL.

Urea nitrogen: [S or P] 8–25 mg/dL (2.9–8.9 mmol/L). Do not use anticoagulant containing ammonium oxalate.

Uric acid: [S or P] Men, 3–9 mg/dL (0.18–0.54 mmol/L); women, 2.5–7.5 mg/dL (0.15–0.45 mmol/L).

Vitamin A: [S] 15–60 µg/dL (0.53–2.1 µmol/L).

Vitamin B$_{12}$: [S] > 200 pg/mL (> 148 pmol/L).

Vitamin D: [S] Cholecalciferol (D$_3$): 25-Hydroxycholecalciferol, 8–55 ng/mL (19.4–137 nmol/L); 1,25-dihydroxycholecalciferol, 26–65 pg/mL (62–155 pmol/L); 24,25-dihydroxycholecalciferol, 1–5 ng/mL (2.4–12 nmol/L).

Volume, blood (Evans blue dye method): Adults, 2990–6980 mL. Women, 46.3–85.5 mL/kg; men, 66.2–97.7 mL/kg.

Zinc: [S] 50–150 µg/dL (7.65–22.95 µmol/L).

HORMONES, SERUM, OR PLASMA

Adrenal:
Aldosterone: [P] Supine, normal salt intake, 2–9 ng/dL (56–250 pmol/L); increased when upright.

Cortisol: [S] 8:00 AM, < 5–20 µg/dL (0.14–0.55 µmol/L); 8:00 PM, < 10 µg/dL (0.28 µmol/L).

Deoxycortisol: [S] After metyrapone, > 7 µg/dL (> 0.2 µmol/L).

Dopamine: [P] < 135 pg/mL.

Epinephrine: [P] < 0.1 ng/mL (< 0.55 nmol/L).

Norepinephrine: [P] < 0.5 µg/L (< 3 nmol/L). See also Miscellaneous Normal Values.

Gonad:
Testosterone, free: [S] Men, 10–30 ng/dL; women, 0.3–2 ng/dL. (1 ng/dL = 0.035 nmol/L).

Testosterone, total: [S] Prepubertal, < 100 ng/dL; adult men, 300–1000 ng/dL; adult women, 20–80 ng/dL; luteal phase, up to 120 ng/dL.

Estradiol (E2): [S, special handling] Men, 12–34 pg/mL; women, menstrual cycle 1–10 days, 24–68 pg/mL; 11–20 days, 50–300 pg/mL; 21–30 days, 73–149 pg/mL (by radioimmunoassay [RIA]). (1 pg/mL = 3.6 pmol/L.)

Progesterone: [S] Follicular phase, 0.2–1.5 ng/mL; luteal phase, 6–32 ng/mL; pregnancy, > 24 ng/mL; men, < 1 ng/mL (by RIA). (1 ng/mL = 3.2 nmol/L.)

Islets:
Insulin: [S] 4–25 µU/mL (29–181 pmol/L).

C-peptide: [S] 0.9–4.2 ng/mL.

Glucagon: [S, fasting] 20–100 pg/mL.

Kidney:
Renin activity: [P, special handling] Normal sodium intake: Supine, 1–3 ng/mL/h; standing, 3–6 ng/mL/h. Sodium depleted: Supine, 2–6 ng/mL/h; standing, 3–20 ng/mL/h.

Parathyroid:
Parathyroid hormone levels vary with method and antibody. Correlate with serum calcium.

Pituitary:
Growth hormone (GH): [S] Adults, 1–10 ng/mL (46–465 pmol/L) (by RIA).

Thyroid-stimulating hormone (TSH): [S] < 10 µU/mL.

Follicle-stimulating hormone (FSH): [S] Prepubertal, 2–12 mIU/mL; adult men, 1–15 mIU/mL; adult women, 1–30 mIU/mL; castrate or postmenopausal, 30–200 mIU/mL (by RIA).

Luteinizing hormone (LH): [S] Prepubertal, 2–12 mIU/mL; adult men, 1–15 mIU/mL; adult women, < 30 mIU/mL; castrate or postmenopausal, > 30 mIU/mL.

Corticotropin (ACTH): [P] 8:00–10:00 AM, up to 100 pg/mL (22 pmol/L).

Prolactin: [S] 1–25 ng/mL (0.4–10 nmol/L).

Somatomedin C: [P] 0.4–2 U/mL.

Antidiuretic hormone (ADH; vasopressin): [P] Serum osmolality 285 mOsm/kg, 0–2 pg/mL; > 290 mOsm/kg, 2–12+ pg/mL.

Placenta:
Estriol (E$_3$): [S] Men and nonpregnant women, < 0.2 µg/dL (< 7 nmol/L) (by RIA).

Chorionic gonadotropin: [S] Beta subunit: Men, < 9 mIU/mL; pregnant women after implantation, > 10 mIU/mL.

Stomach:
Gastrin: [S, special handling] Up to 100 pg/mL (47 pmol/L). Elevated, > 200 pg/mL.

Pepsinogen I: [S] 25–100 ng/mL.

Thyroid:
Thyroxine, free (FT$_4$): [S] 0.8–2.4 ng/dL (10–30 pmol/L).

Thyroxine, total (TT$_4$): [S] 5–12 µg/dL (65–156 nmol/L) (by RIA).

Thyroxine-binding globulin capacity (T_4): [S] 12–28 µg/dL (150–360 nmol/L).

Triiodothyronine (T_3): [S] 80–220 ng/dL (1.2–3.3 nmol/L). Reverse triiodothyronine (rT_3): [S] 30–80 ng/dL (0.45–1.2 nmol/L).

Triiodothyronine uptake (rT_3U): [S] 25–36%; as TBG assessment (rT_3U ratio), 0.85–1.15.

Calcitonin: [S] < 100 pg/mL (< 29.2 pmol/L).

NORMAL CEREBROSPINAL FLUID VALUES

Appearance: Clear and colorless.

Cells: Adults, 0–5 mononuclear cells/µL; infants, 0–20 mononuclear cells/µL.

Glucose: 50–85 mg/dL (2.8–4.7 mmol/L). (Draw serum glucose at same time.)

Pressure (reclining): Newborns, 30–88 mm water; children, 50–100 mm water; adults, 70–200 mm water (avg = 125).

Proteins: Total, 20–45 mg/dL (200–450 mg/L) in lumbar cerebrospinal fluid. IgG, 2–4 mg/dL (0.02–0.04 g/L).

Specific gravity: 1.003–1.008.

RENAL FUNCTION TESTS

ρ-Aminohippurate (PAH) clearance (RPF): Men, 560–830 mL/min; women, 490–700 mL/min.

Creatinine clearance: calculation from serum creatinine:

Men: $\dfrac{(140 - \text{age}) \times (\text{wt in kg})}{72 \times \text{serum creatinine mg/dL}} = \text{creatinine clearanc mL/min}$

Women: calculated value × 0.85

Creatinine clearance, endogenous (GFR): Approximates inulin clearance (see below).

Inulin clearance (GFR): Men, 110–150 mL/min; women, 105–132 mL/min (corrected to 1.73 m^2 surface area).

Maximal glucose reabsorptive capacity (Tm$_G$): Men, 300–450 mg/min; women, 250–350 mg/min.

Maximal PAH excretory capacity (Tm$_{PAH}$): 80–90 mg/min.

Osmolality: On normal diet and fluid intake: Range 500–850 mOsm/kg water. Achievable range, normal kidney: Dilution 40–80 mOsm; concentration (dehydration) up to 1400 mOsm/kg water (at least 3–4 times plasma osmolality).

Specific gravity of urine: 1.003–1.030.

MISCELLANEOUS NORMAL VALUES

Adrenal hormones and metabolites:

Aldosterone: [U] 2–26 µg/24 h (5.5–72 nmol). Values vary with sodium and potassium intake.

Catecholamines: [U] Total, < 100 µg/24 h. Epinephrine, < 10 µg/24 h (< 55 nmol); norepinephrine, < 100 µg/24 h (< 591 nmol). Values vary with method used.

Cortisol, free: [U] 20–100 µg/24 h (0.55–2.76 mmol).

11,17-Hydroxycorticoids: [U] Men, 4–12 mg/24 h; women, 4–8 mg/24 h. Values vary with method used.

17-Ketosteroids: [U] Under 8 years, 0–2 mg/24 h; adolescents, 2–20 mg/24 h. Men, 10–20 mg/24 h; women, 5–15 mg/24 h. Values vary with method used. (1 mg = 3.5 mmol.)

Metanephrine: [U] < 1.3 mg/24 h (< 6.6 µmol) or < 2.2 µg/mg creatinine. Values vary with method used.

Vanillylmandelic acid (VMA): [U] Up to 7 mg/24 h (< 35 µmol).

Fecal fat: Less than 30% dry weight.

Lead: [U] < 80 µg/24 h (< 0.4 µmol/d).

Porphyrins:
Delta-aminolevulinic acid: [U] 1.5–7.5 mg/24 h (11.4–57.2 µmol).
Coproporphyrin: [U] < 230 µg/24 h (< 345 nmol).
Uroporphyrin: [U] < 50 µg/24 h (< 60 nmol).
Porphobilinogen: [U] < 2 mg/24 h (<8.8 µmol).

Urobilinogen: [U] 0–2.5 mg/24 h (< 4.23 µmol).

Urobilinogen, fecal: 40–280 mg/24 h (68–474 µmol).

Index

NOTE: Page numbers in bold face type indicate a major discussion. A *t* following a page number indicates tabular material and an *f* following a page number indicates a figure. Drugs are listed under their generic names. When a drug trade name is listed, the reader is referred to the generic name.

Abacterial (amicrobic) cystitis, 271–272
 tuberculosis differentiated from, 270, 272
Abdomen
 exiting, after laparoscopic surgery, 154
 plain film of, **66–67**, 67*f*, 68*f*, 69*f*. *See also specific disorder*
Abdominal (ureteral) compression devices, for intravenous urography, 70
Abdominal pain, after extracorporeal shock wave lithotripsy, 327
ABH antigens, in bladder cancer, 363
Abscess
 perinephric/perirenal, 249–250
  percutaneous aspiration of, 139, 249, 250
  tuberculous, 271
 prostatic, 256
 renal, 248–249
Absorptive hypercalciuric nephrolithiasis, 294–295
Accelerated hyperfractionation, radiation sensitivity and tolerances and, 474
Accommodation, bladder
 cystometry in evaluation of, 502, 520–521, 522*f*
 pathologic changes in, 525
Acetohydroxamic acid, in urinary stone prevention, 313
N-Acetylcysteine, for stone dissolution, 308
Achilles tendon reflex, 48
Acid-base disorders. *See also* Acidosis
 during laparoscopic surgery, 151
Acid-pyuria, renal tuberculosis causing, 53–54
Acidification of urine, for struvite stones, 308
Acidosis
 in chronic renal failure, 611
 jejunal conduit urinary diversion causing, 438, 445
 renal tubular
  in chronic renal failure, 611

stone formation and, 294, 296, 297*f*, 304
type I, 602, 611
type II, 602
type IV, 611
urinary diversion/bladder substitution and, 445–447
Acorn-tip catheter, 199
Acquired immunodeficiency syndrome (AIDS). *See* HIV infection/AIDS
Acridine-orange staining, for urinary tract infection diagnosis, 58
Acrosome reaction, 756
ACTH, in Cushing syndrome
 dexamethasone suppression of, 557–558, 559*f*
 ectopic production of, 555, 557, 558, 559, 561
 localization of source of excess of, 550
 plasma levels of, 558
Actinomyces (actinomycosis), genitourinary, **273**
 bovis, 273
 israelii, 273
Actinomycin D, for Wilms tumor, 393
Activin, 753
Acute retroviral syndrome, 290
Acute tubular necrosis
 renal failure caused by, 607–608
 in transplanted kidney, 624
Acyclovir, for genital herpes, 286, 286*t*, 697, 698
AD-32, for bladder cancer, 366
Adenocarcinoma
 bladder, 357
 kidney, **380–390**. *See also* Renal cell carcinoma
 prostate, 407. *See also* Prostate cancer
 upper urinary tract, 369
Adenoma, renal, 378
Adjuvant chemotherapy, 465
 for bladder cancer, 468
 for germ cell tumors, 467
Adnexa, male, examination of, **44**
Adrenal adenocarcinoma, 555, 557*f*, 560, 561

Adrenal adenoma, 555, 557*f*, 560
Adrenal androgen excess, in Cushing syndrome, 556–557
Adrenal androgenic syndromes, 45, 556*f*, **561–563**. *See also* Adrenal hyperplasia, congenital
Adrenal cortex
 diseases of, **555–564**
  androgen-producing tumors, **563**
  androgenic syndromes, 556*f*, **561–563**. *See also* Adrenal hyperplasia, congenital
  Cushing syndrome, **555–561**, 556*f*
  hyperplasia. *See* Adrenal hyperplasia
  primary aldosteronism (hypertensive, hypokalemic syndrome), **563–564**, 563*f*, 564*f*
  radionuclide imaging in evaluation of, 190–191, 192*f*
Adrenal enzymes, congenital defects in, androgenic hyperplasia caused by, 561–563, 716–721, 717*f*, 718*t*. *See also* Adrenal hyperplasia, congenital
Adrenal glands, **555–571**. *See also* Adrenal cortex; Adrenal medulla
 anatomy of, **1**, 2*f*
 disorders of, **555–571**, 556*f*
 laparoscopic surgery of, **175–177**, 175*f*, 176*f*
 tumors of
  aldosterone-producing, 564, 564*f*
  androgen-producing, **563**
  computed tomography in evaluation of, 96*f*, 111*f*
  cortisol-producing, 555, 557*f*, 559, 560*f*
  in Cushing syndrome, 555, 557*f*
  localization of, 559, 560*f*
  gradient echo imaging in evaluation of, 111*f*, 112
  hormonal studies in diagnosis of, 59